GRS

Geriatrics Review Syllabus

9th Edition

Syllabus Book 1

EDITORS-IN-CHIEF

Annette Medina-Walpole, MD, AGSF

James T. Pacala, MD, MS, AGSF

Jane F. Potter, MD, AGSF

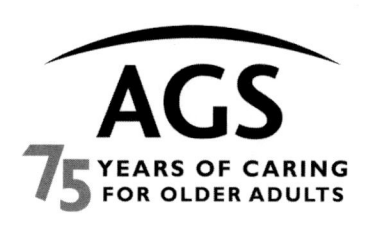

AGS
75 YEARS OF CARING FOR OLDER ADULTS

As new research and clinical experience broaden our knowledge of medicine, changes in treatment and drug therapy are required. This publication is intended to facilitate the free flow of information of interest to the medical community involved in the care of older adults.

No responsibility is assumed by the editors or the American Geriatrics Society, as the Publisher, for any injury and/or damage to persons or property, as a matter of product liability, negligence, warranty, or otherwise, arising out of the use or application of any methods, products, instructions, or ideas contained herein. No guarantee, endorsement, or warranty of any kind, express or implied (including specifically no warranty of merchantability or of fitness for a particular purpose) is given by the Society in connection with any information contained herein. Independent verification of any diagnosis, treatment, or drug use or dosage should be obtained. No test or procedure should be performed unless, in the judgment of an independent qualified physician, it is justified in light of the risk involved.

Inclusion in this publication of product information does not constitute a guarantee, warranty, or endorsement by the American Geriatrics Society (the Publisher) of the quality, value, safety, effectiveness, or usefulness of any such product or of any claim made about such product by its manufacturer or an author.

The Chief Editors were Annette Medina-Walpole, MD, AGSF, James T. Pacala, MD, MS, AGSF, and Jane F. Potter, MD, AGSF. Chapter Editors were Lisa J. Granville, MD, AGSF, G. Michael Harper, MD, AGSF, Melinda S. Lantz, MD, and William L. Lyons, MD; Question Editors were John D. Gazewood, MD, MSPH, Gary J. Kennedy, MD, and Rainier Patrick Soriano, MD. Consulting Editor on Ethnogeriatrics was Sharon A. Brangman, MD, AGSF. Consulting Editor on Pharmacotherapy was Judith L. Beizer, PharmD, CGP, FASCP, AGSF. Special Advisors were Jonathan M. Flacker, MD, AGSF, and James S. Powers, MD, AGSF. Medical Writers were Susan E. Aiello, DVM, ELS, and Dalia Ritter. Indexer was L. Pilar Wyman. Managing Editor was Andrea N. Sherman, MS.

Many thanks to Fry Communications for all production work including typesetting, graphic design, and printing. With more than 70 years in the information industry, Fry offers printing and ancillary services to publishers and other content providers.

Citation: Medina-Walpole A, Pacala JT, Potter JF, eds. *Geriatrics Review Syllabus: A Core Curriculum in Geriatric Medicine*. 9th ed. New York: American Geriatrics Society; 2016.

All rights reserved. Except where authorized, no part of this publication may be reproduced, stored in a retrieval system, or transmitted in any form or by any means, electronic, mechanical, photocopying, recording, or otherwise without prior written permission of the American Geriatrics Society, 40 Fulton Street, 18th Floor, New York, New York, 10038 USA.

Geriatrics Review Syllabus: A Core Curriculum in Geriatric Medicine, 9th Edition. Cataloging in publication data is available from the Library of Congress.
Library of Congress Control Number: 2016931643

Copyright © 2016 by the American Geriatrics Society

ISBN Number Book 1: 978-1-886775-41-1

All rights reserved. Printed in the United States of America. Except as permitted under the United States Copyright Act of 1976, no part of this publication may be reproduced or distributed in any form or by any means, or stored in a database or retrieval system, without the prior written permission of the publisher, the American Geriatrics Society.

Printed in the United States of America

10 9 8 7 6 5 4 3 2 1

TABLE OF CONTENTS

Editorial Board and Staff ix
Introduction xi
Program Guidelines xiii
Acknowledgments xv
Editorial Board xvii
Contributing Chapter Authors xix
Contributing Question Authors xxv
Disclosures of Financial Interests xxx

I. CURRENT ISSUES IN AGING

Chapter 1—Demography 1
Key Points 1
Global Aging Trends and Demographics 1
United States Aging Trends and Demographics 2
References 6

Chapter 2—Biology 7
Key Points 7
Theories of Aging 7
Organ System Changes with Aging 11
Normal Aging 15
Complexity, Homeostenosis, and Integrated Systems . 16
References 17

Chapter 3—Ethics and Law 18
Key Points 18
Approach to Ethical Dilemmas 18
Principles of Medical Ethics 21
Informed Consent and Decisional Capacity 21
Truth Telling 22
Surrogate Decision-Making 23
Promoting Individual Preferences for Future Care . 23
Controversial Procedures at End of Life 25
Moral Distress 26
References 26

Chapter 4—Financing, Coverage, and Costs of Health Care 27
Key Points 27
Major Delivery and Payment Initiatives 27
Medicare 28
Financing of Care at Different Sites 35
Changes in the Federal Financing of Health Care . . 40
References 42

II. APPROACH TO THE PATIENT

Chapter 5—Assessment 43
Key Points 43
The Routine Office Visit 43
Patient-Clinician Communication 43
Physical Assessment 43
Medication Assessment 45
Cognitive Assessment 45
Psychologic Assessment 45
Social Assessment 46
Functional Status 46
Acute Functional Decline 47
Quality of Life 48
References 48

Chapter 6—Multimorbidity 49
Key Points 49
Approach to the Older Adult with Multimorbidity . . 50
Guiding Principles 50
Controversies and Challenges 52
References 52

Chapter 7—Caregiving 54
Key Points 54
What Is Caregiving? 54
Caregiving Interventions 56
Clinical Considerations 56
References 60

Chapter 8—Cultural Aspects of Care 62
Key Points 62
Use of Language and Nonverbal Communication . . 63
History of Traumatic Experiences 64
Issues of Immigration 64
Acculturation, Tradition, and Health Beliefs 65
Unspoken Challenges 65
Approaches to Decision Making 66
Attitudes Regarding Disclosure and Consent 66
Gender Issues 66
Advance Directives and End-of-Life Care 66
Approaches: The Ethnics Mnemonic 67
Spiritual and Religious Issues 67
References 68

Chapter 9—Lesbian Gay Bisexual Transgender Health 70
Key Points 70
Background 70
Asking About Sexual Orientation and Gender Identity 71
Medical Issues of LGBT Older Adults 71
Mental Health, Social, and Economic Issues Affecting LGBT Older Adults 74
Social Supports, Outreach, and Policy Issues 75
References 76

Chapter 10—Physical Activity 78
Key Points 78
Benefits of Physical Activity 78
Recommended Amounts of Physical Activity 79
Promotion of Physical Activity in Older Adults 81

References. 84	Ethnographic Data. 137

Chapter 11—Prevention. 85
Key Points. 85
Cancer Screening Tests Among Older Adults 85
Other Screening Tests and Preventive Measures. . . . 90
Healthy Lifestyle Counseling 93
Geriatric Health Issues. 95
Immunizations. 97
Chemoprophylaxis. 97
Counseling on Cancer Screening and Preventive
   Health 98
References. 99

Chapter 12—Pharmacotherapy 101
Key Points. 101
Age-Associated Changes in Pharmacokinetics. 101
Age-Associated Changes in Pharmacodynamics . . .104
Optimizing Prescribing .104
Adverse Drug Events 106
Drug-Drug Interactions 107
Drug-Disease Interactions. 107
Principles of Prescribing 108
Discontinuing Medications 109
Nonadherence 109
References. 110

**Chapter 13—Complementary and Integrative
   Medicine** 112
Key Points. 112
Safety Issues 113
CIM Efficacy for Managing Illness in Older Adults . .114
References. 119

Chapter 14—Mistreatment 120
Key Points. 120
Risk Factors and Prevention. 120
History 120
Physical Assessment. 121
Psychological Assessment 121
Financial Assessment 122
Self-Neglect 123
The Role of the Older Adult 123
Institutional Mistreatment 123
Intervention 123
The Medical-Legal Interface 124
References. 124

Chapter 15—Perioperative Care. 126
Key Points. 126
Surgical Decision-Making 126
Preoperative Assessment and Management. 126
Perioperative and Postoperative Management of
   Selected Medical Problems 131
References. 134

Chapter 16—Palliative Care 136
Key Points. 136
Overall Care Near Death 136

Ethnographic Data. 137
Palliative Care and Hospice 137
Quality Indicators for Palliative Care 138
Communication 138
Palliation of Symptoms. 140
Death Certificate Completion 145
Health Professional Burnout 146
References. 146

Chapter 17—Pain Management. 147
Key Points. 147
Assessment 148
Assessing and Treating Pain in Cognitively
   Impaired Older Adults 150
Treatment 151
References. 158

III. CARE SYSTEMS

Chapter 18—Hospital Care. 160
Key Points. 160
Hazards of Hospitalization 160
Never Events 162
Assessing and Managing Hospitalized
   Older Patients 164
Daily Evaluation 168
Models of Care for Older Hospitalized Patients 170
Alternatives to Hospital Care 171
Hospital Compare 171
Readmission 172
References. 172

Chapter 19—Transitions of Care. 174
Key Points. 174
The Treachery of Suboptimal Care Transitions 174
Barriers to Safe Transitions 175
Strategies to Improve Transitional Care, and
   Outcomes of Specific Care Models 176
Discharge Destinations and Care Venues 177
The Discharge Medication Regimen 178
Communicating with Patient, Caregivers, and
   Receiving Team. 178
Three Steps to Improve Care Transitions 178
References. 180

Chapter 20—Rehabilitation 181
Key Points. 181
Conceptual Model for Geriatric Rehabilitation 181
Sites of Rehabilitation Care 181
Teams and Roles 184
Impact of Comorbid Conditions 185
Rehabilitation Approaches and Interventions 186
Comprehensive Assessment. 187
Stroke. 187
Hip Fracture 189
Total Hip and Knee Arthroplasty 190
Amputation 191

Cardiac Rehabilitation 192
Pulmonary Rehabilitation 192
Mobility Aids, Orthotics, Adaptive Methods, and
    Environmental Modifications 193
References. 195

Chapter 21—Nursing-Home Care 196
Key Points. 196
The Nursing-Home Population 196
Nursing-Home Availability 197
Nursing-Home Financing 198
Staffing Patterns 198
Factors Associated with Nursing-Home Placement . .201
The Interface of Acute and Long-Term Care 201
Quality Issues and Legislation Influencing Care in
    the Nursing Home. 202
Medical Care Issues 205
Physician Practice in the Nursing Home 206
References. 207

Chapter 22—Community-Based Care 209
Key Points. 209
Home Care 209
Community-Based Services Not Requiring a
    Change in Residence 211
Community-Based Services Requiring a Change of
    Residence. 213
References. 215

Chapter 23—Outpatient Care Systems 216
Key Points. 216
Geriatrics in Primary Care. 216
Geriatric Specialty Care 219
Patient Selection for Outpatient Interventions 220
References. 220

IV. SYNDROMES

Chapter 24—Frailty 222
Key Points. 222
Evidence-Based Findings .222
Evidence as to Cause 224
Assessment of Frailty 225
Prevailing Management Strategies 226
Potential Approaches for Prevention of Frailty 226
Frailty and Failure to Thrive 227
Frailty and Palliative Care 227
References. 227

Chapter 25—Visual Loss and Eye Conditions 229
Key Points. 229
Common Eye Conditions in Older Adults 229
Red Eye 230
Ophthalmic Corticosteroids 232
Refractive Error and Cataracts. 232
Age-Related Macular Degeneration 233
Diabetic Retinopathy 235
Glaucoma 236

Anterior Ischemic Optic Neuropathy 238
Charles Bonnet Syndrome 238
Low-Vision Rehabilitation. 238
References. 239

Chapter 26—Hearing Loss 240
Key Points. 240
Normal Hearing and Age-Related Changes in the
    Auditory System 240
Epidemiology 240
Presbycusis 241
Clinical Presentation and Hearing Loss Detection. . .241
Evaluation of Suspected Hearing Loss 243
Treatment 243
References. 248

Chapter 27—Dizziness .249
Key Points. 249
Classification 249
Evaluation. 251
Management 253
References. 253

Chapter 28—Syncope. .254
Key Points. 254
Natural History: Diagnosis and Prognosis 254
Pathophysiology 255
Evaluation. 256
Treatment 259
References. 260

Chapter 29—Nutrition and Weight 262
Key Points. 262
Age-Related Changes 262
Nutrition Screening and Assessment 263
Nutrition Syndromes 266
Nutritional Interventions .266
Culturally Appropriate Nutritional Care 268
Legal and Ethical Issues .268
References. 269

Chapter 30—Feeding and Swallowing 270
Key Points. 270
Swallowing in Health and Disease 270
Feeding. 272
References. 273

Chapter 31—Urinary Incontinence 274
Key Points. 274
Prevalence and Impact. 274
Risk Factors and Associated Comorbid Conditions . .275
Pathophysiology 275
Evaluation. 277
Treatment and Management 279
Evaluation and Management of UI in Nursing-
    Home Residents 282
Catheters and Catheter Care. 282
References. 283

Chapter 32—Pressure Ulcers and Wound Care ...284
Key Points....284
Chronic Wound Healing....285
Pressure Ulcer Definition and Classification....285
Pressure Ulcer Assessment and Documentation ...286
Pressure Ulcer Prevention 288
Principles of Pressure Ulcer Treatment....290
Infectious Aspects of Pressure Ulcers 293
Palliative Care for Chronic Wounds 293
References....294

Chapter 33—Gait Impairment 296
Key Points....296
Epidemiology....296
Conditions that Contribute to Gait Impairment 296
Assessment 297
Interventions to Reduce Gait Disorders....300
References....302

Chapter 34—Falls....303
Key Points....303
Prevalence and Morbidity 303
Causes 303
Clinical Guidelines....305
Diagnostic Approach 305
Treatment and Prevention 307
References....311

Chapter 35—Osteoporosis 313
Key Points....313
Epidemiology and Impact....313
Bone Remodeling and Bone Loss in Aging 314
Pathogenesis....314
Diagnosis and Prediction of Fracture 316
Prevention and Treatment 319
Vertebral Fracture Management 324
References....324

Chapter 36—Dementia 326
Key Points....326
Epidemiology and Societal Impact....326
Etiology....327
Risk Factors and Prevention....327
Assessment and Differential Diagnosis....328
Differentiating Types of Dementias or
    Neurocognitive Disorders 329
Treatment and Management 332
References....337

**Chapter 37—Behavioral Disturbances in
    Dementia....339**
Key Points....339
Clinical Features 339
Assessment and Differential Diagnosis 340
Treatment Approach 342
Treatments for Specific Disturbances....342
References....347

Chapter 38—Delirium 349
Key Points....349
Incidence and Prognosis....349
Diagnosis and Differential Diagnosis 349
The Spectrum and Neuropathophysiology of
    Delirium 351
Risk Factors 352
Delirium and Dementia 352
Postoperative Delirium....353
Evaluation and Management....353
Quality Measures and Consensus Guidelines 359
References....359

Chapter 39—Sleep Issues 361
Key Points....361
Epidemiology....361
Changes in Sleep with Aging 361
Evaluation of Sleep 362
Common Sleep Problems 362
Changes in Sleep with Dementia 366
Sleep Disturbances in the Hospital 366
Sleep in the Nursing Home 367
Management of Insomnia 367
References....372

V. PSYCHIATRY

**Chapter 40—Depression and Other Mood
    Disorders....373**
Key Points....373
Epidemiology....373
Clinical Presentation and Diagnosis....373
Treatment....376
References....381

Chapter 41—Anxiety Disorders 382
Key Points....382
Classes of Anxiety Disorders....382
Comorbidity 385
Pharmacologic Management 385
Psychologic Management 386
References....387

**Chapter 42—Schizophrenia Spectrum and
    Other Psychotic Disorders....388**
Key Points....388
Schizophrenia and Schizophrenia Spectrum
    Syndromes 388
Psychotic Symptoms 390
Isolated Suspiciousness....391
Isolated Hallucinations....391
Other Psychotic Disorders 392
References....392

**Chapter 43—Personality and Somatic Symptom
    and Related Disorders 394**
Key Points....394
Personality Disorders....394

Somatic Symptom and Related Disorders.........398
References..401

Chapter 44—Addictions....................402
Key Points..402
Definitions of Substance Use Disorders.........402
Magnitude of the Problem........................403
Risks and Benefits of Substance Use...........404
Identifying Substance Use Disorders..........405
Treatment..405
Other Addictions..................................407
References..409

Chapter 45—Intellectual and Developmental Disabilities..................410
Key Points..410
Prevalence..410
Diagnostic and Treatment Issues..............411
Psychiatric and Mental Disorders in Aging Adults with Intellectual Disability..........412
Medical Disorders..................................414
Social Conditions..................................414
Developmental Disabilities and Comorbidity....416
References..416

VI. DISEASES AND DISORDERS

Chapter 46—Dermatology..................417
Key Points..417
Aging and Photoaging............................417
Inflammatory and Autoimmune Skin Conditions...418
Ulcers..422
Infections and Infestations......................423
Benign Growths..................................425
Skin Cancer..426
References..428

Chapter 47—Dentistry and Oral Health.......429
Key Points..429
Aging of the Teeth................................429
Dental Decay......................................429
Diseases of the Periodontium..................430
Toothlessness......................................431
Salivary Function in Aging......................432
Common Oral Lesions............................432
Chemosensory Perception......................435
Common Medical Considerations in Dental Treatment of Older Adults..................436
References..437

Chapter 48—Pulmonology..................438
Key Points..438
Age-Related Pulmonary Changes...............438
Common Respiratory Symptoms and Complaints...438
Major Pulmonary Diseases......................439
References..446

Chapter 49—Cardiology....................448
Key Points..448
Epidemiology......................................448
Effects of Aging on Cardiovascular Function....448
Cardiovascular Risk Factors....................450
Coronary Artery Disease........................451
Acute Coronary Syndromes....................452
Chronic Coronary Artery Disease.............453
Valvular Heart Disease..........................456
Transcatheter Aortic Valve Replacement....456
Infective Endocarditis..........................458
Cardiac Arrhythmias............................458
Peripheral Arterial Disease....................463
References..465

Chapter 50—Heart Failure..................466
Key Points..466
Epidemiology......................................466
Etiology and Pathophysiology..................466
Clinical Features..................................466
Diagnosis..467
Management......................................467
Recurrent Hospitalization......................472
Prognosis..473
End-of-Life Care..................................473
References..474

Chapter 51—Hypertension..................475
Key Points..475
Epidemiology and Physiology..................475
Clinical Evaluation..............................476
Treatment..476
Special Considerations..........................480
References..481

Chapter 52—Gastroenterology..............483
Key Points..483
Disorders of the Esophagus....................483
Disorders of the Stomach......................486
Disorders of the Colon..........................489
References..496

Chapter 53—Nephrology....................497
Key Points..497
Kidney Assessment..............................497
Metabolic and Volume Disorders.............498
Secondary Hypertension and Renal Artery Disease..502
Hematuria and Nephrolithiasis.................503
Acute Kidney Injury............................503
Intrinsic Renal Disease..........................504
Nephrotic Syndrome............................506
Chronic Kidney Disease........................507
End-Stage Renal Disease........................510
References..511

Chapter 54—Gynecology....................512
Key Points..512
History and Physical Examination.............512

vii

Treatment of Menopausal Symptoms 513
Urogenital Atrophy 513
Vulvovaginal Infection and Inflammation. 514
Disorders of the Vulva 514
Disorders of Pelvic Floor Support 516
Postmenopausal Vaginal Bleeding 518
References. 519

Chapter 55—Prostate Disease and Cancer 520
Key Points. 520
Benign Prostatic Hyperplasia 520
Prostate Cancer. 522
Prostatitis 528
References. 528

Chapter 56—Sexuality 530
Key Points. 530
Male Sexuality 530
Female Sexuality 534
References. 537

Chapter 57—Musculoskeletal Pain 538
Key Points. 538
General Principles for Diagnosis 538
Evaluation and Management of Regional
    Musculoskeletal Complaints. 539
References. 547

Chapter 58—Rheumatology 548
Key Points. 548
Osteoarthritis 548
Rheumatoid Arthritis. 550
Gout 551
Calcium Pyrophosphate Dihydrate Deposition
    Disease. 552
Polymyalgia Rheumatica 552
Giant Cell Arteritis 554
Systemic Lupus Erythematosus 554
Sjögren Syndrome 555
Polymyositis and Dermatomyositis 556
Fibromyalgia 557
References. 558

Chapter 59—Podiatry 559
Key Points. 559
The Role of the Primary Care Clinician
    in Foot Care. 559
Common Deformities of the Foot 559
Skin and Nail Disorders 565
Systemic Diseases Affecting the Foot and Ankle . . .566
References. 567

Chapter 60—Neurology 568
Key Points. 568
Epilepsy in Older Adults. 568
Movement Disorders in Older Adults 570
Neuromuscular Disorders, Peripheral
    Neuropathy, and Myelopathy. 575
Headaches. 578

References. 579

Chapter 61—Stroke and Cerebrovascular Disease .580
Key Points. 580
Impact of Cerebrovascular Disease 580
Ischemic Stroke 580
Hemorrhagic Stroke. .584
References. 585

Chapter 62—Infectious Diseases 586
Key Points. 586
Predisposition to Infection 586
Diagnosis and Management of Infections 587
Immunizations 588
Infectious Syndromes. 591
Fever of Unknown Origin 599
References. 600

Chapter 63—Endocrinology 601
Key Points. 601
Thyroid Disorders 601
Disorders of Parathyroid and Calcium Metabolism. .606
Disorders of the Anterior Pituitary 610
Disorders of the Adrenal Cortex 612
Testosterone 615
Estrogen Therapy 617
Growth Hormone 618
Melatonin 618
References. 619

Chapter 64—Diabetes Mellitus 621
Key Points. 621
Pathophysiology of Diabetes in Older Adults 621
Diagnosis and Evaluation 622
Prevention 622
Management 622
Interventions 623
References. 628

Chapter 65—Hematology 629
Key Points. 629
Hematopoiesis 629
Anemia 630
Vitamin B_{12}, Folate, and Homocysteine 638
Platelets and Coagulation 638
Chronic Myeloproliferative Neoplasms 640
References. 641

Chapter 66—Oncology and Hematologic
    Malignancies 642
Key Points. 642
Cancer Biology and Aging 642
Principles of Cancer Management 644
Specific Cancers 650
Hematologic Malignancies, Lymphomas, and
    Multiple Myeloma 655
Principles of Management 656
References. 657

Index 659

EDITORIAL BOARD

Chief Editors, Syllabus
Annette Medina-Walpole, MD, AGSF
James T. Pacala, MD, MS, AGSF

Syllabus Editors
Lisa J. Granville, MD, FACP, AGSF
G. Michael Harper, MD, AGSF
Melinda S. Lantz, MD
William L. Lyons, MD

Special Advisors
Jonathan M. Flacker, MD, AGSF
James S. Powers, MD, AGSF

Chief Editor, Questions
Jane F. Potter, MD, AGSF

Question Editors
John D. Gazewood, MD, MSPH
Gary J. Kennedy, MD
Rainier Patrick Soriano, MD

Consulting Editor for Pharmacotherapy
Judith L. Beizer, PharmD, CGP, FASCP, AGSF

Consulting Editor for Ethnogeriatrics
Sharon A. Brangman, MD, AGSF

EDITORIAL STAFF

Managing Editor
Andrea N. Sherman, MS

Medical Writers
Susan E. Aiello, DVM, ELS
Dalia Ritter

Indexer
L. Pilar Wyman

Question Scoring and Evaluation Service
Program Management Services, Inc.

AGS Staff
Nancy Lundebjerg, MPA, Deputy Executive Vice
   President, Chief Operating Officer
Elvy Ickowicz, MPH, Associate Vice President,
   Product Development and Marketing
Joe Douglas, Managing Editor, GeriatricsCareOnline.org
   and *Geriatrics At Your Fingertips*
Aimee Cegelka, Manager, Special Projects and
   Professional Development
Linda Saunders, MSW, Senior Director, Professional
   Education and Special Projects
Dennise McAlpin, Senior Manager, Professional
   Education and Special Projects

Fry Communications, Inc.
Melissa Durborow, Information Services Manager
Jason Hughes, Technical Services Manager
Rhonda Liddick, Composition Manager
William F. Adams, Compositor
Julie Stevens, Customer Service
Brian Judge, Graphic Designer

INTRODUCTION

The core mission of the American Geriatrics Society (AGS) is to improve the health, independence, and quality of life of all older adults. Since the AGS published the first *Geriatrics Review Syllabus (GRS)* in 1989, the *GRS* has become recognized as the premier geriatric medicine resource for clinicians who wish to stay current and provide evidence-based, high-quality care to older adults. To keep pace with advances in geriatric medicine, the AGS is proud to publish this ninth edition (*GRS9*). Over 180 AGS members, and leaders in the field of geriatric medicine, contributed to the *GRS9* as editors, authors, and question writers.

CONTENTS

The *GRS9* is available as a 3-volume set of books as well as in digital and mobile app formats. Book 1 contains the *Syllabus* of 66 chapters and annotated references that allow the interested reader to pursue topics in greater depth. Book 2 contains 350 case-oriented, multiple-choice questions and Book 3 repeats the questions and contains answers, supporting critiques, and references to aid learner self-assessment. The digital format comprises the entire program.

Choosing Wisely® recommendations have been added to many chapters based on the American Board of Internal Medicine Foundation's *Choosing Wisely®* Campaign.

The *Syllabus* is divided into six sections: Principles of Aging, Approach to the Patient, Systems of Care, Syndromes, Psychiatry, and Diseases and Disorders. *GRS9* highlights developments in geriatric medicine since publication of the eighth edition in 2013.

When discussing specific drugs, the authors and editors verified that the information provided was up-to-date at the time of publication. Any mention of drug uses not specifically approved by the U.S. Food and Drug Administration (ie, "off-label") are tagged as ^{OL}. The majority of medications described in the text are approved in the United States, although authors occasionally note the use of medications that are approved in Europe but not in the United States.

STRENGTH OF EVIDENCE RATINGS

In support of an evidence-based approach to care, authors have included strength-of-evidence (SOE) ratings for key diagnostic, prognostic, and therapeutic information. Authors and editors also have endeavored to present measures of association (between risk factors or therapies and conditions) in terms of absolute risk or numbers needed to treat (NNT), as well as relative risk. Please see the inside cover for further explanation of the SOE rating system.

MULTIPLE CHOICE QUESTIONS

The question editors, using questions drafted by question writers, have developed an entirely new set of 350 case-oriented, best-single-answer, multiple-choice self-study questions. These questions are designed to complement material in the *Syllabus* chapters. The questions draw on the entire knowledge base of geriatric medicine, rather than just material from the *Syllabus* text. Although the content of the questions does not completely overlap with *Syllabus* content, participants will enhance their understanding of questions by reading through the *Syllabus* chapters. Material addressed in the questions that is not discussed in the chapters is discussed in the critiques. The questions have been developed independently of any specialty board and will not be a part of any secure board certification examination.

CONTINUING MEDICAL EDUCATION (CME) AND MAINTENANCE OF CERTIFICATION (MOC)

The *GRS* self-assessment program provides participants the option of applying for *100 AMA PRA Category 1 Credit(s)™* as well as *100 ABIM Medical Knowledge MOC points*. For information on submitting answers for CME and MOC credit, please see the Program Guidelines.

We hope the *GRS9* will meet our goal of enhancing participants' knowledge base and practice patterns when caring for older adults by providing a self-study tool that is current, concise, scholarly, and clinically relevant. We encourage your comments and suggestions, as the AGS continually strives to better serve its members and the older adults they treat.

LEARNING OBJECTIVES

The learning objectives for this activity have been designed to address participant knowledge, competence, performance, and patient outcomes. At the conclusion of this program, participants should be able to:

- Describe the general principles of aging and the biomedical and psychosocial issues of aging (knowledge)
- Discuss legal and ethical issues related to geriatric medicine (knowledge/competence)
- Evaluate the financing of health care for older adults (knowledge/competence)
- Identify the basic principles of geriatric medicine, including assessment, geriatric pharmacotherapy,

- prevention, exercise, palliative care, rehabilitation, and sensory deficits (knowledge/competence)
- Use state-of-the-art approaches to geriatric care while providing care in hospital, office-practice, nursing-home, and home-care settings (performance)
- Diagnose and manage geriatric syndromes, including dementia, delirium, urinary incontinence, malnutrition, osteoporosis, falls, pressure ulcers, sleep disorders, pain, dysphagia, and dizziness (performance)
- Apply relevant information from the fields of internal medicine, neurology, psychiatry, dermatology, and gynecology to the care of older patients (performance)
- Adjust patient care in the light of evidence-based data regarding the particular risks and needs of ethnic, racial, and sexual patient groups (patient outcomes)
- Use quality indicators to assess and improve the care of older adults in their own practices (performance/patient outcomes) and
- Use evidence-based data to increase the effectiveness of teaching geriatrics to all health professionals (performance)

ADDITIONAL AMERICAN GERIATRICS SOCIETY RESOURCES

The intent of the GRS is to provide an up-to-date resource that covers the broad scope of geriatric medicine. Other AGS products designed to complement the *GRS9* in caring for older adults include:

GRS Teaching Slides are available as a subscription through www.geriatricscareonline.org. The slide presentations in Microsoft® Power Point® are based on each of the *GRS* chapters and suitable for faculty and students. Each presentation is designed for approximately a 1-hour seminar and may be used as a stand-alone lecture or as a complement to one's own personal teaching materials.

GRS Audio Companion includes 30-minute audio discussions on over 60 topics based on the *GRS* content with chapter authors and experts in the field. Continuing education credits can be obtained by successfully completing multiple choice questions derived from the audio content.

The Geriatrics Evaluation and Management (GEM) Tools include clinical templates to support clinicians and systems that are caring for older adults with common geriatric conditions.

These and other publications, including resources and clinical practice guidelines, are available at www.geriatricscareonline.org.

Other premier AGS products include:

Geriatrics at Your Fingertips, published annually, provides practical, up-to-date information for clinicians in a pocket-sized format (available in print, digital, and for mobile devices).

Doorway Thoughts: Cross-Cultural Health Care for Older Adults is a series that helps the health practitioner to understand how best to care for an increasingly multicultural patient population.

The Geriatric Nursing Review Syllabus (GNRS) and GNRS Teaching Slides, based on the *Geriatrics Review Syllabus: A Core Curriculum in Geriatric Medicine*, and adapted for advanced practice geriatric nurses.

For more information on the American Geriatrics Society, visit www.americangeriatrics.org.

PROGRAM GUIDELINES

PRE-ACTIVITY ASSESSMENT

To assess changes in participant knowledge and competence, the *GRS9* contains both a pre-activity assessment and a Continuing Medical Education (CME) exam (post-test). The pre-activity assessment is designed to test participant knowledge before reading the *GRS9 Syllabus*. These data will be used to help the American Geriatrics Society (AGS) measure the effectiveness of this CME activity.

Before reading the *GRS9 Syllabus*, please complete the first 10 questions of Book 2 and record your answers on the *GRS9* exam located at www.grs9.org.

CONTINUING EDUCATION CREDITS

ACCREDITATION

The AGS is accredited by the Accreditation Council for Continuing Medical Education (ACCME) to provide continuing medical education for physicians.

CME CREDIT HOURS

American Medical Association (AMA). The AGS designates this enduring material for a maximum of *100 AMA PRA Category 1 Credit(s)*^{TM}. Physicians should claim only the credit commensurate with the extent of their participation in the activity. The credit is available from May 1, 2016 (release date) through April 30, 2019 (expiration date). All U.S. licensing jurisdictions requiring CME recognize the AMA PRA credit system. For information on submitting answers for CME credit, please see the next section.

METHOD OF PARTICIPATION

Based on pilot tests, this activity should take approximately 100 hours to complete. To receive CME credit, participants must complete the pre-activity assessment, read the *GRS9 Syllabus*, and complete the CME exam (post-test) with at least 70% of the questions answered correctly.

SUBMISSION AND NOTIFICATION OF CME EXAMINATION PERFORMANCE

If you have purchased a digital subscription to *GRS9*, submit your answers and print your CME certificate using the self-assessment tab of the *GRS* Digital product on geriatricscareonline.org. For those who have purchased the *GRS* Print Edition only, visit www.mygrs.org to complete the CME exam (post-test).

Go online to www.grs9.org to complete the CME exam (post-test). You do not have to complete the entire exam at one time. You may save your answers, revise, and complete the exam at your own pace. Once your answers are successfully submitted, your exam results will be immediately available and you will be able to download and/or print your CME certificate of completion, check credits earned, and reprint your CME certificate and Personal Performance Results.

USER ELIGIBILITY FOR CME CREDITS

Each copy of the *GRS9* program is valid for CME credits *for only one participant*.

ABIM MEDICAL KNOWLEDGE MAINTENANCE OF CERTIFICATION (MOC)

Successful completion of this CME activity, which includes participation in the evaluation component, enables the participant to earn up to 100 MOC points in the American Board of Internal Medicine's (ABIM) Maintenance of Certification (MOC) program. Participants will earn MOC points equivalent to the amount of CME credits claimed for the activity. It is the CME activity provider's responsibility to submit participant completion information to ACCME for the purpose of granting ABIM MOC credit.

USER EVALUATION

The AGS would appreciate participants' comments about the *GRS9* program through the user evaluation on www.grs9.org. Comments and suggestions will be taken into consideration by those planning the next edition.

CONGRUITY OF CONTENT BETWEEN *SYLLABUS* AND QUESTIONS

Because the *Syllabus* chapters and the questions with critiques are written by different authors, questions may not always correlate directly with the *Syllabus*. In the event that a question's content is not addressed in the correlating chapter, its answer is fully supported in the question critique.

UPDATES AND ERRATA

Errata and important updates, such as medication alerts, will be posted as necessary on the AGS website: geriatricscareonline.org. Please report any errata to info.amger@americangeriatrics.org, Attention: *GRS* Managing Editor.

AGS GERIATRICS RECOGNITION AWARD

The Geriatrics Recognition Award (GRA) was developed by the AGS to encourage health care professionals to acquire special knowledge and keep abreast of the latest developments in geriatrics through continuing education programs. The GRA demonstrates a healthcare professional's commitment to providing quality care to patients by participating in continuing education programs in geriatrics. It provides professional recognition of a health care professional's special knowledge in geriatrics sought by many employers. CME credits earned from successfully completing the *GRS9* may be applied toward the GRA. To receive more information and an application, please provide your mailing address to the American Geriatrics Society, CME Department, 40 Fulton Street, 18th floor, New York, NY 10038, telephone (212) 308-1414, fax (212) 832-8646.

ACKNOWLEDGMENTS

The *Geriatrics Review Syllabus: A Core Curriculum in Geriatric Medicine*, 9th Edition *(GRS9)* is only possible through the collaborative efforts of many talented people. First, we express our gratitude to the Syllabus Editors: Lisa J. Granville, MD, FACP, AGSF, G. Michael Harper, MD, AGSF, Melinda S. Lantz, MD, and William L. Lyons, MD; and to the Question Editors: John D. Gazewood, MD, MSPH, Gary J. Kennedy, MD, and Rainier Patrick Soriano, MD. These editors devoted long hours to editing the chapters and questions which make this program a cutting edge resource for our readers. We also thank our Special Advisors: Jonathan M. Flacker, MD, AGSF, and James S. Powers, MD, AGSF; as well as our Consulting Editors: Sharon A. Brangman, MD, AGSF, and Judith L. Beizer, PharmD, CGP, FASCP, AGSF, for their contributions. Finally, we are very grateful to the contributing authors of chapters and questions for lending us their expertise and time for this publication.

GRS is extremely fortunate to have again the steady hand of Andrea Sherman, MS, *GRS* Managing Editor at the helm to coordinate all aspects of the production, from initial organization through distribution. Andrea's kind but firm guidance has been essential to producing a review program of the highest quality and we give enormous thanks for her assistance. We are grateful also to Susan E. Aiello, DVM, ELS, our medical editor, whose fine hand is evident throughout the *GRS*; to Dalia Ritter for editing the first round of questions and critiques and for helping us to ensure that these are consistent with the style of the questions on Board exams; and to L. Pilar Wyman for her comprehensive index of the *GRS*, which facilitates reader's access to *GRS* content.

We wish to express our appreciation for the strong support of the AGS Board of Directors and AGS staff. Furthermore, this work could not have been accomplished without the efforts of the administrative assistants of the editors and contributing authors. We salute their assistance in preparing drafts of the chapters, questions, and critiques. In addition, we thank our families for their unwavering support during the nights and weekends of this project. Finally, we thank our patients, who continually inform, inspire, challenge, and sustain us.

Annette Medina-Walpole, MD, AGSF
James T. Pacala, MD, MS, AGSF
Jane F. Potter, MD, AGSF

Chief Editors

EDITORIAL BOARD

CO-CHIEF EDITORS, SYLLABUS

Annette Medina-Walpole, MD, AGSF
Professor of Medicine
Acting Chief, Division of Geriatrics and Aging
University of Rochester School of Medicine and Dentistry
Rochester, NY

James T. Pacala, MD, MS, AGSF
Professor and Associate Head
Distinguished University Teaching Professor
Department of Family Practice and Community Health
University of Minnesota Medical School
Minneapolis, MN

CHAPTER EDITORS

Lisa J. Granville, MD, AGSF
Professor and Associate Chair, Department of Geriatrics
Florida State University College of Medicine
Tallahassee, FL

G. Michael Harper, MD, AGSF
Professor of Medicine, University of California San Francisco
Staff Physician, San Francisco Veteran Affairs Medical Center
San Francisco, CA

Melinda S. Lantz, MD
Chief of Geriatric Psychiatry
Beth Israel Medical Center
New York, NY

William L. Lyons, MD
Professor, Division of Geriatrics and Gerontology
Department of Internal Medicine
University of Nebraska Medical Center
Omaha, NE

CONSULTING EDITOR FOR PHARMACOTHERAPY

Judith L. Beizer, PharmD, CGP, FASCP, AGSF
Clinical Professor, College of Pharmacy & Health Sciences
St. John's University
Queens, NY

CONSULTING EDITOR FOR ETHNOGERIATRICS

Sharon A. Brangman, MD, AGSF
Distinguished Service Professor, Division Chief, Geriatrics
SUNY Upstate Medical University
Syracuse, NY

CHIEF EDITOR, QUESTIONS

Jane F. Potter, MD, AGSF
Harris Professor of Geriatric Medicine
Chief, Division of Geriatrics and Gerontology
Department of Internal Medicine
University of Nebraska Medical Center
Director, Home Instead Center for Successful Aging
Omaha, NE

QUESTION EDITORS

John D. Gazewood, MD, MSPH
Harrison Medical Teaching Associate Professor of Family Medicine
Residency Director
University of Virginia Health System
Charlottesville, VA

Gary J. Kennedy, MD
Professor of Psychiatry and Behavioral Science
Albert Einstein College of Medicine
Director, Division of Geriatric Psychiatry and the
  Leslie and Roslyn Goldstein Geriatric Psychiatry Fellowship Program
Montefiore Medical Center
Bronx, NY

Rainier Patrick Soriano, MD
Associate Professor, Medicine, Medical Education, Geriatrics and Palliative Care
Director of Curriculum and Director of Educational Technology
Department of Medical Education
Icahn School of Medicine at Mount Sinai
New York, NY

SPECIAL ADVISORS

Jonathan M. Flacker, MD, AGSF
Professor
Emory University School of Medicine
Atlanta, GA

James S. Powers, MD, AGSF
Associate Professor of Medicine
Vanderbilt University Medical Center
Associate Clinical Director, TVHS GRECC
Nashville, TN

CONTRIBUTING CHAPTER AUTHORS

Marc E. Agronin, MD
Affiliate Associate Professor of Psychiatry and Neurology
University of Miami Miller School of Medicine
Vice President, Behavioral Health and Clinical Research
Miami Jewish Health Systems
Miami, FL

Kathleen M. Akgün, MD, MS
Assistant Professor
VA Connecticut Healthcare System
Department of Internal Medicine, Section of Pulmonary, Critical Care and Sleep Medicine
West Haven, CT
Yale University School of Medicine
Department of Internal Medicine
Section of Pulmonary, Critical Care and Sleep Medicine
New Haven, CT

Douglas A. Albreski, DPM
Assistant Professor, Department of Dermatology
University of Connecticut School of Medicine
Director of the Podiatric Dermatology Clinic
Farmington, CT

Cathy A. Alessi, MD, AGSF
Director, Geriatric Research, Education and Clinical Center
Veterans Administration Greater Los Angeles Healthcare System
Professor, David Geffen School of Medicine at UCLA
Los Angeles, CA

Neil B. Alexander, MD
Director, Mobility Research Center
Professor, Division of Geriatric and Palliative Medicine, Department of Internal Medicine
Research Professor, Institute of Gerontology
University of Michigan
Director, VA Ann Arbor Health Care System GRECC
Ann Arbor, MI

Alicia I. Arbaje, MD, MPH
Assistant Professor of Medicine
Associate Director of Transitional Care Research
Division of Geriatric Medicine and Gerontology
Johns Hopkins University School of Medicine
Baltimore, MD

Priscilla F. Bade, MD, FACP, CMD
Professor of Internal Medicine
Sanford School of Medicine at the University of South Dakota
Rapid City, SD

Cynthia Barton, RN, MSN
Geriatric Nurse Practitioner, Memory and Aging Center
Associate Clinical Professor, School of Nursing
University of California, San Francisco
San Francisco, CA

Joshua I. Bernstein, MD
Renal Medical Associates
Associate Clinical Professor, School of Nursing
San Francisco, CA

Sarah D. Berry, MD, MPH
Assistant Professor of Medicine
Department of Medicine
Beth Israel Deaconess Medical Center and Harvard Medical School
Research Scientist
Institute for Aging Research
Hebrew SeniorLife
Boston, MA

Marc R. Blackman, MD
Associate Chief of Staff for Research & Development
Washington DC VAMC
Assistant Dean for VA Research
Professor of Medicine and Rehabilitation Medicine
Georgetown University School of Medicine
Clinical Professor of Medicine, Biochemistry & Molecular Medicine
George Washington University School of Medicine
Washington, DC

Yara Bonet-Pagan, MD
Department of Geriatric Psychiatry
Montefiore Medical Center
Bronx, NY

Cynthia M. Boyd, MD, MPH
Associate Professor
Division of Geriatric Medicine and Gerontology
Department of Medicine
Johns Hopkins School of Medicine
Baltimore, MD

Cynthia J. Brown, MD, MSPH, AGSF
Professor of Medicine
Director, Division of Gerontology, Geriatrics, and Palliative Care
University of Alabama at Birmingham
Veterans Affairs Medical Center GRECC
Birmingham, AL

Maciej S. Buchowski, PhD
Research Professor of Medicine and Pediatrics
Department of Medicine
Division of Gastroenterology, Hepatology and Nutrition
Vanderbilt University Medical Center
Nashville, TN

Thomas V. Caprio, MD, MPH, MSHPE, FACP, CMD, HMDC, AGSF
Associate Professor of Medicine/Geriatrics, Clinical Nursing, and Public Health Sciences
Program Director, Geriatric Medicine Fellowship
Project Director, Finger Lakes Geriatric Workforce Enhancement Program
Medical Director, Visiting Nurse Service of Rochester
University of Rochester Medical Center
Rochester, NY

Julie C. Chapman, PsyD
Director of Neuroscience
Neurology Service
Veterans Affairs Medical Center
Assistant Professor of Neurology
Georgetown University School of Medicine
Washington, DC

Gurkamal S. Chatta, MD
Professor of Oncology
Roswell Park Cancer Institute
University of Buffalo
Buffalo, NY

Colleen Christmas, MD, FACP
Associate Professor of Medicine
Director, Primary Care Track
Johns Hopkins School of Medicine
Associate Residency Program Director
Johns Hopkins Bayview Medical Center
Divisions of Geriatric Medicine and General Internal Medicine
Baltimore, MD

Leo M. Cooney, Jr., MD
Humana Foundation Professor of Geriatric Medicine
Yale University School of Medicine
New Haven, CT

Grace A. Cordts, MD, MPH, MS
Medical Director
Optum Complex Population Management
Pittsburgh, PA

Steven R. Counsell, MD, AGSF
Mary Elizabeth Mitchell Professor
Director, IU Geriatrics
Scientist, IU Center for Aging Research
Indiana University School of Medicine
Indianapolis, IN

G. Willy Davila, MD
Chairman, Department of Gynecology
Head, Section of Urogynecology and Reconstructive Pelvic Surgery
Cleveland Clinic Florida
Weston, FL

Danielle J. Doberman, MD, MPH
Director, Palliative Medicine Program
George Washington University Hospital
Assistant Professor of Medicine
George Washington University School of Medicine
Washington DC

Catherine E. DuBeau, MD
Professor of Medicine
Division of Geriatric Medicine
Departments of Medicine, Family Medicine and Community Health, and Obstetrics & Gynecology
University of Massachusetts Medical School
UMass Memorial Medical Center
Worcester, MA

Manuel A. Eskildsen, MD, MPH, CMD, AGSF
Associate Clinical Professor
David Geffen School of Medicine at UCLA
Department of Medicine, Division of Geriatrics
Santa Monica, CA

Neal S. Fedarko, PhD
Professor, Division of Geriatric Medicine and Gerontology
Department of Medicine
Co-Director, Biology of Healthy Aging Program
Director, Translational Research Training Program in Gerontology & Geriatrics
Johns Hopkins University
Baltimore, MD

Luigi Ferrucci, MD, PhD
Senior Investigator
NIA Scientific Director
Chief, Longitudinal Studies Section
The National Institute on Aging
National Institute of Health
Baltimore, MD

Kathleen T. Foley, PhD, OTR/L
Associate Professor/Research Coordinator
School of Occupational Therapy
Brenau University
Norcross, GA

Linda P. Fried, MD, MPH, AGSF
Dean and DeLamar Professor of Public Health
Columbia University Mailman School of Public Health
Professor of Epidemiology and Medicine
Senior Vice President, Columbia University Medical Center
New York, NY

Terry Fulmer, PhD, RN, FAAN, AGSF
Dean of the Bouvé College of Health Sciences
Northeastern University
College of Health Sciences
Boston, MA

Elizabeth Galik, PhD, CRNP
Assistant Professor
Robert Wood Johnson Foundation Nurse
Faculty Scholar
University of Maryland School of Nursing
Baltimore, MD

Joseph E. Gaugler, PhD
Associate Professor, McKnight Presidential Fellow
Editor-in-Chief, *Journal of Applied Gerontology*
School of Nursing, Center on Aging, University of Minnesota
Minneapolis, MN

Angela Gentili, MD
Associate Professor of Internal Medicine
Director, Geriatrics Fellowship Training Program
VAMC/Virginia Commonwealth University
Richmond, VA

JoAnn A. Giaconi, MD
Associate Clinical Professor of Ophthalmology
Jules Stein Eye Institute
UCLA David Geffen School of Medicine and the
Veterans Administration of Greater Los Angeles
Los Angeles, CA

Thomas M. Gill, MD
Humana Foundation Professor of Geriatric Medicine
Professor of Medicine, Epidemiology & Investigative Medicine
Yale School of Medicine
New Haven, CT

Suzanne M. Gillespie, MD, RD, CMD, FACP
Associate Professor of Medicine
Division of Geriatrics/Aging
University of Rochester School of Medicine and Dentistry
Rochester, NY

Seth Gordon, MBA
Managing Partner
The Access Group
Berkeley Heights, NJ

Jane M. Grant-Kels, MD
Assistant Dean of Clinical Affairs
University of Connecticut Health Center
Chair, Department of Dermatology
Professor of Dermatology, Pathology and Pediatrics
Dermatology Residency Director
Director of Dermatopathology
Director of the Cutaneous Oncology and Melanoma Program
Farmington, CT

Lisa J. Granville, MD, AGSF, FACP
Professor and Associate Chair
Department of Geriatrics
Florida State University College of Medicine
Tallahassee, FL

David A. Gruenewald, MD
Associate Professor of Medicine
Division of Gerontology and Geriatric Medicine
Department of Medicine
University of Washington School of Medicine
Geriatrics/Extended Care Service
VA Puget Sound Health Care System
Seattle, WA

Ihab Hajjar, MD, MS, FACP, AGSF
Associate Professor of Medicine and Neurology
Division of Geriatrics and General Internal Medicine
Department of Medicine, Emory University
Atlanta, GA

Janna Hardland, MD
UT Southwestern Medical Center
Dallas, TX

Manisha Juthani-Mehta, MD
Associate Professor, Section of Infectious Diseases
Infectious Diseases Fellowship Program Director
Yale University School of Medicine
New Haven, CT

Paul R. Katz, MD, CMD, AGSF
Chair, Department of Geriatrics
College of Medicine
Florida State University
Tallahassee, FL

Philip O. Katz, MD
Clinical Professor of Medicine
Jefferson Medical College
Chairman, Division of Gastroenterology
Albert Einstein Medical Center
Philadelphia, PA

Gary J. Kennedy, MD
Professor of Psychiatry and Behavioral Science
Albert Einstein College of Medicine
Director, Division of Geriatric Psychiatry and the
  Leslie and Roslyn Goldstein Geriatric Psychiatry Fellowship
  Program
Montefiore Medical Center
Bronx, NY

Anne M. Kenny, MD
Professor of Medicine
Department of Medicine
University of Connecticut Health Center
Farmington, CT

Douglas P. Kiel, MD, MPH
Professor of Medicine
Department of Medicine
Beth Israel Deaconess Medical Center and Harvard Medical School
Director, Musculoskeletal Research Center
Institute for Aging Research
Hebrew SeniorLife
Boston, MA

Melinda S. Lantz, MD
Chief of Geriatric Psychiatry
Mount Sinai Beth Israel Medical Center
New York, NY

Sei J. Lee, MD, MAS
Associate Professor
University of California, San Francisco
Senior Scholar, SF VA Quality Scholars Fellowship
Division of Geriatrics
San Francisco, CA

Susan W. Lehmann, MD
Associate Professor
Department of Psychiatry and Behavioral Sciences
Johns Hopkins University School of Medicine
Baltimore, MD

Jeffrey M. Levine, MD, AGSF, CWSP
Assistant Professor of Geriatrics and Palliative Care
The Brookdale Department of Geriatrics and Palliative Care
Icahn School of Medicine at Mount Sinai
Attending, Center for Advanced Wound Care
Mount Sinai Beth Israel Medical Center
New York, NY

Kenneth W. Lyles, MD, AGSF
Professor of Medicine
Director, Medicine Clinical Research Unit
Duke University School of Medicine
VA Medical Center
Durham, NC
Medical Director,
The Carolina's Center for Medical Excellence
Cary, NC

Allison Magnuson, DO
Senior Instructor of Medicine
Geriatric Oncology
University of Rochester Medical Center
Rochester, NY

Una E. Makris, MD, MCS
Assistant Professor, Department of Internal Medicine
Division of Rheumatic Diseases
UT Southwestern Medical Center and Dallas VAMC
Dallas, TX

Edward R. Marcantonio, MD, SM
Professor of Medicine
Harvard Medical School
Section Chief for Research
Director, Aging Research Program
Division of General Medicine and Primary Care
Beth Israel Deaconess Medical Center
Boston, MA

Alvin M. Matsumoto, MD
Professor of Medicine
Acting Head, Division of Gerontology & Geriatric Medicine
Department of Medicine
University of Washington School of Medicine
Associate Director, Geriatric Research, Education, and Clinical Center
VA Puget Sound Health Care System
Seattle, WA

Donovan Maust, MD, MS
Assistant Professor of Psychiatry
University of Michigan
Research Scientist, Center for Clinical Management Research
VA Ann Arbor Healthcare System
Ann Arbor, MI

Matthew K. McNabney, MD, AGSF
Associate Professor of Medicine
Johns Hopkins University
Fellowship Program Director, Geriatrics
Medical Director, Hopkins ElderPlus
Baltimore, MD

Supriya Mohile, MD, MS
Associate Professor of Medicine
Director of Geriatric Oncology
University of Rochester Medical Center
Rochester, NY

Thomas Mulligan, MD, AGSF
Director, Center on Aging
Medical Director, Senior Services
St. Bernards Healthcare
Jonesboro, AR

Daniel L. Murman, MD, MS, FAAN
Director, Behavioral and Geriatric Neurology Program
Professor, Department of Neurological Sciences
College of Medicine
University of Nebraska Medical Center
Omaha, NE

Aman Nanda, MD, AGSF, CMD
Associate Professor of Medicine
Program Director
Geriatric Medicine Fellowship Program
The Warren Alpert Medical School of Brown University
Providence, RI

Judith Neugroschl, MD
Medical Director,
Mount Sinai School of Medicine Alzheimer's Disease Research Center Clinical Core
Co-Director, ADRC Education and Information Transfer Core
New York, NY

David W. Oslin, MD
Chief of Behavioral Health at the Philadelphia VAMC
Director, VISN 4 MIRECC
Professor
Perelman School of Medicine
University of Pennsylvania
Philadelphia, PA

James T. Pacala, MD, MS, AGSF
Professor and Associate Head
Distinguished University Teaching Professor
Department of Family Practice and Community Health
University of Minnesota Medical School
Minneapolis, MN

Vyjeyanthi S. Periyakoil, MD
Clinical Associate Professor
Director, Palliative Care Education & Training
Director, eCampus Geriatrics
VA Palo Alto Health Care System &
Stanford University School of Medicine
Stanford, CA

Edgar Pierluissi, MD
Professor of Medicine, University of California at San Francisco
Medical Director, Acute Care for Elders (ACE) Unit
San Francisco General Hospital
San Francisco, CA

Margaret Pisani, MD, MPH
Associate Professor
Yale University School of Medicine
Pulmonary and Critical Care Medicine
New Haven, CT

James S. Powers, MD, AGSF
Associate Professor of Medicine
Vanderbilt University Medical Center
Associate Clinical Director, TVHS GRECC
Nashville, TN

Michael W. Rich, MD, AGSF
Professor of Medicine
Cardiovascular Division
Washington University School of Medicine
St. Louis, MO

Josette A. Rivera, MD
Associate Professor of Medicine
University of California San Francisco
San Francisco, CA

Theresa A. Rowe, DO
Health Services Research Fellow
Institute for Public Health & Medicine
Instructor of Medicine
Division of General Internal Medicine and Geriatrics
Northwestern University, Feinberg School of Medicine
Chicago, IL

David Sarraf, MD
Clinical Professor of Ophthalmology
Retinal Disorders and Ophthalmic Genetics Division
Jules Stein Eye Institute, UCLA School of Medicine
Veterans Administration of Greater Los Angeles
Los Angeles, CA

Paul Scalzo, BS
NIH Postbaccalaureate IRTA Fellow
The National Institute on Aging
Baltimore, MD

J. William Schleifer, MD
Department of Cardiovascular Diseases
Mayo Clinic Arizona
Phoenix, AZ

Mara A. Schonberg, MD, MPH
Assistant Professor in Medicine
Beth Israel Deaconess Medical Center
Harvard Medical School
Brookline, MA

Todd P. Semla, MS, PharmD, BCPS, FCCP, AGSF
National PBM Clinical Pharmacy Program
Manager–Mental Health & Geriatrics
Pharmacy Benefits Management Services
Department of Veterans Affairs
Associate Professor
Departments of Medicine, and Psychiatry and Behavioral Sciences
The Feinberg School of Medicine
Northwestern University
Evanston, IL

Kenneth Shay, DDS, MS, AGSF
Director of Geriatric Programs
Geriatrics and Extended Care Services
VA Central Office
Washington, DC

Win-Kuang Shen, MD
Professor of Medicine
Mayo Clinic College of Medicine
Chair, Division of Cardiovascular Diseases
Mayo Clinic Arizona
Phoenix, AZ

Mark J. Simone, MD
Associate Program Director-Primary Care
Mount Auburn Internal Medicine Residency Program
Assistant Professor of Medicine
Harvard Medical School
Division of Geriatric Medicine, Mount Auburn
Cambridge, MA

Roy E. Smith, MD, MS
Professor of Medicine
Hematology-Oncology
University of Pittsburgh
Pittsburgh, PA

Peter G. Snell, PhD
Adjunct Associate Professor of Medicine
Department of Internal Medicine
Division of Cardiology
UT Southwestern Medical Center
Dallas, TX

Margarita Sotelo, MD
Associate Clinical Professor
Divisions of Geriatrics and Hospital Medicine
University of California San Francisco
San Francisco, CA

Amir E. Soumekh, MD
Assistant Professor of Clinical Medicine
Jay Monahan Center for Gastrointestinal Health
Weill Cornell Medical College
New York, NY

Richard G. Stefanacci, DO, MGH, MBA, AGSF, CMD
Thomas Jefferson University
College of Population Health
Philadelphia, PA
Chief Medical Officer
The Access Group
Berkeley Heights, NJ

Kristen Thornton, MD, FAAFP, AGSF, CWSP
Assistant Professor of Family Medicine
Highland Family Medicine
Assistant Professor of Medicine
Monroe Community Hospital, Division of Geriatrics & Aging
Co-Director Aging Theme
University of Rochester School of Medicine and Dentistry
Rochester, NY

Alexander W. Threlfall, MD, MA
Associate Chief, CBOC MH
San Francisco VA Medical Center
Acting Director, Mental Health Service Santa Rosa CBOC
Clinical Instructor
Department of Geriatric Psychiatry
University of California, San Francisco
San Francisco, CA

Jay R. Trabin, MD, FACOG
Director, Lower Genital Tract Disorders Clinic
Department of Gynecology
Cleveland Clinic Florida
Weston, FL

Justin M. Vader, MD
Assistant Professor
Cardiovascular Division
Washington University School of Medicine
St. Louis, MO

Elizabeth K. Vig, MD, MPH
Associate Professor, Department of Medicine
Division of Gerontology and Geriatric Medicine
University of Washington
Staff Physician, Geriatrics and Extended Care
VA Puget Sound Health Care System
Seattle, WA

Andrew Warren, MB, BS, DPhil
Psychiatrist
Sheppard Pratt Physicians Association
Baltimore, MD

Loren M. Wilkerson, MD
Medical Instructor
Department of Medicine, Division of Geriatrics
Duke University School of Medicine
Durham, NC

Pui Yin Wong, MD
Attending Geriatric Psychiatrist
Mount Sinai Beth Israel Medical Center
New York, NY

CONTRIBUTING QUESTION AUTHORS

Emaad Abdel-Rahman, MD, PhD, FASN
Professor, Internal Medicine/Nephrology
Director, Kidney Center Clinic and Dialysis Unit
Director, Therapeutic Extra-Corporeal Unit
Head, Section of Geriatric Nephrology
Interim Director, Nephrology Transplant
University of Virginia
Charlottesville, VA

Jonathan S. Appelbaum, MD, FACP, AAHIVS
Laurie L. Dozier, Jr., MD, Education Director and Professor of Internal Medicine
Florida State University College of Medicine
Tallahassee, FL

Michele C. Balas, PhD, RN, APRN-NP, FCCM
Associate Professor
Center of Excellence in Critical and Complex Care
The Ohio State University College of Nursing
Columbus, OH

Matthew Barrett, MD
Assistant Professor
Department of Neurology
Charlottesville, VA

Lisa C. Barry, PhD, MPH
Assistant Professor of Psychiatry
UConn Center on Aging
Farmington, CT

Rachelle Bernacki, MD, MS, AGSF
Director of Quality Initiatives
Adult Palliative Care
Dana Farber Cancer Institute
Division of Aging
Brigham and Women's Hospital
Boston, MA

Michael Bogaisky, MD
Assistant Professor
Division of Geriatrics
Albert Einstein College of Medicine
Bronx, NY

Kenneth Brummel-Smith, MD, AGSF
Health and Aging Policy Fellow
Charlotte Edwards Maguire Professor and Chair,
Department of Geriatrics
Florida State University College of Medicine
Tallahassee, FL

Morgan Carlson, PhD
Research Investigator, Drug Discovery
Genomics Institute of the Novartis Research Foundation
San Diego, CA

Susan Charette, MD
Clinical Professor
Division of Geriatrics
Department of Medicine
Los Angeles, CA

Carl I. Cohen, MD
SUNY Distinguished Service Professor
Professor and Director
Division of Geriatric Psychiatry
SUNY Downstate Medical Center
Brooklyn, NY

Leo M. Cooney, Jr, MD
Humana Foundation Professor of Geriatric Medicine
Yale University School of Medicine
New Haven, CT

Mary Ellen Csuka, MD
Professor
Division of Rheumatology
Department of Medicine
Medical College of Wisconsin
Milwaukee, WI

Della E. Dillard, MD, MBA
Assistant Professor
Donald W. Reynolds Department of Geriatric Medicine
Department of Medicine
University of Oklahoma
Oklahoma City, OK

Ian M. Deutchki, MD
University of Rochester Medical Center
School of Medicine and Dentistry
Assistant Professor
Department of Family Medicine and Department of Medicine
Division of Geriatrics
Rochester, NY

Justin Endo, MD, FAAD
Assistant Professor of Dermatology
University of Wisconsin
Madison, WI

Jerome Epplin, MD, AGSF
Clinical Professor
Southern Illinois School of Medicine
Litchfield Family Practice Center
Litchfield, IL

Daniel E. Forman, MD, FACC, FAHA
Chair, Section of Geriatric Cardiology
University of Pittsburgh Medical Center
Pittsburgh, PA

Susan M. Friedman, MD, MPH, AGSF
Associate Professor of Medicine
Research Director, Geriatric Fracture Center
University of Rochester School of Medicine and Dentistry
Rochester, NY

Shelly L. Gray, PharmD, MS, AGSF
Professor and Vice Chair, Pharmacy
Director, Geriatrics Pharmacy Program
School of Pharmacy
University of Washington
Seattle, WA

Asaff Harel, MD
Department of Neurology
Mount Sinai Medical Center
New York, NY

Elizabeth N. Harlow, MD
Assistant Professor
Geriatrics, Internal Medicine
Omaha, NE

Holly B. Hindman, MD, MPH
Associate Professor of Ophthalmology and Visual Science
Flaum Eye Institute
University of Rochester
Rochester, NY

Lianne Hirano, MD
Acting Assistant Professor
Division of Gerontology & Geriatric Medicine
Harborview Medical Center
Seattle, WA

Ted Johnson, MD, MPH, AGSF
Professor of Medicine and Epidemiology, Emory University
Division Chief, General Medicine & Geriatrics
Atlanta Site Director, Birmingham/Atlanta VA GRECC
Decatur, GA

Fran E. Kaiser, MD, AGSF, FGSA
Adjunct Professor of Medicine
St. Louis University School of Medicine
St Louis, MO
Executive Medical Director
Region Medical Director Program
Merck and Co., Inc
Upper Gwynedd, PA

Helen Kao, MD
University of California, San Francisco
Division of Geriatrics
San Francisco, CA

Anne Kenny, MD
Professor of Medicine
Department of Medicine
University of Connecticut Health Center
Farmington, CT

Tia Kostas, MD
Assistant Professor of Medicine
Section of Geriatrics and Palliative Medicine
University of Chicago
Chicago, IL

Lawrence R. Krakoff, MD
Professor of Medicine
Center for Cardiovascular Health
Mount Sinai Medical Center
New York, NY

Stephen Krieger, MD
Associate Professor of Neurology
Corinne Goldsmith Dickinson Center for MS
Director, Neurology Residency Program
Icahn School of Medicine at Mount Sinai
New York, NY

Lorand Kristof, MD, MSc
Assistant Clinical Professor
McMaster University
Department of Family Medicine
Wise Elephant Family Health Team
Brampton Civic Hospital
William Osler Health System
Brampton, Ontario

Chandrika Kumar, MD, FACP
Director of Resident Geriatric Medical Education
Associate Fellowship Director
Yale University School of Medicine
New Haven, CT
Geriatric Consult Service
West Haven Veterans Administration
West Haven, CT

Mark S. Lachs, MD, MPH
Irene F. and I. Roy Psaty Distinguished Professor of Medicine
Co-chief, Division of Geriatrics and Palliative Medicine
Director of Geriatrics
The New York-Presbyterian Health Care System
New York, NY

Sei J. Lee, MD, MAS
Associate Professor
University of California, San Francisco
Senior Scholar, SF VA Quality Scholars Fellowship
Division of Geriatrics
San Francisco, CA

Michael C. Lindberg, MD, FACP
Chief Medical Officer
Monadnock Community Hospital
Peterborough, NH

Hannah I. Lipman, MD, MS
Associate Director, Montefiore-Einstein Center for Bioethics
Chief, Bioethics Consultation Service
Associate Professor of Medicine
Divisions of Geriatrics and Cardiology
Bronx, NY

Hao Liu, PT, PhD, MD
Associate Professor of Physical Therapy
University of North Texas Health Science Center
Fort Worth, TX

Vera P. Luther, MD, FACP
Associate Professor of Medicine
Director, Infectious Diseases Fellowship
Associate Program Director, Internal Medicine Residency
Department of Internal Medicine
Section on Infectious Diseases
Wake Forest School of Medicine
Winston-Salem, NC

Diana V. Messadi, DDS, MMSc, DMSc
Professor of Dentistry
Associate Dean for Education and Faculty Development
Chair, Section of Oral Medicine and Orofacial Pain
UCLA School of Dentistry
Los Angeles, CA

Leigh Ann Mike, PharmD, BCPS, CGP
Clinical Assistant Professor
Coordinator, Plein Certificate in Geriatric Pharmacy
University of Washington School of Pharmacy
Consultant Pharmacist, UW Pharmacy Cares
Seattle, WA

Karen L. Miller, MD
Adjunct Associate Professor
Department of Obstetrics and Gynecology
University of Utah
Salt Lake City, UT

Irene Moore, MSW, LISW-S, AGSF
Professor, Department of Family & Community Medicine
Assistant Director, Geriatric Medicine Program
University of Cincinnati Geriatric Medicine Program
Cincinnati, OH

Bryan C. Markinson, DPM
Associate Professor of Orthopedic Surgery
Chief, Podiatric Medicine and Surgery
The Leni and Peter W. May Department of Orthopedic Surgery
Icahn School of Medicine at Mount Sinai
New York, NY

Alison A. Moore, MD, MPH
Professor, Departments of Medicine and Psychiatry
David Geffen School of Medicine at UCLA
Division of Geriatric Medicine
Los Angeles, CA

Cynthia X. Pan, MD, FACP, AGSF
Chief, Division of Geriatrics and Palliative Care Medicine
New York Presbyterian Queens
Associate Professor of Clinical Medicine
Weill Cornell Medical College
Flushing, NY

Kourosh Parham, MD, PhD, FACS
Associate Professor of Surgery
Director of Research, Division of Otolaryngology
Department of Surgery
UConn Health
Farmington, CT

Barbara Resnick, PhD, CRNP, FAAN, FAANP, AGSF
Professor
Sonya Ziporkin Gershowitz Chair in Gerontology
University of Maryland School of Nursing
Baltimore, MD

Miriam Rodin, MD, PhD
Professor of Geriatric Medicine
Department of Internal Medicine
St. Louis University School of Medicine
St. Louis, MO

Laurence Z. Rubenstein, MD, MPH, FACP, AGSF
Professor and Chairman
Reynolds Department of Geriatric Medicine
The Donald W. Reynolds Chair in Geriatric Medicine
The University of Oklahoma, Health Sciences Center
Oklahoma City, OK

Alessandra Scalmati, MD, PhD
Department of Psychiatry and Behavioral Sciences
Montefiore Medical Center
The University Hospital of The Albert Einstein College of Medicine
Outpatient Department of Psychiatry
Bronx, NY

Krupa Shah, MD, MPH, AGSF
Assistant Professor
University of Rochester School of Medicine & Dentistry
Division of Geriatrics and Aging
Department of Medicine
Rochester, NY

Nina J. Solenski, MD
Associate Professor in Neurology
Department of Neurology
University of Virginia
Charlottesville, VA

Margarita Sotelo, MD
Associate Clinical Professor
Divisions of Geriatrics and Hospital Medicine
University of California San Francisco
San Francisco, CA

Richard G. Stefanacci, DO, MGH, MBA, AGSF, CMD
Thomas Jefferson University
College of Population Health
Philadelphia, PA
Chief Medical Officer
The Access Group
Berkeley Heights, NJ

Martin Steinberg, MD
Assistant Professor of Psychiatry and Behavioral Sciences
Johns Hopkins Bayview Medical Center
Baltimore, MD

Winnie Suen, MD, AGSF
Medical Director of Geriatrics
Section Chief of Geriatrics
Inova Fairfax Hospital
Falls Church, VA

Dennis H. Sullivan, MD, AGSF
Director, Geriatric Research Education and Clinical Center
Central Arkansas Veterans Healthcare System
Professor and Vice-Chair
Donald W Reynolds Department of Geriatrics
University of Arkansas for Medical Sciences
Little Rock, AR

George E. Taffet, MD, FACP
Professor in Medicine
Chief, Geriatrics
Geriatrics and Cardiovascular Sciences
Robert J. Luchi, MD Chair in Geriatric Medicine
Baylor College of Medicine
Head of the Division of Geriatrics
The Methodist Hospital
Houston, TX

George Taler, MD
Director, Long Term Care
Washington Hospital Center
Professor, Clinical Medicine, Geriatrics and Long Term Care
Georgetown University School of Medicine
Washington, DC

John A. Taylor, III, MD, MS
Associate Professor of Surgery
Division of Urology
Chairman, Cancer Committee
University of Connecticut Health Center
Farmington, CT

Ipsit V. Vahia, MD
Assistant Professor of Psychiatry
Director of Research, Senior Behavioral Health
Stein Institute for Research on Aging
University of California, San Diego
La Jolla, CA

Camille P. Vaughan, MD, MS
Assistant Professor of Medicine, Emory University
Associate Section Chief for Research, Geriatrics and Gerontology
Investigator, Birmingham/Atlanta VA GRECC
Decatur, GA

Fran Valle, DNP, CRNP
Assistant Professor of Nursing
Director of the Post Master's Doctor of Nursing Practice Program
University of Maryland School of Nursing
Baltimore, MD

Dennis T. Villareal, MD, FACP, FACE
Professor, Baylor College of Medicine
Michael E. DeBakey VA Medical Center
Houston, TX

Barbara E. Weinstein, PhD
Professor and Founding Executive Officer
Health Sciences Doctoral Programs and AuD Program
Professor Speech Language Hearing Sciences
The Graduate Center
The City University of New York
New York, NY

Julie Wetherell, MD
Staff Psychologist
VA San Diego Healthcare System
Professor of Psychiatry
University of California San Diego
La Jolla, CA

G. Darryl Wieland, PhD, MPH, AGSF
Senior Research Scientist
Center for Population Health and Aging
Social Science Research Institute
Duke University
Durham, NC

Rebecca Wysoske, MD
Assistant Professor
College of Medicine
Department of Psychiatry
University of Nebraska Medical Center
Omaha, NE

Fariba S. Younai, DDS
Professor of Clinical Dentistry
Oral Medicine and Orofacial Pain
Vice Chair, Division of Oral Biology and Medicine
UCLA School of Dentistry
Los Angeles, CA

Michi Yukawa MD, MPH
Professor of Medicine
Medical Director of Community Living Center
San Francisco VA Medical Center
University of California, San Francisco
San Francisco, CA

Raymond Yung, MD
Professor of Internal Medicine
Chief, Division of Geriatric and Palliative Medicine
University of Michigan
Ann Arbor, MI

Valerie Zamudio, MD
Longterm Care Physician and Faculty
Geriatrics, Palliative Medicine, and Continuing Care Services
Kaiser Permanente Los Angeles Medical Center
Los Angeles, CA

Phyllis C. Zee, MD, PhD
Professor of Neurology
Department of Neurobiology and Physiology
Director Sleep Disorders Center
Chicago, IL

Richard A. Zweig, PhD
Director, Ferkauf Older Adult Program
Associate Professor of Psychology
Ferkauf Graduate School of Yeshiva University
Assistant Professor of Psychiatry
Albert Einstein College of Medicine
Bronx, NY

Jessica L. Zwerling, MD, MS
Assistant Professor
The Saul R. Korey Department of Neurology
Albert Einstein College of Medicine/Montefiore Medical Center
Neurologist and Director of the Memory Disorders Center
Associate Director of the Center for the Aging Brain
Program Director, Geriatric Neurology Fellowship
Montefiore Medical Center
Bronx, NY

GRS9 DISCLOSURES OF FINANCIAL INTERESTS

As an accredited provider of Continuing Medical Education, the American Geriatrics Society continuously strives to ensure that the education activities planned and conducted by our faculty meet generally accepted ethical standards as codified by the ACCME, the Food and Drug Administration, and the American Medical Association. To this end, we have implemented a process wherein everyone who is in a position to control the content of an educational activity has disclosed to us all relevant financial relationships with any commercial interests within the past 12 months as related to the content of their presentations and under which we work to resolve any real or apparent conflicts of interest. Conflicts of interest in this particular CME activity have been resolved by having the presentation content independently peer reviewed before publication by the Editorial Board and Question Review Committee.

The following contributors (and/or their spouses/partners) have reported real or apparent conflicts of interest that have been resolved through a peer review content validation process:

Cathy A. Alessi, MD, AGSF
Dr. Alessi is a paid consultant for Optum Rx, Inc.

Jonathan S. Appelbaum, MD, FACTP, AAHIVS
Dr. Appelbaum is on the advisory board and is a speaker for Merck & Co., Inc.

Priscilla F. Bade, MD, FACP, CMD
Dr. Bade works with the following commercial entities: Golden Living and Hospice of the Hills.

Sarah D. Berry, MD, MPH
Dr. Berry was a paid consultant for Amgen.

Cynthia M. Boyd, MD, MPH
Dr. Boyd is a paid author for *UpToDate*.

Cynthia J. Brown, MD, MSPH, AGSF
Dr. Brown is a paid consultant for Novartis.

Justin Endo, MD, FAAD
Dr. Endo is a shareholder of Actavis, Medtronic, and Amgen.

JoAnn A. Giaconi, MD
Dr. Giaconi is a paid consultant for Allergan, Inc.

Ted Johnson, MD, MPH, AGSF
Dr. Johnson is a paid consultant for Vantia and a paid author for *UpToDate*.

Fran E. Kaiser, MD, AGSF, FGSA
Dr. Kaiser holds significant shares and is an employee of Merck & Co., Inc.

Gary J. Kennedy, MD
Dr. Kennedy receives CME support from Lilly.

Douglas P. Kiel, MD, MPH
Dr. Kiel is a paid consultant for Merck, Novartis, and Amgen. He receives grant support from Merck, Amgen, Lilly, and Policy Analysis, Inc. Dr. Kiel receives royalties for book publishing from Springer and Wolters Kluwer.

Kenneth W. Lyles, MD, AGSF
Dr. Lyles is a paid consultant for UCB Pharmaceuticals. He is founder, president, and equity owner of BisCardia, Inc. He is founder, equity owner, and member of the board of directors for Faculty Connection, LLC.

Alvin M. Matsumoto, MD
Dr. Matsumoto receives grant support from Abbott and GSK.

David Sarraf, MD
Dr. Sarraf has a research grant from Regeneron and has received board consultation fees from Genentech.

Todd P. Semla, MS, PharmD, BCPS, FCCP, AGSF
Dr. Semla receives honoraria from Omnicare, LexiComp, Inc, and the American Geriatrics Society. His spouse is an employee of AbbVie and is a shareholder of Abbott Labs and AbbVie.

George E. Taffet, MD, FACP
Dr. Taffet is a consultant for Novartis Pharmaceutical.

George Taler, MD
Dr. Taler is on the speaker's bureau of Merck & Co., Inc. for a noncommercial educational program.

Phyllis C. Zee, MD, PhD
Dr. Zee is a consultant for Merck and Pernix.

The following contributors have returned disclosure forms indicating that they (and/or their spouses/partners) have no affiliation with, or financial interest in, any commercial interest that may have direct interest in the subject matter of their chapters/questions:

Emaad Abdel-Rahman, MD, PhD, FASN
Marc E. Agronin, MD
Susan E. Aiello, DVM, ELS
Kathleen M. Akgün, MD
Douglas A. Albreski, DPM
Neil B. Alexander, MD
Alicia I. Arbaje, MD, MPH
Michele C. Balas, PhD, RN, APRN-NP, FCCM
Matthew Barrett, MD
Lisa C. Barry, PhD, MPH
Cynthia Barton, RN, MSN
Judith L. Beizer, PharmD, CGP, FASCP, AGSF
Rachelle Bernacki, MD, MS, AGSF
Marc R. Blackman, MD
Michael Bogaisky, MD
Yara Bonet-Pagan, MD
Sharon A. Brangman, MD, AGSF
Cynthia J. Brown, MD, MSPH
Kenneth Brummel-Smith, MD, AGSF
Maciej S. Buchowski, PhD
Thomas V. Caprio, MD, MPH, MSHPE, FACP, CMD, HMDC, AGSF
Morgan Carlson, PhD
Julie C. Chapman, PsyD
Susan Charette, MD
Gurkamal S. Chatta, MD
Colleen Christmas, MD, FACP
Carl I. Cohen, MD
Leo M. Cooney, Jr, MD
Grace A. Cordts, MD, MPH, MS
Steven R. Counsell, MD, AGSF
Mary Ellen Csuka, MD
G. Willy Davila, MD
Ian M. Deutchki, MD
Della E. Dillard, MD, MBA
Danielle J. Doberman, MD, MPH
Catherine E. DuBeau, MD
Jerome Epplin, MD, AGSF
Manuel A. Eskildsen, MD, MPH, CMD, AGSF
Neal S. Fedarko, PhD
Luigi Ferrucci, MD, PhD
Jonathan M. Flacker, MD, AGSF
Kathleen T. Foley, PhD, OTR/L
Daniel E. Forman, MD, FACC, FAHA
Linda P. Fried, MD, MPH
Susan M. Friedman, MD, MPH, AGSF
Terry Fulmer, PhD, RN, FAAN, AGSF
Elizabeth Galik, PhD, CRNP
Joseph E. Gaugler, PhD
John D. Gazewood, MD, MSPH, CAQGM
Angela Gentili, MD
Thomas M. Gill, MD

Suzanne M. Gillespie, MD, RD, CMD, FACP
Seth Gordon, MBA
Lisa J. Granville, MD, AGSF, FACP
Shelly L. Gray, PharmD, MS, AGSF
David A. Gruenewald, MD
Jane M. Grant-Kels, MD
Ihab Hajjar, MD, MS, FACP
Janna Hardland, MD
Asaff Harel, MD
Elizabeth N. Harlow, MD
G. Michael Harper, MD, AGSF
Holly B. Hindman, MD, MPH
Lianne Hirano, MD
Manisha Juthani-Mehta, MD
Helen Kao, MD
Paul R. Katz, MD, CMD, AGSF
Philip O. Katz, MD
Anne M. Kenny, MD
Tia Kostas, MD
Lawrence R. Krakoff, MD
Stephen Krieger, MD
Lorand Kristof, MD, MSc
Chandrika Kumar, MD, FACP
Mark S. Lachs, MD, MPH
Sei J. Lee, MD, MAS
Melinda S. Lantz, MD
Susan W. Lehmann, MD
Jeffrey M. Levine, MD, AGSF, CWSP
Michael C. Lindberg, MD, FACP
Hannah I. Lipman, MD, MS
Hao Liu, PT, PhD, MD
Vera P. Luther, MD, FACP
William L. Lyons, MD
Allison Magnuson, DO
Una E. Makris, MD, MCS
Edward R. Marcantonio, MD, SM
Bryan C. Markinson, DPM
Donovan Maust, MD, MS
Matthew K. McNabney, MD, AGSF
Annette Medina-Walpole, MD, AGSF
Diana V. Messadi, DDS, MMSc, DMSc
Leigh Ann Mike, PharmD, BCPS, CGP
Karen L. Miller, MD
Supriya Mohile, MD, MS
Alison A. Moore, MD, MPH
Irene Moore, MSW, LISW-S, AGSF
Thomas Mulligan, MD, AGSF
Daniel L. Murman, MD, MS, FAAN
Aman Nanda, MD, AGSF, CMD
Judith Neugroschl, MD
David W. Oslin, MD
James T. Pacala, MD, MS, AGSF
Cynthia X. Pan, MD, FACP, AGSF
Kourosh Parham, MD, PhD, FACS
Vyjeyanthi S. Periyakoil, MD

Edgar Pierluissi, MD
Margaret Pisani, MD, MPH
Jane F. Potter, MD, AGSF
James S. Powers, MD, AGSF
Barbara Resnick, PhD, CRNP, FAAN, FAANP, AGSF
Michael W. Rich, MD, AGSF
Dalia Ritter
Miriam Rodin, MD, PhD
Theresa A. Rowe, DO
Laurence Z. Rubenstein, MD, MPH, FACP, AGSF
Alessandra Scalmati, MD, PhD
Paul Scalzo, BS
J. William Schleifer, MD
Mara A. Schonberg, MD, MPH
Krupa Shah, MD, MPH, AGSF
Kenneth Shay, DDS, MS, AGSF
Win-Kuang Shen, MD
Andrea N. Sherman, MS
Mark Simone, MD
Roy E. Smith, MD
Peter G. Snell, PhD
Nina J. Solenski, MD
Rainier Patrick Soriano, MD
Margarita Sotelo, MD
Amir E. Soumekh, MD
Richard G. Stefanacci, DO, MGH, MBA, AGSF, CMD
Martin Steinberg, MD
Winnie Suen, MD
Dennis H. Sullivan, MD
John A. Taylor, III, MD, MS
Kristen Thornton, MD, FAAFP, AGSF, CWSP
Alexander W. Threlfall, MD, MA
Jay Trabin, MD, FACOG
Justin M. Vader, MD
Ipsit V. Vahia, MD
Camille P. Vaughan, MD, MS
Fran Valle, DNP, CRNP
Elizabeth K. Vig, MD, MPH
Dennis T. Villareal, MD, FACP, FACE
Andrew Warren, MB, BS, DPhil
Barbara E. Weinstein, PhD
Julie Wetherell, MD
G. Darryl Wieland, PhD, MPH
Loren M. Wilkerson, MD
Pui Yin Wong, MD
Rebecca Wysoske, MD
Fariba S. Younai, DDS
Michi Yukawa MD, MPH
Raymond Yung, MD
Valerie Zamudio, MD
Richard A. Zweig, PhD
Jessica L. Zwerling, MD, MS

CHAPTER 1—DEMOGRAPHY

KEY POINTS

- The number and proportion of older adults is increasing globally because of the increase in life expectancy and the decline in fertility and mortality.

- Less developed regions are experiencing a greater rate of population aging.

- Noncommunicable/chronic diseases are more prevalent in older adults and cause a greater financial burden than communicable diseases.

- In the United States, the aging of the baby boomer generation is causing a large increase in the number of older adults. The proportion of older adults of a minority racial and ethnic background is increasing.

- Older Americans rely greatly on public programs, such as Medicare and Social Security, and spend more on health care than younger Americans.

GLOBAL AGING TRENDS AND DEMOGRAPHICS

The recent global decline in fertility and mortality, coupled with the increase in life expectancy, has ushered the world into an era of population aging. Population aging can be defined as the change in the age composition toward older ages (≥60 years old), as the number of older adults increases relative to the number of younger people. Although population aging is a global phenomenon, substantial variability exists between geographic areas and population groups. Thus, it is important to note that most of the data presented in this global section of the chapter are medium variant values taken from the *World Population Prospects: The 2012 Revision* (United Nations).

In 2015, the proportion of adults ≥60 years old is estimated to be 23.7% of the population in more developed regions and 9.8% of the population in less developed regions. Of note is that the longitudinal rate of population aging is much steeper in less developed regions. From 1950 to 2015, the number of older adults more than tripled in more developed regions, from 93 to 298 million, and more than quintupled in less developed regions, from 107 to 597 million. In 2050, 21.2% of the global population will be ≥60 years old, and about 80% of this age group will be living in less developed regions. This growth in the old age groups creates a square-shaped population pyramid (Figure 1.1). In 2015, the 3 countries with the greatest number of people ≥60 years old were China (209 million), India (112.3 million) and the United States (67 million). China

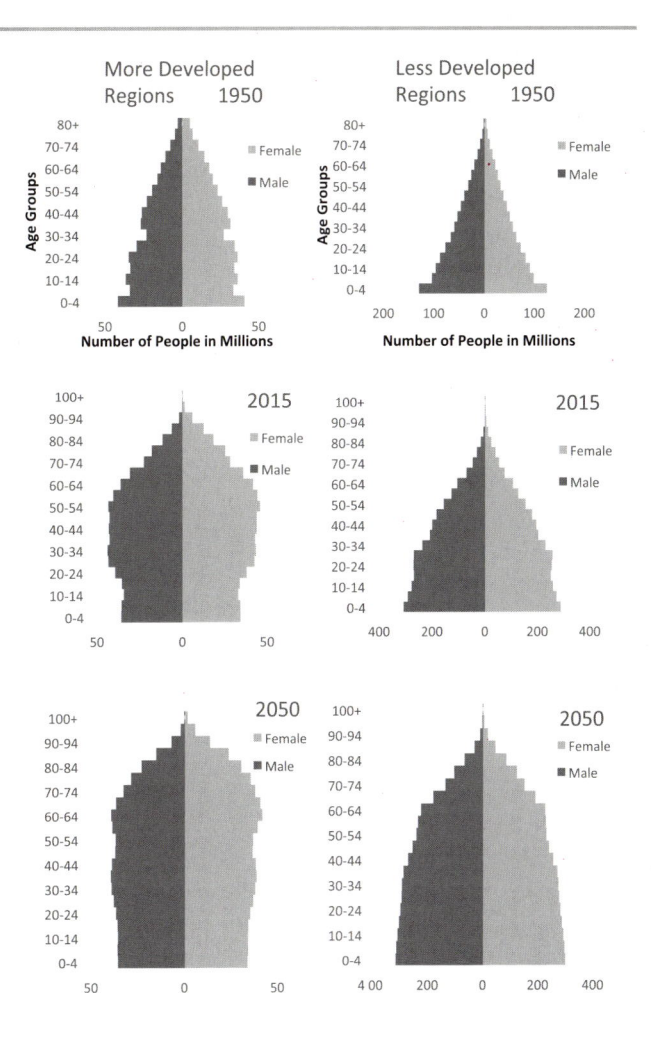

Figure 1.1—Number of People (millions) by Sex, 5-Year Age Group and Degree of Regional Development (all races)

SOURCE: Data from *World Population Prospects: The 2012 Revision*. Projections for Population by Five Year Age Group and Sex (thousands) Medium variant. 1950–2050. http://esa.un.org/unpd/wpp/unpp/panel_indicators.htm (accessed Jan 2016).

will experience the fastest growth of the proportion of people ≥60 years old than any other major country in the world, from 14.9% in 2015 to 32.8% in 2050. In 2015, 23.6% of the population in Europe was ≥60 years old—a higher proportion than any other major area of the world.

According to *World Population Aging 2013* (United Nations), the preeminent cause of the increase in the proportion of older people is a decrease in fertility and the consequent progressive reduction in the proportion of children. Between 1950 and 1955, the average total fertility was 5 children per woman, dropping to approximately half of this value between 2010 and 2015. Total fertility is still relatively high in less developed regions but is projected to fall steadily worldwide in the future. Increase in life expectancy also contributes to global population aging. Between 2010 and 2015, the average life expectancy at birth was 77.7 years in more developed regions and 68.3 years in less developed regions. Under relatively robust assumptions, it is estimated that between 2045 and 2050, the life expectancy at birth will rise to 82.8 years in more developed regions and 74.7 years in less developed regions.

Marital status does not vary considerably by developed regions. Globally, older women are more likely to be widowed than older men because of their longer life span. Living arrangements depend on the social norms of the culture. In general, about 25% of older adults live independently in less developed countries, whereas about 75% of older adults live independently in more developed regions.

Rising median age (the age that divides equal amounts of the population) is a useful indicator of population aging. The median age of the world has been steadily increasing and is projected to continue to increase in the future. Globally, the median age was 23.5 years of age in 1950 and 29.6 years of age in 2015; it is projected to be 36.1 years of age by 2050 and 41.2 years of age by the end of the century. From 1950, more developed regions have experienced a significant increase of 12.4 years in the median age, increasing to 40.9 years of age in 2015; for less developed regions, the median age has increased by only 6.4 years, increasing to 27.8 years of age in 2015. It is estimated that by 2050, less developed regions will experience significant gains in median age compared with more developed regions, 7.1 versus 3.6 years, respectively. This is likely due to the faster growth rate of the numbers of older adults in less developed regions. In 2015, Japan, Germany, and Italy were the 3 countries with the highest median ages (46.5, 46.3, and 45.0 respectively). Japan has the oldest population in the world, with 33.2% of the Japanese population ≥60 years old in 2015; the median age is expected to rise to 53.4 years of age in 2050.

The old-age dependency ratio is a metric used to assess the number of older persons for 100 persons of working age (15–64 years old) in the population, who are assumed to be independent and productive. The utility of this metric is controversial, because an increasing proportion of older adults work past age 65. Also, the old-age dependency ratio is less meaningful in less developed regions, because older adults in these areas are more likely to work past the statutory retirement age. Globally, the dependency ratio has been increasing. From 1950 to 2015, the old-age dependency ratio rose from 12 to 26 older adults (≥65 years old) per 100 productive workers in more developed regions, and it is projected to increase by an additional 18 older adults by 2050. Changes of dependency ratios in less developed regions are less dramatic because of the high number of working-age persons. From 1950 to 2015, the old-age dependency ratio rose from 7 to 10 older adults per 100 productive workers, a figure estimated to increase by 12 in 2050.

According to *World Employment and Social Outlook: Trends 2015* (International Labor Office), the proportion of workers ≥55 years old grew from 10.5% in 1990 to 14.3% in 2014, and by 2030 older workers will account for 18% of the total labor force. Under the assumption that migratory patterns will remain stable, it is likely that the fast rate of population aging will negatively impact the economy of many less developed countries and slow financial growth.

Because aging is a strong risk factor for most chronic diseases and because the management of chronic noncommunicable diseases is costly and long-lasting, the aging of the population is paralleled by expanding health expenditure and health care resource utilization. According to the World Health Organization's 2015 projections, noncommunicable disease accounts for 91.2% of deaths in adults ≥70 years old in developed regions, and for an average of 83.4% of deaths in the same age group in developing countries. In more developed countries, most health care costs for older adults are directly provided and financially covered by national health care systems, whereas in most of the less developed regions, older adults and their families bear most of the financial burden of care without help from the government or a structured pension system. Accordingly, most older adults keep working after the statutory retirement age to support themselves and sometimes their extended families. The reform of social programs is a priority for countries with significant population aging to create a more sustainable and productive work environment for both the younger and older generations.

UNITED STATES AGING TRENDS AND DEMOGRAPHICS

Population Projections

The U.S. population is aging rapidly. The baby boomers (those born between 1946 and 1964) began turning 65 years old in 2011, and in 2029 the youngest of the individuals born during that time will turn 65 years old. The U.S. Census Bureau previously projected that in 2015, 14.9% of the U.S. population would be ≥65 years old and by 2030 one in five Americans, 20.6% of the U.S. population, will be ≥65 years old. In addition, the proportion of the "oldest-old" (those ≥85 years old) will grow significantly. It was previously projected there would be 6.3 million people ≥85 years old in 2015, and by 2050 that number will triple and reach 4.8% of the total population.

As the population grows older, it will also become more diverse. The U.S. Census Bureau has projected that in 2044 the aggregate minority population will surpass in number the current majority of white, non-Hispanic people. In 2014, the racial and ethnic minority population made up about 21.7% of the population aged ≥65 years old: based on self-identification, about 8.7% were black or African-Americans (non-Hispanic), 7.7% were Hispanic, 4.0% were Asian (non-Hispanic), 0.5% were American Indian and Alaska Native (non-Hispanic), 0.1% were Native Hawaiian and Other Pacific Islander (non-Hispanic), and 0.7% identified as being more than one race. In 2014, about 17.7% of the population ≥85 years old was of a racial or ethnic minority. It is estimated that by 2050, "minority" individuals will account for 39.1% of the population ≥65 years old and 29.7% of the population ≥85 years old.

Because women have a longer life expectancy than men, they represent a larger proportion of the older population. In 2015, men were 44.2% of the population ≥65 years old, and 34.6% of the population ≥85 years old.

Life Expectancy

In 2015, at the time of birth men can expect to live an average of 77.1 years and women 81.7 years. Difference in life expectancy between men and women is projected to decline because of the faster rate of growth of life expectancy in men. Specifically, it has been estimated that by 2060 in the United States, men will have gained 6.9 years of life expectancy at birth, whereas women will gain only 5.4 years. White, native Hawaiian and other Pacific Islander men, and native Hawaiian and other Pacific Islander women will have the highest life expectancies at birth compared with other races. Black men and women will have the lowest life expectancy compared with other races. However, if ethnicity were considered, men and women of Hispanic origin have the highest life expectancy among members of the same sex (Figure 1.2).

Health in old age is also improving, although the pace of improved health does not keep up with the increase in life expectancy. The healthy life expectancy (HALE), a statistic created by the World Health Organization, measures years of life expectancy free from morbidity and/or injury. In 2000, for the United States, it was estimated the HALE at birth was 68 years for both sexes, 70 years for women and 66 years for men. HALE tends to increase slowly but steadily over time. In 2013, the HALE at birth for both sexes was 69 years, 71 years for women and 68 years for men.

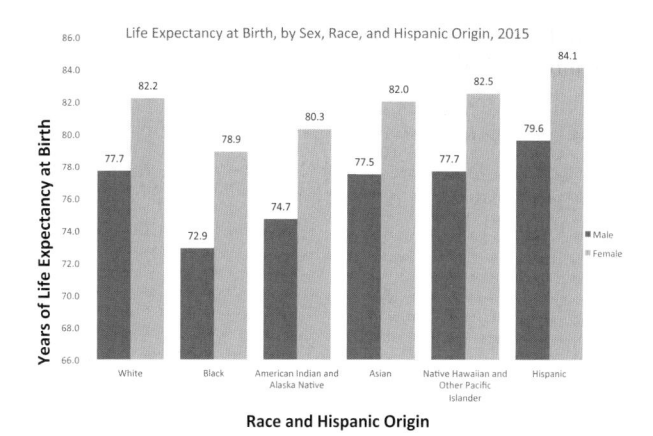

Figure 1.2—Life Expectancy at Birth by Sex, Race, and Hispanic Origin, 2015

SOURCE: Data from United States Census Bureau, Population Division, 2014 National Population Projections as reported in Table 17. www.census.gov/population/projections/data/national/2014/summarytables.html (accessed Jan 2016).

Marital Status and Living Arrangements

The disparity in life expectancy accounts for differences in marital status and living arrangements among older men and women in the United States. In 2014, the U.S. Census Bureau estimated that a larger proportion of men ≥65 years old (72.1%) than women (45.7%) were married and living with their spouse. Differences between sexes in marital status and living arrangements become more accentuated with aging. At the age of ≥85 years, 56.8% of men lived with their spouse, whereas only 16.3% of women lived with their spouse. About 11.4% of men ≥65 years old were widowed, versus 35.2% of women in the same age group. Overall, at the age of ≥65 years, 19.2% of male householders and 35.4% of female householders were not in a family group and lived alone. (For the definition of *householder*, see www.census.gov/cps/about/cpsdef.html.) At the age of ≥85 years, those percentages increased to 29.5% of men and 55.8% of women.

In 2013, about 3.6% of adults ≥65 years old were living in group quarters. Group quarters are defined by the U.S. Census Bureau as places where people stay or live in a group living environment, such as noninstitutional group homes in the form of residential treatment facilities for adults, or institutional group homes such as nursing facilities. About 3% of the population ≥65 years old lived in nursing homes. As can be expected, the proportion of older adults who live in an institution increases dramatically with aging. About 11.1% of those ≥85 years old live in nursing homes. Older adults 65–74 years old make up 14.6% of the resident nursing-home population, those 75–84 years old make up 27.9%, and those ≥85 years old make up

41.4%. Women ≥65 years old make up 70.6% of the ≥65 years old nursing-home population.

The Distribution of Older Adults in the United States

The number of adults ≥65 years old varies greatly among states. In 2014, it was estimated that about 53.7% of the total population of older adults was concentrated in only 10 states: California (5 million), Florida (3.8 million), Texas (3.1 million), New York (2.9 million), Pennsylvania (2.1 million), Ohio (1.8 million), Illinois (1.8 million), Michigan (1.5 million), North Carolina (1.5 million), and New Jersey (1.3 million). California had the highest number of older adults, accounting for 10.8% of the total population of older adults in the United States. In contrast, Alaska had the fewest, accounting for 0.15% of the total population of older adults in the United States. The state with the highest proportion of older adults was Florida, with 19.1% of its state population ≥65 years old. Alaska had the lowest proportion of older adults, accounting for about 9.4% of the state population.

Educational Attainment

The percentages of adults ≥65 years old that have higher education has been increasing for both men and women. In 1950, it was estimated that 17.7% of adults ≥65 years old had completed high school, and 3.6% had a bachelor's degree. In 2014, 83.7% of adults ≥65 years old had a high school or higher degree. The percentage of high school graduates in this population varied by race as follows: 88.1% white (non-Hispanic), 76.4% Asian (non-Hispanic), 73.5% black or African-American (non-Hispanic), and 54% Hispanic. The percentage of adults ≥65 years old who had a bachelor's degree was 26.3%, and according to race were 28.4% white (non-Hispanic), 35.9% Asian (non-Hispanic), 16.6% black or African-American (non-Hispanic), and 12.5% Hispanic. A higher degree usually equates to a higher income.

Income and Labor Force Participation

According to the Social Security Administration, in 2012 about 86% of adults ≥65 years old received some Social Security income, and such income accounted for 50% or more of the total income for 65% of the aged beneficiaries. The major source of aggregate income for older couples and nonmarried people was Social Security benefits, which accounted for 35% of the aggregate income.

According to the Current Population Survey, 2014 Annual Social and Economic Supplement (Bureau of Labor Statistics and the Census Bureau), in 2013 (when all the types of households are considered), the median income of householders who were ≥65 years old was $35,611 (USD). However, this overall figure covers widespread situations. It was estimated that about 27.3% of householders ≥65 years old had a median annual income lower than $20,000, while about 22.4% had a median income of $70,000 and over. There is even wider disparity according to race: white non-Hispanic households ($37,653), Asian ($36,547), black or African-American ($26,641), and Hispanic ($25,315).

According to the Bureau of Labor Statistics, in 2014 about 17.7% of the noninstitutionalized adult population ≥65 years old was employed. A larger percentage of men (21.9%) than women (14.4%) ≥65 years old were working. Older Asians are more likely to work than white and African-American older adults.

Poverty

The poverty threshold income for an adult ≥65 years old in 2013 was set at $11,173. According to the official poverty measure, it was estimated that about 9.5% of older persons (11.6% of women and 6.8% of men) were in poverty. The proportion according to race were black or African-American (17.7%), Asian (13.5%), two or more races (11.2%), American Indian and Alaska Native (8%), white (7.4%), and native Hawaiian and other Pacific Islander (2.7%). A large percentage of older adults of Hispanic origin were also in poverty (19.9%). The proportion of householders ≥65 years old who lived alone and were in poverty was 17.4%, but adding even one more person in the household, the percentage dropped dramatically to about 5.3%, then it gradually went up with the addition of family members until about 11.5% of adults living in a family of 5 or more people.

A more comprehensive method of measuring poverty is using the Supplemental Poverty Measure (SPM). First released in 2011 by the U.S. Census Bureau, the SPM takes into account factors that affect income such as income after taxes, medical out-of-pocket expenses, and cash benefits. According to the SPM, 14.6% of older adults were in poverty in 2013, and it estimates that Social Security keeps 38% of the older population in the United States above the poverty threshold. Expenses that are medical out-of-pocket expenses account for 6.3% of poverty in the older population in the United States.

Health-Related Data

The CDC found that as people age, they are less likely to report their health as excellent or very good. About 84.5% of people 18 years or younger, 64.7% of people 18–64 years old, and 44.9% of those ≥65 years old reported in 2014 their health as excellent or very good.

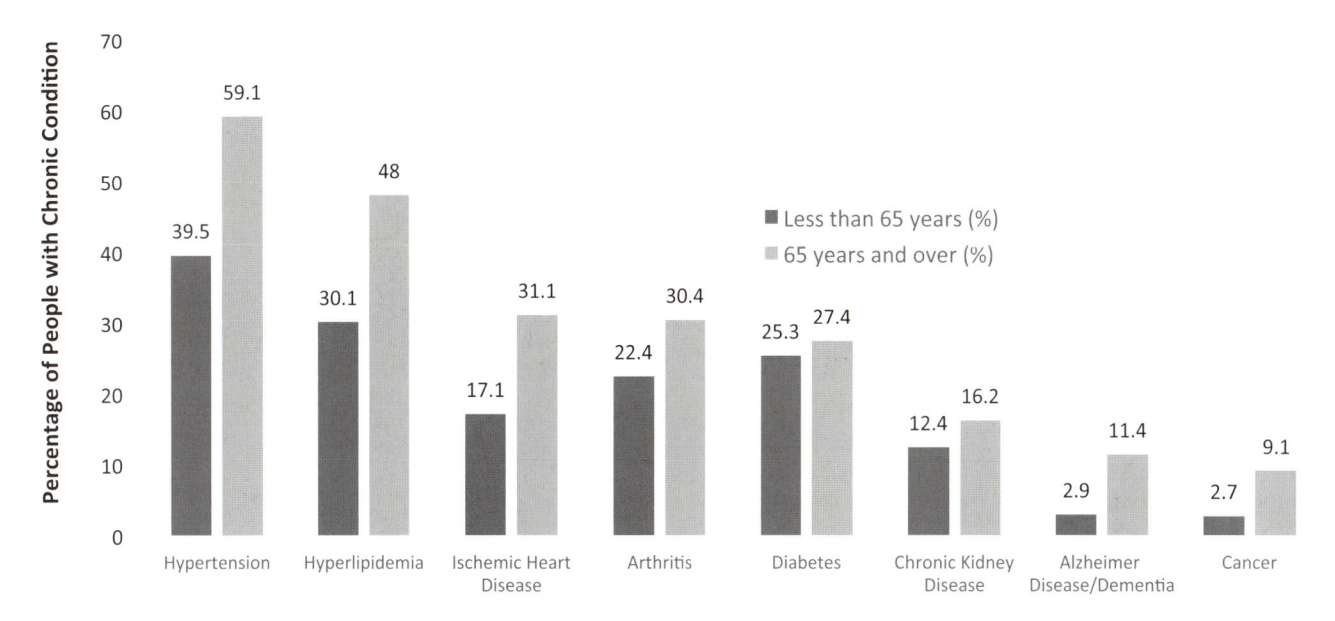

Figure 1.3—Prevalence of Selected Chronic Conditions Among Medicare Beneficiaries by Age Groups, 2012

SOURCE: Data from the Centers for Medicare & Medicaid Services, Research, Statistics, Data & Systems, Chronic Conditions. Prevalence State/County Level: All beneficiaries by Age, 2008–2012. www.cms.gov/Research-Statistics-Data-and-Systems/Statistics-Trends-and-Reports/Chronic-Conditions/CC_Main.html (accessed Jan 2016).

Most chronic diseases are highly prevalent in the older population (Figure 1.3). For example, in 2012, almost 60% of Medicare beneficiaries ≥65 years old had hypertension. Multimorbidity, or being affected by more than one chronic disease, is the most frequent medical condition in older adults. A large proportion, 68.6% of older adults (enrolled in Medicare) had 2 or more chronic conditions.

The prevalence of risk factors for major chronic disease, such as smoking and obesity, change with age. For example, whereas 8.5% of adults aged ≥65 years old are current smokers, an average 18.6% of adults <65 years old reported in 2014 that they currently smoke.

Generally, older adults have less robust immune systems, and there is strong evidence to recommend that older adults receive a flu vaccination annually and a pneumococcal vaccination at least once after age 65. Based on data collected in 2014, the CDC reported that the percentage of adults ≥65 years old who had received the influenza vaccine during the past 12 months was 70%, whereas about 61.3% had received a pneumococcal vaccination in their lifetime.

In 2013, about 36.4% of the population ≥65 years old had some sort of disability; 15.2% had hearing difficulty, 6.8% had vision difficulty, 9.2% had cognitive impairment, 23.3% had difficulty in performing mobility tasks, 8.5% had self-care difficulty, and 15.4% had difficultly living independently.

In 2012, the CMS reported that among Medicare beneficiaries 65–84 years old and older, 24.5% had difficulty walking, 11.8% getting in or out of bed/chair, 8.6% bathing, 6.5% dressing, 4.4% toileting, and 2.9% eating. The percentages of those having difficulty performing specific activities of daily living (ADLs) among beneficiaries ≥85 years old were higher: walking (50.5%), getting in or out of bed/chair (25.0%), bathing (25.8%), dressing (17.0%), toileting (12.8%), and eating (6.9%). The percentage of beneficiaries 65–84 years old who reported having difficulty with ADLs and were receiving help ranged from 19.6% to 61.2% (depending on the ADL), whereas the percentage range was 27.7%–74.4% for beneficiaries ≥85 years old. Therefore, beneficiaries ≥85 years old were more likely to receive help with ADLs than those 65–84 years old.

Figure 1.4—Percentage of Share of Average Annual Health Care Expenditures by Source for Americans ≥65 Years Old, 2013

SOURCE: Bureau of Labor Statistics. Consumer Expenditure Survey. www.bls.gov/cex/ Annual Calendar Year Tables: 2013. Selected age of reference person (accessed Jan 2016).

In 2013, Americans ≥65 years old spent 12.2% of their total average annual expenditures on health care, in contrast to all other younger Americans, who spent an average of 6.7%. For the share of average annual health care expenditures by source for Americans ≥65 years old, see Figure 1.4. It was also found that 98.4% of older adults had some type of health insurance. The majority of this proportion was accounted for by Medicare (93.1%). Private insurance covered 54% of the older adult population, while 1.6% had no health care coverage.

Death rates for the 15 leading causes of death in the United States in 2013 rose with age, sometimes dramatically. The total number of deaths per 100,000 of adults 35–44 years old was 172, but for adults ≥85 years old, that number was 13,660 deaths per 100,000. For most of the top 15 causes of death in the United States, the cause-specific mortality increased exponentially with aging.

In 2013, the 5 leading causes of death and the number of deaths for adults ≥65 years old were cardiac diseases (488,156), malignant neoplasms (407,558), chronic lower respiratory diseases (127,194), cerebrovascular diseases (109,602), and Alzheimer disease (83,786).

REFERENCES

- *An Aging Nation: The Older Population in the United States.* United States Census Bureau; 2014.

   This report presents data and the projected composition of the United States' older population.

- Early Release of Selected Estimates Based on Data from the 2014 National Health Interview Survey. Centers for Disease Control and Prevention, National Center for Health Statistics, Publication and Information Products; 2015. Available at www.cdc.gov/nchs/nhis/released201506.htm (accessed Jan 2016).

   This report contains information on risk factors that contribute to chronic conditions reported in older people, as well as data on vaccinations.

- Life Expectancy Data by Country. Mortality and global health estimates. Global Health Observatory Data Repository. World Health Organization. Available at http://apps.who.int/gho/data/view.main.680?lang=en (accessed Jan 2016).

   This table contains data on healthy years of life expectancy at birth.

- Multiple Chronic Conditions. Centers for Medicare & Medicaid Services. Available at www.cms.gov/Research-Statistics-Data-and-Systems/Statistics-Trends-and-Reports/Chronic-Conditions/MCC_Main.html (accessed Jan 2016).

   This report presents data on the prevalence of multiple chronic conditions among Medicare beneficiaries.

- *Projections of Mortality and Causes of Death, 2015 and 2030.* World Health Organization, Health Statistics and Information Systems. Available at www.who.int/healthinfo/global_burden_disease/projections/en/ (accessed Jan 2016).

   This report contains information on mortality due to noncommunicable diseases in different regions of the world.

- Short K. The Supplemental Poverty Measure; 2013. *Current Population Reports*; 2014.

   This report presents data and information about the supplemental poverty measure.

- *World Employment and Social Outlook: Trends 2015.* International Labor Office, Geneva, Switzerland; 2015.

   This report explains the consequences of an aging labor force and provides data on the participation rates in varying regions.

- *World Population Ageing 2013.* United Nations, Department of Economic and Social Affairs, Population Division. Available at www.un.org/en/development/desa/population/publications/pdf/ageing/WorldPopulationAgeing2013.pdf (accessed Jan 2016).

   This report contains information on the regions of the world and how they will change over time in regards to aging populations.

- *World Population Prospects: The 2012 Revision.* United Nations, Department of Economic and Social Affairs, Population Division. Available at http://esa.un.org/wpp/ (accessed Jan 2016).

   This report contains data and projections used to calculate the numbers of older adults in the world and in different geographic regions.

Paul Scalzo, BS
Luigi Ferrucci, MD, PhD

CHAPTER 2—BIOLOGY

KEY POINTS

- Aging is a loss of homeostasis, or a breakdown in maintenance of specific molecular structures and pathways; this breakdown is the inevitable consequence of the evolved anatomy and physiology of an organism.

- There are three main types of theories of aging: evolutionary (the "why" of aging), psychosocial (the "who" of aging), and physiologic (the "how" of aging).

- The many theories of aging are not competing or mutually exclusive; rather, the theories reflect current understanding of the multiple homeostatic mechanisms that allow us to live as long as we do.

- Some of the molecular and cellular changes that occur with aging are unique to the specific cellular and tissue context of the organ, whereas others occur across a number of organ systems with a common effect on functional capacity when systems are stressed.

- The onset, rate, and extent of the aging process is extremely heterogeneous.

The most visible imprints of aging are loss of hair and pigmentation of hair; diminished height and muscle and bone mass; and increasingly wrinkled, thinned skin. These progressive changes have a biologic basis in altered molecular and cellular structure and function. The rate and extent of aging varies both between individuals and within an individual (eg, asymmetric changes in vision, hearing), increasing the variability with which an older adult presents. Thus, biologic age, based on an individual's functional capacity, and not chronologic age, is the metric for studying the biology of aging. Functional capacity is a direct measure of the ability of cells, tissues, and organ systems to function properly and optimally and is influenced by both genes and environment. Within this context, aging is defined as the progressive decline and deterioration of functional properties at the cellular, tissue, and organ level that lead to a loss of homeostasis, decreased ability to adapt to internal or external stimuli, and increased vulnerability to disease and mortality. Gradual changes in cells, tissues, and organs of the body lead to the eventual breakdown of maintenance processes—an inevitable consequence of the evolved anatomy and physiology of the organism.

THEORIES OF AGING

Evolutionary theories of aging explain historical and evolutionary aspects of aging, addressing why aging exists in living things and how aging may have evolved as a process. Psychosocial theories of aging explain behavioral, cognitive, and social features of aging. Physiologic theories of aging explain structural and functional age changes and elaborate a framework for translating the "what" and "where" of aging from molecules to organ system and homeostasis.

The many theories of aging should not be viewed as competing or mutually exclusive. Rather, the theories reflect our current understanding of the individual maintenance pathways and homeostatic mechanisms that allow us to live as long as we do. The theories also provide pathways for investigating interventions that modify aging. For example, caloric restriction, which increases life span in organisms from worms to mice, may be acting through modulation of energy metabolism, defense against free radicals, and clearance of defective components (autophagy). Similarly, exercise, which can modify the rate and extent of aging, may act through pathways involving energy metabolism, autophagy, and defense against injury.

Evolutionary Theories of Aging

Evolution deals with the impact of natural selection (selective pressure) on the reproductive fitness of a species. An adaptive trait is one in which selection of a mutation improves reproductive fitness, whereas a nonadaptive trait is one in which there is no effect on reproductive fitness and minimal natural selection. There are currently two main evolutionary theories of aging: mutation accumulation theory and antagonistic pleiotropy theory.

Mutation Accumulation Theory

In this theory, aging is viewed as a nonadaptive trait. That is, traits that yield aging are neither selected for nor against. No selective pressure is brought to bear on older, post-reproductive age organisms expressing a mutation that has minimal effects on fitness. Thus, these late-acting genes accumulate over time and yield the aging phenotype.

Antagonistic Pleiotropy Theory

Pleiotropy is when a single gene controls or influences multiple traits. The antagonistic pleiotropic theory considers aging an adaptive trait. Genes that can influence several traits are selected for and affect

Table 2.1—Physiologic Theories of Aging

Homeostasis/Maintenance	Theory	Synopsis
DNA integrity and stability	Targeted DNA damage	Cumulative nuclear DNA deletions, mutations, and translocations contribute to altered functional capacity of proteins and cells.
	Mitochondrial DNA damage	Mutations to mitochondrial DNA occur at higher frequency than to nuclear DNA, altering efficiency of respiration/ATP production and generating more free radicals.
	Telomere	Telomere length and telomerase activity act as clock-and-winding mechanism for continued replication. Senescence is induced by loss of telomerase activity and critical telomere length.
	Transposable element activation	Aging is associated with activation of endogenous transposable elements that results in insertional mutagenesis, DNA damage, and genome rearrangements.
	Epigenetic	Maintaining stable phenotype is epigenetic, dependent on DNA-protein interactions, DNA methylation, and histone acetylation. Phenotypic drift leads to altered gene expression and cellular function.
Synthesis fidelity	Error catastrophe	Cumulative errors in RNA and protein synthesis fidelity reach a critical threshold over time, accelerating loss of function.
Defense against free radicals	Free radicals	Highly reactive oxygen-derived free radicals (generated through respiration) damage protein, lipid, and DNA, leading to altered structure and functional capacity.
Clearance of defective components	Accumulation	Abnormal proteins (cross-linked collagen, amyloid), lipids (lipofuscin), and/or organelles (mitochondria, membranes) are not removed, compromising cellular and tissue functional capacity.
Energy metabolism	Rate of living	Changes in energy availability and in body size and composition act independently and in concert to modify life span.
Physiologic signaling	Endocrine	Age-related changes in the kinetics and levels of secretion of hormones (eg, growth hormone, cortisol, glucocorticoids) cause loss of functional capacity in target organ systems.
Response to pathogens, injury	Immunologic, immunosenescence	Time-acquired deficits in immune response and T-cell function predispose older adults to infections and disease. The accumulation of senescent immune cells increases production of pro-inflammatory cytokines, causing chronic molecular inflammation with systemic effects.
Physical reserves	Stem cell	Stem cell/progenitor cell pools involved in tissue remodeling and repair (eg, adult stem cells in bone, muscle, and brain) or in organ system maintenance (eg, hematopoietic stem cells and the immune system) are depleted over time.

individual fitness in opposite (ie, antagonistic) ways at different stages of life. Pleiotropic genes that have beneficial effects on early fitness components in the young but harmful effects on late fitness components are favored by natural selection. For example, there are inverse relationships between fecundity and life span or between longevity and brood size or metabolic rate.

Psychosocial Theories of Aging

Psychosocial theories explain aging in terms of individual changes in behavior, cognitive function, relationships, roles, and social interactions. These theories present models of what happens to an individual during normal aging. Four of the more common theories are summarized below.

Activity theory highlights the maintenance of and alterations in regular activities, roles, and social pursuits as a coping strategy. *Life-course theory* views aging as the progressive adjustment of older individuals to changes associated with increasing age (declining health and physical strength, retirement and reduced income, death of a spouse or family members, new living arrangements, etc). *Continuity theory*, as the name implies, states that older adults may seek to use familiar strategies in familiar areas of life as an adaptive strategy to deal with changes that occur during normal aging. *Gerotranscendence theory* holds aging as part of a natural progression toward a goal of achieving maturation and wisdom, with a shift in perspective from a materialistic and rational view to a more cosmic and transcendent view.

Physiologic Theories of Aging

Physiologic theories address how we age. Over the past several decades, dozens of physiologic theories have been proposed (see Table 2.1). The major physiologic theories with special emphasis on available supporting evidence are described below. These theories involve protocols for maintaining DNA integrity and stability, synthesis fidelity, defense against free radicals, clearance of damaged/defective components, energy metabolism, systemic physiologic signaling, response to pathogens and/or injury, and physiologic reserves.

Target Theory of Genetic Damage

Underlying the genetic theories of aging is the idea that aging is heavily influenced or caused by genes. The genome is the repository for all genetic material, and the integrity of this information is essential for reproductive fitness and survival. DNA is subject to a number of insults, including spontaneous chemical changes, environmental damage by ionizing radiation, aflatoxin, and alkylating agents, all of which modify DNA structure. Mechanisms of repair rely on the efficiency of many enzymes that in turn depend on fidelity of the information in the encoding DNA. Thus, the target theory of genetic damage states that genes are susceptible to "hits" from radiation or other damaging agents that then alter function of structural, signaling, and/or repair molecules, and that these cumulative hits give rise to an aging phenotype.

The evidence supporting this theory includes observations that whole-body irradiation shortens life span, somatic mutations in human T lymphocytes increase with age, chromosomal abnormalities increase with age, and mutations in genes involved in DNA metabolism are associated with a number of premature aging syndromes (Werner, Hutchinson-Gilford, ataxia telangiectasia, and Cockayne). The observations that DNA damage, mutations, and chromosome abnormalities increase during aging may not be a cause but rather a consequence of aging.

Mitochondrial DNA Damage Theory

Unlike nuclear DNA, mitochondrial DNA (mtDNA) is not protected by proteins (eg, histones, chromatin) and is attached to the inner mitochondrial membrane, where free radicals are produced. Thus, mtDNA damage occurs 10–20 times faster than nuclear DNA damage. In addition, mtDNA cannot repair itself, and some damaged mitochondria replicate faster than undamaged mitochondria, which gives rise to expansion of aberrant mitochondria. As a consequence, genes encoded within the mitochondria are more likely to lose their integrity over time. Damage to mtDNA has more harmful effects than damage to nuclear DNA, because each cell translates almost all its mtDNA genes but only 7% of its nuclear DNA. Nearly any adverse change in mtDNA will have deleterious effects on mitochondrial function. These effects include less energy production, more free-radical formation, reduced control of other cell processes, and accumulation of damaged harmful molecules, leading to aging and certain age-related diseases. The mitochondrial DNA theory of aging is closely allied with the free radical theory of aging.

Telomere Theory

Telomeres are specialized sequences found at the ends of linear chromosomes. The DNA replication machinery cannot make a copy of the the physical end of a chromosome (because the machinery physically occupies space on the DNA). Every time DNA replicates, there is progressive shortening of the telomeres. Once telomeres are reduced beyond a threshold length, cells enter a nonreplicating state. Cellular (replicative) senescence is triggered when cells acquire critically short telomeres. Telomere length provides a mechanism for Leonard Hayflick's mid-20th century observation that mammalian cells are limited in the number of times they can divide ("Hayflick's limit"). The telomere hypothesis of aging proposes that telomere shortening causes aging through inducing replicative senescence. Evidence supporting the telomere theory includes observations that telomere length is directly proportional to cell age, telomeres are lost faster from individuals with progerias, immortal cells such as cancerous cells have a constant telomere length, and restoring telomerase enzyme in somatic cells in vitro causes an increase in replicative life span of these cells. Evidence that is not supportive include observations that telomere length is not related to life span (mouse telomeres are much longer then those in people) and that telomerase protects against replicative senescence but not cellular senescence triggered by other pathways.

Transposable Element Activation

Transposable elements are pieces of DNA that can move from one location in the genome to another, resulting in insertional mutagenesis. The random insertion may favor evolutionary advance, or it may lead to DNA damage and genomic instability. Cells have evolved elaborate mechanisms to repress transposons. The hypothesis that transposable elements may contribute to the aging process through somatic mutation was first proposed in 1992. Recent work has demonstrated that transposition increases in frequency with age in mammals. Activation of transposable elements is proposed to be an important contributor to the progressive dysfunction of aging cells and to induced cell senescence and cell loss. In addition to providing a mechanism for age-associated changes in genetic stability, this theory is supported by observations that increasing transposon activation in *Drosophila* brain resulted in progressive and age-dependent memory impairment, and shortened life span.

Epigenetic Theory

Most cells in the human body are somatic cells. A major mechanism maintaining the appropriate, differentiated phenotype of these cells is epigenetic, dependent on DNA-protein interactions, DNA methylation, and histone acetylation. The epigenetic theory posits that phenotypic drift arising from inappropriate epigenetic modifications leads to altered gene expression and cellular function and the aging phenotype. In general, DNA methylation increases with age, but there can be variation within a tissue. The degree of hypermethylation depends on multiple factors, including age, diet, and exposure to environmental agents/insults (eg, carcinogens, epimutagens, toxins). Epigenetic silencing of repressive transcription factors may contribute to cells switching to a senescent phenotype. The association of epigenetic changes with increasing age provides supportive evidence, although the causal action of these changes in producing the aging phenotype has yet to be demonstrated.

Error Catastrophe Theory

The error catastrophe theory holds that damage is not to the genes themselves but to the RNA and proteins that read the genes and carry out their instructions. The damaged molecules spread, increasing the number of mistakes and causing biologic changes that are seen as "aging." For RNA, there may be issues with transcriptional accuracy, proofreading, mismatch repair, splicing, and transport. For proteins, errors in translating RNA to the correct amino acid sequence or in polypeptide folding and conformation have deleterious effects on protein function. Error catastrophe theory holds that cumulative errors in subsets of proteins involved in transfer of information from DNA to protein are normally below a threshold. Critical errors can destabilize the information transfer machinery, causing an irreversible increase in the error level and accelerating loss of function. This theory has equivocal support, because predictions that senescent cells should contain abnormal protein molecules and that mutations that reduce accuracy of synthesis should accelerate aging have not been consistently demonstrated under experimental conditions.

Free Radical Theory

Free radicals are extremely reactive and unstable and are produced in mitochondria, in oxidative enzymes in the endoplasmic reticulum, in peroxisomes, and by phagocytes. Free radicals are normally policed by enzymes that inactivate them (superoxide dismutase, catalase, glutathione peroxidase), antioxidants that neutralize them (α-tocopherol, ascorbic acid, uric acid), sulfhydryl-containing compounds (cysteine, glutathione, bilirubin, ubiquinol, and carnosine), and β-carotene.

Evidence in favor of this theory include that positive correlations have been observed between metabolic rate and free radical production, age and rate of free radical formation, age and amount of free radical damage, and that abnormal mitochondria increase during aging. Evidence against this theory includes that antioxidant treatment does not reproducibly increase life span and that genetic manipulation of mice to either under- or over-express key components involved in free radical metabolism does not have a consistent effect on life span. Free radicals can act as causative agents in other physiologic theories of aging, including DNA integrity, protein error, accumulation, and rate of living theories.

Accumulation Theories

Accumulation theories posit that aging is associated with accumulation of cellular and extracellular components with altered structure that compromise cellular function. The components can be *molecular,* as in the clinker theory in which lipofuscin (an oxidized lipid), for example, accumulates in lysosomes compromising the organelle's capacity for catabolism. These components can be *macromolecular,* as in the protein modifications theory in which, for example, collagen cross-links in skin and bone, neurofibrillary tangles and plaque formation in the brain, and advanced glycation end products in multiple organ systems alter cellular and tissue functional capacity. Finally, components can be damaged organelles such as mitochondria, lysosomes, peroxisomes, and cell membranes, and the inability to remove functionally compromised organelles through autophagy leads to further loss of function. Whether the accumulation of compromised molecular components or cellular organelles is a cause or a consequence of aging has been difficult to determine.

Rate of Living Theory

The rate of living theory holds that aging is determined by the rate of metabolism, because aerobic metabolism causes damage, primarily through the production of oxygen-free radicals. This theory predicts that the higher the rate of metabolism, the faster the rate of aging and the shorter the life span. Although this is indeed the case in most animals, two major exceptions are mammals and birds, which have life spans longer than their rates of metabolism would predict.

Endocrine Theory

With increasing age, the synthesis and secretion of many hormones change. In addition, cell receptors on target organs can change in number and functional signal transduction. The circadian cycles of certain hormones also become irregular. The endocrine theory of aging posits that changes in hormone levels and signaling are a major cause of loss of homeostasis and that aging arises from dysregulated hormone signaling. For example, deficits in growth hormone or sex steroid hormones impact target organs' size and ability to repair and maintain functional capacity.

Immune Theory

Relatively slow-growing organisms must confront infection by rapidly growing pathogens or parasites, and the immune system has evolved to do this. Homeostasis of the immune system is maintained by innate or nonspecific mechanisms such as humoral mechanisms (complement) and cellular mechanisms (macrophages, neutrophils, natural killer cells), as well as by the specific, acquired immune response involving humoral mechanisms (antibodies) and cellular mechanisms (T and B lymphocytes). The well documented gradual decline in the acquired immune system maintenance ("immunosenescence") has been associated with increased morbidity and mortality in late life. The immune theory of aging posits that immunosenescence contributes to aging by limiting systemic defensive and repair responses that impact the functional capacity of other organ systems. An aging-associated increase in innate imune system activation yielding an elevated pro-inflammatory state marked by increased levels of cytokines (such as interleukin-6) and macrophage activation markers is perhaps a compensatory mechanism for declining acquired immunity. Failure to resolve the repair and remodeling program of inflammation results in an altered tissue structure and cellular organization that can negatively feedback on cellular and organ system function.

Stem Cell/Progenitor Cell Theory

Adult stem cells in the brain, bone marrow, and circulation maintain homeostasis by replenishing depleted reserves. Examples include satellite cells that contribute to muscle mass and repair of muscle tissue, and osteoprogenitor cells that replenish osteoblasts and form bone. Over time, precursor cells become depleted either by phenotypic drift or perhaps by injury, illness, or environmental challenge. Normally, adult bone mesenchymal stem cells can produce cells in the osteoblastic, myoblastic, or adipocytic lines. Aging is associated with osteopenia, sarcopenia, and an increase in fat content in bone marrow and muscle. These age-related changes may arise from a shift in the pathway commitment of bone mesenchymal stem cells (away from bone and muscle cells) toward the adipocytic cell line.

ORGAN SYSTEM CHANGES WITH AGING

Aging nerves, muscle, skin, hair, cartilage and bone, vasculature, and other organs exhibit changes at the molecular and cellular level. Some molecular changes with aging are shared between tissue types and organ systems, whereas others are unique. For example, in skin, bone, and cartilage, increases in cross-links (both enzymatic and nonenzymatic) alter compressibility and resiliency, and decreases in structural components (eg, proteoglycans and glycosaminoglycans) alter tissue hydration and function. In contrast, changes in the immune system (eg, diminished ability of dendritic cells to present antigen) are unique to the specific cell type, organ system, and function. A brief overview of significant age-related changes in the major organ systems follows below and in Table 2.2. These changes represent biologic processes common to everyone, although they progress at different rates.

Nerves

On average, with increasing age, both the number and functioning of sensory neurons decline. The number of motor neurons decreases, reducing the number of muscle cells that can be stimulated, decreasing the maximal strength of contraction. The speed of action potentials in their axons decreases slightly, such that impulses arrive over an increasingly long period, contractions of muscle cells are spread out over a longer period, and the slower transmission results in further delay in starting a motion. Neurons remaining in the brain have less fluid and stiffer cell membranes, internal membranes that become irregular in structure and accumulate lipofuscin, and tangled neurofibrils. The ability of neurons to grow branches of both axons and dendrites decreases, reducing fine motor control. Changes in motor neuron cell membranes, myelin, or blood vessels within the nerves reduce blood flow in nerves, decreasing the supply of nutrients and the elimination of wastes, which contribute to the slower action potentials and spreading of muscle cell contraction. The slower contraction, lower peak strength of contraction, and slower relaxation reduce maximal muscle strength when performing quick movements.

Muscle

Lean body mass decreases, caused in part by loss of muscle tissue. The rate and extent of muscle changes seem to be genetically determined. Average rates of muscle mass decline are 15% per decade at ages 50–60 and increase up to 30% after age 60. Lipofuscin and fat are deposited in muscle tissue. There is selective loss of type II (fast twitch) muscle fibers, and remaining

Table 2.2—Physiologic Changes of Aging

Body System	Change	Consequences
Nervous	↓ Number of neurons ↓ Action potential speed ↓ Axon/dendrite branches	↓ Muscle innervation ↓ Fine motor control
Muscle	Fibers shrink ↓ Type II (fast twitch) fibers ↑ Lipofuscin and fat deposits	Tissue atrophies ↓ Tone and contractility ↓ Strength
Skin	↓ Thickness ↑ Collagen cross-links	Loss of elasticity
Skeletal	↓ Bone density Joints become stiffer, less flexible	Movement slows and may become limited

Cardiovascular
  Heart
 	
  Vasculature
	
	↑ Left ventricular wall thickness
	↑ Lipofuscin and fat deposits
	↑ Stiffness
	↓ Responsiveness to agents
		
		Stressed heart is less able to respond

Pulmonary	↓ Elastin fibers ↑ Collagen cross-links ↓ Elastic recoil of the lung ↑ Residual volume ↓ Vital capacity, forced expiratory volume, and forced vital capacity	↓ Effort dependent and independent respiration (quiet and forced breathing) ↓ Exercise tolerance and pulmonary reserve
Eyes	↑ Lipid infiltrates/deposits ↑ Thickening of the lens ↓ Pupil diameter	↓ Transparency of the cornea Difficulty in focusing on near objects ↓ Accommodation and dark adaptation
Ears	↑ Thickening of tympanic membrane ↓ Elasticity and efficiency of ossicular articulation ↑ Organ atrophy ↓ Cochlear neurons ↓ Number of neurons in the utricle, saccule, and ampullae ↓ In size and number of otoliths	↑ Conductive deafness (low-frequency range) ↑ Sensorineural hearing loss (high-frequency sounds) ↓ Detection of gravity, changes in speed, and rotation
Digestive	↑ Dysphagia ↑ Achlorhydria Altered intestinal absorption ↑ Lipofuscin and fat deposition in pancreas ↑ Mucosal cell atrophy	 ↓ Iron absorption ↓ B_{12} and calcium absorption ↑ Incidence of diverticula, transit time, and constipation
Urinary	↓ Kidney size, weight, and number of functional glomeruli ↓ Number and length of functional renal tubules ↓ Glomerular filtration rate ↓ Renal blood flow	↓ Ability to resorb glucose ↓ Concentrating ability of kidney
Immune	↓ Primary and secondary response ↑ Autoimmune antibodies ↓ T-cell function, fewer naive and more memory T cells Atrophy of thymus	↓ Immune functioning ↓ Response to new pathogens ↓ T lymphocytes, natural killer cells, cytokines needed for growth and maturation of B cells
Endocrine	↑ Atrophy of certain glands (eg, pituitary, thyroid, thymus) ↓ Growth hormone, dehydroepiandrosterone, testosterone, estrogen ↑ Parathyroid hormone, atrial natriuretic peptide, norepinephrine, baseline cortisol, erythropoietin	Changes in target organ response, organ system homeostasis, response to stress, functional capacity

muscle fibers shrink. Muscle tissue is replaced more slowly, and lost muscle tissue may be replaced with a tough fibrous tissue. This is most noticeable in the hands, which may appear thin and bony. Changes in muscle tissue, combined with normal aging changes in the nervous system, lead to reduced muscle tone and contractility. Muscles can become rigid with age and can lose tone even if exercised regularly, leading to changes in strength and endurance.

Skin

Cellular changes in the skin include thinning of the epidermis with a reduced mitotic rate in epidermal basal cells, shortened and attenuated rete ridges, reduced epidermal appendages, and fewer fibroblasts and capillaries in the dermis. Melanocytes in both exposed and unexposed skin decrease with age, while those remaining become larger but produce less melanin. At the molecular level, the dermal thickness decreases as the collagen content per unit area of the skin decreases. Loss of skin elasticity (caused by increased collagen cross-links and decreased elastin) leads to skin sagging and wrinkling. Hair follicles atrophy, and hair density and color decrease uniformly in both men and women. Hair turns gray, because melanocytes are lost at the base of the hair follicles. Eyebrows, ear, and nasal hair coarsen and get longer, especially in men. Linear nail growth slows, and nail thickness and strength decrease. Nails become brittle, dull, opaque, and yellowish.

Bone

Bone mass (or density) is lost, especially in women after menopause, and bones become more brittle and can break more easily. Height decreases, primarily caused by shortening of the trunk and spine as the intervertebral discs gradually lose fluid and become thinner, and vertebrae lose some of their mineral content, making each bone thinner. The spinal column becomes curved forward and compressed. The foot arches become less pronounced, contributing to slight loss of height. The long bones of the arms and legs, although more brittle because of mineral losses, do not change length, making the arms and legs look longer in relation to the shortened trunk. The joints become stiffer and less flexible. Fluid in the joints may decrease, and the cartilage may begin to rub together and erode. Minerals may deposit in some joints. Hip and knee joints may begin to lose structure because of degenerative changes. The finger joints lose cartilage, and the bones thicken slightly. Inflammation, pain, stiffness, and deformity can result from breakdown of the joint structures. The posture can become progressively stooped, and the knees and hips more flexed. The neck may become tilted. The shoulders may narrow, while the pelvis may become wider. Movement slows and may become limited. The gait becomes slower and shorter. Walking may become unsteady, with less arm swing.

Cardiovascular System

The heart increases in size and weight. The increasing thickness of the left ventricular wall is thought to be a compensatory mechanism to increased afterload caused by decreased central arterial compliance and increased peripheral resistance. The myocardium thickens, and there are increased lipofuscin deposits, fatty infiltration, and fibrosis, resulting in ventricular stiffness. The endocardium undergoes diffuse thickening, and valves may become thickened and calcified. Fibrosis, myocyte hypertrophy, and calcium deposition can impact the rest of the conduction system, which may manifest as prolongation in the PR and QRS intervals on electrocardiography and right bundle-branch block.

Pacemaker cells are lost at a rate of 10% per decade and can result in sinus arrest or tachy–brady syndrome. Heart rate variability is diminished, and hypertrophy, especially in older women, may actually result in an increased (hyperdynamic) resting ejection fraction. The arteries become dilated, and the vessels increase in length, become more rigid, and lose their sensitivity to receptor-mediated agents. The intima and basement membrane progressively thicken, while endothelial cells become irregular in size and shape. Smooth muscle cells and macrophages infiltrate, followed by increased matrix synthesis (ie, intimal sclerosis). In the media, internal elastic lamina becomes thinner and straighter, and elastin fibers are replaced by collagen, causing decreased elasticity; calcification increases, and lipids accumulate intra- and extracellularly.

Pulmonary System

The costal cartilages undergo calcification, there is kyphosis, and the compliance of the chest wall decreases. Elastin fibers in the parenchymal framework decrease with increasing cross-linkage between these fibers, which decreases elastic recoil of the lungs. Decreased recoil can lead to reduced intrathoracic negative pressure and airway collapse. Collagen levels also decrease. Alveolar duct volume increases at the expense of the alveolus (ductectasia). The surface area of the lung decreases, residual volume increases by 20 mL/year, vital capacity decreases, and forced expiratory volume and forced vital capacity decrease by 30% by 80 years of age. Effort-independent respiration (ie, quiet breathing) decreases due to decreased elastic recoil and airway collapse in the lower lung zones. Effort-dependent respiration (ie, forced breathing) decreases with decreasing respiratory musculature. All the above factors can contribute to decreased arterial partial pressure of oxygen, exercise tolerance, and pulmonary reserve.

Eyes

Loss of periorbital fat produces sunken eyes and laxity of eyelids. Transparency of the cornea decreases as lipid infiltrates/deposits (ie, arcus senilis) accumulate. The anterior chamber becomes progressively shallower because of the thickening of the lens. Pupil diameter decreases progressively. Increasing fibrosis of the iris reduces accommodation and slows dark adaptation. On average, the eye needs double the illumination every 13 years to maintain recognition in subdued light. The lens increases in size and becomes more rigid because of the constant formation of new central epithelial cells at the front of the lens. Consequences of these changes include presbyopia (ie, difficulty in focusing, especially on near objects due to lens rigidity), general decline in transparency with an increase in yellow pigment, reduced metabolic activity, and increased cataract formation (due to a progressive increase in the annular layers of the lens and a compression of central components that become hard and opaque).

In the retina, rods constantly produce pigment membranes, but with age less phagocytosis of the pigment membranes leads to buckling and kinking of rods. Cones show a major deterioration of membranes with age, and a decline in numbers that is particularly marked after age 40. Pigment epithelial cells become full of debris that they try to extrude through Bruch's membrane, forming yellow or white plaques (termed drusen) that are visible through an ophthalmoscope. Macrophages migrate in and break up Bruch's membrane, allowing blood vessels to invade, which can lead to visual impairment. The lens, cornea, and macula exhibit increased yellow pigment with increasing age.

Ears

The pinna continues to grow, and ear wax accumulates and hardens. In the middle ear, the tympanic membrane thickens, with a loss of both elasticity and efficiency of ossicular articulation. These changes may lead to conductive hearing loss, which affects predominately low-frequency sounds. In the inner ear, a gradual bilaterally symmetrical sensorineural hearing loss predominately affects high-frequency sounds. With aging, the extent of hearing loss varies greatly. Significant hearing loss is defined as presbycusis. The multiple forms of presbycusis include sensory (atrophy of the hair cells in the organ of Corti), neural (loss of cochlear neurons in the basal part of the spiral ganglion), metabolic (patchy atrophy of the stria vascularis over the middle and apical regions of the cochlea, restricting blood supply to the neurosensory receptors), and mechanical (changes in the motion mechanics of the cochlear duct, such as that caused by increasing stiffness of the basilar membrane). The auditory canal narrows progressively. On average, the inner ear experiences a decrease in the number of sensory cells in the saccule, utricle, and ampullae; the number of neurons transmitting from ear to brain; and the size and number of otoliths, which impacts sensing of gravity, speed, and rotation.

Digestive System

In general, with increasing age, the tongue develops varicosities, and decreased saliva production predisposes the mouth to oral infections. An increase in nonperistaltic spontaneous contractions of the esophagus produces difficulty in swallowing (ie, dysphagia). Swallowing is often not followed by the primary peristaltic wave, nonpropulsive contractions increase relaxation, and the lower esophageal sphincter is uncoordinated resulting in presbyesophagus. Diverticulae and herniation are common in older adults. In the stomach there is variable atrophy of the mucosa and muscularis mucosae, and inflammation and loss of gastric glands. The incidence of achlorhydria increases; pepsin activity decreases, whereas plasma gastrin levels increase. Gastric emptying is delayed after fatty meals.

The proximal jejunal villi become broader and shorter. Cell production in jejunal crypts decreases, incidence of diverticula increases, and chronic intestinal ischemia due to atheroma in supply vessels also increases. Intestinal fat absorption is delayed and reduced because of delayed gastric emptying and decreased lipase production. Vitamin B12 absorption and calcium absorption decrease; iron absorption also decreases in the presence of achlorhydria. In the pancreas, there is duct hyperplasia, increased cyst formation, deposition of lipofuscin granules in acinar cells, and increased fatty deposition. In the large intestine, mucosa cells atrophy. There is cellular infiltration of the lamina propria and mucosa and hypertrophy of the muscularis mucosae. Atrophy of other muscle layers leads to an increase in connective tissue, development of diverticula, increased transit time, and constipation.

Urinary System

Kidney size and weight decreases. The number of functional glomeruli decreases, and the number of abnormal and sclerotic glomeruli increases. The number of functional renal tubules decreases, and these tubules decrease in length. These changes lead to an increase in tubular diverticula and an increase in tubular basement membrane thickness; impaired permeability decreases the ability to resorb glucose. The glomerular filtration rate (GFR) declines. Renal blood flow falls as a consequence of altered vascular pattern, atherosclerotic changes, altered arteriole-glomerular flow, and focal ischemic lesions. Filtration fraction (GFR/renal plasma flow) increases; therefore, renal plasma flow must decline relatively more than GFR. The concentrating ability of the kidney declines. In the bladder, there is edema, lymphocyte infiltration, trabeculae and diverticula, prolapse, and urethral mucosal atrophy.

Immune System

The general effects of aging on the immune system include a variable but gradual average decline in acquired immune functioning. The immune system requires more stimulus and more time to become activated, produces less primary and secondary responses, and loses memory cells faster. Autoimmune antibodies also increase. T-cell function decreases gradually, and fewer naive and more memory T cells reduce the ability to mount an immune response when new exposures to pathogens occur. B-cell function decreases gradually, as does the response by naive B cells to newly introduced antigens. Aging B cells also increase production of abnormal antibodies. Atrophy of the thymus reduces function and production of T lymphocytes, proliferation of natural killer cells, and production of cytokines needed for growth and maturation of B cells. Loss of self-renewal capacity by hematopoietic stem cells contributes to immune-cell dysfunction.

Endocrine System

Age-related changes in the endocrine system vary with the individual gland and can involve changes in hormone levels, in receptor numbers on target cells, or in signal-transducing pathways. The concentration of certain hormones decreases with increasing age, including growth horomone, prolactin, melatonin, total serum calcitonin, aldosterone, serum cortisol, insulin (in some populations), thymosin, renin, dehydroepiandrosterone (DHEA) and its more abundant sulfated form (DHEA-S), pregnenolone, testosterone, estrogen, progesterone, and leptin. In contrast, the concentration of other hormones increases with increasing age, including norepinephrine, parathyroid hormone, atrial natriuretic peptide, and erythropoietin. There is an evolving debate over whether TSH levels change with normal aging, or whether levels associated with hypothyroidism in older adults reflect a change in the set point of this hormone.

Age-related changes in the endocrine system can also include delayed negative feedback after a stressor (eg, impaired restoration of ACTH and cortisol to unstimulated levels), loss of major gland/hormone unmasking secondary gland/hormone activity (eg, loss of ovarian estrogen with continued adrenal production of androgens promoting masculinization after menopause), and changes in signaling at the target cell level (eg, decreased insulin receptors and cellular glucose transporters). A number of hormones exhibit an altered two-hormone synchrony. For example, older men secrete luteinizing hormone (LH) and testosterone more irregularly and more asynchronously. Other hormone pairs that exhibit age-related asynchronous secretion include insulin and growth hormone, ACTH and cortisol, LH and prolactin, and LH and follicle-stimulating hormone.

NORMAL AGING

All of the above changes accompany advancing age but occur at different rates in individuals. Variability in onset, rates, and extent of aging suggest complex interactions between genetic predisposition, environmental exposure, and biologic and behavioral coping mechanisms in the etiology of aging. Despite these age-related changes, the different organ systems continue to maintain function, although their ability to maintain homeostatic conditions under times of stress diminishes. These changes may also be magnified by the impact of organic disease. The greater incidence of certain pathologies or diseases with increasing age (Table 2.3) reflects, in part, diminution of immune and other defense systems, increased exposure to disease-causing factors, and greater time for development of slow-progressing pathologies. Age-dependent increases in frequency of diseases such as diabetes, atherosclerosis, thrombosis, hypertension, cancer (especially of the breast, prostate, and colon), coronary heart disease, stroke, osteoporosis, and Alzheimer disease may characterize a synergy between aging and chronic disease in dysregulating homeostasis. Although age-related chronic disease can be viewed as promoting an advanced biological age, a distinction between normal aging and pathology is that in disease, compromised function is evident in the resting (nonstressed) state. Normal aging involves cumulative diminution in molecular and cellular properties and processes that exhibit physiologic effects only when internal or external stressors, or both, perturb homeostasis.

Changes at the molecular, cellular, and organ system levels that accompany advancing age can also be exacerbated by modifiable cultural factors, activity, or environmental exposures. For example, sun-induced skin aging (photoaging) depends on the degree of sun exposure and innate skin pigmentation. Photoaging may overlay and compound age-related changes in skin. Collagen levels in dermis are decreased, and cyclooxygenase-2 expression, collagen-degrading enzymes, and reactive oxygen species are upregulated in both aging and photoaging. In contrast, elastin fibers

Table 2.3—Organ System Age-Related Pathologies

Body System	Pathologies or Diseases that Increase in Incidence with Increasing Age
Nervous	Stroke, dementias
Muscle	Sarcopenia
Skin	Pressure ulcers, fungal infections (especially toenails) Neoplasms (basal and squamous cell carcinomas, melanoma)
Skeletal	Osteoporosis Rheumatoid arthritis, osteoarthritis

Cardiovascular
  Heart
  Vasculature
	Hypertension, thrombosis, anemia
	Congestive heart failure, myocardial infarction
	Coronary artery disease, atherosclerosis, varicose veins, hemorrhoids

Pulmonary	Chronic bronchitis, emphysema, pneumonia, pulmonary embolism Sleep apnea, stertorous breathing Lung cancer
Eyes	Entropion, ectropion, cataracts, age-related macular degeneration, glaucoma Diabetic retinopathy
Ears	Presbycusis Tinnitus, dizziness, vertigo
Digestive	Esophageal strictures, hiatal hernia Atrophic gastritis, acute gastritis, peptic ulcer, diverticulitis Fecal incontinence, cirrhosis, gall stones, pancreatitis Cancer
Urinary	Urinary incontinence Benign prostatic hyperplasia
Immune	Autoimmune disorders (multiple sclerosis, myasthenia gravis) Leukemias
Endocrine	Diabetes Grave disease

decrease in normal skin aging, but their deposition is increased in photoaging. Thus photoaging does not recapitulate an aging of skin. Other modifiable factors associated with facets of an accelerated aging phenotype include alcohol consumption and smoking.

COMPLEXITY, HOMEOSTENOSIS, AND INTEGRATED SYSTEMS

The changes that occur with aging contribute to systems-wide dysregulation and loss of maintenance. Additionally, the complexity in the dynamics of interacting physiologic systems decreases with age, resulting in a loss of integrated physiologic homeostasis. Loss of complexity occurs at the anatomic level (eg, neuron structure, bone trabeculae) and in the dynamics of physiologic processes (eg, heart rate, blood pressure). Reduced system complexity is associated with loss of ability to adapt to extrenal or internal stresses. The term *homeostenosis* is used to describe the narrowing of reserve capacity that contributes to a decreased ability to maintain homeostasis under stress. An increasing proportion of physiologic reserves is devoted to maintaining homeostasis as the individual ages. This encumbering of physiologic reserves results in eventual loss of homeostasis and increased vulnerability to disease. Loss of complexity and homeostenosis provide frameworks for understanding the heterogeneity in aging, disease presentation and susceptibility, and integration of interacting systems.

The physiologic parameter of body temperature maintenance can be used to explore systems-wide aging effects. With increased age, biologic changes to structures (loss of fat and thinning of skin, loss of sweat glands, decreased number of blood vessels and blood flow to skin surface, decreased muscle mass) have discrete molecular correlates and contribute to decrements in the functional capacity to maintain body temperature. Also, with increased age, biologic changes to negative feedback pathways (eg, nervous system changes such as fewer nerve cells that monitor/sense temperature and weakly functioning remaining nerve cells) also impinge on thermal regulation. Thus, aging is associated with a decreased detection and response to thermal variance, placing individuals at greater risk of hypo- and hyperthermia.

Geriatric syndromes such as delirium, dementia, depression, dizziness, failure to thrive, malnutrition, falls, frailty, functional dependence, and gait disorders are composites of dysregulation in multiple domains. For example, with malnutrition, in addition to the well-known, age-related changes in the digestive system that affect nutrition (eg, decreased absorption of vitamins A, D, and K, and zinc in the small intestines, decreased vitamin D production by skin and activation by kidneys causing reduced calcium) and age-related changes in other organ systems also contribute. Aging in the nervous system leads to a decreased sense of smell; altered flavor preferences lead to an altered diet. Decreased sensory function and coordination, muscle weakness, and changes in cartilage and in bone mobility and stability can make it more difficult to obtain, prepare, and eat nutritionally adequate food. In the circulatory system, thicker blood vessels reduce blood flow through the digestive system, causing reduced digestion and absorption of various nutrients. In the respiratory system, decreased compliance and capacity can also lead to difficulty in obtaining, preparing, and eating a proper diet. Similarly, domains contributing to the geriatric syndrome of gait impairment include age-related changes in cartilage, bone, muscle, nerves, circulation, and vision.

Thus, the biologic changes that occur with aging act across multiple systems and create expanding perturbations to homeostasis and functional capacity. The challenge for the geriatrician is to provide care to an ever-increasing older patient population in the context of numerous subtle and not-so-subtle primary aging-related physiologic changes, along with increasing comorbid medical conditions, frailty and other geriatric conditions, and disability.

REFERENCES

- De Cecco M, Criscione SW, Peterson AL, et al. Transposable elements become active and mobile in the genomes of aging mammalian somatic tissues. *Aging (Albany NY)*. 2013;5(12):867–883.

    This study provides evidence for activation of retrotransposable elements in late life, associating with disruption of genetic integrity and loss of homeostasis in mammalian cells.

- Moskalev AA, Aliper AM, Smit-McBride Z, et al. Genetics and epigenetics of aging and longevity. *Cell Cycle*. 2014;13(7):1063–1077.

    This paper reviews the evolutionary theories of aging with reference to molecular pathways and genetic and epigenetic components that associate with an aging phenotype.

- Shega JW, Dale W, Andrew M, et al. Persistent pain and frailty: a case for homeostenosis. *J Am Geriatr Soc*. 2012;60(1):113–117.

    This paper describes a clinical study of the association between self-reported pain and the presence of frailty, indicating that persistent pain could act as a homeostenosis stressor.

- Sleimen-Malkoun R, Temprado JJ, Hong SL. Aging induced loss of complexity and dedifferentiation: consequences for coordination dynamics within and between brain, muscular and behavioral levels. *Front Aging Neurosci*. 2014;6:140.

    This paper discusses neuromusculoskeletal system changes in cross-level and cross-domain interactions during aging, developing a predictive model integrating coordination dynamics, and loss of complexity.

Neal S. Fedarko, PhD
Matthew K. McNabney, MD, AGSF

CHAPTER 3—ETHICS AND LAW

KEY POINTS

- Ethical dilemmas arise out of conflicts in values or from uncertainty about the right thing to do in a given situation. Clinicians should be familiar with current perspectives on ethics topics and adopt a framework for working through these situations.

- Four guiding ethical principles of American medical practice are respect for autonomy, nonmaleficence, beneficence, and justice. Ethical dilemmas often result from conflicts between these principles. No priniciple is absolute, although autonomy is valued more in the United States than in some other countries.

- Decisional capacity is a patient's ability to accept or refuse a treatment. Capacity is decision-specific and may change over time. Determining if a patient has decisional capacity usually hinges on an assessment of four decision-making abilities: understanding, appreciation, reasoning, and choice.

- Patients who lack decision-making capacity need someone to make medical decisions on their behalf. The identified legal surrogate is tasked with making health care decisions that they believe the patient would have made through applying substituted judgment.

- Fully informed patients with decisional capacity have the right to forgo or terminate life-sustaining treatments. Advance directives include living wills, which provide information about an individual's end-of-life care preferences, and Durable Powers of Attorney for Health Care, which designate someone to be an individual's legal decision-maker should that individual lose decisional capacity.

- Untreated moral distress can have devastating impacts on patient care, individual clinicians, and institutions; thus, recognition is an important first step toward mitigating its damaging effects.

APPROACH TO ETHICAL DILEMMAS

Health care professionals frequently encounter ethical dilemmas in working with older patients across a variety of care settings. Ethical dilemmas can be stressful and contribute to burnout for health care professionals. Clinicians should be familiar with current perspectives on ethics topics and adopt a framework for working through these situations.

Ethical dilemmas arise out of conflicts in values or from uncertainty about the right thing to do in a given situation. For example, a primary care clinician may not be sure how to respond when a patient with oxygen-dependent COPD also continues to smoke. Should the oxygen be discontinued to protect the patient and others from a risk of fire? Can the oxygen prescription be renewed only if the patient agrees to stop smoking? Can the patient be forcibly moved from his or her home to a safer environment where there is no access to cigarettes? What are the ethically justifiable options for managing the patient's COPD?

Table 3.1 gives examples of some ethical dilemmas that occur in different geriatric health care settings, identifies stakeholder values and ethical principles that may be in conflict, and provides references for further information.

Different approaches for evaluating ethical dilemmas exist, but many share the same elements. One approach, developed by the National Center for Ethics in Health Care at the Veterans Administration, is the CASES approach (see Table 3.2). The first 3 steps of this approach can be helpful when encountering an ethical dilemma. The last 2 steps are more relevant to those engaged in ethics consultation.

The first step is to identify whether the dilemma is about ethics or something else, such as the law. Ethical dilemmas stem from cases in which there is uncertainty or conflict in values between stakeholders about the right thing to do in a situation. Values are defined as an individual's strongly held beliefs or principles. In the case of the patient who uses oxygen and continues to smoke, the conflict is between the patient, who believes that smoking contributes significantly to his or her quality of life and that he or she has a right to continue smoking, and the clinician prescribing the oxygen who is concerned about the patient's health, as well as the safety of the patient and his or her neighbors if the oxygen catches on fire. The clinician also may be concerned about liability.

The second step is to identify what information is needed to fully understand the situation. This may include information about the patient's medical condition, the patient's values and care preferences, and the preferences of others involved such as family and clinicians. It also may involve investigation for additional relevant information such as precedent cases, published literature, clinical guidelines, legal cases, institutional policies, and professional codes of ethics. For example, in considering the literature related to the above case, one would learn that the risk of fire both to the patient and to others nearby is less than might have been anticipated.

Table 3.1—Sample Ethical Dilemmas in Geriatric Medicine, Uncertainty or Conflict in Values, and Resources

Situation	Values (Ethical Principle)	Additional Resources
A hospitalized patient wants to go home, but the medical team feels this is unsafe and wants to discharge patient to a skilled-nursing facility for rehabilitation.	Patient believes he or she has the right to be in her own home (autonomy). Medical team wants to promote patient health and safety (beneficence).	Carrese, J. Refusal of care: patients' well-being and physicians' ethical obligations "But Doctor, I Want to Go Home." *JAMA*. 2006;296(6): 691–695.
A patient does not want to start dialysis, but the medical team feels that initiating dialysis will help the patient live a better life.	Patient/family do not feel that the benefits of dialysis outweigh the burdens (autonomy). Medical team believes that dialysis will help the patient live longer and better (beneficence).	Lam DY, O'Hare AM, Vig EK. Decisions about dialysis initiation in the elderly. *J Pain Symptom Manage*. 2013;46(2):298–302.
A patient's spouse asks the patient's primary care provider (PCP) not to disclose the diagnosis of dementia to the patient.	Patient's spouse wants to protect patient from any suffering related to knowing dementia diagnosis (nonmaleficence). The PCP feels that he or she has a duty to share the diagnosis with the patient (autonomy, informed consent).	van den Dungen P, van Kuijk L, van Marwijk H, et al. Preferences regarding disclosure of a diagnosis of dementia: a systematic review. *Int Psychogeriatr*. 2014;26(10):1603–1618.
A patient who is a convicted sex offender requests a prescription for sildenafil; the PCP is concerned about the risk to others and liability if he or she writes the prescription.	Patient believes that he has a right to have his erectile dysfunction treated similarly to any other patient (justice). The PCP is concerned that giving the prescription could enable the patient to abuse new victims and create liability (nonmaleficence).	www.ethics.va.gov/docs/net/ NET_Topic_20040526_Treating_ ED_In_Patients_with_STDs.doc (accessed Jan 2016)
A PCP is concerned about a patient's continued ability to drive but is uncertain about reporting the patient to the Department of Motor Vehicles (DMV).	Patient believes he or she has a right to continue driving to maintain independence (autonomy). The PCP is concerned about potential risk to others, potential liability, and impairing the clinician-patient relationship if the patient is reported to the DMV (nonmaleficence, confidentiality).	Reuben DB, Silliman RA, Traines M. The aging driver: medicine, policy, and ethics. *J Am Geriatr Soc*. 1988;36(12):1135–1142.
Nursing home staff want to hide a patient's medications in his or her food to ensure that the patient takes it.	Patient refuses to take medication (autonomy). Staff want to promote patient's health (beneficence).	McCullough LB, Coverdale JH, Chervenak FA, et al. Constructing a systemic review for argument-based clinical ethics literature: the example of concealed medications. *J Med Philos*. 2007;32:65–76.
Nursing home administrators are concerned about receiving poor marks from state regulators if the prevalence of weight loss in patients with advanced dementia is too high in their facility.	Administration values facility receiving high marks for quality of care (beneficence). The Medical Director believes that weight loss and risk of pressure ulcers is part of the normal course of dementia progression, and believes that ensuring a facility's quality marks should not be part of families' decision-making about feeding tubes (nonmaleficence).	Palecek EJ, Teno JM, Casarett DJ, et al. Comfort feeding only: a proposal to bring clarity to decision-making regarding difficulty with eating for persons with advanced dementia. *J Am Geriatr Soc*. 2010;58:580–584.
An investigator wonders whether he or she can include patients with dementia in a new research study.	Investigator wants to include patients in a research study to see if they respond to an intervention differently than people without dementia but is uncertain about whether it is ethical to expose people who do not fully understand the risks of participating to an intervention (autonomy, informed consent, nonmaleficence, justice).	Johnson RA, Karlawish J. A review of ethical issues in dementia. *Int Psychogeriatr*. 2015;27(10):1635–1647.

The third step is to analyze the information gathered, evaluating the benefits and risks of each potential solution and its likely consequences. For the patient with oxygen-dependent COPD who smokes, the consequences and implications of 2 potential options should be weighed. If oxygen is discontinued, the patient has a high chance of dying prematurely and the patient's preferences are ignored. If oxygen is continued, the chance of starting a significant fire is relatively small. If the patient has decisional capacity, it is neither ethical nor legal to forcibly move the patient from his or her residence to a more structured environment. Additionally, the clinician's duty to maintain the patient's privacy prohibits informing neighbors of the (minimal) risk without his permission.

In these difficult cases, creative solutions can often be found when considering more than 2 possible outcomes. In the case of the smoker who continues

Table 3.2—The CASES Approach to Ethical Dilemmas, Applied to the Case of Smoking and Using Oxygen

Step	Information Gathered
1. Clarify: 　Is there an ethics concern? 　Is there a conflict in values?	Conflict in values between ■ Patient believes it is his or her right to continue smoking. ■ Oxygen prescriber believes it is his or her duty to promote health and prevent injury to others. *Ethics question:* Given that this patient believes he or she has a right to continue to smoke, and the patient's geriatrician is concerned about the safety of the patient and his or her neighbors, if the patient starts a fire, what are the ethically appropriate options for prescribing oxygen?
2. Assemble the relevant information: 　Medical facts 　Patient preferences and interests 　Other parties' preferences and interests 　Ethics knowledge: 　　■ Codes of ethics, guidelines 　　■ Published literature 　　■ Precedent cases 　　■ Institutional policies 　　■ Laws	In the case of the patient who smokes and uses oxygen, it would be important to understand: ■ How severe is the patient's lung disease? How necessary is the oxygen supplementation? ■ Is the patient truly informed of the risks of smoking while using oxygen? ■ Does the patient have decisional capacity? ■ What is the patient's living situation (does he live with others, are there others nearby)? ■ Does the oxygen supplier have any concerns or relevant policies, etc? ■ What are the statistics on fires resulting from patients who use oxygen and smoke? Is there literature about the ethics of smoking and using oxygen? Is there literature on other issues with similar conflicts in values? ■ National Center for Ethics in Health Care, Report – Ethical Considerations That Arise When a Home Care Patient on Long Term Oxygen Therapy Continues to Smoke, March 2010. Available at www.ethics.va.gov/docs/necrpts/NEC_Report_20100301_Smoking_while_on_LTOT.pdf (accessed Jan 2016)
3. Synthesize the information: 　Apply different approaches to ethical analysis 　Weigh claims and counterclaims 　Review ethically justifiable options	Continuing oxygen　　　　　　　　　Withholding oxygen ■ Honors patient preferences　　　■ Disregards patient preferences ■ Keeps him alive　　　　　　　　■ Patient dies ■ Small risk to others　　　　　　　■ Prevents risks to others Are there other options that have not been considered?
4. Explain the synthesis	Share analysis and pertinent resources/information with involved others.
5. Support the process	Are there systems issues contributing to this problem? Would an institutional policy about oxygen and smoking by patients be of use?

to use oxygen, a creative option would be to attach a special valve to the oxygen tubing that will stop the flow of oxygen if fire is detected. This would allow the patient to continue to smoke while reducing the risk of fire.

In weighing all the relevant information in this case, one might determine that withholding the patient's oxygen or forcing the patient to move to a facility where smoking is closely monitored is not ethically justifiable on grounds of violating the patient's autonomy. By using the special smoke-detecting valve, the already small risk of fire is reduced further. This option would serve to minimize risk to the patient and others while honoring the patient's preference to continue smoking.

Another complementary approach is to evaluate the case through different ethical lenses. One commonly used approach is principlism, ie, the weighing of different ethical principles that are in conflict (see next section). The prima facie principles of autonomy, beneficence, nonmaleficence, and justice are often applied in this process (see Table 3.1). Other ethical lenses include casuistry (comparing the case to other similar ones), utilitarianism/consequentialism (evaluating which outcomes maximize the greatest good), and deontological/rights-based (determining which outcome honors universally held principles).

It can be beneficial for the clinician to share the relevant information and the analysis with others involved, providing an opportunity for further discussion. For the example of the patient who is smoking while using oxygen, the staff involved in the patient's care would gain a better understanding of why discontinuing oxygen is not ethically justifiable and is also reasonably safe. The group also may want to consider whether any systems-level interventions could prevent future cases, such as development of an institutional policy.

For particularly difficult situations, a formal ethics consultation can be obtained. There is indirect evidence on the positive effects of guidance from ethics consultants. Studies have found that ethics consultation is associated with increased patient and provider satisfaction, and with decreased unwanted treatments, leading to decreased lengths of stay.

Principles of Medical Ethics

The four guiding principles of American medical ethics most often cited are respect for autonomy, nonmaleficence, beneficence, and justice. Ethical dilemmas often arise when there is a conflict between these principles, as illustrated in Table 3.1. When there is an ethical dilemma, these ethical principles can be weighed against each other to help determine the ethicality of different proposed options.

The primacy of individual autonomy is a foundation of American culture, from the early pioneers to modern medical practice. Early court cases, such as Schloendorff vs. Society of NY Hospital in 1914, established the importance of patient autonomy by ruling that informed consent was essential prior to treatments and procedures, or they could be considered battery. Respect for individuals' autonomy includes allowing individuals to defer medical decision-making to others. In many cultures, family structure dictates who will be the decision maker for individuals within that family, and that person is deferred to even when the individual involved has the cognitive ability to make his or her own decisions. However, it is unethical to automatically defer decision making to an adult child of an older patient who is capable of making decisions for himself or herself if that older person wants to make his or her own decisions.

Beneficence, doing more good than harm, is largely determined by each individual's reactions and needs as well as culture. The weighing of benefits, risks, and burdens (ie, how much would someone be willing to go through for what chances of what outcomes) is the mainstay of decision making in older adults whose wishes are unclear or unobtainable.

Nonmaleficence is often interpreted as "do no harm" but is better represented by the phrase "do not intend to do harm." Definitions or perceptions of harm differ widely between cultures and between individuals within cultures. A frequently cited medical conflict between mainstream culture and subculture perspectives is blood transfusions for a Jehovah's Witness. For a Jehovah's Witness, blood transfusion may be thought to cause more harm than good, even if the outcome of not having the transfusion might be death. Understanding the values of subcultures within our society may provide clues to the spectrum of values that underlie an individual's perspective on harm.

Finally, the concept of justice in the context of health care in our society remains ambiguous. There is not a recognized right to health care in the United States. The distribution of health care benefits and the use of health care technologies continue to be uneven and reflect biases regarding gender, age, race, and ethnic origin. Researchers have frequently excluded older adults in their study populations, and the lack of knowledge on the relative effectiveness of interventions when they are used for older adults can lead to the under- or overuse of interventions in this age group. Furthermore, assumptions that equate age with chronic illness and comorbidity can deny beneficial treatment to healthy older adults. Patients from groups that have long been denied many of the benefits of our society may be more reluctant than more historically privileged patients to step back from aggressive treatments because of a perception of continued prejudice.

Informed Consent and Decisional Capacity

In the United States, the right to patient autonomy is longstanding. Beginning in the early 20th century, a series of legal cases gave rise to the concept of informed consent, enabling patients to have a say in the types of medical care they receive. To give informed consent, patients need to hear about the condition at hand and the associated risks, benefits, and alternatives of each therapeutic option. Decisions are then made voluntarily without coercion. Patient autonomy is prominently valued when deliberating an ethical dilemma. Patients who are deemed to have decisional capacity (see below) and who are fully informed of the risks, benefits, and alternatives of a given treatment have the right to refuse that treatment, even if refusal of treatment may shorten life.

Medical decision-making has evolved from a historically paternalistic approach to encourage more patient engagement in decision-making. More recently, the concept of shared decision-making has become increasingly popular. In shared decision-making, the medical professional shares the relevant medical information with the patient, and the patient, in turn, shares information about his or her values and preferences. The clinician and patient then make the best decision together by weighing all relevant information and options.

Before undergoing procedures or treatments, patients need to give informed consent and must have decisional capacity to do so. Decisional capacity is a patient's ability to accept or refuse a treatment. Capacity is decision-specific and may change over time. Refusal of recommended treatments does not necessarily indicate lack of decisional capacity. Capacity can be assessed by any qualified provider, including geriatricians. In challenging or complex situations, psychiatrists should be called on to determine decisional capacity. Although clinicians determine patients' capacity, the courts determine if a person is *competent* to make his or her own decisions. Table 3.3 lists several common myths about decision-making capacity.

Determining if a patient has decisional capacity usually hinges on an assessment of 4 decision-making abilities: understanding, appreciation, reasoning, and

Table 3.3—Some Myths About Decision-Making Capacity

- Lack of decision-making capacity can be presumed when patients go against medical advice.
- There is no need to assess decision-making capacity unless patients go against medical advice.
- Decision-making capacity is an "all or nothing" phenomenon.
- Cognitive impairment equals lack of decision-making capacity.
- Patients with certain psychiatric disorders lack decision-making capacity.
- Lack of decision-making capacity is a permanent condition.
- Only mental health experts can assess decision-making capacity.

SOURCE: www.ethics.va.gov/docs/necrpts/NEC_Report_20020201_Ten_Myths_about_DMC.pdf (accessed Jan 2016)

Table 3.4—Sample Questions to Assess Decisional Capacity

- What's your main medical problem right now?
- What treatment has been recommended?
- If you receive this treatment, what will happen?
- If you don't receive this treatment, what will happen?
- Why have you decided to/not to receive this treatment?

SOURCE: Courtesy of Dr. Mark Siegler, used with permission.

choice. The MacArthur Capacity Assessment Tool, an instrument that has been primarily used in research settings to assess capacity, can also be helpful in the clinical setting. Table 3.4 lists 5 questions that can be used to assess decisional capacity.

The first step in determining if a patient can make a given medical decision is to review the decision at hand, including the associated risks, benefits, and alternatives. The patient then explains this back to the clinician in his or her own words, which comprises his or her **understanding** of the relevant information. Simply asking a patient if he or she understands the risks and benefits associated with a given treatment is not adequate. Patients who do not understand may not feel comfortable asking their clinician to review the relevant information.

The second step is to assess whether the patient has an **appreciation** of the fact that the decision being made will affect his or her body. For example, a patient in denial about a diagnosis may be able to repeat back the relevant information (and have a good understanding) but may not be able to apply this information to his or her specific situation.

The third step is to assess **reasoning**, including how well the patient is able to take in the information, weigh the options against his or her own values, and make a choice. Reasoning and choice should be consistent with previous decisions the patient has made over time. As the patient explains the rationale for his or her choice, he or she may demonstrate comparative and/or consequential reasoning.

Finally, the patient makes a **choice**, consistent with his or her values and preferences and maintains this choice over time. If a patient is delirious, for example, he or she may not have decisional capacity when the delirium waxes but may have capacity when it wanes. Thus, assessing decisional capacity when cognition is at its best is important to honor patient autonomy.

Assessment of decision-making capacity can be modified, based on the seriousness of the decision and its consequences. For example, before allowing a patient to stop a life-sustaining treatment such as dialysis, an in-depth assessment of capacity is needed. An assessment of capacity to refuse a routine blood draw would be appropriately much less stringent.

Patients with cognitive impairments such as dementia may still be able to make some of their own decisions and should be allowed to do so. Studies have documented that up to 70% of nursing-home residents, 50% of residents of adult family homes, and 75% of hospitalized older patients may lack decisional capacity for most or all medical decisions. Although lack of decisional capacity is more prevalent in those with lower scores on cognitive tests such as the Montreal Cognitive Assessment (MOCA), St. Louis University Mental Status (SLUMS), and Mini–Mental State Examination (MMSE), incapacity does not automatically occur at a given test score. When patients can no longer give consent, their legal surrogate decision-makers make these decisions (discussed below). However, efforts should still be made to obtain assent from the patient.

Patients who have decisional capacity have the right to defer decision-making to others. As they have aged, some members of past generations have done this. As the baby boomers age, however, they may be less inclined to defer decision-making to others, preferring to maintain the locus of control.

TRUTH TELLING

Clinicians have not always routinely informed patients of serious diagnoses such as cancer. Some clinicians still do not routinely inform their patients of dementia diagnoses, feeling that this information could be emotionally upsetting to patients. Similarly, family members may want their loved ones protected from hearing information about poor prognoses and diagnoses such as dementia.

Research has found that most patients want to be informed of diagnoses, even if effective treatments do not exist. This allows patients to attend to unfinished business and be involved in planning in case of future decline. A recent systematic review found that nearly 91% of people would want to know if they had dementia, and 85% of people attending memory clinics or with dementia diagnoses would want to know if they had dementia. Although learning that one has dementia may be distressing, people with cognitive impairments may already sense that something is wrong and be relieved that there is a reason for their difficulties. Before giving patients a new diagnosis, it is best to check with them about whether they want this information or whether they want it shared with someone else. Asking for patient preferences about sharing results when testing is initiated rather than when the testing has been completed is preferable.

SURROGATE DECISION-MAKING

Patients who lack decision-making capacity need someone to make medical decisions on their behalf. Most states and the Veterans Health Administration have laws or policies designating a hierarchy of legal surrogate decision-makers for incapacitated patients. A legal guardian is usually the first on the list of legal surrogates, followed by a designated decision-maker or health care agent through a Durable Power of Attorney for Health Care (see below). If neither of these individuals have been appointed or are unavailable, the designated decision-maker is usually the spouse, followed by other family members. Checking with one's own state laws is recommended, because states have different hierarchies. Some states require consensus of all members of a category, such as adult children, whereas other states require only majority agreement. The oldest child is not automatically the legal decision-maker. Table 3.5 illustrates one state's legal hierarchy of surrogates.

The identified legal surrogate is tasked with making health care decisions. Surrogates are expected to make decisions they believe the patient would have made through applying substituted judgment. When a surrogate is uncertain what a patient would want, the decision that is felt to be the patient's best interests is invoked.

Surrogates are often close family members who are emotionally attached to the patient. Research has shown that surrogates sometimes make decisions for others based on their own personal preferences. Although this may appear to disregard the patient's preferences, there also is research showing that patients often allow their surrogates leeway in following their preferences. Patients are concerned about burdening loved ones and recognize that their loved ones may need to make decisions that they can live with, even if these decisions go against what patients would have wanted. Thus, when surrogates appear to be making decisions that are different from what the patient would have wanted, it is best to ask surrogates for their rationale and offer support before assuming that surrogates have nefarious reasons behind their choices.

Although a clinician's primary duty is to his or her patients, he or she also should consider the impact of decisions and decision-making on the surrogate and

Table 3.5—Sample State Hierarchy of Surrogates (Washington State Law)

- The appointed guardian of the patient, if any
- The individual, if any, to whom the patient has given a durable power of attorney that encompasses the authority to make health care decisions
- The patient's spouse or state registered domestic partner
- Children of the patient who are ≥18 years old
- Parents of the patient
- Adult siblings of the patient

SOURCE: RCW 7.70.065. Informed consent—Persons authorized to provide for patients who are not competent (http://app.leg.wa.gov/rcw/default.aspx?cite=7.70.065 [accessed Jan 2016]).

other family members. Researchers who have studied the impact on surrogates of making medical decisions, especially end-of-life decisions, for loved ones, found that symptoms of posttraumatic stress disorder were present in approximately a third of all surrogates 6 months after their loved ones were in ICUs and in up to 80% of surrogates who made end-of-life decisions. In light of this, clinicians can support decision-makers by providing them with recommendations that are based on the clinician's knowledge of the patient's preferences.

When patients lose decisional capacity and do not have family to fill the role of decision-maker, clinicians can petition the courts to obtain a legal guardian for the patient. Initially, the courts appoint a guardian ad litem, who is tasked with gathering information about the patient and his or her situation. This information is presented to the courts and, if deemed necessary, a permanent guardian is then appointed. Guardians have variable levels of experience and training requirements. State laws differ on what decisions guardians can make with and without returning to the courts.

PROMOTING INDIVIDUAL PREFERENCES FOR FUTURE CARE

Advance Directives

Fully informed patients with decisional capacity have the right to forgo or terminate life-sustaining treatments. This was not true in the past. Life-sustaining medical technologies were developed in the latter half of the 20th century, raising the possibility that patients could be kept alive against their wishes. Karen Ann Quinlan and Nancy Cruzan were two young women in persistent vegetative states after catastrophic events, whose families requested cessation of life-sustaining treatments. When their medical teams refused those requests, the families petitioned the courts to obtain permission to withdraw life-sustaining treatments, arguing that these women would not have wanted their lives prolonged in their conditions.

Table 3.6—Documents and Other Important Information to Compile to Help Loved Ones or Surrogates with Decision-Making

- Durable Power of Attorney (for health care, finance, or other)
- POLST form
- Living will
- Last Will and Testament
- Physician names and contact information
- List of medications
- Organ donation preferences
- Bank accounts and other financial funds
- Insurance information (health, life, vehicle, house, other)

These court cases inspired the development of advance directives. In the late 1970s, California was the first state to pass a law creating living wills (the Natural Death Act), with all other states following suit. In 1990, the Patient Self-Determination Act was passed, which encouraged facilities receiving funds from Medicare and/or Medicaid to offer patients information about completing an advance directive on admission.

Advance directives include living wills, which provide information about an individual's end-of-life care preferences, and Durable Powers of Attorney for Health Care, which designate someone to be an individual's legal decision-maker should that person lose decisional capacity. Durable Power of Attorney (DPOA) documents can vary by category of decision-making. Some designate a proxy for medical decisions, some identify a surrogate for financial decisions, and some establish a surrogate for both financial and medical decisions. Some DPOA documents give surrogates the power to make medical decisions even if the patient has not lost decisional capacity. Because of these differences, health care providers should review their patients' DPOA documents.

Advance Care Planning

Advance care planning is the process by which patients and their clinicians engage in discussions about future goals of care and care preferences at the end of life. As people age and develop chronic conditions, advance care planning is important to ensure they receive the type of care they desire. The older population is heterogeneous in end-of-life care preferences, with some older adults desiring to forgo any life-sustaining treatments and others wanting any and all treatments to prolong life regardless of condition. Clinicians should not presume to know a patient's preferences without talking to the patient, and advance care planning is rarely completed in one session. In one study, primary care physicians did no better than chance at estimating their patients' preferences for resuscitation.

One outcome of advance care planning can be completion of a living will. Research has demonstrated the benefit of living wills in preventing patients from receiving unwanted care, especially undesired aggressive care at the end of life. Living wills have also been shown to provide surrogate decision-makers guidance in making decisions and to reduce their stress and decisional regret. Living wills, however, also have limitations and can be vague and difficult to interpret. Some believe that once a living will is completed, the patient's preferences will be clearly outlined to all. For example, a patient with heart failure may have a living will stating that he or she does not want life-sustaining measures if "terminally ill." When that patient is admitted to the hospital with an exacerbation of congestive heart failure, it may be unclear if the patient is actually terminally ill, casting into doubt the applicability of the preferences in the living will.

In addition to engaging in advance care planning with their clinicians, patients should also be encouraged to discuss care preferences with their loved ones, especially those they have designated as their surrogate decision-makers through DPOA documents. Decision-making is easier for surrogates who are familiar with their loved ones' preferences. Individuals also can reduce stress for loved ones and surrogates by compiling important documents and information in one place (see Table 3.6).

As patients approach the end of life, many decisions need to be made, and patients should be involved in this decision-making as much as they want and can be. Engaging in discussions about the patient's preferred goals of care may be helpful in framing treatment decisions through a shared decision-making process. For example, consider the case of a patient who highly values her independence and has previously voiced that she would never want to live in a nursing home dependent on others to help with her activities of daily living. If this patient suffers a large stroke from which she is not expected to regain her previous functioning, her clinician can use this information when talking to her family about decisions, such as placement of a feeding tube and discharge to a nursing home. The clinician may even want to make care recommendations that are based on knowledge of the patient's values, because this is consistent with a shared decision-making process.

More recently, some states have passed laws authorizing forms that identify a patient's preferences about such treatments as resuscitation, feeding tubes, and antibiotics. These forms serve as physician orders that are active outside the hospital and are honored by paramedics. The POLST (Physician Orders for Life-Sustaining Treatment) form was originally developed in Oregon to help convey the preferences of nursing-home residents being transferred across health care sites. Research has shown that these forms help promote patient preferences at the end of life. Names of these forms vary across states, eg, MOLST (Medical Orders for Life-Sustaining Treatment), MOST (Medical Orders for Scope of Treatment), and POST (Physician Orders for Scope of Treatment).

CONTROVERSIAL PROCEDURES AT END OF LIFE

In addition to the myriad difficult decisions that may arise as patients approach the end of life, certain procedures are considered to be controversial by some clinicians and family members. These procedures include palliative sedation, physician-assisted suicide, and euthanasia. The ethicality of these procedures has been greatly debated.

Palliative sedation is a procedure of last resort used to promote comfort at the end of life in individuals with intractable suffering. It may be an appropriate procedure for patients who are terminally ill, have comfort-focused goals, and have endured reasonable efforts by their medical teams to promote comfort using other palliative care therapies. When palliative sedation is undertaken, patients are purposely given medications, such as barbiturates or benzodiazepines, at the minimal doses to ensure their comfort, but not necessarily until they become unconscious. Although a recent systematic review indicated that palliative sedation does not hasten death, this concern remains prevalent. The use of palliative sedation for patients with intractable suffering due to existential concerns is more controversial than using it to palliate physical symptoms, such as pain or nausea.

The doctrine of double effect often has been used to justify palliative sedation. Under this doctrine, if a procedure has both potentially good and bad effects, it can be justified if the action itself is good, if the intent is for the good effect, and if the good effect is not achieved through the bad effect. For example, in considering a terminally ill patient with a primary goal of comfort, large doses of opioids may be required, which could cause respiratory depression and hasten death. The double effect would ethically justify prescribing large doses of opioids if the clinician's primary intent was for patient comfort and if suppressing respiration was not essential to provide comfort.

Physician aid-in-dying (PAD), also referred to as physician-assisted suicide and physician-assisted death, is currently legal in a few states in the United States. In 1997, the Supreme Court heard 2 cases about the legality of PAD. The court ruled that suicide is not a fundamental right and that state laws prohibiting assistance with suicide are not unconstitutional. However, these rulings did not establish that the U.S. Constitution forbids all types of suicide or participation in suicide events by others. Oregon was the first state to legalize the practice in 1998.

Before the legalization of PAD, concerns were voiced that patients would seek it because of poorly managed physical symptoms. Data from Oregon and Washington show that >70% of those who request lethal medications are already receiving hospice care. Most patients who seek PAD do so out of concerns about loss of control and dignity, not because of uncontrolled symptoms. Data from these states on the reasons that patients request PAD indicate that the top 3 reasons are "loss of autonomy," "less able to enjoy life," and "loss of dignity" (cited in >80% of requests).

In the Oregon and Washington state laws, patients interested in pursuing death with dignity must take several steps to qualify. Patients must have decisional capacity and a terminal prognosis to make a request (2 oral and 1 written request), and they must be evaluated by 2 attending physicians. They also must be able to self-administer the medications. Because of this requirement, patients with end-stage dementia are not eligible to participate. Patients with other conditions, such as amyotrophic lateral sclerosis, also may not be eligible. Of those patients who make requests and receive medication, about a third of them do not take the lethal medication before death. Patients may want the medication available in case life becomes too difficult or unacceptable, and some may die before needing to take the medication.

Clinicians should recognize that some patients ask about PAD to begin a conversation about death and dying, not because they are ready to request lethal medications. Even if a patient lives in a state where the practice is illegal, or if the physician cannot or will not participate, the physician's initial response to requests should be to inquire about the patient's intractable sources of suffering, rather than to suppress a dialogue about dying. An ensuing conversation can cover alternatives to PAD such as hospice care and appropriate referral to a chaplain or psychologist to address existential suffering.

One legal alternative to PAD is the voluntary cessation of eating and drinking by terminally ill patients with decisional capacity. Some living wills stipulate that the patient not be fed or given fluids if he or she develops dementia that progresses to a specified stage. Because of liability concerns, staff at assisted living, group homes, and nursing homes may not be able to honor requests to withhold food and water from residents with dementia.

The practice of euthanasia, in which a clinician purposely acts to cause the death of a terminally ill patient (eg, with injection of a lethal medication) is legal in Belgium and the Netherlands but not in the United States. It differs from PAD because of the role that the physician takes (administering the lethal medication versus writing the prescription). Some believe that palliative sedation is a form of euthanasia, although most literature and medical societies consider them to be different.

MORAL DISTRESS

Moral distress occurs when health care professionals are unable to do what they think is morally right because of obstacles. For example, nurses may experience moral distress when providing aggressive care that they believe to be futile to a critically ill patient. In this situation, nurses may believe that the goal of care should be maximizing comfort and feel as if they are actually contributing to patient suffering by providing life-prolonging treatment. Different aspects of a patient's case may cause moral distress for different clinicians. For example, one nurse might experience moral distress when trying to suction a patient who she believes is dying, whereas another might experience moral distress when observing physicians painting an overly optimistic prognosis to the patient and family.

Although studied most in nursing, moral distress also has been noted in nearly every other health care profession, including health care managers. Risk factors for moral distress include the following:

- Clinical factors, such as continuing life-prolonging care in cases of perceived futility, inadequately managing pain, providing false hopes, and working with incompetent colleagues
- Institutional factors, such as poor administrative support, poor staffing ratios, policies that impact patient care, and poor communication between disciplines
- Individual factors, such as sense of powerlessness, lack of assertiveness, lack of understanding about the pertinent ethical issues, and lack of understanding of all aspects of a given case

Untreated moral distress can have devastating impacts on patient care, individual clinicians, and institutions. Clinicians may be haunted by disturbing cases for their entire careers. The effect of being exposed to cases causing moral distress is hypothesized to build up over time as morally complex cases accrue during the course of a clinician's career. The residue of moral distress remains after each case resolves, and the accumulation of moral residue can lead to patients receiving substandard care, to clinicians leaving their jobs or professions, and to institutions having difficulty recruiting new staff.

Recognizing moral distress is an important first step toward mitigating its damaging effects. Interventions have been developed to help clinicians understand their sources of moral distress and the relevant ethical tenets. Resources for managing moral distress are available at the website of the American Association of Critical-Care Nurses (www.aacn.org/WD/Practice/Content/ethic-moral.pcms?menu=Practice [accessed Jan 2016]).

REFERENCES

- Appelbaum PS. Clinical practice. Assessment of patients' competence to consent to treatment. *N Engl J Med.* 2007;357(18):1834–1840.

    This article uses a case to illustrate how clinicians determine if a patient has decisional capacity to consent to treatment. It contains a table listing the different decision-making abilities, sample questions to assess each, and additional information linked to each decision-making ability.

- Bernacki R, Block S. Communication about serious illness care goals: a review and synthesis of best practices. *JAMA Intern Med.* 2014;174(12):1994–2003.

    This article reviews goals-of-care conversations between clinicians and their seriously ill patients. It includes a guide with specific steps and questions to help clinicians engage in such conversations with their patients.

- Billings JA, Churchill LR. Monolithic moral frameworks: how are the ethics of palliative sedation discussed in the clinical literature? *J Palliat Med.* 2012;15(6):709–713.

    This article examines the ethics of palliative sedation from many different ethical perspectives. Looking at ethical dilemmas through different lenses can be helpful in considering the most appropriate ethical action.

- Hamric AB, Borchers CT, Epstein EG, et al. Development and testing of an instrument to measure moral distress in healthcare professionals. *AJOB Primary Research.* 2012;3(2):1–9.

    This article describes moral distress and the results of a study that identified those situations that cause the most moral distress for physicians and nurses.

- Houben CH, Spruit MA, Groenen MR, et al. Efficacy of advance care planning: a systematic review and meta-analysis. *J Am Med Dir Assoc.* 2014;15(7):477–489.

    This article reviews advance care planning interventions with adults from the past 50 years. Successful outcomes of advance care planning are identified.

- Johnson RA, Karlawish J. A review of ethical issues in dementia. *Int Psychogeriatr.* 2015;27(10):1635–1647.

    This article gives an overview of ethical issues that can arise when a person has dementia, including whether to share dementia diagnoses with patients, including people who have dementia in research, and challenges with driving and voting.

- VA IntegratedEthics site on Ethics Consultation. http://www.ethics.va.gov/integratedethics/ecc.asp (accessed Jan 2016)

    The VA's National Center for Ethics in Health Care site for ethics consultants includes links to a detailed primer about an approach to thinking about ethical dilemmas, transcripts from national conference calls on ethics topics, and other resources.

Elizabeth K. Vig, MD, MPH

CHAPTER 4—FINANCING, COVERAGE, AND COSTS OF HEALTH CARE

KEY POINTS

- Medicare comprises 4 benefits: Medicare Parts A, B, C, and D.

  - Medicare Part A covers hospital, skilled nursing-home, home-health, and hospice services.

  - Medicare Part B covers physicians, nurse practitioners, social workers, psychologists, therapists, laboratory tests, and durable medical equipment.

  - Medicare Part C provides the benefits offered under Medicare Parts A and B through Medicare Advantage (MA) plans, which are managed care plans. Most MA plans also offer Medicare Part D benefits.

  - Medicare Part D covers some of the cost of prescription medications.

- Medigap supplemental insurance plans are available that cover Medicare Part A and Part B deductibles and co-insurance costs, as well as preventive care and other health-related goods and services.

- Medicaid is a joint federal and state program that provides health insurance (including long-term custodial care in nursing homes) to people of all ages who have low incomes and limited savings.

MAJOR DELIVERY AND PAYMENT INITIATIVES

With the enactment of the 2010 Patient Protection and Affordable Care Act (the ACA), new delivery models are continually being tested and implemented to improve quality and lower costs for older Americans. In particular, coordinated care models such as accountable care organizations (ACOs) and the patient-centered medical home (PCMH), as well as bundled payment arrangements, have grown out of the need to improve health outcomes for older Americans while decreasing costs.

The ACA established the Center for Medicare & Medicaid Innovation (CMI), charged with reducing costs in Medicare, Medicaid, and the Children's Health Insurance Program while preserving or enhancing quality of care. CMI has been tasked with developing, testing, and supporting new delivery models to increase coordination of care and improve quality, along with new payment systems to encourage more value-based care and move away from fee-for-service payment.

Accountable Care Organizations (ACOs)

ACOs are groups of doctors, hospitals, and other health care providers who come together voluntarily to give coordinated high-quality care to patients. The goal of coordinated care is to ensure that Medicare beneficiaries, especially the chronically ill, get the right care at the right time, while avoiding unnecessary duplication of services and preventing medical errors. When an ACO succeeds in both delivering high-quality care and spending health care dollars more wisely, it will share in the savings it achieves for the Medicare program. Currently, Medicare offers several ACO programs:

- Medicare Shared Savings Program—a program that helps Medicare fee-for-service program providers become an ACO

- Advance Payment ACO Model—a supplementary incentive program for selected participants in the Shared Savings Program

- Pioneer ACO Model—a program designed for early adopters of coordinated care

Bundled Payments for Care Improvement

Historically, Medicare has made separate payments to providers for each service they perform for beneficiaries during a single illness or course of treatment. This approach, commonly referred to as fee-for-service (FFS), results in fragmented care with minimal coordination across providers and health care settings. Rather than incentivizing quality, the FFS system rewards the quantity of services offered. Bundled payments have been shown to align incentives for providers (hospitals, postacute care providers, physicians, and other practitioners). This system of reimbursement allows providers to work closely together across all specialties and settings. As a result, in the beginning of 2013, to provide higher quality and more coordinated care at a lower cost to Medicare, the Centers for Medicare & Medicaid Services (CMS) introduced the Bundled Payments for Care Improvement initiative. The initiative includes 4 innovative new payment models focused on financial and performance accountability for episodes of care (see Table 4.1):

Table 4.1—Bundled Payment Models

	Model 1	Model 2	Model 3	Model 4
Episode of care	All acute patients, all DRGs	Selected DRGs, hospital plus postacute period	Selected DRGs, postacute period only	Selected DRGs, hospital plus readmissions
Services included in the bundle	All Part A services paid as part of the MS-DRG payment	All nonhospice Part A and B services during the initial inpatient stay, postacute period, and readmissions	All nonhospice Part A and B services during the postacute period and readmissions	All nonhospice Part A and B services (including the hospital and physician) during initial inpatient stay and readmissions
Payment	Retrospective	Retrospective	Retrospective	Prospective

SOURCE: www.cms.gov/Newsroom/MediaReleaseDatabase/Fact-sheets/2014-Fact-sheets-items/2014-01-30-2.html (accessed Jan 2016)

- Model 1 focuses on the acute care inpatient hospitalization. Awardees agree to provide a standard discount to Medicare from the usual Part A hospital inpatient payments.

- Models 2 and 3 involve a retrospective bundled payment arrangement in which actual expenditures are reconciled against a target price for an episode of care.

- Model 4 involves a prospective bundled payment arrangement, in which a lump sum payment is made to a provider for the entire episode of care (http://innovation.cms.gov/initiatives/Bundled-Payments).

Other ACA Changes

- Partial closure of the coverage gap in the Medicare Part D prescription drug benefit, which began in 2011, with 50% of the cost of branded pharmaceuticals covered during the coverage gap

- Extended coverage for preventive care services, as well as elimination of the co-payment requirements for some services

- Expansion of Medicaid (beginning in 2014), in which many more Medicare beneficiaries have been qualified as dually eligible, eliminating much of their out-of-pocket expenditures

- Changes in provider reimbursement, including decreases for Medicare Advantage Plans and increases in reimbursement to primary care physicians through Medicare and Medicaid

Appreciation of these changes starts with an examination of the beginning of the current health care system for older adults. This foundation began in 1965, the year that the U.S. government passed legislation designed to improve access to acute health care for old, disabled, or poor people. During the decades that followed, the resulting Medicare and Medicaid programs expanded, evolved, and spawned thousands of supplemental commercial insurance plans. Today, a complex and often confusing array of personal payments, public programs, and private insurance plans (see Figure 4.1) pays for, and thereby determines, much of the health care that older Americans receive.

MEDICARE

Medicare is a federal insurance program run by CMS, which pays health professionals and organizations to provide primarily acute health care for Americans who are ≥65 years old, disabled, or suffering from end-stage renal disease. As originally enacted, Medicare comprises two separate FFS plans (Part A and Part B), each of which pays predetermined amounts for specified health-related goods and services that are needed by its beneficiaries. More than 47 million Americans are covered by both plans, which is 15% of the total U.S. population. The net federal Medicare outlays in 2013 were $492 billion, which represented 14% of the federal budget (Figure 4.2). Concerns are centered around the large outlay of dollars by the federal government, because this is expected to reach $858 billion in 2024 (Figure 4.3).

Parts A and B

The Medicare FFS program, the nation's largest health insurance plan, is administered by private organizations under contract to CMS. Called Medicare Administrative Contractors, they enroll providers, educate them about coverage and appropriate billing, answer beneficiary and provider inquiries, and detect fraud and abuse. However, the primary task is prompt and accurate payment of the 4.4 million claims submitted daily for Medicare-covered services, costing more than $1 billion per day.

Older Americans (and their spouses) who have had Medicare taxes deducted from their paychecks for at least 10 years are entitled to coverage through Part A without paying premiums. Others may be able to purchase Part A coverage (for up to $411/month in

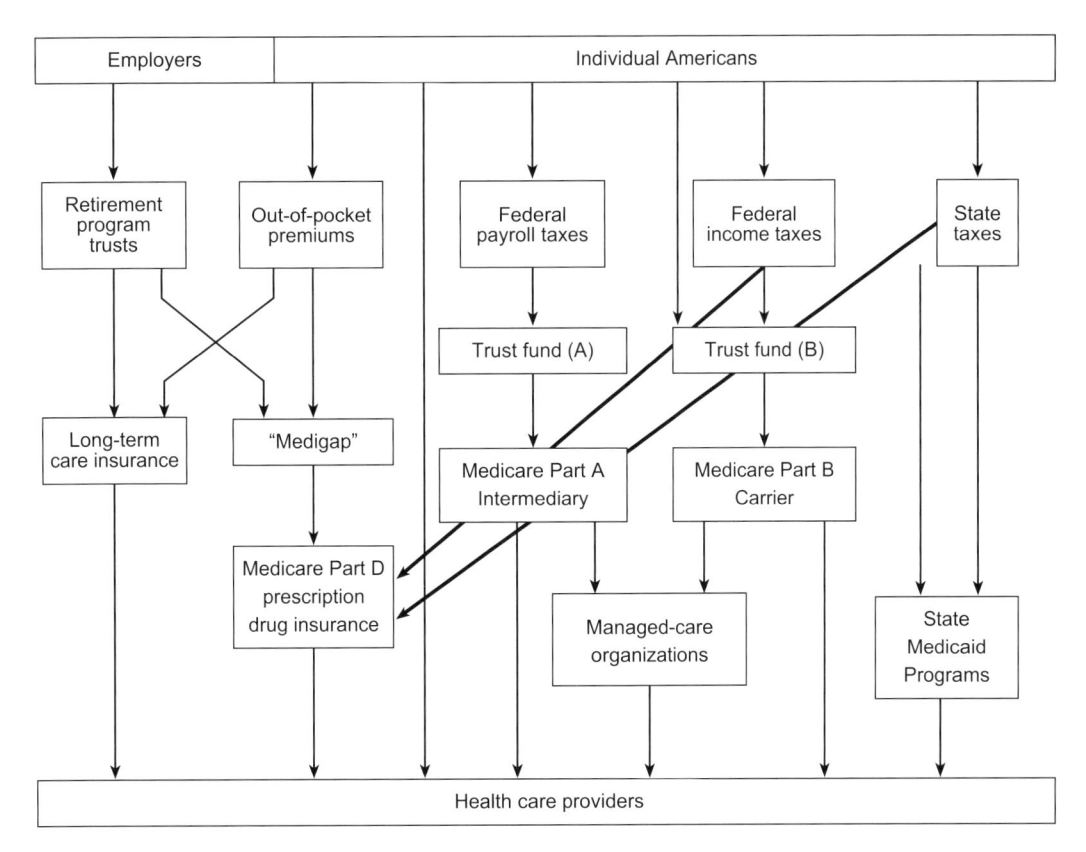

Figure 4.1— The Flow of Funds for the Health Care of Older Americans

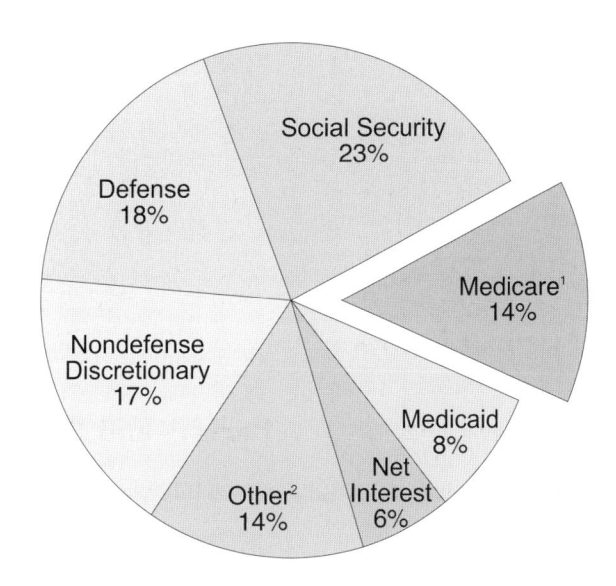

Total Federal Outlays, 2013 = $3.5 Trillion
Net Federal Medicare Outlays, 2013 = $492 Billion

NOTE: All amounts are for federal fiscal year 2013. [1]Consists of Medicare spending minus income from premiums and other offsetting recipts. [2]Other category includes spending on other mandatory outlays minus income from offsetting receipts.
SOURCE: Congressional Budget Office, Updated Budget Projections: 2014 to 2024 (April 2014)

Figure 4.2—Medicare as a Share of the Federal Budget, 2013

Reference: http://kff.org/medicare/fact-sheet/medicare-spending-and-financing-fact-sheet/ (accessed Jan 2016)

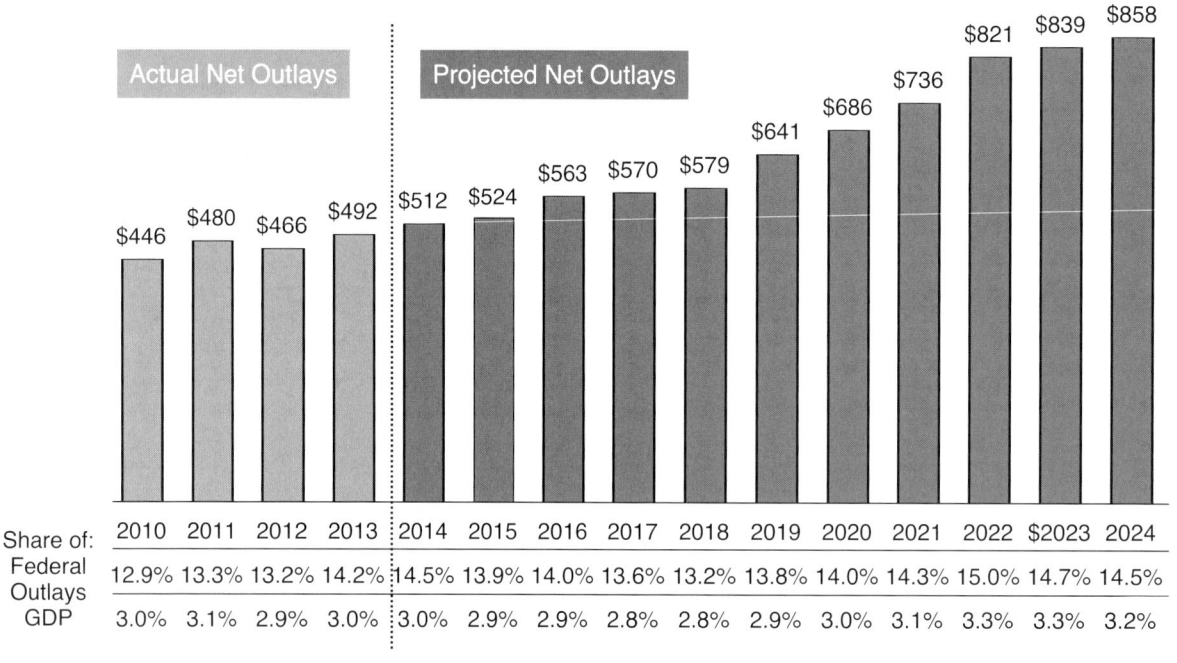

	Actual Net Outlays				Projected Net Outlays										
	2010	2011	2012	2013	2014	2015	2016	2017	2018	2019	2020	2021	2022	2023	2024
Net Outlays (billions)	$446	$480	$466	$492	$512	$524	$563	$570	$579	$641	$686	$736	$821	$839	$858
Share of Federal Outlays	12.9%	13.3%	13.2%	14.2%	14.5%	13.9%	14.0%	13.6%	13.2%	13.8%	14.0%	14.3%	15.0%	14.7%	14.5%
GDP	3.0%	3.1%	2.9%	3.0%	3.0%	2.9%	2.9%	2.8%	2.8%	2.9%	3.0%	3.1%	3.3%	3.3%	3.2%

NOTE: All amounts are for federal fiscal years; amounts are in billions and consist of Medicare spending minus income from premiums and other offsetting receipts.
SOURCE: Congressional Budget Office, Updated Budget Projections: 2014 to 2024 (April 2014); The 2014 Long-Term Budget Outlook (July 2014)

Figure 4.3—Net Medicare Spending, 2010–2024

Reference: http://kff.org/medicare/fact-sheet/medicare-spending-and-financing-fact-sheet/ (accessed Jan 2016)

2016, depending on how long they had Medicare taxes deducted from their paychecks).

Medicare Part B uses other regional insurance companies ("carriers") to pay physicians, nurse practitioners, social workers, psychologists, rehabilitation therapists, home-care agencies, ambulances, outpatient facilities, laboratory and imaging facilities, and suppliers of durable medical equipment for the Medicare-covered goods and services they provide.

At age 65, older adults become eligible for Part B coverage if they are entitled to Part A coverage or if they are citizens or permanent residents of the United States. To obtain this coverage, eligible older adults must enroll in Part B and pay premiums, usually by agreeing to have these amounts deducted from their monthly Social Security checks.

Physicians must choose among three options for participating in the FFS Medicare program: participation, nonparticipation, and private contracting. For each Medicare-covered service provided, a participating physician submits a claim to the Part B carrier, accepts Medicare's fee for the service (80% of its preestablished "allowed" amount), and bills the patient or the patient's secondary insurer for no more than a 20% co-insurance payment. Physicians electing nonparticipation status can bill patients directly for up to 15% more than 95% of Medicare's allowed amounts. The patients pay the physicians and then submit their requests to Medicare for partial reimbursement (ie, for 80% of 95% of the allowed amounts). For services not covered by Medicare, the physician may bill the patient, if the patient agrees in advance in writing.

A small minority (<1%) of physicians choose to "opt out" of Medicare altogether and enter into "private contracts" (also known as "concierge practice") with their older patients. Such opt-out decisions apply to all their patients; they may not be made on a case-by-case or patient-by-patient basis. Under private contracts, Medicare carriers (and Medigap insurance plans) pay nothing, and patients pay physicians the full amount of the fees specified by the contracts. Private contracts must meet specific requirements:

- The physician must sign and file an affidavit agreeing to forego receiving any payment from Medicare for items or services provided to any Medicare beneficiary for the following 2-year period.
- Medicare does not pay for the services provided or contracted for.
- The contract must be in writing and must be signed by the beneficiary before any item or service is provided.
- The contract cannot be entered into at a time when the beneficiary is facing an emergency or an urgent health situation.

Table 4.2—Health Insurance Coverage for Older Americans 2015

	Fee-For-Service Medicare Supplemental Coverage		Supplemental Coverage			
	Part A	Part B	Medicaid[a]	Part D	Medigap Insurance	Medicare Advantage Insurance (Part C)
Covers the cost of:						
Hospitals	100%[c]	—	100%[c]	—	$550–$1,100	100%
Postacute care in skilled-nursing facility	100%[d]	—	—	—	—	100%
Hospice	100%[e]	—	—	—	—	—
Home care ("medically necessary")	100%	100%	—	—	—	100%
Durable medical equipment	80%[f]	80%[f]	20%	—	20%	100%
Diagnostic laboratory tests	—	100%	—	—	—	100%
Diagnostic imaging tests	—	80%	20%	—	20%	100%
Physicians, nurse practitioners	—	80%	20%	—	20%	100%
Outpatient PT, OT, ST	—	80%	20%	—	20%	100%
Outpatient services, supplies	—	80%	20%	—	20%	100%
Emergency care	—	80%	20%	—	20%	100%
Ambulance services	—	80%	20%	—	20%	100%
Preventive services		[g]	20%		20%	[g, h]
Outpatient mental health care		50%	50%	—	50%	100%
Custodial care in nursing home	—	—	100%	—	—	—
Hearing, vision services	—	—	[i]	—	[i]	[i]
Outpatient medications	—	—	[i]	50%–95%[j]	[i]	[i]
Additional costs to patient:						
Deductibles	$1,260[k]	$147[l]	—	$320	[i]	[i]
Monthly premiums	—	$105–$335	—	$33[m]	[i]	[i]

NOTE: PT = physical therapy; OT = occupational therapy; ST = speech therapy

[a] Under the Balanced Budget Act of 1997, state Medicaid programs were given the option whether or not to pay deductibles and co-insurance costs.
[b] Some Medicare Advantage plans require members to pay deductibles and co-payments.
[c] After the beneficiary or secondary insurer pays the Part A deductible plus $315 per day for days 61–90 of each benefit period
[d] For the first 20 days of care in a skilled-nursing facility after a hospital stay of at least 3 days: $144.50 per day for days 21–100 of each benefit period
[e] Patient makes co-payments of $5.00 per outpatient prescription and 5% of cost of respite care.
[f] When patient is receiving Medicare-covered home care
[g] 100% of allowed cost of fecal occult blood test, Pap smear interpretation, prostate-specific antigen test, blood tests for diabetes and cardiovascular disease, and influenza and pneumococcal vaccinations; 80% of allowed cost of mammograms and clinical examination of breast and pelvis (no deductible applies); after the annual Part B deductible has been paid, 80% of allowed cost of a general physical examination at age 65, glaucoma screening, sigmoidoscopy or colonoscopy or barium enema, digital rectal examination (men), measurement of bone mass, hepatitis B vaccination, and diabetic education and equipment (coverage subject to change by health reform legislation)
[h] Some Medicare Advantage plans cover additional preventive services.
[i] Benefits and costs vary widely among Medigap insurance plans, state Medicaid plans, prescription drug plans, and Medicare Advantage Plans.
[j] Starting in 2011, the coverage gap ("doughnut hole") will gradually be closed over the next 10 years. In 2015, anyone reaching the donut hole receives a 55% discount on brand-name formulary drugs while in the coverage gap.
[k] Per benefit period (first 60 days after hospital admission)
[l] Annually
[m] Basic premium for 2015; premiums vary by plan. In addition, there is an additional program required for those with individual incomes >$85,000 (joint >$170,000), which is an additional payment on top of the standard monthly premium.

In addition, the contract must state unambiguously that by signing the private contract, the beneficiary:

- Gives up all Medicare payment for services furnished by the "opt-out" physician.

- Agrees not to bill Medicare or ask the physician to bill Medicare.

- Is liable for all of the physician's charges, without any Medicare balance billing limits.

- Acknowledges that Medigap or any other supplemental insurance will not pay toward the services.

- Acknowledges that he or she has the right to receive services from physicians for whom Medicare coverage and payment would be available.

To opt out, a physician must file an affidavit that meets the above criteria and is received by the carrier at least 30 days before the first day of the next calendar quarter. There is a 90-day period after the effective date of the first opt-out affidavit, during which physicians may revoke the opt out and return to Medicare. Once physicians have opted out of Medicare, however, they cannot submit claims to Medicare for any of their patients for a 2-year period. Physicians who opt out of Medicare still have their Medicare Part D medications covered through that program. It is the office visit and related charges for services provided directly by that physician that are not covered by Medicare.

Neither Part A nor Part B of the Medicare program covers routine dental or foot care, hearing aids, eyeglasses, orthopedic shoes, cosmetic surgery, care in foreign countries, or custodial long-term care at home or in nursing homes. Part B covers some preventive services (see Table 4.2).

Beneficiaries pay out-of-pocket for the following (rates are for 2016):

- Monthly premiums for Part B (standard premium is $104.90 but can be as high as $335.70, depending on income)

- Part B annual deductible ($166)

- Part A deductible ($1,288 per benefit period)

- Co-insurance payments (usually 20%) for goods and services for which Medicare or other insurance pays only a portion

- The full cost of those goods and services not covered by Medicare or other insurance

Although most retirees who signed up for Medicare Part B in 2016 paid $104.90 each month, premiums for wealthier retirees ranged from $170.50 for individuals earning between $85,000 and $107,000 annually to $389.80 monthly for single tax filers with incomes greater than $214,000 annually.

Part C

As an alternative to traditional FFS Parts A, B, and D, Medicare beneficiaries can instead elect to enroll in a Medicare managed-care plan, an option known as Part C or Medicare Advantage (MA). MA plans, operated by private insurers, hold contracts with CMS specifying that for each Medicare beneficiary they enroll, they will provide at least the standard Medicare Part A, B, and D benefits in return for fixed monthly capitation payments. Plans operate on a risk-adjusted basis for each member based on the ICD diagnoses that are provided. As a result, plans are paid more for individuals with more diagnoses that require a higher level of care. Effective October 2015, ICD-10 diagnosis codes went into effect.

To attract enrollees, most MA plans also cover additional benefits and charge low or no premiums, deductibles, and co-payments. The average premium in 2016 was $32.50 per month. The plans achieve cost savings by managing their enrollees' use of services within their networks of providers, with whom they negotiate price discounts in return for patient volume. Each January, MA plans have the option of changing their premiums, benefits, and provider networks—or of discontinuing their plans altogether.

There are several types of MA plans:

- Medicare Health Maintenance Organizations (HMOs)—insurance companies that accept capitation payments from CMS and provide or purchase Medicare-covered health services

- Preferred provider organizations (PPOs)—alliances of providers that accept capitation payments and deliver Medicare-covered health services to their enrolled patients

- Provider-sponsored organizations (PSOs)—partnerships of physician groups and hospitals that accept capitation payments and deliver Medicare-covered health services to their enrolled patients

- Private FFS plans—plans that may charge beneficiaries a premium, that pay providers more liberally than the original Medicare FFS program does, and that allow physicians to charge their patients co-payments of up to 15%

- Special needs plans (SNPs)—plans designed for patients with certain chronic diseases or other special needs, such as those who have both Medicare and Medicaid or who live in certain institutions

- Medical savings accounts—accounts into which Medicare beneficiaries can make tax-deductible contributions and out of which they can withdraw funds to purchase routine health-related goods (including medications) and services (including long-term care insurance) from any Medicare provider; linked to the medical savings account is a catastrophic insurance policy that limits the individual beneficiary's out-of-pocket expenses for health care to $6,000/year.

Between October 15 and December 7, beneficiaries covered by Medicare Part A and Part B have the option of joining any MA plan operating in their area; they cannot be denied enrollment because of any health problems except end-stage renal disease. Between January 1 and February 14, beneficiaries enrolled in an MA plan can switch to original Medicare. Enrollees must continue to pay their monthly Medicare Part B premiums to Medicare, plus any additional premium that the MA plan charges to cover additional services, and they must obtain their health care services from the plan's provider network. They have the option of leaving the plan at any time and returning to the FFS Medicare program.

The ACA was passed in 2010. By August 2014, MA premiums fell 10% and enrollment increased 38% to more than 15 million beneficiaries, with almost 30% of Medicare beneficiaries enrolled in an MA plan.

Part D

In 2003, the U.S. Congress passed and President George W. Bush signed a sweeping Medicare reform bill that included an option (Medicare Part D) for beneficiaries to purchase insurance coverage for outpatient prescription medications. The Part D option is open to all Medicare beneficiaries, whether enrolled in traditional FFS or MA. Part D benefits can be purchased as stand-alone policies or as sponsored by MA plans. For most Medicare beneficiaries, there is a dizzying array of plans from which to choose, with premiums, deductibles, co-payments, and formularies differing from plan to plan. CMS set up a Medicare Prescription Drug Plan Finder (www.medicare.gov/find-a-plan/questions/home.aspx [accessed Jan 2016]), in which enrollees can enter their location and medications to compare Part D options available to them.

Part D coverage policies create further confusion for many beneficiaries by having different levels of coverage apply to cumulative yearly prescription drug expenditures. Many plans have a relatively small deductible; the maximal allowable deductible by law in the standard 2016 Medicare Part D benefit is $360, an increase of $40 from the 2015 deductible. Some plans may have a lower deductible or no deductible at all.

As originally implemented, Part D provided no coverage when prescription drug costs exceeded a specified yearly amount, a policy known as the "coverage gap" or "doughnut hole." Under the ACA, Medicare gradually began closing the doughnut hole, including giving a $250 rebate to all Part D beneficiaries who entered the doughnut hole in 2010, providing discounts on brand-name drugs and generic drugs in the doughnut hole beginning in 2011, and phasing in additional discounts for brand-name and generic drugs to close the doughnut hole completely by 2020. In 2016, anyone reaching the donut hole ($4,850 maximum out-of-pocket amount in 2016) receives a 55% discount on brand-name formulary drugs; after this point, the plans cover 95% of the ensuing additional drug costs. Moving forward, the coverage gap cost-sharing levels for the beneficiary will be reduced annually until 2020, when the level is then set at 25%, which is consistent with cost-sharing levels of coverage before hitting the gap.

It is important for prescribers to appreciate that the standard Medicare Part D benefit changes each year. Some aspects (eg, the initial deductible and period of time before getting to the catastrophic point) change, such that patients experience an increase in their out-of-pocket expense. This could result in adherence issues as patients are forced to pay more out of pocket at different times during the year.

Hospice

Hospice is a benefit under Medicare Part A, providing a wide range of medical coverage for patients deemed to be within 6 months of death. Medicare hospice beneficiaries can receive drug coverage under the hospice benefit or under Part D, the circumstances for which were clarified by CMS in 2013. Hospice is responsible for covering all drugs for the palliation and management of the terminal and related conditions. Drugs covered under the Medicare Part A per diem payment to a hospice program, therefore, are excluded from coverage under Part D. Part D covers prescription drugs for problems unrelated to the terminal condition.

There may be some drugs that were for treatment of the terminal illness and/or related conditions before the hospice election that will be discontinued upon hospice election, having been determined by the hospice interprofessional group, after discussions with the hospice patient and family, that those medications may no longer be effective in the intended treatment, and/or may be causing additional negative symptoms in the individual. These medications would not be covered under the Medicare hospice benefit, because they would not be reasonable and necessary for palliation of pain and/or symptom management; they would not be covered by Part D either, because of the hospice group's determination that they are not medically necessary for palliation.

In 2014, CMS issued revised guidance stating that it expects Part D sponsors to use hospice prior authorization only on 4 categories of drugs (analgesics, antiemetics, laxatives, and antianxiety drugs) identified as nearly always covered under the hospice benefit. Careful review of medications and communication with the hospice and Medicare Part D plan is critical to assure timely access and appropriate coverage for medications for hospice patients.

Medigap

Medigap supplemental plans fill some of the holes in the insurance coverage provided by Medicare Part A and Part B. Private insurance companies offer FFS Medigap plans of 12 types (A through L), classified according to the benefits they offer. For new Medicare beneficiaries at age 65, the premiums for A-level (basic) plans across the United States vary considerably. These policies cover a person's Part A and Part B co-insurance costs, eg, 20% of Medicare's allowed fees for durable medical equipment and physicians' services. B-level plans cover Part A and Part B co-insurance, plus the Part A deductible. Each successive level of Medigap policy provides additional benefits and costs more. J-level plans cover co-insurance, deductibles, care in foreign countries, and preventive services. Less expensive Medigap coverage can be obtained by purchasing plans that require the insured to pay high deductibles (F- and J-level plans only) or plans that cover the services of only selected physicians and hospitals ("Medicare SELECT" policies). Medigap policies do not cover long-term care, dental care, eyeglasses, hearing aids, or private-duty nursing. They also do not cover out-of-pocket costs for MA plans.

Within 6 months of their initial enrollment in Medicare Part B, beneficiaries are entitled to purchase any Medigap policy on the market at advertised prices. After this open enrollment period, Medigap insurers can refuse to insure individual beneficiaries or charge them higher premiums because of their past or present health problems.

Medicaid

Medicaid is a joint federal and state program that provides health insurance to people of all ages who have low incomes and limited savings. The exact criteria for Medicaid eligibility and the benefit packages provided by Medicaid programs vary considerably from state to state. For persons qualifying for both Medicaid and Medicare, known as *dual eligibles*, most Medicaid programs pay for Medicare Part B premiums and some pay for Medicare deductibles and co-insurance costs. Most important, Medicaid pays for long-term custodial care in nursing homes for those who qualify. Several states offer fixed capitation payments to managed-care organizations that are willing to provide Medicaid and Medicare benefits to residents who are dually eligible (ie, for Medicaid and Medicare).

In 2016, the cost of medications for beneficiaries who qualify for Medicaid is $2.95 for generic products and $7.40 for branded ones. The dual-eligible beneficiaries have no premium or coverage gap; in fact, beneficiaries who are nursing-home eligible have no out-of-pocket expense for any Part D–covered medication.

The ACA extended the opportunity for states to expand Medicaid coverage to all nonelderly individuals with incomes below 133% of the federal poverty level in 2014. The Supreme Court ruled that this expansion of Medicaid is optional rather than mandatory. In states electing to expand Medicaid, the federal government pays 100% of the cost for newly eligible individuals from 2014 through 2016. The reimbursement rate to those states declines to 95% in 2017 and will be reduced gradually to 90% after 2019.

Dual Eligibles

Medicare and Medicaid, which were initially developed in 1965 as two distinct programs, jointly provide benefits to 9 million dual eligibles because their circumstances qualify them for both programs. Despite the notable differences between Medicare and Medicaid, the line separating the programs has become blurred over the years. For example, Medicaid used to provide prescription drug coverage for dual eligibles, but the Medicare Part D provision of the Medicare Modernization Act of 2003 shifted that responsibility to Medicare as of January 2006.

Although eligible for benefits, many low-income individuals do not receive Medicaid. Some do not meet their state's income and asset eligibility criteria, and others are likely eligible but have trouble navigating the application process. Poor health literacy is an especially common problem among dual eligible, who often do not understand their plan or its benefits.

Women, African-Americans, Hispanics, and disabled Medicare beneficiaries <65 years old make up a relatively large share of the dual-eligible population. Dual eligibles tend to have more functional and cognitive limitations and correspondingly greater medical need than beneficiaries enrolled in Medicare or Medicaid alone. As a result, they account for a disproportionate share of Medicare and Medicaid spending. Constituting just 15% of the Medicaid population, dual eligibles account for 39% of total Medicaid spending. They make up 21% of the Medicare population, yet are responsible for 36% of Medicare spending.

Considering the significant level of need and the limited resources of dual eligibles, it is perhaps not surprising that long-term care expenses account for an overwhelming share of medical expenses on behalf of this population, with dual-eligible individuals spending 70% of their Medicaid dollars on long-term care services.

Despite the high level of need that dual eligibles typically have, they are all too often subjected to uncoordinated payment systems in Medicare and Medicaid. To address this dysfunction and to improve coordination between Medicare and Medicaid, the ACA established the Federal Coordinated Health Care Office within the CMS. The ACA also created CMI to develop and implement innovative payment and service delivery models for recipients of Medicare, Medicaid, and the Children's Health Insurance Program, including those who are dually eligible.

One possible approach to integrating Medicaid and Medicare financially is to give each state a yearly block grant intended to fund all services used by state residents who are enrolled in either or both programs. States that spend less on Medicaid and Medicare services than the amount funded through the block grant would be permitted to keep the difference, but states that spend more on Medicaid and Medicare services than the amount of the block grant would be obligated to make up the difference. Another suggested approach is to have Medicare bear full financial responsibility for dual-eligible beneficiaries.

While the Federal Coordinated Health Care Office has begun its work, other measures and programs have been enacted with the purpose of improving care for dual eligibles. For example, Section 3309 of the ACA contains provisions for eliminating cost-sharing for certain full-benefit, dual-eligible individuals. In addition, effective January 1, 2012, all cost-sharing under Medicare Part D is waived for full-benefit, dual-eligible individuals who would require institutionalization if not for access to home-based and community-based services.

Extensive information about all the options is available to consumers at each state's medical assistance office, at 1-800-MEDICARE (1-800-633-4227) or 1-877-486-2048 for hearing-impaired TTY users, and at the Medicare Personal Plan Finder (www.medicare.gov).

Veterans Administration (VA) Benefit

The VA provides a medical benefits package to all enrolled veterans. This comprehensive plan provides a full range of preventive outpatient and inpatient services within the VA health care system. Also, once enrolled in the VA's health care system, veterans can be seen at any VA facility across the country.

Those VA facilities include a system comprising 153 medical centers, 773 ambulatory care and community-based outpatient clinics, 260 vet centers, 136 nursing homes, 45 residential rehabilitation treatment programs, and 92 comprehensive home-based care programs—all providing medical and related services to eligible veterans. These facilities provide inpatient hospital care, outpatient care, laboratory services, pharmaceutical dispensing, rehabilitation for a variety of disabilities and conditions, mental health counseling, and custodial care. They employ about 200,000 full-time–equivalent employees, including more than 13,000 physicians and nearly 55,000 nurses. Although the VA system is a closed system—meaning that all care is provided through VA facilities and providers—there are some exceptions. Veterans who are Medicare beneficiaries can use the Medicare system as well. In addition, the VA is increasing partnering with outside providers to extend the services available to veterans.

FINANCING OF CARE AT DIFFERENT SITES

This section describes, through the eyes of both patients and providers, how the various programs influence the day-to-day care of older adults. It illustrates their effects during a year in the life of Mrs. Rose Murat, an imaginary 79-year-old retired schoolteacher who lives with her 83-year-old husband in a small, older home. Mrs. Murat has hypertension, coronary artery disease, and mild heart failure, for which she takes hydrochlorothiazide, metoprolol, lisinopril, and nitroglycerin, with total drug costs of $1500 per year. She is covered by traditional Medicare Parts A and B. Mrs. Murat has also purchased a Part D drug plan, for which she pays annual premiums ($383), deductibles ($360), and co-insurance (25% of her remaining medication expenses = $285). As a result, her total out-of-pocket medication costs were reduced 34% from $1,500 to $1028 per year (from $125 to $83 per month). For the primary advantages and disadvantages of each of Mrs. Murat's coverage options, see Table 4.3.

Outpatient Care

Mrs. Murat sees her physician quarterly for monitoring of her chronic conditions.

Fee for Service

Under the Medicare FFS system, providers obtain the fairest possible reimbursement by understanding and

Table 4.3—Advantages and Disadvantages of Four Types of Health Insurance

Type of Insurance	Primary Advantages	Primary Disadvantages
Fee-for-Service Medicare (Parts A, B, and D)	Traditional Medicare benefits, choice of any provider that participates in the Medicare program, partial coverage for prescription medications	Cost of co-insurance, deductibles, noncovered goods and services (eg, eyeglasses, hearing aids)
Medicaid	Coverage of co-insurance, deductibles, and some benefits[a] not covered by Medicare	Choice of providers restricted to a single network in some states
Medigap insurance	Coverage of co-insurance, deductibles, and some benefits[b] not covered by Medicare	Out-of-pocket monthly premiums may be expensive, depending on the coverage provided by the policy purchased
Medicare Advantage plan (ie, Part C)	Traditional Medicare benefits plus coverage of additional goods and services[b]	Choice of providers restricted to a network; potential for changes in premiums, co-payments, deductibles, benefits, and providers at the discretion of the plan

[a] Under the Balanced Budget Act of 1997, state Medicaid programs were given the option whether or not to pay deductibles and co-insurance costs.
[b] Some Medicare Advantage plans require members to pay deductibles and co-payments.

Table 4.4—Eligibility and Coverage for Nursing-Home Services

	Eligibility	Room and Board Coverage	Coverage for Physician Services	Medication Coverage
Subacute	For Medicare beneficiaries requiring skilled-nursing care after a 3-day acute hospitalization	Part A	Part B or C	Part A or C
Nursing care	ADL/IADL needs	Medicaid, long-term care insurance, private payment	Part B or C	Part D

following CMS's payment system, which is based on evaluation and management (E&M) codes.

For each Medicare-covered service provided, the provider submits to the regional Medicare carrier the appropriate E&M code and the ICD code that indicates the diagnosis for which the service was provided. Entries in the medical record, which are subject to audit, must document that the data collection and medical decision-making aspects of the service conform to standards established for the E&M code submitted. By providing and documenting services efficiently, providers can maximize their FFS reimbursements within the limits imposed by the Medicare fee schedules.

Were Mrs. Murat newly enrolled in Medicare, she would be eligible for a preventive visit. The "Welcome to Medicare" preventive visit, also known as the Initial Preventive Physical Examination, is offered free of charge to all new Medicare beneficiaries within their first 12 months of Medicare as a means for individuals to develop a personalized plan to prevent disease, improve their health, and help stay well. During this visit, physicians are responsible for the following:

- Recording and evaluating medical and family history, current health conditions, and prescriptions

- Checking blood pressure, vision, weight, and height (to get a baseline)

- Making sure each patient is up-to-date with preventive screenings and services, such as cancer screenings and shots

- Ordering further tests, depending on general health and medical history

After Mrs. Murat has been enrolled in Medicare Part B for longer than 12 months, she is eligible for a yearly Medicare Annual Wellness Visit to develop or update a prevention plan based on current health and risk factors. This visit is covered once every 12 months.

At the end of her quarterly office visit, Mrs. Murat asks for advice on joining a managed care organization that has been marketing an MA plan in her county. She is impressed by the MA plan's offer of free eyeglasses, hearing aids, and preventive check-ups, all of which she has purchased out-of-pocket in the past. Her options are as follows: staying with traditional FFS Medicare as her only coverage, keeping FFS Medicare and applying for either Medicaid or supplemental (Medigap) coverage, or exchanging her FFS Medicare coverage for membership in the MA plan (see Table 4.2). Depending on the Murats' income, savings, and state of residence, they may also qualify for a Medicare assistance program that pays for some combination of their Medicare premiums, deductibles, and co-insurance costs. Some older Americans may have additional health insurance options through the federal Department of Veterans Affairs or through their (or their spouses') present or previous employer or union.

Managed Care

Mrs. Murat's primary care provider, knowledgeable about her health and prognosis, can help her choose the plan(s) that will cover the goods and services she needs, both now and in the future. If she can obtain what she is likely to need from the MA plan's network of providers, joining the plan might be her best option, because it will likely cover eyeglasses, hearing aids, and preventive services, and she can avoid paying the usual Medicare deductibles and co-insurance. Data about the quality of care and satisfaction of enrollees in local MA plans are available at the Medicare Personal Plan Finder.

If Mrs. Murat needs health care that is not available from the MA plan's network, or if she is reluctant to change providers, retaining the flexibility of her traditional FFS Medicare coverage (which covers her use of any provider that participates in the Medicare program) might be a better choice, especially if she also qualifies for Medicaid or buys a Medigap policy. Information from Medicare's information line or from the Medicare Personal Plan Finder would help her compare the prices and coverage of the Medigap policies available in her area.

The primary care provider's recommendations to Mrs. Murat are likely to be influenced by the characteristics of the different plans she is considering. For instance, if the primary care provider is not in the MA plan's service network, he or she would likely point out to Mrs. Murat that her enrollment in the MA plan would require her to select a new primary care provider. If the primary care provider is in the MA plan's network, Mrs. Murat's enrollment might change (ie, probably reduce) the payment for her care. The payments would depend on the type of plan involved. If it is a group or independent practice association model, the MA plan may pay providers "discounted FFS," ie, possibly less than Medicare Part B would pay for each service, or it may pay primary providers a fixed capitation amount each month to cover specified services. If these services are limited to primary ambulatory care, the capitation amount will be relatively small. Plans may choose to reward primary care providers with bonus payments for efficient and effective use of resources for the patients for whom they are responsible. If the covered services also include specialty and inpatient care, the capitation amounts will be considerably larger, and the provider will have incentives to use these services judiciously because he or she will have to pay for them, at least in part.

Regardless of the payment mechanism, the crucial question is whether the amount of payment suffices to support high-quality care. For example, if capitation rates are below the aggregate cost of the services they are intended to cover, the provider will feel pressure to take on more patients and to limit the amount of service that each patient receives. Similarly, if FFS amounts are too small, the provider will feel pressure to schedule more visits and procedures and to reduce the time devoted to each patient. Each provider should, therefore, monitor carefully and continually the many changing elements in the practice environment (eg, payment schedules, covered services, expenses, patients' and families' expectations, population demographics) to help determine the numbers and types of services appropriate for each older patient.

Inpatient Care

Four months later, Mrs. Murat awakes dysarthric and unable to feel her left hand. Her face is asymmetric, and her left arm and left leg are weak. Her husband calls 911. The ambulance rushes her to the nearest emergency department, where the physician on duty diagnoses a right hemispheric stroke and admits her to the hospital. Mrs. Murat may qualify for the Community Care Transitions Program, which provides transition services to high-risk Medicare beneficiaries. In addition, she may fall under a program monitoring hospital readmissions. This program directs CMS to track hospital readmission rates for certain high-volume or high-cost conditions, while using financial incentives to encourage hospitals to undertake reforms needed to reduce preventable readmissions.

Fee for Service

If Mrs. Murat had retained traditional Medicare as her only health insurance, she would have to pay Medicare's required deductibles (in 2016, $147 per year under Part B for the ambulance and the emergency medical care, plus $1,260 under Part A for the hospital admission) and co-insurance amounts (20% of Medicare's allowed charges by physicians and the ambulance service). She would also have to pay any ambulance charges in excess of Medicare's approved fee. If she had supplemented her Medicare coverage, her Medicaid or private Medigap coverage would cover some of these deductibles and co-insurance payments, and she would not be transferred to another hospital for insurance reasons.

When Mrs. Murat is admitted to a hospital, the hospital would submit its claim for emergency and inpatient care, which would be based on the diagnosis-related group (DRG) of her discharge diagnosis, to Medicare's Part A regional intermediary insurance company. The involved physicians and the ambulance service would submit their E&M-coded claims to Medicare's Part B regional insurance carrier. The intermediary and the carrier would pay their shares of these costs and, if Mrs. Murat had supplemental coverage, they would forward requests for payment of the balances to the state Medicaid program or to Mrs. Murat's Medigap insurance company. Ultimately, CMS would reimburse the intermediary from the Medicare Part A Trust Fund and the carrier from the Medicare Part B Trust Fund.

Managed Care
If Mrs. Murat had joined the MA plan, the MA plan would pay for the ambulance, emergency, and physician services; in most cases, it would pay the hospital a prenegotiated lump sum or a per diem fee to cover all of her inpatient care. The amount of this lump sum would be determined by the DRG of her discharge diagnosis, in this case, stroke. If the admitting hospital had no contract with her MA plan, Mrs. Murat would probably be transferred to a hospital in the plan's provider network as soon as she was medically stable. Depending on the MA plan's benefit package, she might be responsible for co-payments and deductibles for some of these services.

Postacute Rehabilitation

After 4 days of stabilization, evaluation, and rehabilitation, Mrs. Murat is deemed stable enough for discharge from the acute care hospital. She has improved somewhat, but she is still mildly hemiparetic and dysarthric, and she is apathetic and easily fatigued. Because her days in the hospital are fewer than the average number of hospital days associated with the DRG of her discharge diagnosis (ie, 5.9 days), CMS regards her "early" discharge as a "transfer." This permits CMS to reduce the amount it pays the hospital for her care. The consulting neurologist advises Mrs. Murat and her husband that her progress during the next few weeks will determine her potential for functional recovery. Mr. Murat asks the neurologist to recommend a rehabilitation facility for his wife.

Fee for Service
If Mrs. Murat could participate in rehabilitative therapy, Medicare Part A would pay for 20 days of postacute rehabilitation, in either a rehabilitation facility or a transitional (postacute) care unit of a nursing home. Mrs. Murat's admission to either type of postacute care unit would be reimbursed by Medicare under the Prospective Payment System (PPS). The Medicare PPS was implemented under the Balanced Budget Act of 1997 to control the increasing costs of subacute care. The PPS payment rates are adjusted for case mix and geographic variation in wages and cover all costs of providing covered skilled-nursing facility services (routine, ancillary, and capital-related costs). Per diem payments for each admission are case-mix adjusted using a resource utilization group system (RUGS) based on data from resident assessments and relative weights developed from staff time data. In addition, rates are based on geographic adjustment—the labor portion of the federal rates is adjusted for geographic variation in wages using the hospital wage index as well as an annual update; payment rates are increased each federal fiscal year using a skilled-nursing facility market basket index.

Mrs. Murat's RUGS category would determine the daily rate that Medicare Part A would pay the facility for the first 2 weeks of her care as long as she was demonstrating progress in rehabilitation. After 2 weeks, a nurse would reevaluate her status, update her plan of care, and adjust her RUGS category, thereby adjusting Medicare's payments to the facility for the next 2 weeks. Under this prospective payment system, the facility would be responsible not only for Mrs. Murat's nursing, rehabilitative, and social services but also for the costs of her medications, laboratory tests, and visits to an emergency department not resulting in admission to the hospital.

Using nursing-home rates, Medicare Part B would pay 80% of the allowed charges for the postacute medical care provided by Mrs. Murat's physician. Any postacute care related to an inpatient surgical procedure would be the responsibility of the surgeon, who would receive a "global fee" to cover the surgery and all postoperative surgical care. The Murats would need to satisfy Medicare Part B's $147 annual deductible and then make 20% co-insurance payments for the physician's care. Their out-of-pocket expenses would be reduced or eliminated by any Medicare supplements in effect, such as Medicaid, Medigap, or long-term care coverage.

Managed Care
If Mrs. Murat had joined the MA plan, her insurance coverage would include postacute rehabilitative care, probably at a nursing home in the MA plan's provider network rather than at a rehabilitation facility. Some nursing homes concentrate such high-acuity patients in transitional (or postacute) care units and provide them with coordinated rehabilitative (physical, occupational, and speech), social, and nursing services. Most homes, lacking such units, offer only custodial care supplemented by rehabilitative services as needed. The MA plan would also cover the physician's postacute services, but the Murats may be responsible for a deductible and co-payments.

More than 3 million Americans have long-term care insurance policies, but these policies pay for <2% of all nursing-home care. The high premiums for these policies, combined with consumers' uncertainty about needing long-term care in the future and their doubts about the policies' ability to cover the costs of long-term care in the future, have limited the growth of the long-term care insurance sector. Many middle-aged Americans believe they will retain good health and independence into old age; they appear to be relying on a combination of good fortune, social insurance (ie, Medicaid), and their personal assets to see them through their later years.

Home-Health Care

During the first 10 days of rehabilitative therapy, Mrs. Murat regains her ability to speak, and her left arm becomes stronger. During the next 8 days, however, she makes few additional gains. After 18 days, she is still unable to walk, cook, bathe, or dress herself without help. Her lack of continued progress toward functional independence will probably make her ineligible for coverage of additional rehabilitative services in either the MA plan or the FFS Medicare program. The Murats will have to pay for any future physical or occupational therapy on their own.

To obtain long-term care for Mrs. Murat's functional deficits, the Murats will need to choose between a home-health agency and a custodial nursing home. If Mrs. Murat returns home, neither the FFS Medicare program nor the MA plan will be likely to pay for a home-health aide unless she is homebound and requires the services of a registered nurse or rehabilitation therapist. However, local community agencies may be able to offer assistance. The Murats' choice of a home-health agency could be informed by comparisons of their local agencies' recent clinical performance, available at Home Health Compare (www.medicare.gov/HomeHealthCompare).

Fee for Service

In the FFS environment, if Mrs. Murat were homebound and dependent on skilled professional services, then traditional Medicare Part A would pay any Medicare-certified home-health agency a fixed fee to provide her with the services and equipment necessary to treat her primary diagnosis. Medicare Part B would pay her primary care physician 80% of the allowed charges for house calls, office visits, and care plan oversight services. In addition, Medicare Part B would pay her physician for home-health certifications and recertifications. The Murats would be responsible for the Part B annual deductible ($147) and the 20% co-insurance payments, unless they had supplemental coverage through Medicaid, a Medigap policy, or a long-term care policy.

Managed Care

If Mrs. Murat's condition made her homebound and dependent on skilled professional services, her MA plan probably would pay a home-health agency a fixed fee to provide her with the services and equipment necessary to treat her primary diagnosis. The MA plan would also provide her with the services of a primary care physician.

Program for All-inclusive Care of the Elderly (PACE)

If a health care organization in the area had contracted with CMS and the state Medicaid agency to create a Program for All-inclusive Care of the Elderly (PACE), it could provide community-based long-term care for dual eligibles whose disabilities qualified them for custodial care in a nursing home. If she were eligible for Medicaid and she enrolled in PACE, Mrs. Murat would attend an adult day health care center several days each week and receive comprehensive outpatient, inpatient, acute, and long-term care from a salaried interprofessional team composed of a physician, a nurse practitioner or physician assistant, a nurse, a social worker, rehabilitation therapists, and other members of the PACE staff.

Nursing-Home Care

Three months after Mrs. Murat returns home, Mr. Murat, now 84 years old, suffers a myocardial infarction and is no longer able to care for his wife at home. Their daughter logs on to Nursing Home Compare (www.medicare.gov/NursingHomeCompare) to shop for a nursing home. After comparing the local facilities' nurse-to-resident ratios, results of recent quality-of-care inspections, and rates of pressure ulcers and behavior problems, she arranges for her mother to enter a high-quality nursing home in her neighborhood, at least until Mr. Murat recovers.

Fee for Service

The FFS Medicare program would pay 80% of the allowed charges submitted by Mrs. Murat's physician for visits to the nursing home. The Murats would be responsible for the Medicare Part B annual deductible ($147) and the 20% co-insurance payments. Medicare would not cover any of the nursing home's per diem charges. See Table 4.4.

Managed Care

If Mrs. Murat had joined the MA plan, one of the MA plan's physicians would provide her primary care in the nursing home. However, unless she was covered by Medicaid or a long-term care policy, she and her husband would be responsible for the nursing home's per diem charges for room, board, and other basic services (about $200/day). After "spending down" their savings at this rate, the Murats might become sufficiently impoverished to qualify, if they had not qualified previously, for Medicaid coverage. If the Murats owned their house, some states would put a lien on it to recover some of its payments to the nursing home when the house was eventually sold.

End-of-Life Care

After residing in the nursing home for 6 months, Mrs. Murat suffers a massive stroke that leaves her physiologically stable but in a persistent vegetative state. Her husband reports that she had always said she would not want to go on living in such a condition if there were little hope of recovery. Mrs. Murat is unable to swallow thin liquids, and her husband says she would not want to be fed through any sort of tube. Her physician says that, with oral feeding, she is likely to live for several weeks. Her husband agrees to enroll Mrs. Murat in a hospice program with the understanding that she will receive palliative care without life-prolonging interventions.

Optimally, a discussion of end-of-life care should occur before this change in condition. In fact, since the Patient Self-Determination Act (PSDA) was passed by the U.S. Congress in 1990, hospitals, nursing homes, home-health agencies, hospice providers, HMOs, and other health care institutions are required to provide information about advance directives to adult patients on their admission to the health care facility. Despite this, physicians can still provide discussions regarding advance directive planning as part of any physical examination, and health care facilities are required under PSDA to include this information on entry into their facilities.

After an end-of-life discussion, Mrs. Murat can be enrolled in hospice. Enrollment in hospice would require the traditional FFS Medicare program (Part A) to pay a Medicare-certified hospice program a daily fee that would cover all palliative care for the terminal diagnosis, including home care, medications, equipment, respite, counseling, and social services even if Mrs. Murat had enrolled in (and remained in) the MA plan.

If Mrs. Murat had remained in the FFS Medicare program, Part B would pay her primary care physician 80% of the allowed charges for home or office visits and care-plan oversight services. Mr. Murat would be responsible for the 20% co-insurance and small co-payments for outpatient prescription medications, as well as for respite care.

CHANGES IN THE FEDERAL FINANCING OF HEALTH CARE

The complex and evolving combinations of coverage and programs create difficult choices for older Americans and powerful incentives for the providers of their health care. The U.S. Congress and CMS continue to revise the Medicare program, making it important to stay alert for changes.

The Balanced Budget Act of 1997 (BBA 97)

BBA 97 required CMS to adjust capitation amounts according to enrollees' risk of requiring expensive health care. This resulted in higher capitation payments for high-risk enrollees and lower payments for low-risk enrollees. This risk-adjustment method is based on the diagnoses associated with beneficiaries' health care during a recent 12-month period.

BBA 97 provisions for improving the quality of health care for older Americans included the following:

- The Quality Improvement System for Managed Care (QISMC)

- The Healthcare Employers' Data Information System (HEDIS), which requires MA plans to monitor and report to CMS their rates of compliance with selected processes and outcomes of health care (eg, mammography and immunization against influenza)

- The Medicare Health Outcomes Survey, which requires MA plans to contract with third parties to survey a sample of their members and report information to CMS about their health status, functional ability, and satisfaction with their recent health care

CMS summarizes the information generated by all 3 systems and makes it available at the Medicare Personal Plan Finder to help older Americans make informed choices about Medicare's FFS program and its various managed care options.

Balanced Budget Revision Act of 1999

Within the first 18 months of the enactment of BBA 97, the quality of health care for older Americans began to erode, and the decreases in payments to providers proved to be steeper than projected. For example, Medicare payments for home-health care decreased by

45% between 1997 and 1999. In response, Congress passed the Balanced Budget Revision Act at the end of 1999. This legislation restored some of the budget cuts made 2 years earlier, including $4.5 billion to MA plans.

Medicare Modernization Act of 2003

The Medicare Prescription Drug Improvement and Modernization Act of 2003 required dramatic changes in the nature and scope of the Medicare program, including the following:

- The creation of the Medicare Part D program covering prescription medications
- Subsidies for employers who continue to provide their retirees with insurance that covers prescription medications
- Elimination of coverage for prescription medications by Medicaid
- Competition between traditional FFS Medicare and MA plans
- Higher premiums for Medicare Part B to be paid by beneficiaries with higher incomes
- Expanded coverage for preventive services
- Increased reimbursement rates to physicians and hospitals in rural areas

The American Recovery and Reinvestment Act of 2009

As part of the American Recovery and Reinvestment Act, funds were allocated with an aim to modernize the U.S. health care system through a new federal health care information technology leadership structure. Through incentive payments, providers are eligible for maximal payments of $63,750 for those primarily involved in Medicaid and of $44,000 for those in Medicare to adopt, implement, upgrade, or demonstrate certified electronic health record technology. To qualify, the electronic health record must meet or exceed the "Meaningful Use" standard, which includes clinical decision support, e-prescribing, exchange of health information, and quality reporting.

The Affordable Care Act of 2010

The areas of the ACA affecting older adults and those providing their care primarily were focused on increasing access and changing the current FFS reimbursement system. In the area of access, the ACA increased access to Medicare beneficiaries by eliminating out-of-pocket expenditures for many preventive screening studies, reducing the Medicare Part D coverage gap, and expanding Medicaid coverage, which increased the number of dual eligibles. The ACA also moved to change reimbursement from the current FFS system to systems that improve outcomes, such as those delivered through coordination of Medicare and Medicaid for dual eligibles, bundling reimbursement, and pay-for-performance. The CMI is dedicated to developing and implementing these new payment systems, likely to be delivered through organizations such as Accountable Care Organizations and Patient Centered Medical Home models.

The Future of Medicare and Medicaid

The CMI is evaluating many programs designed to improve the quality and outcomes of care for beneficiaries with chronic conditions. In most of these, CMS is paying provider and managed-care contractors capitated monthly fees for providing case-management or disease-management services to beneficiaries with specified chronic conditions, such as heart failure, diabetes mellitus, or other "special needs." Many of these are based on the principle of "pay for performance," which stipulates that CMS will pay the capitation fees only to the extent that the contractor attains pre-agreed on standards of performance, eg, performing certain diagnostic tests, reducing Medicare's overall FFS payments, and satisfying beneficiaries with the services they provide.

Another Pay-for-Performance program is the Physician Quality Reporting System (PQRS), to be replaced by the Merit-Based Incentive Payment System (MIPS) in 2019. Physicians and other health care providers who report data about the quality of their care when they submit their bills to their Medicare carriers may earn bonuses of up to 1.5% of their total Medicare payments. CMS also sends them personal reports comparing their PQRD/MIPS data to that of peers nationwide. In 2015, there were 285 quality measures that could be reported, but some are specific to certain specialties. Incentive payments for each program year are issued separately as a single consolidated incentive payment in the following year. In January 2015, the U.S. Department of Health and Human Services established a goal of tying 30% of fee-for-service Medicare payments to value- or quality-based payment structures such as ACOs or bundled payments by the end of 2016, and a goal of increasing this percentage to 50% by the end of 2018.

The aging of the baby-boom generation, technology-driven increases in health care spending, and a decline in the number of workers per Medicare beneficiary will contribute to serious financial challenges for the Medicare program in the years ahead. Similarly, imminent sharp increases in the number of older Americans with serious disabilities will soon surpass states' ability to pay for their long-term care. To meet these challenges, the nation needs visionary geriatric providers able to develop and implement efficient and effective delivery systems to care for our older adults.

REFERENCES

- Centers for Medicare and Medicaid Services, Department of Health and Human Services. *Medicare and You Handbook*. www.medicare.gov/Publications/Pubs/pdf/10050.pdf (accessed Jan 2016).

    This informative handbook is written and distributed annually to all Medicare beneficiaries. It contains information on all the Medicare programs, which includes Parts A, B, C, and D.

- Centers for Medicare and Medicaid Services. *2015 Medicare Costs*. www.medicare.gov/Publications/Pubs/pdf/11579.pdf (accessed Jan 2016).

    This site describes 2015 Medicare Part A, B, and D beneficiary costs and coverages.

- Kaiser Family Foundation. *Medicare Spending and Financing*. www.kff.org/medicare/upload/7305-07.pdf (accessed Jan 2016).

    This very good resource for providers describes where Medicare funds come from and go to.

- Kaiser Family Foundation. *Medicaid Benefits*. http://kff.org/data-collection/medicaid-benefits/ (accessed Jan 2016).

    This very good resource for providers describes the Medicaid program.

- Stefanacci RG. Improving the care of "dual eligibles"—what's ahead. *Clin Geriatr*. 2011;19(9):28–32.

    The Affordable Care Act establishes programs to improve the care coordination between Medicare and Medicaid for the 9 million individuals who are eligible for both insurances; these individuals are commonly referred to as "dual eligibles."

Richard G. Stefanacci, DO, MGH, MBA, AGSF, CMD
Seth Gordon, MBA

CHAPTER 5—ASSESSMENT

KEY POINTS

- Geriatric assessment is a multifaceted approach to the care of older adults, with the goal of promoting wellness and independent function.

- Assessment of function includes physical, cognitive, psychologic, and social domains.

- Time-efficient, valid tools are available for use in a variety of settings to evaluate the status of older adults in all these domains.

- Time tends to be a less important element than the skills of the clinician in successful communication with older adults.

The scope of the assessment of any individual depends on the goals of care, the site of care, the patient's level of frailty, time constraints, and the availability of an interprofessional team. The essential aspects of geriatric assessment should be performed routinely in all sites of care, including the ambulatory setting, the emergency department, the hospital, the nursing home, and the home. Whenever possible, assessments should be performance based. An informant, ideally a caregiver or family member who lives with the patient, is often required to provide or to verify pertinent historical information about the older adult's day-to-day functioning.

THE ROUTINE OFFICE VISIT

Incorporating geriatric assessment into routine office practice requires use of efficient strategies, which can be facilitated by use of the electronic medical record through prompts, checklists, and templates. One such stepped approach entails rapid screening of targeted areas (Table 5.1), followed by comprehensive assessment in areas of concern. Many of the initial screens can be completed by trained office staff; some can be completed by the patients themselves while seated in the waiting area or at home before the visit. Attention to several components of geriatric assessment, including functional status, nutrition, cognitive impairment and depression, is required as part of Medicare's Annual Wellness visit. Alternatively, the use of a "rolling" assessment, which targets at least one area for screening during each office visit, should be considered. Finally, in the absence of specific target symptoms, parts of the routine examination, such as auscultation of the chest and palpation of the abdomen, can be replaced by aspects of geriatric assessment, such as observation of gait, balance, and transfers. However, office-based screening for common geriatric conditions has not been shown to improve patient outcomes (SOE=A).

PATIENT-CLINICIAN COMMUNICATION

Because of the demands of a busy clinical practice, the time available for office visits is often constrained. However, time tends to be less important than the skills of the clinician in successful communication. For several simple strategies that can be used to enhance communication, see Table 5.2. To accommodate the high prevalence of sensory deficits among older adults, particular attention should be given to the environment of the examination room. The use of simple, inexpensive amplification devices with lightweight earphones can be especially effective, even for those with severe hearing impairment. During the course of the interview, the clinician should go beyond the customary clinical inquiries by asking open-ended questions such as, "What would you like me to do for you?" Finding out what the patient wants can be a prime mechanism for solving potential problems, generating trust, and improving mutual satisfaction in the patient-clinician relationship. A National Institute on Aging booklet offers practical strategies to facilitate communication with older patients; this invaluable resource is available at www.nia.nih.gov/health/publication/talking-your-older-patient-clinicians-handbook (accessed Jan 2016).

Effective communication can be compromised by low health literacy—the diminished ability to obtain, process, and understand basic health information and services needed to make appropriate health decisions. Increasing evidence suggests that low health literacy, which has been documented in about one of every four community-living older adults, has deleterious effects on health and survival, at least in part because of deficiencies in self-management skills, poor adherence, and inadequate use of preventive services (SOE=A). Helpful information on low health literacy, including strategies to enhance communication, is available at http://healthlit.fcm.arizona.edu/HealthLitPlayer.html (accessed Jan 2016).

PHYSICAL ASSESSMENT

The importance of an appropriately detailed physical examination cannot be overstated. Many older adults cannot see well enough to report signs of disease, or have cognitive impairment that prevents them from being able to accurately report symptoms. The clinician cannot assume that "no news is good news" in the

Table 5.1—Rapid Screening Followed by Assessment and Management in Key Domains

Domain	Rapid Screen	Assessment and Management
Functional status	Answers "Yes" to one or more of the following: Because of a health or physical problem, do you need help to: ■ take a bath or shower? ■ walk across the room? ■ prepare meals? ■ manage medications? ■ manage the household finances?	Assess all other ADLs listed in Table 5.3. Evaluate cognitive function and mobility using performance-based tests. Assess social support. Consider use of adaptive equipment.
Mobility	"Timed Up and Go" test: unable to complete in <15 sec Usual gait speed: unable to walk 50 feet in <20 sec	Treat underlying musculoskeletal or neurologic disorder. Consider referral to physical therapy.
Nutrition	Unintentional weight loss of ≥5% in prior 6 months (or BMI <20 kg/m^2)	Monitor weight and consider referral to nutritionist.
Vision	If unable to read a newspaper headline and sentence while wearing corrective lenses, test each eye with Snellen chart; unable to read greater than 20/40	Use effective strategies to enhance communication and consider referral to ophthalmology.
Hearing	Acknowledges hearing loss when questioned or unable to perceive a letter/number combination whispered at a distance of 2 feet	Use effective strategies to enhance communication and consider referral to audiology.
Cognitive function	3-item recall: unable to remember all 3 items after 1 min Mini-Cog: recall = 0 or recall <3 and abnormal clock	Administer Montreal Cognitive Assessment (MoCA) or Saint Louis University Mental Status examination (SLUMS).
Depression	Answers "Yes" to either of the following: In the past month, have you often been bothered by: ■ feeling down, depressed, or hopeless? ■ having little interest or pleasure in doing things?	Administer 15-item Geriatric Depression Scale or 9-item Patient Health Questionnaire.

Table 5.2—Effective Strategies to Enhance Communication

- Use a well-lit room and avoid backlighting.
- Minimize extraneous noise and interruptions.
- Face the patient directly, sitting at eye level.
- Speak slowly.
- Inquire about hearing deficits; raise the volume and lower the tone of your voice accordingly.
- If necessary, write questions in large print.
- Allow sufficient time for the patient to answer.
- Provide patient education materials that are appropriate for individuals with low health literacy.

care of older adults. The physical examination should routinely include measurement of blood pressure, weight, and BMI, followed by additional evaluations individualized based on symptoms, underlying medical conditions, effects of disease progression, and adverse effects of treatments. Gait and sensory impairment are particularly common and should be periodically assessed (described below).

Vision and Hearing

Although visual impairment from cataracts, glaucoma, macular degeneration, and abnormalities of accommodation usually worsens with age, older adults are often unaware of their visual deficits. Asking about difficulty with driving, watching television, or reading may uncover a problem with vision. A brief performance-based screen can be accomplished by asking an older adult to read (using corrective lenses, if applicable) a short passage from a newspaper or magazine (SOE=C). Significant visual impairment can be confirmed through use of a Snellen chart or Jaeger card; visual acuity worse than 20/40 is the standard criteria for visual impairment.

The high prevalence of hearing loss among older adults and its association with depression, dissatisfaction with life, and withdrawal from social activities make it an important target for assessment. Hearing loss is usually bilateral and in the high-frequency range. Older adults who acknowledge hearing loss in the absence of cerumen impaction should be referred directly for formal audiometric testing. For those who deny hearing loss, further screening with the whisper-voice test is indicated (SOE=B). Inability to perceive a letter/number combination whispered at a distance of 2 feet is considered abnormal and warrants a discussion about referral for formal audiometric testing.

Nutrition

Poor nutrition in older adults can reflect concurrent medical illness, depression, dementia, inability to shop or cook, inability to feed oneself, or financial hardship. Aside from visual inspection for signs of malnutrition, older adults should have their weight and height measured routinely. Unintentional weight loss of ≥5% in 6 months or a low BMI (ie, <20 kg/m²) suggests poor nutrition and requires further evaluation (SOE=A).

MEDICATION ASSESSMENT

Time should be dedicated at each office visit to review both prescribed and OTC medications. Polypharmacy, which is common in older adults, can be the cause of many adverse reactions and contribute to the onset of new symptoms. Suspected treatment failure may be related to medication nonadherence. Exploring issues around nonadherence is important to discern whether the cause is related to finances, fear of being overmedicated, or lack of understanding of the need for a medication.

COGNITIVE ASSESSMENT

The prevalence of dementia doubles every 5 years after the age of 65 and approaches 40%–50% at age 90. Many patients with dementia do not complain of memory loss or volunteer symptoms of cognitive impairment unless specifically questioned. Older adults with cognitive impairment, even in the absence of dementia, are at increased risk of accidents, delirium, medical nonadherence, and disability. Therefore, an important feature of every assessment of an older adult, especially those ≥75 years old, is a brief cognitive screen (SOE=C). Before cognitive testing, clinicians should determine the patient's native language and be aware of any vision and hearing deficits.

Because short-term memory loss is typically the first sign of dementia, the best single screening question is recall of three words after 1 min. Anything other than perfect recall should lead to further testing. The clock-drawing test is valuable, because it assesses executive control and visual-spatial skills, two domains of cognition with profound effects on daily function. In the clock-drawing test, the patient is asked to draw the face of a clock and to place the hands correctly to indicate 2:50 or 11:10. The clock-drawing test is combined with the three-item recall in the Mini-Cog Assessment Instrument for Dementia, a validated screening test that takes about 3 min to administer. The Mini-Cog has an advantage over many other instruments of being relatively uninfluenced by level of education or language differences. As another quick screen of executive function, the patient can be asked to name as many four-legged animals as possible in 1 min. Fewer than 10 animals or repetition of the same animals is abnormal and suggests the need for further evaluation.

For many years, the most commonly used instrument for formal testing of cognition has been the Folstein Mini–Mental State Examination (MMSE). Because the MMSE is now proprietary and has several limitations, other validated tools are being used more commonly to assess cognition, including the Montreal Cognitive Assessment (MoCA) and Saint Louis University Mental Status Examination (SLUMS). These two instruments assess a comparable set of cognitive domains, including memory, executive function, abstract thinking, attention, calculation, and visual-spatial skills. The MoCA, which also assesses concentration, language, and orientation, takes about 10 minutes to complete. The total possible score is 30 points; a score of ≥26 is considered normal. The SLUMS takes about 7 minutes to complete. The total possible score is 30 points; a score ≥27 or above is considered normal. However, the results of cognitive testing should be interpreted in the context of the patient's educational attainment and literacy.

PSYCHOLOGIC ASSESSMENT

Although the prevalence of major depressive disorder among community-dwelling older adults is only about 1%–2%, the rate is much higher—up to 10%—in those seen in primary care settings. A large number of older adults, moreover, suffer from significant symptoms of depression below the severity threshold of major depression as defined by the *Diagnostic and Statistical Manual of Mental Disorders, Fifth Edition*. These subthreshold depressive symptoms, which often include somatic complaints such as poor sleep and fatigue, increase the risk of physical disability and slower recovery after an acute disabling event (SOE=A). They are also associated with a significant increase in the cost of medical services, even after accounting for the severity of chronic medical illness (SOE=A). Hence, clinicians should have a high index of suspicion for depressive symptoms and a low threshold for treatment. The best single question to ask is, "Do you often feel sad or depressed?" An affirmative response warrants further evaluation of other depressive symptoms, perhaps through the use of a standardized instrument such as the 15-item Geriatric Depression Scale or the 9-item Patient Health Questionnaire (SOE=B). The PHQ-2 is a very short, validated instrument for depression screening as well.

Anxiety and worries are also important symptoms in older adults and are often a manifestation of an underlying depressive disorder. Finally, because older adults are particularly likely to experience the loss of a loved one, special efforts should be made to recognize and manage the consequences of bereavement.

Table 5.3—Activities of Daily Living

Self-care
- Bathing
- Dressing
- Transferring from bed to chair
- Toileting
- Grooming
- Feeding oneself

Instrumental
- Using the telephone
- Preparing meals
- Managing household finances
- Taking medications
- Doing laundry
- Doing housework
- Shopping
- Managing transportation

Mobility
- Walking from room to room
- Climbing a flight of stairs
- Walking outside one's home

SOCIAL ASSESSMENT

A social assessment consists of evaluation of several elements, including ethnic, spiritual, and cultural background; availability of a personal support system; need for a caregiver, his or her role, and presence of caregiver burden; safety of the home environment; economic well-being; possibility of mistreatment; and the patient's advance directives. Although a comprehensive social assessment may not be feasible in a busy office practice, clinicians caring for older adults should be mindful of these aspects of their patient's lives. Clinicians can uncover important clues to unmet needs by inquiring about the availability of help in case of an emergency. For frail older adults, particularly those who lack social support, referral to a visiting nurse or physical therapist may help assess home safety and level of personal risk.

FUNCTIONAL STATUS

Functional status refers to the person's ability to perform activities of daily living (ADLs), which are listed in Table 5.3. When assessing function, clinicians should ask whether the patient is independent or requires the help of another person to complete ADLs. Bathing is typically the self-care ADL with the highest prevalence of disability, and needing assistance with bathing is often the reason for home aide services (SOE=A). Disability in ADLs may occur when there is a gap or mismatch between personal capabilities (eg, balance, muscle strength, cognition) and environmental demands. For example, an older adult with quadriceps weakness might require assistance to stand from a deeply cushioned, low-lying chair but have no difficulty standing from a hard-back kitchen chair. To identify patients with "preclinical" disability, ie, those who do not yet require personal assistance but who are at risk of becoming disabled, clinicians should ask about perceived difficulty with the tasks and whether the patient has changed the way he or she completes the task because of a health-related problem or condition (SOE=A). Use of any assistive devices, such as a cane or walker, as well as duration and circumstances of use, should also be assessed.

Outside a rehabilitation setting, performance-based testing of most self-care and instrumental ADLs is not practical. Hence, performance-based testing of functional status focuses primarily on mobility, including transfers, gait, and balance. The patient should be asked to stand from a seated position in a hard-backed chair while keeping his or her arms folded. Inability to complete this task suggests leg (quadriceps) weakness and is highly predictive of future disability (SOE=A). Once the patient is standing, he or she should be observed walking back and forth over a short distance, ideally with the usual walking aid. Abnormalities of gait include path deviation; diminished step height or length, or both; trips, slips, or near falls; and difficulty with turning. The tasks of rising from the chair, walking 10 feet (3 meters), turning around and returning to the chair, turning, and then sitting back down in the chair make up the "Timed Up and Go" test. Individuals who take ≥15 sec have an increased risk for falls and require further evaluation (SOE=B).

If time permits completion of only one performance test, gait speed should be measured. Gait speed is the single strongest predictor of future disability and death (SOE=A). A gait speed of 0.8 meters/sec allows for independent community ambulation; a speed of 0.6 meters/sec allows for community activity without use of a wheelchair. These norms indicate that older adults who can walk 50 feet in an office hallway in ≤20 sec should be able to walk independently in normal activities.

Balance can be tested progressively by asking the older adult to stand first with his or her feet side by side, then in semitandem position, and finally in tandem position. Difficulty with balance in these positions predicts an increased risk of falling (SOE=A). Although standardized instruments, such as the Performance-Oriented Mobility Assessment, can be used to quantify impairments in gait and balance, a qualitative assessment is usually sufficient to make recommendations about the need for an assistive device, such as a cane or walker. When assessing gait and balance, particularly in older women, clinicians should observe for use of proper footwear, ie, flat, hard-soled shoes.

Useful functional information can also be gleaned by observing older adults as they complete simple tasks such as undressing or dressing, picking up a pen and writing a sentence, touching the back of the head with both hands, and climbing up and down from an examination table.

Assessing life space (Table 5.4), offers a complementary strategy for distinguishing among different levels of mobility, not only in community-living older adults but also in nursing-home patients. Life space can be viewed rather simply as a series of concentric areas radiating from the room where a person sleeps to more distant locations, such as beyond one's town (for community-living older adults) or outside the facility (for nursing-home patients). The frequency of movement to various locations and the need for assistance are also assessed by formal life space instruments. For older adults with low life space, the ability to get in and out of a bed should be assessed.

Assessing the Older Driver

Evaluating the older driver is a difficult challenge. The automobile is the most important—and often the only—source of transportation for older adults. Yet a variety of age-related changes, chronic conditions, and medications place older adults at risk of automobile accidents. Although the absolute number of crashes involving older drivers is low, the number of crashes per mile driven and the likelihood of serious injury or death are higher than for any age group other than those 16–24 years old.

The vast majority of older adults make prudent adjustments in their driving behaviors by avoiding rush hour or congested thoroughfares or by not driving at night or during adverse weather conditions. Nonetheless, impaired older adults who continue to drive are a hazard not only to themselves but also to other drivers, passengers, and pedestrians. Pertinent risk factors for automobile accidents include poor visual acuity (less than 20/40) and contrast sensitivity; dementia, particularly deficits in visual-spatial skills and visual attention; impaired neck and trunk rotation; and poor motor coordination and speed of movement (SOE=A). Alcohol and medications that adversely affect alertness, such as narcotics, benzodiazepines, antihistamines, antidepressants, antipsychotics, sedatives, and muscle relaxants, can impair driving skills and increase accident risk. Hence, caution is warranted when starting or adjusting the dosage of these medications, and patients should be warned about potential adverse effects on driving safety.

Any report of an accident or moving violation should trigger an assessment of an older adult's driving ability. Safety concerns should be discussed honestly with the older driver, and ideally with a partner or other family member as well, particularly when the older driver lacks insight into his or her driving limitations. Alternative modes of transportation should be considered. Recommendations to stop driving, however, should not be proffered lightly, because driving cessation can lead to a decreased activity level and increased depressive symptoms (SOE=B). Referral for a formal driving evaluation by a skilled occupational therapist may be helpful in confirming unsafe driving behaviors, or perhaps in suggesting interventions such as adaptive equipment to correct for specific physical disabilities. In the interest of public safety, clinicians should know their state's law on reporting impaired drivers. In most states, clinicians are encouraged, and in some states mandated, to report their concerns to the licensing agency. To assist clinicians caring for older drivers, an excellent resource has been developed by the American Medical Association in cooperation with the National Highway Traffic Safety Administration: *The Clinician's Guide to Assessing and Counseling Older Drivers* (http://geriatricscareonline.org/ProductAbstract/clinician's-guide-to-assessing-and-counseling-older-drivers/B022) (accessed Jan 2016).

Table 5.4—Assessing Life Space

During the past 4 weeks, have you been to:
- rooms of your home other than the room where you sleep?
- an area outside your home such as your porch, deck, patio, or garage, or hallway of an apartment building?
- places in your neighborhood, other than your own yard or apartment building?
- places outside your neighborhood but within your town?
- places outside your town?

ACUTE FUNCTIONAL DECLINE

An acute decline in functional status is usually precipitated by illness or injury. Most new disability episodes are attributable to illnesses or injuries leading to hospitalization (SOE=A). The most severe forms of disability commonly arise from a relatively small number of acute conditions, including hip fracture, stroke, heart failure, and pneumonia. The adverse functional consequences of hospitalization reflect not only the disabling effects of these and other serious conditions but also the hazards of immobility and hospital-acquired complications. Up to 20% of new disability episodes are attributable to less serious illnesses or injuries that lead to restriction of activity but not to hospitalization. These restrictions are usually caused by several concurrent health-related problems, although a fall or injury is most likely to result in disability. Among older adults who are physically frail, about a third of new disability episodes occur insidiously, ie, in the absence of a discernable illness or injury. These episodes may be attributable to relatively subtle perturbations in physiologic status or to the loss of compensatory strategies among highly vulnerable older adults with relatively little reserve capacity. Most older adults who become newly disabled recover independent function within 6 months

(SOE=A). However, these individuals are at high risk of subsequent disability.

QUALITY OF LIFE

During the past two decades, *quality of life* has been embraced as a convenient "catch phrase" to denote important patient outcomes other than death and traditional physiologic measures of morbidity. Although a gold standard does not exist, most instruments designed to measure quality of life include various aspects of physical, cognitive, psychological, and social function. Perhaps the most commonly used instrument is the Short Form-36 Health Survey (SF-36), which includes 36 items organized into 8 domains: physical function, role limitations due to physical health, role limitations due to emotional health, bodily pain, social functioning, mental health, vitality, and general health perceptions. The SF-36 has been tested extensively among community-living adults and hospitalized patients, but it may not be suitable for use among the oldest-old group, especially those who are frail, because of floor effects and insensitivity to clinically important changes in health status.

When assessing quality of life, clinicians should ask about patient preferences regarding medical care and goals of care. Goals can be multiple, diverse, and sometimes conflicting. Older adults exhibit striking heterogeneity with respect to physiologic function, health status, belief systems, cultural and ethnic backgrounds, values, and personal preferences. The successful management of chronic conditions, such as diabetes mellitus, arthritis, and heart failure, requires that patients, families, and clinicians work collaboratively to define the specific problems, to elicit personal preferences, and to establish the goals of care. Patients' cultural and ethnic heritages have an important role in their understanding of their illness, its meaning in their lives, and their response to it. It is crucial, therefore, for the clinician to have an appreciation of that heritage and the role it plays in the patient's understanding of health and illness. Treatment plans that include patient preferences enhance adherence, increase satisfaction, and have the potential to improve patient outcomes.

REFERENCES

- Lin FR, Yaffe K, Xia J, et al. Hearing loss and cognitive decline in older adults. *JAMA Intern Med*. 2013;173(23):293–299.

    The prevalence of hearing loss increases with age, approaching 50% for those 70–79 years old and exceeding 75% for those ≥80 years old. In this study of nearly 2,000 nondemented, community-living older adults, aged 74–83 years, hearing loss, defined objectively using an audiometer, was strongly and independently associated with clinically meaningful declines in global and executive cognitive function over the course of 6 years. Because hearing loss may be amenable to rehabilitative interventions, establishing the mechanisms for this association could inform potential treatments to slow the rate of cognitive decline among older adults.

- Lin JS, O'Connor E, Rossom RC, et al. Screening for cognitive impairment in older adults: a systematic review for the U.S. Preventive Services Task Force. *Ann Intern Med*. 2013;159(9):601–612.

    Despite its high prevalence, cognitive impairment among older adults is often not recognized by primary care clinicians. Based on this systematic review, the authors conclude that brief instruments to screen for cognitive impairment can adequately detect dementia, but there is no empirical evidence that screening for or early diagnosis of cognitive impairment improves decision-making or important patient, caregiver, or societal outcomes.

- Quinn TJ, McArthur K, Ellis G, et al. Functional assessment in older people. *Br Med J*. 2011;343:d4681.

    This article provides a comprehensive review of functional assessment in older adults for use by generalist clinicians. The authors suggest a process of functional evaluation based on a structured history and examination, supplemented with standardized assessment tools. A series of tips are provided to facilitate an effective and efficient assessment of functional abilities. A hypothetical case study of an older woman with multiple chronic conditions illustrates how the practical application of assessment tools can inform interventions designed to enhance independent function.

- Studenski S, Perera S, Patel K, et al. Gait speed and survival in older adults. *JAMA*. 2011;305(1):50–58.

    Because it can be readily assessed in most clinical settings, gait speed has been proposed as a possible vital sign in older adults. In this pooled analysis of individual data from 9 selected cohorts, the investigators evaluated the relationship between gait speed and survival. For both men and women 65–95 years old, life expectancy increased monotonically as gait speed increased, from 0.2 to 1.6 meter/sec. At age 75, predicted 10-year survival across the range of gait speeds ranged from 19% to 87% in men and from 35% to 91% in women. As an integrative measure of known and unrecognized disturbances in multiple organ systems, gait speed is a simple and accessible indicator of health in older adults.

- Swenor BK, Ramulu PY, Willis JR, et al. The prevalence of concurrent hearing and vision impairment in the United States. *JAMA Intern Med*. 2013;173(23):312–313.

    Sensory impairments often have adverse functional consequences. In this study, nationally representative data from the National Health and Nutrition Examination Surveys (NHANES) were used to estimate the prevalence of objective impairments in hearing and vision for men and women within 10-year age groups starting at age 20. The prevalence of concurrent impairments in hearing and vision was <1% among those younger than 70 years and only 2.2% among those 70–79 years, but increased to 11.3% among those ≥80 years old. For this oldest subgroup, only 19% remained free of having any sensory impairment.

Thomas M. Gill, MD

CHAPTER 6—MULTIMORBIDITY

KEY POINTS

- More than 50% of older adults have 3 or more chronic diseases, or multimorbidity.

- Multimorbidity is associated with increased rates of death, disability, adverse treatment effects, institutionalization, use of health care resources, and decreased quality of life.

- Older adults with multimorbidity are heterogeneous in terms of illness severity, functional status, prognosis, personal priorities, and risk of adverse events, necessitating flexible approaches to care.

One of the greatest challenges in geriatrics is providing optimal care for older adults with multiple chronic conditions, or *multimorbidity* (Table 6.1). More than 50% of older adults have ≥3 chronic diseases, with distinctive cumulative effects for each individual.

Multimorbidity is associated with increased rates of death, disability, adverse treatment effects, institutionalization, use of health care resources, and decreased quality of life. Comprehensive strategies and interventions for common syndromes and organization of care for this population show promise, but the best clinical management approaches remain unclear.

Most clinical practice guidelines (CPGs) focus on management of a single disease, but CPG-based care may be cumulatively impractical, irrelevant, or even harmful for individuals with multimorbidity. CPG deficiencies are not based solely on shortcomings of guideline development and implementation. Older adults with multimorbidity are regularly excluded or underrepresented in trials and observational studies. This translates to less representation of older adults in meta-analyses and systematic reviews and guidelines, and affects appropriate interpretation of results.

Clinical management is defined here as representing all types of care for chronic conditions, including pharmacologic and nonpharmacologic treatment and interventions (eg, referral to specialists, physical and occupational therapy, use of pacemakers), as well as screening, prevention, diagnostic tests, follow-up, and advanced illness care. Currently, the best strategies for prioritizing specific aspects of this management spectrum in a particular older adult with multimorbidity are unknown.

Clinicians need a management approach that will consider the issues particular to each individual, including the often limited available evidence, interactions among conditions or treatments, the patient's own preferences and goals, prognosis, multifactorial geriatric issues and syndromes, and the feasibility of proposed management approaches and their implementation.

Older adults with multimorbidity are heterogeneous in terms of illness severity, functional status, prognosis, personal priorities, and risk of adverse events, even when diagnosed with the same pattern of conditions. Not only do the individuals themselves differ but also their treatment options differ, necessitating more flexible approaches to care of this population. Depending on how the definition is used, even older adults without serious illness may be considered to have multimorbidity. Older adults with multiple chronic conditions when there are condition-condition, condition-treatment, or treatment-treatment interactions may benefit from this approach even when they do not meet the criteria for serious illness. This chapter should be viewed as complementary to the chapter on palliative care.

Table 6.1—Terms Used to Describe Older Adults Who Need a Geriatric Approach to Care

Multimorbidity	The presence of multiple chronic conditions in one individual, at times, referred to as ≥2 or ≥3 conditions. The number of conditions considered affects who meets this definition. Similarly, the phrase "multiple chronic conditions" is often used, particularly because the term multimorbidity may have negative associations for older adults and their families. In some contexts, multimorbidity implies that no single condition is primary or dominant. Depending on how the definition is used, even older adults without serious illness may be considered to have multimorbidity. Older adults with multiple chronic conditions who have condition-condition, condition-treatment, or treatment-treatment interactions may benefit from this approach even when they do not meet the criteria for serious illness.
Comorbidity	The presence of an additional condition in relation to an index condition in one individual.
Complexity	The overall impact of different conditions in an individual, taking into account their severity as well as other health-related attributes, such as serving in a caregiver role, cultural background, etc.
Frailty	A condition of reduced strength, endurance, and physiologic reserve, characterized by an enhanced vulnerability to minor stressors. (However, specific definitions of frailty vary.)
Disability	An impairment that results in activity limitations (eg, affecting mobility, manual dexterity, continence, and other ADL functions) or restricted participation in life. It reflects the interaction between a person and his or her social and physical environment.

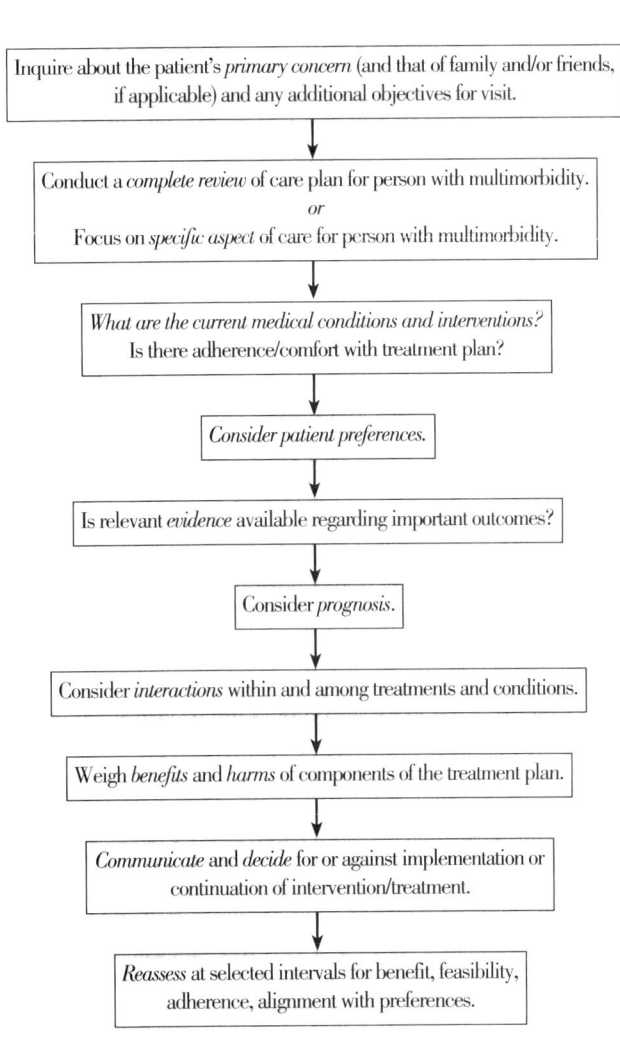

Figure 6.1—Approach to the Evaluation and Management of the Older Adult with Multimorbidity

SOURCE: American Geriatrics Society Expert Panel on the Care of Older Adults with Multimorbidity. Guiding principles for the care of older adults with multimorbidity: an approach for clinicians. *J Am Geriatr Soc.* 2012;60(10):E1–E25.

APPROACH TO THE OLDER ADULT WITH MULTIMORBIDITY

Clinicians treating older adults with multimorbidity face many challenges, including complex clinical management decisions, inadequate evidence base, and time constraints and reimbursement structures that hinder provision of efficient quality care. For a useful approach for optimal management of these individuals, see Figure 6.1.

Five domains are relevant to the care of older adults with multimorbidity: patient preferences, interpreting the evidence, prognosis, clinical feasibility, and optimizing therapies and care plans. The 5 domains apply at various steps in the process, and because differing approaches for addressing this population have not been compared, there is no justification for insisting on a particular sequence. Patient preferences, for example, are often best elicited in the context of a discussion of prognosis, rather than as an initial subject of inquiry.

GUIDING PRINCIPLES

The principles below are intended to help guide the clinician in management of older adults with multimorbidity to improve health care and outcomes in this challenging population. Patients should be evaluated, and care plans designed and implemented, according to individual needs. Researchers have yet to rigorously evaluate all approaches related to these guiding principles. Therefore, just as failure to strictly adhere to CPGs for single diseases should not imply medical liability or malpractice, neither should failure to adopt these principles for multimorbidity management.

Patient Preferences Domain

The guiding principle of this domain is to elicit and incorporate patient preferences into medical decision-making for older adults with multimorbidity.

Care provided in accordance with CPGs may not adequately address patients' individual preferences, a key aspect of medical decision-making. Older adults with multimorbidity should be presented the opportunity to evaluate choices and to prioritize their preferences for care, within personal and cultural contexts. Clinicians can engage patients in these dialogues using an approach that emphasizes advance care planning. In this approach, clinicians ask patients to clarify values about possible outcomes of treatment, with consideration given to matters such as the ability to live independently, symptoms, cognitive and physical function, and life expectancy. Patients can be encouraged to use their own stories to clarify values and priorities, while recognizing that these may change over time.

Example: An 80-year-old woman with atrial fibrillation has an indication for warfarin therapy by traditional algorithms. She does not wish to undergo regular blood monitoring and does not feel safe taking newer anticoagulants. She understands the trade-offs and elects to take daily aspirin.

Interpreting the Evidence Domain

The guiding principle of this domain is to recognize the limitations of the evidence base and to interpret and apply the medical literature specifically to older adults with multimorbidity.

CPGs evaluate the best current evidence from many types of studies, but most focus on only one or two clinical conditions. Comorbidities are typically addressed in limited ways, if at all. However, different conditions in the same patient may interact, changing the risks associated with each condition and its treatments. Consequently, determining whether a given individual is likely to benefit from a particular treatment is complicated.

Thoughtful standardized approaches for interpretation of the medical literature ("evidence-based medicine") provide tools for clinicians to evaluate the evidence base. However, one element of such methodologies that must not be neglected is whether uncovered information applies to the individual under consideration. Clinicians should be aware that significant evidence gaps exist concerning condition and treatment interactions, particularly in older adults with multimorbidity.

Example: An 84-year-old man with hypercholesterolemia has no history of any vascular (cardiac, cerebral, peripheral) events. He has been on a statin for 12 years. You examine the evidence and advise him that he can stop taking the statin, if he wishes, because of lack of evidence that he will benefit from this medicine in primary prevention.

Prognosis Domain

The guiding principle of this domain is to frame clinical management decisions within the context of risks, burdens, benefits, and prognosis (eg, remaining life expectancy, functional status, quality of life) for older adults with multimorbidity.

Clinical management decisions for the multimorbid population necessitate the evaluation of prognosis to inform patient preferences and to adequately assess risks, burdens, and benefits. Important prognostic variables include remaining life expectancy, likelihood of functional disability, and future quality of life. Clinicians also need to evaluate risks for specific conditions (eg, GI hemorrhage with aspirin use for primary prevention of cardiovascular disease in men) as prognosis is considered.

The prognosis for each patient informs, but does not dictate, clinical management decisions within the context of his or her preferences. Often the time horizon to benefit for a treatment may be longer than the individual's projected life span, raising the risk of polypharmacy and drug-drug and drug-disease interactions, particularly in older adults with multimorbidity. Screening tests (eg, colonoscopy) may not be beneficial or even harmful if the time horizon to benefit exceeds remaining life expectancy, especially because associated harms and burdens increase with age and comorbidity.

A discussion about prognosis can serve as an introduction to difficult conversations, facilitating decision-making and advance care planning, and allowing exploration of patient preferences, treatment rationales, and therapy prioritization. For example, the prognosis of a cancer patient with a solid tumor and poor performance status usually worsens with chemotherapy. At the same time, progression through first- and second-line therapies predicts a low likelihood of third-line treatment response. A discussion about hospice, however, may offer the patient options for improved home support, better quality of life, and possibly prolonged survival. A candid and individualized review of prognosis early on may allow for introduction of hospice as an attractive alternative to chemotherapy.

Example: A 79-year-old woman has diabetes, heart failure, and stage IV renal failure. Her daughter is pushing her to get her regular colonoscopy; she is reluctant. Using the Web-based resource www.eprognosis.org indicates that her estimated life expectancy is <10 years, and she is not likely to experience overall benefit from screening colonoscopy.

Clinical Feasibility Domain

The guiding principle of this domain is to consider treatment complexity and feasibility when making clinical management recommendations for older adults with multimorbidity.

Some guideline organizations, such as the Grading of Recommendations Assessment, Development and Evaluation (GRADE) Working Group, now encourage routine consideration of burden of treatment when making recommendations for clinical management. However, the definition of these concepts has been inconsistent.

One practical approach is to break down treatment complexity and burden into individual components that can then be evaluated separately. This can help to identify particularly burdensome components of the process and more specific methods to resolve challenges. The Medication Regimen Complexity Index also identifies factors that need to be considered when assessing medication regimen complexity.

The more complex a treatment regimen, the higher the risk of nonadherence, adverse reactions, decreased quality of life, increased economic burden, and increased strain and depression among caregivers. Medication adherence also changes according to situational factors and perceptions of need, cost, or current symptoms.

Treatment-related education and assessments must be ongoing, multifaceted, and individualized, and are best delivered via a variety of methods and settings, because patients often recall only a small fraction of what is discussed with clinicians. Cognitive impairment frequently impacts on adherence as well.

Example: An 87-year-old man complains of fatigue and feels he takes too many medications. He has dementia, heart failure, osteoarthritis, osteoporosis, insomnia, diabetes, and prostate disease. He is prescribed 16 medications as well as other treatments. He often forgets to take his evening doses and does not monitor his blood glucose. After using tools to assess medication complexity and discussions with the patient and his daughter, you decide to stop 5 of his medications, to modify times of administration, and to recommend a pill box.

Optimizing Therapies and Care Plans Domain

The guiding principle of this domain is to use strategies for choosing therapies that maximize benefit, minimize harm, and enhance quality of life.

Older adults with multimorbidity are at risk of polypharmacy, suboptimal medication use, and potential harms from various interventions. Treatments and interventions must be prioritized to assure adherence to the most essential pharmacologic and nonpharmacologic therapies, minimize risk exposure, and maximize benefit. Polypharmacy is associated with therapeutic omissions, reduced benefit from otherwise beneficial medications, and even net harm in this population. Nonpharmacologic interventions (eg, implantable cardiac electronic devices) may prove more burdensome than beneficial if inconsistent with patient preferences.

Older adults with multimorbidity take more medications and have greater likelihood of adverse drug reactions, exacerbated by age-related changes in pharmacokinetics and pharmacodynamics. Reducing the number of medications, particularly high-risk ones, can lower the risk of adverse drug reactions.

Example: A 92-year-old widowed man with advanced Alzheimer disease returns home to the care of his daughter, after a hospitalization for systolic heart failure. A cardiologist has proposed implantation of an automatic cardioverter-defibrillator, but the patient's daughter points out that her father is unable to leave the home without experiencing intense anxiety. You broach the subject of quality of life and ask the daughter if her father—if he were able to speak for himself—would choose an invasive intervention designed only to prolong his life.

CONTROVERSIES AND CHALLENGES

Implementing this patient-centered approach in older patients with multimorbidity is challenging, especially given the dynamic health status of such individuals and the involvement of multiple clinicians and settings. Even with appropriate decision tools and skilled communication, the need to make multiple simultaneous decisions makes it difficult to explain information and uncertainties about benefits and harms. This may prevent individuals, families, and friends from fully participating in treatment decisions, communicating preferences, and prioritizing outcomes. Satisfactory evidence for clinical management of individuals with multimorbidity is scarce, as are reasonable prognostic measures, and different prognostic tools often yield conflicting results for the same patient. Treatments meant to improve one outcome (eg, survival) may worsen another (eg, function). Many clinical management regimens are also simply too complex to be feasible in this population, yet as clinicians attempt to reduce polypharmacy and unnecessary interventions, they may fear liability regarding underuse of therapies. Use of the strategies put forth in this chapter may help alleviate these concerns. However, some patient-centered approaches may simply be too time-consuming for an overwhelmed clinician working within the current reimbursement structure and without the support of an interprofessional team. Vigorous advocacy efforts are needed to address these resource issues. Fortunately, new models of care such as the VA GERI-PACT (patient-aligned care teams) model and other interdisciplinary care models for older outpatients are being evaluated through the Affordable Care Act. Clinicians caring for multimorbid older adults should closely watch the geriatrics and gerontology literature for reports on these innovations.

REFERENCES

- American Geriatrics Society Expert Panel on the Care of Older Adults with Multimorbidity. Guiding Principles for the Care of Older Adults with Multimorbidity: An Approach for Clinicians. *J Am Geriatr Soc.* 2012;60(10):E1–E25.

    This work provides guiding principles and a framework by which clinicians can move away from the single-disease-at-a-time approach to care and toward more patient-centered care in older adults with multimorbidity. It includes useful references and highlights challenges and future research needed to advance the care of older adults with multimorbidity. An executive summary is available *at J Am Geriatr Soc* 2012;60(10):1957–1968.

- Boyd CM, Darer J, Boult C, et al. Clinical practice guidelines and quality of care for older patients with multiple comorbid diseases: implications for pay for performance. *JAMA.* 2005;294(6):716–724.

    This work demonstrates the limited applicability of clinical practice guidelines to the care of older adults with multimorbidity. Guideline-defined "appropriate care" for each condition may lead to dangerous medication interactions and adverse events, as well as a complex daily routine.

- Sudore RL, Fried TR. Redefining the "planning" in advance care planning: preparing for end-of-life decision making. *Ann Intern Med.* 2010;153(4):256–261.

    This paper describes an approach to focus on preparing patients and surrogates to make the best possible in-the-moment medical decisions and outlines practical steps clinicians can take to achieve this in the outpatient setting. The authors' approach can be useful in exploring the patient preferences domain discussed in this chapter.

- Valderas JM, Starfield B, Sibbald B, et al. Defining comorbidity: implications for understanding health and health services. *Ann Fam Med*. 2009;7(4):357–363.

    This paper describes definitions of terms and a framework for thinking about the coexistence of multiple conditions.

- Yourman LC, Lee SJ, Schonberg MA, et al. Prognostic indices for older adults: a systematic review. *JAMA*. 2012:307(2):182–192.

    This systematic review describes the currently available prognostic indices, including a detailed summary of 16 validated general prognostic indices for older adults. Importantly, none of the indices are "disease specific" and therefore may be useful to consider for populations of older adults with multimorbidity. Several useful and readable tables are also included.

Cynthia M. Boyd, MD, MPH
Matthew K. McNabney, MD, AGSF

CHAPTER 7—CAREGIVING

KEY POINTS

- Caregiving is defined as assistance or help provided to someone because of a health need.

- Family members provide needed help to 85%–90% of all older adults; 18.9%, or 43.5 million Americans, care for someone ≥50 years old. Over half (58%) of family caregivers assist someone with at least one activity of daily living.

- The most common negative aspects of family care provision are exhaustion, and caregivers having too much to do and too little time for themselves. Family caregivers indicate significantly higher rates of depression and stress than non-caregivers.

- The most effective family caregiver interventions are those that are more intensive and delivered over longer periods of time, flexible and tailored to the needs of caregivers and care recipients, and multidimensional.

- Clinical engagement based on robust assessment principles, iterative treatment strategies, and ongoing information and referral can help to address the challenges faced by many family caregivers.

Family caregivers are a cornerstone of geriatric care, particularly for older adults who continue to live at home. Understanding the challenges of family caregiving, assessing caregivers efficiently during routine clinical encounters, and intervening on behalf of family caregivers to provide education, support, and referral are all areas geriatric professionals must master to provide optimal care not only to family caregivers but also to their older care recipients.

Various estimates suggest that 85%–90% of all older adults receive needed help from family members, commonly a spouse or adult daughter. This family help comes in many forms, such as helping a relative understand a diagnosis, coordinating appointments or finances, completing house work, adhering to medication regimens, and assisting with activities of daily living (ADLs). In other instances, an older patient may be providing help to another relative.

Even though family caregiving is very common, it is not clear how well family caregiving is integrated into the more formal medical care of older adults. The extent to which family caregivers are involved in medical decisions made by a primary care provider is inconsistent, and given the short time period of most clinical encounters, providers may not even identify whether a family caregiver for an older adult is available or able to offer ongoing help at home. This is problematic because transitions from home to hospital to residential care and back can occur throughout the course of chronic disease in late life, and family caregivers are often the ones who coordinate and arrange care for the older adult. Therefore, ensuring that the family caregiver is included as a core component of any geriatric care strategy is critical. Otherwise, older adults in need may not receive optimal management of acute or chronic disease conditions, regardless of the intensity of the medical intervention.

WHAT IS CAREGIVING?

Who is a caregiver? There is no established clinical definition of a caregiver, and attempts to identify who caregivers are range from objective measures (eg, someone who provides at least help with one ADL) to subjective appraisals (eg, relying on individual caregivers to identify themselves as such). Identification of caregiving is further complicated by the care recipient's disease context: the types of help a family member provides to someone with Alzheimer disease, for instance, are much different than what a husband provides to a wife with breast cancer. Caregiving is perhaps best defined as assistance or help provided to someone because of a health need, with "health" broadly construed. An important distinction is that the care provided in family caregiving goes beyond the normal bounds of support between two individuals.

A particularly important clinical issue to explore is that many individuals do not consider the help they provide as "caregiving" but instead as what should "just be done." To some, there is reluctance to be called a "caregiver," because this label may suggest requiring help in addition to providing it. Understanding what caregiving is and offering the opportunity for family members and/or older adults themselves to discuss their situation is important. Assessing the care someone provides is more straightforward; it is more complicated to help someone understand that he or she is a caregiver, as well as to develop a clinical plan for information, education, and resources for the future that will help both the family caregiver and the older adult. When beginning such discussions, clinicians can rely on tools such as the website www.whatisacaregiver.org/ (accessed Jan 2016), which is part of a public awareness campaign to help individuals realize that what they are doing is indeed "caregiving."

Caregiving Prevalence

In 2009, the National Alliance of Caregiving and the American Association of Retired Persons (NAC/AARP) conducted a telephone survey of a representative sample of family caregivers in the United States (www.aarp.org/livable-communities/learn/health-wellness/info-12-2012/Caregiving-in-the-us-2009.html) (accessed Jan 2016). More recently, the 2011 National Health and Aging Trends Study/National Survey of Caregiving (NHATS/NSOC) was conducted to offer additional information on family caregivers. The NHATS/NSOC is an annual survey of Medicare beneficiaries ≥65 years old living outside of nursing homes (http://aspe.hhs.gov/daltcp/reports/2014/NHATS-ICes.cfm) (accessed Jan 2016). Key characteristics of family caregivers from these surveys and other nationally representative sources of data include the following:

- 18.9%, or 43.5 million Americans, care for someone ≥50 years old; 66% of family caregivers are women.

- On average, family caregivers are 61 years old and have been providing assistance for 4.6 years.

- 72% of family caregivers are white, 13% are African-American, 2% are Hispanic, and 2% are Asian-American.

- Spouses make up 20% of caregivers and provide close to 1/3 of all assistance, whereas adult children provide nearly half of all informal (ie, unpaid) help.

- 74% of caregivers live within 20 minutes of the care recipient.

- The average amount of family care provided on a weekly basis ranges from 17.3 to 20.4 hours. Spouses, caregivers who live with the care recipient, and those helping recipients with higher needs tend to provide considerably more hours of care per month.

- On average, care recipients are close to 80 years of age, and close to 70% are women. Close to half of care recipients are widowed, while approximately 40% live alone.

- Care recipients with the greatest health needs require extensive family care; the 31% of caregivers assisting care recipients with at least self-care or mobility tasks account for nearly half of all informal care hours, whereas the 33% of caregivers assisting someone with dementia account for 40% of informal care hours.

Extent of Family Care Provision

In addition to the large number of family members who provide care to older adults, national surveys also demonstrate the extent of this care. This has led many in the field to emphasize that families are at the front lines of providing long-term care in the United States. When the economic value of family care is estimated, it becomes apparent that families overwhelmingly provide the bulk of assistance to older adults when compared with home-health or residential long-term care.

The NAC/AARP 2009 survey reported the following: Over half (58%) of family caregivers assist a care recipient with at least one ADL. Family caregivers provide a wide range of ADL support (43% help a relative transfer from beds and chairs, 32% help with dressing, and approximately 25% help with bathing, showering, or toileting.). Close to 1 in 5 caregivers help to feed a relative or help a relative with incontinence-related challenges (19% each). All respondents of this survey assisted an adult care recipient with at least one instrumental ADL.

A topic that has garnered attention in public media and research is the "sandwich generation," or those caregivers who help parents and children simultaneously. According to the NAC/AARP 2009 survey, 2/3 of family caregivers provide assistance to one relative, and the remaining 1/3 provide assistance to more than one relative. Such findings may reflect 2 trends: one of sandwich caregiving, and the other of the general aging of the population and concurrent prevalence of chronic disease, in which a baby-boomer caregiver is helping a parent as well as a spouse in need of long-term care.

The Effects of Family Caregiving

The relationship between stress and provision of care has long been studied. A particular outcome of interest since the early 1980s is "burden," or the emotional, psychological, social, financial, and physical stress related to the provision of care. Since then, a number of additional outcomes related to family caregiving have been considered, resulting in multiple meta-analyses of the various health implications of family care provision. The following represents a synthesis of these results and national survey data.

As indicated by the NSOC, the most common negative aspects of family care provision are exhaustion, and caregivers having too much to do and too little time for themselves. Family caregivers indicate significantly higher rates of depression and stress than non-caregivers. The amount of care provided and the care recipient's physical impairments are positively correlated with caregiver burden and depression. Negative consequences are the most substantial for caregivers who provide more intensive assistance, who assist individuals with dementia, or who are struggling with health challenges themselves. Uplifts, or perceived positive aspects of caregiving, are positively associated with the well-being of family caregivers, whereas caregiving stress is linked to depressive symptoms. Interestingly, the NSOC reports that 68% of caregivers report positive aspects of caregiving, whereas 10% indicate substantial negative consequences. Depressive symptomatology is associated with negative perceptions of health among family caregivers. Behavior problems on the part of care recipients are also associated with poorer health of family caregivers, as is older age, lower socioeconomic status, and less social support among caregivers. Family caregivers are more likely than non-caregivers to suffer from clinical depression and anxiety, less social support, greater physical impairments and disabilities, poorer self-rated health, and acute and chronic medical conditions. Ethnically and racially diverse family caregivers are more likely to be of lower socioeconomic status, younger, receive informal support, have stronger filial obligation beliefs, and experience worse physical health and depression. They are less likely to be a spouse. There is substantial diversity in caregiving experience and outcomes across various racial and ethnic groups; more attention to cultural beliefs, values, and norms is needed.

CAREGIVING INTERVENTIONS

The extensive care contributions of families to older adults with health needs has led to the development and implementation of various support strategies to help reduce distress on the part of family caregivers as well as improve outcomes for care recipients (eg, reduced health service utilization). Various meta-analyses and systematic reviews have grouped interventions into specific types, although the categorization of interventions remains inconsistent. These include informational and referral (eg, case management) strategies, support groups, psychoeducational interventions, psychotherapy/counseling, self-care and relaxation approaches, respite, and multicomponent interventions that tend to combine multiple intervention modalities (eg, individual and family counseling with support groups). Outcomes most commonly considered include burden, caregiver's appraisals of stress, depression, anxiety, and self-efficacy/sense of competence. Care recipient outcomes often include symptom severity and health care service utilization (eg, time to nursing-home admission).

Although specific disease contexts tend to feature interventions with different clinical content, family caregiver protocols tend to evolve in similar fashion across diseases. Initial interventions focus on providing education and support as well as respite, or relief, from care demands. Building on the strengths and limitations of these initial approaches, interventions then rely on more rigorous theoretical and conceptual models (eg, the stress process) and outcome measurement to test controlled or randomized controlled intervention protocols. Subsequent phases then attempt to test these rigorous approaches in multisite, diverse samples. The final phase of evolution progresses to the translation/implementation of evidence-based interventions into clinical and community-based care contexts, either as stand-alone services or in collaboration with other disease management models.

The evolution of caregiver interventions is not consistent across disease contexts. For example, caregiver interventions have been tested more extensively in Alzheimer disease to the point of translation via several national initiatives. The same has yet to be done for other disease contexts such as stroke, cancer, or cardiovascular heart disease. In general, the quality of evidence available remains limited by small sample sizes, short follow-up times, inconsistent measurement, and other methodologic issues. Effective interventions are generally more intensive and delivered over longer periods of time, flexible and tailored to the need of caregivers and care recipients via the clinical content delivered, and often include multiple components to meet the needs of caregivers. In part because of the many health transitions that occur over the long periods of chronic disease, individualizing intervention content to meet the diverse needs of families that may have their own complex histories and dynamics is important when attempting to achieve positive outcomes for both caregivers and care recipients.

Table 7.1 highlights select interventions across disease contexts that have used high-quality, randomized controlled research designs. These interventions have the potential for implementation in various clinical settings and community organizations or have already undergone translation (SOE=A).

CLINICAL CONSIDERATIONS

It is critical to incorporate the scientific advances that have emerged in caregiving research into everyday clinical encounters with older adults and their families. A useful clinical framework includes the following components: assessment, treatment, cultural considerations, and information/referral support. These elements can be used to guide clinical encounters with family caregivers.

Assessment

Before conducting an assessment, key principles relevant to caregiving are important to consider. The following principles, developed by the Family Caregiver Alliance (www.caregiver.org/

Table 7.1—Select Family Caregiver Interventions Evaluated in Randomized Controlled Trials for Specific Conditions (SOE=A)

Condition	Methods/Intervention(s)	Findings/Outcomes
Cancer[a]	Cognitive-behavioral therapy/stress-coping skills therapy Three 90-minute monthly joint home visits alternating with 2 joint telephone calls (30 minutes each) for 13 weeks Follow up of 12 months N=263	Treatment led to improved communication/less uncertainty in caregivers, improved quality of life
End-of-life[b]	The Family COPE intervention, which included hospice care and a coping skills intervention N=354	Caregivers' quality of life increased, burden decreased
Chronic pain/arthritis[c]	Patient education, support, and coping Dyadic education and support with up to 5 monthly booster telephone sessions 6 month follow-up N=242	Caregivers reported greater decreases in stress and depressive symptoms and increases in mastery. Care recipients reported improved function and spousal support.
Heart failure[d]	Usual care and integrated dyad psychosocial care (3 sessions of counseling, online, and written educational materials) at 2, 6, and 12 weeks 12 months follow-up N=155	Care recipients' perceived control increased; no caregiver effects
Stroke[e]	Caregiver problem-solving intervention 6-month follow-up N=255	Statistically significant changes in depression, life change, and health at 3 months, but faded by 6 months
Alzheimer disease[f]	Multicomponent: combination of individual, family, and ad hoc counseling with support groups Follow-up of approximately 14 years N=406	Significant decreases in caregiver stress, depressive symptoms; increases in social support and caregiver health; prevention and delay of care recipient nursing-home admission

[a] Northouse LL, Mood DW, Schafenacker A, et al. Randomized clinical trial of a family intervention for prostate cancer patients and their spouses. *Cancer*. 2007;110(12):2809–2818.

[b] McMillan SC, Small BJ, Weitzner M, et al. Impact of coping skills intervention with family caregivers of hospice patients with cancer: A randomized clinical trial. *Cancer*. 2006;106(1):214–222.

[c] Martire LM, Schulz R, Keefe FJ, et al. Couple-oriented education and support intervention for osteoarthritis: Effects on spouses' support and responses to patient pain. *Fam Syst Health*. 2008;26(2):185–195.

[d] Ågren S, Evangelista LS, Hjelm C, et al. Dyads affected by chronic heart failure: A randomized study evaluating effects of education and psychosocial support to patients with heart failure and their partners. *J Card Fail*. 2012;18(5):359–366.

[e] King RB, Hartke RJ, Houle T, et al. A problem-solving early intervention for stroke caregivers: One year follow-up. *Rehabil Nurs*. 2012;37(5):231–243.

[f] Mittelman MS, Haley WE, Clay OJ, Roth DL. Improving caregiver well-being delays nursing home placement of patients with Alzheimer disease. *Neurology*. 2006;67(9):1592–1599.

caregivers-count-too-s3-fundamental-principles) (accessed Jan 2016), are recommended: Because family caregivers are a core part of health care and long-term care, it is important to recognize, respect, assess, and address their needs. Caregiver assessment should embrace a family-centered perspective, inclusive of the needs and preferences of both the care recipient and the caregiver. Caregiver assessment should result in a care plan (developed collaboratively with the caregiver) that indicates the provision of services and intended measurable outcomes, be multidimensional in approach and periodically updated, and reflect culturally competent practice. Effective caregiver assessment requires assessors to have specialized knowledge and skills, including understanding the caregiving process and its impact, as well as the benefits and elements of an effective caregiver assessment.

Family caregiving may emerge during the clinical encounter in several ways. For example, an older adult who presents during a clinical encounter may have complex care needs that necessitate family involvement or care. Alternatively, the older adult seen is a caregiver themselves (in such instances, it is possible that the stress related to care provision is a major reason for the visit, although the older adult may not raise this as an issue). For these reasons, the first step in the assessment process is to determine whether the older adult is actually serving as a family caregiver or is a primary caregiver. A primary caregiver is the person who identifies himself or herself as the individual most responsible for providing help to someone because of a health need. Primary caregivers may have difficulty differentiating between caregiving and normal supportive exchanges provided in health challenge, and caregiving may compound their health problems. Other issues that may emerge include family conflicts with adult children or siblings that may complicate legal and financial planning.

This type of clinical encounter with an older adult may branch onto one of two paths: if the older adult is a caregiver, then the subsequent assessment recommendations become important to consider. If the older adult is receiving care from a family member and that caregiver is having challenges and difficulties, it may be important for the clinician to refer the caregiver to important informational and service resources (see Table 3.2). However, in this latter case, the caregiver may be the clinical provider's "patient," so it is important for the clinician to realize the significance of the family caregiver's well-being to the older adult's health. For this reason, engaging family caregivers and ensuring their connection to relevant education and services is necessary.

In instances when the presenting older adult is a caregiver, the next step of the assessment process is to identify what about care provision has led to the visit, and to allow the caregiver to tell his or her story. Although this can be time-consuming, it is a critical aspect of the clinical encounter—it not only builds rapport and comfort with the caregiver but also may allow the clinician to obtain insights about the caregiving context and reveal information that can complete key elements of a more formal, structured assessment protocol (as described below). Some recommendations to guide this process include a determination of the health needs of the caregiver and care recipient, the disease trajectory of the care recipient (onset, course, duration, and severity), whether the caregiver has had to quit working to provide help, and similar queries.

It is then important to conduct a more structured assessment of the caregiver. A number of resources and tools can help inform specific assessment elements, including The Family Caregiver Alliance/National Center on Caregiving (https://caregiver.org/national-consensus-report-caregiver-assessment-volumes-1-2) and the American Psychological Association (http://apa.org/pi/about/publications/caregivers/practice-settings/assessment/index.aspx) (accessed Jan 2016). Regardless of the specific tools selected, questionnaires or structured interviews should collect information on the following areas: background of the caregiver and the caregiving situation, care recipient's medical history, the caregiver's perception of the health and functional status of the care recipient, the caregiver's values and preferences, the health and well-being of the caregiver, the consequences of caregiving on the caregiver, care provision requirements, and resources to support the caregiver.

Some of the information on the structured assessment may already be available from the caregiver's story. If time is an issue, the structured assessment could be sent home via a form or online survey, which the caregiver can complete and return at the next visit or via mail or e-mail. Nonetheless, assessment should be seen as a process rather than a discrete event, because the domains above may change over time. Although the scientific quality of measures included is important (eg, reliability, validity, accuracy), brief, clinically relevant measures for family caregivers that are easy to administer are also necessary.

Treatment

A key element in any clinical treatment approach is to use the assessment process to determine how support could be strengthened for the family caregiver. Essentially, the clinician attempts to determine who is providing what kind of help (eg, personal care, household care, money, communication, and activities) to the care recipient. This could be ascertained through the use of a matrix or similar tool to determine whether there are gaps in the care provided to the care recipient, and if so, whether other members of the caregiver's support network or other sources of support are available to supplement the assistance that that caregiver currently provides to meet the needs of the care recipient.

A problem list is another tool used to identify what problems occur for the caregiver and at what time of day, as well as the surrounding circumstances. A matrix, table, or similar tool can be used to generate this problem list, which can help both the caregiver and clinician determine the extent of challenges and potential triggering events faced by the family caregiver, as well as how the caregiver copes with or attempts to adapt to such problems. In this manner, the clinician can offer suggestions to the caregiver to manage or avoid stimuli that may help prevent the problem, or to generate a solution list that may help enhance or improve the caregiver's reaction to a problem once it occurs.

As with much of chronic disease and geriatric care, offering direct clinical intervention to a family caregiver is one of trial and error, and "failures" are to be expected in how the caregiver copes with or manages the many complicated issues that may arise in providing help to an older adult with care needs. From a clinical standpoint, it is important to remember that these "failures" can serve as the basis for new solutions and strategies for the caregiver to implement. Moreover, a trial and error perspective can help to reduce caregivers' feelings of disappointment and frustration that the

Table 7.2—Resources and Tools for Caregivers

Resource	Organization/Website	Comments
Area Agency on Aging	To find a local area agency on aging, see http://n4a.org/about-n4a/?fa=aaa-title-VI.	Family caregiver information and/or support services; family caregiver support specialists are also available.
Advocacy organizations for persons with specific diseases and their families	*Examples:* Alzheimer's Association (www.alz.org) American Cancer Society (www.cancer.org) American Heart Association (www.heart.org) American Stroke Association (www.strokeassociation.org)	Robust caregiver information and support, including for disease-specific symptoms
National Institutes of Health consumer-oriented sites	*Examples:* National Institute on Aging's Alzheimer's Disease Education and Referral (www.nia.nih.gov/alzheimers) National Cancer Institute (www.cancer.gov)	Information for family caregivers across disease contexts
Family Caregiver Alliance	http://caregiver.org	Family caregiving resources and information, including online support groups
Family Caregiver Navigator	https://caregiver.org/family-care-navigator	State-by-state resources and services for family caregivers
National Adult Day Services Association	www.nadsa.org	Help family caregivers find a local adult day service program
Eldercare Locator	www.eldercare.gov	Help family caregivers find additional respite services
The Caregiving Resource Center from the American Association of Retired Persons	www.aarp.org/home-family/caregiving/	Various planning resources for family caregivers
"The Caregiver's Briefcase" from the American Psychological Association	www.apa.org/pi/about/publications/caregivers/practice-settings/index.aspx	Overviews of assessments, interventions, information on cultural diversity in care, and other tools
Rosalynn Carter Institute for Caregiving	www.rosalynncarter.org/caregiver_intervention_database/	Information and resources for family caregivers, a comprehensive list of caregiving interventions, and a variety of clinical tools
Ottawa Hospital Research Institute	http://decisionaid.ohri.ca	Decision-making tools, many of them evidence-based, to help families navigate complex health-related decisions as chronic disease progresses
Medicare Basics for Caregivers	http://nihseniorhealth.gov/medicareandcaregivers/managingmedicalconditions/01.html	Educational resources and tools for family caregivers
Center for Medicare and Medicaid Services' Nursing Home Compare tool	www.medicare.gov/nursinghomecompare/search.html	Provides detailed quality of care information about every Medicare- and Medicaid-certified nursing home in the United States
Medline Plus and PubMed	www.nlm.nih.gov/medlineplus/healthtopics.html www.ncbi.nlm.nih.gov/pubmedhealth/	Information portals for families interested in various diseases and other public health topics
Apps for mobile devices	Enter "caregiver apps" in a web browser search tool.	Many apps are not free, and there is little documentation of their efficacy (SOE=D), but they may offer an important supplement to more intensive clinical services.

Note: Above websites accessed Jan 2016.

situation is not immediately improving. (In various high-quality, evidence-based intervention models such as those summarized in Table 7.1, caregivers' distress often increases or does not decrease in the initial months of participation; however, as caregivers acquire skills and strategies and implement them effectively, clinical benefits are evident later.) An iterative, "try it" approach is appropriate because of the number of community-based resources and services available to assist family caregivers (see below) and because the unique histories, backgrounds, and family dynamics of each caregiver make it unlikely that a single solution will always be successful throughout the caregiving trajectory.

Cultural Considerations

Cultural diversity offers another layer of opportunity and complexity for clinicians. Family caregiving in many cultures is not recognized as a stand-alone concept but is instead integrated into the broader notion of family and familiar responsibility (eg, *familismo* in Latino cultures). With this in mind, clinicians should not assume that the term "caregiving" is necessarily understood or even accepted among families and older adults of diverse cultural origin. Chronic diseases, particularly those with mental health aspects, may carry particular stigma in certain cultures. Thus, it is imperative that clinicians speak the cultural "language" of caregiving to better tailor their collaborations with diverse families. With increasing immigration, issues pertaining to the acculturation of immigrant caregivers who have lived in the United States for longer periods of time than those who have recently entered the country and the cross-generational tensions that may occur are emerging areas to understand and acknowledge.

Establishing trust, rapport, and open communication with diverse caregivers is a process that likely requires considerable relationship-building; in some instances, a de-emphasis on professional hierarchy is required to do so. For example, distrust of medical and social health care based on historical precedent and tragedy continue to resonate powerfully in many communities (eg, the Tuskegee experiment among African-American communities, immigrants from war-torn countries, displacement of Native Americans). Such history can present significant barriers in establishing clinical relationships. To this end, geriatric care providers who serve family caregivers from diverse cultures must constantly appraise their assumptions and when necessary place such assumptions on hold to build relationships with caregiving families. Certain behaviors in diverse families may appear counterproductive according to Western/European ideas of care regimens (eg, reliance on traditional healing methods), but make perfect sense within the greater cultural context of that particular family. Identifying a key family contact, such as a first-generation child, who can serve as the liaison for the clinician and family may help to facilitate the clinical process. Also, building clinical care activities around what the family is willing to accept and working in tandem with cultural health traditions are other steps to consider when working with diverse caregivers and their aging family members.

Some additional strategies to consider adopting include the following. First, differences in care goals should be recognized, acknowledged, and reviewed throughout the care process. Discerning how decisions are made within a family is important; decision making may not be shared or adhere to the concept of autonomy inherent in European cultures. More specifically, decisions may be made in concert and not by any one person, nor by the person expected (eg, the oldest adult daughter). Clinicians should also be aware that certain clinical recommendations may be unacceptable in certain cultures (eg, advance directives, hospice, or other end-of-life recommendations). In addition, remaining open to alternative health care methods valued in various cultures may help build rapport with the caregiver and family. Although these options may not meet high-quality, evidence-based thresholds, it is possible to use such approaches in concert with evidence-based approaches. Finally, relying on other members of the care team may allow better "connection" and more effective communication with the family, because the lead clinician may be viewed more as a distant authority figure.

Information and Referral for Family Caregivers

It is not possible for clinical care providers to offer direct intervention to family caregivers in all situations. Nevertheless, geriatric care providers should be familiar with local organizations, services, and sources of information for family caregivers. Clinical collaboration with family caregivers is an ongoing process, and information and referral is no different. As opposed to simply providing a list of resources to family caregivers with no follow-up, clinical providers should ensure a "warm handoff" by arranging connections with appropriate community-based or other services. Family caregivers are often under considerable stress, and providing information or service resources in a passive fashion could result in less use of needed services.

Table 7.2 details resources and tools used in various community outreach efforts that offer excellent information and services as a starting point for family caregivers.

REFERENCES

- Adelman RD, Tmanova LL, Delgado D, et al. Caregiver burden: A clinical review. *JAMA*. 2014;311(10):1052–1060.

    This paper highlights the need to assess and address caregiver burden in patients and outlines a number of relevant clinical considerations.

- Burgio LD, Gaugler JE, Hilgeman M. *Family Caregiving for Adults and Elders with Chronic Conditions*. New York, NY: Oxford University Press; 2015.

    This book summarizes the state-of-the-art of caregiving interventions and services across a range of chronic conditions that are most prevalent among older adults (eg, cancer, stroke, dementia, cardiovascular disease) and highlights how these protocols can be translated into routine clinical practice.

- Callahan CM, Kales HC, Gitlin LN, et al. The historical development and state of the art approach to delivery of dementia care services. In: de Waal H, Ames D, O'Brien J, et al, eds. *Designing Dementia Care Services*. John Wiley & Sons, Ltd.: West Sussex, UK; 2013:43–62.

    This chapter provides both a historical overview of dementia care services (including family caregiver interventions) and insights into their clinical delivery (eg, integration of dementia care management alongside traditional care models).

- Gaugler JE, Potter T, Pruinelli L. Partnering with caregivers. *Clin Geriatr Med*. 2014;30(3):493–515.

    This paper provides a detailed overview of the definitions of family caregiving, prevalence and clinical correlates, evidence-based intervention approaches, how to clinically partner with caregiving families, and information and resource supports for family caregivers.

- Gitlin LN, Hodgson N. Caregivers as therapeutic agents in dementia care: The evidence-base for interventions supporting their role. In: Gaugler JE, Kane RL, eds. *Family Caregiving in the New Normal*. Philadelphia, PA: Elsevier, Inc.; 2015.

    This chapter traces the development and evolution of dementia caregiving interventions, provides an evidence-based synthesis of existing interventions, and identifies a number of issues related to implementation and translation of high-quality, evidence-based dementia caregiver interventions.

- Zarit J. Assessment and intervention with family caregivers. In: Qualls SH, Zarit SH, eds. *Aging families and caregiving*. Hoboken, NJ: John Wiley & Sons, Inc.; 2009:241–268.

    This reference largely informed the Clinical Considerations section of this chapter. It provides a superb framework to work with family caregivers during clinical encounters.

Joseph E. Gaugler, PhD

CHAPTER 8—CULTURAL ASPECTS OF CARE

KEY POINTS

- Culture and faith/spiritual beliefs have a significant impact on patients' world views, interpretation of health and illness, and their health-related behaviors.

- Clinicians should remain alert to the differences among individual patients from a given culture or faith/spiritual tradition and guard against stereotyping.

- Communication and clinical care are enhanced when health care providers make an effort to simplify medical messages and negotiate with patients a common understanding of causation, diagnosis, and treatment, while maintaining respect for the beliefs and constructs of both the provider and the patient.

As the cultural and religious/spiritual diversity of older Americans continues to grow, it is increasingly important for clinicians to develop an approach to working with older adults from a broad range of cultural and faith groups. The United States is projected to become a minority-majority nation by 2044 and by 2050, one of every three older Americans will be of "minority" status. In addition, it is currently estimated that more than one in three Americans has low health literacy. Data show that older adults and ethnic minorities have a particular proclivity toward lower health literacy status. Clinicians must be sensitive to the possibility that culture and religious/spiritual beliefs may affect relationships with individual patients and families. It also influences a patient's willingness or ability to engage in a therapeutic relationship, participate in shared decision making, and accept and adhere to the care plan. Health literacy certainly affects the patient's ability to comprehend and act on health messages.

The quality of any encounter between a clinician and a patient from different cultural or religious backgrounds depends on the clinician's skill and sensitivity in gauging cultural practices and considering any possible literacy gap that needs to be overcome. Questions about the individual patient's cultural attitudes, beliefs, and practices should be incorporated naturally and carefully into the clinical interview so that the care provided is both respectful and responsive and perceived as such.

There is no single or standard definition of cultural competence. Most definitions emphasize a careful coordination of individual behavior, organizational policy, and system design to facilitate mutually respectful and effective cross-cultural and interfaith interactions. Cultural competence combines attitudes, knowledge base, acquired skills, and behaviors that demonstrate an awareness of and respect for the patient's beliefs and behaviors. Ideally, it is a nuanced understanding of the role that culture plays in all of our lives and of the impact culture has on every health care encounter, for both the clinician and the patient.

This chapter is intended to help clinicians gain an initial understanding of the key issues in cross-cultural and interfaith patient encounters, so that they can create a self-directed training plan to develop and implement culturally competent behaviors. Readers are also referred to the *Doorway Thoughts* series, published by the American Geriatrics Society (see annotated references), which demonstrate how the general approaches outlined here in each topic relate to working with patients from a variety of cultural or religious groups. It is important to keep in mind that the information presented in this chapter and in *Doorway Thoughts* is accurate in general, but that the attitudes, beliefs, traditions, customs, and preferences of individuals in all cultural and religious groups vary widely. Clinicians should never assume that any person's cultural or religious background will dictate his or her health choices or behavior. They should remain alert to the differences among individual patients and families from a given culture or religious tradition, and guard against stereotyping older adults on the basis of their cultural or religious/spiritual affiliation. It is also neither necessary nor possible to know all the information about every cultural and faith group. Clinicians need to be able to take a learning stance to gently and respectfully elicit required information from the patient and family.

Clinicians have their own personal cultural identity and beliefs, which can implicitly or explicitly affect the manner in which they provide clinical care. Therefore, in reality, each cross-cultural and interfaith encounter is an opportunity for clinicians to engage in self-reflection on their own personal beliefs and biases and how this may potentially influence their perception of the patient. In addition to self-reflection, it is recommended that clinicians work in conjunction with the interprofessional health care team, including administrators, to promote diffusion of cultural competence in the health care organizations in which they practice.

Use of Language and Nonverbal Communication

Preferred Terms for Cultural or Religious Identity

The terms referring to specific cultural, ethnic, or religious groups can change over time, and individuals in any one group do not always agree on appropriate terminology. It is helpful to learn the term that the individual patient prefers for his or her cultural or religious identity, and to use that terminology in conversation with the patient, as well as in his or her health records.

Formality

Attitudes regarding the appropriate degree of formality in a health care encounter differ widely among cultural groups. Learning a patient's preferences with regard to formality and allowing those preferences to shape the relationship is always advisable. Initially, a more formal approach is likely to be appropriate.

For example, when addressing the patient, the patient's correct title (eg, Dr., Reverend, Mr., Mrs., Ms., Miss) and his or her surname should be used unless and until he or she specifically requests a more casual form of address. Another important issue is to determine the correct pronunciation of the person's name, as well as the appropriate ordering of names; in a variety of countries, the family name is given first, followed by the individual's given name.

Addressing the Health Care Provider

It is also important to learn how the patient would prefer to address the clinician and to allow his or her preference to prevail. For example, in some cultures, trust in the clinician depends on his or her assuming an authoritative role, and informality would undermine the patient's trust. This is an aspect of the clinical relationship in which the clinician's personal preferences may need to be relinquished.

Language and Literacy

The following questions should be considered before an encounter.

- What language does the patient feel most comfortable speaking?
- Will a medical interpreter be needed?
- Does the patient read and write English? Another primary language? If so, which one(s)?
- If the patient has low health literacy, does he or she have access to someone who can assist at home with written instructions?

It is best to deliver health messages at a basic health literacy level, because patients may be reluctant or too embarrassed to admit to their inability to comprehend complex health messages.

It is worthwhile to consider these questions early in the process of establishing a therapeutic relationship to ensure that communication with the patient is effective. Even those who speak English fluently may wish to discuss complicated issues in their native language. It is the clinician's responsibility to explain medical terms and to ask the patient for explanations of any cultural or foreign terms that are unfamiliar.

Health Literacy Concerns

Health literacy is defined as "the degree to which individuals have the capacity to obtain, process, and understand basic health information and services needed to make appropriate health decisions." According to the U.S. Department of Health and Human Services, only 12% of the U.S. adult population has been determined to be at the "proficient" level of health literacy. Adults ≥65 years old were more likely to have below basic or basic health literacy skills than younger populations. More than two-thirds of older adults ≥75 years old had below basic or basic health literacy. Also, older adults who are uninsured or enrolled in both Medicare and Medicaid are at higher risk of having below basic or basic level of health literacy. It is prudent to screen all patients for low health literacy. Ideally, clinicians should simplify their verbal communication and avoid medical jargon with *all* patients.

Key Communication Techniques

- Speak clearly and slowly (many older adults may have hearing deficits but may be too embarrassed to voice their difficulties) and explain things in plain English, while avoiding jargon.

- Emphasize not more than three key points during each visit, and write these out in large print size in capitals and give to the patient as a handout.

- Offer to repeat the information until you are comfortable that the patient has grasped the main messages and knows exactly what he or she is supposed to do to adhere to the care plan.

- Encourage patients to ask questions; use an open-ended approach.

- Use the teach-back method to verify patient understanding. This method can be useful to confirm the patient's understanding of the medical visit by asking the patient to recall or explain in his or her own words what has been discussed. Consider use of demonstration skill, if needed. For example, the clinician may say "I always ask my patients to repeat things back to me to make sure I explained it clearly. I'd like you to tell me exactly when and how you're going to take the new medicine we discussed today."

Use of Medical Interpreters

Medical interpreters are trained professionals who can facilitate the communication between clinicians and patients (and families) who speak different languages. Interpreters relay concepts and ideas between languages in a culturally sensitive way by listening attentively and then repeating the original message accurately and completely in another language. They are ethically bound to repeat everything and are obligated to maintain patient privacy and confidentiality. All clinicians caring for patients with limited English proficiency should be skilled in working with medical interpreters to communicate effectively with these patients and their families. For specific guidelines and resources about how best to work with medical interpreters, see https://geriatrics.stanford.edu/medical-interpreters.html (accessed Jan 2016).

Respectful Nonverbal Communication

Body position and motion is interpreted differently from one cultural group to another. Specific hand gestures, facial expressions, physical contact, and eye contact can hold different meanings in different cultures. The clinician should watch for particular body language cues that appear to be significant and that might be linked to cultural norms that are important to the patient, in an effort to cultivate sensitivity to the conditions that facilitate and improve communication.

Conservative body language is advisable early in a relationship with a patient or when in doubt about a patient's background or preferences; clinicians should assume a calm demeanor and avoid expressive extremes (eg, very vigorous handshakes, a loud and hearty voice, many hand gestures, an impassive facial expression, avoidance of eye contact, standing at a distance). Clinicians should remain alert for signals of the patient's level of comfort. Directly asking the patient questions about body language may also help. Making negative judgments about a patient that are rooted in unconscious cultural assumptions about the meaning of his or her gestures, facial expressions, or body language should be avoided.

The physical distance from others that individuals find comfortable varies, depending in part on their cultural background. The clinician should determine what distance seems to be the most comfortable for each patient and, whenever practicable, allow the patient's preference to establish the optimal distance during the encounter. Before doing a physical examination, it is prudent to request the patient's permission to do so. In doing sensitive procedures like a breast or genitalia examination, some patients may have a strong preference for a provider of the same gender. If this is not possible, it may be advisable to have a family member of the patient close at hand to support the patient while still respecting the patient's privacy. For example, in doing a rectal exam of an older South Asian woman, a male provider may want to have a female nurse in the examination room or invite a female family member of the patient to stay in close proximity during the examination while protecting the patient's personal privacy by use of a screen.

HISTORY OF TRAUMATIC EXPERIENCES

Is the patient a refugee or survivor of violence or genocide? Are family members missing or dead? Have patients or family members been tortured? Such experiences could negatively affect the health care encounter without the clinician's knowledge unless relevant questions are included among standard questions about the patient's history. Clinicians should remember that in some historical periods and jurisdictions, health care providers have participated in torture and genocide (eg, Nazi medical personnel in World War II). The methods and tools of torture used have sometimes resembled legitimate clinical procedures and tools. Patients who have survived such experiences may not feel safe in medical or governmental settings, and contact with any clinician may invoke feelings of vulnerability, fear, panic, or anger. Great sensitivity is necessary in providing health care for these individuals.

ISSUES OF IMMIGRATION

Immigration Status

Some individuals may be living in North America without appropriate immigration documents. Clinicians may wish to assure each patient that information given within the medical encounter will be kept confidential.

History of Immigration or Migration

The history of the movements of a large portion of a religious or cultural group can affect the attitudes and behavior of an individual in that group even when he or she has not immigrated to North America from another country. In addition, understanding an individual's specific migration history often provides insight into the key life transitions informing his or her outlook. Knowing how a person came to live in North America can be important. The time and effort the clinician invests in learning more about a cultural or religious group's history and current situation can be repaid not only in a better relationship with the individual patient but also in an enhanced appreciation of the factors affecting clinical relationships with other patients from that group.

ACCULTURATION, TRADITION, AND HEALTH BELIEFS

Acculturation is a process in which members of one cultural group adopt the beliefs and behaviors of another group. Acculturation of a group may be evidenced by changes in language preference, adoption of common attitudes and values, evolution of religious practices, or gradual loss of separate ethnic identification. Although acculturation typically occurs when a minority group adopts the habits and language patterns of a dominant group, acculturation may also be reciprocal between groups.

It is essential to keep principles of acculturation in mind during any cross-cultural or interfaith health encounter. Beginning by determining how long a person has lived in North America and whether he or she was born here is helpful. However, remember that the degree to which the person is acculturated to North American customs and attitudes is the consequence of many factors and not just of the number of years since he or she immigrated. Older adults who follow the traditions of their cultural or religious group may have been born outside of the United States, may be recent arrivals to the continent, or may even be lifelong North American residents.

A patient's level of cultural or spiritual shifting can impact not only his or her health behavior but also preferences in end-of-life planning and decision-making. Acculturation can also be an issue dividing family members, and a person's resistance to or ease of acculturation may be a matter of pride or of shame and guilt. Developing sensitivity about the issues of acculturation for one's older minority patients is a key element in effective cross-cultural health care. Asking patients directly about their adherence to cultural and spiritual traditions can be useful.

People from a variety of cultural groups may not conceive of illness in North American terms. Some may have highly developed concepts of the causes of health and disease that are incompatible with the concepts that form the foundations of North American medicine. Some other paradigms of wellness and illness include beliefs that illnesses have spiritual causation, are the result of imbalance among bodily humors, or are caused by a person's actions in past lives, to name but a few. Patients may make unexamined assumptions that are based on traditional beliefs, and these can cause confusion or create misunderstanding. The more the clinician knows about specific cultural and religious traditions, the better he or she can promote effective clinical communication.

In addition, patients from any cultural background may be using alternative remedies (eg, rituals, herbal preparations) that they do not mention. Therefore, it is prudent to routinely ask all patients about the use of complementary and alternative treatments as part of their history. It is unrealistic to expect that a patient will simply "adapt" to North American approaches to health and health care, just as it is impractical to expect the clinician to accept a new conception of wellness and disease. Clinical communication and efficacy will be enhanced when patients and health care providers make an effort to negotiate a common understanding of causation, diagnosis, and treatment for a specific health problem, while maintaining respect for the beliefs and constructs of both individuals.

UNSPOKEN CHALLENGES

Clinicians should remain alert to the possibility of issues that are critical to the success of the health care encounter that the patient may not voice. Examples include the following:

- Lack of trust in health care providers and the health care system

- Fear of medical research and experimentation

- Fear of medications or their adverse events

- Unfamiliarity or discomfort with the Western biomedical belief system

Some patients may feel uncomfortable or uneasy in customary North American health care settings for a variety of reasons, including lack of familiarity with Western practices, dissatisfying previous encounters with the health care system, or the belief that insensitivity or discrimination is inevitable for anyone in the cultural or religious group. Such feelings may result from having been stereotyped or treated insensitively or even unfairly by clinicians in the past. Sensitive exploration of these issues with patients is often both worthwhile and necessary. In general, sensitivity to the possibility that such issues are in play is advised in all patient encounters.

APPROACHES TO DECISION MAKING

Western bioethics emphasizes individual autonomy in all health decisions, but for many other cultures, decision-making is family or community centered. Autonomy principles allow competent individuals to involve others in their health decisions or to cede those rights to a proxy decision maker. The clinician should ask patients if they prefer to make their own health decisions or if they would prefer to involve or defer to others. Some may wish to assign the decision-making authority wholly to another individual or a group. In some cultures, the definition of family may include "fictive kin." In families in which the degree of acculturation of the generations differs, the older adult may defer to or depend on younger relatives, even though the tradition might suggest that the reverse would occur.

Many studies have documented the impact of religious and spiritual beliefs on preferences regarding end-of-life practices and decision-making. Some religious traditions characterize health outcomes as divinely willed and emphasize acceptance in the face of adversity. Other traditions stress the religious obligation for individuals to save or extend life at almost any cost.

Establishing an understanding of each patient's decision-making construct and preferences early in the clinical relationship will, in most instances, promote better communication and avoid the difficulties inherent in trying to address the issues at a time of crisis. When the patient's and clinician's cultural or religious backgrounds differ, careful exploration of the issues is all the more important, because the clinician cannot proceed if he or she and the patient are not starting from common assumptions.

ATTITUDES REGARDING DISCLOSURE AND CONSENT

Cultural attitudes toward truth telling and disclosure of terminal diagnoses vary widely. In some cultures, it is commonly believed that patients should not be informed of a terminal diagnosis, because this may be injurious to health or hasten death. Obtaining informed consent from patients with this belief may prove difficult. There is no consensus in bioethics concerning the rigorous application of full clinical disclosure in every situation. However, it is generally agreed that incorporating a patient's beliefs concerning disclosure and truth telling into clinical planning whenever possible is desirable. Some patients may prefer not to know if they are terminally ill and ask that family members or other caregivers receive all diagnostic information and make all treatment decisions. It is advisable to explore each patient's preferences regarding disclosure of serious clinical findings early in the clinical relationship and to reconfirm these wishes at intervals.

GENDER ISSUES

Culture and religion intertwine in describing traditions and structures with regard to gender roles. Societies seemingly based on the same patriarchal or matriarchal model may vary widely in their expressions of the model. A person's gender influences the sorts of experiences he or she has had, not only within the family but also in the community and health care system. Another level of complexity may be added to health care encounters when an older adult's group struggles with conflicting traditional and contemporary views on gender roles. Cultural norms for men and women can influence their health behavior, and such norms for the genders vary widely from one culture to another. Gender-based norms may also affect how patients choose a health care provider and make health decisions, as well as how they form their preferences for disclosure and consent.

The clinician is strongly advised to explore each patient's attitudes regarding the interplay among gender, choice of health care provider, autonomy, and personal decision making early in the patient-provider relationship; to confirm the patient's preferences at intervals; and to follow the individual patient's wishes whenever possible.

ADVANCE DIRECTIVES AND END-OF-LIFE CARE

The use of advance directives and health care proxies has become more common over the past 25 years, but research indicates that the use of written directives may be more common among older adults in the dominant North American culture than among older adults in minority cultural groups (SOE=A). Most clinicians struggle in conducting end-of-life conversations with ethnic patients. The most common barriers reported by physicians include language and medical interpretation issues; patient/family religious/spiritual beliefs about death and dying; physicians' lack of knowledge of patients' cultural beliefs, values, and practices; patient/family's cultural differences in truth handling and decision making; patients' limited health literacy; and patients' mistrust of doctors and the health care system.

In cross-cultural situations, when discussing attitudes and beliefs regarding written directives with a patient, clinicians should be sensitive to the possibility that some minority older adults will prefer to use alternatives (eg, verbal directives or directives dictated to family members or others), whereas others will avoid any such discussion so as to observe proscriptions against talking about death. In view of the fact that preferences for care intensity may also differ according to cultural and religious backgrounds, patients should also be given the opportunity to indicate the interventions they *do* want as well as those they do not want in any written or verbal directive used.

Cultural, religious, and spiritual beliefs are an important influence in a person's formation of his or her attitudes toward supportable quality of life, approach to suffering, and beliefs about medical feeding, life-prolonging treatments, and palliative care. Some cultures and religious traditions value a direct struggle for life in the face of death, and both patients and families expect an intensive approach to treatment. Others avoid personal confrontation of death and dying and prefer to leave such decisions to the clinician. Still others take a direct approach to death and dying but reject too aggressive an approach.

Research has shown that clinicians and patients from shared cultural and religious backgrounds have similar values in these areas (SOE=B); the implications of such findings for clinicians and patients from differing backgrounds are obviously important. Both clinicians and patients bring their own attitudes and beliefs to any clinical encounter. Clinicians should be aware of their personal views, cultural values, and religious beliefs when discussing end-of-life plans with patients, and respect patients' beliefs and preferences even when they are different from their own.

In negotiating end-of-life decisions with a patient whose background is different from his or her own, the clinician must listen especially carefully to the patient's goals and concerns and exert every effort to avoid making assumptions that do not apply. For example, the assumption that "no one would want to live in that condition" or that "everyone would want treatment in this situation" is likely to be faulty. To ensure that end-of-life plans and decisions reflect an individual's rights and wishes, the clinician must strive to understand the older adult's overall approach to life and death and, as far as possible, provide care that is consistent with that approach.

APPROACHES: THE ETHNICS MNEMONIC

The ETHNICS mnemonic is a tool to facilitate effective health interviews and care planning in cross-cultural settings. Rather than serving as a prescribed outline of questions to ask, the ETHNICS mnemonic (below) provides a framework in which to ascertain a wide variety of information and to negotiate effective therapeutic next steps, all within a routine 15-minute clinical session.

- **Explanation:** Ask patients to describe what they think is happening to them in their own words.
- **Treatments:** Inquire as to which treatments patients have used for their health problem(s) before the interview. Clinicians should specifically ask about biomedical interventions, as well as any complementary and alternative treatments.
- **Healers:** Respectfully inquire about other healers involved in a patient's care; many patients seek treatment from alternative practitioners or traditional healers, as well as from conventional health care providers. Incorporating this information into the health care encounter is important to overall care planning and efficacy.
- **Negotiate:** Negotiate with each patient and/or his or her designated caregiver(s) as to which treatments the patient will accept and participate in.
- **Intervene:** Put together a care plan that is acceptable from the perspectives of both the provider and the patient. This frequently incorporates a blending of "scientific" explanations of wellness and disease, as well as each individual patient's concept of his or her health status and acceptable approaches to addressing concerns.
- **Collaborate:** Focus on building a trusting and resilient relationship with each older patient. Incorporating formal and informal caregivers into a broader team alliance is also critical to the success of health care for all older adults.
- **Spirituality:** Inquire respectfully about patients' spiritual beliefs, and how these might impact their health care preferences and behavior, particularly at the end of life.

SPIRITUAL AND RELIGIOUS ISSUES

In some cultural groups, most individuals share one religious heritage; in others, there is a great deal of religious and spiritual diversity. As a result, the relative impact of religion and culture on health behavior and decision making for older adults may be subtle and complex, warranting respectful exploration on the part of the clinician.

Several studies have documented that most patients either prefer or would accept clinicians asking them about their spiritual beliefs and the impact such beliefs might have on their world view, health behavior, and health decision making (SOE=A). Questions regarding religion and spirituality should be incorporated sensitively and early in the patient-provider relationship and reexplored when significant health problems arise. The acronym FICA (for faith and belief, importance, community, and address in care) can help health care providers to structure questions in taking a spiritual history (https://smhs.gwu.edu/gwish/clinical/fica/spiritual-history-tool [accessed Jan 2016]).

Religious and spiritual beliefs and practices affect how patients interpret health, illness, and suffering. Koenig and colleagues found that among 838 older hospitalized patients, religiousness and spirituality consistently predicted greater social support, fewer depressive symptoms, better cognitive and physical function, less severe illness and comorbidity, and better general health. The Joint Commission on Accreditation of Healthcare Organizations requires that both spiritual and cultural assessments be performed and integrated into care plans. Religion is "a more formal system that provides meaning to life through a common set of beliefs, rituals and practices. It provides the structure for spiritual beliefs for most people."

Spirituality has been defined "as the aspect of humanity that refers to the way individuals seek and express meaning and purpose and the way they experience their connectedness to the moment, to self, to others, to nature, and to the significant or sacred." Data show that spirituality and religion tend to play more pronounced roles in lives of older adults than in the general population. Patients use religion and spirituality to cope with illness-related suffering. More than 50% of older adults report frequent attendance at religious events (with little variation by gender or race), which has been a lifelong practice rather than a late-life development (SOE=A). A number of studies have demonstrated positive associations between religiousness, typically measured as regular attendance in organized religious activities, and a variety of health markers (eg, blood pressure) and mental health (eg, depression). There is evidence that regular attendance at religious services is associated with a lower composite measure of allostatic load among older women but not men (SOE=B). The literature suggests that religious participation may be beneficial, in part, because it promotes social interaction; however, one study suggests evidence that the effect is independent of social interaction. In addition, a number of studies have found that the beneficial effects of religious participation are not universal, and there is a suggestion that it may be most beneficial for those with the least social resources, eg, women and minorities (SOE=B).

One benefit of this growing body of literature is an increasing clarity of the distinction between the two elements. Although religion and spirituality are in no way mutually exclusive, neither do they necessarily overlap. In particular, the literature emphasizes the individualized quality of spirituality, portraying it in terms of practices through which a person seeks to establish or strengthen a link with a higher power or truth. In studies that have focused more on spirituality, findings generally indicate that such practices (eg, meditation or daily spiritual experiences) also are associated with better health and mental health (SOE=B). One study characterized the distinction between religion and spirituality as having positive associations for well-being related, in the case of religiousness, to positive social linkages and a sense of community service and, in the case of spirituality, to a sense of personal growth.

There are myriad religious and spiritual belief systems, and it is neither necessary nor feasible for clinician to be familiar with them all. However, it is very important for clinicians to recognize the important role that faith plays in the lives of many patients. It is also important that clinicians assess the patient's spiritual needs and be able to support them. Patients with complex spiritual needs should be referred to chaplains and faith leaders who may be better able to assist them.

REFERENCES

- American Geriatrics Society Ethnogeriatrics Committee. Achieving High-Quality Multicultural Geriatric Care. *J Am Geriatric Soc*. 2016; Jan 25. Epub ahead of print.

    This article and position statement, developed by the American Geriatrics Society Ethnogeriatrics Committee, outlines a vision for the case of ethnically diverse older adults by identifying the minimum quality indicators that health care organizations and providers should adopt. Topics covered include population diversity, provider awareness and communication skills, ethnicity and health disparities, preferred language, use of an interpreter, and areas for future research and education.

- American Geriatrics Society. Brangman S, Periyakoil VS, eds. *Doorway Thoughts: Cross-Cultural Health Care for Older Adults;* 2014. Available at http://alpha.ags.impelsys.com/ProductAbstract/doorway-thoughts-cross-cultural-health-care-for-older-adults/B016 (accessed Jan 2016).

    Doorway Thoughts addresses the health care issues raised by the increasingly multicultural state of North American society. It focuses on the ways clinicians who care for older adults can develop an understanding of various ethnic and cultural groups to enhance their ability to care for older minority patients.

- Best M, Butow P, Olver I. Doctors discussing religion and spirituality: a systematic literature review. *Palliat Med*. 2015 Aug 12 (epub ahead of print).

    This review states that physician enquiry into the religion and/or spirituality of patients is inconsistent in frequency and nature and that to meet patient needs, barriers to discussion need to be overcome.

- Connolly A, Sampson E, Purandare N. End-of-life care for people with dementia from ethnic minority groups: a systematic review. *J Am Geriatr Soc*. 2012;60(2):351–360.

    This thorough review of the literature examines issues surrounding the relationship between ethnic minority status and provision of end-of-life care for people with dementia.

- Feinberg F, Reinhard SC, Houser A, et al. Valuing the invaluable: 2011 update. The growing contributions and costs of family caregiving. AARP Public Policy Institute. Available at http://assets.aarp.org/rgcenter/ppi/ltc/i51-caregiving.pdf (accessed Jan 2016).

    Family support is a key driver in remaining in one's home and in the community, but it comes at substantial costs to the caregivers themselves, to their families, and to society. This paper gives an excellent national overview of caregiver issues.

- Kwak J, Haley WE. Current research findings on end-of-life decision making among racially or ethnically diverse groups. *Gerontologist*. 2005;45(5):634–641.

    This paper provides an excellent overview of the peer-reviewed literature on diverse cultural groups in the United States.

- Periyakoil VS, Stevens M, Kraemer H. Multicultural long-term care nurses' perceptions of factors influencing patient dignity at the end of life. *J Am Geriatr Soc*. 2013;61(3):440–446.

    This mixed-methods study reviews how long-term care nurses' cultural and religious backgrounds influenced their perceptions of what constitutes dignity-conserving care. This study highlights that the cultural background of clinicians can influence the care they provide to patients.

- Stanford Ethnogeriatrics Portal: http://geriatrics.stanford.edu (accessed Jan 2016).

    This portal hosts ethnogeriatric resource materials to educate health care professionals on the cultural issues associated with aging and health. There are 13 ethnic-specific peer-reviewed modules that provide free, full text, detailed information about common groups of ethnic older adults in the United States. There are also other resources on ethnogeriatrics, as well as information about how to work with medical interpreters.

Vyjeyanthi S. Periyakoil, MD

CHAPTER 9—LESBIAN GAY BISEXUAL TRANSGENDER HEALTH

KEY POINTS

- Lesbian gay bisexual transgender (LGBT) older adults face the same health challenges as other older adults but have additional medical, psychological, and social needs.

- LGBT older adults are often underserved by the health care system. LGBT adults may have difficulty in disclosing sexual orientation because of prior negative experiences in the health care system and/or as a result of experiencing and fearing societal discrimination. Lack of disclosure can lead to poor access to care and sometimes inappropriate care. Health care providers may also be less likely to explore the sexual health of older adults and more likely to incorrectly assume heterosexuality.

- As transgender adults age, they may be more likely to encounter health issues that correspond to their biological sex; these patients may need help in coping with a disease or condition associated with their prior gender.

- LGBT older adults are more likely to live alone, be single, and not have children. They may rely more on extensive networks of friends rather than family. As they age, they may be at greater risk of isolation.

- Health care providers should provide appropriate support and resources that address and are sensitive to the needs of LGBT older adults.

LGBT older adults are at risk of experiencing disparities in physical and mental health. The Institute of Medicine's 2011 report about LGBT health disparities highlights the health care needs and inequalities of LGBT adults. The cohort of LGBT older adults has specific needs and experiences different from those of both the general LGBT population and the general older population. For example, LGBT older adults report higher rates of disability, poor mental health, smoking, and excessive drinking than heterosexual older adults. Lesbian and bisexual women report higher rates of cardiovascular disease and obesity and are less likely to have screening mammography than heterosexual women. Gay and bisexual men report higher rates of poor physical health and living alone than heterosexual men.

Some of these disparities are linked to the lasting effects of discrimination faced by the older LGBT generation throughout most of their lives. Although societal views about homosexuality have changed rapidly over recent years, it is important to recognize that LGBT older adults have experienced a lifetime of widespread discrimination, forcing them for much of their lives to hide their sexual orientation or transgender identity from their health care providers, their families, their employers, and sometimes even from themselves. Despite recent advances, LGBT older adults continue to be affected by past and ongoing social stigmata, governmental policies, and health care inequalities, which have important effects on their health, social supports, financial security, long-term housing options, and advance care planning. They also often lack access to clinicians trained in the health needs of and sensitivity to LGBT older adults.

BACKGROUND

Currently, an estimated 1 to 2 million LGBT older adults are living in the United States. By 2030, these numbers are expected to rise considerably along with the overall aging U.S. population. The exact number of LGBT people is unknown and probably underrepresented because of a lack of data, differing estimates by experts in related fields, and stigma that prevents LGBT people from identifying as such on surveys.

LGBT older adults came of age during a time in the United States when being a sexual or gender minority was viewed in an especially negative light. The experiences of LGBT older adults are influenced in part by whether they are part of the baby boomer generation (born 1946–1964) or were born before 1946. Those born before 1946 lived much of their lives in a society in which expression of their sexual orientation was criminalized by the government and considered pathological by the medical community. For instance, it was not until 1962 that the first state decriminalized private, consensual homosexual acts, and it was not until 2003 that the last antisodomy laws were struck down. Being gay was considered not only a crime but also a mental illness until 1973, when the American Psychiatric Association stopped designating homosexuality as a disorder that could be treated and cured. As a result, LGBT persons could have been involuntarily hospitalized or treated against their will, leading to a decrease of this older generation's ability to trust the medical profession and seek psychiatric care. Given widespread discrimination, LGBT older adults are likely to have kept, and continue to keep, their sexual orientation and/or transgender identity hidden.

Table 9.1—Examples of Medical and Psychosocial Concerns of LGBT Older Adults

Medical concerns with increased risk and/or prevalence
- Cardiovascular disease
- Anal cancer
- Prostate cancer
- Breast cancer
- Cervical cancer
- HIV/AIDS
- Palliative care needs
- Advance care planning needs

Mental health concerns with increased risk and/or prevalence
- Anxiety
- Depression
- Substance abuse

Social supports and resources
- Isolation and invisibility
- Fragile and/or small social networks and support systems
- Housing concerns
- Long-term care discrimination
- Lack of financial security

Society's views of homosexuality did not begin to change until the late 1960s and 1970s, and then only slowly. The Stonewall Riots of 1969, a series of violent demonstrations by LGBT people in New York City opposing ongoing police harassment, is considered to be the beginning of the modern gay civil rights movement in the United States. Baby boomers came of age during this social unrest of the 1960s and, as such, have benefited from the gay civil rights movement. To varying degrees, they have been more likely to disclose their sexual orientation than prior cohorts. For example, a marketing survey of about 1,000 LGBT individuals in the baby boomer generation in 2009 indicated that 74%–76% of lesbian and gay respondents were "completely or mostly out [of the closet]," while 16% of bisexual and 39% of transgender respondents were "completely or mostly out." Although many baby boomers have lived openly, many have still experienced acts of homophobia and transphobia. Among older adults who are open about their sexuality, some are faced with the decision to return to hiding their sexual orientation because of fear of discrimination, isolation, or mistreatment by staff or other residents when faced with the need for long-term care in an assisted-living facility or nursing home.

LGBT older adults are more likely to have experienced homophobia in health care situations and are therefore much less likely to disclose their sexual orienation with health care providers. In a 2014 survey, 40% of LGBT adults aged 60–70 years reported that their health care providers do not know their sexual orientation; 23% were reluctant to discuss certain issues for fear of being judged, and 65% of transgender adults also felt there will be limited access to health care as they age. Studies suggest that nondisclosure of sexual orientation can be associated with lower life satisfaction, lower self-esteem, depression and suicide, substance abuse, delay in seeking medical treatment, and increase in risk of illness (SOE=B). Medical mistrust is cited as a major reason why gay people, especially lesbians, do not always receive appropriate preventive care. Fear of culturally incompetent or discriminatory health care providers can also result in LGBT people avoiding care until they have reached a crisis level.

ASKING ABOUT SEXUAL ORIENTATION AND GENDER IDENTITY

An important part of offering appropriate, targeted health care requires providers to ask their older patients about their sexual orientation and gender identity. To optimize care for LGBT older adults, it is important to create an environment that allows this population to feel respected and safe to disclose their sexual orientation and identity. Because LGBT older adults may be unwilling to risk disclosing their sexual orientation or transgender identity to their health care providers, even when asked directly, it is important for providers to be sensitive when asking these questions. LGBT older adults are also much less likely to identify as LGBT, so it is best not to use labels or force individuals to disclose such information. A helpful tip for inquiring into sexual orientation is to ask more general questions about living situation, current or past relationships, and sources of support, which can generate a conversation that often leads to this information.

MEDICAL ISSUES OF LGBT OLDER ADULTS

Although LGBT older adults can experience the same geriatric syndromes as their heterosexual counterparts, and as a result need much the same health promotion and maintenance, certain issues require particular attention (see Table 9.1).

Disease Risk in Older Gay and Bisexual Men

Cardiovascular Disease

Cardiovascular disease, despite a decline in incidence, still kills more men than cancer. Mitigating or removing traditional cardiac risk factors is key to prevention. Data pooled from 2001–2010 from the NHANES study found that bisexual men had an increased risk of cardiovascular disease. The ratio of vascular to chronological age was significantly higher for bisexual men than for heterosexuals (8.1%, 95% CI, 1.3%–15%), indicating that bisexual men were at increased risk of developing cardiovascular disease. This is likely due to higher rates of smoking, hypertension, diabetes, and hard drug use in this population in the study. Also, because gay men have an increased rate of recreational drug use and smoking, attention to traditional cardiovascular risk factors is important. The combination of smoking and HIV infection is particularly deadly; in a cohort of mostly men, all-cause mortality was 4 times higher in HIV-infected smokers than those who had never smoked. More than 12 life-years were lost from smoking compared with 5.1 life-years lost from HIV infection alone (SOE=A).

Anal Cancer

Anal cancer, like cervical cancer, is caused by infection with human papillomavirus. Anal human papillomavirus infection disproportionately affects men who have sex with men (MSM) compared with the general population of men. The prevalence of anal human papillomavirus infection in HIV-positive MSM is extremely high, ranging between 72% and 90%; in HIV-negative MSM, the prevalence is 57%–61%. Risk factors for anal cancer include receptive anal intercourse and degree of immunosuppression, such as nadir CD4 count and higher HIV viral load. Although there are no recognized guidelines for routine anal cancer screening, some organizations have proposed annual anal cytology for HIV-infected MSM, and screening every 2 years for HIV-uninfected MSM (SOE=C).

Prostate Cancer

There are no data on the incidence of prostate cancer in gay and bisexual men, but prostate cancer is the second leading cause of cancer deaths among men in the general population. Among gay couples, there is a 28% chance that prostate cancer will be diagnosed in one partner and a 3% chance that both partners will get the disease. Prostate cancer can also affect the sexual health of gay and bisexual men in ways that are different from those in heterosexual men (SOE=C). The prostate gland is involved in the sexual response to receptive anal intercourse, and treatment options (eg, surgical vs radiation) may lead to differences in ability to maintain insertive and receptive anal intercourse.

Disease Risk in Older Lesbian and Bisexual Women

Cardiovascular Disease

Cardiovascular disease is the number 1 killer of women in the United States. Higher rates of cardiovascular disease risk factors have been observed in older lesbian and bisexual women. Rates of smoking appear to be higher in the general lesbian population, and older lesbian women are twice as likely to report being heavy smokers than heterosexual women (SOE=A). Obesity is also an independent risk factor for cardiovascular disease in women. Lesbian and bisexual women, on average, have a higher BMI than heterosexual women, and in women, the risk of cardiovascular disease is more than 3 times higher with a BMI >29 kg/m^2 (SOE=B).

Cervical Cancer

Cervical and breast cancer screening rates have historically been lower among lesbian than heterosexual women. Fear of discrimination and not disclosing sexual orientation are associated with decreased likelihood for Pap screening. Lesbian and bisexual women remain at risk of cervical cancer, partly because many have had intercourse with a man at some point in their lives, and therefore need to be screened according to guidelines for all women.

Breast Cancer

The primary risk factor for breast cancer is age; other risk factors include family history, obesity, smoking, alcohol use, and nulliparity. Although some studies report that lesbian women may have greater risk factors for breast cancer, no prospective study has definitively shown an increased risk. However, older lesbian women may receive fewer mammograms than heterosexual women, and studies suggest higher rates of obesity and alcohol use among lesbian women.

Medical Needs of Older Transgender Men and Women

Cardiovascular Disease

Transgender adults have higher rates of smoking than cisgender adults, which therefore increases the risk of cardiovascular disease and other smoking-related illness. In addition, the pharmacologic use of sex hormones is thought to increase the risk of cardiovascular disease. For instance, estrogen has the potential to increase the risk of venous thromboembolism, blood pressure, and blood glucose and to cause water retention. Some studies suggest a possible increase in cardiovascular risk over time for transgender women taking feminizing hormones, although transgender men taking testosterone do not appear to have an increased risk of cardiovascular disease (SOE=C).

Cancer Screening in Transgender Older Adults

As transgender adults age, they may encounter health issues that correspond to their biological sex.

Therefore, the major concern relates to appropriate health screening for biological sex, such as prostate examinations in transgender women (male-to-female) and pelvic examinations in transgender men (female-to-male). For instance, a person who was born male and transitioned to a woman may develop prostate cancer if the prostate was not removed. Similarly, a person who was born female and transitioned to a man may develop uterine cancer if the female sexual organs were not removed. These patients may feel significant distress in coping with a disease or condition associated with their prior gender. Hormone-related cancer in transgender persons is very rare (there are, however, case reports of breast cancer in male-to-female transgender patients).

Sexual Health of LGBT Older Adults

It is important for health care providers to address sexual function and sexual health in all LGBT older adults, most of whom can benefit from routine sexual history taking and risk-reduction counseling.

Prevention of HIV and Sexually Transmitted Infection in LGBT Older Adults

More than half of older adults 65–75 years old report being sexually active, and one quarter of those 75–85 years old are sexually active. Sexually active older adults are much less likely to use condoms than younger adults and less likely to have been tested for HIV, even in the presence of HIV risk factors. Older adults also report receiving little information about sexual health, HIV infection, and other sexually transmitted infections (STIs) from their health care providers. There are reports of increasing rates of syphilis and chlamydia in older adults and in counties with a high number of retirees.

For all these reasons, health care providers need to take routine and thorough sexual and substance use histories from their older patients, regardless of sexual orientation or gender identity. Prevention of HIV and STI transmission also requires that clinicians provide counseling on safer sex practices and offer, when appropriate, information on HIV prophylaxis (both before and after exposure).

Barriers to optimal prevention and detection of HIV and other STIs in older adults (which providers should attempt to address) include the following:

- Lack of knowledge about HIV/AIDS by older adults
- Underestimation of risk by health care providers
- Misdiagnosis and/or delay in diagnosis of HIV/AIDS
- Stigma about HIV in older adults
- Nondisclosure of sexual orientation or sexual behavior

Sexual Risk in Older Gay and Bisexual Men

Gay, bisexual, and other MSM remain the group at greatest risk of acquiring HIV infection, with MSM >50 years old accounting for almost half of all new HIV infections. Older adults who are racial/ethnic minorities appear to be at greater risk of death from HIV/AIDS (SOE=A).

According to CDC guidelines, sexually active MSM who engage in high-risk sexual behavior should be routinely assessed for risk of gonorrhea, chlamydia, syphilis, herpes simplex virus, and human papillomavirus. Although the CDC's universal screening recommendations only go up to 64 years of age, providers should also screen MSM who are > 65 years old based on individual risk behaviors.

Sexual Risk in Older Lesbian and Bisexual Women

Many lesbian and bisexual women have been sexually active with both women and men. Therefore, taking a complete sexual history and providing sensitive risk-reduction counseling is recommended. Lesbian and bisexual women can develop the same STIs as heterosexual women. In addition, lesbian women have a higher incidence of bacterial vaginosis and can transmit candidiasis and *Trichomonas vaginalis* to their female partners. The use of barriers ("dental dams") is recommended for oral-vaginal and oral-anal contact.

Women who are exclusively sexually active with other women have a low risk of acquiring HIV infection, but because many lesbian and bisexual women have had heterosexual experiences, current HIV screening recommendations should be followed. Older women who have sex with men may be at increased risk of HIV because of age-related vaginal thinning and dryness. In addition, older women starting a new sexual relationship after many years of being in a monogamous relationship may find it difficult to initiate discussions about risks and the use of barriers.

Sexual Risk in Transgender People

HIV risk is high among transgender women, and frequent screening is important. Transgender women who engage in sex work and injection drug use are at extremely high risk of STIs and HIV infection. A study in San Francisco found that 35% of transgender women respondents were HIV positive, with black Americans having an even higher rate of HIV infection. The black American transgender community has one of the highest prevalence rates of HIV infection in the United States, highlighting the increased risk based on both racial minority status and being transgender (SOE=B).

HIV/AIDS Treatment and Care

Among older adults, HIV/AIDS tends to be diagnosed much later in the course of infection, primarily because the diagnosis is not considered and because older people are less likely to get tested. HIV/AIDS-related symptoms and associated diseases can be easily mistaken for other problems typically seen in older adults. In addition, because aging naturally weakens the immune system and comorbid conditions are more likely to exist, AIDS may progress more rapidly in older adults. In one study, older patients presenting with advanced HIV infection were 14 times more likely to die within a year of diagnosis than older adults in whom infection was not diagnosed at a late stage (SOE=B).

At the same time, patients >50 years old who take antiretroviral medications seem to respond virologically as well as younger patients do, but they do not have as robust a return of their immune system. Treating older patients with HIV/AIDS is complex because many of these patients have other underlying illnesses, take several medications, and may additionally be dealing with some of the issues of aging (such as sensory loss, frailty, and dementia). For additional information about the care of older adults with HIV/AIDS, see "Recommended Treatment Strategies for Clinicians Managing Older Patients with HIV," a compendium of recommended treatment approaches published by the American Academy of HIV Medicine, the American Geriatrics Society, and the AIDS Community Research Initiative of America (http://aahivm.org/Upload_Module/upload/HIV%20 and%20Aging/Aging%20report%20working%20 document%20FINAL%2012.1.pdf [accessed Jan 2016]). The latest set of HIV treatment guidelines advises early treatment, regardless of baseline CD4 count, and that treatment protects against spread of this disease.

MENTAL HEALTH, SOCIAL, AND ECONOMIC ISSUES AFFECTING LGBT OLDER ADULTS

Mental Health

The link between mental health disorders and discrimination in LGBT populations is well documented. Discrimination is present in health care, as well as in employment, housing, civil rights, federal laws, and organizational policies, all of which must be accounted for in addressing the psychosocial needs of LGBT older adults. For an LGBT older adult, who may have lived most of his or her life in a hostile or intolerant environment, disclosing sexual orientation can induce significant stress and contribute to lower life satisfaction and self-esteem. For older adults, managing social stressors such as prejudice, stigmatization, violence, and internalized homophobia over long periods can result in higher risks of depression, suicide, risky behavior, and substance abuse. LGBT adults are one and a half to two times as likely as heterosexuals to report lifetime prevalence of mood and anxiety disorders, but little is known about the prevalence of mental health disorders in LGBT older adults (SOE=B). In studies that do exist, rates of current or lifetime mood and anxiety disorders have been increased among LGBT older adults, with rates highest among transgender people. Among MSM, depression and emotional distress were associated with being single, experiencing antigay harassment or violence, feeling alienated from the gay community, or not identifying as gay. Depression is linked to disability and poor general health, with internalized stigma and lifetime victimization predicting poor outcomes, whereas social supports and social network size have protective effects.

Suicide rates are alarmingly high in LGBT young persons, and suicidality may persist throughout adulthood into old age. A self-administered survey of 416 LGB adults 60–91 years old in 2001 found that 29% of participants rarely considered suicide, 12% had suicidal thoughts in the past year, 8% sometimes considered suicide, and 2% often considered suicide. Most, however, did not relate their suicidal thoughts to their sexual orientation. Notably, better mental health was predicted in part by a higher percentage of people who knew about the participants' sexual orientation, including their health care provider.

Transgender persons may experience mental health problems, such as adjustment disorders, anxiety disorders, post-traumatic stress disorder, depression, and substance abuse, which are similar to those experienced by other persons who endure major life changes and discrimination. A survey of transgender adults found that 13% reported abusing alcohol or drugs as a means to cope with mistreatment, and 16% had attempted suicide at least once in their lifetimes.

Substance Use

Although LGBT youth have higher rates of alcohol and tobacco use than their heterosexual peers, some of those behaviors differ on the basis of sexual orientation and may not persist in older age. For instance, older lesbian women and bisexual men are more likely to be current smokers than heterosexuals of the same gender after age 50, whereas there is no difference in smoking for older gay men and bisexual women than for heterosexuals. Alcohol use in LGB older adults is similar to that in heterosexuals, with the caveat that binge drinking behavior is more common in older lesbian women and less likely in gay men than in heterosexuals. In contrast, a different survey found that all LGB older adults, regardless of gender, were more likely to smoke and drink excessively than older heterosexuals. Transgender adults also have higher rates of alcohol, smoking, and substance abuse.

Concerns About Aging

LGBT adults may approach the aging process differently from their peers, and this approach may also differ by gender. Although some theories state that LGBT adults are better able to cope with aging than heterosexuals because of the development of adaptive skills and the reconstruction of their identities during the process of disclosing sexual orientation, a study published in 2005 found that 88% of younger gay men and 73% of older gay men felt that gay society viewed aging as a negative process. Lesbian women, however, felt that lesbian society viewed aging in a positive manner. This difference may be because of the influence of youth and physical attraction in gay male subculture, thus subjecting older gay men to ageism from within their own community.

Lesbian and gay older adults generally have the same concerns about aging (eg, loneliness, health, and income) as their heterosexual counterparts, with the additional fears of rejection by their children and grandchildren, uncertain support, and concerns of discrimination in health care, employment, housing, and long-term care. About one-third of gay men and one quarter of lesbian women identified discrimination against their sexual orientation as their greatest concern about aging.

Palliative Care Needs

Minority stress, internalized homophobia, stigma, and misconceptions can all affect the mental health needs of LGBT older adults at the end of life. These issues may be magnified if the LGBT older adult is struggling with issues of disclosure of sexual orientation, fear of discrimination, and estrangement from family when approaching death. Disenfranchised grief, another important concern, refers to the ignored and unrecognized needs of a surviving same-sex spouse if that relationship is not recognized and validated by family, health care providers, or the legal system. For instance, a surviving same-sex partner may be excluded (intentionally or unintentionally) from making funeral arrangements if not legally married. They may also not feel welcome in support groups or community agencies and, as a result, may experience additional grief.

SOCIAL SUPPORTS, OUTREACH, AND POLICY ISSUES

Social Supports and Family Structure

LGBT older adults often find themselves without traditional spousal, familial, and social supports to help with age-related needs. Compared with heterosexual older adults, gay or bisexual men are twice as likely to be living alone, and lesbian or bisexual women are one-third more likely to be living alone. Moreover, LGBT older adults are half as likely to have a significant other, half as likely to have close relatives to call for help, and 3 to 4 times more likely to not have children (SOE=B). A 2014 survey found that 32% of LGBT older adults are very or extremely concerned about being lonely and growing old alone, versus 19% of non-LGBT older adults; 30% are very or extremely concerned about not having someone to take care of them, versus 16% of non-LGBT older adults. LGBT older adults may also have strained relationships with their extended family or children as a result of either the lack of acceptance of their sexuality or the attempt to continue to conceal their sexual orientation.

These diminished social connections lead to higher rates of isolation and loneliness among LGBT older adults than among their non-LGB peers, and LGBT older adults are likely to have unmet needs for basic support. Diminished social supports have been correlated with a wide range of health problems that can have serious consequences, including premature institutionalization and early death.

LGBT adults are sometimes able to rely on "nontraditional" family structures. For example, some form "families of choice," a term used to describe diverse family structures that include close friends, partners, or significant others who are a source of social and caregiving support although not biologically or legally related. However, families of choice pose some difficulties, because they are not recognized by law. For example, a chosen family member cannot make care decisions for a patient unless he or she has been named in an advance directive.

Given these issues, it is vital for health care providers to recognize families of choice, be aware of the possibility of isolation and severe loneliness, and have referral points set up to assist LGBT older adults with targeted services and culturally competent care in traditional service settings.

Housing, Home Care, and Long-Term Care

Surveys show that LGBT older adults fear rejection and discrimination by both staff and other older adults in long-term care facilities. LGBT older adults report an increased frequency of mistreatment incidents, including verbal or physical harassment from other residents and/or staff, refused admission or attempted discharge from facilities, denial of medical treatment, restriction of visitors, staff refusal to accept medical power of attorney, and/or staff refusal to refer to transgender residents by preferred name or pronoun. In an attempt to address such concerns, there have been legislative initiatives to mandate training; for example, California passed a law that requires health care staff in senior care settings to be trained in LGBT culturally competent care. Despite some advances, most states do not require such training.

Some surveys of LGBT older adults indicate that they prefer to age alongside other LGBT older adults if unable to age in place at home, citing safety as the main reason. The idea of LGBT-targeted housing for older adults has resonated conceptually, although there are few such places across the country. However, not all LGBT older adults wish to live in an LGBT-targeted facility, and some older adult residential settings have sought training in providing LGBT culturally competent care so that LGBT older adults' real and perceived fears of mistreatment may be alleviated.

Challenges with Financial Security

LGBT older adults are more likely to live in poverty than their heterosexual counterparts. The rate of poverty is 4.6% among older heterosexual couples, compared with 4.9% for older gay male couples and 9.1% for older lesbian couples (SOE=C). LGBT older adults were more likely to have lived their productive years during a time when discrimination was more common, potentially equating to lower earnings and reduced savings compared with their heterosexual peers. Older lesbian couples are likely poorer than senior gay couples, in part because of gender wage disparities in the general population. A 2014 study found that 51% of LGBT middle-aged and older adults worry about financial security versus 36% of heterosexuals.

Historical unequal access to benefits programs can also affect the financial security of LGBT older adults. Some of this has changed recently with landmark Supreme Court rulings, most notably the 2015 decision in Obergefell v. Hodges granting equal marriage rights to all LGBT adults throughout the nation. In the preceding several years leading up to this ruling, there was a rapid increase in the number of individual U.S. states recognizing marriage equality, beginning with Massachusetts in 2004. Without legal recognition of marriage, disparities continued to exist in states where same-sex couples were not allowed to marry. Disparities also existed at the federal level, which did not recognize same sex marriages even if the individual state did. In 2013, the Supreme Court repealed a key portion of the Defense of Marriage Act (DOMA), allowing for federal recognition of same-sex marriage where recognized at the state level, thus allowing same-sex married couples to receive protections such as Social Security survivor and spousal benefits, Veterans Administration spousal benefits, and preferred tax treatment of health insurance and retirement savings. Before these rulings, couples in states without marriage equality experienced disparities in the adjudication of certain state benefits (such as inheritance benefits) as well as Medicaid benefits. Because the states and the federal government jointly administer Medicaid, states without marriage equality could impose unequal treatment to LGBT couples, affecting the ability of LGBT partners to pass along property, negatively affecting their ability to become eligible for Medicaid. It is also important to note that many LGBT older couples may have never had the opportunity to legally marry, perhaps because of advanced illness or the death of a spouse before marriage became legal, therefore denying the surviving spouse access to protections and benefits such as social security, pensions, and other spousal benefits.

REFERENCES

- American Geriatrics Society Ethics Committee. American Geriatrics Society Care of Lesbian, Gay, Bisexual, and Transgender Older Adults Position Statement. *J Am Geriatr Soc.* 2015;63(3):423–426.

    This position statement of the American Geriatrics Society Ethics Committee raises awareness about the needs of older LGBT adults and outlines specific steps that can be taken to ensure that they receive the care that they need.

- Fredriksen-Goldsen KI, Kim HJ, Emlet CA, et al. The Aging and Health Report: Disparities and Resilience among Lesbian, Gay, Bisexual, and Transgender Older Adults. Seattle: Institute for Multigenerational Health; 2011. http://depts.washington.edu/agepride/wordpress/wp-content/uploads/2012/10/Executive_Summary10-25-12.pdf (accessed Jan 2016).

    This report highlights results of a comparison of key health indicators for LGBT older adults and heterosexual peers. Areas focused on include health disparities (eg, disability, mental health disorders, smoking, and isolation) and the risk and protective factors impacting LGBT older adults. The report also highlights the impact of health care discrimination and describes needed change in policy, services, education, and research.

- LGBT Movement Advancement Project and SAGE (Services and Advocacy for Gay, Lesbian, Bisexual and Transgender Elders). *Improving the Lives of LGBT Older Adults.* March 2010. www.lgbtagingcenter.org/resources/resource.cfm?r=16 (accessed Jan 2016).

    This 2010 report outlines why and how LGBT older adults face additional obstacles to successful aging and lays the groundwork for solutions that address the unique barriers and inequalities affecting the health and well-being of LGBT older adults. Three key elements of successful aging are emphasized: financial security, good health and health care, and social support and community engagement.

- National Resource Center on LGBT Aging. http://lgbtagingcenter.org (accessed Jan 2016).

  This national resource center seeks to improve the quality of services and supports offered to LGBT older adults. Established in 2010 through a federal grant from the U.S. Department of Health and Human Services, the National Resource Center on LGBT Aging provides training, technical assistance, and educational resources to aging providers, LGBT organizations, and LGBT older adults. The center is led by Services & Advocacy for GLBT Elders (SAGE) in collaboration with 18 leading organizations from around the country.

- Services & Advocacy for Gay, Lesbian, Bisexual, & Transgender Elders (SAGE). www.sageusa.org (accessed Jan 2016).

  SAGE is the country's largest and oldest organization dedicated to improving the lives of LGBT older adults. SAGE offers services and programs to LGBT older people nationwide. Among other roles, SAGE also trains aging providers and LGBT organizations on the best ways to support LGBT older people in their long-term care settings, and advocates at the federal, state and local level.

- Simone MJ, Appelbaum JS. Addressing the needs of older lesbian, gay, bisexual and transgender adults. *Clin Geriatr.* 2011;19(2):38–45.

  This review article explores the unique needs of LGBT older adults, focusing on the impact of a lifetime of discrimination and its effects on past and current health, including health disparities and mental health needs. The article also explores social needs unique to this group.

- Simone MJ, Meyer H, Eskildsen MA, et al. Caring for LGBT Older Adults. In: Makadon H, Mayer K, Potter J, et al, eds. *The Fenway Guide to Lesbian, Gay, Bisexual and Transgender Health, 2nd Edition.* Philadelphia: American College of Physicians; 2015:133–156.

  This textbook, a comprehensive resource written by experts in LGBT health, addresses important issues facing patients and providers and includes a chapter specific to the needs of LGBT older adults.

- UCSF Center of Excellence for Transgender Health. www.transhealth.ucsf.edu/trans?page=home-00-00 (accessed Jan 2016).

  The Center of Excellence for Transgender Health (CoE) combines the unique strengths and resources of the Pacific AIDS Education and Training Center and the Center for AIDS Prevention Studies, both of which are housed at the University of California San Francisco. The ultimate CoE goal is to improve the overall health and well-being of transgender individuals by developing and implementing programs in response to community-identified needs.

- Working Group for the HIV and Aging Consensus Project. Recommended Treatment Strategies for Clinicians Managing Older Patients with HIV. 2012. http://aahivm.org/Upload_Module/upload/HIV%20and%20Aging/Aging%20report%20working%20document%20FINAL%202012.1.pdf (accessed Jan 2016).

  This expert review of HIV in older adults provides recommended treatment strategies for clinicians caring for older adults with HIV/AIDS.

Mark J. Simone, MD
Manuel A. Eskildsen, MD, MPH, CMD, AGSF

CHAPTER 10—PHYSICAL ACTIVITY

KEY POINTS

- Regular physical activity provides numerous and substantial health benefits for older adults.

- The health benefits of physical activity accrue independently of other risk factors. Greater amounts of physical activity, within limits, have greater health benefits.

- To obtain substantial health benefits of physical activity, older adults should do at least 30 minutes of moderate-intensity aerobic activity on ≥5 days each week. If they cannot do this intensity or amount of activity, they should do the amount that is possible according to their abilities, so as to avoid inactivity.

- Older adults should also engage in light-moderate muscle-strengthening activity daily or at least 2 days each week and include balance training regularly.

- When possible, obese people and those with osteoarthritis or balance problems should perform aerobic and resistance exercise using water.

- Promoting physical activity is one of the most important and effective preventive and therapeutic interventions in older adults. The clinician's recommendation for exercise (and other lifestyle habits) for their patients carries more weight than any other source of advice. Counseling by a health care provider is an important way of promoting physical activity in clinical settings. Referral of patients to community resources, particularly evidence-based programs, is also important.

Physical activity in the context of public health refers to all muscular activity either at work or during leisure time, ranging from light to high vigorous as shown in Table 10.1. Its benefits arise from the adaptation of multiple body systems to the muscular demand for oxygen, and generally these benefits may be considered proportional to the absolute intensity of the exercise or the mass of muscle activated by the exercise coupled with the duration of the exercise. The term *relative exercise intensity* refers to the percentage of the individual's maximal capacity that is utilized. Thus, a weaker person will activate fewer muscle fibers than a stronger person at the same relative intensity. In this sense, being physically fit allows the individual to perform more vigorous physical activity.

Another important concept is the exercise volume, which in population studies is defined as the product of exercise intensity in METS and duration in hours. Thus, a person who walks briskly (4–5 METS) for 30 minutes 4 times a week achieves an exercise volume of 8–10 MET-hours, which is considered medium volume. See Table 10.1.

BENEFITS OF PHYSICAL ACTIVITY

Preventive Health Benefits

Regular physical activity in adults and older adults improves cardiorespiratory and muscular fitness (SOE=A). It reduces the risk of many diseases, including coronary heart disease, stroke, hypertension, some lipid disorders, type 2 diabetes, colon cancer, breast cancer, osteoporosis, and depression (SOE=A). It also reduces the risk of unhealthy weight gain and assists in weight loss (SOE=A). In older adults, physical activity reduces the risk of falls (SOE=A) and sarcopenia, and regularly active older adults have a lower risk of hip fracture (SOE=B). The evidence that physical activity reduces the risk of cognitive impairment is growing and substantial (SOE=B). There is some evidence that physical activity can reduce the risk of lung cancer, endometrial cancer, osteoarthritis, sleep problems, and anxiety disorders (SOE=B).

Consistent with its broad physiologic effects, regular physical activity decreases both cardiovascular and noncardiovascular mortality in older adults. This benefit is large. The risk of premature mortality is estimated to be 40% less in adults who are active ≥7 hours each week than in those who are active for <0.5 hours each week (SOE=B). Although this estimate is based on cohort studies that determined amounts of physical activity from questionnaires, one study of older adults determined level of physical activity objectively using doubly labeled water. In this study, adults in the highest tertile of energy expenditure per day had a 67% lower mortality rate than adults in the lowest tertile of energy expenditure (SOE=B).

In general, greater amounts of physical activity have greater health benefits, although the relationship between the amount of physical activity and the amount of benefit appears nonlinear for many health conditions. That is, the absolute increase in benefit is greatest at low levels of activity, and less at high levels of activity. The "dose-response" relationship varies by disease in a manner that is incompletely understood. Risk of cardiovascular disease decreases with amount of aerobic activity over a wide range of dose. Blood pressure shows little dose-response effect, with most of the effect of physical activity on blood pressure occurring at low to medium levels of activity.

Table 10.1—Exercise Intensity and Exercise Volume

Exercise intensity, in METS	
Light	= 2.5; walking (approx ~2.2 mph)
Moderate	= 4–5; brisk walking (3.4–3.9 mph)
Moderate–vigorous	= 6.5; jogging (4 mph)
High vigorous	= 8.5; running (5.4 mph)
Duration of physical activity (also known as exercise volume, ie, intensity × duration), in MET-hours per week	
Inactive	<3.75
Low volume	3.75–7.5
Medium volume	7.6–16.5
High volume	16.6–25.5
Very high volume	>25.5

1 MET = 3.5 mL O_2/kg/min = 210 mL O_2/kg/hr = 1 kcal/kg/hr (1 L O_2 = 5 kcal)

The health benefits of physical activity accrue independently of risk factors. For example, sedentary smokers experience health benefits of increasing physical activity even if they continue to smoke. The health benefits of physical activity are also generally independent of body weight: overweight and obese adults obtain benefits from physical activity even if it does not promote weight loss.

Strong, consistent observational evidence indicates that regularly active older adults are at reduced risk of moderate or severe functional limitations and role limitations (SOE=B). One review estimated that moderate amounts of aerobic physical activity reduced risk of functional decline by 30%. There appears to be a dose-response relationship, with greater amounts of physical activity producing more benefit.

Therapeutic Benefits

Physical activity is commonly recommended in clinical practice guidelines as therapy for specific conditions. Clinical practice guidelines identify a substantial therapeutic role for physical activity in coronary heart disease, peripheral vascular disease, hypertension, type 2 diabetes, osteoarthritis, osteoporosis, some lipid disorders, obesity, claudication, and COPD. Physical activity also has a role in the management of depression, anxiety disorders, pain, heart failure, syncope, sleep disorders, stroke, dementia, back pain, and constipation, and in the prevention of venous thromboembolism.

In a systematic review, there was solid evidence from controlled trials that physical activity has a beneficial effect on functional limitations in older adults with existing mild, moderate, or severe limitations (SOE=A).

Economic Benefits

Regularly active adults are consistently reported to have lower medical expenditures than sedentary adults (SOE=B). In one study comparing older adults who remained sedentary with those who became active ≥3 days each week, medical expenditures of the active group were lower by about $2,200 per year. In one managed-care plan that offered a physical activity benefit consisting of paying per-visit costs for Medicare-eligible enrollees who participated in an exercise program called EnhanceFitness, participants adjusted total costs were $1,186 lower per year than those of nonparticipants by year two.

RECOMMENDED AMOUNTS OF PHYSICAL ACTIVITY

A public health recommendation for ≥20 minutes of vigorous aerobic activity on ≥3 days per week was developed in the 1980s. In 1995, the CDC and the American College of Sports Medicine (ACSM) developed a moderate-intensity recommendation: "Every US adult should accumulate 30 minutes or more of moderate-intensity physical activity on most, preferably all, days of the week." In 2007, the ACSM and the American Heart Association (AHA) updated the 1995 recommendation by issuing separate recommendations for adults and for older adults. In 2008, the U.S. Department of Health and Human Services issued the first national guidelines for physical activity, the *2008 Physical Activity Guidelines for Americans*. For recommended types and amounts of physical activity, see Table 10.2.

Aerobic Activity

An older adult can achieve recommended levels of aerobic activity by doing either moderate-intensity aerobic physical activity for at least 150 minutes each week, or vigorous-intensity activity for at least 75 minutes each week. This corresponds to a walking pace of 20–24 minutes per mile (see Table 10.1). However, overweight and older adults should judge their effort at 5 or 6 out of 10 (on a 10-point scale) while being able to talk but not sing or feel breathless. Doing a combination of moderate- and vigorous-intensity activity is also acceptable. Aerobic activity should be spread throughout the week, preferably on ≥3 days per week. Doing at least 30 minutes of aerobic activity on ≥5 days each week remains an appropriate way for older adults to obtain the health benefits of activity. Studies using objective measures of physical activity have shown that most adults do not adhere to these recommendations, suggesting that an approach based on reducing inactivity may be more beneficial.

Several comments help clarify this recommendation. First, episodes of moderate-intensity activity of ≥10 minutes count toward meeting the recommendation. Second, the recommendation does not refer to just leisure activity or exercise. Occupational activity (eg,

Table 10.2—Recommended Types and Amounts of Physical Activity

Type of Exercise	Frequency/Duration	Examples of Activities	Examples of Targeted Conditions
Aerobic	≥150 minutes of moderate-intensity activity each week, spread throughout the week; ≥75 minutes of vigorous-intensity activity each week, spread throughout the week	Walking, running, swimming, bicycling, rowing, or aerobic exercise machines (eg, ellipticals, stair steppers); walking 30 minutes/day, 5–6 days/week, or 10,000 steps/day using a pedometer	Many conditions, including cardiovascular disease, cancer, diabetes, osteoarthritis, and depression; low physical work capacity
Muscle strengthening	≥2 days each week for 20–30 minutes	Resistance training (eg, using weight machines) or floor exercises using body weight against gravity (eg, abdominal "crunches," push-ups off knees or against a table, climbing stairs); pool exercises against water resistance	Falls, frailty, sarcopenia, osteoporosis
Flexibility	10 minutes stretching daily to maintain range of motion	Stretching, gentle yoga, Pilates	Osteoarthritis, joint stiffness
Balance training	≥3 days/week	Backward walking, heel-to-toe walking, Tai Chi exercise, standing on one foot	Falls, osteoporosis

carpentry), domestic activity (eg, mowing the grass), and transportation activity (eg, walking to the store) all count toward meeting recommendations. Third, participation in physical activity above the minimum recommended levels results in greater health benefits. Some physical activity is clearly preferable to none for those who are unable to meet these targets. Older adults should be strongly encouraged to avoid an inactive lifestyle, even if they do not (or cannot) obtain recommended amounts of activity. Finally, as indicated earlier, the recommended activity is in addition to routine (baseline) activity of light-intensity or of short duration (<10 minutes). This is supported by a large clinical trial in which men and women ≥60 years old had a 14% lower risk of all-cause mortality with 15 minutes of moderate exercise per day. Each additional 15 minutes of exercise a day reduced the risk by a further 4%. This finding may reduce the barriers to individuals who attempt to meet the recommendation of 30 minutes a day of moderate exercise in the *2008 Physical Activity Guidelines for Americans*.

Muscle-Strengthening Activity

ACSM/AHA recommendations and the *2008 Physical Activity Guidelines for Americans* state that older adults should perform muscle-strengthening activities of the major muscle groups (arms, shoulder, legs, hip, back, chest, and abdomen) on ≥2 days each week. A typical routine for older adults involves 2 or 3 nonconsecutive days each week. These activities can be done at home; popular exercises include sit-ups and push-ups, modified to reduce the strength required to perform them. For example, push-ups may be done off the knees or against a wall, and sit-ups may be done in reverse by lowering the torso to the point where it can be raised again without excessive strain.

For adults who choose resistance training (eg, weight machines), one set of 8 to 10 different exercises is sufficient, with 10 to 15 repetitions per set. Moderate-intensity or high-intensity training is recommended, in which level of effort of moderate intensity is 5 or 6 on a 0 to 10 scale (0=no movement and 10=maximal effort). High-intensity is 7 or 8 on the same scale and should be done with caution with at least one day between each session.

Flexibility Activity

Flexibility activity is recommended for older adults as a means of maintaining the range of motion needed for regular physical activity and daily life. Stiffness of ligaments, tendons, and other connective tissue occurs after soft-tissue injury and through the gradual glycosylation of collagen fibers with age. This process can be ameliorated with regular stretching to the point of tightness and holding the position for a few seconds. Yoga is a good activity for older adults because it combines strengthening and stretching, and classes for all abilities are widely available. Caution is advised to avoid injury by trying to achieve positions that may be too difficult.

Balance Training

Balance training is recommended for all older adults especially those at risk of falls, including adults with frequent falls or mobility problems. This can be done throughout the day in a variety of situations. Walking backward, and standing on one foot for several seconds and then the other while using gentle support initially, are simple examples. Balance can be thought of as any other motor skill, which requires practice, muscle coordination, and adequate strength.

Several effective interventions to prevent falls that included balance training on ≥3 days per week have been studied. Hence, it is preferable that older adults do standardized balance exercises from a program demonstrated to reduce falls. There is moderate evidence that Tai Chi exercise is effective in fall prevention, although the optimal amount and forms of Tai Chi are unclear (SOE=B).

Management of Body Weight

Most weight-loss studies conclude that exercise enhances the effectiveness of dietary restriction in achieving a healthy body weight beyond what might be expected from calculations of caloric balance. The amount of exercise to metabolize the 3,500 kcals of energy in a pound of fat is substantial. Walking a mile at 1.5–4 mph requires about 1.25 kcals/kg body weight/mile, or 100 kcal for a person weighing 175 lbs. Therefore, 5 miles of daily walking, which for most older adults would take 2 hours, is required to lose 1 lb of fat per week. This fact emphasizes the need for other forms of energy expenditure throughout the day, and especially to minimize the time spent sitting.

A reasonable approach for physical activity and weight management in older adults is to follow the *2008 Physical Activity Guidelines for Americans*. Overweight and obese older adults should first achieve minimal recommended levels of physical activity (150 minutes of moderate-intensity aerobic activity per week). If a healthy weight is not achieved with this level of activity, then caloric intake should be controlled, physical activity increased gradually, and body weight monitored. Physical activity can be increased to the point that is individually effective in controlling weight.

When older adults lose weight, they lose not only fat mass but also muscle mass and bone mass. Because physical activity, particularly muscle-strengthening activity, acts to preserve bone and muscle mass, older adults should not attempt to lose weight by diet alone. Exercises should include non-weight-bearing muscle groups of the arms, torso, and shoulders.

Screening

Rather than advise older adults to consult a health care provider before starting to increase physical activity, ACSM/AHA recommends that health care provider consultation about physical activity should occur regardless of whether an adult currently plans to increase physical activity. One quality of care measure for older adults ascertains whether older adults discuss physical activity with a health care provider at least once a year. At the time of a consultation about physical activity, the clinician should ensure that the patient does not have any undiagnosed symptoms and is up-to-date on preventive care, and that medical conditions are stable. Further, the clinician should assess if and how the patient should limit his or her activity because of chronic conditions.

Thus, "screening" older adults can be used to match them to an activity plan appropriate for their abilities. Most, if not all, studies of exercise in people with disabilities have assessed potential participants to ensure the exercise intervention is appropriate. These study populations have included adults with osteoarthritis, lower limb loss, cerebral palsy, multiple sclerosis, muscular dystrophy, Parkinson disease, spinal cord injury, stroke, traumatic brain injury, dementia, intellectual disability, and mental illness. A review concluded that the benefits of physical activity for such people with disabilities clearly outweigh the risks.

It is appropriate for providers of exercise programs to ask new participants (who are not referred after an examination by a health care provider) to complete a symptom checklist. People with undiagnosed symptoms should seek medical care before starting an exercise program.

The Physical Activity Guidelines Advisory Committee concluded, after a systematic review of the literature, that "the protective value of a medical consultation for persons with or without chronic diseases who are interested in increasing their physical activity level is not established." The U.S. Preventive Services Task Force (USPSTF) does not recommend any type of routine pre-exercise screening of healthy asymptomatic adults. Specifically, for adults at increased risk of coronary heart disease, the USPSTF finds insufficient evidence for and routine screening with resting ECG, exercise treadmill test, or electron-beam CT scanning for coronary calcium for adults at low risk of heart disease.

PROMOTION OF PHYSICAL ACTIVITY IN OLDER ADULTS

The public health approach to promotion of physical activity is based on a socioecologic model that recognizes the interrelationship that exists between the individual and his or her environment. This involves action at all levels of society: individual, interpersonal, organizational, community, and public policy. To illustrate the logic of the model, consider that counseling an older adult to walk regularly (individual level intervention) is more effective if the person lives in a neighborhood with good access to parks and other safe places to walk (a community level intervention). A referral to an exercise program (an individual level intervention) is more likely to succeed if the costs of the exercise program are subsidized by a health plan (organizational level intervention). Physical activity promotion in clinical settings occurs in this broader context. The Task Force on Community Preventive Services has identified 8 evidence-based community approaches for promoting physical activity (www.thecommunityguide.org).

Clinical Settings

A system is needed in each clinical setting for routinely assessing levels of physical activity in patients, for providing patients with a recommendation about physical activity, for helping patients achieve recommended levels, and for evaluating the effectiveness of the system in promoting physical activity. An example of an evidence-based system is the Green Prescription in New Zealand. In brief, after their level of physical activity has been assessed, patients are given the option of requesting a prescription from a primary care provider. The provider provides a written "green" prescription, typically for walking or other home-based activity. A copy is faxed to the local sports foundation, which contacts patients and offers them assistance by telephone or face-to-face counseling, or peer group support. In a randomized trial of this approach, the intervention group averaged 35–40 more minutes of physical activity each week (SOE=A).

Assessing Physical Activity

The importance of routine assessment of physical activity is emphasized by the Exercise is Medicine Initiative of the ACSM. This initiative advocates for physical activity as a vital sign to be checked each visit. Tools have been developed to provide quick assessments of the physical activity level of older adults, such as the Rapid Assessment of Physical Activity, a 9-item questionnaire in which patients self-rate their strength, flexibility, and frequency and intensity of exercise. Both the amount of aerobic activity and the amount of muscle-strengthening activity should be assessed.

Emerging evidence indicates that how we spend our time during daily living may be important. In a large prospective study of U.S. adults enrolled by the American Cancer Society, time spent sitting was independently associated with total mortality, regardless of physical activity level. Similar results were found in a more recent meta-analysis of 47 studies of outcomes for cardiovascular disease and diabetes, cancer, and all-cause mortality for which physical activity data was available. Prolonged sedentary time was associated with deleterious health outcomes independently from physical activity.

Recommendations for physical activity should include advice on ways to avoid excessive time spent sitting and in bedrest. Caregivers should be aware that doing too much for those in their care may not be in the best interests of the patient. At particular risk are workers who sit in front of computers all day without hourly walking breaks and older adults with or without limited mobility, who spend excessive time laying down.

Providing an Activity Prescription

For older adults, especially those with chronic conditions, the ACSM/AHA recommends development of an activity plan in consultation with primary care providers. The activity plan should integrate public health preventive recommendations (summarized above) with any therapeutic use of physical activity recommended, eg, by clinical practice guidelines. Older adults should understand if, and how, chronic conditions limit the amounts and types of activity they can do.

The activity prescription is considered part of a broader approach of developing the physical activity plan. The plan considers individual preferences, individual abilities and fitness, chronic conditions and activity limitations, risk of falls, strategies for decreasing risk of injury, and behavioral strategies to increase adherence to the plan. Essentially, the plan provides specific guidance on how to meet physical activity guidelines. A resource for developing the plan is ACSM's *Exercise Management for Chronic Diseases and Disabilities*. This book covers issues in exercise management for some 40 different conditions. Some guidelines for developing a plan include the following:

- The plan will commonly emphasize walking, which is a popular and safe activity in older adults. However, for many people with knee osteoarthritis, swimming, pool exercise, and non-weight-bearing activities such as cycling and rowing, which can be done on machines, may be preferred.

- The plan should emphasize the importance of gradually increasing physical activity over time (see below). It can be appropriate for older adults to spend weeks or months at activity levels below recommended levels.

- The less active an adult is currently and the less experience he or she has with physical activity, the more appropriate it is to recommend starting in a supervised, evidence-based program (see below).

- Providing social support for physical activity is important. Social support can be provided by classes, formal mall walking groups, telephone counseling, and informal arrangements in which people simply meet to go for a walk.

Providing Assistance in Increasing Physical Activity

In 2002, the USPSTF concluded that the evidence is insufficient to recommend for or against behavioral counseling in primary care settings to promote physical activity. However, some clinic-based systems of promoting physical activity have been carefully studied and reported to increase physical activity, such as the "Green Prescription" system mentioned above. A reasonable conclusion is that a clinic can implement either an existing evidence-based approach, or implement and evaluate a new approach tailored to the clinical situation based on principles of behavior change and building on existing approaches. The many negative studies of physical activity counseling in clinical settings emphasize the importance of evaluating any new approaches.

Particularly for adults with some functional limitations, an appropriate way to provide assistance is to make a referral to an evidence-based program. Resources, such as the National Council on Aging website (www.ncoa.org), can help identify evidence-based programs that have been tested in research studies and translated into versions that work in the community. For example, Active Living Every Day and Active Choices are two programs that were originally tested in research studies and subsequently translated into programs appropriate for community settings. A recent study demonstrated that the community versions of these programs were effective in large samples of older adults who were substantially more ethnically, economically, and functionally diverse than the samples in the original research studies.

A longstanding resource for older adults from the National Institute on Aging is *Exercise: A Guide from the National Institute on Aging*. This publication is updated periodically.

Management of Risks of Physical Activity

The most important recommendation for avoiding activity-related injuries is to increase physical activity gradually over time (SOE=B). Observational evidence is strong that the risk of injury is directly related to the size of the gap between a person's usual level of activity and their new level of activity. A series of small increments in activity, each followed by a period of adaptation, is associated with lower rates of musculoskeletal injury. The safest method for increasing activity has not been established by intervention studies. For reasonably healthy adults, adding a small amount of light- to moderate-intensity activity (eg, walking 5–15 minutes per session, 2 to 3 times per week) has low risk of musculoskeletal injury and no known risk of sudden cardiac events (SOE=B).

In contrast, during vigorous-intensity activity, all individuals are at higher risk of sudden adverse cardiac events. However, regularly active adults are at much less risk than inactive adults who abruptly engage in vigorous activity.

In older adults, cardiovascular adaptation to a target level of physical activity can take as long as ≥20 weeks. This suggests that activity levels should be increased once per month instead of once per week.

Other factors also affect injury risk. The risk of injury is higher with vigorous exercise, with greater amounts of exercise, and with activities that involve frequent contact (eg, soccer, basketball) or purposeful collision (eg, football). The risk of injury is less with a higher level of fitness, supervision, protective equipment such as bike helmets, and in well-designed environments. To illustrate the safety of walking, one community-based study estimated 0.2 injuries per 1,000 hours of walking for transportation. In contrast, in 1,000 hours of participation, dancing had 0.7 injuries, gardening 1.0 injuries, and running 3.6 injuries.

Older Adults with Low Fitness or Low Functional Ability

In the lifestyle interventions and independence for elders (LIFE) pilot study, a randomized trial in which older adults (70–89 years old) with chronic diseases and reduced functional ability who were at substantial risk of mobility disability were enrolled, regular exercise improved measures of physical function without appreciably increasing risk of adverse events. This trial affirmed that older adults with functional impairments can achieve benefits from exercise (SOE=A). Similarly, an older study of resistance exercise in frail nursing-home residents demonstrated improvements in strength and function (SOE=A).

Regardless, in such older adults with low fitness or low functional ability, it is more challenging to match abilities with types and amounts of activity. Sometimes referrals can be made to specific rehabilitation programs, such as pulmonary rehabilitation, for assessment, exercise prescription, and medically supervised exercise. Assessment by a physical therapist is generally appropriate, and the therapist can design and tailor an exercise program to the specific limitations of the patient. This assessment can also confirm that a patient is capable of participating in a specific community exercise program (eg, a water exercise program designed for adults with arthritis). Given that the care of such patients often involves a geriatric team and consultants, methods should be in place to ensure the activity recommendation is communicated to all the health care providers.

REFERENCES

- Jansen FM, Prins RG, Etman A, et al. Physical activity in non-frail and frail older adults. *PLoS One*. 2015;10(4):e0123168.

    In this careful analysis of physical activity using accelerometers and GPS-devices, almost none of the participants (65–89 years old) engaged in moderate to vigorous physical activity recommended in many consensus guidelines. Furthermore there were no differences in physical activity between frail and non-frail adults. These results emphasize the need for enjoyable activities that these adults can do and so avoid excessive sedentary behavior.

- Matthews CE, George SM, Moore SM, et al. Amount of time spent in sedentary behaviors and cause-specific mortality in US adults. *Am J Clin Nutr*. 2012;95(2):437–445.

    A very large cohort from the NIH-AARP Diet and Health Study provides evidence for a strong relationship between sedentary behavior, as determined by time spent watching television, and all-cause and cardiovascular mortality. Participation in high levels of moderate to vigorous physical activity did not fully mitigate health risks associated with prolonged time watching television. The trend persisted even among those engaged in high levels of moderate to vigorous physical activity.

- Pahor M, Figural JM, Ambrosius WT, et al. Effect of structured physical activity on prevention of major mobility disability in older adults: the LIFE study randomized clinical trial. *JAMA*. 2014;311(23):2387–2396.

    The LIFE study is one of the largest and most recent randomized trials of exercise in sedentary older adults. It has provided important evidence that physical activity in older adults with chronic diseases and impaired physical performance is safe and has a beneficial effect on performance. In this report, older adults at high risk of mobility disability but able to walk 400 meters were enrolled in a structured physical activity program and followed for 2.6 years. Compared with a control group participating in a health education program, the structured program participants increased their time in moderate intensity walking and weight training activities by 104 minutes/week, and this was associated with significantly reduced mobility disability as defined by inability to walk 400 meters. This provides further evidence that structured programs enhance adherence to appropriate physical activity, which in turn improves mobility.

- Rejeski WJ, Brubaker PH, Goff DC Jr., et al. Translating weight loss and physical activity programs into the community to preserve mobility in older, obese adults in poor cardiovascular health. *Arch Intern Med*. 2011;171(10):880–886.

    This 18-month study demonstrated the effectiveness of existing community infrastructures in delivering lifestyle interventions to enhance mobility in older adults in poor cardiovascular health. Subjects were randomized to 3 groups: control, physical activity, and physical activity plus weight loss. The control groups had 18 educational meetings over the duration of the study and the other groups had 48 meetings, which included supervised diet and exercise programs. After 6 months, all three groups improved on the primary outcome measure of walk time, which was maintained over 18 months.

- Tse MM, Wan VT, Ho SS. Physical exercise: does it help in relieving pain and increasing mobility among older adults with chronic pain. *J Clin Nursing*. 2011;20(5–6):635–644.

    This study addresses the important issue of chronic pain, which hinders ADLs and the desire of older adults to participate in exercise and social programs.

- US Department of Health and Human Services. 2008 Physical Activity Guidelines for Americans. www.health.gov/paguidelines/pdf/paguide.pdf (accessed Jan 2016).

    This comprehensive guide to physical activity includes specific recommendations for children, adults, and older adults >65 years old. The guidelines cover the type of exercise—aerobic, resistance, flexibility, and balance—and the total amount of exercise per week in terms of frequency, duration, and intensity. Tips are given on how to achieve the guidelines and deal with chronic debilitating conditions.

- Waters DL, Ward AL, Villareal D. Weight loss in obese adults 65 years and older: a review of the controversy. *Exp Gerontol*. 2013;48(10):1054–1061.

    This review supports the position that moderate weight loss associated with strengthening exercise to ameliorate loss of bone and muscle mass has multiple metabolic and functional benefits for older adults.

Peter G. Snell, PhD

CHAPTER 11—PREVENTION

Key Points

- It is important to consider a patient's remaining life expectancy, comorbidities, and cognitive and functional status when deciding which preventive health measures to offer. If the natural history of the disease is greater than the individual's expected life span, screening is not indicated.

- Many preventive health measures are underused among older adults, including immunizations (eg, flu shots, pneumococcal vaccinations), exercise counseling, depression screening, and counseling on geriatric health issues (eg, safety, falls prevention, incontinence), whereas cancer screening tests are overused among older adults in poor health.

- Tools are available to help clinicians estimate life expectancy to appropriately target cancer screening to those with adequate remaining life expectancy.

- Medicare is increasingly covering preventive services and wellness visits.

Many preventive health measures are available to older adults, including screening tests (eg, colonoscopy), counseling about a healthy lifestyle (eg, exercise) and/or geriatric health issues (eg, incontinence), immunizations (eg, flu shot), and chemoprophylaxis (eg, aspirin). Ideally, older adults should receive preventive health measures from which they are most likely to benefit based on their health and remaining life expectancy. In this era of patient-centered practice, recommendations should incorporate patient preferences as well.

Remaining life expectancy decreases uniformly with age, but it can vary from one individual to the next according to illness burden and functional status. Predicted remaining life expectancy, cognition, and function are important determinants to consider when offering preventive services to older adults. In vulnerable older adults, screening and prevention should focus on evidence-based interventions that minimize functional limitations and increase the number of healthy years lived.

This chapter reviews the preventive health measures available to older adults and discusses which measures are appropriate based on remaining life expectancy. Table 11.1 provides an overview of measures available and their recommended use in different populations of older adults, including those with ≥10 years of remaining life expectancy, those with 5–10 years of remaining life expectancy, those with moderate dementia, and those near the end of life. The recommendations given in Table 11.1 are based on reports from geriatric expert panels, as well as on guidelines from the American Geriatrics Society (AGS) and the United States Preventive Services Task Force (USPSTF), and include information on whether each service is cost-effective. A service that costs less than $50,000 per life-year saved is generally considered cost-effective, while those that cost more than $100,000 per life-year saved are generally not. This chapter focuses mainly on primary (ie, disease avoidance) and secondary (ie, early detection and treatment of asymptomatic disease) prevention rather than on tertiary prevention (ie, preventing functional decline from established illness). Effective ways to counsel older adults about preventive health measures are also discussed.

Several criteria should generally be met before recommending disease screening: 1) The condition being screened for must be serious and prevalent in the population being tested. 2) The disease should have a significant asymptomatic phase that can be detected by the screening test. 3) The screening test must be safe, sensitive, and specific to limit false-positive and false-negative tests. 4) Effective treatment must be available for use early in the natural course of the disease that results in a better prognosis than treatment given after symptoms develop. 5) The costs of screening should be acceptable. 6) Ideally, the screening test should have been found effective in a randomized controlled trial (RCT). Few older adults have been included in RCTs that evaluate screening measures, especially frail older adults; therefore, recommendations are often based on indirect evidence. Geriatricians are encouraged to consider the effect of preventive health measures not only on quantity of life but also on quality of life, satisfaction with life, and in maintaining independence. Preventive health recommendations for older adults need to be individualized based on patient health, function, risk of disease, and preferences.

Cancer Screening Tests Among Older Adults

The main potential benefit of screening is reducing cancer mortality experienced by individuals whose cancer is detected early and that otherwise would have resulted in serious morbidity or death if the cancer was not treated early. The potential harms of screening include complications from screening tests or diagnostic evaluations after false-positive test results, false reassurance from false-negative test results, detection and treatment of disease that never would have become clinically significant during a person's lifetime (overdiagnosis), and psychological distress.

Cancer screening research is subject to three main types of bias: lead time, length, and selection biases. These biases can make a test appear to be effective when it actually is not. Lead-time bias occurs when screening results in earlier identification without altering the time to death. Thus, the person spends more time as a patient, but the course of the disease is basically unaltered.

Length bias occurs when screening increases the number of identified clinically slowly progressive or nonprogressive diseases that would never have become a symptomatic problem. Screening for prostate cancer is affected by length bias. Increased levels of prostate-specific antigen can detect cancers that may never cause the patient's death. This leads to overdiagnosis, or the detection of "disease" that is of no consequence, also called *pseudodisease*.

Selection bias is based on the observation that people willing to be screened for cancer may not reflect the population as a whole. Volunteers may be more health conscious or have other personal habits that favorably influence prognosis. Thus, their outcome from screening may be better than what would be seen in a random population.

Prospective RCTs are the only method of documenting the value of screening while effectively eliminating these sources of bias. Study populations must be followed for many years to document the cancer cause–specific survival advantage, if any, for the screened group. However, few cancer screening RCTs have included individuals ≥70 years old.

Breast Cancer

Because the mammography screening trials did not include women >74 years old, it is unknown whether screening mammography helps older women live longer. The USPSTF states that there is insufficient evidence on whether to screen women ≥75 years old. The AGS Choosing Wisely® list states not to recommend breast cancer screening to older women without considering their life expectancy, because women with <10 years of remaining life expectancy are exposed to immediate harms of screening with little chance of benefit. These recommendations are based on a 10-year remaining life expectancy, because a meta-analysis of the RCTs on mammography screening found that on average it takes around 10 years before one death from breast cancer is prevented for 1,000 patients screened (SOE=A). In terms of the benefits of screening, modeling studies estimate that 2 fewer breast cancer deaths are seen per 1,000 women in their 70s who continue biennial screening for 10 years instead of stopping screening at 69. However, harms of screening older women longer than 10 years include false-positive mammograms, which occur in approximately 200 of 1,000 women screened, and overdiagnosis, which occurs in approximately 13 of 1,000 women screened. Ideally, older women will consider their risk of breast cancer, life expectancy, and their preferences around the risks and benefits of screening in deciding whether to continue mammography screening. A promising peer-reviewed decision aid to help women ≥75 years old decide whether or not to continue being screened is being tested in a larger trial. As for breast self-examination (BSE) and clinical breast examinations (CBEs), two large RCTs of women of all ages found no benefit of BSE compared with no breast cancer screening, and no trials have compared CBE alone to no screening. The AGS recommends that CBEs be performed periodically and neither endorses nor discourages BSEs. Similarly, the USPSTF found insufficient evidence to recommend for or against CBEs and recommends against teaching BSE, because BSE may lead to unnecessary biopsies and is not associated with a survival benefit (SOE=B).

Colorectal Cancer (CRC)

Adenomatous polyps develop in 30%–50% of Americans >50 years old; 1%–10% of these polyps will progress to cancer in 5–10 years. Fortunately, several tests are considered effective for CRC screening among adults 50–75 years old, including colonoscopy every 10 years, home-based high-sensitivity fecal occult blood tests (FOBT) annually, and flexible sigmoidoscopy every 5 years with high-sensitivity FOBTs every 3 years. Although air-contrast barium enemas every 5 years were previously considered for screening, this test has not been subject to screening trials, has lower sensitivity than other screening strategies, and is thus not commonly used. Colonoscopy is the most sensitive (95%) and cost-effective screening test for colorectal cancer and has specificity similar to that of flexible sigmoidoscopy (90%). However, there are known risks of colonoscopy. Among Medicare enrollees >65 years old, 0.6 per 1,000 experienced perforation after colonoscopy, 2.1 per 1,000 experienced gastrointestinal bleeding (even when no polypectomy was performed), and 10 per 1,000 experienced cardiovascular events; the risks rose with age and comorbidity. In addition, although bowel preparation with polyethylene glycol electrolyte lavage solution is commonly used and considered safe for older adults, complaints of dizziness, abdominal pain, fecal incontinence, and nausea are common. Therefore, it is important for clinicians to consider patient life expectancy before recommending CRC screening to older adults, because adults with <10 years of remaining life expectancy are thought to have little chance to benefit.

Before screening older adults with FOBT, clinicians should be sure to ask if the patient is willing to consider colonoscopy, because one study found that 58% of veterans ≥70 years old did not receive a complete colon evaluation within 1 year after a positive FOBT. In 43% of these cases, there was a lack of acknowledgement of the positive FOBT, 26% refused colonoscopy, 10% were in poor health, and the others had scheduling difficulties or difficulties with the prep. Decisions about first-time screening after age 75 need to be made in the context of patient health. In patients with no comorbid disease, initial screening colonoscopy up to age 83 may be cost-effective. The USPSTF recommends against routinely screening adults >75 years old and against ever screening adults ≥85 years old because the risks outweigh the benefits. The Choosing Wisely® campaign recommends not screening adults with <10 years of life expectancy. These recommendations do not apply to adults who have had previous adenomas on colonoscopy and are undergoing surveillance. Guidelines are not available as to when to stop testing these individuals for CRC cancer.

Cervical Cancer

Although screening for cervical cancer with cytology is recommended every 3 years or every 5 years if combined with human papilloma virus (HPV) testing (a test for the presence of >2 high-risk or carcinogenic types), guidelines recommend stopping screening after age 65 for women who have had adequate prior screening *regardless of sexual history or new sexual partners* and are not otherwise at high risk of cervical cancer (no history of a high-grade precancerous cervical lesion in the past 20 years, no exposure in utero to diethylstilbestrol, not immunocompromised). Three consecutive negative cytology results or 2 consecutive negative HPV results within 10 years before cessation of screening, with the most recent test within 5 years, is considered adequate prior screening. These recommendations are based on evidence that shows that the incidence of high-grade cervical lesions significantly declines after middle age (SOE=A) and that the risk of false-positive tests resulting in invasive procedures is increased. Of note, positive screening results are more common with screening strategies that include HPV testing; 2.6% of women 60–65 years old will be HPV positive despite normal cytology, and follow-up testing is recommended. Older women who have undergone total hysterectomy with removal of the cervix and who do not have a history of cervical intraepithelial neoplasia grade 2 or 3 or cervical cancer should not be screened (SOE=A). Approximately half of cervical cancers diagnosed in the United States occur among women never screened, and an additional 10% occur among women not screened in the past 5 years; therefore, an older woman who has never been screened or has been inadequately screened should be screened every 2–5 years, ending at age 70 or 75.

Prostate Cancer

Prostate cancer is the most commonly diagnosed non-skin cancer in U.S. men, with a lifetime risk of 16%. Two large RCTs have evaluated the effectiveness of measuring prostate-specific antigen (PSA) levels for prostate cancer screening. The Prostate, Lung, Colorectal, and Ovarian Cancer Screening Trial was a multisite U.S. trial that included men 55–74 years old without a history of prostate, colon, or lung cancer. Men randomized to the intervention were screened annually with PSA for 6 years and a digital rectal examination for 4 years. Because men in the control group received standard care, there was high contamination of the controls (approximately 50% of the controls underwent PSA screening compared with 85% of those in the intervention group), which may explain why no reduction in mortality was found for PSA screening after 7–10 years follow-up. The European Randomized Study of Screening for Prostate Cancer (ERSCP) trial randomized men 50–74 years old to PSA screening every 2–4 years. In this study, the control group did not receive PSA screening. The ERSCP trial found a 20% reduction in prostate cancer mortality at 9 years for men 55–69 years old in the intervention group but no reduction in mortality for men ≥70 years old and no overall reduction in mortality for men of any age. The ERSCP trial concluded that 1,410 men 55–69 years old would need to be screened and 48 treated to prevent 1 death from prostate cancer. However, men who were screened in this trial were more likely to be treated with radical prostatectomy than those who were not screened, which may explain the reduction in mortality found. Both trials documented detection of numerous clinically insignificant tumors (17%–50% of all cancers detected). The American Cancer Society and American Urological Society recommend that clinicians discuss the potential benefits of PSA screening (modest reduction of morbidity and mortality from prostate cancer) and the possible harms (false-positive results [80% of positive PSAs are false-positives when thresholds of 2.5–4 mcg/L are used], unnecessary biopsies [15%–20% of those screened longer than 10 years], overdiagnosis/overtreatment, and possible complications of treatment [eg, erectile dysfunction, urinary incontinence, and even death from surgery]) among men ≥50 years old with at least 10 years remaining life expectancy. The USPSTF recommends against PSA-based screening for prostate cancer regardless of a man's age (SOE=A).

Table 11.1—Preventive Health Measures Available for Older Adults and Recommended Use

Procedure	≥10 years remaining life expectancy	5 to <10 years remaining life expectancy	Moderate dementia	Near end of life	SOE	Cost-effectiveness
Cancer screening						
Mammography	Every 2 years	Not recommended	Not recommended	Not recommended	A/C[b]	Somewhat cost-effective for women <80 years old, may be cost-effective for women ≥80 years old in top quartile of life expectancy.
Pap smear	Stop after age 65	Not recommended	Not recommended	Not recommended	B	Cost-effective to stop
Prostate-specific antigen	Consider discussing pros/cons if remaining life expectancy >10 years	Not recommended	Not recommended	Not recommended	B	Uncertain
Colon cancer screening						
Fecal occult blood test	Yearly, may stop at age 75	Not recommended	Not recommended	Not recommended	A/C[c]	Cost-effective
Colonoscopy	Every 10 years, may stop at age 75	Not recommended	Not recommended	Not recommended		
Low-dose CT for lung cancer screening	Consider annually in those at risk[d], stop at age 80	Consider in those at risk[d], stop at age 80	Not recommended	Not recommended	A	Uncertain
Other screening tests						
DEXA screening for osteoporosis	At least once after age 65, or age 60 if high risk	Consider if not done previously	Not recommended	Not recommended	A	Cost-effective
Blood glucose	Screen when results would affect cardiovascular disease prevention (lipids, aspirin use)[e]	Not recommended	Not recommended	Not recommended	C	Uncertain
Cholesterol screening	Consider for those with additional risk factors[f]	Not recommended	Not recommended	Not recommended	C	Uncertain
Ultrasonography for abdominal aortic aneurysm	Once for men 65–75 years old who ever smoked	Consider	Not recommended	Not recommended	A	Cost-effective
Thyrotropin	Every 2–5 years	Every 2–5 years	Every 3 years	Consider	C	Uncertain
HIV	Consider for those at high risk	Consider for those at high risk	Consider for those at high risk	Not recommended	A	Cost-effective
Hepatitis C	One time for those born between 1945–1965	One time for those born between 1945–1965	One time for those born between 1945–1965	Not recommended	B	Cost-effective
Blood pressure	Consider each visit	Consider each visit	Consider each visit	Consider each visit	A	Uncertain
Height	Once a year	Once a year	Consider	Consider	C	Uncertain
Weight	Each visit	Each visit	Each visit	Each visit	C	Uncertain
Immunizations						
Influenza	Annually	Annually	Annually	Annually	A	Cost-effective
Pneumococcal series	Once after age 65[g]	Once after age 65[g]	Once after age 65[g]	Once after age 65[g]	A	Cost-effective
Tetanus	Booster every 10 years	Booster every 10 years	Booster every 10 years	Not recommended	C	Cost-effective (a single booster at age 65)
Herpes zoster	Once after age 60	Once after age 60	Once after age 60	Once after age 60	A	Cost-effective

Table 11.1—Preventive Health Measures Available for Older Adults and Recommended Use (continued)

Procedure	≥10 years remaining life expectancy	5 to <10 years remaining life expectancy	Moderate dementia	Near end of life	SOE	Cost-effectiveness
Healthy lifestyle counseling						
Smoking cessation	Every visit	Every visit	Discuss with caregiver	Not recommended	A	Telephone quit lines and counseling are cost-effective.
Exercise	Annually	Annually	Consider annually	Consider	C	Uncertain
Alcohol misuse	Annually	Annually	Annually	Recommended initially, then if symptomatic	A	Screening and brief behavioral counseling interventions for alcohol abuse are cost-effective.
Driving assessment	Consider	Consider	Routinely	Consider	A	Uncertain
Sexual function	Annually	Annually	Consider annually	Not recommended	D	Uncertain
Geriatric health issues						
Urinary incontinence screening	Annually	Annually	Annually	Annually	C	Uncertain
Visual acuity testing[h]	Consider annually	Consider annually	Consider annually	Not recommended	C	Population screening is not cost-effective; however, targeted screening of high-risk groups may be.
Hearing impairment screening[h,i]	Consider annually	Consider annually	Consider annually	Not recommended	C	A simple systematic screen, using an audiometric screening instrument, may be cost-effective for those 55–74 years old.
Cognitive impairment screening[i,j]	If symptomatic	If symptomatic	If symptomatic	If symptomatic	C	Uncertain
Gait and balance screening	Annually	Annually	Annually	Annually	C	Uncertain
Depression screening[h,i]	Annually	Annually	Annually	Annually	C	Uncertain
Falls risk assessment[i]	Annually	Annually	Annually	Annually	C	Uncertain
Advance directives completion[k]	Complete and update as needed	Complete and update as needed	Complete and update as needed	Complete and update as needed	C	Uncertain
Chemoprevention						
Aspirin	See below[l]	See below[l]	See below[l]	See below[l]	A	
Calcium	Not recommended	Not recommended	Not recommended	Not recommended	A	
Vitamin D	Consider 800 IU in adults >70 years old	Consider 800 IU in adults >70 years old	Consider 800 IU in adults >70 years old	Consider 800 IU in adults >70 years old	A	
Multivitamin	Not recommended	Not recommended	Not recommended	Not recommended	D	
Hormone therapy (women)	Not recommended	Not recommended	Not recommended	Not recommended	A	

SOURCE: Adapted with permission from Flaherty JH, Morley JE, Murphy DJ, et al. The development of outpatient clinical glidepaths. *J Am Geriatr Soc.* 2002;50(11):1886–1901.

[a] Cost-effectiveness is the ratio of costs of a test/procedure compared with the benefits of the test/procedure. It is expressed as the cost per year of life saved or the cost per quality-adjusted-life-year saved. Less than $50,000 per life-year gained is considered cost-effective.
[b] A for women up to age 74 years, C otherwise
[c] A remaining life expectancy >10 years, C otherwise
[d] Adults aged 55–80 years old who have a 30 pack-year smoking history and currently smoke or have quit within the past 15 years. www.uspreventiveservicestaskforce.org/Page/Document/UpdateSummaryFinal/lung-cancer-screening (accessed Jan 2016)
[e] Optimal screening interval unknown
[f] Examples: smoking, diabetes, hypertension
[g] If vaccinated with the 23-valent pneumococcal polysaccharide vaccine (PPSV23) before age 65, PPSV23 should be administered again 5 years later and at least 1 year after the 13-valent pneumococcal conjugate vaccine (PCV13).
[h] Required element of Medicare Initial Preventive Physical Examination
[i] Required element of Medicare First Annual Wellness Visit
[j] Required element of Medicare Subsequent Annual Wellness Visits
[k] With patient's consent, end-of-life planning is a required element of the Medicare Initial Preventive Physical Examination
[l] Men: 45–79 years old when benefit from myocardial infarction reduction outweighs risk of GI hemorrhage; coronary heart disease risk estimation tool: http://cvdrisk.nhlbi.nih.gov/calculator.asp (accessed Jan 2016)
Women: 55–79 years old when benefit from ischemic stroke reduction outweighs risk of GI hemorrhage; stroke risk estimation tool: http://stroke.ucla.edu/body.cfm?id=66#calculaterisk (accessed Jan 2016)
Those ≥80 years old (men and women): insufficient data for recommendation

Lung Cancer

Lung cancer is the third most common cancer and the leading cause of cancer death in the United States. Smoking results in 85% of U.S. lung cancer cases, and 37% of U.S. adults are current or former smokers. Annual screening for lung cancer with low-dose computed tomography (LDCT) in adults 55–74 years old (American Cancer Society) or 55–80 years old (USPSTF) who have a 30 pack-year smoking history and currently smoke or have quit within the past 15 years is now recommended (SOE=A). Screening should stop when a patient has not smoked for 15 years or life expectancy has declined such that curative lung surgery would not be performed. These recommendations are based on data from the National Lung Screening Trial (NLST), which found that 3 annual LDCTs resulted in a 20% reduction in lung cancer mortality (which translates to 3 or 4 fewer lung cancer deaths per 1,000 participants who had LDCT screening over 6 years) and a 6.7% reduction in all-cause mortality after 6.5 years follow-up. The NNS to prevent one death from lung cancer was 320 (245 in adults 65–74 years old). LDCT was found to have a sensitivity of 93.8% and a specificity of 73.4% in this trial. Harms of LDCT include false-positive tests (95% of positive results do not lead to a lung cancer diagnosis, but further imaging can usually resolve most false positive results; 2.5% require invasive diagnostic procedures), overdiagnosis (estimated at 10% of screen-detected tumors), and radiation exposure. Both the benefits (more lung cancer deaths avoided) and harms of lung cancer screening (eg, false positive tests) were greater in the NLST among adults 65–74 years old than among adults 55–64 years old. LDCT may be of most benefit to adults at the highest risk of lung cancer, and a decision tool for lung cancer screening based on patient risk is available at http://nomograms.mskcc.org/Lung/Screening.aspx (accessed Jan 2016). Three small European trials found no benefit to LDCT, but they were not powered to detect a survival difference; additional trials are underway. Medicare recently proposed to pay for an annual LDCT to screen adults 55–74 years old at high risk (30 pack-years, current smoker, or quit in the past 15 years) for lung cancer.

Other Cancers

The USPSTF states there is insufficient evidence to recommend whole-body skin examination by a primary care clinician for early detection of skin cancer or to counsel older adults about sun protection. There is also insufficient evidence to assess the benefits and harms of screening for oral cancer, bladder cancer, and thyroid cancer (the American Cancer Society does recommend screening for thyroid cancer by palpation annually). In addition, screening for ovarian cancer with CA-125, transvaginal ultrasound, or pelvic examination did not reduce ovarian cancer mortality in a large RCT of women 55–74 years old at average risk and is not recommended. Screening pelvic examinations in asymptomatic women are also not recommended, because the examination is not associated with improved health outcomes. Table 11.2 lists the diseases that the USPSTF does not recommend screening for in asymptomatic older adults.

OTHER SCREENING TESTS AND PREVENTIVE MEASURES

Thyroid Disease

Because of the low cost of screening, the increasing risk of subclinical and clinical hyperthyroidism and hypothyroidism with age, and the low risks of treatment (particularly for hypothyroidism), screening older adults for thyroid dysfunction by measurement of thyroid-stimulating hormone every 2–5 years is recommended by some clinical experts. Screening those ≥60 years old in the clinical setting detects previously unsuspected hyperthyroidism in 0.1%–0.9% and hypothyroidism in 0.7%–2.1%. However, the USPSTF states there is insufficient evidence to recommend for or against screening for thyroid disease in high-risk patients, including older adults. Instead, the USPSTF states that clinicians should remain alert for subtle or nonspecific symptoms of thyroid dysfunction when examining older patients and maintain a low threshold for diagnostic evaluation of thyroid function.

Hypertension

Strong indirect evidence supports screening for hypertension. Randomized trials have confirmed that treatment of isolated systolic hypertension in patients >60 years old with pharmacologic therapy reduces the risk of stroke, coronary disease, and total mortality (SOE=A). Evidence is lacking to recommend an optimal interval for screening adults for hypertension, and recommendations range from as frequently as each visit to biennially. Because of the variability in individual blood pressure measurements, it is recommended that hypertension be diagnosed only after ≥2 increased readings are obtained on at least 2 visits over a period of a week to several weeks.

Diabetes

The incidence of diabetes increases with age until about 65 years old and then levels off. Although a history of retinopathy is more common in older adults with middle-age onset diabetes than those with older-age onset, there is no difference in prevalence of cardiovascular disease or peripheral neuropathy by age of onset. Older adults

Table 11.2—Tests Not Recommended by the USPSTF for Screening Asymptomatic Older Adults for Disease

USPSTF recommends against screening an asymptomatic adult for:	With these tests:
Asymptomatic bacteriuria	Urinalysis
Coronary artery disease in adults with few or no risk factors	ECG, exercise treadmill test, or electron-beam CT
Carotid artery stenosis	Duplex ultrasonography
Cervical cancer in women ≥65 years old who have had adequate prior screening or among women who have had a hysterectomy with removal of the cervix for benign disease	Pap smear
Colon cancer in adults ≥85 years old (Screening may be modestly beneficial in adults 76–85 years old with long remaining life expectancy and no or few comorbidities.)	Fecal occult blood test/sigmoidoscopy/colonoscopy
COPD	Spirometry
Ovarian cancer	Transvaginal ultrasonography, CA-125, or pelvic examination
Pancreatic cancer	Ultrasonography, abdominal palpation, or serologic markers
Prostate cancer	PSA and/or digital rectal examination
USPSTF states the evidence is insufficient to assess the balance of benefits and harms of screening an asymptomatic adult for:	**With these tests:**
Bladder cancer	Urinalysis, bladder tumor antigen measurement, NMP22 urinary enzyme immunoassay, or urine cytology
Breast cancer in women ≥75 years old	Mammography
Chronic kidney disease	Creatinine-derived estimates of glomerular filtration rate, urine testing for albumin
Oral cancer	Systematic clinical examination of the oral cavity
Peripheral arterial disease	Ankle-brachial index
Skin cancer	Whole-body skin examination
Coronary artery disease in adults at intermediate or high risk	ECG or exercise treadmill test
Thyroid cancer	Palpation
Thyroid disease	Thyroid stimulating hormone
Type 2 diabetes in asymptomatic adults with blood pressure of 135/80 mmHg or lower	Fasting plasma glucose, 2-hour postload plasma, hemoglobin A_{1c}

are at high risk of development of type 2 diabetes due to increasing insulin resistance and impaired pancreatic islet cell function with aging. However, no RCT of screening for diabetes has been performed, and the magnitude of benefit of initiating tight glycemic control during the preclinical phase of diabetes is unknown. In one RCT, intensive lifestyle modification in people with prediabetes delayed progression to clinical diabetes, particularly for adults ≥60 years old, but it is unknown whether early treatment affects micro- or macrovascular outcomes of diabetes or decreases mortality. Based on indirect evidence on the benefits of treatment of type II diabetes, the American Diabetic Association recommends that all adults ≥45 years old be screened in the clinical setting every 1–3 years with a fasting plasma glucose, hemoglobin A_{1c}, or oral glucose tolerance test (SOE=C). A consensus panel recommends screening older adults for diabetes if the patient will be likely to benefit, noting that adults with <10 years of life expectancy are unlikely to benefit from intensive glucose control and are subject to harms associated with hypoglycemia.

Abdominal Aortic Aneurysm (AAA)

AAAs are found in 4%–7% of older men and around 1% of older women. Although AAAs may be asymptomatic for years, as many as 1 in 3 eventually rupture, and rupture is associated with death in 75%–90% of cases. In a meta-analysis, screening men 65–75 years old and surgical repair of those with AAAs ≥5.5 cm was associated with a significant reduction in AAA-related mortality (odds ratio 0.6 [0.5–0.7]) but no significant difference in all-cause mortality (SOE=A). Because the prevalence of AAAs was very low among men who never smoked, and because screening and early treatment are associated with significant harms (increased number of surgeries with associated clinically significant morbidity and mortality), the USPSTF concluded that the balance between the benefits and harms of screening for AAAs was too close to make a general recommendation; however, the USPSTF does recommend 1-time screening of men 65–75 years old who have ever smoked (defined as ≥100 cigarettes in lifetime) with a conventional abdominal duplex ultrasonography (sensitivity 94%–100% and specificity 98%–100%). No significant reduction in AAA-related mortality was found among women, and screening is not recommended. Medicare offers coverage of this screening test only as part of a "welcome-to-Medicare visit" for all men and for women with a family history of AAA.

Osteoporosis

Four of every ten white U.S. women ≥50 years old will eventually experience a hip, spine, or wrist fracture. Over half of women ≥80 years old have osteoporosis (T score less than or equal to −2.5). No clinical trials have evaluated the effectiveness of screening older women for osteoporosis. However, age-based screening is supported by prevalence data. The NNS to prevent one hip fracture ranges from 731 for women 65–69 years old to 143 for women 75–79 years old. Routine screening (ie, measurement of bone mineral density through dual x-ray absorptiometry) is recommended by the USPSTF for all women ≥65 years old and for women ≥60 years old at high risk. The USPSTF assessed fracture risk using the FRAX tool, which considers patient age, BMI, parental fracture history, and tobacco and alcohol use (www.shef.ac.uk/FRAX/ [accessed Jan 2016]). An appropriate interval for screening has not been determined; however, a study found that osteoporosis would develop in 10% of women >65 years old with normal bone mineral density (BMD) or mild osteopenia (T score −1.01 to −1.49) within 15 years follow-up, within 5 years for women with moderate osteopenia (T score −1.50 to −1.99), and within 1 year for women with advanced osteopenia (T score −2.00 to −2.49). In another study, among women (mean age 75) untreated for osteoporosis, a second bone density test did not meaningfully improve the prediction of hip or major osteoporotic fracture after 4 years. Medicare currently reimburses BMD screening every 2 years regardless of previous test results. When to stop screening is also a matter of controversy. In the Fracture Intervention Trial, the benefit of treatment emerged 18 to 24 months after initiation of treatment.

The USPSTF concludes that the current evidence is insufficient to assess the balance of benefits and harms of screening for osteoporosis in men. However, screening men ≥65 years old with a prior clinical fracture and all men ≥80 years old has been shown to be cost-effective, and several organizations recommend that clinicians assess older men, such as those undergoing androgen therapy, for osteoporosis risk and screen those at increased risk who are candidates for drug therapy.

Hyperlipidemia

Data are limited on the benefits of cholesterol-lowering medications for primary prevention of cardiovascular disease among adults >75 years old. Therefore, initiation of statins for primary prevention of atherosclerotic cardiovascular disease (ASCVD) in individuals >75 years requires consideration of patient life expectancy, risks and benefits, and patient preferences. Although there is no agreed-upon life expectancy at which to stop screening for hyperlipidemia, most of the RCTs that evaluated statins for primary prevention showed that statins reduced cardiovascular events after 5 years in middle-aged adults. The PROSPER trial showed that pravastatin reduced cardiovascular events after 3 years in adults 70–82 years old at high risk (SOE=A). The 2013 American College of Cardiology and the American Heart Association recommend that individuals 40–75 years old with LDL-C of 70–189 mg/dL who do not have ASCVD or diabetes, but have an estimated 10-year ASCVD of ≥7.5% begin moderate- or high-intensity statin therapy. High-intensity statin therapy is recommended for all adults with LCL-C ≥190 mg/dL. RCT evidence supports use of an initial fasting lipid panel for screening (total cholesterol, triglycerides, HDL-C and calculated LDL-C). Direct LDL-C testing, which does not require a fasting sample measurement, is available; however, calculated LDL (which requires fasting) is the validated measurement used in trials for risk assessment and treatment decisions. Based on these new guidelines, among adults 60–75 years old without ASCVD not on statins, 87% of men and 54% of women would now be eligible. However, risks of statin therapy include statin myopathy, diabetes, and drug-drug interactions. Risks may be greater for adults >75 years old and those with multiple comorbidities.

Hepatitis C

Hepatitis C virus (HCV) is the most common chronic blood-borne pathogen in the United States and a leading cause of complications from chronic liver disease, and HCV-related end-stage liver disease is the most common indication for liver transplant in U.S. adults. The prevalence of the anti-HCV antibody in the United States is ≥50% in high-risk persons (eg, those with past or current injection drug use) and is 3-4% in U.S. adults born between 1945 and 1965 (which may be from blood transfusions before screening was implemented in 1992). Most with chronic HCV are unaware. In patients at high-risk, anti-HCV antibody testing is associated with high sensitivity (>90%) and NNS of <20 persons to identify

1 case of HCV infection. Identifying infected patients at earlier stages of disease may reduce complications from liver damage, because antiviral regimens are effective. Therefore, the USPSTF recommends offering 1-time screening for HCV infection to adults born between 1945 and 1965 and those at high risk.

Other Diseases

The USPSTF does not recommend routine screening for chronic kidney disease, for asymptomatic carotid artery stenosis, or for peripheral artery disease (Table 11.2). Because there is inadequate evidence that treatment of asymptomatic, screen-detected vitamin D deficiency improves health outcomes, no primary care organization recommends screening adults for vitamin D deficiency.

HEALTHY LIFESTYLE COUNSELING

Physical Activity

Physical inactivity is recognized as a risk factor for many diseases (eg, coronary artery disease, diabetes, and obesity). Increasing physical activity in sedentary older adults reduces morbidity and mortality and improves psychological health, promotes functional independence, and prevents falls. Almost all older adults can engage safely in a program of moderate physical activity (such as walking) or lifestyle modification, without special screening. Stress testing is recommended for any older adult who intends to begin a vigorous exercise program (eg, strenuous cycling, jogging). The U.S. Department of Health and Human Services recommends that older adults get at least 150 minutes per week of moderate-intensity or 75 minutes per week of vigorous-intensity aerobic physical activity, as well as muscle-strengthening activities (eg, weight training) twice per week and balance training (eg, tai chi, dance) ≥3 times per week for those at high risk of falls. Clinicians are encouraged to counsel patients about the importance of exercise and to consider patient-specific goals and barriers for exercise, as well as encourage patients to expand current exercise habits as needed. An exercise prescription should address the type, frequency, duration, and intensity of physical activity for each fitness component.

Nutrition

The weight of older adults should be obtained at each visit, and height measured annually and BMI (in kg/m^2) calculated. The USPSTF recommends that obese (BMI ≥30) adults be offered intensive counseling and behavioral interventions to promote sustained weight loss. However, ideal BMI may be higher for older adults than middle-aged adults. In fact, BMIs between 25–29 are associated with the lowest mortality risk for adults ≥70 years old, which may be because of benefits from greater nutritional reserve. In general, higher BMI values are associated with smaller relative mortality risk in older adults than in younger adults. However, weight loss, especially when combined with exercise, may improve physical function and ameliorate frailty among obese older adults (SOE=A). On the other end of the spectrum, malnutrition and undernutrition are common yet frequently unidentified problems in the geriatric population; 15% of older outpatients are malnourished. Nutritional health screens generally include questions on meal frequency, unintentional weight loss, dental health, alcohol intake, money for food, and on the ability to shop, cook, and feed oneself. However, limited data are available on the effectiveness of nutritional screening in primary care.

Alcohol Misuse

Approximately half of the population ≥65 years old drinks alcohol, and many may experience health risks from consuming alcohol or from the combination of alcohol use with medications; approximately 2%–4% have abuse or dependence. Conversely, light to moderate alcohol consumption in middle-aged or older adults has been associated with some health benefits, such as reduced risk of coronary heart disease. Moderate drinking is defined as 1 drink or less per day for adults >65 years old.

The AGS recommends that all older adults ≥65 years old be asked annually about their alcohol use to detect abuse. Those who report alcohol use in the past year should be given the Alcohol Use Disorders Identification Test (AUDIT), the abbreviated AUDIT-Consumption, or a single question screening "How many times in the past year have you had 4 or more drinks in a day?" (SOE=A). The well-known CAGE questionnaire has lower sensitivity than these instruments in detecting risky or hazardous drinking in older adults. Those who report misuse may benefit from behavioral counseling interventions (eg, behavioral strategies such as action plans, drinking diaries, stress management, or problem solving). Brief behavioral counseling interventions are effective in reducing heavy drinking episodes in adults with risky or hazardous drinking.

Smoking Cessation

Smoking cessation at any age decreases rates of COPD, many cancers, and coronary artery disease. Clinicians should ask all adults about tobacco use. If an adult uses tobacco, he or she should be counseled to quit. Once he or she is ready to quit, there should be documentation of a quit date, discussion of therapies to aid cessation, and

Table 11.3—Components of Medicare Wellness Visits

	Initial Preventive Physical Examination (IPPE)[a]	First Annual Wellness Visit[b]	Subsequent Annual Wellness Visits[c]
History			
Past medical/surgical history	✓	✓	✓
Current medications (including calcium and vitamins)	✓	✓	✓
Family history	✓	✓	✓
Alcohol, tobacco, and illicit drug use	✓	HRA	HRA
Diet	✓	HRA	HRA
Physical activities	✓	HRA	HRA
Review risk factors for depression (eg, past history) and depression screen	✓	✓	✓
Review functional ability (ADLs)	✓	✓	✓
Fall risk	✓	✓	
Home safety	✓	✓	
Hearing impairment	✓	✓	
Examination			
Vital signs, including weight, height, blood pressure, BMI	✓	✓	✓
Visual acuity screen	✓		
Other based on history	✓	✓	✓
Counseling and referral			
Based on history and examination	✓		
End-of-life planning, provide verbal or written information[d]	✓		
Preventive services plan			
Includes a brief written plan of appropriate screenings and other preventive services (eg, checklist) to be given to the beneficiary	✓	Establish a written schedule based on USPSTF and ACIP[e]	Update written schedule
Laboratory tests	None included	None included	
Health Risk Assessment[f]			
Demographic data (age, gender, race, ethnicity)		✓	Update
Self-assessment of health status		✓	Update
Psychosocial risks (depression, life satisfaction, stress, anger, loneliness/social isolation, pain, and fatigue)		✓	Update
Behavioral risks (tobacco use, physical activity, nutrition and oral health, alcohol consumption, sexual health, motor vehicle safety [seat belt use]), and home safety		✓	Update
ADLs and IADLs		✓	Update
List of providers/suppliers		Establish list	Update
Cognitive function			
Direct observation combined with patient report and concerns of family and others		✓	✓

Table 11.3—Components of Medicare Wellness Visits (continued)

	Initial Preventive Physical Examination (IPPE)[a]	First Annual Wellness Visit[b]	Subsequent Annual Wellness Visits[c]
Establish list of risk factors and conditions for which primary, secondary, or tertiary interventions are recommended or underway		For example: mental health conditions, or conditions identified through IPPE	Update
Provide personalized advice and referral to health education or preventive counseling services			
Examples: weight loss, physical activity, tobacco cessation, fall prevention, nutrition	✓	✓	✓

NOTE: HRA = health risk assessment; ADLs = activities of daily living; IADLs = instrumental activities of daily living
[a] Initial Preventive Physical Examination (IPPE) is available to all newly enrolled Medicare beneficiaries within the first 12 months after the effective date of their first Medicare Part B coverage period (a one-time benefit).
[b] Medicare covers an annual wellness visit (AWV) for beneficiaries who are no longer in the first 12 months of their Part B coverage period. Medicare pays for only one *first* AWV per lifetime.
[c] Medicare pays for one subsequent AWV per year.
[d] End-of-life planning includes the beneficiary's ability to prepare an advance directive and whether the provider is willing to follow the beneficiary's wishes as expressed in the advance directive.
[e] May be a checklist for the next 5–10 years as appropriate, based on recommendations of the USPSTF and the Advisory Committee on Immunization Practices (ACIP) and the individual's health status, screening history, and age-appropriate preventive services covered by Medicare.
[f] For an example HRA, see www.howsyourhealth.org/MEDICAREAAFPPACKAGE.pdf (accessed Jan 2016).

follow-up in person or by phone within 3–7 days of the quit date and monthly for the first 3 months (SOE=A).

Sexual Dysfunction and Sexually Transmitted Infections

Increasingly, Americans ≥50 years old are afflicted with sexually transmitted infections (STIs) and HIV. Nationally, approximately 20% of patients with HIV are >50 years old. The USPTSF recommends routine screening of adults up to age 65, and screening adults >65 years old who are at increased risk. A recent cost-effective analysis found that one-time HIV screening is cost-effective for patients age 65–75 years old (<$60,000 per quality-adjusted life year gained) if the tested population has an HIV prevalence ≥0.1%, the screened patient has a partner at risk, and counseling is streamlined (abbreviated pretest counseling).

Although the prevalence of sexual activity declines with age (73% among adults 57–64 years old versus 26% among adults 75–85 years old) and is significantly less common among women than men, many older adults are sexually active. The USPSTF recommends high-intensity behavioral counseling to prevent STI for all sexually active adults at increased risk of STIs.

GERIATRIC HEALTH ISSUES

Although there are little data examining the effectiveness of screening or counseling about geriatric health issues, expert panels generally recommend clinicians screen for these conditions annually. Assessing for geriatric health issues is also an essential component of Medicare's wellness exams (Table 11.3). The elements of a comprehensive geriatric assessment (CGA) include assessment of medications, cognitive status, functional status, nutritional status, hearing, vision, affect, social support, gait, and balance. CGA has been associated with improvements in general well-being, life satisfaction, instrumental activities of daily living, and fewer clinic visits (SOE=A). Although the benefits of cancer screening tests may not be achieved for 10 years, the benefits of diagnosing and treating older adults with geriatric health issues can be immediate. Therefore, screening for these conditions should be of high priority in frail older adults with limited life expectancy.

Falls

Falls are the leading cause of injury in adults ≥65 years old, and the AGS recommends that clinicians ask patients about falls, balance, or gait problems annually. Around 30%–40% of noninstitutionalized older adults fall each year, and the annual incidence of falls approaches 50% in those >80 years old. Increasing age, a history of falls, mobility problems, and poor performance on the "Timed Up and Go test" are important risk factors for falls. Extrinsic factors that contribute to falls include poor lighting, obtrusive furniture, inadequate footwear, slippery floors, loose floor coverings, and bathrooms without handrails or grab bars. A multifactorial risk assessment for falls, which incorporates a focused medical history, physical examination, functional assessments, and review of extrinsic factors, is recommended by AGS for older adults with 2 falls in the past year or 1 fall if combined with gait or balance problems assessed by a standardized gait and balance test. The AGS recommends several primary care–based interventions to prevent falls (eg, exercise and physical therapy, vitamin D supplementation, adaptation or modification of home environment, withdrawal or minimization of psychoactive or other medications, management of postural hypotension, and management of foot problems/footwear).

Incontinence

Incontinence is estimated to affect 30%–60% of older adults. Continence problems, which have major social and emotional consequences, are frequently treatable, but only 30%–45% of women with incontinence seek care. Because of the high prevalence of undiagnosed incontinence, older women should be specifically asked about urinary incontinence as part of a review of systems, particularly those who have had children, who have comorbid conditions associated with increased risk of urinary incontinence (ie, diabetes, neurologic disease, obesity), and who are >65 years old. The following screening questions have been suggested: Do you ever leak urine when you don't want to? Do you ever leak urine when you cough, laugh, or exercise? Do you ever leak urine on the way to the bathroom? Do you ever use pads, tissue, or cloth in your underwear to catch urine?

Cognitive Status

The USPSTF concluded that evidence is insufficient to recommend screening older adults for dementia. However, early detection and diagnosis of dementia through the assessment of patient-, family-, or physician-recognized signs and/or symptoms was not considered screening by the USPSTF and was not the focus of that group's recommendations. Meanwhile, a Medicare annual wellness visit must include detection of cognitive impairment by direct observation with due consideration of concerns raised by the patient, family, or others. Medicare does not require use of a standardized tool for assessment of cognitive function. However, brief assessment tools, such as the Mini-Cog (clock drawing test combined with a three-item recall test), the Memory Impairment Screen, and the General Practitioner Assessment of Cognition may be helpful. All require <5 minutes to administer; are easily administered by staff who are not physicians; and are relatively free of educational, language, and/or culture bias (all are available at www.nia.nih.gov). Early detection of dementia may lead to improved symptom control, help patients maintain independence, and help reduce caregiver stress and depression.

Depression

Studies report a 1%–2% prevalence of a major depressive disorder, 2% prevalence of dysthymia, and 13%–27% prevalence of subsyndromal depression among community-dwelling older adults. However, depression is often missed by primary care physicians. The USPSTF recommends that clinicians screen adults for depression as long as they work in practice settings equipped to treat and follow patients with this disease; annual screening is covered by Medicare. The Geriatric Depression Scale, the one-question screen "Do you often feel sad or depressed?", or the Patient Health Questionnaire-2 ("Over the past 2 weeks, have you felt down, depressed, or hopeless?"and "Over the past 2 weeks, have you felt little interest or pleasure in doing things?") are effective screening tools. A positive response should be followed by a fuller assessment of severity and duration of symptoms. Because of high suicide rates, particularly in older white men, older adults who screen positive should be specifically asked about these symptoms.

Vision

Approximately, 9% of adults ≥60 years old have impaired visual acuity (best-corrected vision of 20/40 or worse). The most common causes are presbyopia, cataracts, glaucoma, diabetic retinopathy, and age-related macular degeneration. Data from three RCTs show that screening for vision impairment in older adults in primary care settings is not associated with improved visual or other clinical outcomes. Based on these data, the USPSTF found insufficient evidence to recommend for or against visual acuity screening by primary care clinicians. However, a visual exam is a necessary component of a Medicare initial preventive physical examination. The USPSTF also found insufficient evidence to recommend screening adults for glaucoma; however, Medicare does cover annual glaucoma screening for those at high risk.

Hearing

The prevalence of hearing loss is 20%-40% in adults ≥50 years old and more than 80% for those ≥80 years old. Causes of hearing loss in older adults include presbycusis, genetic factors, exposure to loud noises or ototoxic agents, history of ear infections, and presence of systemic diseases (eg, diabetes). Although one large (N=2,305) randomized trial found that screening for hearing loss was associated with increased hearing aid use at 1 year, screening was not associated with improvement in hearing-related function. The USPSTF states there is insufficient evidence to assess the balance of benefits and harms of screening for hearing loss. However, screening for hearing impairment is a necessary component of Medicare's wellness exam. Although pure-tone audiometry is the gold standard for screening hearing, a whispered voice test at 2 feet has a positive predictive value of approximately 75%.

Mistreatment of Older Adults

Estimates of mistreatment of older adults range from 3% to 14%. Older adults who present with contusions, burns, bite marks, genital or rectal trauma, pressure ulcers, or BMI ≤17.5 kg/m² with no clinical explanation should be asked about possible mistreatment or referred to social work for assessment. Although multiple instruments have been developed to test for different types of mistreatment in older adults (eg, psychological, physical, and/or financial abuse), few have been tested in primary care. The paucity of data led the USPSTF to conclude there is insufficient evidence to recommend routine screening for mistreatment of older adults.

Safety and Preventing Injury

Older adults should be advised to keep a list of emergency numbers by each phone, to check their smoke detectors and carbon monoxide detectors, and to not set their hot water heaters >120°F. Because older adults do not adjust as well to sudden changes in temperature (sometimes because of illness or medicines that impair the body's ability to regulate its temperature), it is important to remind older adults to take precautions against heat stroke. Recommendations include drinking cool/nonalcoholic beverages, resting, taking a cool bath or shower, seeking an air-conditioned environment, and wearing lightweight clothing when the weather is hot.

In addition, older adults should be encouraged to wear seat belts and to undergo regular driving tests. One study found that 75% of adults 75–84 years old, and 70% of adults ≥85 years old were current drivers. Drivers >75 years old have more traffic violations and nonfatal collisions than younger drivers, and some states are considering legislation that would tighten license renewal requirements for older drivers. However, older adults who are forced to stop driving rely more on their families, reduce their social activities, and often become depressed. There is not currently one effective, easily administered test (or series of tests) to evaluate driving competence. However, driving refresher courses and on-the-road evaluations of older adults are available in many communities. Specific questions about driving should be included in the assessment of older adults: How did the older patient get to the primary care visit? How often and under what circumstances does he or she drive? Any traffic violations, accidents, or close calls within the past 6 months, 1 year, 2 years? Any episodes of getting lost while driving? Does the patient feel comfortable and want to continue driving?

Older adults are also encouraged to develop an advance directive and determine a health care proxy.

IMMUNIZATIONS

Several immunizations are currently recommended for older adults. An annual influenza vaccination is recommended for adults ≥50 years old without contraindications (eg, egg allergy). Despite these recommendations, many older adults, especially those of racial and ethnic minorities, do not receive the influenza vaccine. Adults ≥65 years old may receive the standard or high-dose influenza vaccine; however, the intranasally administered live-attenuated influenza vaccine has not been approved for adults ≥50 years old. Although the CDC has not made a recommendation favoring the high-dose influenza vaccine over the standard-dose influenza vaccine, the high-dose vaccine has been demonstrated in an RCT to reduce the rate of laboratory-confirmed influenza by 24.2% compared with the standard-dose influenza vaccine. The rates of serious adverse events were similar in both groups.

Adults ≥65 years old should also receive immunization against pneumococcus (*Streptococcus pneumonia*). The CDC recommends administering the 13-valent pneumococcal conjugate vaccine (PCV13) and 23-valent pneumococcal polysaccharide vaccine (PPSV23) in series. Immunocompetent adults ≥65 years old who have never received PPSV23 should first receive PCV13 followed at least 1 year later by PPSV23. Those who have previously been vaccinated with PPSV23 should receive PCV13 at least 1 year after their most recent dose of PPSV23. For those who received their first dose of PPSV23 before the age of 65 and who will require a second dose, PPSV23 should be administered at least 1 year after PCV13 is given and at least 5 years after the most recent PPSV23.

The Td (tetanus, diphtheria) booster is recommended every 10 years. Adults ≥65 years old may get the Tdap (tetanus, diphtheria, and acellular pertussis) instead. The Tdap is specifically recommended for adults ≥65 years old who have close contact with an infant <12 months old. Herpes zoster vaccine is recommended for those ≥60 years old. In an RCT, the vaccine reduced the incidence of post-herpetic neuralgia by 67% after 3 years in patients ≥60 years old (median age 69).

CHEMOPROPHYLAXIS

Aspirin

In a meta-analysis of prospective RCTs on the sex-specific benefits of aspirin (dosage range 100 mg q48h to 500 mg q24h), among women aspirin significantly reduced the risk of cardiovascular events combined (strokes, myocardial infarctions, or death from either cause) and ischemic strokes but there was no significant effect on myocardial infarctions or cardiovascular mortality. Among men, aspirin therapy reduced the risk of cardiovascular events combined and myocardial infarction but had no significant effects on ischemic strokes or cardiovascular mortality. Aspirin therapy increased the risk of bleeding by approximately 70% in both men and women. The USPSTF recommends aspirin for primary prevention for men with a 10-year risk of coronary heart disease of ≥4% for those aged 45–59 years old, ≥9% for those 60–69 years old, and ≥12% for those 70–79 years old; and for women with a 10-year stroke risk of ≥3% for those 55–59 years old, ≥8% for those 60–69 years old, and ≥11% for those 70–79 years old. See Table 11.1 for websites where individual patient data can be entered to calculate these risks. The ARR depends on the individual risks of cardiovascular disease and gastrointestinal bleeding for men and on individual risks of stroke and gastrointestinal bleeding for women (to calculate ARR for an individual, see www.uspreventiveservicestaskforce.org/Page/Document/RecommendationStatementFinal/aspirin-for-the-prevention-of-cardiovascular-disease-preventive-medication#fig4 [accessed Jan 2016]).

Calcium, Vitamin D, and Multivitamins

The USPSTF recommends against daily supplementation with ≤400 IU of vitamin D_3 and ≤1,000 mg of calcium for primary prevention of fractures, because supplementation at these levels does not prevent incident fractures and increases the incidence of renal stones (NNH=273 over 7 years; SOE=A). The USPSTF also states the evidence is insufficient to recommend combined vitamin D (>400 IU) and calcium supplementation (>1,000 mg) for the primary prevention of fractures or other diseases. In a meta-analysis published after the USPSTF review, high-dose supplementation of vitamin D (≥800 IU daily) was associated with prevention of hip and nonvertebral fractures in adults ≥65 years old (SOE=A). According to the Institute of Medicine (IOM), assuming minimal sun exposure, the recommended daily allowance to meet or exceed the vitamin D needs for 97.5% of the population is daily dietary intake of 600 IU in adults 50–70 years old and 800 IU in adults >70 years old. Most adults can reach these targets through sun exposure or dietary intake (such as fatty fish, cod liver oil, dairy products, fortified beverages and foods); however, the targets may be difficult for some adults ≥70 years old, and vitamin D supplementation should be considered. The IOM also recommends dietary intake of 1,200 mg/d of calcium in women >50 years old and men >70 years old, and 1,000 mg/d for men 51–70 years old. A rough method of estimating dietary calcium intake is to multiply the number of dairy servings consumed per day by 300 mg. The USPSTF also concludes there is insufficient evidence to recommend a multivitamin for prevention of cardiovascular disease or cancer. The 2010 Dietary Guidelines for Americans suggest that nutrients should come primarily from eating a diet rich in fruits, vegetables, whole grains, fat-free and low-fat dairy products, and seafood.

Other

Hormone therapy for chemoprophylaxis is not recommended, because the Women's Health Initiative Trial showed that it (ie, estrogen plus progesterone) increased the risk of ischemic stroke, coronary artery disease, venous thrombosis, pulmonary embolism, decline in cognitive function, urinary incontinence, and invasive breast cancer among older women. The USPSTF recommends that clinicians engage in shared, informed decision making with women ≥35 years old with a 5-year projected risk of breast cancer of ≥3% (calculated using the Breast Cancer Risk Assessment Tool [www.cancer.gov/bcrisktool, accessed Jan 2016] or other models) for whom the potential benefits of risk-reducing medications (eg, tamoxifen, raloxifene) outweigh the potential risks (considering a woman's age [data on risk/benefit ratio available for women up to age 79], comorbid conditions, presence of a uterus, and risks of thromboembolic or medication-related adverse events).

COUNSELING ON CANCER SCREENING AND PREVENTIVE HEALTH

Delivery of preventive health services to older adults can be challenging for many reasons. First, many preventive health services are available, and primary care clinicians are often relied on to deliver or at least discuss most of these services. Second, there is little reimbursement for counseling about screening tests or geriatric health issues, and time during clinic visits often needs to be spent caring for older adults' acute or chronic medical conditions. Third, experts increasingly recommend that clinicians consider a patient's remaining life expectancy when deciding which screening tests to recommend; however, estimating remaining life expectancy may be difficult, and discussing remaining life expectancy with patients may be uncomfortable. Few studies have addressed ways to discuss life expectancy with patients in the context of clinical decision-making around preventive services. Finally, many older adults suffer from comcomitant disorders that encompass multiple risk factors; this presents a challenge to clinicians to synthesize the evidence and in turn make individual recommendations to patients for primary, secondary, and tertiary screening measures.

Several tools are available to help clinicians estimate patients' remaining life expectancy to guide screening decisions. One available prognostic index includes 11 questions (eg, history of diabetes, difficulty walking several blocks) that patients can answer during an office visit to help predict their risk of 5-year or 9-year mortality. In another framework, clinicians are first asked to estimate whether an individual patient is in the top quartile of health, the bottom quartile of health, or in average health, for his or her age group. Then, clinicians are referred to life expectancy tables stratified by age and health. Additional tools to help clinicians prognosticate are available at www.eprognosis.org (accessed Jan 2016).

When discussing cancer or other screening tests with older adults, clinicians should indicate whether any data suggest that the screening test improves older adults' quality or quantity of life. Clinicians should also discuss the risks of screening, including discomfort from undergoing the test itself, anxiety, potential complications from diagnostic procedures resulting from a false-positive test, false reassurance from a false-negative test, and overdiagnosis/diagnosis of tumors that are of no threat and that may result in overtreatment. Furthermore, clinicians may want to explain that overdiagnosis is thought to increase with age because of decreasing life expectancy, competing mortality risks, and slower-growing tumors among older adults. Older adults should be asked how they view the potential benefits and harms of different screening tests, so that their values and preferences are considered in screening decisions. Health maintenance discussions among older adults with limited remaining life expectancies should focus on measures that have benefits likely to be achieved in a short time frame (eg, counseling on home safety, falls prevention, immunizations).

Medicare recently began covering wellness visits for those who have had Part B coverage for >12 months in addition to a "Welcome to Medicare" visit that must be completed within the first 12 months of enrollment (Table 11.3). These visits offer clinicians the opportunity to discuss the pros and cons of many screening tests with older adults and to offer appropriate preventive health measures.

REFERENCES

- Gourlay ML, Fine JP, Preisser JS, et al; Study of Osteoporotic Fractures Research Group. Bone-density testing interval and transition to osteoporosis in older women. *N Engl J Med.* 2012; 366(3):225–233.

  This study aimed to investigate the interval before 10% of women with normal bone mineral density (BMD) or osteopenia developed osteoporosis (before fracture occurrence or initiation of osteoporosis treatment). This was a prospective cohort study that included 4,957 women >67 years old and followed them up to 15 years. The study found that for women with normal BMD (T score −1.00 or greater) or mild osteopenia (T score −1.01 to −1.49), osteoporosis developed by 15 years for 10% of women. For women with moderate osteopenia (T score −1.50 to −1.99), osteoporosis developed by 5 years. For women with advanced osteopenia (T score −2.00 to −2.49) osteoporosis developed in 1 year. These data suggest that longer screening intervals (up to 15 years) than what is typically covered by Medicare (every 2 years) may be appropriate for women with initial normal BMD or mild osteopenia.

- Institute of Medicine (IOM). Dietary reference intakes for calcium and vitamin D. Washington DC: National Academy of Sciences; 2010. Available at https://iom.nationalacademies.org/~/media/Files/Report%20Files/2010/Dietary-Reference-Intakes-for-Calcium-and-Vitamin-D/Vitamin%20D%20and%20Calcium%202010%20Report%20Brief.pdf (accessed Jan 2016).

  In 2010, the IOM published specific recommendations about calcium and vitamin D intake by age. The IOM recommended calcium intake of 1,200 mg/d for women >50 years old and for men >70 years old. For men 50-70 years old, the IOM recommended 1,000 mg/d of calcium. The IOM also recommended 600 IU/d of vitamin D for adults 50–70 years old and 800 IU/d for adults >70 years old.

- Lee SJ, Boscardin WJ, Stijacic-Cenzer I, et al. Time lag to benefit after screening for breast and colorectal cancer: meta-analysis of survival data from the United States, Sweden, United Kingdom, and Denmark. *Brit Med J.* 2013;346:e8441.

  The authors performed a meta-analysis of survival data from population based, randomized controlled trials that compared populations screened and not screened for breast or colorectal cancer. The study aimed to determine an estimate of the length of time needed after breast or colorectal cancer screening before a survival benefit is observed. For breast cancer screening, it took on average 10.7 years before one death from breast cancer was prevented for

---

Choosing Wisely® Recommendations

Prevention

- Do not use PET/CT for cancer screening in healthy individuals.

- Do not recommend screening for breast, colorectal, or prostate cancer (with the PSA test) without considering life expectancy and the risks of testing, overdiagnosis, and overtreatment.

- Measurement of PSA is controversial but should not be measured if remaining life expectancy is <10 years.

- Do not repeat colorectal cancer screening (by any method) for 10 years after a high-quality colonoscopy is negative in average-risk individuals.

- Do not perform routine cancer screening for dialysis patients with limited life expectancies without signs or symptoms.

Prevention/Cancer Screening Tests Among Older Adults

- Do not recommend screening for breast, colorectal, or prostate cancer (with the PSA test) without considering remaining life expectancy and the risks of testing, overdiagnosis, and overtreatment.

1,000 women screened. For colorectal cancer screening, it took on average 10.3 years before one death from colorectal cancer was prevented for 1,000 patients screened with fecal occult blood testing. The authors concluded that screening for breast and colorectal cancer is most appropriate for patients with a remaining life expectancy of >10 years.

- National Lung Screening Trial Research Team. Reduced lung-cancer mortality with low-dose computed tomographic screening. *N Engl J Med.* 2011:365(5):395–409.

    This randomized controlled trial compared annual low-dose CT for 3 years and chest radiography in adults 55–74 years old with a smoking history of ≥30 pack-years who had smoked within the past 15 years. The study found a 20% decrease in lung cancer mortality and a 6.7% decrease in all-cause mortality.

- Schonberg MA, Hamel MB, Davis RB, et al. Development and evaluation of a decision aid on mammography screening for women 75 years and older. *JAMA Intern Med.* 2014;174(3):417–424.

    Because guidelines encourage shared decision-making around mammography screening for older women, this study aimed to develop and evaluate a decision aid on mammography screening for women ≥75 years old. The pamphlet decision aid includes information on breast cancer risk, life expectancy, competing mortality risks, possible outcomes of screening, and a values clarification exercise; it is written at a sixth-grade reading level. It was tested among 45 women 75–89 years old in a pretest/posttest trial and was found to improve older women's knowledge of the benefits and risks of screening. In addition, fewer participants intended to be screened after reading the decision aid, especially those with a remaining life expectancy of <10 years. Most women found the decision aid helpful.

- Yourman LC, Lee SJ, Schonberg MA, et al. Prognostic indices for older adults: a systematic review. *JAMA.* 2012;307(2):182–192.

    This systematic review assesses the quality and limitations of prognostic indices for mortality in older adults. The study identified 16 indices that predict risk of mortality from 6 months to 5 years for older adults in the community, nursing home, and hospital. The authors concluded that future studies need to independently test the accuracy of the indices in heterogeneous populations and their effect on clinical outcomes before widespread use can be recommended. Ideally, mortality indices could be used to help target clinical services (eg, cancer screening) to older adults who may benefit.

Mara A. Schonberg, MD, MPH

CHAPTER 12—PHARMACOTHERAPY

KEY POINTS

- Risk factors associated with inappropriate prescribing and overprescribing include having more than one prescriber, poor record keeping, and using more than one pharmacy.

- Evidence suggests that underprescribing of indicated medications for older adults is a bigger problem than the prescribing of inappropriate medications.

- Cardiovascular drugs, diuretics, NSAIDs, hypoglycemics, second-generation antipsychotics, anticoagulants, and antiplatelet agents are the drug classes most often associated with preventable adverse drug events.

- Age-associated changes in body composition, metabolism, and pharmacodynamics make benzodiazepine use by older adults especially hazardous.

- Collaboration with pharmacists and access to up-to-date drug information can help to minimize the total number of medications and dosages prescribed for individual patients and to avoid important drug-drug and drug-disease interactions.

Adults ≥65 years old are prescribed the highest proportion of medications relative to their percentage of the U.S. population. Currently, approximately 13% of the U.S. population is ≥65 years old; this age group purchases 33% of all prescription drugs. These figures are expected to increase to 25% and 50%, respectively, by the year 2040.

Drugs are the most common treatment for acute and chronic diseases. They are also used to prevent many diseases and disorders experienced by older adults. Successful pharmacotherapy requires the correct medication at the correct dosage, for the correct disease or condition, for the correct patient. Unfortunately, achieving these goals is not simple or easy. Many other factors come into play, including the patient's other disease states, other medications, adherence, beliefs, functional status, physiologic changes due to aging and disease, and ability to afford the medication. The basic principle of prescribing for older patients—briefly, "start low, go slow"—is repeated often. However, even when this principle is adhered to, some patients will have negative outcomes from one or more of their medications.

Although the principles of pharmacotherapy have not changed significantly during the past 20 years, drug treatment has become much more complex. More medications are available every year, some with a new pharmacologic profile or mechanism of action. In addition, many available agents have expanded indications, some of which are approved by the FDA and some of which are off-label. Additional complicating factors include frequent changes in the managed-care formulary, scientific advances in the understanding of drug-drug interactions, the change of many medications from prescription to nonprescription, and the boom in an unregulated third class of medications called nutriceuticals, including nutritional supplements, alternative medicines, and herbal preparations. Finally, very little information is available about use of these unregulated medications in older adults, particularly in sick older patients on other medications.

AGE-ASSOCIATED CHANGES IN PHARMACOKINETICS

Pharmacokinetic studies define the time course of a drug and its metabolites throughout the body with respect to absorption, distribution, metabolism, and elimination. The effects of aging on each of these four parameters have been studied, with the resulting generalizations incorporated into the principles of prescribing for older adults.

Absorption

Aging does not affect the extent of drug absorption via the GI tract to any clinically significant degree, although the rate of absorption may be slowed. Consequently, the peak serum concentration of a drug in older patients may be lower and the time to reach it delayed, but the overall amount absorbed *(bioavailability)* does not differ in younger and older patients. Exceptions include drugs that undergo an extensive first-pass effect (eg, nitrates); they tend to have higher serum concentrations or increased bioavailability, because less drug is extracted by the liver as a consequence of decreased hepatic size and blood flow.

Factors that have a greater impact on drug absorption include the way a medication is taken, what it is taken with, and a patient's comorbid illnesses. For example, the absorption of many fluoroquinolones (eg, ciprofloxacin) is reduced when they are taken with divalent cations such as calcium, magnesium, and iron, which are found in antacids, sucralfate, dairy products, or vitamins. Enteral feedings interfere with the absorption of some drugs (eg, levothyroxine, phenytoin). An increase in gastric pH from proton-pump inhibitors,

H₂ antagonists, or antacids can increase the absorption of some drugs, such as nifedipine and amoxicillin, and decrease the absorption of other drugs, such as the imidazole antifungals, ampicillin, cyanocobalamin, and indinavir. Agents that promote or delay GI motility, such as stimulant laxatives and metoclopramide, can, in theory, affect a drug's absorption by increasing or decreasing the time spent in the segment of the GI tract necessary for dissolution or absorption. Another mechanism that can increase or decrease drug absorption is the inhibition or induction of enzymes in the GI tract (see drug interactions, below).

Distribution

Distribution refers to the locations in the body a drug penetrates and the time required for the drug to reach those locations. Distribution is expressed as the volume of distribution (Vd), with units of volume (eg, liters) or volume per weight (eg, L/kg).

Age-associated changes in body composition can alter drug distribution. In older adults, drugs that are water soluble *(hydrophilic)* have a lower volume of distribution, because older adults have less body water and lean body mass. Examples include ethanol and lithium. Digoxin, which distributes and binds to skeletal muscle, has been reported to have a reduced volume of distribution in older adults because of their reduced muscle mass. Drugs that are fat soluble *(lipophilic)* have an increased volume of distribution in older adults, because fat stores are greater in older than in younger people. Thus, in older adults, lipophilic drugs take longer to reach a steady-state concentration and longer to be eliminated from the body. Examples of fat-soluble drugs include diazepam, flurazepam, and trazodone.

The extent to which a drug is bound to plasma proteins also influences its volume of distribution. Albumin, the primary plasma protein to which drugs bind, is often decreased in older adults; thus, a higher proportion of drug is unbound (free) and pharmacologically active. Drugs that bind to albumin and that have an increased unbound fraction in older adults include ceftriaxone, diazepam, lorazepam, phenytoin, valproic acid, and warfarin. Normally, additional unbound drug is eliminated; however, age-related decreases in the organ systems of elimination can result in accumulation of unbound drug in the body. Phenytoin provides an example of the way an increase in unbound drug can lead to an unnecessary and potentially harmful dosage increase. A patient with a low serum albumin (≤3 g/dL) whose phenytoin dosage is increased because his or her total phenytoin concentration is subtherapeutic can develop symptoms and signs of phenytoin toxicity after a dosage increase, because the concentration of free phenytoin is increased.

Metabolism

The liver is the most common site of drug metabolism, but metabolic conversion also can occur in the intestinal wall, lungs, skin, kidneys, and other organs. Aging affects the liver by decreasing hepatic blood flow as well as by decreasing hepatic size and mass. Consequently, the metabolic clearance of drugs by the liver may be reduced in older adults. Drug clearance is also reduced with aging for drugs that are subject to the phase I pathways or reactions, which include hydroxylation, oxidation, dealkylation, and reduction. Most drugs metabolized through phase I pathways can be converted to metabolites of lesser, equal, or greater pharmacologic effect than the parent compound (eg, diazepam). Drugs metabolized through the phase II pathways are converted to inactive compounds through glucuronidation, conjugation, or acetylation (eg, lorazepam). Medications subject to phase II metabolism are generally preferred for older adults, because their metabolites are not active and do not accumulate.

The effect of aging on the cytochrome P-450 system and the clinical implications for prescribing have not been completely determined. Cross-sectional data have shown that cytochrome P-450 content declines incrementally, once in the fourth decade and again after age 70. In vitro microsomal activity of cytochrome (CYP) 3A4 is not altered by aging, but in vivo age- and gender-related reductions in drug clearance have been found for the CYP3A4 substrates erythromycin, prednisolone, verapamil, alprazolam, nifedipine, and diazepam. CYP3A4 accounts for 30% of the P-450 content in the liver and is also prominent in the intestinal tract. This isozyme is involved in the metabolism of >50% of medications on the market and can be induced by drugs such as rifampin, phenytoin, and carbamazepine, and inhibited by many drugs, including the macrolide antibiotics, nefazodone, itraconazole, and ketoconazole, as well as grapefruit juice. The isozyme CYP2D6 is involved in the metabolism of 25%–30% of marketed medications and has been associated with only minimal age-related changes. CYP2D6 is involved in the metabolism of many psychotropic drugs and can be inhibited by many agents. In addition, approximately 10% of white people are deficient in CYP2D6 (called poor metabolizers [PMs]) and have reduced ability to clear and increased sensitivity to CYP2D6 substrates. This has been established with venlafaxine whose PMs have a 7-fold and 5-fold increase in serum concentration and adverse effects, respectively, than "normal" extensive metabolizers. The difference in PMs is magnified when adjusted for age; PMs >70 years old are reported to have serum concentrations 8-fold those of PMs <40 years old. Clinically, these patients and those taking CYP2D6 inhibitors (eg, quinidine, paroxetine, fluoxetine) cannot convert codeine and tramadol to their active metabolites and, therefore, have a reduced analgesic response to these agents.

Age and gender differences also have been reported. For example, oxazepam is metabolized faster in older men than in older women. The reason is unknown. Zolpidem's peak serum concentrations and exposure (area under the curve) have been reported to be 44.6% and 40.4% greater in older women, respectively, with only modest differences found between older and younger men.

In drug metabolism, factors other than aging can exaggerate or override the effects of aging. For example, hepatic congestion due to heart failure decreases the metabolism of warfarin, resulting in an increased pharmacologic response. Smoking stimulates monooxygenase enzymes and increases the clearance of theophylline, even in older adults.

Elimination

Elimination refers to a drug's final route(s) of exit from the body. For most drugs, this involves elimination by the kidneys as either the parent compound or as a metabolite(s). Terms used to express elimination are a drug's *half-life* and its *clearance*.

A drug's half-life is the time it takes for its plasma or serum concentration to decline by 50% (eg, from 20 mcg/mL to 10 mcg/mL). Half-life is usually expressed in hours. Steady state is reached when the amount of drug entering the systemic circulation is equal to the amount being eliminated. For a drug administered on a regular basis, 95% of steady state in the body is achieved after 5 half-lives of the drug.

Clearance is usually expressed as volume per unit of time (eg, L/h or mL/min) and represents the volume of plasma or serum from which the drug is removed (ie, cleared) per unit of time. Clearance can also be expressed as volume per weight per unit of time (L/kg/h). Half-life and clearance can also refer to metabolic elimination.

The effects of aging have been studied to a greater extent on kidney function than on liver function. Glomerular filtration declines as a consequence of a decrease in renal size and blood flow and a decrease in functioning nephrons. On average, kidney function begins to decline when people reach their mid-30s, with an average decline of 6–12 mL/min/1.73 m² per decade. Follow-up studies (conducted in men only) over 10–15 years found 3 normally distributed groups: those whose creatinine clearance declined to the extent that it was clinically significant, those whose creatinine clearance declined to the extent that it was statistically but not clinically significant, and those whose creatinine clearance did not change. Renal tubular secretion also declines with age. Frailty may be responsible for a fraction of reduced renal clearance of medication as is the case with gentamicin accounting for 12% lower clearance.

Serum creatinine is not an accurate reflection of creatinine clearance in older adults. Because of the age-related decline in lean muscle mass, production of creatinine is reduced in older adults. The decrease in glomerular filtration rate (GFR) counters the decreased production of creatinine, and serum creatinine stays within the normal range, not revealing the change in creatinine clearance.

The conservative approach in treating older adults is to calculate the appropriate dosage for renally eliminated medications as if the patient's kidney function actually has declined with aging. Measuring a patient's 24-hour creatinine clearance is the most accurate way to determine the appropriate dosage, but doing so is unrealistic because it requires an accurate 24-hour urine collection. An 8-hour urine collection time has been shown to be accurate but has not been widely accepted.

The Cockcroft-Gault equation (C-G) can be used to initially estimate a patient's creatinine clearance (CrCl) (SOE=B in older adults for dosage adjustment):

$$CrCl = \frac{(140 - age)(weight\ in\ kg)(0.85\ if\ female)}{72(stable\ serum\ creatinine\ in\ mg/dL)}$$

Note: serum creatinine in mg/100 mL; 85% less in women

The equation is widely applied, but it has limitations. First, not all patients experience a significant age-related decline in renal function, and for them, the equation underestimates creatinine clearance. Second, for patients whose muscle mass is reduced beyond that of normal aging, the creatinine clearance is overestimated. This would apply to individuals whose serum creatinine is less than normal, ie, <0.7 mg/dL. It has been suggested that 1 mg/dL be substituted for a low serum creatinine. However, normalizing the serum creatinine has not been shown to be a precise estimate, and it generally underestimates the actual creatinine clearance.

Another method for estimating glomerular filtration rate (eGFR) is the Modification of Diet in Renal Disease (MDRD), which is endorsed by the National Kidney Foundation in its Kidney Disease Outcomes Quality Initiative (KDOQI) and the NIH National Kidney Disease Education Program for identifying and staging individuals with chronic kidney disease. The MDRD has not been validated in adults ≥70 years old or in racial or ethnic groups other than white and black Americans. The routine appearance of eGFR on laboratory reports has created confusion about its use to adjust medication dosages, and it is not recommended by KDOQI for this purpose (SOE=A). Analysis of data from the Baltimore Longitudinal Study on Aging recently confirmed that the C-G was the least biased estimate of kidney function compared with the MDRD and Chronic Kidney Disease Epidemiology Collaboration (CKD-EC) equations using measured CrCl as the reference. Both MDRD and CKD-EC significantly overestimate CrCl in older adults. Such an overestimation can result in dosing errors that place patients at increased risk of adverse effects, eg, bleeding with dabigatran, rivaroxaban, and edoxaban.

FDA-labeled dosing is based on the C-G estimated CrCl and the drug's pharmacokinetic characteristics. Substituting eGFR for estimated CrCl can result in suboptimal dosing, especially in patients with Stage 2 chronic kidney disease as their GFR approaches 60 mL/min/1.73 m^2.

In cases in which the patient's kidney function may be impaired but estimates of function are uncertain, the clinician should consider the following:

- Avoid drugs that depend entirely on renal elimination and for which accumulation would result in toxicity (eg, imipenem).
- If the use of such an agent cannot be avoided, obtain an accurate measure of kidney function (eg, an 8- or 24-hour creatinine clearance).
- Monitor serum or plasma concentrations of the drug (eg, aminoglycosides).

AGE-ASSOCIATED CHANGES IN PHARMACODYNAMICS

The pharmacodynamic action of a drug, ie, its time course and intensity of pharmacologic effect, can change with increasing age. An excellent example of such pharmacodynamic changes in older adults has been demonstrated with the benzodiazepines. After a single dose of triazolam, older adults experience more sedation and lower performance on a psychomotor test than younger adults. These differences are attributed to pharmacokinetic changes, ie, to significantly higher plasma triazolam concentrations that are due to reduced clearance in older adults. However, a different pattern has been found for nitrazepam, an intermediate-acting benzodiazepine similar to lorazepam: the pharmacokinetics of nitrazepam were found to be no different in young and older individuals after a single 10-mg dose; yet, 12 hours and 36 hours after a 10-mg dose, older adults made significantly more mistakes on a psychomotor test than when they had taken placebo. Younger individuals did not demonstrate significant impairment at any time. In addition, even with short-term use, young older adults can experience impaired balance and posture after a single dose of a benzodiazepine (SOE=A).

It is uncertain whether the age-associated pharmacokinetic changes of morphine account for the increased level and prolonged duration of pain relief experienced by older adults. Morphine has a smaller volume of distribution, higher plasma concentrations, and longer clearance in older adults than in younger adults. Older adults experience pain relief at least equivalent to that experienced by younger patients at half the intramuscular dose, and the pain relief lasts longer. Thus, the dose or frequency, or both, of morphine given intramuscularly or by intravenous infusion should be lower, at least initially, in older adults.

Pharmacodynamic and pharmacokinetic changes, alone or together, generally result in an increased sensitivity to medications in older adults. In some patients, particularly those who are frail, the use of lower doses, longer intervals between doses, and longer periods between changes in dose are ways to successfully manage drug therapy and to decrease the chances of medication intolerance or toxicity. Disease- and drug-specific monitoring are also necessary to ensure a successful outcome.

OPTIMIZING PRESCRIBING

Optimizing drug therapy for older adults means achieving the balance between prescribing what is indicated to treat the patient's diseases and symptoms, while being consistent with the patient's goals. Overprescribing of drug therapies refers to the use of multiple medications coupled with a lack of appropriateness in medication selection, dosage, or use. In one survey, 40% of nursing-home residents had an order for at least one potentially inappropriate medication. Analyses of national medication use surveys in the ambulatory setting have consistently shown that >20% of older adults received at least one potentially inappropriate medication, with at least one potentially inappropriate medication prescribed at approximately 8% of office visits. Furthermore, nearly 4% of office visits and 10% of medical hospital admissions resulted in a prescription for one or more medications classified as "never" or "rarely appropriate" for older adults. Identification of a potentially inappropriate medication in a patient's regimen is a signal for additional prescribing problems with other medications not considered potentially inappropriate. The potential consequences of overprescribing include adverse drug events, drug-drug interactions, duplication of drug therapy, decreased quality of life, and unnecessary costs. Medications frequently deemed unnecessary based on lack of indication, lack of efficacy, or therapeutic duplication are often from the same medication classes

Table 12.1—Common Inappropriate/ Overprescribed and Underprescribed Medications or Classes

Inappropriate/Overprescribed
- Androgens/testosterone
- Anti-infective agents
- Anticholinergic agents
- Urinary and GI antispasmodics
- Antipsychotics
- Benzodiazepines and nonbenzodiazepine hypnotics (eg, zolpidem, zaleplon, eszopiclone)
- Digoxin (not a first-line drug for atrial fibrillation or heart failure)
- Dipyridamole
- H_2-receptor antagonists
- Fecal softeners
- Insulin, sliding scale
- NSAIDs
- Proton-pump inhibitors
- Sedating antihistamines (H_1-receptor antagonists, eg, diphenhydramine)
- Skeletal muscle relaxants
- Tricyclic antidepressants
- Vitamins and minerals

Underprescribed
- ACE inhibitors for patients with diabetes and proteinuria
- Angiotensin-receptor blockers
- Anticoagulants
- Antihypertensives and diuretics as evidenced by uncontrolled hypertension
- β-blockers for patients after myocardial infarction or with heart failure
- Bronchodilators
- Proton-pump inhibitors or misoprostol for GI protection from NSAIDs
- Statins
- Vitamin D and calcium for patients with or at risk of osteoporosis

Table 12.2—Factors Associated with Inappropriate Prescribing or Overprescribing

Patient Factors
- Advanced age
- Female gender
- Lower educational level
- Rural residence
- Belief in using "a pill for every ill"
- Multiple health problems
- Use of multiple medications
- Use of multiple pharmacies

System Factors
- Multiple prescribers for individual patient
- Poor record keeping
- Failure to review a patient's medication regimen at least annually

Table 12.3—Risk Factors for Adverse Drug Events in Older Adults
- Age >85 years
- Low body weight or BMI
- Six or more concurrent chronic diagnoses
- An estimated CrCl <50 mL/min
- Nine or more medications
- Twelve or more doses of medications per day
- A prior adverse drug event

as those considered inappropriate or overprescribed (Table 12.1). In studies in the U.S. Veterans Administration, 44% of veterans at hospital discharge and 57%–59% of outpatients had prescriptions for one or more unnecessary medications.

For factors associated with inappropriate prescribing or overprescribing, see Table 12.2. Simply limiting the number of medications for a given patient is not always possible or desirable. For example, a patient with heart failure may be appropriately treated with 3 or 4 drugs: a diuretic, an ACE inhibitor, a β-blocker, and perhaps digoxin. If this patient has hyperlipidemia and diabetes mellitus, another 2 or 3 medications could be required. Hence, such a patient would be taking 5–7 indicated medications for major medical conditions alone.

One source to identify potentially inappropriate medications has been the American Geriatrics Society (AGS) Beers criteria. The intent of the AGS Beers criteria is to improve drug selection and reduce exposure to potentially inappropriate medications in older adults. Recommendations are evidence based and appear in 5 categories: drugs to avoid, drugs to avoid in patients with specific diseases or syndromes because the drug can worsen the disease or syndrome, drugs to use with caution, selected drugs whose dose should be adjusted based on kidney function (Table 12.5), and selected drug-drug interactions (DDIs) that have been associated with harmful outcomes in older adults (Table 12.6). A detailed description of the updated 2015 American Geriatrics Society Beers criteria for potentially inappropriate medication use in older adults, including evidence tables, useful clinical tools, and patient education materials, is available at the Geriatrics Care Online website (www.geriatricscareonline.org).

The underprescribing of medications to older adults is also of concern. Underprescribing can result from an effort to avoid overprescribing, a complex medication regimen, or adverse events. It can also result from the thinking that older adults will not benefit from medications intended as primary or secondary prevention, or from aggressive management of chronic conditions, such as hypertension and diabetes mellitus. Underuse of medications was found in 64% of 125 veterans attending a veteran's outpatient clinic. Medications to treat cardiovascular conditions (including hypertension, anticoagulants, and lipid-lowering agents), GI conditions, diabetes, osteoporosis, and COPD were commonly omitted. For other medications often cited as underprescribed in older adults, see Table 12.1.

Table 12.4—Common Adverse Drug Events of Selected Medications

Adverse Drug Event	Medications
Cardiovascular effects	
Decreased heart rate	Cholinesterase inhibitors, β-adrenergic blockers, diltiazem, verapamil, digoxin
Hypotension	Antihypertensives, diuretics, nitrates, phosphodiesterase type 5 inhibitors, α-blockers, tricyclic antidepressants, trazodone
CNS effects	
Delirium	Anticholinergic agents, antiparkinson agents, antidepressants, antipsychotics, opioids, glucocorticoids, benzodiazepines, first-generation antihistamines (eg, diphenhydramine), H$_2$-receptor antagonists, drug withdrawal (eg, benzodiazepines, ethanol)
Depression	β-Adrenergic blockers, benzodiazepines, central-acting antihypertensives
Dizziness	SSRIs, cholinesterase inhibitors
Parkinsonism	Antipsychotics, metoclopramide
Sedation	Antidepressants, antipsychotics, first-generation antihistamines (eg, diphenhydramine), opioids, anticonvulsants, benzodiazepines
Falls	Benzodiazepines, tricyclic and SSRI antidepressants, antipsychotics, sedatives/hypnotics, anticonvulsants, opioids, diuretics, antihypertensives, anticholinergic agents, antiarrhythmics
GI effects	
Bleeding/ulceration	NSAIDs, aspirin, glucocorticoids, bisphosphonates, antiplatelet agents, anticoagulants (eg, warfarin, apixaban, edoxaban, dabigatran, rivaroxaban)
Constipation	Opioids, iron- or calcium-containing antacids, calcium channel blockers, anticholinergic agents, cholestyramine
Diarrhea	Magnesium-containing antacids, SSRIs, cholinesterase inhibitors
Nausea/vomiting	Digoxin, cholinesterase inhibitors, bisphosphonates
Kidney or electrolyte effects	
Hyperkalemia	ACE inhibitors, angiotensin-receptor blockers, potassium supplements, potassium-sparing diuretics
Hypokalemia	Diuretics
Kidney impairment	NSAIDs, triamterene
SIADH/hyponatremia	Carbamazepine, SSRIs, diuretics
Urinary retention	Agents with anticholinergic properties, opioids, calcium channel blockers, α-adrenergic agonists

ADVERSE DRUG EVENTS

An adverse drug event (ADE) is defined as an injury resulting from the use of a drug. Preventable ADEs are among the most serious consequences of inappropriate drug prescribing among older adults. An adverse drug reaction (ADR) is a type of ADE; it refers to harm that is directly caused by a drug at usual dosages. For a listing of risk factors for ADEs in older patients, see Table 12.3.

ADEs are estimated to be responsible for 5%–28% of acute geriatric medical admissions; the estimated annual incidence rate is 26 per 1,000 beds for hospitalized patients. One study estimated there were nearly 100,000 emergency hospitalizations of older adults for ADEs annually in the United States. Adults ≥80 years old accounted for 48% of hospitalizations. Two-thirds of hospitalizations were attributed to warfarin, oral antiplatelet agents, insulin, and oral hypoglycemic drugs. The most common type of ADE was an unintentional overdose (67%). It has been estimated that in the nursing home, for every dollar spent on medications, $1.33 in health care resources is consumed in the treatment of drug-related morbidity and mortality. A cohort study of all long-term care residents in 18 nursing homes in Massachusetts demonstrated that ADEs are common and often preventable in nursing homes. During 28,839 resident-months of observations, 546 ADEs were identified. Overall, 51% of these ADEs were judged to have been preventable. Most of the errors occurred at the ordering and monitoring stages. In a cohort study of residents of 2 long-term care facilities, the overall rate of ADEs was 9.8 per 100 resident-months. Second-generation antipsychotics, anticoagulants, and diuretics were the drug classes most frequently associated with ADEs.

In the ambulatory setting, the ADE rate has been reported to be 50.1 per 1,000 person-years, and the preventable ADE rate to be 13.8 per 1,000 person-years. Cardiovascular drugs, diuretics, NSAIDs, hypoglycemics, and anticoagulants are the drug classes found to be most often associated with preventable ADEs. Again, errors occurred most often at the time of prescribing or were related to inadequate monitoring. Most ADEs (≥95%) experienced by older adults are considered to be predictable. For examples of common ADRs experienced by older adults and the medications that frequently cause them, see Table 12.4.

Table 12.5—Adverse Drug Interactions That Increase the Risk of Harm

Combination	Risk
ACE inhibitor + potassium-sparing diuretic	Hyperkalemia
Anticholinergic + anticholinergic (ie, concurrent use of ≥2 drugs with anticholinergic effects)	Cognitive decline
Calcium channel blockers + erythromycin or clarithromycin	Hypotension and shock
Concurrent use of ≥3 CNS active drugs (antipsychotics, benzodiazepines, nonbenzodiazepine receptor agonist hypnotics, tricyclic antidepressants, SSRIs, and opioids)	Falls and fractures
Digoxin + erythromycin, clarithromycin, or azithromycin	Digoxin toxicity
Lithium + loop diuretics or ACE inhibitor	Lithium toxicity
Peripheral alpha$_1$ blockers + loop diuretics	Urinary incontinence in women
Phenytoin + SMX/TMP	Phenytoin toxicity
Sulfonylureas + SMX/TMP, ciprofloxacin, levofloxacin, erythromycin, clarithromycin, azithromycin, and cephalexin	Hypoglycemia
Tamoxifen + paroxetine (other CYP2D6 inhibitors)	Prevention of converting tamoxifen to its active moiety, resulting in increased breast cancer–related deaths
Theophylline + ciprofloxacin	Theophylline toxicity
Trimethoprim (alone or as SMX/TMP) + ACE inhibitor or angiotensin receptor blocker or spironolactone	Hyperkalemia
Warfarin + SMX/TMP, ciprofloxacin, levofloxacin, gatifloxacin, fluconazole, amoxicillin, cephalexin, and amiodarone	Bleeding
Warfarin + NSAIDs	GI bleeding

Note: SMX/TMP = sulfamethoxazole/trimethoprim
SOURCE: Data from Hines L, Murphy JE. Potentially harmful drug-drug interactions in the elderly: a review. *Am J Geriatr Pharmacother*. 2011;9:364–377; Antoniou T, Gomes T, Juurlink DN, et al. Trimethoprim-sulfamethoxazole-induced hyperkalemia in patients receiving inhibitors of the renin-angiotensin system: a population-based study. *Arch Intern Med*. 2010;170(12):1045–1049; Antoniou T, Gomes T, Mamdani MM, et al. Trimethoprim-sulfamethoxazole induced hyperkalaemia in elderly patients receiving spironolactone: nested case-control study. *BMJ*. 2011;343:d5228; Antoniou T, Hollands S, Macdonald EM, et al; Canadian Drug Safety and Effectiveness Research Network. Trimethoprim-sulfamethoxazole and risk of sudden death among patients taking spironolactone. *CMAJ*. 2015;187(4):E138–143; and American Geriatrics Society 2015 Beers Criteria Update Expert Panel. American Geriatrics Society 2015 Updated Beers Criteria for Potentially Inappropriate Medication Use in Older Adults. *J Am Geriatr Soc*. 2015;63:2227–2246.

A common pathway for ADEs and polypharmacy has been described as the "prescribing cascade." One form of this cascade occurs when a medication results in an ADE that is mistaken as a separate diagnosis and treated with more medications, which puts the patient at risk of additional ADEs and more medications. Examples that have been studied include metoclopramide-induced parkinsonism and the subsequent prescribing of antiparkinson medications, and calcium channel blockers that result in peripheral edema and subsequent use of diuretics.

DRUG-DRUG INTERACTIONS

A drug-drug interaction (DDI) is defined as the pharmacologic or clinical response to the administration of a drug combination that differs from that anticipated from the known effects of each of the two agents when given alone. DDIs can take many forms. For example, absorption can be altered, drugs with similar or opposite pharmacologic effects can result in exaggerated or impaired effects, and drug metabolism can be inhibited or induced. DDIs are important because they may lead to ADEs. The likelihood of DDIs increases as the number of medications a patient is taking increases. Among prescription drugs, cardiovascular and psychotropic drugs are most commonly involved in DDIs. A positive correlation exists between the number of potential DDIs and the number of adverse events experienced by hospitalized older patients. The most common adverse events are neuropsychologic (primarily delirium), arterial hypotension, and acute kidney failure. For drug combinations that are reported to result in increased risk of harmful outcomes in older adults, see Table 12.6. Risk factors associated with DDIs include the use of multiple medications, receiving care from several prescribing clinicians, and using more than one pharmacy.

DRUG-DISEASE INTERACTIONS

Drug-disease combinations common in older adults can affect drug response and lead to ADEs, including exacerbation of existing conditions. Obesity and ascites

Table 12.6—2015 American Geriatrics Society Beers Criteria for Non-Anti-Infective Medications That Should Be Avoided or Have Their Dosage Reduced with Varying Levels of Kidney Function in Older Adults

Medication Class and Medication	Creatinine Clearance (mL/min) at Which Action Is Required	Rationale	Recommendation
Cardiovascular or hemostasis			
Amiloride	<30	Increased potassium and decreased sodium	Avoid
Apixaban	<25	Increased risk of bleeding	Avoid
Dabigatran	<30	Increased risk of bleeding	Avoid
Edoxaban	30–50 <30 or >95	Increased risk of bleeding	Reduce dose Avoid
Enoxaparin	<30	Increased risk of bleeding	Reduce dose
Fondaparinux	<30	Increased risk of bleeding	Avoid
Rivaroxaban	30–50 <30	Increased risk of bleeding	Reduce dose Avoid
Spironolactone	<30	Increased potassium	Avoid
Triamterene	<30	Increased potassium and decreased sodium	Avoid
Central nervous system and analgesics			
Duloxetine	<30	Increased GI adverse effects (nausea, diarrhea)	Avoid
Gabapentin	<60	CNS adverse effects	Reduce dose
Levetiracetam	≤80	CNS adverse effects	Reduce dose
Pregabalin	<60	CNS adverse effects	Reduce dose
Tramadol	<30	CNS adverse effects	Immediate release: reduce dose Extended release: avoid
Gastrointestinal			
Cimetidine	<50	Mental status changes	Reduce dose
Famotidine	<50	Mental status changes	Reduce dose
Nizatidine	<50	Mental status changes	Reduce dose
Ranitidine	<50	Mental status changes	Reduce dose
Hyperuricemia			
Colchicine	<30	GI, neuromuscular, bone marrow toxicity	Reduce dose; monitor for adverse effects
Probenecid	<30	Loss of effectiveness	Avoid

alter the volumes of distribution of lipophilic and hydrophilic drugs, respectively. Patients with dementia can have increased sensitivity or paradoxical reactions to drugs with CNS or anticholinergic activity. Patients with renal insufficiency or impaired hepatic function due to cirrhosis or hepatic congestion have impaired detoxification and excretion of drugs.

PRINCIPLES OF PRESCRIBING

For principles of prescribing for older adults, see Table 12.7. This basic approach applies primarily to medications that are used to treat chronic conditions for which an immediate, complete therapeutic response is not necessary. Dosage adjustment may still be needed for medications used to treat conditions requiring an immediate response (eg, when prescribing antibiotics for a patient with impaired kidney function). Medications that have been newly approved by the FDA should be used cautiously in treating older adults. Such medications are likely to be more expensive, and information about their use in older adults is often limited.

Overprescribing can be prevented by reviewing a patient's medications on a regular basis and each time a new medication is started or a dosage is changed. The importance of maintaining accurate records of all medications taken by the patient cannot be overemphasized. It is crucial to know and document in the patient's record all medications being taken by the patient, including those prescribed by others and those the patient is taking on his or her own. Many patients do not consider vitamins, herbal preparations, or OTC medications (even aspirin) to be medications, so clinicians should be specific when inquiring about a patient's use of other medications.

It is best if the patient brings all medications to the review, including OTC medications, vitamins, and any herbal preparations or other types of supplements (a "brown-bag" evaluation). Examining the containers and labels and asking what each medication is for and how and when it is taken can provide insight into the patient's understanding and adherence to his or her medication regimens. Any medication for which there is no longer an indication for its continued use should be stopped.

Table 12.7—Principles of Prescribing for Older Adults

The basics:
- Start with a low dosage.
- Titrate the dosage upward slowly, as tolerated by the patient.
- Try not to start two medications at the same time.

Determine the following before prescribing a new medication:
- Is the medication necessary? Are there nonpharmacologic ways to treat the condition?
- What are the therapeutic end points, and how will they be assessed?
- Do the benefits outweigh the risks of the medication?
- Is one medication being used to treat the adverse events of another?
- Is there one medication that could be prescribed to treat two conditions?
- Are there potential drug-drug or drug-disease interactions?
- Will the new medication's administration times be the same as those of existing medications?
- Do the patient and caregiver understand what the medication is for, how to take it, how long to take it, when it should start to work, possible adverse events that it might cause, and what to do if such events occur?

At least annually:
- Ask the patient to bring all medications (prescription, OTC, supplements, and herbal preparations) to the office; for new patients, conduct a detailed medication history.
- For prescription medications, determine whether the label directions and dosage match those in the patient's chart; ask the patient how he or she is taking each medication.
- Ask about medication adverse events.
- Note if other medications are being prescribed (by other health care providers) for the patient, and what the medications are and their indications.
- Look for medications with duplicate therapeutic, pharmacologic, or adverse event profiles.
- Screen for drug-drug and drug-disease interactions.
- Eliminate unnecessary medications; confer with other prescribers if necessary.
- Simplify the medication regimen; use the fewest possible number of medications and doses per day.
- Always review any changes with the patient and caregiver; provide the changes in writing.

A new complaint or worsening of an existing condition should prompt consideration of whether or not it could be drug-induced. When considering treatment for a new medical condition, nonpharmacologic approaches should always be considered first. If drug therapy is still indicated, a medication that minimizes the risk of an ADE should be selected.

When initiating therapy, the basic principle should be "start low and go slow." Although the FDA requires that labeling for new medications regarding dosing in older adults not be extrapolated from another patient population (eg, patients with kidney impairment), it does not require that a drug be studied explicitly in older adults. Older adults are included in phase I and II dose tolerability and pharmacokinetic and pharmacodynamic studies of many drugs, but the older adults chosen for these studies are usually healthy and free of concomitant illnesses. Much of what is known about medications and how to use them in sick older patients, particularly those who are frail, is learned only after a medication has been available for several years.

Finally, before prescribing a new medication or renewing a prescription, the clinician should consider the patient's life expectancy, time required to achieve therapeutic benefit, goal of treatment, and treatment targets.

DISCONTINUING MEDICATIONS

Discontinuing medications or de-prescribing is as complicated as starting a new medication, sharing many of the same tasks: recognizing an opportunity such as a care transition or annual review; planning; communicating and coordinating the change with the patient, caregiver, and other healthcare providers; and adequate monitoring and follow-up for withdrawal reactions, disease worsening, and adverse effects (Table 12.4).

NONADHERENCE

Adherence is the extent that medication administration coincides with instructions. Nonadherence and poor adherence to medication regimens is a huge and often unrecognized problem. It is estimated that nonadherence among older adults may be as high as 50%. Patients may be reluctant to admit they are not taking medications or not following directions. Because there are many possible reasons for nonadherence, there is no simple screen. Predictors of nonadherence include asymptomatic disease, inadequate follow-up, patient's lack of insight or perception of the value of treatment, missed appointments and transportation difficulties, and a poor provider–patient relationship. If nonadherence is suspected, clinicians should inquire about difficulties taking medication and adverse events; they should also ask (in a nonjudgmental manner) patients to review which medications they are taking and how they are taking them. Measuring a drug's serum concentration is one way to assess adherence, but assays are available for only a small percentage of medications. Measuring a physiologic or therapeutic response such as blood pressure, heart rate, intraocular pressure, hemoglobin A_{1c}, or a change in hormone concentration is possible for many medications to treat chronic conditions. Other measures include pill counts, refill history, and confirmation by a caregiver. All these measures have limitations, and none is foolproof. The clinician needs to consider the patient's financial, cognitive, and functional status, as well as his or her beliefs about and understanding of medications and diseases.

Prescription drug costs have increased substantially, and supplemental prescription drug benefit plans are expensive. Some plans may still leave a patient with a co-payment that he or she cannot afford or with only a fixed dollar amount for the year. Clinicians should avoid prescribing expensive new medications that have not been shown to be superior to less expensive generic alternatives.

A systematic review of interventions to improve medication compliance in older, community-dwelling adults concluded that multifaceted, tailored interventions to individual barriers were more effective than single interventions (SOE=B). Medication reviews and counseling can be used to identify individual barriers, simplify regimens, and provide education. Telephone call reminders have demonstrated improved compliance in patients with heart failure or cognitive impairment. Reminder charts and calendars have been shown to be less effective. Interactive technology is available in some areas to supervise, remind, and monitor drug adherence. This usually relies on a telephone or Internet connection, which reduces availability for many older adults. This technology has not undergone extensive scientific analysis.

Combination products, ie, those containing more than one medication, offer the advantages of decreased pill burden and increased adherence. Potential disadvantages include exposure to higher dosages than necessary, patients not recognizing that there is more than one medication in the product, and increased cost. Before starting a combination product, it needs to be determined that both medications are necessary and that the fixed doses in the product are appropriate for the patient.

Cognitive impairment can also cause nonadherence, because patients may forget to take medications or confuse them. Simplifying the regimen and involving a caregiver to oversee medication management can be helpful approaches. Medication trays also can help with organization, and they are very useful for patients who have difficulty remembering when they last took a medication.

The older adults' ability to read labels, open containers, or pour medications or even a glass of water may be impaired, so functional assessment can be useful. Some patients may need additional education or reinforcement about the purpose of a medication, especially those used to treat conditions that are usually asymptomatic, such as hypertension and diabetes mellitus. Older adults also may need reassurance regarding the safety and possible adverse events of certain medications, particularly newly prescribed medications or those associated with serious adverse events, such as anticoagulants.

CHOOSING WISELY® RECOMMENDATIONS

Pharmacotherapy

- Do not prescribe a medication without conducting a drug regimen review.

REFERENCES

- American Geriatrics Society 2015 Beers Criteria Update Expert Panel. American Geriatrics Society Updated Beers Criteria for Potentially Inappropriate Medication Use in Older Adults. *J Am Geriatr Soc*. 2015;63(11):616–631.

    A 13-member interdisciplinary panel updated the 2012 AGS Beers Criteria applying a modified Delphi method to an evidence-based systematic review. Recommendations were graded based on the quality of the evidence and benefit-to-harm risk ratio (strength of recommendation). The 2015 AGS Beers Criteria encompass >40 medications or drug classes considered potentially inappropriate (PIMs) for adults ≥65 years old. The criteria are divided into PIMs to avoid, PIMS to avoid in certain diseases and syndromes, PIMS to use with caution, 13 combinations of medications known to cause harmful drug-drug interactions, and medications to avoid or dose-adjust based on kidney function. Two companion papers "How to Use the American Geriatrics Society Updated Beers Criteria – A Guide for Patients, Clinicians, Health Systems, and Payors" and "Alternative Medications for Medications in the Use of High-Risk Medications in the Elderly and Potentially Harmful Drug–Disease Interactions in the Elderly Quality Measures," are available online at http://geriatricscareonline.org/toc/american-geriatrics-society-updated-beers-criteria-for-potentially-inappropriate-medication-use-in-older-adults/CL001

- Dowling TC, Wang ES, Ferrucci L, et al. Glomerular filtration rate equations overestimate creatinine clearance in older individuals enrolled in the Baltimore Longitudinal Study on Aging: Impact on renal drug dosing. *Pharmacotherapy*. 2013;33(9):912–921.

Using data from 269 randomly selected men and women participants from the Baltimore Longitudinal Study of Aging, investigators conducted a cross-sectional analysis comparing the bias and precision performance and dose discordance of equations commonly used to estimate kidney function. Measured 24-hour creatinine clearance (mCrCl) was used as the comparison standard. The Modification of Diet in Renal Disease (MDRD) and Chronic Kidney Disease Epidemiology Collaboration (CKD-EPI) equations significantly overestimated creatinine clearance compared with mCrCl, while the Cockcroft-Gault (CG) equation was the least biased and underestimated mCrCl. Rounding participants with a serum creatinine <1 mg/dL up to 1 mg/dL resulted in significantly lower CG estimates; therefore, this practice should be avoided. The median dosing discordance relative to the CG for 10 drugs requiring renal dose adjustment was 28.6% and 22.9% for the MDRD and CKD-EPI, respectively. The analysis provides further evidence that unless specifically stated in a drug's label information, the CG is the least biased equation for estimating renal function when adjusting drug doses.

■ O'Mahoney D, O'Sullivan D, Byrne S, et al. STOPP/START criteria for potentially inappropriate prescribing in older people: version 2. *Age Ageing*. 2014;44(2):213–218.

Nineteen experts from 13 countries convened to update the 2008 STOPP/START (Screening Tool of Older Peoples Prescriptions/Screening Tool to Alert to Right Treatment). The update includes 80 STOPP and 34 START criteria. Like the 2015 AGS Beers Criteria, the STOPP/START criteria are principally explicit criteria requiring varying amounts of individual patient information.

■ Tannenbaum C, Martin P, Tamblyn R. et al. Reduction in inappropriate benzodiazepine prescriptions among older adults through direct patient education. The EMPOWER cluster randomized trial. *JAMA Intern Med*. 2014;174(6):890–898.

The Eliminating Medication Through Patient Ownership of End Results (EMPOWER) trial evaluated the effectiveness of personalized patient education on benzodiazepine dose reduction or discontinuation in patients ≥65 years old. Chronic benzodiazepine users were randomized to an intervention of personalized education on the harms of benzodiazepines and a 21-week step-wise tapering protocol (n=148), while the control group (n=155) received usual care. After 6 months, benzodiazepines had been discontinued by 27% in the intervention group compared with 5% in the control group. Another 11% and 6% achieved a ≥25% dose reduction, respectively. The number needed to treat was equal to 4. This study is an example of how a personalized patient intervention can be used to successfully discontinue benzodiazepines.

Todd P. Semla, MS, PharmD, BCPS, FCCP, AGSF

CHAPTER 13—COMPLEMENTARY AND INTEGRATIVE MEDICINE

KEY POINTS

- The use of complementary and integrative medicine (CIM) appears to be on the rise in all adult age groups, including the older population.

- Herbal products and dietary supplements are among the most frequently used CIM therapies by older adults. Most adults ≥50 years old report they have not discussed CIM with their healthcare providers. Thus, it is imperative that healthcare providers ask patients about CIM practices at *every visit*.

- More research is needed to determine the effectiveness and safety of many widely used CIM treatments for common conditions in older adults.

In 2014, Congress changed the name of the National Center for Complementary and Alternative Medicine (NCCAM) of the National Institutes of Health to the National Center for Complementary and Integrative Health (NCCIH) to better reflect practices already in use by the U.S. population. Alternative medicine refers to unproven approaches substituted for traditional Western medicine. Extensive surveys have found that use of alternative medicine is rare; thus, many in the field have begun using the term integrative medicine. In practice and at NCCIM, the terms "complementary medicine" and "integrative medicine" are frequently used interchangeably. Although scientific evidence accumulates for some complementary and integrative medicine (CIM) treatments, key questions remain that must be answered through well-designed research studies—questions that address the safety and efficacy of certain CIM therapies for the diseases or medical conditions for which they are used.

NCCIM has condensed the categorization of CIM modalities from prior years:

- Natural products, including herbal medicines, botanicals, vitamins, minerals, probiotics and other dietary supplements

- Mind and body practices, such as massage therapy, meditation, yoga, acupuncture, chiropractic/osteopathic manipulation, hypnotherapy, tai chi, qi gong, healing touch, relaxation exercises

- Other complementary health approaches, including indigenous healing practices, Chinese medicine, Ayurvedic medicine, homeopathy, naturopathy

The list of what constitutes the practice of CIM is continually evolving, as interventions that are proved to be safe and effective become adopted as components of conventional, or allopathic, medicine and as new approaches to health care emerge.

The use of CIM is increasing within the U.S. adult population, particularly among middle-aged adults. The 2007 National Health Interview Survey, a nationally representative sample of over 31,000 U.S. adults ≥18 years old, found that 36% of those interviewed used some of 27 different CIM modalities during the previous 12 months. When CIM was defined to include self-prayer for health reasons, usage increased to 62%.

Studies consistently demonstrate that, with the exception of self-prayer, older adults use CIM less frequently than do adults 50–59 years old, the largest CIM user group. However, it is logical to predict that, as middle-aged adults grow older, they will continue the CIM practices begun in earlier decades of life. See Table 13.1 for more details.

The use of CIM by older adults is beginning to be more closely studied, in part to help design safer and more efficacious treatments specific to the needs of this rapidly expanding segment of the population. A 2010 telephone survey by the American Association of Retired Persons and NCCIM asked 1,013 participants ≥50 years old about their CIM use; 53% reported some lifetime use of CIM, and 47% reported CIM use within the last 12 months. Within that time period, the consumption of herbal product or dietary supplements was most frequently reported (37%), with the receipt of massage, chiropractic, or other bodywork services ranking second (22%). Of concern, 67% had not discussed CIM use with their healthcare provider, because their healthcare provider had not inquired (42%) or because the patient did not know it should be discussed (30%). Respondents reported their primary sources of CIM information as family/friends (26%); Internet (14%); physician (13%); magazines, newspapers, or books (13%); and radio/television (7%). These data confirm and extend similar observations reported in previous small-scale studies.

CIM use can vary depending on ethnic group. An analysis of 2002 National Health Interview Study data revealed the patterns shown in Table 13.1 and demonstrated that CIM was used by ethnic minority groups more than previously reported. Socioeconomic status and degree of acculturation may be important factors in the use and specific choice of CIM modalities by individuals belonging to certain ethnic minority groups. For example, Mexican curanderos may be the first line of health care for impoverished individuals of Mexican descent. Curanderos are community "healers"

Table 13.1—Complementary and Integrative Medicine Usage Patterns in Adults

Modality	Older Adults Usage (n=5,837) % / Mean (SE)	All Adults Usage (n=30,802) % / Mean (SE)	Most Frequent Users (All Adults) By Ethnicity
Self-prayer	56.20 (0.78)	42.92 (0.40)	Black
Biologically based method (eg, herbal medicines, vitamins)	15.59 (0.57)	22.01 (0.30)	Asian
Mind-body (eg, meditation, acupuncture)	11.68 (0.48)	18.45 (0.32)	Asian
Manipulative and body-based methods (eg, therapeutic massage, chiropractic manipulation)	7.57 (0.39)	10.91 (0.24)	White
Alternative medical system (eg, traditional Chinese medicine, homeopathy)	1.41 (0.18)	2.74 (0.14)	Asian
Energy therapy (eg, bioelectromagnetic-based therapies)	0.34 (0.09)	0.74 (0.06)	Asian

NOTE: SE = standard error
Data from Grzywacz JG, Suerken CK, Neiberg RH, et al. Age, ethnicity, and use of complementary and alternative medicine in health self-management. *J Health Social Behav.* 2007;48(1):84–98.

who believe that illness can result from natural, as well as spiritual, causes. They often use herbal remedies in the form of teas, baths, or poultices, depending on the symptoms. Similarly, Native Americans may mix modern and traditional medicines, sometimes using "white man's medicine" to treat "white man's diseases." Traditional Native American medicine covers a broad range of interventions, including ceremony, fasting, sweating, herbal and/or animal medicines, or avoidance or inclusion of specific foods. Some Western pharmaceuticals were derived from Native American herbal medicines.

SAFETY ISSUES

Most CIM practices have not been regulated, and licensure and certification among CIM practitioners can vary among practices and by geographic location. There is substantial potential for adverse reactions with the use of herbal preparations and of botanical and dietary supplements in older adults (see Table 13.2).

As mentioned above, 67% of CIM users ≥50 years old in the United States do not discuss their use of CIM modalities with their healthcare providers. This statistic is of particular concern in the care of older adults because of the increased risk of adverse interactions between conventional drugs and various CIM biologic agents. Moreover, aging impacts the metabolism of numerous prescriptions and OTC medications, and possibly that of many herbal preparations, botanicals, and dietary supplements. Age-related alterations in hepatic and renal function contribute importantly to these phenomena, both in the absence and presence of disease.

Older adults report using herbal/dietary products and bodywork services most frequently, both of which can pose health risks. Negative outcomes from chiropractic interventions, albeit uncommon, have included stroke, transient ischemic attack, and other focal neurologic signs. Additionally, recently reported data suggest that older adults are ill informed about the dangers associated with herbal/dietary products. In one study (n=267) of older adults in the central United States, the following percentages of respondents inaccurately believed that herbal/dietary products were regulated by the FDA (60%), were routinely tested by the FDA (70%), and posed no risk to the general population (66%).

Under the Dietary Supplement Health and Education Act (DSHEA) of 1994, the FDA is not authorized to evaluate or regulate the use of dietary supplements, and manufacturers of such products are not required to prove that the advertised ingredients provide the health benefits or safety they claim. Multiple studies have found that dietary supplements often can contain little, none, or more of what the product labels claim, as well as contaminants or adulterants with unlisted products and prescription drugs. In November 2004, the FDA announced initiatives to monitor and evaluate ingredient quality, safety, and labeling of herbal and dietary products, thus attempting to assure the reliability of "what's in the bottle." Since 2004, the FDA has introduced multiple nonbinding recommendations and guidelines for manufacturers to follow in the production and labeling of these supplements and the reporting of adverse events.

Without knowledge of what these products contain in their entirety, or the consequences of their use, consumers and healthcare professionals must increase communication while continued research is conducted to provide accurate evaluations. It is imperative that clinicians ask patients specifically about their use of dietary supplements and biologic products and look

Table 13.2—Safety Issues Related to Dietary Supplements Used by Older Adults

Supplement	Adverse Effects	Interacts With
Coenzyme Q_{10}	Infrequent nausea, emesis, epigastric pain, headaches >300 mg/day linked to increased liver transaminase	Warfarin
Dehydroepiandrosterone (DHEA)	Women: weight gain, voice changes, facial hair, headaches Men: prostatic hyperplasia, possible increase in hormone-sensitive tumors	Calcium channel blockers, sildenafil
Echinacea	Allergic reactions, hepatitis, asthma, vertigo, anaphylaxis (rare)	Immunosuppressants
Ginkgo biloba	All rare: serious bleeding, seizures, headaches, dizziness, vertigo	Anticoagulants
Glucosamine	Nausea, diarrhea, heartburn	Hypoglycemic drugs (reduce effectiveness)
Melatonin	Daytime sleepiness, headache, dizziness	Anticoagulants, immunosuppresants, diabetes medications, birth control pills
Omega-3 fatty acids	Belching, halitosis, increased blood glucose	Antiplatelets, anticoagulants, antihypertensives
SAM-e (S-adenosyl-methionine)	Nausea, vomiting, diarrhea, anxiety, restlessness	Tricyclics, SSRIs
Saw palmetto	All rare: constipation, diarrhea, decreased libido, headaches, hypertension, urine retention	None described
St. John's wort	Nausea, allergic reactions, dizziness, headache, photosensitivity (rare)	Anticoagulants, antivirals, SSRIs

at the ingredients in those supplements. Older adults also consistently indicate willingness to receive more information about CIM treatments; thus, it is important for healthcare providers to disseminate such information.

CIM EFFICACY FOR MANAGING ILLNESS IN OLDER ADULTS

The aging of the baby-boomer generation is contributing to the already established largest group of healthcare consumers—older adults. Demographic considerations assure that the needs of the expanding aging population for medical services will continue to increase, and it is reasonable to predict that specific interest in, and use of, CIM modalities will expand as well.

Anecdotal reports or claims of the efficacy of diverse CIM modalities are numerous; however, scientific efficacy and safety must be established through careful study. Studies examining the effectiveness and safety of CIM interventions continue to accumulate. However, as the research efforts summarized in this chapter demonstrate, the current evidence base is hindered by studies lacking the appropriate design and methodology, number of participants, duration of investigation, and/or standardization of product or practice. Investigators planning trials of CIM modalities can improve their study design by verifying that the planned research meets the criteria for scientific quality and acceptability by reviewing resources such as those provided by the Cochrane Collaboration.

Musculoskeletal Disorders

Osteoarthritis

Osteoarthritis is the most common musculoskeletal disorder and one of the most common chronic diseases affecting older adults. Very small statistically significant but clinically irrelevant results were found for acupuncture versus sham acupuncture in the treatment of osteoarthritis of the knee and hip (SOE=C). A Cochrane Collaboration review of transcutaneous electrical nerve stimulation (TENS) for osteoarthritis of the knee was inconclusive because of the poor methodologic and reporting quality of extant studies (SOE=C). A review of electromagnetic field therapy studies for osteoarthritis found an absolute improvement in pain of 15% (95% CI; 9.08 to 21.13) after 4–26 weeks of treatment but no significant effect on physical function (absolute improvement of 4.5% [95% CI; –2.23 to 11.32]) after 12–26 weeks, or on quality of life (absolute improvement of 0.09% [95% CI; –0.36 to 0.54) after 4–6 weeks (SOE=B). A systematic review comparing chondroitin (with or without glucosamine or other supplement) with placebo for knee osteoarthritis showed a modest decrease in pain in studies <6 months in duration. Participants who received chondroitin rated their pain on average 10 points lower on a 0–100 scale compared with participants receiving placebo (95% CI; 15% to 6% lower). However, there was no improvement in function when chondroitin was compared with placebo or active control with conventional pain medications (SOE=B). Viscosupplementation of hyaluronic acid in the treatment of osteoarthritis has increased in clinical practice over recent years, but its effectiveness and safety are debated. Although a 2013 review and meta-analysis concluded that it resulted in small but clinically irrelevant benefit and considerable complication risks, a 2015 eight-member European expert panel concluded that it was an effective treatment for mild to moderate knee osteoarthritis.

Osteoporosis

Recent studies have highlighted gender and racial disparities favoring white women in the diagnosis and treatment of osteoporosis after a fracture. Over their lifetime, one in five men >50 years old will sustain an osteoporotic fracture, and their mortality rates associated with hip fracture are higher than those for women. Thus, increased scrutiny of potential osteoporosis in men and in black Americans is warranted.

Many of the available studies of osteoporosis examine women's responses to interventions, such as phytoestrogen and soy products. The inconsistent findings from trials likely result from the use of differing soy products (ie, food versus tablets of varying strengths and combinations therein) in various populations. At this time, evidence is insufficient to recommend their use for the prevention or treatment of osteoporosis in peri- or postmenopausal women. Moreover, there is controversy regarding the safety of their use in women with estrogen-sensitive diseases such as breast or endometrial cancer.

Dehydroepiandrosterone (DHEA) is the most abundant circulating steroid hormone, reaching peak levels in early adulthood and then declining progressively with age. This decline coupled with the correlation between low DHEA sulfate and osteoporosis and frailty has led to the use of DHEA supplements in an attempt to improve bone density, muscle mass, and physical functioning in older adults. Small-scale trials of DHEA supplementation in older adults have produced conflicting results regarding its effects to moderately enhance bone density, and further studies are needed to determine its possible use in preventing or treating osteoporosis in older adults. These same trials have shown DHEA to have no effect on muscle mass or physical performance.

Rheumatoid Arthritis and Inflammatory Bowel Disease

Omega-3 polyunsaturated fatty acid (PUFA) supplementation may reduce inflammatory joint pain from rheumatoid arthritis and inflammatory bowel disease (SOE=B). A recent meta-analysis examining placebo-controlled studies of omega-3 PUFA supplementation in rheumatoid arthritis and found that omega-3 groups used significantly less NSAIDs than placebo groups. However, specific pain indicators and physical function were not significantly different between groups. An older Cochrane Collaboration review of omega-3 PUFA use for rheumatoid arthritis or inflammatory bowel disease found significant results for reduced NSAID consumption, pain indicators, and physical function in the omega-3 group versus the placebo group. A meta-analysis of specific diet plans (vegetarian, Mediterranean, elemental, and elimination diets), including fasting, for rheumatoid arthritis pain generally found no evidence of improved patient-oriented outcomes (SOE=B). However, the risk of bias and inadequate data reporting inherent in the reviewed studies supports the need for better designed future research. Finally, a recent Cochrane Collaboration review reported that 2 high-quality studies have found that omega-3 polyunsaturated fatty acids were not effective in maintaining remission in Crohn disease and may cause GI upset (SOE=A).

Low Back Pain

Acupuncture, spinal manipulation therapy (including muscle energy techniques) or massage, and herbal medicine are all used in treatment of lower back pain. Although the examined studies were of limited quality, acupuncture appeared to provide clinically meaningful and significant reduction in self-reported chronic pain when compared with sham acupuncture and improved function when compared with no treatment (SOE=B). Acute lower back pain reduction with acupuncture is more inconsistent (SOE=B). Randomized controlled trials using spinal manipulation therapy and massage have been of low quality and have produced little evidence to support these modalities. Herbal medicines are also used to treat lower back pain. A Cochrane Collaboration review found that *Capsicum frutescens* (cayenne) probably reduces chronic lower back pain better than placebo (SOE=B). This review also reported that, although study quality was limited, short-term pain improvements were found for *Harpagophytum procumbens* (devil's claw), *Salix alba* (white willow bark), and *Symphytom officinale L.* (comfrey root extract) (SOE=C).

Cardiovascular Disorders

In the United States, 69.1% of men and 67.9% of women 60–79 years old have cerebrovascular disease. In Americans aged ≥80 years old, these rates climb to 87.4% in men and 85.9% in women. Of particular relevance is the higher incidence of cardiovascular disease occurring in obese patients or those with type 2 diabetes mellitus. Healthy diet and aerobic exercise are the first nonpharmacologic recommendations to manage high blood pressure and dyslipidemia. A heart-healthy diet includes limiting processed meats, red meat (beef, lamb, and pork), sodium, refined sugar, and saturated fat, while increasing amounts of complex carbohydrates, vegetables, and fruits. In the Dietary Approach to Stop Hypertension (DASH) trial, nearly 70% of participants following the healthy diet decreased both systolic and diastolic blood pressure measurements.

Ten randomized clinical trials (RCTs) and 6 meta-analyses have evaluated the efficacy of fish oil for cardiovascular outcomes and reported results in high-impact journals. Only one of the trials and one of the meta-analyses found any benefit from use of fish oil supplements on primary endpoints. Based on the overall negative findings, the use of fish oil supplements for cardiovascular disease cannot be recommended (SOE=A). To reduce the risk of developing hypertension and obesity, aerobic exercise, such as swimming or brisk walking, for at least 30 minutes 3 times a week is recommended. Data suggest that even mild to moderate increases in physical activity, such as walking slowly or gardening, have beneficial cardiovascular effects. Increased blood pressure can also be associated with inadequate sleep.

Relaxation therapy has resulted in a small, but statistically significant, decrease in both systolic and diastolic blood pressure. However, the quality of included studies was considered poor, and the authors concluded that this finding could have been due to therapeutic factors (eg, patient-provider relationship) other than the relaxation therapy.

Studies of the use of biofeedback to reduce hypertension have suffered from poor study design and heterogeneous treatments. In a systematic (nonquantitative) review of 52 RCTs, no difference was found between biofeedback and the comparison (placebo, no intervention, other behavioral treatments) in 24, biofeedback was favored over comparators in 16, medication or other behavioral treatments were favored over biofeedback in 4, and comparative data were not reported in 8. The term "favored" usually, but not always, referred to statistically significant results.

Psychiatric Disorders

Depression is one of the most common and debilitating major public health problems, and its incidence increases with advancing age. Although depression is more common in women, increasing attention is focused on the issue of depression in men, in whom it is more often unrecognized or untreated. There is an alarming prevalence of depression and suicide in widowed men ≥70 years old. CIM use by older patients may assist in management of mild to moderate depression. However, adequate treatment of severe depression often incorporates use of psychotherapy and antidepressants to prevent or decrease morbidity and mortality. Research suggests that depression is also a systemic disease and is accompanied by an increased incidence of sleep disorders, osteoporosis, obesity, insulin resistance, and immune dysfunction. The impact of CIM modalities on these "extrabehavioral" outcomes is unclear.

A healthy diet can be one of the first recommendations to assist with improving mood. Dietary intake that includes complex carbohydrates can improve serotonin levels. Increasing essential fatty acids and protein intake may increase alertness and mood. Of equal importance is discontinuing excess alcohol, caffeine, and tobacco, which can contribute to depression and irritability.

A Cochrane Collaboration review evaluating exercise for the treatment of mild to moderate depression has shown very small benefits from which clinical meaningfulness is difficult to gauge. Currently, it is unclear whether such small improvements can be attributed to a biochemical response to exercise, the social activation (getting out of the house and being around others) that may accompany exercise, or both.

The botanical *Hypericum perforatum*, commonly known as St. John's wort, has received strong evidence of efficacy for mild depression when compared with placebo or antidepressants (SOE=A). Adverse effects of St. John's wort include GI upset, hypomania, insomnia, and photosensitivity. Special attention should be paid to the interactions of St. John's wort with the hepatic P-450 enzyme system that induces the metabolism of many drugs, which can cause clinically significant adverse interactions and therapeutic failure with various antiretroviral, anticoagulant, immunosuppressant, antidepressant, and chemotherapeutic drugs.

Neurologic Disorders

Alzheimer Disease

Some studies have investigated the use of supplements for treatment of dementia from Alzheimer disease and vascular insufficiency. Studies of *Ginkgo biloba* extract (EGb 761) for cognitive decline in older adults have produced inconsistent results (SOE=B) overall and no significant benefit over placebo (SOE=A). Brain tissue studies and spinal fluid abnormalities in Alzheimer patients also offer some rationale for supplementing with various antioxidants, including vitamins A, C, and E, and selenium. A 2014 RCT in older veterans with mild to moderate Alzheimer disease taking an acetylcholinesterase inhibitor compared placebo with alpha tocopherol (vitamin E), memantine, or the combination to prevent functional decline. Only the alpha tocopherol group had a slower functional decline (19% slower per year) and less caregiver time (SOE=A). No differences in effectiveness were found for the memantine or for the memantine plus alpha tocopherol groups. The only differences in safety and all-cause mortality occurred as greater frequencies in the infections and infestations category of serious adverse events for the memantine and the combination of memantine and alpha tocopherol groups.

Parkinson Disease

Studies have shown that Parkinson disease patients have reduced brain levels of glutathione, an antioxidant involved in neuroprotective functions. Parkinson patients also have deficiencies in coenzyme Q_{10}. In very small, unblinded clinical trials, supplementation with these two naturally occurring substances may have slowed the progression of disease and reduced the severity of symptoms. Acupuncture, music therapy, and physical therapy are used by Parkinson patients to attempt to reduce disabilities and improve cognitive, emotional, and social functioning (SOE=B).

Sleep Disorders

Sleep disorders are common in older adults, affecting both sleep quality and quantity. Studies suggest that abnormalities in slow-wave and rapid-eye-movement sleep may be linked to psychologic, endocrine-metabolic, and immune system dysfunctions. However, in older adults with primary insomnia, age-related changes in circadian rhythms (earlier morning awakenings and earlier evening drowsiness) appear to play a role. Nutritional and exercise modifications are among the safest recommendations when working with older patients with sleep disorders. Milk, bananas, brown rice, and turkey are examples of foods containing tryptophan, which is a precursor of serotonin. Endogenous melatonin is a major circadian regulator of the sleep-wake cycle. Due to the short half-life of exogenous melatonin, extended-release formulations have been developed. The limited extant studies have investigated mainly short-term use, finding some evidence of improved sleep parameters (SOE=B). Longer-term studies are currently needed to bolster such results. Evidence for the use of valerian root to improve sleep quality, quantity, or next-day functioning has been mixed (SOE=C). Aerobic exercise in the early evening has been shown to contribute to improved sleep quality. However, exercise later in the evening can be too stimulating and hinder restful sleep. Other CIM modalities purported to improve sleep include aromatherapy combined with a warm bath and relaxing music.

Menopause

Perceptions about menopause have become more realistic in recent years, with this transition becoming less frequently viewed as a pathologic process than as a natural progression in the life cycle. In addition, concerns about the safety of long-term conventional estrogen use have increased. These changes have influenced the use of alternatives, such as nutritional, nonpharmacologic supplements, and exercise, for symptom management. Approximately 80% of menopausal women report using one or more CIM modalities, such as natural and plant estrogens and other herbal preparations.

Alternative treatments under current study for menopausal symptoms consist primarily of herbal and phytoestrogen remedies. Although very popular, black cohosh has not been found to reduce patient- or disease-oriented symptoms in good quality clinical trials (SOE=A). Phytoestrogens are naturally occurring sources of estrogen found in plant foods. Isoflavones, such as daidzein and genistein, are found in soy products and have been studied as alternatives to conventional estrogen therapy. The current evidence supports the efficacy of soy over placebo, especially soy extracts, but this conclusion must be tempered by methodologic concerns in some of the studies (SOE=B). Both aerobic exercise and mind-body relaxation techniques are also helpful in decreasing irritability, restlessness, and anxiety.

Urinary incontinence and vaginal dryness are common symptoms in postmenopausal women, increase with advancing age after menopause, and negatively impact quality of life. Evidence is inconclusive on the effectiveness of local estrogens on urinary incontinence, but they may improve vaginal dryness. Information is insufficient as to whether use of any CIM natural products or other modalities provide any relief of symptoms of urinary incontinence and vaginal dryness.

Benign Prostatic Hyperplasia

Symptomatic benign prostatic hyperplasia affects more than 40% of men ≥70 years old approximately equally among racial groups. In recent decades, men in the United States have begun to self-treat this condition with saw palmetto, which has become the fifth leading medicinal herb consumed in the United States. A review of randomized controlled trials comparing saw palmetto to placebo or other conventional medications found no evidence of efficacy. Other supplements (eg, *Hypoxis rooperi*, stinging nettle, pumpkin seed extracts, rye pollen, African plum) have been studied but need more rigorous scientific investigation. The American and European Association of Urology does not currently recommend plant extracts in treatment of benign prostatic hyperplasia.

Diabetes Mellitus

Type 2 diabetes mellitus, a major public health problem, is associated with increased incidence and prevalence of obesity, hypertension, dyslipidemia, and macro- and microvascular disease. Normal aging is associated with increased insulin resistance and glucose intolerances, and increased risk of developing type 2 diabetes mellitus. In one survey, approximately 50%–60% of diabetic patients reported the use of CIM interventions, including folk remedies in ethnic populations.

There is considerable interest in examining the potential benefit of various CIM biologic agents (eg, omega-3-fatty acids, chromium, vitamin C, other dietary antioxidants) or other modalities (eg, stress-reduction techniques), in combination with dietary modifications, exercise, and weight management, in the treatment of patients with diabetes. In this regard, omega-3 polyunsaturated fatty acids have not been shown to improve glycemic control or fasting insulin.

Cancer

Approximately 30%–50% of cancer patients in one survey noted they were using CIM interventions to manage their specific cancer. Cancer CIM therapies purportedly can be used to strengthen the body's innate immune systems as well as to manage the adverse effects of conventional treatments, such as chemotherapy and radiation. One of the most important benefits for many cancer patients who use CIM modalities is the experience of being more empowered while dealing with the challenges of cancer. This has been substantiated by numerous studies examining various indices of health-related quality of life. The CIM therapies most frequently used are herbal preparations, exercise, and spiritual and energy modalities (such as qi gong, therapeutic touch, Reiki, polarity, healing touch, or Johrei).

Controversy remains regarding the role of diet as a possible risk factor for developing breast cancer. Of particular importance is the link between obesity and its associated increase in estrogen levels that are thought to contribute to de novo breast cancer development and recurrence after early-stage disease. In contrast, consumption of a high-fiber, low-fat diet with fruits, vegetables, whole grains, fish, and legumes is associated with decreased risk of disease. Biologic agents, herbal preparations, and vitamins have all been tried by patients; however, most of these modalities have not undergone much scientific study. In contrast, lifestyle changes, including exercise and stress management techniques, have been helpful in managing mood and energy changes associated with breast cancer.

Prostate cancer usually develops slowly in older men, and CIM use in combination with conventional treatment has been reported to reduce associated discomforts and improve the quality of life. Risk of death in this population is higher from heart disease than from prostate cancer per se. Exercise and healthy diet remain the safest CIM recommendations to assist with the management of adverse effects and improvement of quality of life in these patients.

Lung cancer has been strongly linked to smoking. The possible associations of lung cancer risk to excess dietary intake of dairy products, red meats, and saturated fats has been raised, but the evidence is inconclusive. In addition, preliminary research has suggested that ingestion of vitamin A by those who smoke may be harmful, whereas vitamin A intake in those who do not smoke may be beneficial. Dietary changes as well as mind-body interventions may assist patients with lung cancer to manage emotional distress and the adverse effects of treatment. Cancer patients using relaxation and stress-management techniques have been able to manage cravings when pursuing tobacco cessation. These mind-body techniques are also effective in managing the emotional and physical distress associated with diagnosis and with the adverse effects of treatment.

Currently, there are no herbal preparations or botanical supplements that appear to be useful in the prevention or management of patients with colon cancer. A fiber-rich diet has been postulated to possibly prevent the onset of colon cancer; however, studies are inconclusive. Lutein, which is present in broccoli, carrots, oranges, and spinach, was found in one study to be beneficial for colon cancer prevention.

Medical Cannabis and Cannabinoids

Twenty-three states and the District of Columbia have enacted laws that allow for the medicinal use of marijuana (*Cannabis sativa*). Although epidemiologic data confirm that older adults are using cannabis and cannabinoids to treat a variety of symptoms and ailments, the exact prevalence is not known. In Colorado, approximately 16% of registered medical marijuana users are ≥61 years old.

Marijuana exerts its psychoactive and therapeutic effect through cannabinoids, which act predominantly on receptors in the CNS. Two synthetic cannabinoids (dronabinol and nabilone) are FDA-approved for treatment of chemotherapy-induced nausea and vomiting that has not responded to other antiemetics. Dronabinol has an additional indication for AIDS-related anorexia and weight loss. Studies of herbal cannabis and cannabinoids have demonstrated effectiveness in treatment of chronic pain, neuropathic pain, and spasticity caused by multiple sclerosis (SOE=A). Most studies to date have included very few older adults, limiting the ability to make sweeping recommendations. Further, frail older adults would be at high risk for some of the common adverse effects (dizziness, disorientation, confusion, loss of balance, fatigue, drowsiness and hallucinations).

REFERENCES

- American Association of Retired Persons & National Centers for Complementary and Alternative Medicine Survey Report. *Complementary and Alternative Medicine: What People Aged 50 and Older Discuss With Their Health Care Providers.* https://nccih.nih.gov/research/statistics/2010 (accessed Jan 2016).

    AARP and NCCAM interviewed 1,013 patients ≥50 years old about their use of complementary and alternative medicine. This telephone survey examined the patterns of use, sources of information, and communication with health care providers.

- Cooney GM, Dwan K, Greig CA, et al. Exercise for depression. *Cochrane Database Syst Rev.* 2013 Sep 12;9.

    In this systematic review, the authors analyze data from 39 randomized controlled trials comparing exercise with a variety of treatments for depression, including placebo. Exercise was found to have a moderate effect compared with control interventions in reducing symptoms of depression.

- Dysken MW, Sano M, Asthana S, et al. Effect of vitamin E and memantine on functional decline in Alzheimer disease. *JAMA.* 2014;311(1):33–44.

    This randomized controlled trial compared vitamin E, memantine, and the combination with placebo in 613 patients with mild to moderate Alzheimer disease. Subjects who received vitamin E had a statistically significant slower functional decline on the Alzheimer's Disease Cooperative Study/Activities of Daily Living Inventory. Memantine and the combination of vitamin E and memantine were no better than placebo.

- Grey A, Bolland M. Clinical trial evidence and use of fish oil supplements. *JAMA: Intern Med.* 2014;174(3):460–462.

    This research letter discusses the factors that may influence the growing use of fish oil to treat a variety of conditions despite robust clinical trial evidence demonstrating no consistent benefit.

- Lam M, Galvin R, Curry P. Effectiveness of acupuncture for nonspecific chronic low back pain: a systematic review and meta-analysis. *Spine.* 2013;38(24):2124–2138.

    In this systematic review, 32 randomized controlled trials of acupuncture were assessed for their efficacy in treating nonspecific low back pain. Compared with sham, acupuncture reduced self-reported levels of pain, but compared with medications and usual care, the benefits were too small to be considered clinically meaningful.

- Oltean H, Robbins C, van Tulder MW, et al. Herbal medicine for low-back pain. *Cochrane Database Syst Rev.* 2014 Dec 23;12:CD004504.

    This systematic review of 14 randomized controlled trials of herbal medicine for treatment of low-back pain concluded that *Capsicum frutescens* (cayenne) reduced pain compared with placebo. The quality of evidence for additional herbal medicines was considered moderate at best.

Julie C. Chapman, PsyD
Marc R. Blackman, MD

CHAPTER 14—MISTREATMENT

KEY POINTS

- Mistreatment of older adults affects 11.4% of those ≥60 years old.

- Forms of mistreatment include financial, physical, sexual, emotional, caregiver neglect, and self-neglect. Screening for mistreatment of older adults is important and most effective when conducted in a sensitive manner.

- Indicators of mistreatment of older adults range from dramatic (eg, bruising, fractures) to subtle (eg, withdrawn behavior, dehydration).

Mistreatment of older adults is referred to by the National Research Council in its report on elder mistreatment as "(a) intentional actions that cause harm or create a serious risk of harm (whether or not harm is intended) to a vulnerable elder by a caregiver or other person who stands in a trust relationship to the elder or (b) failure by a caregiver to satisfy the elder's basic needs or to protect the elder from harm." The Center of Excellence on Elder Abuse & Neglect website (www.centeronelderabuse.org) provides an evidence-based approach to the assessment and detection of elder mistreatment with cases, multimedia resources, and results from an ongoing program of research that is led by experts in the field and provides the best current resource for those practicing in geriatrics. Mistreatment can manifest itself in a variety of ways, including physical or emotional abuse, intentional or unintentional neglect, self-neglect, financial exploitation, abandonment, or a combination of these. Research suggests that the U.S. national incidence of mistreatment of older adults is approximately 450,000 annually. Given these estimates, routine screening for mistreatment is an appropriate part of primary care for older adults.

Research conducted in the context of a longitudinal aging cohort study sought to determine mortality related to mistreatment. In a pooled logistic regression analysis that adjusted for demographics, chronic disease, functional status, social networks, cognitive status, and depressive symptoms, the risk of death remained higher for cohort members experiencing either mistreatment or self-neglect (SOE=A). To date, no intervention studies have evaluated the impact of screening on health outcomes, and such studies are needed. However, screening for mistreatment appears warranted, given the findings of case studies and longitudinal studies that document risk factors, as well as the information in databases of adult protective services organizations across the country.

RISK FACTORS AND PREVENTION

Risk factors for mistreatment include poverty, dependency of older adults for caregiving needs, age, race, functional disability, frailty, and cognitive impairment (SOE=B). Some factors may actually be proxies for other variables. For example, lower socioeconomic status is often associated with fewer resources to meet caregiving demands; mistreatment may be as high as 47.3% in this group. Research has shown that demented older adults who are victims of crime have the ability, in certain circumstances, to provide testimony about criminal events (SOE=B).

Frail, debilitated older adults may need a level of care that at times exceeds caregiver ability. In particular, the demented person who exhibits disturbing behaviors (eg, hitting, spitting, screaming) poses immense challenges to caregivers. Caregiver stress can give way to any of the forms of mistreatment, and a careful assessment of caregiver stress can identify opportunities to prevent mistreatment. Minority older adults may be preferentially targeted for health care fraud by unscrupulous home care organizations and/or durable medical equipment suppliers. For factors that indicate a risk of development of inadequate or abusive caregiving, see Table 14.1.

HISTORY

An interdisciplinary approach to assessment and care planning is optimal. Comprehensive interdisciplinary geriatric assessment that includes the physical, psychosocial, and financial domains of older adults should detect potential or any alleged mistreatment. The mistreatment history, provided by both the older adult and caregiver(s), should be conducted in private so that all individuals can speak freely and frankly. Studies suggest that the different cultures of racial and ethnic groups may define abuse and neglect very differently; thus, cultural sensitivity is important. The older adult or caregiver from a culture different than the clinician's may be offended by some mistreatment screening questions; wording questions carefully can avoid alienating the older adult or caregiver, which could abolish any further opportunity to help the patient and family.

If the older adult's responses to the mistreatment questions indicate that mistreatment may be occurring, progressively focused follow-up questions are indicated. For example, the clinician might first ask, "Is there any difficult behavior in your family you would like to tell me about?" If the answer is positive, possible questions to follow include: "Has anyone tried to hurt or hit you?"

"Has anyone made you do things that you did not want to do?" "Has anyone taken your things?" Obtaining such information requires sensitive clinical interviewing skills similar to those needed when asking about sexual orientation, alcoholism, or substance abuse.

Private interviews with caregivers can detect not only abusive or neglectful behavior but also signs of stress, isolation, or depression in the caregiver, in which case help for the caregiver can also be provided. Caregivers may be reluctant to discuss their own problems in the presence of the older adult who depends on their care. Because caregivers can range from registered professionals to well-intended neighbors, it is important to know and document the caregiver's skill level, as well as his or her understanding of the situation. The latter is an essential factor in evaluating the underlying intention of any mistreatment of a dependent older adult. For example, a registered nurse in a nursing home is held to a different level of accountability than a frail spouse providing care in the home setting.

Identification of shortcomings in the older adult's care can be the most elusive aspect of a comprehensive assessment. The symptoms and signs of incomplete, inadequate, or neglectful caregiving can be subtle (eg, when an older adult does not do as well as expected on a given regimen) or attributable to the older adult's physical or emotional disorders (eg, weight loss in an older adult with a history of depression).

Effective assessment detects mistreatment without placing undue suspicion on well-meaning caregivers or undermining a family's ability to care for an older adult with appropriate support and counseling.

For examples of symptoms and signs that indicate a particularly high level of risk of mistreatment, see Table 14.2. A number of assessment instruments have been developed to help clinicians screen for and assess mistreatment, although none has been fully validated yet, and research is ongoing.

PHYSICAL ASSESSMENT

Medical implications of elder abuse have been well described (SOE=B), and differences among disease, physiology, and mistreatment indicators are important to distinguish and document. Key signs of mistreatment include physical indicators that are incongruent with the history; examples are bruises and welts in unusual places or in various stages of healing. Bilateral bruises on the upper torso are rarely the result of falls and warrant follow-up. Other indications of possible mistreatment include frequent, unexplained, or inconsistently explained falls and injuries, multiple visits to the emergency department, delays in seeking treatment, inconsistent follow-up, or serial switching among physicians. The clinician should search for unusual patterns or marks, such as bruises on

Table 14.1—Risk Factors for Inadequate or Abusive Caregiving

- Cognitive impairment in patient, caregiver, or both
- Functional decline in patient, caregiver, or both
- Dependency of the caregiver on the older patient, or vice versa
- Family conflict
- Family history of abusive behavior, alcohol or drug misuse or abuse, mental illness, or intellectual disability
- Financial stress or lack of funds to meet new health demands
- Isolation of the patient, caregiver, or both
- Living arrangements inadequate for the needs of the ill person
- Stressful events in the family, such as death of a loved one or loss of employment

inner arms or thighs; cigarette, rope, chain, or chemical burns; lacerations and abrasions on the face, lips, and eyes; or marks on areas of the body usually covered by clothes. Head injuries, hair loss, or hemorrhages beneath the scalp as a consequence of hair pulling are significant markers. Cachectic states can be the result of malnutrition that is a consequence of neglect. Unusual discharges, bruising, bleeding, or trauma around the genitalia or rectum raise concern of possible sexual abuse, prompting gynecologic and rectal examination. See www.centeronelderabuse.org (accessed Jan 2016).

The behavior of the older adult when in the presence of the suspected abuser may be significant. A victim of mistreatment may avoid eye contact, or dart his or her eyes continually. He or she may sit a distance away from an abusive caregiver, cringe, back off, or startle easily as if expecting to be struck. The caregiver may be nervous and fearful, or quiet and passive. The older adult may defer excessively to the caregiver, who may invariably answer for the older adult or even try to prevent a private interview with or examination of the older adult. Dubious explanations may be given to explain the older adult's injuries.

The emergency department is an important setting for assessment of mistreatment. The emergency department may see older adults in crisis, and every effort should be made not to simply treat and release patients whose domestic situation merits further assessment. Astute emergency personnel can identify cases in which there may be serious safety problems in the caregiving situation.

PSYCHOLOGICAL ASSESSMENT

Mistreatment is not invariably or entirely physical. Psychological abuse or neglect is generally more

Table 14.2—Screening for Mistreatment of Older Adults

Assessment Domain	Key Indicators
General	■ Clothing: inappropriate dress, soil, or disrepair ■ Hygiene (including appearance of hair and nails) ■ Nutritional status ■ Skin integrity
Abuse	■ Anxiety, nervousness, especially toward caregiver ■ Bruising, in various healing stages, especially bilateral or on inner arms or thighs ■ Fractures, especially in various healing stages ■ Lacerations ■ Repeated emergency department visits ■ Repeated falls ■ Signs of sexual abuse ■ Statements about abuse by the patient
Neglect	■ Contractures ■ Dehydration ■ Depression ■ Diarrhea ■ Failure to respond to warning of obvious disease ■ Fecal impaction ■ Malnutrition ■ Medication under- or overuse or otherwise inappropriate use ■ Poor hygiene ■ Pressure ulcers ■ Repeated falls ■ Repeated hospital admissions ■ Urine burns ■ Statements about neglect by the patient
Self-neglect	■ Older age ■ Cognitive impairment ■ Functional decline ■ Depression ■ Weak social network ■ Low social engagement
Exploitation	■ Evidence of misuse of patient's assets ■ Inability of patient to account for money and property or to pay for essential care ■ Reports of demands for money or goods in exchange for caregiving or services ■ Unexplained loss of Social Security, pension checks ■ Statements about exploitation by the patient
Abandonment	■ Evidence that patient is left alone unsafely ■ Evidence of sudden withdrawal of care by caregiver ■ Statements about abandonment by the patient

SOURCE: Data in part from Fulmer T. Elder mistreatment assessment. *Try This: Best Practices in Nursing Care to Older Adults*. 2015;15 (www.consultgerirn.org/ [accessed Jan 2016]).

difficult than physical abuse to detect and confirm, but it can be equally dangerous to the dependent older adult. The behavior of both the older adult and the caregiver can provide important clues about the quality of their relationship and of the care the older adult is receiving. Factors that suggest a poor or deteriorating social and emotional situation are an important focus of assessment for mistreatment.

Psychological abuse includes taunting, name-calling, promoting regressive behaviors by infantilization, making painful jokes at the expense of the older adult, or other demeaning activities. The caregiver's style of communication can provide important clues. Impatience, irritability, and demeaning statements may indicate a pattern of verbal abuse. However, psychological neglect or mistreatment by the caregiver can also take more subtle forms. For example, not providing social or emotional stimulation, or restricting or preventing normal activities can result in total social isolation of the older adult.

The older adult's demeanor and emotional status can suggest the presence of psychological neglect or abuse. For example, ambivalence or high levels of anxiety, fearfulness, or anger toward the caregiver indicate the need for further assessment. Unexpected depression (ie, no obvious pathophysiologic or psychological reason for new onset, such as death in family) or uncharacteristic withdrawal also merits follow-up. Other high-risk behaviors include lack of adherence with treatment recommendations, frequent requests for sedating medication, or frequently canceled appointments.

Cognitive impairment, dementia, and depression are prevalent in older adults referred for evaluation for possible mistreatment. It is therefore appropriate to check any older adult presenting with cognitive impairment, dementia, or depression for symptoms and signs of neglect or mistreatment. Aggressive behaviors associated with dementia can trigger abusive responses in caregivers.

FINANCIAL ASSESSMENT

Financial exploitation includes unauthorized use of the older adult's funds, possessions, or property. Financial mistreatment by family members is estimated to have a prevalence of 5.2%. Fiscal neglect consists of the failure to use the older adult's funds and resources to provide for his or her needs. Signs that an older adult is being mistreated financially include the following (SOE=C):

■ A recent marked disparity between the older adult's living conditions or appearance and his or her assets

■ A sudden inability to pay for health care or basic needs

- An unusual interest on the part of caregivers in the older adult's assets
- The sudden acquisition of expensive possessions by a caregiver who has apparently limited financial assets
- Unwillingness of a caregiver to allow access to the home of an older adult

SELF-NEGLECT

For some older adults, especially those who live in isolation or who choose to accept and endure mistreatment, self-neglect may be an issue. Self-neglected older adults reported to Adult Protective Services have multiple sociodemographic, health-related, and psychosocial characteristics that are different from those of older adults who do not get reported. Lower levels of social network and social engagement have been determined to be risk factors for self-neglect. Further, self-neglect is associated with an increased rate of 30-day hospital readmissions. Successful management in such cases requires an assessment of the older adult's capacity to understand the risks and benefits of the situation, as well as the consequences of allowing the circumstances to continue. These are complex situations, but the older adult's right to autonomy and self-determination must be honored. Paternalistic viewpoints regarding what the older person "should do" need to be avoided. In self-neglect cases, the clinician may need support when coming to terms with the requirement to respect the decisionally capable older adult's wishes when this involves his or her choosing to remain in an abusive or neglectful situation. (The clinical dilemma resembles that confronting clinicians who treat battered women.) Intervention contrary to the decisionally capable older adult's choice is generally inappropriate, as well as being uncomfortable for the clinician. The Diogenes syndrome, in which an older adult suffers from severe self-neglect, is still poorly understood, and evidence is primarily from case studies. Home assessment is crucial, along with a meticulous functional assessment; the Kohlman Evaluation of Living Skills is particularly useful in cases of self-neglect.

THE ROLE OF THE OLDER ADULT

The relationship of the older adult with caregivers can be very complex, and a dysfunctional relationship between a dependent older adult and a caregiver may not be entirely the fault of the caregiver. To approach such situations with the idea that the older adult is inevitably the victim infantilizes the person and is unfair to caregivers. Situations in which older adults are mistreated fall along a spectrum from victimization to mutual abusiveness to relationships in which the older adult can be viewed as a witting cause of the mistreatment. Of course, there are many cases in which the older adult and his or her caregivers are making the best of a tragic situation.

To determine the best possible approach for ameliorating if not solving a dysfunctional caregiving relationship, the clinician needs to make every effort to determine the facts in the situation, including the motives of the people involved. Consultation with social workers, psychologists, or psychiatrists can be useful. Legal reporting requirements are not limited in any way by these considerations. If an older man hits his son and the son strikes back, clinicians in most states are required to report the latter hitting.

INSTITUTIONAL MISTREATMENT

Mistreatment in the setting of home care by family or friends has been the focus of much of the discussion so far, but detecting and intervening to prevent mistreatment in the institutional setting is also important. Several factors in this setting could aggravate the problem, including poor working conditions, low salaries, inadequate staff training and supervision resulting in poor motivation, and prejudiced attitudes. Disruptive or insulting behavior by the older adult can also be a factor.

The Omnibus Budget Reconciliation Act of 1987 set a new standard for care in nursing homes. The clinician who is alert to the possibility of abuse and neglect in any institutional setting plays an important role in protecting vulnerable older adults. Equally important is the clinician's readiness to use the resources available through the institution itself or through state regulatory agencies to investigate and intervene when appropriate. In cases of suspected institutional mistreatment, the challenge is to balance the rights of staff members with the rights of residents. State departments of public health are usually responsible for investigating cases of abuse and neglect in nursing homes. Evidence is growing (SOE=B) regarding the phenomenon of resident-to-resident mistreatment in long-term care facilities, which warrants careful attention. In such cases, residents may assault, rob, or psychologically abuse other residents, and this will be an important area for further research.

INTERVENTION

The clinician who suspects mistreatment can use the following questions to guide intervention:

- How safe is the older adult if he or she returns to the current setting? Does he or she need to be removed to a safe environment?

- What services or resources are available locally to support the care of the older adult?
- Are there any caregivers who have health problems of their own that need attention?
- Does this situation need the expertise of others (eg, medicine, nursing, social work), and if so, who would best serve the older adult's needs?

Successful intervention in cases of mistreatment can become complex. Factors governing the clinician's course of action include the exact nature and degree of the mistreatment, and whether the patient and/or caregiver(s) can or will cooperate with evaluation and intervention.

Local resources in support of interventions for mistreatment vary, but information is readily available. Consultation with the social work staff of the hospital, nursing home, or local health department can be a useful early step. Each state's Adult Protective Services can provide relevant information as well as direct assistance. However, this essential service has limitations, given the older adult's willingness to participate in the system and the constraints on available resources. Websites of the National Adult Protective Services Association (www.napsa-now.org) and the National Center on Elder Abuse (www.ncea.aoa.gov) both provide a convenient starting point in the search for information and resources. The website of the Elder Justice Roadmap (www.justice.gov/elderjustice/research/roadmap.html [accessed Jan 2016]) is also exceptionally helpful for identifying resources, support, evidence for interventions, and ongoing efforts to eradicate mistreatment.

THE MEDICAL-LEGAL INTERFACE

It is important to know state laws applicable to cases of mistreatment of older adults; 46 states have a reporting mechanism for mistreatment, either through Adult Protective Services or state agencies associated with aging. Here, again, the Elder Justice Roadmap is extremely helpful. Clinicians need to be familiar with the reporting mandates in their area. In some states, neglect by others must be reported, whereas reports of self-neglect are not required. Adult children can be charged with neglect of the older parent if a caregiving relationship can be proved and it can also be proved that care has been precipitously withdrawn without substitute services. In states where self-neglect is reportable, this category represents the largest number of cases. Finally, states can mandate reports for self-neglect but may not provide any services unless the older adult agrees to accept them.

Clinicians are in a key position to assess and report suspected mistreatment of older adults, and most states require such reporting. Although clinicians are appropriately wary of acting precipitously, they should be willing to enlist the help of government agencies and the courts when mistreatment is clearly dangerous for an older adult. Penalties can be assessed against a nonreporter in some regions. Reports of mistreatment of older adults are confidential, and as is the case with reports of child abuse, the clinical reporter is protected from litigation unless it can be proved that the report was made maliciously. The home page for the National Center on Elder Abuse (www.ncea.aoa.gov [accessed Jan 2016]) provides one means for reporting information.

Especially when a case is to be reported, photographs and body charts may be required to document the findings on physical examination. Risk management personnel can provide guidance in documentation and assist the clinician when evidence suggests a possible need for police or court action. In any case in which the clinician is called to court to discuss his or her findings, documentation is an important part of testimony. Cases of mistreatment are often extremely complicated, and it is likely that experts in several fields will need to work with clinicians and administrators to avoid under- or overreporting of mistreatment of older adults and to provide the best outcomes for the mistreatment victims.

REFERENCES

- Acierno R, Hernandez MA, Amstadter AB, et al. Prevalence and correlates of emotional, physical, sexual, and financial abuse and potential neglect in the United States: the national elder mistreatment study. *Am J Public Health*. 2010;100(2):292–297.

    Estimates of prevalence and correlates of emotional, physical, sexual, and financial mistreatment and potential neglect were determined from a randomly selected national sample. Using random digit dialing across geographic strata, the authors used computer-assisted telephone interviewing. Data from 5,777 respondents were analyzed. The 1-year prevalence was 4.6% for emotional abuse, 1.6% for physical abuse, 0.6% for sexual abuse, 5.1% for potential neglect, and 5.2% for current financial abuse by a family member.

- Dong XQ. Elder abuse: systematic review and implications for practice. *J Am Geriatr Soc*. 2015;63(6):1214–1238.

    This review article is based on the lecture for the 2014 American Geriatrics Society Outstanding Scientific Achievement for Clinical Investigation Award. The article provides an overview of the epidemiology of elder abuse including its prevalence, risk factors, and consequences. It highlights gaps in research and policy issues and addresses implications for researchers, health professionals, and social service providers.

- Dong X, Simon MA. Elder self-neglect is associated with an increased rate of 30-day hospital readmission: findings from the Chicago health and aging project. *Gerontology*. 2015;61(1):41–50.

    The objective of this study was to examine the prospective relationship between reported elder self-neglect and the rate of 30-day hospital readmission in a community population. Using the Chicago Health and Aging Project data, consisting of 7,219 community-dwelling older adults, a subset of 1,228 participants was reported to the social services agency for suspected elder self-neglect. The primary predictor was elder self-neglect reported to the social services agency. The outcome of interest was the annual rate of 30-day hospital readmission calculated from the CMS hospitalization data from 1993 to 2009. Poisson regression models were used to assess these relationships. The average annual rate of 30-day hospital readmission for those without elder self-neglect was 0.2 (SD 0.7) and for those with reported elder self-neglect was 0.9 (SD 2.8). After adjusting for sociodemographic and socioeconomic characteristics, medical comorbidities, cognitive function, physical function, and psychosocial well-being, elders who reported self-neglect had a significantly higher rate of 30-day hospital readmission. Greater self-neglect was associated with increased annual rates of 30-day hospital readmission.

- Gibbs LM, Mosqueda L. Medical implications of elder abuse and neglect. *Clin Geriatr Med.* 2014;30(4):xv–xvi.

  This excellent edition of *Clinics in Geriatric Medicine* focuses on the medical implications associated with diagnosing and treating elder mistreatment. Fifteen chapters cover critical content related to assessment and intervention in these cases, providing an outstanding synthesis of the interdisciplinary issues that must be addressed. Of particular note are chapters on medical and laboratory indicators for mistreatment and on the distinctions among physiology, disease, and elder mistreatment. Helpful flow charts and tables are provided to guide the practitioner.

- Mosqueda L, Dong X. Elder abuse and self-neglect: "I don't care anything about going to the doctor, to be honest..." *JAMA.* 2011;306(5):532.

  Elder mistreatment encompasses a range of behaviors, including emotional, financial, physical, and sexual abuse, neglect by other individuals, and self-neglect. This article discusses the range of elder mistreatment in community-living older adults, associated factors, and consequences. Although self-neglect is not considered a type of abuse in many research definitions, it is the most commonly reported form of elder mistreatment and is associated with increased morbidity and mortality. The case on which this article is based describes a 70-year-old woman who neglects herself and dies despite multiple contacts with the medical community. Although significant research gaps exist, enough is known to guide clinical practice. This article presents the practical approaches a health care professional can take when a reasonable suspicion of elder mistreatment arises. Public health and interdisciplinary team approaches are needed to manage what is becoming an increasing problem with the increasing number of older adults worldwide.

Terry Fulmer, PhD, RN, FAAN, AGSF

CHAPTER 15—PERIOPERATIVE CARE

KEY POINTS

- Operative therapy is an important option for many health problems affecting older adults.

- The preoperative evaluation should include an appraisal of the patient's medical conditions, functional status, and risk of cardiac and other perioperative complications, as well as recommendations for preoperative testing and therapy to minimize surgical risk.

- Risk indices and practice guidelines for common cardiac, pulmonary, and neuropsychiatric problems assist in decision making and management of older surgical patients.

- Although age is a risk factor for perioperative and postoperative complications, these problems can be minimized with appropriate proactive assessment and management.

Surgery is a common form of treatment for older adults; currently >55% of all operative procedures are done in patients ≥65 years old, and this proportion is expected to grow. Many of the chronic conditions that increase in prevalence with advancing age—cataracts, arthritis, vascular occlusions, and cancers—are amenable to surgery. Over half of all malignancies are seen in patients ≥65 years old, and the primary treatment for many tumors is surgical. Advances in surgical, anesthetic, and medical care have lowered surgical risks and shifted the risk-benefit ratio to favor surgery in increasingly older patients with more complex conditions. Nevertheless, although older patients account for just over half of all surgical procedures, they suffer three-quarters of the postoperative mortality, as well as a disproportionate majority of the postoperative morbidity.

Many of the physiologic changes accompanying normal aging impact the perioperative management of older surgical patients. For example, altered body composition, and decreased kidney function, hepatic blood flow, and hepatic enzyme activity all contribute to changes in the pharmacokinetics of drugs. Cardiac and vascular stiffening complicate fluid management and optimization of intravascular volume. Both volume overload and volume depletion occur commonly in the perioperative setting and are poorly tolerated by many older adults. Stiffening of the thoracic cage and diminished ciliary function contribute to decreases in pulmonary reserve and heightened risk of postoperative pneumonia. Because of decreased thermoregulation, the older surgical patient is at particular risk of perioperative hypothermia. Finally, by mechanisms that are not yet fully elucidated, changes in the brain that accompany aging make older adults exquisitely susceptible to postoperative cognitive changes.

It is well recognized that the aging process is extremely variable from person to person and that within one individual not all organ systems age at the same rate, producing dramatic heterogeneity even among healthy older adults. Older individuals may have several chronic conditions that can impact on perioperative care, either directly or through the medications being used to treat those conditions. The heterogeneity in physiologic aging combined with the potential for multiple comorbidities means that older patients require a more comprehensive and individualized preoperative evaluation. They often benefit from a multidisciplinary approach to perioperative care and recovery.

SURGICAL DECISION-MAKING

Geriatric providers should assist in the process of deciding on surgery. As with any prospect of a medical or surgical intervention, the patient's goals of care should be elicited first. Goals should be elucidated in the context of patient preferences for care, overall functional status, comorbidities, decision-making capacity, and life expectancy. When establishing goals of care with the patient and family, the geriatrician should particularly address conditions of cognitive impairment, frailty, malnutrition, and functional dependence, all of which are risk factors for adverse surgical outcomes such as mortality, institutionalization, and functional decline. Surgical consultation should be pursued only if surgery is potentially consistent with patient-oriented goals. If referral results in a decision to proceed with surgery, the next role of the geriatric provider is often to preoperatively assess and minimize the patient's risks of surgery.

PREOPERATIVE ASSESSMENT AND MANAGEMENT

Clinicians are commonly asked to perform preoperative evaluations with the goals of reducing complications and death and optimizing patient outcomes. The goal of such a consultation should not be to "clear" the patient for surgery but rather to maximize the possibility of a good outcome from surgery. This consultation should appraise the patient's medical, cognitive, and functional status, assess risk of perioperative and postoperative complications, and provide recommendations for preoperative interventions to minimize potential complications. Preoperative assessment should include

Table 15.1—American Society of Anesthesiologists Classification of Physical Status

Class	Description of Patient
I	Healthy
II	Mild systemic disease
III	Severe systemic disease
IV	Severe systemic disease that is a constant threat to life
V	Moribund; not expected to survive without surgery
VI	Declared brain-dead; organs being harvested for donor purposes

NOTE: There is no additional information to help further define these categories.
SOURCE: Data from American Society of Anesthesiologists. ASA Physical Status Classification System. Available at www.asahq.org/resources/clinical-information/asa-physical-status-classification-system (accessed Jan 2016).

evaluation of the patient's cardiovascular, respiratory, renal, metabolic, and neuropsychiatric status, as well as the patient's risk of iatrogenic problems. Usually, the preoperative assessment can be accomplished with only a history and physical examination for low-risk procedures, eg, ambulatory, breast, cataract, endoscopic, or superficial surgery (SOE=B). For patients undergoing procedures that are not low risk, or in whom the history and physical examination have uncovered other potential risks, further assessment and testing are indicated.

Cardiovascular System

It is estimated that 25%–30% of postoperative deaths are from cardiac causes, and the likelihood of postoperative cardiac events is directly related to age. Cardiac risk assessment is the most fully developed and widely investigated portion of the preoperative medical assessment. The American Society of Anesthesiologists classification of patient physical status relies heavily on clinical judgment and is not specific for cardiovascular morbidity and mortality (see Table 15.1). This system has been used by anesthesiologists for years and has consistently been shown to be useful in predicting postoperative outcomes. Several indices and algorithms for specifically assessing cardiac risk in noncardiac surgery have been published since the 1970s. In 2014, the American College of Cardiology and the American Heart Association (ACC/AHA) published an algorithm for preoperative cardiac assessment (Figure 15.1). The guideline calls for consideration, in order, of the following clinical factors:

1. Urgency of surgery; if emergent, proceed to surgery if consistent with patient's overall goals (SOE=C). Depending on those goals, broaching the subject of a palliative approach may be appropriate.

2. Presence of active major cardiac risk factors, eg, unstable angina or recent MI, decompensated heart failure, dyspnea, or moderate or severe valvular disease; if present, assess and correct these conditions before reconsidering surgery (SOE=B).

3. Type of surgery; if low-risk procedure, proceed to surgery (SOE=B).

4. Patient's functional capacity; if good, proceed to surgery (SOE=B).

5. Poor or unknown functional capacity; if present, assess utility of further quantification of cardiac risk and patient willingness to undergo testing for cardiac ischemia before surgery (SOE=B).

6. Calculation of cardiac risk and preoperative testing for cardiac ischemia; perform if they will change management (SOE=B). Several scales for further quantification of cardiac risk are available including the Revised Cardiac Risk Index (www.mdcalc.com/revised-cardiac-risk-index-for-pre-operative-risk/) and 2 risk calculators from the American College of Surgeons (www.riskcalculator.facs.org and www.surgicalriskcalculator.com/miorcardiacarrest [accessed Jan 2016]).

Aside from a careful history and physical examination to determine the presence of active major cardiac risk factors and to assess functional capacity, supplemental cardiac testing or therapy should be considered in only a few specific circumstances. ECG testing is not necessary in asymptomatic patients undergoing low-risk procedures (SOE=B). A preoperative ECG can provide useful information, mostly as a baseline for comparing postoperative cardiac complications, in patients with known coronary artery disease, significant arrhythmia, peripheral arterial disease, prior stroke or transient ischemic attack (TIA), or significant structural heart disease who are undergoing non-low-risk surgery (SOE=B). ECG findings suggestive of ischemia, left ventricular hypertrophy, QT prolongation, or bundle-branch blocks portend a higher risk of cardiac complications and death. Measurement of left ventricular function using echocardiography, radionuclide studies, or contrast ventriculography should be considered in patients with dyspnea of uncertain cause (SOE=C). When newly diagnosed heart failure is determined to be the cause of unexplained dyspnea, it should be maximally treated before surgery. The utility of detecting and treating asymptomatic heart failure preoperatively is unknown. A preoperative echocardiogram should be obtained in patients with moderate or worse valvular stenosis or regurgitation who have not had an echocardiogram in the previous year (SOE=C).

If noninvasive cardiac stress testing will change management, eg, postponement or cancellation of

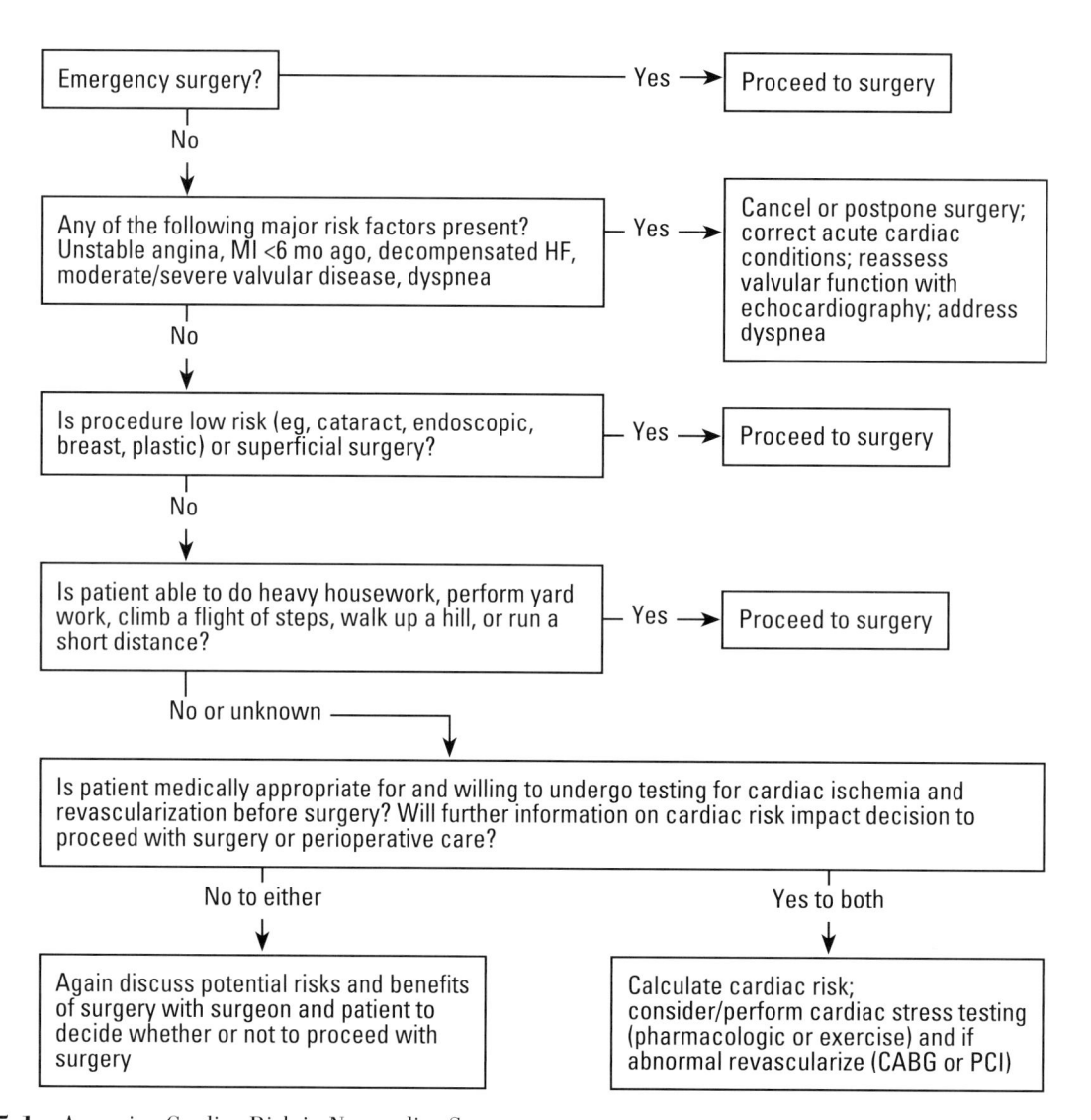

```
Emergency surgery? ──Yes──> Proceed to surgery
       │
       No
       ▼
Any of the following major risk factors present?
Unstable angina, MI <6 mo ago, decompensated HF,    ──Yes──> Cancel or postpone surgery;
moderate/severe valvular disease, dyspnea                    correct acute cardiac
       │                                                     conditions; reassess
       No                                                    valvular function with
       ▼                                                     echocardiography; address
                                                             dyspnea
Is procedure low risk (eg, cataract, endoscopic,
breast, plastic) or superficial surgery?            ──Yes──> Proceed to surgery
       │
       No
       ▼
Is patient able to do heavy housework, perform yard
work, climb a flight of steps, walk up a hill, or run a  ──Yes──> Proceed to surgery
short distance?
       │
       No or unknown
       ▼
Is patient medically appropriate for and willing to undergo testing for cardiac ischemia and
revascularization before surgery? Will further information on cardiac risk impact decision to
proceed with surgery or perioperative care?

      No to either                                    Yes to both
          ▼                                                ▼
Again discuss potential risks and benefits      Calculate cardiac risk;
of surgery with surgeon and patient to          consider/perform cardiac stress testing
decide whether or not to proceed with           (pharmacologic or exercise) and if
surgery                                         abnormal revascularize (CABG or PCI)
```

Figure 15.1—Assessing Cardiac Risk in Noncardiac Surgery

SOURCE: Fleisher LA, Fleischmann KE, Auerbach AD, et al. 2014 ACC/AHA Guideline on Perioperative Cardiovascular Evaluation and Management of Patients Undergoing Noncardiac Surgery: Executive Summary: A Report of the American College of Cardiology/American Heart Association Task Force on Practice Guidelines. *J Am Coll Cardiol*. 2014;64(22):2373–2405.

surgery, it should be considered in patients with clinical risk factors who are undergoing intermediate- or high-risk procedures, and have unknown or poor functional capacity (SOE=B). It is under comparatively rare circumstances that coronary revascularization (with coronary artery bypass graft surgery or percutaneous coronary intervention) should be performed before noncardiac surgery to decrease risk of cardiac complications (SOE=A), and as medical therapies continue to advance, the benefit of surgery relative to medical therapy even for these indications has narrowed. For indications for perioperative revascularization, see Table 15.2 (SOE=A).

Certain medications given before or after surgery reduce cardiac and vascular complications of surgery (Table 15.3). In general, prior antiplatelet therapy can be safely continued in patients undergoing neuraxial anesthesia, cutaneous surgery, dental procedures, diagnostic endoscopy, ophthalmologic procedures, and peripheral vascular surgery (SOE=C). For patients already on an anticoagulant, its protective benefits need to be weighed against the risk of perioperative hemorrhage. Anticoagulation therapy does not need to be withheld (as long as the INR is therapeutic) for cutaneous surgery (SOE=C), dental extractions and minor oral procedures (SOE=B), or cataract surgery (SOE=C). For other surgical procedures, cessation of warfarin, with or without bridging therapy with low-molecular-weight heparin (LMWH), can be based on the patient's risk factors for thromboembolism (Table 15.4). For patients receiving bridging therapy, LMWH can generally be restarted 24 hours after surgery, longer in cases of major surgery with increased risk of major bleeding. The indications for infective endocarditis prophylaxis were dramatically reduced with the publication of guidelines by the American Heart Association in 2007.

Finally, management of patients with coronary stents requires particular attention. Cohort studies identify substantially increased risk of major adverse cardiac events when surgery is performed soon after a coronary stent is placed, particularly for drug-eluting stents. The optimal timing for elective surgery is not before 30 days after a bare metal stent is placed and not before 365 days after a drug eluting stent is placed (SOE=B). Urgent or emergent surgeries that must be performed before those time frames require careful consideration of the added adverse cardiac risks they entail. Similarly, continuation of antiplatelet medications given to reduce stent thrombosis must be carefully weighed against the risk of significant postoperative bleeding incurred, and consideration of individual risk factors and preferences related to those competing risks must be considered.

Respiratory System

Postoperative pulmonary complications, most commonly atelectasis, pneumonia, and prolonged mechanical ventilation, occur more often in older adults than in younger age groups. The impact of these complications is more costly than the cardiovascular complications of surgery in older adults (SOE=A). Pulmonary complications are predictive of increased short- and long-term mortality in older adults and have been reported to prolong the hospital stay by an average of 1–2 weeks in this age group. A comprehensive review published by the American College of Physicians (ACP) in 2006 found that age is a powerful independent risk factor for postoperative pulmonary complications (SOE=A). Other patient-associated major risk factors include COPD, ASA Class II or greater (see Table 15.1), heart failure, deficit in ADLs, and a serum albumin <3.5 g/dL (SOE=A). Minor patient-associated risk factors include acute confusion or delirium, alcohol use, smoking, weight loss, pulmonary findings on physical examination, and an increased BUN concentration (SOE=B). The following procedures are associated with increased pulmonary complications: emergency surgery; prolonged (>3 hour) surgery; repair of abdominal aortic aneurysm (AAA); neurosurgery; and thoracic, abdominal, head and neck, or vascular surgery (SOE=A). General anesthesia is also a risk factor (SOE=A).

In 2007, the ACP published a guideline for risk assessment and perioperative management of pulmonary complications associated with noncardiothoracic surgery. It calls for preoperative assessment of pulmonary risk by appraising the above predictive factors through history, physical examination, and modest laboratory testing. Routine chest radiography is not recommended, but imaging can be helpful for detection and management of pulmonary conditions in patients with known cardiac or pulmonary disease who are undergoing thoracic, upper abdominal, or surgery for AAA. Spirometry should be reserved for evaluating lung function in patients suspected of having undiagnosed COPD after history and physical examination, based on findings such as dyspnea or wheezing. The question of whether treatment of newly discovered COPD changes outcomes after surgery has not been well studied. Preoperative pulmonary function testing is also routine before lung reduction surgeries. In recent years, several tools to predict the risk of postoperative respiratory failure and postoperative pneumonia have been published. The type of surgery, whether the surgery is emergent, the albumin level, BUN level, functional status, presence of COPD, and age are all components of the Veterans Administration Surgical Quality Improvement Program respiratory failure risk index (SOE=B). The same group validated a risk index to predict postoperative pneumonia using largely clinical information (SOE=B).

Table 15.2—Major Indications for Revascularization in the Perioperative Period (2011 ACC/AHA Guidelines)

- Significant unprotected left main vessel disease
- 3-Vessel disease
- 2-Vessel disease with proximal left anterior descending disease
- Survivors of sudden cardiac death with presumed ischemic ventricular tachycardia

The ACP guideline primarily recommends postoperative lung expansion therapy, which has been associated most consistently with reduced pulmonary complications of atelectasis, pneumonia, bronchitis, and severe hypoxemia (SOE=A). Lung expansion therapy can be accomplished through deep breathing exercises, incentive spirometry, and/or continuous positive-airway pressure. Use of a nasogastric tube for management of postoperative nausea and vomiting, inability to tolerate oral feeding, or abdominal distention can also be helpful for minimizing pulmonary complications (SOE=B). The evidence is also good for using short-acting neuromuscular blocking agents (as opposed to long-acting agents) to reduce complications (SOE=B). Less clear are the benefits of preoperative smoking cessation, use of laparoscopic versus open procedures, epidural versus general anesthesia, and epidural analgesia.

Kidneys and Metabolism

Glomerular blood flow decreases with age as does muscle mass, such that an apparently normal serum creatinine can be misinterpreted as indicating normal kidney function. The glomerular filtration rate (GFR) can be estimated by calculating the creatinine clearance using the Cockcroft-Gault equation or by relying on the Modification of Diet in Renal Disease study (MDRD

Table 15.3—Perioperative Medical Therapy to Reduce Cardiovascular Complications of Surgery

Medication	Target Conditions To Be Prevented	Dosage	Indications	SOE
β-Blocker	Myocardial infarction, ischemia, death	Usual dosage if already on a β-blocker.	Continue usual dosage if already on a β-blocker.	B
		β-Blocker therapy begun 2–30 days before surgery, titrated to achieve resting heart rate of 60–70 bpm and continued throughout postoperative period. Heart rate and blood pressure must be meticulously monitored to avoid bradycardia or hypotension, which significantly increase risk of ischemic stroke.	Consider initiating in patients with ≥3 cardiovascular risk factors or evidence of significant myocardial ischemia on preoperative testing.	C
Statin	Myocardial infarction, ischemia, death	Uncertain timing, specific drug, and dosage; one randomized trial used atorvastatin 20 mg/d po begun an average of 30 d before surgery	Continue usual dosage if already on a statin.	B
			Consider in all patients undergoing vascular surgery.	B
			Consider in patients with >1 clinical risk factor undergoing intermediate- or high-risk surgery.	C
Aspirin	Coronary events, transient ischemic attack, stroke	81–325 mg/d po	For patients already on aspirin, consider not withdrawing it before surgery unless patient is undergoing tonsillectomy, prostate surgery, or intracranial surgery.	B
			Data do not support initiation of aspirin in the preoperative period for noncardiac surgery patients.	
			Begin <24 hours after coronary artery bypass surgery.	A
Anticoagulant	Deep-vein thrombosis, pulmonary embolus	Enoxaparin, dalteparin, fondaparinux, unfractionated heparin, warfarin at dosages that depend on patient's risk of thromboembolism and bleeding complications	Begin postoperatively for patients >60 years old undergoing most types of surgery.	A
Antibiotic	Infective endocarditis	Amoxicillin 2 g po 30–60 min before procedure	Patients with selected cardiac conditions undergoing selected dental, respiratory tract, infected skin, or infected musculoskeletal tissue procedures	C

Table 15.4—Cessation of Anticoagulation Before Elective Surgery in Older Adults[a]

Thromboembolic Risk	Patient Conditions Determining Risk	Recommendations for Cessation of Anticoagulation
Low	No VTE in past 12 months; AF with $CHADS_2$ score of 0–2; bileaflet mechanical aortic valve without AF, prior TIA/stroke, or stroke risk factors	If INR therapeutic, stop warfarin 5 days before surgery, earlier if INR is supratherapeutic or >3.
Moderate	VTE in past 3–12 months; recurrent VTE; active malignancy (treated within 6 months or palliative); AF with $CHADS_2$ score of 3 or 4; bileaflet mechanical aortic valve with AF, prior TIA/stroke, or any stroke risk factors; nonsevere thrombophilia	Stop warfarin 5 days before surgery and begin LMWH 3 days before surgery at therapeutic (preferred) or prophylactic (optional) dosage; give last preoperative dose of LMWH 24 hours before surgery.
High	VTE within past 3 months; TIA/stroke within 6 months with mechanical heart valve or within 3 months with AF; rheumatic heart disease with AF; AF with $CHADS_2$ score of 5 or 6; mechanical mitral valve or ball/cage or tilting disc mechanical aortic valve; severe thrombophilia	Stop warfarin 5 days before surgery and begin LMWH 3 days before surgery at therapeutic dosage; give last preoperative dose of LMWH 24 hours before surgery.

VTE = venous thromboembolism; AF = atrial fibrillation; TIA = transient ischemic attack; INR = international normalized ratio; LMWH = low-molecular-weight heparin; $CHADS_2$ score = 1 point each for heart failure, hypertension, age >74 years, diabetes; 2 points for history of stroke

[a] SOE=C

SOURCE: Data from Douketis JD, Berger PB, Dunn AS, et al. The perioperative management of antithrombotic therapy. American College of Chest Physicians Evidence-Based Clinical Practice Guidelines. *Chest*. 2012;141(2Suppl);e326S.

method) that some laboratories use to automatically calculate GFR. Because many drugs administered during the perioperative period may require dosage adjustments in patients with diminished renal function, accurate estimation of GFR is important.

Also, because of decrements in the ability of the kidney to appropriately conserve salt or to maximally concentrate or dilute urine in response to intravascular volume or osmolality, the use of intravenous fluids needs to be monitored carefully. The combination of pain in a patient who is receiving nothing by mouth while receiving intravenous 5% dextrose in 0.45% normal saline may result in hyponatremia.

Neuropsychiatric Concerns

Delirium is a common event in the postoperative period. The type of surgery appears to be an important determinant of delirium, with incidence rates ranging from about 4%–5% in cataract or urologic procedures to 50%–60% in some series of patients with infrarenal AAA repair or hip fracture surgery. Both preoperative and intraoperative factors have been evaluated as risk factors for delirium. Preoperative assessment is focused on identifying factors in patients undergoing surgery that predispose to postoperative delirium, including age ≥70 years; cognitive impairment; limited physical function; a history of alcohol abuse; abnormal serum sodium, potassium, or glucose; intrathoracic surgery; and AAA surgery. Preoperative assessment should include clear assessment and documentation of mental status, so that postoperative assessments have a baseline for comparison. The most important intraoperative factor found to be associated with delirium is volume of intraoperative blood loss. Patients with a postoperative hematocrit <30% have an increased risk of delirium irrespective of the presence or absence of preoperative risk factors (SOE=B). Undertreatment of pain postoperatively is a significant risk factor for the development of delirium, at least in patients who were cognitively intact at baseline (SOE=B). When preoperative risk factors are present, the clinician can identify patients at greatest risk of developing delirium and can be vigilant about correcting fluid, electrolyte, and metabolic derangements; optimizing replacement of blood loss; maintaining circadian rhythms (by getting patients out of bed during the day and minimizing sleep interruptions at night); and prescribing medications cautiously while assuring adequate pain control. In particular, medications with CNS effects and especially those with anticholinergic adverse effects should be used with caution in the perioperative period, because they may precipitate delirium.

In recent years, the concept of postoperative cognitive decline (POCD) has emerged, but this syndrome is as yet poorly understood. Currently there is no consensus on the definition of POCD and whether it is an entity distinct from delirium in the perioperative period. This lack of sharp definition has resulted in incidence rate estimations that vary widely from 5% to 50%. Similarly, the duration and impact of POCD remains to be determined.

Iatrogenic Complications

Untoward effects of well-intentioned interventions are common among older hospitalized adults. Some of the more common pitfalls to be avoided include mobility restriction, excessive use of catheters, inattention to nutrition and hydration status, and inappropriate use of medications. Few disease states benefit from bed rest. It is important to maintain mobility and function as much as possible by encouraging time out of bed and avoiding restraints. The risks of skin breakdown, muscle atrophy, joint stiffness, and bone loss can be reduced by preserving mobility (SOE=C). Although bladder catheters can sometimes be critical in accurately measuring urine output, prolonged use of an indwelling catheter carries substantial risk of infection. Indwelling catheters can also contribute to restricted mobility and should be removed as soon as possible. Restricted diets and lack of access to water can contribute to compromise in nutrition and hydration. Studies demonstrate that the traditional practice of nothing-by-mouth beginning the night before surgery to reduce the risk of aspiration is not more beneficial than nothing by mouth for 6 hours except water, with the latter approach more comfortable for the patient and less likely to cause volume depletion (SOE=B). Conversely, continued administration of intravenous fluids after the patient is able to maintain hydration orally can result in volume overload and impaired oxygenation. A regular review of medication administration can avoid unnecessary drug use and inappropriate dosing.

PERIOPERATIVE AND POSTOPERATIVE MANAGEMENT OF SELECTED MEDICAL PROBLEMS

Surgery in older adults often results in destabilization of chronic, coexistent medical conditions. Additionally, because of the diminished physiologic reserve common in older adults, new medical problems can arise in the postoperative period. Some of the most common medical issues to contend with postoperatively are discussed here.

Cardiovascular Problems

The most common cardiovascular problems that arise in older adults after surgery are hypertension, rhythm disturbances, and heart failure. Postoperative hypertension should initially prompt a search for a noncardiovascular cause, such as pain or urinary retention. Next, it is important to assess volume status, review fluid administration records, and note whether antihypertensive medications were mistakenly omitted before the procedure. To treat uncontrolled essential hypertension, parenteral formulations are available in several classes of medications: β-blockers, calcium channel blockers, ACE inhibitors, and drugs that block both α- and β-adrenergic receptors. Topical agents, such as topical nitroglycerin, could also be considered useful when the patient is unable to take medications by mouth.

Cardiac rhythm disturbances are a concern, because they can lead to myocardial ischemia and heart failure. Supraventricular tachycardia, commonly seen in older adults, is associated with a history of prior supraventricular dysrhythmias, asthma, heart failure, and premature atrial complexes on a preoperative ECG. This rhythm disturbance is also more common in patients who have had vascular, abdominal, or thoracic procedures. Early restoration of sinus rhythm, or at least controlling the ventricular rate, can be attempted with an infusion of adenosine, a β-blocker, or a calcium channel blocker. If the rhythm is atrial fibrillation, conversion to sinus rhythm can be attempted with electrical cardioversion or by an infusion of amiodarone if the atrial fibrillation is poorly tolerated and the risk of thromboembolism is low. Because spontaneous reversion to sinus rhythm often occurs by 6 weeks after surgery, long-term use of an antidysrhythmic such as amiodarone may not be necessary. Persistent atrial fibrillation beyond 24–48 hours is associated with an increased risk of thromboembolism, and consideration should be given to anticoagulation therapy to reduce the risk of stroke (SOE=A).

Cardiac reserve is often compromised among older adults, especially those with chronic hypertension or coronary artery disease. Heart failure can develop as a result of excessive fluid administration, new cardiac ischemia, or a rhythm disturbance. It can be extremely challenging to ensure optimal ventricular filling pressures based on the clinical assessment of volume status in older adults by physical examination and standard laboratory parameters alone. Although some have recommended the use of pulmonary artery catheters in high-risk patients, studies have not shown a decreased mortality rate for this intervention, and most authorities advise against this approach (SOE=C).

Most older adults who are undergoing surgery should receive prophylaxis for deep venous thrombosis and pulmonary embolism.

Kidney and Electrolyte Disorders

Impaired preoperative kidney function increases the risk of postoperative kidney failure. The impaired reserve makes the aging kidney more susceptible to the effects of even transient reductions of cardiac output or brief exposure to nephrotoxic medications. When kidney damage has been sustained, early clinical manifestations include oliguria, isosthenuria, and an increase in serum creatinine. When impaired renal blood flow is the cause, the urine sodium will typically be <40 mEq/L and the urine-to-plasma creatinine ratio will be greater than 10:1. In contrast, if acute tubular necrosis is the mechanism of injury, the urine sediment may have granular or epithelial cell casts, and the urine sodium will be >40 mEq/L with a urine-to-plasma creatinine ratio of less than 10:1. When acute tubular necrosis is suspected, vigorous efforts should be made to preserve kidney function by withholding all potentially nephrotoxic medications and meticulously maintaining a euvolemic state.

Another important mechanism of postoperative kidney failure is obstructive nephropathy, especially in older men with prostatic hyperplasia. The partial outflow obstruction combined with immobility, frequent constipation, and exposure to medications with anticholinergic effects compromising detrusor function can easily precipitate acute urinary retention. In addition to oliguria and an increase in serum creatinine, the bladder is typically palpable because of distention. Treatment consists of insertion of a bladder catheter to reduce the risk of hydronephrosis and lasting kidney dysfunction. Commonly, men with prostatic hyperplasia who develop postoperative obstruction are unable to void immediately after catheter removal and may need α-blocking medications and continued use of the catheter for 2–4 weeks, when another voiding trial can be attempted (SOE=C).

Gastrointestinal Concerns

Constipation is quite common postoperatively, as a consequence of the combined effects of altered diet, immobility, and frequent use of narcotics and other constipating medications. At times, ileus and obstipation can be severe and produce significant anorexia, nausea, delirium, and even vomiting. Postoperative iron therapy, commonly prescribed for anemia, is an unproven but likely contributor to postoperative constipation. Given the common co-occurrence of these risk factors for constipation in the postoperative period, a reasonable approach is to simultaneously order a laxative and a fecal softener every time a narcotic is prescribed, particularly if the patient has a history of constipation or if it is reasonably anticipated that mobility will be reduced for longer than a day. Prunes or prune juice, applesauce, and bran can all also have promotility effects.

Postoperative diarrhea should raise concern for fecal impaction and antibiotic-associated or *Clostridium difficile* diarrhea in the setting of recent antibiotic use.

Checking manually for fecal impaction and testing fecal specimens for leukocytes and *C difficile* toxin may be appropriate. Management must focus carefully on volume resuscitation and treating the underlying cause. Use of antimotility agents, while effective in reducing fecal incontinence from diarrhea, is very risky in older adults in the postoperative period, because they significantly increase the risk of delirium, constipation, and toxic megacolon.

Finally, nausea is not uncommon in the postoperative period, often as a result of narcotic, anesthetic, and other medications; new infection; or slowed gut motility.

Managing Common Endocrine Abnormalities

Type 2 diabetes mellitus is a common comorbid condition of many older adults. Usually, given the long half-life of oral hypoglycemic agents and the nothing-by-mouth status for surgery, oral diabetes medications are withheld the day of surgery. It may be especially important to withhold metformin, given the potential (although quite low) additional risk of metabolic acidosis arising from use of this medication during a time of stress. To optimize glucose control, an intravenous solution containing glucose can be administered at a constant rate while blood glucose by fingerstick assay is closely monitored; subcutaneous insulin should be administered as necessary to control glucose concentrations until the patient is able to resume eating. For a patient with type 2 diabetes who uses insulin, insulin should be withheld on the day of surgery and sliding-scale insulin given (SOE=C). Once the patient is able to start eating, usually half the outpatient dosage of diabetes medications are administered the first day of oral intake, with additional sliding-scale insulin coverage as needed; full doses are resumed as the patient consumes a usual diet.

Perioperative hyperglycemia among diabetic and nondiabetic patients is associated with morbidity and mortality in medical and surgical ICU patients (SOE=B), and in patients undergoing coronary artery bypass grafting (SOE=C) or carotid endarterectomy (SOE=B). Maintaining glucose concentrations of <150 mg/dL with intravenous insulin in the perioperative period for patients undergoing vascular or major noncardiac surgery with planned ICU admission has reduced morbidity and mortality (SOE=B). However, maintaining tight glycemic control (≤110 mg/dL) among ICU patients has been associated with increased occurrence of hypoglycemia and no reduction in mortality (SOE=B); therefore, moderate glucose control in these patients is advised. The value of strict glycemic control in other surgical or medical inpatient populations has not been demonstrated.

Patients taking supplemental corticosteroids require special consideration during the perioperative period. Those taking prednisone at dosages >20–30 mg/d for longer than a week or with known adrenal insufficiency should be given "stress doses" of steroids after surgery (SOE=C). A single preoperative measurement of cortisol, if increased, is useful to assess the hypothalamic-pituitary axis (HPA) in patients who chronically use steroids when the function of the HPA is in question. If the cortisol level is not high, a 30-minute adrenocorticotropic hormone (ACTH) stimulation test may be useful. The dosage of steroids to use is debated, but some authorities advise 25 mg of hydrocortisone equivalents the day of surgery only for minor procedures, 50–75 mg of hydrocortisone equivalents daily (eg, hydrocortisone 20 mg q8h IV) for 1–2 days for moderate surgical stress, and 100–150 mg of hydrocortisone equivalents daily (eg, hydrocortisone 50 mg q8h IV beginning within 2 hours of surgery) continuing for 2–3 days after surgery for high surgical stress. Other authorities simply recommend continuing usual dosages of steroids for elective, uncomplicated surgeries, or doubling or tripling the outpatient dosage by giving hydrocortisone at dosages up to 100–150 mg/d IV for higher-risk or anticipated complicated operations.

Delirium and Postoperative Cognitive Decline

Delirium is one of the most common postoperative complications, and certainly the one for which a geriatrician is most likely to be consulted. In a randomized study, a multicomponent intervention that focused on reducing sleep interruptions, minimizing medications and immobility, enhancing sensory input, and reducing dehydration reduced the rate of developing delirium by one-third over standard care for hospitalized medical patients (SOE=A). This approach, although not specifically studied in the postoperative setting, is likely to be beneficial for these patients as well (SOE=C). For the postoperative geriatric surgical patient, undertreated pain, constipation, electrolyte abnormalities, and perioperative myocardial infarction must be particularly considered as possible precipitants of delirium.

Postoperative cognitive dysfunction, characterized by abnormalities in learning and memory, can be subtle or dramatic and is considered to be a syndrome distinct from delirium. It has been reported most commonly after cardiac surgery but is experienced by patients undergoing procedures that do not involve extracorporeal circulation. Although the symptoms are often short-lived, they persist for many months in 10%–30% of patients. Efforts to define the cause of the syndrome have not yet been successful; studies have not been able to demonstrate links with hypotension, hypoxemia, or type of anesthesia. Because a better understanding of the pathophysiology is lacking, treatment efforts are supportive.

Pain Management

Management of postoperative pain remains a challenge, particularly in patients with dementia, delirium, or both. The oldest-old and cognitively impaired patients appear to be at highest risk of undertreatment of pain, so they deserve particular attention. Undertreatment of pain, at least in nondemented individuals, appears to be a more powerful predictor for development of postoperative delirium than narcotic use (SOE=A).

Most postsurgical pain requires narcotic analgesia. Cognitively intact patients may have improved pain relief and overall lower use of narcotics if administered by patient-controlled analgesia pump (SOE=A). Individuals with less severe pain may be able to tolerate scheduled acetaminophen (not to exceed 4 g/d) with only as-needed use of narcotic analgesics, if they are able to ask for them. Patients with pain who are unable to communicate effectively should be given standing orders for narcotic analgesics, with guidelines as to when to withhold the medications, and should be frequently assessed for medication effect. NSAIDs are best avoided because of the potential for GI bleeding, delirium, fluid retention, nephrotoxicity, and cardiovascular risks. Because narcotic analgesics can precipitate constipation, concomitant use of laxatives and fecal softeners is generally advised. A small body of literature is accumulating supporting the benefits of "preemptive" analgesia to reduce anticipated pain and total doses of narcotic required to control pain postoperatively, but this has yet to be studied in older adults. For comprehensive, up-to-date information on pain medications and dosing, see www.geriatricsatyourfingertips.org.

Nonpharmacologic therapies, such as ice packs, heating pads, massage, and relaxation techniques, can be useful adjuncts to therapy and are often underused.

Choosing Wisely® Recommendations

Perioperative Care

- Do not perform stress cardiac imaging or advanced noninvasive imaging as a preoperative assessment in patients scheduled to undergo low-risk noncardiac surgery.
- Patients who have no cardiac history and good functional status do not require preoperative stress testing before noncardiac thoracic surgery.
- Do not perform preoperative medical tests for eye surgery unless there are specific medical indications.
- Avoid echocardiograms for preoperative/perioperative assessment of patients with no history or symptoms of heart disease.
- Do not order coronary artery calcium scoring for preoperative evaluation for any surgery, irrespective of patient risk.
- Do not initiate routine evaluation of carotid artery disease before cardiac surgery in the absence of symptoms or other high-risk criteria.
- Before cardiac surgery, there is no need for pulmonary function testing in the absence of respiratory symptoms.
- Do not obtain preoperative chest radiography in the absence of clinical suspicion for intrathoracic pathology.

REFERENCES

- American College of Surgeons National Surgical Quality Improvement Program (NSQIP) and the American Geriatrics Society. *Optimal Perioperative Management of the Geriatric Patient: Best Practices Guideline from ACS NSQIP®/American Geriatrics Society*; 2016. http://geriatricscareonline.org/toc/optimal-perioperative-management-of-the-geriatric-patient/CL022/ (accessed Jan 2016)

   The American College of Surgeons partnered with the American Geratrics Society to publish this set of guidelines, which are divided into four parts: immediate preoperative management, intraoperative management, postoperative management, and care transitions. While the entire guideline set will be of value to the geriatrician, the latter two sections will have more applicability to clinical services delivered primarily in geratrics practice.

- Chow WB, Rosenthal RA, Merkow RP, et al. Optimal preoperative assessment of the geriatric surgical patient: a best practices guideline from the American College of Surgeons National Surgical Quality Improvement Program and the American Geriatrics Society. *J Am Coll Surg*. 2012;215(4):453–466.

   This article reflects the work of a 21-member expert panel composed of members of the American College of Surgeons National Surgical Quality Improvement Program and the American Geriatrics Society. This literature review included papers relating to preoperative care of older surgical patients of trials published between January 1990 and December 2011. Evidence-based recommendations are made relating to care of patients with cognitive impairment, decision-making capacity, depression, delirium, alcohol and substance abuse, cardiac and pulmonary evaluation, functional status and mobility, frailty, nutritional status, medication management, patient counseling, and preoperative testing.

- Devereaux PJ, Mrkobrada M, Sessler DI, et al for the POISE-2 Investigators. Aspirin in patients undergoing noncardiac surgery. *N Engl J Med*. 2014;370(16):1494–1503.

   In this prospective randomized trial of >10,000 adults undergoing noncardiac surgery and with at least one risk factor for vascular complications, there was no impact on the composite of MI or death at 30 days with either low-dose aspirin or placebo, although major bleeding was increased in the aspirin group (SOE=A). In this study, 52% of the patients were ≥70 years old, and patients with drug-eluting coronary stents placed in the year before surgery, or bare metal stents placed within 6 weeks of surgery, were excluded. This study suggests that in patients for whom anticoagulants are used in the perioperative period, the addition of aspirin probably adds no benefit and likely increases the risk of significant bleeding.

- Devereaux PJ, Sessler DI, Kurz LA, et al for the POISE-2 Investigators. Clonidine in patients undergoing noncardiac surgery. *N Engl J Med.* 2014;370(16):1504–1513.

    The POISE-2 study also contained an arm that randomized patients to clonidine 0.2 mg daily versus placebo started just before surgery and continued for 72 hours total based on the results of smaller studies suggesting potential benefit. Low-dose clonidine was associated with more harm than benefit in this study: significant hypotension and nonfatal cardiac arrest were both increased in the treatment groups and there was no difference between groups in the combined outcome of death or MI in 30 days after surgery.

- Douketis JD, Spyropoulos AC, Spencer FA, et al. Perioperative management of antithrombotic therapy and prevention of thrombosis. American College of Chest Physicians Evidence-Based Clinical Practice Guidelines (9th Ed). *Chest.* 2012;141(2 Suppl):e326S–350S.

    Geriatricians often face the question of whether or not to discontinue antiplatelet agents or anticoagulants in patients undergoing surgery. This comprehensive guideline presents the evidence for hemorrhagic risk of continuing these agents, and the thromboembolic risk of stopping these agents in patients with prior stroke. The authors provide evidence-based schemes for classifying patients into thromboembolic risk categories with specific recommendations for anticoagulation/antiplatelet management before and after surgery.

- Fleisher LA, Fleischmann KE, Auerbach AD, et al. 2014 ACC/AHA guideline on perioperative cardiovascular evaluation and management of patients undergoing noncardiac surgery. *Circulation.* 2014;130(24):e278–e333.

    The ACC and AHA guidelines provide a comprehensive review of the current state of the evidence around perioperative cardiac evaluation and management, including a scholarly discussion about the nuanced evidence related to the use of β-blockers in the perioperative time frame. This is considered the authoritative reference for the perioperative management of cardiac diseases and risk.

- Nadelson MR, Sanders RD, Avidan MS. Perioperative cognitive trajectory in adults. *Br J Anaesth* 2014;112(3):440–451.

    This is a comprehensive review of the state of evidence around the impact of surgery on cognition in older adults. In particular, the authors provide a scholarly discussion about the emerging concept of postoperative cognitive decline, highlighting the need for a consensus definition of the syndrome to better understand risk factors for and impact of the phenomenon.

- Oresanya LB, Lyons WL, Finlayson E. Preoperative assessment of the older patient: a narrative review. *JAMA.* 2014;311(20):2110–2120.

    This is a scholarly review of the literature published in 2000–2013, focused entirely on issues related to surgery in older patients. In this review, the authors are especially thorough in their discussion about the evidence around risk factors for mortality and functional dependence, as well as for geriatric-specific syndromes and complications. A useful set of sample questions is provided to help readers elicit patients' treatment goals, priorities, and insights. Cognitive impairment was associated with a higher risk of death after surgery in most studies, arguing strongly that cognitive status should be a routine part of preoperative assessment in older adults. Functional decline after surgery was substantial, ranging from 24% at 1 year to 61% at 2 years, and cognitive impairment conferred a high risk of functional decline. Notably, frailty was associated with a 3- to 13-fold increase in being discharged to a facility rather than to home. This paper is a very practical and useful reference when contemplating surgery in frail older adults.

- Qaseem A, Snow V, Fitterman N, et al for the Clinical Efficacy Assessment Subcommittee of the American College of Physicians. Risk assessment for and strategies to reduce perioperative pulmonary complications for patients undergoing noncardiothoracic surgery: a guideline from the American College of Physicians. *Ann Intern Med.* 2006;144(8):575–580.

    This concise, evidence-based guideline debunks many previously common practices regarding preoperative testing and postoperative management of pulmonary complications. A detailed set of risk factors (including advanced age) for postoperative pulmonary complications is presented. The recommendations for postoperative management are more brief, reflecting the relative lack of evidence supporting risk-reducing therapies.

Colleen Christmas, MD
James T. Pacala, MD, MS, AGSF

CHAPTER 16—PALLIATIVE CARE

KEY POINTS

- Palliative care, an interdisciplinary activity, aims to relieve physical and emotional suffering, optimize function, and assist with decision making for patients with advanced disease and their families. Palliative services may be provided regardless of whether the patient is receiving curative or disease-modifying treatment. It is distinct from hospice. Hospice is a comprehensive care system for patients expected to live ≤6 months; its sole focus of care is on comfort and relief of suffering for individuals at life's end.

- For many older adults, dying is characterized by inadequately treated physical distress; fragmented care systems; poor or absent communication among clinicians, patients, and families; and enormous strain on family caregivers and support systems.

- The experiences of dying individuals are affected by geographic variations in practice patterns and services available, religious beliefs, economic status, medical diagnoses, gender, and cognitive function.

- Loss of appetite is almost a universal symptom at the end of life; often it is more distressing to loved ones than to the patient.

In the United States, the overwhelming majority of deaths occur among the older adult population. Older adults typically die slowly of chronic diseases, with multiple coexisting problems, progressive dependency on others, and heavy personal care needs, which are met mostly by family members. Many of these deaths become protracted processes for patients, family members, and clinicians, who must make difficult decisions about the use or discontinuation of life-prolonging treatments. Abundant evidence indicates the quality of life during the dying process is often poor. For many older adults, dying is characterized by inadequately treated physical distress; fragmented care systems; poor or absent communication among clinicians, patients, and families; and enormous strains on family caregivers and support systems.

Although Americans usually spend most of their final months at home, their deaths typically occur in the hospital or nursing home. The experience of dying varies greatly from one part of the country to another. For example, in Portland, Oregon, 35% of adult deaths occur in hospitals, but in New York City >80% occur there, a difference associated in part with variations in regional hospital bed supply and availability of community support for the dying. Social and medical variations also account for these differing patterns. The need for paid caregivers or institutionalization in the last months of life is much higher among poor individuals and women. Similarly, older adults suffering from cognitive impairment and dementia are much more likely than cognitively intact individuals to spend their last days in a nursing home.

OVERALL CARE NEAR DEATH

The Hospitalized Elderly Longitudinal Project (HELP) and the Choices, Attitudes, and Strategies for Care of Advanced Dementia at the End-of-Life (CASCADE) are two studies that examined the end of life for older adults. The HELP study characterized the last 6 months of life and dying in 1,266 adults ≥80 years old. Investigators showed that people tend to overestimate their chances of survival near the end of life (SOE=A). Patients who died within 1 year of enrollment had significant functional impairment in activities of daily living (ADLs) and expressed strong preferences for no resuscitation attempts and for comfort care (SOE=A). The number of patients reporting severe pain increased toward the end of life, with one in three reporting severe pain within 3 months of death (SOE=A). The CASCADE study described the course of 323 nursing-home residents with advanced dementia. Researchers showed that pneumonia, eating problems, and fevers were the events most associated with 6-month mortality (SOE=A). Patients in the study commonly experienced pain and dyspnea, with prevalence of these symptoms comparable to those of dying cancer patients (SOE=A). Patients with advanced dementia were under-recognized to be at high risk of death and received suboptimal palliative care. The results of these two studies highlight the need for clinicians to talk with patients early about their preferences and to provide better symptom control and palliative measures at the end of life.

One of the challenges in providing excellent end-of-life care stems from the difficulty to accurately prognosticate, particularly for patients with chronic diseases such as heart failure and COPD, in which exacerbations and remissions are common and unpredictable. Fortunately, prognostic tools are increasingly available. Historically, prognostic inventories focused on single disease states, such as the BODE index for COPD or the New York Heart Association Classification for heart failure. Functional status figures prominently in worthy prognostic tools. The Palliative Performance Scale (www.npcrc.org/files/news/palliative_performance_scale_PPSv2.pdf

[accessed Jan 2016]), for example, embraces self-care function, as well as ratings of mobility, activity level, oral intake, and level of consciousness, and can be used for people with multiple comorbidities. Various online tools and smart phone applications are available to help providers to prognosticate. The online site http://eprognosis.ucsf.edu is a repository of validated geriatric prognostic indices helpful in clinical practice. *"Hospice in a Minute"* is a free application for smart phones that includes a section on hospice eligibility criteria for several diseases.

ETHNOGRAPHIC DATA

Ethnographic studies show that a patient's and family's ethnic, cultural, and religious heritage can influence their responses to serious illness, desire for aggressive care, death, grief, and mourning (SOE=B).

In many Asian cultures, for example, filial piety implies strong devotion to the dying person, with the oldest child expected to accompany the parent through the final stage of life. Discussions of death may be thought to bring it about or speed its advance, so clinicians should be careful when entering into discussions about end-of-life issues. Families may request the diagnosis not be shared directly with patients. Health care decisions are generally viewed as family decisions in Asian cultures, so it is especially important for clinicians to determine who should be present for delivery of bad news or discussion of care goals. Although this is good advice regardless of ethnic and cultural background, the negative consequences of not doing so may be more pronounced in Asian cultures.

Studies of blacks show that as a group, spirituality plays a dominant role in how end of life is experienced and interpreted (SOE=A). Data indicate that blacks are more likely to pray for a miracle rather than accept death, to believe in the omnipotence of God, to believe that God (rather than medical treatment or the lack of it) determines the timing of death, to view the clinician as God's instrument, and to believe God is able to perform miracles (SOE=A).

It is important to remember that not all patients and families from a particular background will respond and make choices in a similar manner. Assuming patients and families will do so can lead to misunderstanding. One useful way to introduce the subject is for the clinician to begin by asking, "Is there anything about your culture or your beliefs that would be helpful for me to know as we plan together for the future?"

PALLIATIVE CARE AND HOSPICE

Palliative care is interdisciplinary care that aims to relieve physical and emotional suffering, improve quality of life, optimize function, and assist with decision making for patients with advanced illness and their families. It is offered simultaneously with all other disease-modifying medical treatments, either by the primary medical team or in conjunction with a palliative care consultant. In contrast, hospice is specialized palliative care limited to patients who meet two criteria: their life expectancy is <6 months if their disease takes its natural course, and they (or their proxies) have elected to focus on comfort measures and forgo curative treatment.

Table 16.1—Hospice Services

- Care provided by an interprofessional team: nurse/care manager, social worker, chaplain, aides, volunteers, physical therapist, occupational therapist, speech therapist, dietitian, physician supervision and services
- Case management by a hospice nurse
- Access to a hospice physician
- Medications at no cost, as long as they are related to the terminal diagnosis and are palliative, as determined by the hospice plan of care
- Tests and other treatments at no cost, as long as they are related to the terminal diagnosis and are palliative, as determined by the hospice plan of care
- Durable medical equipment
- Bereavement services for 13 months after a death

Hospice, established as a Medicare benefit in 1982, can be provided at home or in institutional settings. Initially, hospice coverage was made available through an expanded Medicare benefit; now it is supported through Medicare and Medicaid, the Veterans Affairs Medical System, and most commercial insurance policies. The benefit is a highly regulated, fully capitated health care arrangement, which is now implemented through >3,000 hospice agencies. Hospice is primarily a home-care program, with access to skilled inpatient beds for the infrequent management of acute problems, such as severe pain, dyspnea, or agitation. Hospice programs receive one of four daily rates for reimbursement, based on four levels of care: routine home care, inpatient level of care, continuous care (short term, nursing-intensive crisis management of symptoms in the home), and respite care. For a summary of the services hospice provides, see Table 16.1.

To enroll in hospice services, two physicians—the hospice medical director and the patient's referring physician—must certify that they believe the patient has a remaining life expectancy of ≤6 months if the disease runs its expected course. Both physicians must sign a "Certificate of Terminal Illness" attesting to this assessment. Medicare guidelines require that the patient be recertified hospice-eligible every few months. This is similar to the recertification required for

Medicare skilled rehabilitation and skilled home-care services. If the patient is no longer judged to have a remaining life expectancy of <6 months, then he or she must be discharged from hospice. The patient can also revoke the hospice benefit at any time, for example, if a decision is made to resume curative treatments.

On January 1, 2011, CMS enacted a new regulation on hospices requiring a "face-to-face" visit for all patients entering their third certification period (at 6 months of hospice services) and every 60-day certification period thereafter. These face-to-face visits may only be completed by a physician affiliated with the hospice or by a nurse practitioner who is a W2 employee of the hospice. The purpose of this bedside evaluation is for a trained clinician to assess the patient's ongoing eligibility for hospice services and to deliberately reevaluate a patient's prognosis. Anecdotal evidence suggests the face-to-face visit has not resulted in a dramatic increase in live discharges from hospice.

QUALITY INDICATORS FOR PALLIATIVE CARE

Hospice and palliative care leaders have recognized the need to ensure the delivery of high-quality care in their programs. The National Consensus Project for Quality Palliative Care was convened in 2001 to develop practice guidelines that would improve the quality of palliative care. The first guidelines were published in 2004, the most recent in 2013. The revised guidelines emphasize the need for collaboration across health care settings and incorporate the growing evidence base in palliative care. These guidelines have been adopted by the National Quality Forum, along with preferred practices for hospice and palliative care programs. The guidelines (outlined in Table 16.2) describe high-quality palliative practices in 8 core domains.

Research demonstrates palliative care improves quality of life for patients and their families (SOE=A). A landmark controlled clinical trial showed that patients with metastatic non-small-cell lung cancer who received palliative care had improved quality of life with less depression and anxiety, received less aggressive care, had resuscitative preferences documented, had longer stays in hospice, and even had longer survival (SOE=A). This study based the intervention on the National Consensus Project standards of care for palliative care. Expert opinion recommends the use of quality indicators and guidelines in palliative and end-of-life care (SOE=D) for other disease states.

COMMUNICATION

Skillful communication by clinicians is essential to the delivery of high-quality palliative care. Most patients under care are dying from a progressive chronic illness (or more than one) like heart disease, cancer, cerebrovascular disease, chronic lung disease, dementia, or chronic liver disease. Many face recurrent exacerbations of illness and have to make difficult decisions about treatment options. To accompany patients and families through the process of diagnosis, evaluation of treatment options, and eventual death, clinicians need skills in discussing serious news, prognosis, and transitions of care; clarifying treatment goals; dealing with emotions of patients and families; and facilitating family meetings. Effective communication in end-of-life care improves patients' and families' satisfaction and experience of care (SOE=B).

Clinicians have historically received little formal training in communication skills. As a result, some may feel unprepared to deal with these emotionally charged discussions, and others may fear these discussions will adversely affect the patient and the family, or the clinician-patient relationship. A systematic approach to communication can foster collaboration among the patient, the family, and the clinician (SOE=C). Effective discussions can enhance the patient's and the family's ability to plan for the future, set realistic goals, and support one another emotionally.

A key skill to enhance communication is recognizing and responding to emotions. Patients' emotional responses may interfere with their ability to digest information and thus impede decisions about next steps. Patients often report not hearing anything more after receiving notice of a life-threatening condition. Responding to emotions may help patients to process them, a step that often must precede the assimilation of information about prognosis or treatment options. Clinicians' response to emotions also demonstrates empathy and openness to further discussion, and signifies to patients they are understood. One recommended approach to responding to emotions is, first, to recognize that the patient has had an emotional response; next, to name the emotion; and finally to explicitly respond to the patient in a way that acknowledges the emotion. The recognition can be verbal or nonverbal. Data show that how patients are told about serious information (such as a new cancer diagnosis) impacts patient outcomes (SOE=B).

Communication about serious illness is enhanced when clinicians spend sufficient time getting to know their patients and adopting a goal of exploring their patients' life values and aims. Discussing a patient's preferences and goals of care will help guide treatment recommendations. Clinicians need to understand what is important to the patient, including determining if and how they want information given to them, and how they want to participate in decision making about their care. Although most Americans say they want to be fully informed about their illnesses, a minority may

Table 16.2—National Consensus Guidelines:* 8 Core Palliative Care Domains

Domain	Guideline	Comments
1	Structure and Process	Describes the interprofessional team engagement with patients and families, with emphasis on individual preferences
2	Physical Aspects	Describes the assessment and management of physical symptoms with validated tools and a multidimensional approach to management
3	Psychological and Psychiatric Aspects	Describes the collaborative assessment of psychological concerns and psychiatric diagnoses to enhance care; outlines requirement for a bereavement program for patients, families, and staff
4	Social Aspects	Identifies the essential elements of palliative care social assessment and emphasizes identifying and supporting family strengths
5	Spiritual, Religious, and Existential Aspects	Describes the assessment of these concerns through the disease course and the importance of evaluation by the interprofessional team
6	Cultural Aspects	Defines cultural competence for the interprofessional team
7	Care of the Patient at the End of Life	Describes communication and documentation of signs and symptoms of the dying process with the family
8	Ethical and Legal Aspects	Describes advance care planning, ethics of palliative care, and legal issues

* http://nationalconsensusproject.org (accessed Jan 2016)

Table 16.3—Discussing Serious News: A 6-Step Framework

1. Prepare for the meeting	Have all medical facts available. Prepare an appropriate environment.
2. Establish the patient's understanding	Explore the patient's understanding of the illness. Ask "What do you understand about your illness?" or "What have the doctors told you about your illness?"
3. Determine how much the patient wants to know	Not all patients want to know about their medical situation; data suggest this may be true for certain ethnic groups. Ask "Would you like me to tell you the full details of your condition? If not, is there someone else you would like me to talk to?"
4. Tell the patient	Deliver information in a sensitive, straightforward manner, avoiding technical language or euphemisms. Check for understanding. Phrasing that includes a warning helps prepare patients for bad news. For example: "The report is back, and it's not as we had hoped. It showed that there is cancer in your colon."
5. Respond to feelings	Acknowledge the patient's emotion.
6. Plan and follow up	Organize a therapeutic plan that incorporates a follow-up visit and information on how to reach the clinician if additional questions arise.

not want to know the full details or may prefer to have another family member informed. Although data suggest that these preferences may vary among certain ethnic groups, there is no way to know how much a given patient wants to know or be involved in decision making without asking directly. Patients with serious illness and their families also may have different communication needs from each other, and it is important to determine this early. Asking, "Are you the type of person who is comforted by details and test data?" or "Would it be helpful to discuss prognosis now?" both allows the patient to remain in control as well as determines the amount of information to which they are exposed.

Discussing serious news with patients may provoke anxiety in the clinician. The literature offers several frameworks, all with similar steps, and each based on a shared decision-making paradigm. Use of a framework can minimize stress by serving as a procedural checklist. For one 6-step framework that can be used as a guide for these difficult conversations, see Table 16.3.

One key to these dialogues is determining if patients, their families, or both, understand the current medical situation. It is then important to assess patients' and families' willingness to talk about what to do next. A clinician might first inquire if the patient has thought about what he or she would do at this point in the disease, or what he or she is hoping for or worried about. Based on these discussions, a provider may offer to make a recommendation for care that is seen as consistent with the goals and values a patient has expressed. This often will include the suggestion to enroll in hospice or make a referral to palliative care. After making the recommendation, the clinician may explore what the patient and family think about the proposal. The provider might emphasize the expertise of a palliative care team to improve symptom management and to help address the physical and practical changes brought on by the disease. When discussing hospice, it is important to specifically describe what hospice can do to meet the patient's articulated goals and needs.

Providers should also emphasize their continued involvement with the patient regardless of hospice and/or palliative care involvement, because patients with advanced illness often fear abandonment by their providers at end of life. Patients and families also often have misconceptions about hospice and palliative care, which should be elicited and addressed to ensure that the goals and procedures of hospice and palliative care are understood.

After patients' preferences for end-of-life care are elicited (perhaps through surrogates), they must be faithfully communicated. Often, these preferences are documented in advance directives or written orders about cardiopulmonary resuscitation. Studies show that these documents and orders are often ineffective in determining end-of-life treatment (SOE=B). The Physician Orders for Life Sustaining Treatment (POLST) program was developed initially in Oregon to address the inadequacies of communicating end-of-life preferences, and over the past decade use of these forms has spread to many other states. The forms may go by slightly different names, depending on the jurisdiction. These forms constitute medical orders reflecting preferences for cardiopulmonary resuscitation, medical interventions, antibiotics, and artificial hydration. Importantly, these orders transfer across care settings. For example, a patient with widely metastatic colon cancer who elects a "do-not-attempt-resuscitation" status at his or her cancer center can have a POLST form completed for his ambulance ride to a local hospice facility. The POLST orders would be immediately active on arrival, before evaluation by the receiving hospice clinician. If a cardiac arrest were to transpire en route or on arrival, the POLST would exempt emergency personnel from attempting "heroic measures." Research on the POLST program has shown a decreased rate of unwanted hospitalization and better documentation of preferences (SOE=B).

PALLIATION OF SYMPTOMS

As with all clinical evaluations in geriatric medicine, the first step in a palliative-focused, symptom assessment is determination of the patient's goals of care. Next, the clinical evaluation incorporates an assessment of the patient's functional status, physical ability to tolerate different treatment modalities and routes of medication administration, and overall prognosis. Clinical data are then merged with patient and family goals, values, and cultural norms through a process of shared decision making to develop a care plan that is individualized to each patient. For example, medications that may ordinarily be eschewed elsewhere in geriatric care, such as benzodiazepines, may have their use in the care of a dyspneic patient whose life expectancy is <72 hours and whose family is gathered at bedside, sitting vigil, and wishing for a peaceful death.

Pain

Pain management in older adults with serious and life-limiting illness is no different than it is for other patients. It begins with a thorough assessment of the pain, formulation of the causes of the pain, and deliberation of management strategies to treat the pain. The key to good pain management is reassessment of interventions for their effectiveness in providing relief. It is often helpful to conceptualize pain as acute versus chronic, and with qualities that define it as somatic, visceral, or neuropathic. This is helpful in guiding what treatments might be effective. Patients who have cognitive impairment have not been shown to feel pain any less acutely than others, but they may exhibit their discomfort by withdrawing from surroundings (eg, lack of appetite or participation) or by increasing agitation and resistance to daily care. In patients at the very end of life, oral administration of medication may not be possible, and alternative routes of delivery (eg, via suppositories, transmucosal formulations, or subcutaneous injection) may need to be explored.

Constipation

Constipation is one of the most common and distressing symptoms seen in terminally ill patients. Many medications, including opioid pain medications, significantly contribute to constipation, which is further exacerbated by the reduced mobility and poor fluid intake that accompanies most life-limiting illnesses. Although other unwanted effects of opioids generally diminish over time, constipation usually persists, requiring ongoing bowel management as long as opioid therapy is used (SOE=D). Patients on opioids should receive prophylactic laxatives consisting of a fecal softener (eg, docusate sodium) and a bowel stimulant (eg, senna, bisacodyl), unless diarrhea has already been a problem. If these measures are not effective, then an osmotic laxative (eg, sorbitol, lactulose, or polyethylene glycol) should be added. If a patient has had no bowel movement for ≥4 days, an enema should be considered. Patients presenting with constipation should be evaluated for bowel obstruction or fecal impaction. In cases of impaction, manual disimpaction or enemas should be used before starting laxative therapy. Methylnaltrexone bromide is specifically approved for treatment of opioid-induced constipation in patients with advanced illness, in whom usual treatment (as outlined above) has not been effective. Methylnaltrexone antagonizes opioid binding to the peripheral μ-opioid receptors in the gastrointestinal tract. It does not cross the blood-brain barrier and has no effect on the central analgesic effects

Table 16.4—Medications for Nausea

Class	Predominant Site of Action	Examples	Comments
Dopamine antagonists	Chemoreceptor trigger zone	Haloperidol[OL] 0.5–2 mg po, IV, or SC q6h, then titrate Prochlorperazine 10–20 mg po q6h, or 25 mg pr q12h, or 5–10 mg IV q6h Promethazine 12.5–25 mg IV, or 25 mg po or pr q4–6h Perphenazine 2–8 mg po q6h	Haloperidol is an effective antinausea medication. Promethazine and perphenazine can cause sedation, urinary retention, and delirium in frail older adults.
Serotonin antagonists	Chemoreceptor trigger zone, GI tract	Ondansetron 8 mg po q8h Granisetron 1 mg po q24h or q12h	Effective for chemotherapy-induced nausea; expensive
Neurokinin-1 receptor antagonist	Chemoreceptor trigger zone	Aprepitant 125 mg po then 80 mg/d po	Recommended for resistant cases of chemotherapy-induced nausea
Prokinetic agents	GI tract	Metoclopramide 5–20 mg po q6h	Useful if nausea is secondary to dysmotility
Antacids	GI tract	H_2-receptor antagonists: cimetidine, famotidine, ranitidine Proton-pump inhibitors: omeprazole, lansoprazole	Useful if nausea is caused by gastritis
Corticosteroids	GI tract, cerebral cortex	Dexamethasone 6–10 mg po loading dose followed by 2–4 mg po q6–12h Prednisone 4–10 mg/d po	Useful for nausea from hepatic capsular distention and increased intracranial pressure; monitor for adverse effects, including altered mood, psychosis
Synthetic somatostatin analogue	GI tract	Octreotide 100–200 mcg SC bid to qid or a continuous infusion	Useful in nausea from bowel obstruction
Antihistamines	Vestibular	Diphenhydramine 25–50 mg po q6h Meclizine 25–50 mg po q6h Hydroxyzine 25–50 mg po q6h	Can cause sedation, urinary retention, and delirium in frail older adults
Anticholinergics	Vestibular	Scopolamine 0.1–0.4 mg SC or IV q4h, or 1 to 3 transdermal patches q72h, or 10–80 mcg/h by continuous IV or SC infusion	Useful when cause of nausea is from vestibular apparatus
Benzodiazepines	Cerebral cortex	Lorazepam up to 2mg po night before chemotherapy and up to 2 mg po after chemotherapy	Helpful for anticipatory nausea and vomiting from chemotherapy; can cause agitation in older adults
Cannabinoids	Cerebral cortex	Dronabinol 2.5 mg po to a maximum total dose of 50 mg po qd	Can cause dysphoria, hallucinations; evidence is poor for effectiveness

of opioids. It is contraindicated in known or suspected mechanical intestinal obstruction. Lubiprostone is a chloride channel activator also approved for use in opioid constipation, as well as idiopathic constipation. Like methylnaltrexone, it is contraindicated in bowel obstruction.

Nausea and Vomiting

The incidence of nausea and vomiting is estimated to be 40%–70% in patients with advanced cancer (SOE=B). Nausea is a subjective sensation mediated through the stimulation of the gastrointestinal lining, the chemoreceptor trigger zone, the vestibular apparatus, and the cerebral cortex. Vomiting is a neuromuscular reflex. Symptoms can be caused both by disease and its treatment. Because nausea involves multiple neurotransmitters, numerous agents are used for treatment, and often more than one medication is needed for control. The key to successful management involves identifying the likely cause of the nausea, selecting a medication that works on the cause, and giving around-the-clock medication if the nausea is constant (SOE=D). For medications useful in treatment of nausea, see Table 16.4. Although many providers have used topical lorazepam, diphenhydramine, and haloperidol gel (aka "ABH") for treatment of nausea, evidence has shown it is not effective and should not be used to treat nausea (SOE=A). This is a recommendation of The Choosing Wisely® Campaign.

Diarrhea

Diarrhea affects 7%–10% of patients with cancer who are admitted to hospice (SOE=C). Diarrhea is defined as the passage of more than three unformed bowel movements within a 24-hour period. A common cause of diarrhea in palliative medicine is excessive laxative administration, especially after upward dose adjustments intended to clear an impaction. These diarrheal episodes respond to temporary cessation of laxatives, and delayed reintroduction at a lower dosage.

The clinician should be alert to the possibility of fecal impaction that presents as watery diarrhea, particularly in immobile older adults on opioids. The treatment of impaction should begin with manual disimpaction and tap water enemas, followed, if unsuccessful, by high colonic enemas. Laxatives should not be administered until the impaction is cleared because of the risk of bowel perforation. Untreated fecal impaction can be life threatening.

Radiotherapy involving the abdomen and pelvis commonly causes diarrhea, peaking during the second or third week of therapy. This typically responds to cholestyramine[OL] at 4–12 g q8h (SOE=C). Cholestyramine is also helpful in treating diarrhea occurring as a complication of ileal resection. Diarrhea caused by fat malabsorption (eg, from pancreatic insufficiency or small-bowel disease) responds to pancreatic enzymes such as pancreatin (SOE=B). Secretory diarrhea generally responds to octreotide.

Gastrointestinal Obstruction

In older adults, causes of bowel obstruction include direct intraluminal obstruction by tumor, malignant infiltration of the bowel wall, external compression of the bowel wall (eg, from bulky lymphadenopathy), dysmotility, fecal impaction, adverse effects of radiation treatment, volvulus, and adhesions from previous surgeries. The upper portions of the gastrointestinal tract, such as the esophagus, stomach, and duodenum, and portions of the pancreaticobiliary systems can also become obstructed directly by tumors or infiltrating masses or externally compressed by malignancy or abscess. Patients diagnosed with malignant bowel obstruction have a poor prognosis, with a median survival of 3 months. The incidence of bowel obstruction can be up to 50% in ovarian and gastrointestinal cancers.

The symptom burden from bowel obstruction is significant and can include hyper-salivation, nausea, vomiting, colicky abdominal pain, and anorexia and weight loss. The evaluation and management of bowel obstruction depends on the functional status of the patient, goals of care, and expected survival. General treatment options include radiation therapy, surgical correction (palliative versus definitive), stenting, venting gastrostomy or jejunostomy tubes, and pharmacologic management. There is a scarcity of randomized control trials to guide optimal treatment.

Surgical management to resect the site of blockage has limited evidence for benefit in terms of quality of life and survival for most patients with bowel obstruction and limited life expectancy (ie, ≤3 months). Surgery may be beneficial for patients with a good performance status, an operable lesion, and an expected survival of 2–6 months. In addition to open laparotomy for construction of venting gastrostomies or jejunostomies, palliative surgical measures may involve laparoscopic approaches, or the fashioning of diverting ostomies that allow for bypass around strictures or blockages.

Advances in endoscopic techniques and self-expanding metallic stents have allowed for a nonsurgical approach to bowel obstruction. Stents have been used for esophageal, gastric outlet, small-bowel, and colonic obstructions, as well as in the pancreaticobiliary system. They are most beneficial for patients with a single point of obstruction or locally extensive disease. Stents are contraindicated in patients with perforation and peritonitis and are not well tolerated if the lesion is within 2 cm of the anal margin. Radiation treatments may be considered in conjunction with stent placement, especially in esophageal cancers, or as a sole therapeutic option.

The mainstay of treatment for bowel obstruction is medical management. In most patients, symptoms can be alleviated by combination therapy with opioids, antispasmodic medications, antiemetics, antisecretory agents, and corticosteroids. Opioids can be given subcutaneously, intravenously, sublingually, and transdermally, and should be titrated for relief of abdominal pain. For antispasmodic and antisecretory medications helpful in bowel obstructions, see Table 16.5. Corticosteroids have been used for bowel obstruction as antiemetics and as analgesics, and to reduce peritumor edema. Generally, they are given for a trial period of 4–5 days and discontinued if there is no response. If medical management is not effective, a venting gastrostomy may be considered.

Nasogastric tubes are often placed when a patient is admitted to the hospital with a bowel obstruction. These tubes should be temporary measures only while a decision about surgery is considered or medications to control symptoms are started. Nasogastric tubes are associated with pain, sinusitis, aspiration, and erosions in the nose and esophagus.

Anorexia and Cachexia

Loss of appetite or anorexia is almost a universal symptom of patients with serious and life-threatening illness. Anorexia in those who are actively dying and

Table 16.5—Medications Used for Bowel Obstruction

Drug	Dosage	Comments
Glycopyrrolate	0.2–0.4 mg SC q2–4h	Antisecretory; less centrally mediated adverse events because does not penetrate blood-brain barrier
Scopolamine	0.1–0.2 mg SC or IV q6–8h Transdermal patch every 3 days	Antispasmodic and antisecretory; transdermal patch does not have immediate effect
Hyoscyamine	0.125 mg SL q4–8h	Antispasmodic; may cause urinary retention and confusion
Octreotide	12.5 mcg/h SC or IV continuous infusion, or 200–600 mcg SC or IV intermittently; maximum of 900 mcg in 24 hours	Antisecretory; well tolerated and effective in decreasing GI secretions

who do not express a desire to eat need not be treated. Families and significant others, however, can be very distressed when their loved one does not eat; providing food is often equated with showing love. The clinician needs to evaluate for and treat reversible causes of anorexia and cachexia (eg, thrush, nausea) if the patient's goals and prognosis warrant. Symptoms of dry mouth can be alleviated with ice chips, popsicles, moist compresses, or artificial saliva. Lemon glycerin swabs should not be used, because they irritate dry and cracked mucosa. Megestrol acetate and corticosteroids[OL] have been found to enhance appetite, cause weight gain (primarily fat), and improve quality of life in some patients with anorexia (SOE=B). However, these agents do not prolong survival or improve function or treatment tolerance of cancer therapies, and are associated with adverse events (SOE=B). The Choosing Wisely® Campaign does not recommend using prescription appetite stimulants or high-calorie supplements to treat anorexia or cachexia in older adults based on these findings. In general, patients should be encouraged to eat whatever is most appealing without regard to dietary restrictions. Often, it is preferable to provide patient and family education regarding the normalcy of anorexia as a part of the end-of-life process.

Enteral feedings are often used in chronically ill and dying patients because of families' and clinicians' perceived need to provide nutrition. There is no evidence to support the use of such feedings in this situation. Enteral feedings are not associated with improved quality of life or survival in this context and are associated with increased frequency of aspiration and other complications. An inability to maintain oral nutrition in patients with chronic life-limiting disease is best regarded as a marker of dying, not a problem solvable by artificial nutrition. The Choosing Wisely® Campaign does not recommend the placement of enteral feeding tubes in patients with advanced dementia but instead recommends offering oral-assisted feeding.

Nevertheless, enteral feeding may enhance quality and quantity of life in a few situations; examples include patients with good functional status and proximal gastrointestinal obstruction; patients receiving chemotherapy or radiation involving the proximal gastrointestinal tract; and patients with amyotrophic lateral sclerosis (SOE=B).

Delirium

Delirium is common in terminally ill older patients and is distressing to both patients and family members. It is thought that up to 50% of delirium in palliative care is reversible. Efforts to identifying potentially reversible causes (eg, infection, impaction, uncontrolled pain, urinary retention, medications, dehydration, and hypoxia) should be based on the patient's current goals of care and disease trajectory. Nonpharmacologic and pharmacologic approaches are used to treat delirium. Nonpharmacologic approaches include minimizing noise, using an orientation board, mounting a visible clock in the room, using simple communication, and minimizing disruptions. Antipsychotics such as haloperidol[OL] or risperidone[OL] in low dosages are effective treatments for both hypoactive and hyperactive delirium. Medications are indicated either to ensure the patient's safety or if the delirium is causing distress. Actively dying patients who are nonambulatory and who experience terminal delirium often appear less distressed with use of sedating antipsychotics such as chlorpromazine[OL]. Because benzodiazepines are often associated with paradoxical agitation and worsening of the delirium in older adults, careful consideration should precede their use.

Dyspnea

Dyspnea, the subjective experience of breathlessness, is one of the most distressing symptoms experienced by dying individuals and families. Self-reporting by the patient is the only reliable measure of dyspnea. Respiratory rates, pulmonary congestion, hypoxia, or hypercarbia do not correlate with breathlessness. Clinicians may mistakenly fear that treating dyspnea in patients close to the end of life is associated with unacceptably high risks, leading some to withhold treatment and others to prescribe inadequate dosages of medications.

Because breathlessness has many causes (eg, anxiety, airway obstruction, bronchospasm, hypoxemia, pneumonia, cachexia from advanced disease), symptomatic management should begin immediately while the underlying cause is being investigated. Like pain, dyspnea is mediated through the interaction of complex pathophysiologic processes with poorly defined psychologic factors. The optimal therapy for dyspnea is to treat its underlying cause. When this is not possible, one of a number of agents that have been evaluated for treatment of intractable dyspnea is used. The goal of treatment is the subjective improvement of breathlessness, rather than lowering the respiratory rate to normal. Often, patients report improvement in breathlessness yet still breathe rapidly.

The most effective agents for treatment of dyspnea are opioids[OL]. Opioids are believed to act centrally by decreasing the perception of dyspnea, and peripherally on opioid receptors in the lung without affecting respiratory drive. In randomized controlled trials, both oral and parenteral formulations were effective (SOE=A). There is no consensus on starting dosages, but in frail opioid-naive older adults it is best to start low and titrate upward. For dyspneic patients already on opioids, increasing the dosage by 25%–50% is recommended (SOE=D). Nebulized opioids for intractable dyspnea have been used, but evidence of benefit is scarce. Nebulized morphine has not been shown to be helpful, but small studies of fentanyl have shown effectiveness (SOE=C). The theoretical advantages of nebulized opioids include the avoidance of systemic absorption (with resulting constipation, hypotension, sedation, respiratory depression, and hypercapnia), rapid and efficient absorption because of the large surface area of the lung parenchyma, and ease of administration. This route of administration should be reserved for patients who experience intolerable adverse effects from opioids administered by other routes.

Oxygen is considered by many to be an important component of any regimen for dyspnea. It is used and paid for by hospice, regardless of a patient's oxygen saturation. An international study showed that ambient air delivered by nasal cannula was just as effective in relieving breathlessness as oxygen in patients with oxygen saturation >90% (SOE=A). Cool air moving across the face (eg, from fans or an open window) can treat dyspnea by stimulating the second branch of the fifth cranial nerve, which has a central inhibitory effect on the sensation of breathlessness (SOE=C).

Benzodiazepines are beneficial in controlling anxiety associated with dyspnea, but they have not improved breathlessness in randomized controlled trials in which nonanxious persons with COPD were enrolled (SOE=A). These medications should be used only in breathless patients with accompanying anxiety. Bronchodilators and corticosteroids are useful in patients with bronchospasm. Diuretics can help in care of patients with pulmonary congestion.

Cough

The prevalence of cough has been reported in the palliative care literature as ranging from 29% to 83%. Normally, cough maintains the patency and cleanliness of the airways and thus should be treated only when it causes distress. Cough can be caused by the production of excessive amounts of fluids (eg, blood, mucus), inhalation of foreign material, or stimulation of irritant receptors in the airway. Additionally, patients with neuromuscular disorders may be unable to swallow saliva because of the involvement of bulbar cranial nerves. Pooling saliva then triggers cough as it trickles into the larynx or trachea.

Underlying causes of cough should be investigated when feasible and treated (eg, with diuretics for heart failure, antibiotics for infection, anticholinergics for aspiration of saliva resulting from motor neuron disease). However, resolving the underlying cause may be impossible. Opioids can be useful in these situations.

Dextromethorphan is structurally related to opioids and has central cough-suppressant action with few sedative effects (SOE=D). Codeine and hydrocodone, usually in the form of elixirs, are also good first-line choices (SOE=D). Methadone syrup can also be helpful when taken as a single daily dose because of its longer duration of action (SOE=D).

Cough due to a pharynx irritated by local infection or malignancy may be helped by nebulized anesthetics (SOE=D). Nebulized lidocaine up to four times daily has been reported, anecdotally, to offer relief.

Loud Respiration

Inability to clear secretions from the oropharynx often results in noisy or "rattling" respirations at the end of life. This occurs as secretions oscillate up and down during inspiration and expiration. Although there is no indication that this causes discomfort for patients, it often produces anxiety in family and caregivers. Best management includes preparing the family and caregivers for its occurrence and meaning. Anticholinergic medications reduce secretions and may be used if this symptom is distressing to the family. Because anticholinergic agents do not dry up secretions already present, it is important to ask the family to notify clinicians at the first sign of rattling. Scopolamine[OL] patches can be effective and also have a sedative effect. Hyoscyamine, glycopyrrolate, or atropine eye drops^{OL} also effectively dry up secretions; unfortunately, these drugs contribute to dry mouth, constipation, delirium, and mucous plugging, so careful monitoring is necessary.

Depression

Depression is under-recognized and undertreated, both in older adults and terminally ill patients. It may be underdiagnosed because of clinicians' mistaken belief that it is either a normal consequence of aging or appropriate in the context of a terminal illness. Depression must also be distinguished from anticipatory grief and routine emotional response to bad news. Depression and psychological distress diminish quality of life, amplify pain and other symptoms, and impair a patient's ability to deal with the emotions involved in saying good bye. Depression is a major risk factor for suicide and for requests to clinicians to hasten death.

The diagnosis of depression in palliative care settings presents challenges. Standard neurovegetative symptoms described in the *Diagnostic and Statistical Manual of Mental Disorders* (eg, insomnia, anorexia, weight change, fatigue) are often not reliable indicators for depression near life's end, because their cause is often the terminal disease itself. Instead, clinicians should watch for change in mood, hopelessness, helplessness, worthlessness, loss of interest, and suicidal ideation. Suicidal ideation should be openly discussed, including any symptoms that are contributing to the patient's suffering, which may be influencing his or her consideration of suicide. Suicidal thoughts should be assessed immediately, and appropriate referrals considered. Aggressive treatment of symptoms, antidepressant therapy, cognitive-behavioral therapy, and psychiatric consultation are all appropriate initial responses. Involvement of clergy or pastoral care representatives may be helpful. Continued discussion with the patient about a wish to hasten death often reveals a change of mind over time.

Standard antidepressant therapy is effective, but most agents have a delayed onset of action of 2–6 weeks. Psychostimulants (eg, methylphenidate^{OL}, dextroamphetamine^{OL}) are well-tolerated, safe, and effective short-term treatments for medically ill, depressed patients (SOE=B). Additionally, they can have a rapid onset and beneficial effect on energy, mood, appetite, and mental alertness. Methylphenidate is started at 2.5 mg in the morning and given concurrently with standard antidepressants; it should not be taken in the evening hours because of its harmful effect on sleep. Electroconvulsive therapy is an effective, safe method of rapidly treating depression and may be considered for those who are severely depressed. The American Psychiatric Task Force Report advocates consideration of electroconvulsive therapy as a first-line treatment when rapid response is needed (SOE=D). The presence of space-occupying CNS lesions is a contraindication.

Table 16.6—Completing a Death Certificate: Points to Remember

- Do not delay completion of the certificate. The burial or disposition of the remains cannot proceed until a correctly completed death certificate is accepted by the state.
- Print clearly or type using black ink.
- Do not use abbreviations.
- Spell out the month.
- Use a 24-hour clock.
- Complete all items, do not leave blanks. If necessary, use "unknown."
- Do not complete the medical information if another available physician has more knowledge of the circumstances.
- Do not alter the document or erase any part of it.

Cognitive-behavioral therapy and active listening are helpful for patients and families at end of life, whether the cause of distress is anticipatory grief, depression, or the mental fatigue of early dying. One form of brief, focused psychotherapy is dignity therapy. This therapy invites patients to reflect and discuss what is important to them, and how they wish to be remembered. The sessions are transcribed and edited. The final version is presented back to the patient who may wish to distribute it to family and/or friends.

The chaplain and social work members of hospice and palliative care teams typically serve to assist patients and families in working toward closure and resolution. Palliative care physician Ira Byock has written that dying patients need to say and hear four things to feel complete before death: "please forgive me, I forgive you, thank you, and I love you."

DEATH CERTIFICATE COMPLETION

Proper completion of a death certificate is a physician's responsibility. Death certificates are needed for personal, legal, and public health purposes. Accurate documentation of the cause of death and communication with the family may help family members with closure and peace of mind. Death certificates are also necessary for burial and settlement of the decedent's estate. In addition, they are used for state and national mortality statistics. These compilations help to assess the general health of the population, determine prevalence of diseases, and guide research priorities and funding.

Unfortunately, physicians are rarely trained in the proper completion of death certificates, leading to errors in their completion. Physicians are responsible for completing the medical portion of the death certificate, the "Cause of Death" section and usually the pronouncement of death. The Cause of Death section has two parts. Part 1 lists the immediate cause of death and the sequential chain of events that led to the death. Physicians should use their best medical opinion in assigning the immediate cause of death. A common error in this section is to list a mechanism of death (such as cardiac or respiratory arrest) rather than a disease (pulmonary embolism, COPD, Alzheimer dementia). It is important to be as specific as possible. Part 2 asks for other conditions that contributed to the death but not in a clearly causal chain. For a detailed and complete discussion about completing a death certificate, including examples, see www.cdc.gov/nchs/data/misc/hb_cod.pdf (accessed Jan 2016). Important points to remember when filling out a death certificate are outlined in Table 16.6.

HEALTH PROFESSIONAL BURNOUT

Health care providers caring for patients and families at the end of life are exposed to distressing emotional situations and suffering. This may lead to burnout, especially for providers who are not cognizant of their emotional responses to these situations. Symptoms of burnout include irritability, insomnia, forgetfulness, resentment, mental and physical fatigue, social withdrawal, increased alcohol use, apathy, and/or chronic sadness. Burnout at work has both personal and professional consequences. It is important for providers to be aware of and address their responses to emotional situations to prevent burnout. Many activities can contribute to self-care and burnout prevention, including journaling, yoga, meditation, and other stress reduction activities; attending to health with regular exercise and a nutritious diet; and debriefing highly emotional events as a team. If these activities do not help, it is important to seek professional counseling.

CHOOSING WISELY® RECOMMENDATIONS

Palliative Care and Hospice

- Do not use topical lorazepam, diphenhydramine, or haloperidol gel for nausea.
- Do not recommend percutaneous feeding tubes in patients with advanced dementia; instead offer oral assisted feeding.
- Avoid using prescription appetite stimulants or high-calorie supplements for treatment of anorexia or cachexia in older adults; instead, optimize social supports, provide feeding assistance and clarify patient goals and expectations.

REFERENCES

- End of Life Online Curriculum (a joint project of the U.S. Veterans Administration and Stanford University Medical School). http://endoflife.stanford.edu/M11_pain_control/intro_m01.html (accessed Jan 2016).

    This site provides a Web-based curriculum in palliative care, with modules describing pain management and methods for opioid conversion.

- Fast Facts. www.mypcnow.org/#!fast-facts/c6xb (accessed Jan 2016).

    Fast Facts are concise, peer-reviewed, and evidenced-based summaries on numerous topics in hospice and palliative medicine.

- Five Wishes®. https://fivewishesonline.agingwithdignity.org/ (accessed Jan 2016).

    Several online forms are available for advance directives. Five Wishes® is a person-friendly living will available in 23 languages. It can be given to patients to complete to inform their family and medical team about how they want to be treated if they have a serious illness. It meets the legal requirements for an advance directive in the District of Columbia and 42 states.

- Goldstein NE, Morrison RS, eds. *Evidence-Based Practice of Palliative Medicine*. Philadelphia: Saunders; 2013.

    This book has chapters on symptom management, communication, specific diseases topics, caregivers, financial aspects of care, palliative care emergencies, and models for delivering care by well-known researchers in the field of palliative care.

- Mitchell SL, Black BS, Ersek M, et al. Advanced dementia: state of the art and priorities for the next decade. *Ann Intern Med*. 2012;156(1):45–51.

    Dementia is one of the leading causes of death in the United States. This article reviews the current understanding of advanced dementia and outlines the needs of patients dying of this disease.

- Temel JS, Greer JA, Muzikansky A, et al. Early palliative care for patients with metastatic non-small-cell lung cancer. *N Engl J Med*. 2010;363(8):733–742.

    This is the first randomized clinical controlled trial to show benefits of palliative care. The study demonstrated improved quality of life, less depression, more frequent documentation of resuscitative preferences, less aggressive care at the end of life, longer length of stay in hospice, and longer survival in the group that received palliative care along with standard care.

- U.S. Department of Health and Human Services. Centers for Medicare and Medicaid Services. *Medicare Hospice Benefits*. CMS Publication No. 02154. Revised August, 1, 2013. www.medicare.gov/publications/pubs/pdf/02154.pdf (accessed Jan 2016).

    This guide, written in lay language, is useful to help patients and their loved ones understand hospice.

Grace A. Cordts, MD, MPH, MS
Danielle J. Doberman, MD, MPH

CHAPTER 17—PAIN MANAGEMENT

Key Points

- Effective management of pain begins with a thorough assessment to determine its source, severity, and impact on functioning and well-being.

- Persistent pain constitutes a distinct pathology and causes changes throughout the nervous system that may worsen over time. It has significant psychological and cognitive correlates as well.

- Multiple pain scales are available to help quantify the severity of pain. The selection of a pain scale should be based on the cognitive and communication abilities of the patient.

- A stepped approach to the treatment of pain is advised, including local therapies and nonpharmacologic approaches.

- Often, systemic analgesics are needed in the treatment of older adults with moderate to severe persistent pain.

- Physical tolerance generally develops to the respiratory depression, fatigue, and sedating effects of opioid analgesics but not to their constipating effect.

- Given the diverse effects of persistent pain, interprofessional assessment and treatment may produce the best results for older adults who continue to have moderate or severe persistent pain despite optimal medical management.

- Effective management of persistent pain requires a collaborative and ongoing partnership between the clinician, the patient, and family.

Relief of pain and suffering, and promotion of functional status and quality of life are primary tenets of geriatric medicine. Pain is a distressing symptom that is not just physical but involves and influences the mood and even the personality of a person, thereby affecting behavior, social life, and interactions. Dame Cicely Saunders, the founder of the modern hospice movement, coined the term "total pain" to describe the multifaceted effect of pain on the "whole person including the bio-psycho-socio-spiritual-cultural impact." The contribution of each of these facets is both dynamic (varies over time) and specific to each patient.

Persistent pain, ie, pain that is persistent or recurrent for at least 3–6 months, affects at least 116 million U.S. adults at an estimated cost of almost $650 billion annually in direct medical treatment costs and lost productivity.

Pain is particularly common in adults ≥ 65 years old. Studies have revealed that 25%–50% of community-dwelling older adults and 45%–80% of nursing-home residents have substantial pain. Studies further show that the ability to tolerate severe pain decreases with age. Common causes of pain in older adults include osteoarthritic pain, degenerative bone diseases, postsurgical pain, nocturnal leg pain, and pain associated with various chronic illnesses. Shingles and resultant post-herpetic neuralgia are more common in older adults, with half the cases of shingles occurring in adults ≥ 60 years old.

Pain is also commonly underdiagnosed and undertreated in older adults who are cognitively impaired, a group shown to receive less analgesic medication than younger, cognitively intact cohorts. The undertreatment of pain among the older population is probably due to a variety of factors. Some older adults tend to underreport or do not report their pain because of cognitive impairment, limited health literacy, or an erroneous perception that pain is a part of the normal aging process. Clinicians may be overwhelmed in caring for older adults who frequently have several comorbid illnesses, and thus fail to regularly and systematically assess for and manage pain during busy clinic visits. Even when pain is identified, clinicians may be reluctant to manage it effectively because of the lack of adequate knowledge of pain management strategies, as well as misperceptions about narcotic medications. The paucity of older adults as subjects in clinical trials for analgesic therapies may contribute to clinicians' challenges in pain management. Patients, too, may fear addiction to opioid analgesics, and commonly choose to live with pain to avoid taking these agents.

Pain is an unpleasant sensory and emotional experience associated with actual or potential tissue damage, or described in terms of such damage. Pain is subjective and idiosyncratic, beyond objective measure; its intensity and character are what the patient says they are. Pain is certainly a sensation in a part or parts of the body, but it is also by definition unpleasant and therefore also an emotional experience. *Acute pain* is of sudden onset and expected to last a short time and is clearly linked to a specific bodily insult or injury. *Chronic* or *persistent pain*, by contrast, is defined as pain without apparent biologic purpose that has persisted beyond the normal tissue healing time, variously defined as 3–6 months. Persistent pain endures as the pain signals keep firing in the nervous system for weeks, months, or even years after the initial insult or injury. Some people suffer persistent pain even in the absence of any past injury or evident body damage.

Table 17.1—Terms Commonly Used in Care of Patients in Pain

Term	Definition
Addiction	Continued use of a substance (eg, an opioid analgesic) despite harmful consequences
Allodynia	Pain caused by a stimulus that does not normally provoke pain
Analgesia	Absence of pain in response to a noxious stimulus
Central pain	Pain initiated or caused by a primary lesion or dysfunction in the CNS (eg, pain after stroke, phantom limb pain)
Dysesthesia	An unpleasant abnormal sensation, whether spontaneous or evoked
Hyperalgesia	Increased sensitivity to a noxious stimulus
Hyperpathia	A syndrome in which pain-provoking stimuli result in magnified levels of pain
Hypoalgesia	Decreased sensitivity to a noxious stimulus
Nociceptor	A nerve fiber preferentially sensitive to a noxious stimulus or to a stimulus that would become noxious if prolonged
Noxious stimulus	A stimulus that is capable of activating receptors for tissue damage
Pseudoaddiction	A situation in which a patient with significant unrelieved pain adopts behaviors (eg, theatricality in pleas for relief) similar to those of truly addicted patients
Wind-up pain	Pain sensitization caused by repetitive noxious stimulation of peripheral nerve fibers; may cause perceived magnitude of pain to gradually increase

Persistent pain can become so debilitating that it affects basic and instrumental activities of daily living, causes psychological distress (depression or anxiety), disturbs sleep, and negatively impacts social and personal relationships. For additional terms used in care of patients in pain, see Table 17.1.

Risk factors for transition from acute to persistent pain in older adults include lower socioeconomic status, vivid memory of childhood trauma, obesity, low level of physical fitness, overuse of joints and muscles, chronic illnesses, lack of social support, and abuse.

ASSESSMENT

A thorough assessment is necessary to formulate a plan to successfully treat persistent pain. The International Association for the Study of Pain (IASP) has developed a helpful taxonomy for the classification of pain that identifies 5 axes:

- Axis I: anatomic regions
- Axis II: organ systems
- Axis III: temporal characteristics, pattern of occurrence
- Axis IV: intensity, time since onset of pain
- Axis V: etiology

A major barrier to effective pain treatment is inadequate assessment. Beyond the limited scope of the above 5 axes, assessment should also include an exploration of the effects of pain on functional status and sleep, as well as on emotional and social well-being. Because of its subjective nature, clinicians must rely on the patient's or caregiver's description of the pain, in addition to the findings of a thorough physical examination. Assessment is complicated by several factors, including underreporting of symptoms by many older adults, the existence of multiple medical comorbidities exacerbating the pain and impairing function, and the increased prevalence of cognitive impairment with age. When assessing pain in patients with cognitive impairment, it is important to remember that such patients may be unable to report their pain, much less its history. They may instead present with depression or agitation, and these secondary behaviors often serve as important clues to the presence of underlying pain.

Pain intensity can be quantified using pain intensity scales. Three commonly used, validated scales are the Numeric Rating Scale, the Faces Pain Scale (www.iasp-pain.org/Education/Content.aspx?ItemNumber=1519 [accessed Jan 2016]), and the Verbal Descriptor Scale. These scales are referred to as one-dimensional, because they ask the patient to rate the intensity of a single characteristic of the symptom—in this case the intensity of the pain. The patient is asked to rate his or her pain by assigning a numerical value (with 0 indicating no pain, and 10 representing the worst pain imaginable), a verbal description ("no pain" to "pain as bad as it could be"), or a facial expression corresponding to the pain. The choice of scale depends on the preference of a particular language or presence of sensory impairment. For example, if a patient does not speak English well, the faces scale may be the best choice, because it relies on pictures alone. The Wong-Baker FACES Pain Rating Scale with Foreign Translations is useful for non-English speaking patients (www.wongbakerfaces.org/public_html/wp-content/uploads/2013/11/TranslationsAll.pdf [accessed Jan 2016]). The same scale should be used at follow-up examinations to evaluate how the pain has changed since the initial assessment. Scales such as the McGill Pain Questionnaire and the Pain Disability Scale measure pain in a variety of domains, including intensity, location, and affect. Although time intensive,

Table 17.2—Types of Pain, Examples, and Treatment

Type of Pain and Examples	Source of Pain	Typical Description	Effective Drug Classes and Nonpharmacologic Treatments (SOE)
Nociceptive: somatic			
Arthritis, acute postoperative, fracture, bone metastases	Tissue injury, eg, bones, soft tissue, joints, muscles	Well localized, constant; aching, stabbing, gnawing, throbbing	Acetaminophen (A), opioids (B), NSAIDs (A) Physical and cognitive-behavioral therapies (B)
Nociceptive: visceral			
Renal colic, constipation	Viscera	Diffuse, poorly localized, referred to other sites, intermittent, paroxysmal; dull, colicky, squeezing, deep, cramping; often accompanied by nausea, vomiting, diaphoresis	Treatment of underlying cause, acetaminophen (C), opioids (B) Physical and cognitive-behavioral therapies (C)
Neuropathic			
Cervical or lumbar radiculopathy, post-herpetic neuralgia, trigeminal neuralgia, diabetic neuropathy, post-stroke syndrome, herniated intervertebral disc, drug toxicities	Peripheral or central nervous system	Prolonged, usually constant, but can have paroxysms; sharp, burning, pricking, tingling, electric shock–like; associated with other sensory disturbances, eg, paresthesias and dysesthesias; allodynia, hyperalgesia, impaired motor function, atrophy, or abnormal deep tendon reflexes	Tricyclic antidepressants (A), serotonin-norepinephrine reuptake inhibitor antidepressants (A), anticonvulsants (A), opioids (B), topical anesthetics (C) Physical and cognitive-behavioral therapies (C)
Undetermined			
Myofascial pain syndrome, somatic symptom pain disorders, fibromyalgia	Poorly understood	No identifiable pathologic processes or symptoms out of proportion to identifiable organic pathology; widespread musculoskeletal pain, stiffness, and weakness	Antidepressants (B), antianxiety agents (C) Physical (B), cognitive-behavioral (B), and psychological therapies (B)

SOURCE: Adapted with permission. Reuben DB, Herr KA, Pacala JT, et al. *Geriatrics At Your Fingertips*, 17th ed. New York: American Geriatrics Society; 2015:232.

such scales measuring multiple domains can provide a wealth of information about the patient's unique experience of pain. However, patients in pain may be unable or unwilling to use scales that take much time. Patients with cognitive impairment may not be able to use complex pain assessment tools.

Before the physical examination, the patient can be asked to describe the location of the pain using a drawing of a human figure, called a pain map. The patient indicates the locations on the figure that correspond to his or her pain. Pain maps may enhance reliability in repeated assessment of pain in cognitively intact patients. In some cultures, it may be easier for patients to use a pain map to indicate pain in sensitive areas like the genitalia.

If the patient's pain pattern is erratic and diffuse, or does not conform to an anatomic distribution, a referral to a mental health specialist may help in uncovering an underlying disorder that is complicating or contributing to the complex pain presentation.

The physical examination should include careful scrutiny of the reported site of the pain and any part of the body that may be a source of referred pain. (For example, occipital pain should prompt examination of the neck, and knee pain examination of the hip and lumbar region.) The initial evaluation should include a complete musculoskeletal examination, recognizing the common findings of musculoskeletal disorders such as fibromyalgia, osteoarthritis, and myofascial pain, as either the primary source of pain or exacerbating processes. Accurate diagnosis of these disorders is a critical part of formulating the correct therapeutic plan. Fibromyalgia, which may be underrecognized in older adults, is characterized by multiple tender points, sleep disturbance, fatigue, generalized pain (often with a strong axial component), and morning stiffness. Myofascial pain is present in many patients with persistent pain and is diagnosed by the presence of taut bands of muscles and *trigger* points (ie, pain that may radiate distally when firm pressure is applied to a muscle, as opposed to *tender* points, in which radiation of pain is absent).

Pain syndromes can be divided into at least 3 types: nociceptive, neuropathic, and undetermined (Table 17.2). Nociceptive pain describes pain due to the activation of nociceptive sensory receptors by noxious stimuli resulting from inflammation, swelling, and injury to tissues. It can be defined further as either somatic or visceral pain. Somatic pain is well localized in skin, soft tissue, and bone. Patients may describe it

Table 17.3—Common Pain Behaviors in Cognitively Impaired Older Adults

Behavior	Examples
Facial expressions	Slight frown; sad, frightened face Grimacing, wrinkled forehead, closed or tightened eyes Any distorted expression Rapid blinking
Verbalizations, vocalizations	Sighing, moaning, groaning, grunting, chanting, calling out Noisy breathing Asking for help Verbal abusiveness
Body movements	Rigid or tense body posture, guarding Fidgeting Increased pacing, rocking Restricted movement Gait or mobility changes
Changes in interpersonal interactions	Aggressive, combative, resists care Decreased social interactions Socially inappropriate, disruptive Withdrawn
Changes in activity patterns or routines	Refusing food, appetite change Increase in rest periods Change in sleep or rest pattern Sudden cessation of common routines Increased wandering
Mental status changes	Crying or tears Increased confusion Irritability or distress

NOTE: Some patients demonstrate little or no specific behavior associated with severe pain.
SOURCE: American Geriatrics Society Panel on Persistent Pain in Older Persons. The management of persistent pain in older persons. *J Am Geriatr Soc.* 2002;50(6 Suppl):S211. Reprinted with permission.

as throbbing, aching, and stabbing. Visceral pain, often due to cardiac, GI, or lung injury, is not well localized and can be difficult to describe, but patients may use words like crampy, tearing, dull, and aching. Either type of nociceptive pain is often adequately treated with common analgesics.

Neuropathic pain derives from the irritation of components of the central or peripheral nervous systems. Patients typically report burning, numbness with "pins-and-needles" sensations, and shooting pains. Common causes of neuropathic pain include diabetic neuropathy and post-herpetic neuralgia, whereas central pain after stroke, and phantom limb pain experienced after amputation, occur less often. Confusion between neuropathic pain and myofascial pain is possible, because patients may describe both as "burning." Careful physical examination may help to differentiate these disorders (ie, taut bands and trigger points with myofascial pain, and allodynia or hyperalgesia with either disorder); both may be present in the same patient. Neuropathic pain responds unpredictably to opioid analgesia. It may respond well to nonopioid therapies such as anticonvulsants, tricyclic antidepressants, and antiarrhythmic medications.

Mixed or unspecified pain has characteristics of both nociceptive pain and neuropathic pain, such as chronic headache of unknown cause. Older adults often have mixed pain syndromes, the complexity of which frequently poses management challenges. Lower back pain, for example, often results from a combination of spinal malalignment, myofascial pathology, and neurologic impingement. Complex Regional Pain Syndrome (CRPS), is characterized by pain or sensory changes (allodynia or hyperalgesia), with some combination of edema, regional sweating abnormality, changes in blood flow to the skin, and trophic features (shiny, thin skin; altered hair or nail growth on an extremity). Treating patients with mixed or unspecified pain syndromes with trials of different medications or with combinations of medicines may be necessary, and interprofessional collaboration (physical therapy, occupational therapy, psychology) is often beneficial.

ASSESSING AND TREATING PAIN IN COGNITIVELY IMPAIRED OLDER ADULTS

Although able to speak, patients with dementia may be unable to report and localize their pain. Patients with severe cognitive impairment who are unable to verbally express pain pose a challenge to the clinicians who care for them. Not only are such patients unable to describe their pain or request analgesia, but clinicians may be hesitant to administer pain medications, fearing that pharmacologic treatment will worsen the patients' mental status. Clinicians must rely on observing these patients for pain-related behaviors, as well as on eliciting observations from caregivers. For common pain behaviors in cognitively impaired older adults, see Table 17.3. Validated scales such as the Hurley Discomfort Scale and the Checklist of Nonverbal Pain Indicators have been developed but require trained evaluators to complete properly. Experts suggest empirically providing analgesic therapy during procedures and conditions known to be painful. Trials of analgesia should also be considered for patients exhibiting potentially pain-related behaviors, which might include otherwise unexplained "agitation."

TREATMENT

Nonpharmacologic Therapy

A comprehensive review of nonpharmacologic therapies for persistent pain is beyond the scope of this chapter, but specific therapies are worth mentioning. Many of the strategies mentioned below are appropriate considerations for treatment plans for all patients, and they highlight the importance of an interprofessional approach to pain treatment.

Patient education and involvement in treatment decisions are essential components of all treatment plans for persistent pain. Patients should be taught how to take medications properly and how to use assessment instruments. Studies also suggest that providing partner-guided pain management training to caregivers can decrease discomfort and improve psychological and social function experienced by older adults (SOE=B).

Psychological interventions such as cognitive-behavioral therapy (CBT) can be important tools for treatment of persistent pain (SOE=B). Recognition of depression, anxiety, or other mood disturbances should prompt early consultation with a mental health professional. In CBT, patients are asked to track their pain and record the thoughts associated with the pain experience to identify maladaptive coping strategies. By conscientiously replacing maladaptive coping strategies with constructive ones, patients can increase control over pain and self-efficacy, leading to decreased perception of pain. CBT can be particularly useful in helping patients learn to cope with the stresses of persistent pain. When possible, family members and other caregivers should be included in the therapy.

Regular physical activity has been shown to decrease pain scores, improve mood, boost functional status, and stabilize gait (SOE=A). Referral to the Arthritis Foundation or to community resources such as senior centers for exercise, Tai Chi, and water aerobics (for continent patients) classes can be beneficial for many patients. Frail older adults may require closely monitored rehabilitation services. For patients with advanced illness who are bedbound, regular repositioning, passive range-of-motion exercises, and gentle massage are key interventions. Treatment goals (beyond reduced pain) should include improvements in flexibility, strength, endurance, function, and overall quality of life.

Referral to a pain clinic geared toward an interprofessional team approach to treatment may be useful for patients who suffer from complex pain syndromes or who have shown previous poor response to first-line treatments. Data support the use of many physical modalities such as massage therapy, acupuncture, heat/cold therapy, and transcutaneous electrical nerve stimulation (TENS) units (SOE=B). Interprofessional team members may also incorporate cognitive techniques into the treatment plan, such as hypnosis, aromatherapy, biofeedback, music and pet therapy, and systematic desensitization. A subset of patients may require referral for major interventions, such as radiation therapy for bone metastases or palliative surgical procedures for bowel obstruction. Suboptimal treatment response should not be viewed as a permanent condition but as an opportunity for input from specialists who have additional expertise in treating these difficult problems.

Pharmacologic Therapy

For selected analgesics, with their starting dosages and common adverse effects, see Table 17.4.

Pharmacologic therapy for patients with persistent pain should be viewed not only as a means to reduce suffering but also as a method to promote improved function and enhanced adherence with rehabilitation efforts. When starting pharmacologic therapy in older adults, the risks and benefits of the treatment should be considered and balanced carefully. If appropriate, nonsystemic therapies should be tried first. For example, patients with isolated knee pain may respond to intra-articular corticosteroid injections, avoiding the need for systemic analgesics. (However, convincing data supporting the use of intra-articular injections for knee pain are lacking.) Patients with myofascial pain often respond to local treatments such as massage, gentle stretching exercises, ultrasound, and trigger-point injections (SOE=B). Topical preparations such as capsaicin or diclofenac gel[OL] or lidocaine patches can be effective as primary or adjunctive therapy for treating neuropathic or myofascial pain syndromes (SOE=C). If these local therapies are ineffective and a decision is made to begin systemic therapy, older adults need to be monitored closely to ensure that the treatment is effective and to minimize adverse effects.

Table 17.4—Systemic Pharmacotherapy for Persistent Pain Management

Medication	Starting Dosage[a]	Usual Effective Dose (Maximal Daily Dosage)	Titration	Comments
NONOPIOIDS				
Acetaminophen (Tylenol)	650 mg q4h to 500 mg q6h	2–4 g/d (4 g)	After 4–6 doses	Reduce maximal dosage 50%–75% in patients with hepatic insufficiency or history of alcohol abuse.
Anticonvulsants				
Carbamazepine[OL] (Tegretol)	100 mg/d	800–1,200 mg/d (2,400 mg)	After 3–5 days	Monitor liver enzymes, CBC, BUN/creatinine, electrolytes, and carbamazepine levels. Approved only for trigeminal neuralgia and glossopharyngeal neuralgia; not approved for any other types of pain. Multiple drug interactions.
Clonazepam[OL] (Klonopin)	0.25–0.5 mg hs	0.5–1 mg q8h (20 mg)	After 3–5 days	Monitor sedation, memory, CBC.
Gabapentin (Neurontin)	100 mg hs	300–900 mg q8h (3,600 mg)	After 1–2 days	Monitor sedation, ataxia, edema. Approved for post-herpetic neuralgia; not approved for any other types of pain.
Gabapentin extended-release (Gralise, Horizant)	300 mg hs	(1,800 mg)		
Pregabalin (Lyrica)	50 mg hs	300 mg/d (450 mg)	After 7 days	Monitor sedation, ataxia, edema.
Antidepressants				
Tricyclic antidepressants:[b] desipramine[OL] (Norpramin), nortriptyline[OL] (Pamelor)	10 mg hs	25–100 mg hs (variable, but older adults rarely tolerate doses >75–100 mg)	After 3–5 days	Significant risk of adverse events in older adults; anticholinergic effects
Duloxetine (Cymbalta)	20 mg/d	60 mg/d (120 mg)	After 7 days	Monitor blood pressure, dizziness, cognitive effects and memory; multiple drug-drug interactions. FDA approved for diabetic neuropathy.
Milnacipran (Savella)	12.5 mg/d	50 mg q12h (200 mg)	See package insert for titration recommendations; discontinuation requires tapering.	Reduce dosage by 50% with CrCl <30 mL/min. Common reactions include nausea, constipation, hot flashes, hyperhidrosis, palpitations, dry mouth, hypertension. Contraindicated with MAOIs and narrow-angle glaucoma. FDA approved only for fibromyalgia.
Venlafaxine[OL] (Effexor, Effexor XR)	37.5 mg/d (immediate or extended-release)	75–225 mg/d (225 mg)	After 4–7 days	Associated with dose-related increases in blood pressure and heart rate
Mexiletine[OL] (Mexitil)	150 mg q12h	150 mg q6–8h (variable)	After 3–5 days	Avoid use in patients with conduction block, bradyarrhythmia; monitor ECG at baseline and after dose stabilization.

Table 17.4—Systemic Pharmacotherapy for Persistent Pain Management—Continued

Medication	Starting Dosage[a]	Usual Effective Dose (Maximal Daily Dosage)	Titration	Comments
NSAIDs				Use with caution in older adults, if at all.
Celecoxib (Celebrex)	100 mg/d	100–400 mg/d (400 mg)		Higher dosages associated with higher incidence of GI, cardiovascular adverse events. Patients with indications for cardioprotection require aspirin supplement; therefore, older adults still require concurrent gastroprotection.
Diclofenac sodium	50 mg q12h or 75 mg extended release daily	100–150 mg/d (150 mg)		May be associated with higher cardiovascular risk than other traditional NSAIDs owing to its relative cyclooxygenase-2 inhibitor selectivity
Ibuprofen	OTC: 200 mg q8h Rx: 400 mg q6–8h	400–800 mg q6–8h (3,200 mg)		FDA indicates concurrent use with aspirin inhibits aspirin's antiplatelet effect, but the true clinical import of this remains to be elucidated, and it remains unclear whether this is unique to ibuprofen or true with other NSAIDs.
Ketorolac	15 mg q6h IV or IM 10 mg q4–6h	(60 mg/d) (40 mg)		Not recommended; high potential for GI and renal toxicity; inappropriate for long-term use
Nabumetone (Relafen)	1 g/d	1–2 g/d (2 g)		Relatively long half-life and minimal antiplatelet effect (>5 days)
Naproxen sodium	OTC: 220 mg q12h Rx: 250 mg q6–8h	OTC: 440–660 mg/day (660 mg) Rx: 250–500 mg q8–12h (1,000 mg)		Several studies implicate this agent as having less cardiovascular toxicity than other NSAIDs.
Salsalate (eg, Disalcid)	500–750 mg q12h	1,500–3,000 mg/d (3,000 mg)	After 4–6 doses	In frail patients or those with diminished hepatic or renal function, checking salicylate levels during dosage titration and after steady state is reached may be important.
OPIOIDS				
Hydrocodone (eg, Lorcet, Lortab, Vicodin, Norco, Vicoprofen)	2.5–5 mg q4–6h	5–10 mg (see comments)	After 3–4 doses	Useful for acute recurrent, episodic, or breakthrough pain; daily dose limited by fixed-dose combinations with acetaminophen or NSAIDs. NSAIDS should be used with caution in older adults, if at all.
Hydrocodone sustained-release	10–20 mg q12–24h	Variable	After 3–5 days	Available as a once-every-24-hour extended-release formulation (Hysingla ER) and once every 12 hours extended-release formulation (Zohydro ER). For patients with renal dysfunction, start at lowest dosage and titrate up slowly.
Hydromorphone (Dilaudid) Hydromorphone extended-release (Exalgo)	1–2 mg q3–4h 8 mg	Variable (variable) Variable	After 3–4 doses After 3-4 days	For breakthrough pain or around-the-clock dosing

Table 17.4—Systemic Pharmacotherapy for Persistent Pain Management—Continued

Medication	Starting Dosage[a]	Usual Effective Dose (Maximal Daily Dosage)	Titration	Comments
Morphine, immediate-release (eg, MSIR, Roxanol)	2.5–10 mg q4h	Variable (variable)	After 1–2 doses	Oral liquid concentrate or tablet recommended for breakthrough pain
Morphine, sustained-release (eg, MS Contin, Kadian)	15 mg q8–24h (see dosing guidelines in package insert for each specific formulation)	Variable (variable)	After 3–5 days	Usually started after initial dose determined by effects of immediate-release opioid; toxic metabolites of morphine can limit usefulness in patients with renal insufficiency or when high-dose therapy is required; continuous-release formulations may require more frequent dosing if pain returns regularly at end of dose. Significant interactions with food and alcohol.
Oxycodone, immediate-release (OxyIR, Roxicodone, Percocet, Percodan, Tylox)	2.5–5 mg q4–6h	5–10 mg (see comments)	After 3–4 doses	Useful for acute recurrent, episodic, or breakthrough pain. Daily dose limited with fixed-dose combinations containing acetaminophen or NSAIDs; can obviate using oxycodone-only formulations. NSAIDs should be used with caution in older adults, if at all.
Oxycodone, sustained-release (OxyContin)	10 mg q12h	Variable (variable)	After 3–5 days	Usually started after initial dose determined by effects of immediate-release opioid. Although intended for 12-hour dosing, some individuals may need shorter (every 8 hours) or longer (daily) dosing.
Tapentadol (Nucynta)	50–100 mg q4–q6h	50–100 mg q4–6h prn (600 mg)		Avoid concurrent use of serotonergic agents (SSRIs, SNRIs, tricyclic antidepressants).
Tapentadol extended-release (Nucynta ER)	50 mg q12h	100–250 mg q12h (500 mg)	After 3 days	
Tramadol (Ultram)	12.5–25 mg q4–6h	50–100 mg (300 mg)	After 4–6 doses	Mixed opioid and central neurotransmitter mechanism of action; monitor for opioid adverse events, including drowsiness, constipation, and nausea. Exert caution when used with another serotonergic drug, and observe for symptoms of serotonergic syndrome. Lowers seizure threshold.
Transdermal fentanyl (Duragesic)	12–25 mcg/h patch q72h	Variable (variable)	After 2–3 patch changes	Usually started after initial dose determined by effects of immediate-release opioid; currently available lowest dose patch (12 mcg/h) recommended for patients who require <60 mg/24-h oral morphine equivalents; peak effect of first dose takes 18–24 hours. Duration of effect is usually 3 days but may range from 48–96 hours. May take 2 or 3 patch changes before steady state blood levels are reached.

NOTE: DEA = U.S. Drug Enforcement Agency; hs = at bedtime; NA = not applicable; CrCl = creatinine clearance; MAOI = monoamine oxidase inhibitor
[a] Oral dosing unless otherwise specified.
[b] Amitriptyline is not recommended.
SOURCE: Adapted with permission from American Geriatrics Society Panel on the Pharmacologic Management of Persistent Pain in Older Persons. Pharmacological management of persistent pain in older persons. *J Am Geriatr Soc.* 2009;57(8):1331–1346.

Table 17.5—Interconverting Opioids and Delivery Routes

Drug	Opioid Equivalent Dosages		Conversion Ratio to Oral Morphine
	Oral Route	*Parenteral Route*	
Morphine sulfate	30 mg	10 mg	Parenteral morphine is 3 times as potent as oral morphine.
Oxycodone	20 mg	NA	Oral oxycodone is about 1.5 times as potent as oral morphine.
Hydrocodone	30 mg	NA	Oral hydrocodone has about the same potency as oral morphine.
Hydromorphone	7.5 mg	1.5 mg	Oral hydromorphone is about 4–7 times as potent as oral morphine. Parenteral hydromorphone is 20 times as potent as oral morphine.

The pain ladder from the World Health Organization illustrates an excellent approach toward stepwise analgesic management. (www.who.int/cancer/palliative/painladder/en/ [accessed Jan 2016]). According to the WHO ladder, the first step in treating pain is to start the patient on nonopioid medications with or without adjuvants. If the pain persists or increases, the next step is to start a weak opioid (eg, hydrocodone with acetaminophen) and adjuvants. If the pain still persists or increases despite these efforts, then the patient will likely need strong opioids (eg, morphine, hydromorphone, or others) with or without nonopioid analgesics and adjuvants. Choice of initial dose and rate of titration depends on the individual patient's physiology, which varies considerably among older adults. When using acetaminophen for alleviating chronic pain, it is most effective if scheduled regularly rather than as needed. Acetaminophen provides adequate analgesia for many mild to moderate pain syndromes, particularly musculoskeletal pain from osteoarthritis, and is recommended as first-line therapy for persistent pain. The preferred maximal dose in older adults is approximately 3 grams over a 24-hour period and, given the risk of hepatotoxicity at higher doses, should not exceed 4 grams in patients even with normal hepatic and renal function. Patients at risk of liver dysfunction, particularly those who have a history of heavy alcohol intake, should be treated cautiously; in these patients, the dosage should be decreased by 50%, or acetaminophen should be avoided entirely. Acetaminophen should be administered every 6 hours for patients with a creatinine clearance of 10–50 mL/min, and every 8 hours for patients with a creatinine clearance of <10 mL/min. Acetaminophen is commonly contained in many OTC and prescription products; therefore, knowledge of all medications that a patient is taking is critical to avoiding acetaminophen toxicity.

NSAIDs tend to be more effective than acetaminophen in chronic inflammatory pain but pose significant threats to older adults. They must be used judiciously if at all, should be used only after acetaminophen has been tried, and then only in highly select individuals. Significant adverse events, including renal dysfunction, GI bleeding, platelet dysfunction, fluid retention, exacerbation of hypertension or heart failure, and precipitation of delirium, limit the use of NSAIDs in treatment of persistent pain in older adults. The FDA has issued a particular caution against using ibuprofen with aspirin, owing to an interaction that blocks the antiplatelet effect of the aspirin. COX-2 inhibitors were developed to decrease the risk of GI bleeding by acting on a more selective receptor, but the risk of renal complications and hypertension remains the same as with other NSAIDs, and the degree to which longer-term GI toxicity is reduced is not clear. Several studies have confirmed increased cardiovascular risks associated with COX-2 inhibitors, which is now believed to be a class effect. Thus, COX-2 inhibitor use should be considered with great caution, if at all, in older adults. Misoprostol, a prostaglandin analogue, or a proton-pump inhibitor can be co-prescribed to reduce the risk of NSAID-induced GI bleeding, but these drugs do not reduce the risks of renal disease, hypertension, fluid retention, or delirium. Alternatively, nonacetylated salicylates such as salsalate and trisalicylate may have less renal toxicity and antiplatelet activity than other NSAIDs and therefore may be preferable in older adults, but evidence supporting this theory is sparse. Topical NSAIDs appear to be safe and effective in the short term, but longer-term studies are lacking.

Moderate to severe pain, or pain that requires chronic treatment, often requires opioid medications for sufficient relief, although evidence evaluating their role in managing persistent noncancer pain is scant. In general, it is prudent to start opioid therapy at the lowest dosage possible and to titrate up slowly. That said, opioid dosing should be titrated progressively to achieve the level of analgesia needed, and aggressively rapid titration with frequent monitoring is required for patients in a pain crisis.

Continuous pain should generally be treated with medications in long-acting or sustained-release formulations after total opioid requirements have been estimated by an initial trial of a short-acting agent. Fast-onset medications with short half-lives may be added to the long-acting regimen to cover episodes of breakthrough pain. Typically, a patient is offered approximately 5%–15% of the total daily dose every 2–4 hours orally for breakthrough pain. In general, different opioids provide similar analgesic efficacy. Cost and route of delivery can help guide the choice of medication.

Most opioids are metabolized by the liver and excreted by the kidneys. In renal dysfunction, the active metabolites of morphine, including morphine-6-glucuronide and morphine-3-glucuronide, can accumulate, increasing the risk of prolonged sedation and possible neurotoxicity. When using morphine to treat patients with kidney disease, the dosing intervals should be increased and the dosage decreased to reduce this risk. Hydromorphone has fewer adverse effects in patients with renal failure and, therefore, is many experts' first choice for this population (SOE=C). Some experts and limited data suggest that oxycodone is also safer than morphine in patients with kidney failure because its metabolism results in fewer active metabolites, but this remains controversial (SOE=C).

For suggestions on how to interconvert between different opioids or different routes of administration, see Table 17.5.

Barriers to Using Opioids in Older Adults

Older adults may have concerns about long-term opioid use that keep them from accepting adequate treatment for their pain. They may fear that taking opioid therapy for their current level of pain will result in the medication losing its effectiveness in the future when pain becomes more severe. Fear of addiction is another major obstacle to prescribing medications for older adults. A frank discussion of these concerns may help alleviate these fears.

Providers should be aware that patients who use pharmacies in urban neighborhoods may have difficulty accessing opioids, because many urban pharmacies do not routinely keep these medications in stock. Several studies indicate that there are opioid treatment disparities in black Americans. Cultural barriers also exist when evaluating pain, especially in patients who do not speak English. Providers should become familiar with the patient's cultural and religious context for pain, how pain is expressed, and expectations for treatment.

Physical dependence is an expected change in a patient's physiology that develops while a patient is taking opioid medications for an extended period. If opioids are discontinued suddenly, patients who are physically dependent experience a withdrawal syndrome that may include restlessness, tachycardia, hypertension, fever, tremors, and lacrimation. Symptoms of withdrawal can be avoided by tapering opioids carefully over days to weeks. *Tolerance* refers to a change in physiology resulting in the need to increase opioid dosages over time to achieve adequate analgesic effect. Experts note that tolerance to analgesia, as opposed to tolerance to sedation and respiratory depression, develops slowly in stable disease. If medicines must be titrated rapidly to reduce pain, a search for the cause of the exacerbation should be undertaken, and nonphysical contributors should be considered as well.

There is partial cross-tolerance between different opioids. Therefore, when switching a patient from one agent to another (eg, morphine to oxycodone), the clinician should reduce the amount (suggested range of 50%–65%) of the theoretical equianalgesic dose to reduce the risk of inadvertent overdose. It is important to note that liberal, as-needed, short-acting opioids should be made available during the transition period, so that the patient has access to adequate analgesic medications for treating breakthrough pain. Careful monitoring for pain exacerbation because of inadequate dose, or adverse effects due to the new opioid, is strongly recommended. Patient and caregiver education is vital in successful opioid management, especially during the transition process until a new steady state is reached and the patient's pain is well controlled.

Psychological *dependence*, or true *addiction*, refers to a state defined by compulsive drug seeking and drug using *with disregard for adverse social, physical, and economic* consequences. It is very rare for patients who have persistent pain to become addicted to opioids, but opioid abuse can become a problem in certain individuals, and the potential for abuse should be carefully discussed in those with a prior history of addiction. Although opioid abuse is less common in older adults, clinicians should carefully monitor for misuse of these medications. Addiction must be distinguished from *pseudoaddiction*, which refers to a situation in which a patient with significant unrelieved pain adopts behaviors (eg, theatricality in pleas for relief) similar to those of truly addicted patients.

Adverse Effects of Opioids

The most common adverse effect of opioid treatment is constipation, and tolerance to this toxicity does not occur. Opioid-induced constipation is due to multiple mechanisms, including dehydration, decreased GI tract secretions, and decreased intestinal motility. Because constipation usually complicates opioid use for the duration of treatment, education regarding the probable need for long-term laxative treatment is recommended for all patients when opioid therapy is started. Many experts recommend starting therapy with a stimulant laxative (such as bisacodyl or senna); however, these should be avoided in any patient with signs or symptoms of bowel obstruction. Bulking agents such as fiber and psyllium should be avoided in inactive, seriously ill patients and frail older adults with poor oral fluid intake because of the risk of fecal impaction and obstruction. All patients should be encouraged to exercise, as they are able, and to stay well hydrated. For patients who develop opioid-induced constipation despite laxative therapy, treatment with methylnaltrexone (a mu-opioid-receptor antagonist) or lubiprostone (a chloride channel activator) may relieve constipation without precipitating withdrawal symptoms or pain crisis (SOE=B).

Nausea and vomiting are common adverse effects of opioids. These agents have a direct effect on the chemoreceptor trigger zone, the part of the brain associated with the sensation of nausea. Other common causes of nausea and vomiting in patients taking opioids include gastroparesis, constipation, and metabolic disorders such as renal and hepatic failure. Although opioid-induced nausea and vomiting usually resolve spontaneously after the first few doses, some patients experience chronic nausea. After evaluation for reversible causes of nausea such as constipation, some patients benefit from changing to an alternative opioid (SOE=D). Others may need to be treated with scheduled antiemetics, although the high prevalence of adverse events, including drowsiness, delirium, and other anticholinergic effects, needs to be recognized in older adults treated with these medications.

Respiratory depression is the most serious potential adverse effect associated with opioid use, but tolerance to this effect develops quickly. Older adults and individuals with a history of respiratory dysfunction are at particular risk when opioid dosages are increased rapidly or when another sedative is taken concomitantly. Naloxone, an opioid-receptor antagonist, can reverse opioid-induced respiratory depression; however, when given to a patient who has been treated chronically with opioids, it can precipitate a pain crisis and acute withdrawal symptoms. Experts suggest withholding naloxone and placing the patient under careful observation unless respiratory rate decreases to <8 breaths per minute or the oxygen saturation drops to <90%. When needed, naloxone should be titrated carefully, using the lowest dosage possible.

Older adults can experience sedation, fatigue, and mild cognitive impairment with opioid treatment. These symptoms are common during dosage adjustment. Patients typically overcome the fatigue and sedation within days to weeks as they become tolerant to the medication. They need to be warned of the risks of increased falls and counseled not to drive or operate heavy equipment when the medication is started. A small subset of patients treated with opioids experience incessant fatigue or excessive sedation that significantly limits their function. A limited course of a stimulant such as low-dose methylphenidate may justifiably be tried in this situation (SOE=D). Rotation to a different opioid is an alternative strategy used to alleviate opioid-induced fatigue.

Nonopioid Adjuvant Analgesics

A nonopioid or adjuvant medication can be used as the sole agent or in combination with opioids. These medications can be particularly useful in treating patients with neuropathic pain or mixed pain syndromes.

Although tricyclic antidepressants (TCAs) are the most extensively studied medications for neuropathic pain, none has been FDA approved for this purpose, and their inclusion on the Beers Criteria list signals their potential for excessive risk when prescribed to older persons. Their efficacy in the treatment of post-herpetic neuralgia and diabetic neuropathy has been shown in numerous placebo-controlled studies (SOE=A). Unfortunately, they are associated with significant anticholinergic adverse events in older adults, including constipation, urinary retention, dry mouth, cognitive impairment, tachycardia, and blurred vision. Of note, desipramine[OL] and nortriptyline[OL] may have fewer adverse events than amitriptyline[OL]; thus, amitriptyline should be avoided in older adults.

Clinical depression in patients with persistent pain requires treatment to achieve optimal analgesia and quality of life. Other classes of antidepressants (eg, SSRIs) have generally been less studied than TCAs as analgesics, but older adults typically tolerate these agents better than TCAs when used in antidepressant doses. Duloxetine, a serotonin and norepinephrine reuptake inhibitor (SNRI), is approved both as an antidepressant and for treatment of pain from diabetic neuropathy, and it may offer a more favorable adverse-event profile than the TCAs. Venlafaxine[OL], another SNRI, has been used in similar applications.

Anticonvulsant medications such as carbamazepine, gabapentin, pregabalin, and clonazepam[OL] are commonly used as treatments for neuropathic pain. Gabapentin and pregabalin have demonstrated clinical efficacy in treatment of post-herpetic neuralgia and have fewer adverse events than TCAs, but they cost more. The main adverse events of gabapentin and pregabalin are sedation and dizziness, which frequently limit dosage increases, and peripheral edema commonly occurs as well. Gabapentin doses must be limited in patients with renal dysfunction.

Corticosteroids are useful adjuvants to treat pain associated with swelling, inflammation, and tissue infiltration, as well as neuropathic pain (SOE=C). In addition to their analgesic properties, they also can increase appetite and improve energy, although weight gained is predominantly fluid and fat rather than muscle. Adverse effects seen with short-term use of steroids include psychosis, fluid retention, hair loss, loss of skin integrity, hyperglycemia, insomnia, and immunosuppression. Corticosteroid use should be limited to treatment of inflammatory conditions and metastatic bone pain, and even then these agents should be used with caution.

Intravenous bisphosphonates can substantially reduce pain from malignant bone metastases (SOE=B). Bisphosphonates have been associated with the rare occurrence of osteonecrosis of the jaw, particularly when administered to patients undergoing dental surgery.

Tramadol both binds to opioid receptors and inhibits the reuptake of norepinephrine and serotonin. It can lower the seizure threshold and is therefore not recommended for patients who have a history of seizures or who take other medications known to lower the seizure threshold. Caution should also be exercised in patients taking other medications that have serotonergic properties, to avoid precipitating serotonin syndrome (characterized by myoclonus, agitation, abdominal cramping, hyperpyrexia, hypertension, and potentially death). Tapentadol is a synthetic, oral mu-opioid-receptor agonist approved for management of moderate to severe acute pain and chronic pain in adults. Tapentadol also has SNRI properties and is structurally and pharmacologically similar to tramadol. It is cleared by the liver and excreted by the kidney and consequently should be avoided in patients with severe renal and hepatic impairment. Significant adverse effects include nausea, vomiting, constipation, dizziness, and somnolence. Because patients may experience withdrawal, the extended-release formulation should be titrated downward gradually.

Medications to Avoid in Older Adults

In prescribing analgesics for older adults, it is important to "start low and go slow." Most often, the dosage of analgesics is limited by their adverse effects and drug-drug interactions. In older adults who live alone, it is important to regularly assess cognitive status, because this may influence their ability to take analgesics as prescribed. Mixed agonist-antagonists such as nalbuphine and butorphanol have the potential to cause restlessness and tremulousness and, therefore, should be avoided in older adults. Meperidine should also be avoided in older adults, because it can cause agitation, confusion, delirium, and disorientation.

Interventional Pain Management

Interventional approaches play a complementary role to traditional pharmacologic and nonpharmacologic approaches managing chronic pain. Two commonly used approaches in older adults with chronic pain are described below.

Trigger Point Injection

Trigger points are focal tender areas in soft tissues, muscles, ligaments, periosteum, tendons, and pericapsular areas. Often, there is a small triggering injury that, after healing, forms scar tissue that can entrap and damage nerves. Pain is typically elicited when local pressure is applied to the trigger point. Trigger point injections are indicated in patients with acute and chronic muscle pain often associated with underlying bone or nerve pathology. Local anesthetic (eg, 1% lidocaine) is injected once or more into the trigger point. Although the effect of the local anesthetic is temporary, the mechanical disruption of the scar tissue by the needle results in increased perfusion at the trigger point and theoretically washes away sensitizing noxious substances that accumulate locally. Injections are given once or twice a week until pain relief is attained.

Pulsed Radiofrequency (PRF) Treatment of Chronic Pain

PRF is being increasingly used to treat various types of pain, including cervical radicular pain, trigeminal neuralgia, sacroiliac joint pain, facet arthropathy, shoulder pain, postsurgical pain, radicular pain, and myofascial pain conditions. PRF applies short pulses of radiofrequency (RF) signals from an RF generator to the neural tissue. RF generators provide a pulse frequency of 2 Hz and a pulse width of 20 ms, and the target tissue is subjected to low- or moderate-strength electric fields and localized warming. The electric fields and the heat are thought to reduce pain signals generated by the nerves from that local area, resulting in pain relief. After injecting local anesthetic to numb the skin, a thin needle is inserted into the painful area guided by radiographic imaging. A microelectrode is then inserted through the needle, and an RF current is passed through the electrode. Many patients experience at least some pain relief and, for some, the analgesia lasts for months. Common adverse effects include pain and swelling at the treatment site.

REFERENCES

- American Geriatrics Society Panel on the Pharmacologic Management of Persistent Pain in Older Persons. Pharmacological management of persistent pain in older persons. *J Am Geriatr Soc.* 2009;57(8):1331–1346. Available at www.americangeriatrics.org/files/documents/2009_Guideline.pdf (accessed Jan 2016).

    This excellent review on persistent pain provides information about assessment and management, as well as a review of the strength of evidence for various treatment modalities. It is an invaluable resource for any clinician caring for older adults.

- Cooper JW, Burfield AH. Assessment and management of chronic pain in the older adult. *J Am Pharm Assoc.* 2010;50(3):e89–99.

    The authors provide guidelines on assessing pain in cognitively intact and impaired older adults, as well as strategies for providing patients with analgesia while reducing the risk of increasing drug-related morbidity and mortality.

- Kane CM, Hoskin P, Bennett MI. Cancer induced bone pain. *BMJ*. 2015;350:h315.

    When treating cancer induced bone pain, maintenance of function should be given high priority alongside pain relief. Early recognition, intervention with functional aids, and behavior modification, combined with initial titration of analgesics (commonly, strong opioids) are important first steps.

- Makris UE, Abrams RC, Gurland B, et al. Management of persistent pain in the older patient: a clinical review. *JAMA*. 2014;312(8):825–836.

    Treatment planning for persistent pain in later life requires a clear understanding of the patient's treatment goals and expectations, comorbidities, and cognitive and functional status, as well as the coordination of available community resources and family support. A combination of pharmacologic, nonpharmacologic, and rehabilitative approaches, in addition to a strong therapeutic alliance between the patient and clinician, are essential in setting, adjusting, and achieving realistic goals of therapy.

- Mossey JM. Defining racial and ethnic disparities in pain management. *Clin Orthop Relat Res*. 2011;469(7):1859–1870.

    Racial/ethnic minority patients with pain need to be empowered to accurately report pain intensity levels, and clinicians who treat such patients need to acknowledge their own belief systems regarding pain and to develop strategies to overcome unconscious, potentially harmful, negative stereotyping of minority patients.

- Palliative Care Curriculum 2015 (a joint project of the U.S. Veterans Administration and Stanford University Medical School). Available at https://palliative.stanford.edu/opioid-conversion/ (accessed Jan 2016).

    This site provides a Web-based curriculum in palliative care, with modules describing pain management and methods for conversion among opioids.

Vyjeyanthi S. Periyakoil, MD

CHAPTER 18—HOSPITAL CARE

KEY POINTS

- Adults ≥65 years old make up 13% of the population and account for 36% of acute care hospital admissions and nearly 50% of hospital expenditures for all adults.

- Older adults experience high rates of adverse events during hospitalization, including loss of activities of daily living (ADLs) and development of delirium; they are also at high risk of adverse drug events.

- Older hospitalized adults should be routinely assessed for a limited number of common geriatric problems regardless of their admission diagnosis.

- Specific system changes in providing care to hospitalized older adults have resulted in improved patient outcomes.

Older adults are at disproportionate risk of becoming seriously ill and requiring hospital care, whether in an emergency department, on a medical or surgical ward, or in a critical care unit. Adults ≥65 years old make up 13% of the U.S. population but account for 36% of acute care hospital admissions and nearly 50% of hospital expenditures for adults. The most common principal diagnoses in hospitalized older adults are heart failure, pneumonia, cardiac dysrhythmia, and acute coronary syndromes.

Hospital use rates vary as much as 3-fold for Medicare beneficiaries with the same illnesses across different regions of the United States. There is no evidence that these differences in practice patterns are explained by differences in disease rates or severity. Hospital use and the use of hospital resources is much lower among those enrolled in capitated insurance plans than among those enrolled in fee-for-service plans; this difference in resource use has not been systematically linked to differences in patient outcomes.

Disparities in hospital care exist. Minority patients are significantly less likely than whites to be treated at high-volume hospitals for services for which high volume is associated with better outcomes. The differences were largest for cancer surgeries and cardiovascular procedures. Hospitals in the bottom quintile on most quality measures served a significantly higher percentage of minority patients than hospitals in the top quintile.

During hospitalization, older adults tend to receive less costly care than younger patients. For example, in the Study to Understand Prognoses and Preferences for Outcomes and Risks of Treatments (SUPPORT), seriously ill patients in their 80s received fewer invasive procedures and less resource-intensive, less costly hospital care than similarly ill younger patients (SOE=A). This preferential allocation of hospital services to younger patients was not based on differences in severity of illness or general preferences for life-extending care and is consistent with evidence regarding outpatient care. Differences in the aggressiveness of care have not been shown to explain differences between older and younger patients in survival or other outcomes. Moreover, patients' families and clinicians commonly underestimate older patients' desire for aggressive care (SOE=A). The best guides to assessment and management of any older hospitalized patient are the clinical circumstances and the patient's preferences, irrespective of age.

In a study of vulnerable older adults hospitalized on the medical service of an academic medical center, the quality of care provided was examined by measuring adherence to the third phase of Assessing Care of Vulnerable Elders (ACOVE-3) quality indicators. Adherence to indicators was significantly greater for general medical care (such as for heart failure or diabetes) than for geriatric conditions (such as delirium or pressure sores) (SOE=A). Yet, adherence to 16 ACOVE geriatric-specific quality indicators in the acute care setting may be associated with lower 1-year mortality in vulnerable older hospitalized patients. This chapter is intended to assist providers in the acute setting to adhere to effective geriatric care processes, regardless of the general medical problems of their patients.

HAZARDS OF HOSPITALIZATION

Hospital-Associated Disability

Once hospitalized, older patients are at high risk of loss of independence and institutionalization. Among hospitalized medical patients ≥70 years old, approximately one-third are discharged with a disability that was not present 2 weeks before admission, a condition referred to as hospitalization-associated disability (HAD) (SOE=A). In addition, hospitalization accounts for 50% of new-onset disability in frail older adults. Patients at risk of HAD are easily identified on admission. A recently validated clinical index identified risk factors (age, number of dependencies in ADLs and instrumental activities of daily living [IADLs], mobility 2 weeks before admission, metastatic cancer or stroke, severe cognitive impairment, and hypoalbuminemia) for new-onset disability in hospitalized patients ≥70 years old. Higher risk scores predicted more severe disability, greater likelihood of nursing-home placement, and worse survival.

The ability to perform ADLs and IADLs is necessary for older adults to live independently, and functional dependence is associated with worse quality of life, shortened survival, and increased resource use. The older adult's ability to perform ADLs and IADLs, determined at the time of admission, can serve as a useful baseline. If functional dependence is found, the causes should be explored (eg, dependence in IADLs is often associated with dementia), and strategies to maintain and improve functional ability can be started (eg, physical and occupational therapy). The clinician plays a critical role in educating patients and families regarding the harmful effects of limited activity and the need to engage in function-promoting activity to avoid functional decline.

Delirium

Delirium is present in 10%–15% of hospitalized older adults on admission, and it develops in up to 30% during the course of hospitalization on a general medical ward (SOE=A). Certain subgroups of hospitalized older patients have higher incidence of delirium, with rates of 15%–53% in postoperative patients and 70%–87% in ICU patients. The diagnosis of delirium should be considered when any of the following is observed: acute onset of change and fluctuation in mental status or behavior, inattention, disorganized thinking, and altered consciousness. The Confusion Assessment Method (CAM) is a screening tool that incorporates all four of these features, with a positive screen consisting of both of the first two features plus one or both of the latter two. Three psychomotor behavioral subtypes are currently recognized: hypoactive, hyperactive, and mixed. Hyperactive delirious patients are restless, agitated, and hyperalert (and this diagnosis is rarely missed), whereas hypoactive delirious patients often have decreased movement, paucity of speech, and reduced responsiveness. Hypoactive patients are often not identified in the hospital, or misdiagnosed as having depression or dementia. Delirium arising during the course of hospitalization is associated with prolonged hospital stay, nursing-home placement, increased mortality, and worsening cognitive function. Symptoms of delirium can persist for months after hospital discharge.

Prevention is the best strategy; roughly one-third of cases of delirium can be prevented by appropriately managing 6 risk factors for delirium: cognitive impairment, sleep deprivation, immobility, visual impairment, hearing impairment, and dehydration (SOE=A). Although the benefits of interventions to prevent delirium are well established, interventions for treating established delirium have not demonstrated improved outcomes (SOE=C). Once the diagnosis is made, measures should be taken to identify the medical condition causing the delirium by reviewing recently added medications and by investigating for likely causes such as infection, electrolyte abnormalities, and ischemia. Measures to prevent or ameliorate delirium include avoiding medications associated with delirium (such as benzodiazepines, anticholinergics, and opiates) whenever possible; treating pain, infection, and fever; detecting and correcting urinary retention, fecal impaction, and metabolic abnormalities; frequently orienting patients with cognitive or sensory impairment; limiting room changes; and avoiding excessive bed rest, restraints, and unnecessary tethers (eg, in-dwelling bladder and intravenous catheters, oxygen lines, and telemetry leads).

Suboptimal Pharmacotherapy

Pharmacotherapy involves prescribing, communicating orders, dispensing, administering, and monitoring. There is potential for error at each step. Other factors that contribute to the complexities of pharmacotherapy for older patients in the acute care setting include polypharmacy, multiple prescribing providers, restrictive hospital formularies that require careful medication reconciliation during care transitions, barriers to medication reconciliation, and significant turnover of the medication regimen with many old medications discontinued and new ones introduced. In one study, 40% of medications prescribed before admissions were discontinued during hospitalization, and 45% of medications prescribed at discharge were started during hospitalization. In another study, 88% of older hospitalized patients had at least one clinically significant problem related to prescribing, and 22% had at least one potentially serious and life-threatening problem (SOE=B).

Adverse drug events (ADEs) are a significant source of hospital hazard for older patients. In one meta-analysis, the in-hospital incidence of ADEs was 6.7%. Patients at risk of developing an ADE can be identified using an index that includes the number of drugs, history of ADEs, heart failure, liver disease, presence of ≥4 conditions, and renal failure. Inappropriate medication use likely contributes to the risk of ADEs. The Beers Criteria and the screening tool of older persons' potentially inappropriate prescriptions (STOPP) are two common-sense, evidence-based approaches to reducing inappropriate prescribing.

A hospital admission is an ideal time to completely review a patient's medication regimen and to discontinue or change medications that are unnecessary, have low therapeutic value (eg, sedative-hypnotics), are prescribed at the wrong dose or frequency, are duplicative, interact with another medication, or are prescribed despite a known allergy. In addition, a medication review at admission can evaluate whether medical conditions are being maximally treated. Review of medications should include both prescription and nonprescription medications. Consultation by clinical pharmacists can improve appropriate prescribing and improve the older patient's adherence to prescribed therapy (SOE=A). These changes should be undertaken in consultation with the outpatient provider.

Sleep Disturbance

Over one-third of older patients have difficulty sleeping in the hospital. Sleep deprivation is important to prevent, recognize, and address, because it is associated with increased risk of delirium. Sources of sleep disruption in hospitalized older adults include intrinsic (eg, underlying medical illness, medications, drug withdrawal) and extrinsic factors (eg, noise, measuring vital signs, phlebotomy, medication administration, and beeping medical monitors). Sedative-hypnotic medications are prescribed to one-third of older hospitalized patients despite the associated risks of delirium, falls, hip fractures, and rebound insomnia, as well as their poor benefit-to-harm ratio (SOE=A). Therefore, sleep deprivation in the hospital is best managed nonpharmacologically. One protocol using nighttime noise reduction strategies, including warm drinks, soothing music, massage treatments, and rescheduled medication administration and measurement of vital signs to avoid sleep interruption, significantly reduced the use of sedative-hypnotics in the hospital.

Nutrition

Serious deficiencies of macro- and micronutrients are common in hospitalized older patients. On admission, severe protein-calorie malnutrition is present in approximately 15% of adults ≥70 years old, and moderate malnutrition is present in another 25%. Moreover, 25% of older patients suffer further nutritional depletion during hospitalization. Even after controlling for underlying acute illness, its severity, and comorbid illnesses, malnutrition is associated with increased risk of complications, dependence, institutionalization, and death.

In addition, deficiencies of vitamins (especially vitamin D) and electrolytes are common among older hospitalized patients. In one large hospital, nearly two-thirds of patients ≥65 years old were found to be deficient in vitamin D. Vitamin D deficiency was nearly as common in patients without a risk factor for vitamin D deficiency and in those taking multivitamins as in other patients (SOE=B).

Assessing patients' nutritional health is essential. Patients who receive nutritional assessment in the hospital are less likely to experience short-term functional decline or die 1 year after hospital discharge. Nutritionally at-risk older patients randomized to individualized in-hospital dietary treatment plus 3 home visits demonstrated higher serum albumin and lower mortality at 6 months than those randomized to 1 in-hospital dietitian visit or usual care. Beyond considering supplements, clinicians should assess malnourished older hospitalized patients for remediable factors such as difficulty chewing, need for dentures, dysphagia, medications that impair appetite, overly restrictive prescribed diet, or insufficient time or physical ability to eat.

Another contributor to poor oral intake in the hospital is constipation. Elimination records should be reviewed regularly, and patients who have not moved their bowels in more than a couple of days may benefit from an oral or rectal stimulant (eg, senna, bisacodyl) or an osmotic (eg, polyethylene glycol) laxative, in addition to provision of adequate fluid and fiber intake and mobility.

The maintenance of water and electrolyte balance requires special attention in older adults during and after fluid administration because of their decreased ability to achieve and maintain homeostasis. Initial efforts can be directed toward achieving euvolemia and correcting electrolyte abnormalities. Subsequent efforts to maintain fluid and electrolyte balance are based on estimates of daily metabolic requirements.

NEVER EVENTS

Medicare payment for inpatient care is based on diagnoses and procedures that are assigned diagnosis-related group (DRG) codes. Prior to October 2008, hospitals received greater reimbursement for the care of a patient who developed complications that led to a costlier DRG. Concerned that this was a disincentive to improving patient safety, in October 2008, the CMS mandated non-payment for so-called "never events," conditions that met 3 criteria: 1) are high cost and/or high volume, 2) result in reassignment to a higher reimbursed DRG when designated as secondary diagnosis, and 3) are reasonably preventable through application of evidence-based interventions. This rule applied to the following conditions: surgical object left in patient, air embolism, blood incompatibility, catheter-associated urinary tract infection (CAUTI), hospital-acquired pressure ulcer (HAPU), vascular catheter-associated infection, mediastinitis after coronary artery bypass grafting, and falls.

The financial impact of this policy, using 2006 hospital discharge data from California, was estimated to be negligible.

Some stakeholders argue that the new rule may penalize hospitals that treat high-risk patients, such as frail older adults. Three conditions designated "never events" for which older hospitalized adults are known to be at greater risk of developing (and the number of Medicare cases in 2006) are falls (2,591), HAPU (322,946), and CAUTI (11,780).

Falls

The falls rate in the hospital range from 3 to 13 per 1,000 patient-days. Among older adults, the rates are higher at 6 to 15.9 per 1,000 patient-days. A fall leads to an incremental cost of approximately $4,000 per hospitalization. Although hospital falls meet the first 2 criteria for conditions that ought never to develop after admission, evidence-supported strategies that prevent falls in the acute care setting are limited, and falls with or without injury occur despite delivery of appropriate care.

It is helpful to assess the patient's gait, balance, lower extremity strength, ability to get up from bed, cognition, and mood during the initial physical examination. Individuals able to walk independently should be encouraged to do so frequently during hospitalization. Immobility during hospitalization leads rapidly to diminished strength and subsequent difficulty walking (SOE=A). Those able to walk but unable to do so safely and independently can receive assistance from hospital staff while walking several times daily. Formal physical therapy can yield additional benefits.

The initial physical examination is also a good time to assess a patient's risk of falling by inquiring about a history of falls (SOE=A) and by careful musculoskeletal and neurologic examinations. Strategies to promote mobility and reduce falls include avoiding restraints and tethers, decluttering the environment, minimizing use of medications associated with falls, providing walking assistance for those who walk with difficulty, attending to patient's toileting needs, addressing sensory impairments, and providing physical therapy for those with weakness or gait abnormalities. Multifactorial interventions targeting specific individual risk factors for falls (eg, impairment in gait, balance, or strength; medications; environment; vision) significantly reduced the risk and rates of falls in older patients in the nursing-home and acute/subacute hospital settings. A randomized controlled trial of an information technology-based, nursing-led, patient education and communication falls prevention toolkit reduced both the rate of falls and the proportion of fallers in an acute-care hospital (SOE=A).

During the 27-month period before implementation of the "Never Events" rule, analyzing data from 1,263 National Database of Nursing Quality Indicators (NDNQI) hospitals nationwide, rates of total and injurious falls were trending downward at −0.4% per quarter and −1% per quarter, respectively. The impact of the rule on the trend of hospital fall rate remains to be seen.

Hospital-Acquired Pressure Ulcers

Although there has been an overall decrease in HAPUs since 2004, studies of frail older adults or high-risk individuals report the median incidence of pressure ulcers (PU) in the acute care setting to be 15.7%. Within the first 2 days of hospitalization on a medicine service, as many as 6.2% of patients ≥65 years old will develop one or more PUs. Most PUs are on the sacrum and heels; they are painful, associated with longer hospitalizations and delayed return of function, and costly ($37,800–$70,000 per case, or an estimated $11 billion nationally in 2009). Older age, low body weight, physical and cognitive impairment, incontinence, malnutrition, and conditions that impair circulation are risk factors for developing PUs. The two most commonly used PU risk-assessment scales are the Braden and Norton scales. Patients at risk should have their skin inspected at least daily, focusing on areas of bony prominences.

Most trials on preventive interventions focused on evaluating support surfaces. For patients at higher risk, more advanced static mattresses and overlays were better than standard mattresses for preventing PUs. Although there is a good evidence base for repositioning, the optimal interval for repositioning remains to be determined.

Urinary Catheter Use and Catheter-Associated Urinary Tract Infection

Urinary catheters (UC) are often inappropriately inserted and are associated with adverse outcomes. UCs are 1 of 5 precipitating factors for delirium identified in a prospective study of medical inpatients ≥70 years old. A similar cohort of patients admitted to a general medicine service with no medical indication for a UC were followed prospectively for insertion of a catheter within 48 hours of hospital admission. A catheter was inserted in 14% of the cohort who had no indication for the catheter. Although these patients were older and more likely to have been admitted because of a "geriatric condition" ("altered mental status," fall without hip fracture, urinary tract infection, "failure to thrive"), their admission characteristics were, otherwise, not different from those of matched controls. After adjusting for potential confounders, those who had a UC were more likely to die during hospitalization and within 90 days of discharge. UC use was also associated with longer hospitalization but not with new decline in function or admission to a nursing home.

Older age is a risk factor for urinary catheter–associated bacteriuria. The most important modifiable risk factor is duration of indwelling catheterization; the reported incidence of bacteriuria is 3%–8% per catheter-day. Accordingly, the most effective way to reduce catheter-associated urinary tract infections (CAUTI) is to limit urinary catheterization to those with a clear indication and to remove the catheter as soon as it is no longer necessary. Appropriate indications for a bladder catheter include acute urinary retention or bladder outlet obstruction, perioperatively for selected procedures, open sacral or perineal wounds in incontinent patients, prolonged immobility due to unstable thoracic, lumbar, pelvic fractures, and for comfort at end-of-life as needed. Inserting a catheter to measure urinary output is inappropriate in most cases. Reminder systems are useful; more than 25% of the time, clinicians are unaware that their patients have an indwelling catheter, and those catheters that have no indication are more likely to be overlooked. Evidence-based practices for CAUTI prevention include education and training of health care personnel, appropriate insertion and care, consideration of alternatives to catheter use, and early removal through reminder systems. It has been estimated that 25%–75% of CAUTI cases are preventable with use of multimodal strategies.

ASSESSING AND MANAGING HOSPITALIZED OLDER PATIENTS

Assessment on Admission

Many of the serious illnesses disproportionately experienced by older adults require hospital care for optimal management. The benefits of hospitalization can be remarkable: correcting serious physiologic derangements, repairing vascular obstructions and broken bones, and using highly technical biomedical advances to treat life-threatening illnesses. However, while in the hospital, older adults also commonly experience deteriorating functional status, adverse events from medication, or delirium. A systematic approach to assessing and managing hospitalized older adults offers the best chance of reducing the risk and consequences of these common problems.

The initial assessment should include an evaluation of function at the level of the organ system, the whole person, and the person's environment. This assessment can identify needs for which targeted interventions can improve function or reduce risk of adverse outcomes. This approach complements the traditional medical assessment by highlighting problems that are common in hospitalized older patients, and it is similar in concept to geriatric assessment conducted in other settings.

For suggestions on when assessment of these common geriatric problems can be incorporated into the routine of a hospital admission history and physical examination, see Table 18.1.

For commonly overlooked hazards and opportunities in older hospitalized patients, see Table 18.2. These problems have been selected based on their importance relative to other clinical issues, the quality of relevant evidence, and their specificity to older adults.

Two types of evidence suggest that these interventions are a good use of clinician time. First, for each problem, evidence supporting the proposed intervention is compelling, either because the efficacy of the intervention is well established (eg, prophylaxis of deep-vein thrombosis) or because the associated problem is common, often overlooked, and can be improved with a safe and inexpensive intervention. Second, compared with patients receiving usual care, patients ≥65 years old receiving care in acute geriatric units, in defined physical locations and structures, and managed by specialized interprofessional teams had lower risk of functional decline at discharge and were more likely to be discharged to home.

Cognitive Impairment

Adults >65 years old with dementia are hospitalized at more than 3 times the rate of those without dementia. In one systematic review, the prevalence of dementia among older patients in the acute hospital ranged from 13% to 63%. Patients with dementia were older and more undernourished before hospitalization. In hospital, they required more hours of nursing care, had longer hospitalizations, and were more likely to suffer delirium and functional decline and to be discharged to a nursing home than patients without dementia. Preexisting cognitive impairment is also a risk factor for falls, use of restraints, nonadherence to therapy, and feeding tube placements.

Despite its importance, documentation of a dementia diagnosis is often absent in hospital records. Recognizing an underlying cognitive impairment early

Table 18.1—Systematic Assessment of Older Adults on Hospital Admission

Step	Assessments
Past medical history	Ask about vaccination history.
Medications review	Assess indications for each medication, appropriateness of dosing, potential interactions.
	Assess for medication effects contributing to acute illness.
	Determine patient's or caregiver's method for assuring adherence (eg, pill boxes).
Social history	Ask about help needed (and who provides) for ADLs and IADLs.
	Ask about social support.
	Ask if patient feels safe.
	Ask about treatment goals and preference in event of cardiorespiratory arrest.
Review of systems	Ask about weight loss in preceding 6 months.
	Ask about dietary change.
	Ask about anorexia, nausea, vomiting, diarrhea.
	Ask about incontinence.
	Ask about problems with memory or confusion.
	Ask about falls or difficulty walking.
	Ask about difficulties with vision or hearing.
Physical examination	Take pulse (confirm arrhythmias with ECG).
	Check orthostatic blood pressures in patients with falls, presyncope, syncope.
	Assess for weight change, loss of subcutaneous fat, muscle wasting, edema, ascites, prevalent pressure ulcer.
	Screen for cognitive function.
	Assess vision and hearing.
	Assess gait.
	Use a depression screen.

Table 18.2—Common Hazards and Opportunities to Address during an Older Adult's Hospital Stay

Problem	Possible Interventions
Functional impairments	Assess ADLs on admission, physical therapy, occupational therapy, engage social resources.
Immobility and falls	Avoid restraints, remove in-dwelling bladder catheters, encourage ambulation in hospital and physical therapy, avoid sedating medications.
Sensory impairment	Use eyeglasses, hearing aids; remove cerumen impaction.
Depression	Treat with pharmacotherapy, cognitive therapy, or both.
Cognitive impairment	Evaluate for dementia or delirium, assess social environment, reorientation.
Suboptimal pharmacotherapy	Review all medications at admission and discharge, modify prescriptions, involve clinical pharmacists as medical team members, consider use of explicit appropriateness criteria.
Nutrition	Supplement water, calories, protein; assess social environment and medical factors that contribute to poor oral intake.
Immunization status	Vaccinate against influenza, pneumococcus.
Pressure ulcer prevention	Reposition frequently and use specialized support surfaces, manage moisture and incontinence, encourage ambulation.
Sleep disturbance	Address intrinsic and extrinsic causes, use nonpharmacologic protocols.
Venous thromboembolism prevention	Use prophylactic anticoagulation for patients with ≥1 risk factors for venous thromboembolism, mechanical thromboprophylaxis for high bleeding risk, encourage ambulation.

enables the health care team to implement preemptive measures to prevent these hazards. Cognitive function can be assessed by use of an established test of cognitive function, such as the Montreal Cognitive Assessment or the Mini-Cog test. Exposure to the hospital environment may be disorienting for patients with cognitive impairment because of frequent room changes, noise, and poor way-finding cues. Creating a unit with a home-like ambiance that allows unrestricted mobility, provides meaningful daytime activities, encourages the presence of family, promotes sleep through nonpharmacologic protocols, and addresses nutritional needs are prudent ways of making the hospital environment safer for patients with dementia.

Cognitive impairment may complicate the assessment and treatment of pain in the hospital. As a consequence, pain is often undertreated. Most patients with mild to moderate dementia can comprehend at least one pain assessment scale, but fewer than half of those with severe dementia can do so. Cognitively impaired patients may be unable to recognize their pain trajectory or to differentiate improving pain from new or worsening symptoms. Orders for patient-controlled analgesia pumps and as-needed pain medication should be avoided in patients with impaired recall. Scheduled analgesia should be considered, especially if pain occurs frequently. Nonpharmacologic approaches to pain should be part of the treatment plan. Patients may be unable to report adverse effects from the analgesics, and detection of complications (eg, fecal impaction or delirium) may be delayed. Anticipating and preventing common adverse effects (eg, initiating a bowel regimen whenever opiates are prescribed) is one way of avoiding complications. When patients with dementia develop delirium, looking for untreated pain as a possible cause is appropriate.

Patients with end-stage dementia hospitalized with a hip fracture or pneumonia have poor prognoses (6-month mortality [55% and 53%, respectively]), and many hospital interventions used to treat these conditions may be particularly burdensome to those unable to understand the nature of their illness or express their needs. Clinicians should educate surrogate decision-makers of the patient's prognosis and establish treatment goals that optimize the palliation of symptoms.

Sensory Deficits

Most hospitalized older adults have impairments in vision or hearing, which are risk factors for falls, incontinence, delirium, and functional dependence. The combination of both sensory impairments is associated with IADL loss. Although eyeglasses or hearing aids readily correct most visual and hearing impairments, they are often forgotten or inaccessible in the hospital.

Hospitalized older adults can be screened for sensory impairment by routinely asking if they have difficulty with seeing or hearing and whether they use eyeglasses or hearing aids. Physical examination, including a test of visual acuity (eg, with a pocket card of the Jaeger eye test) and the whisper test of hearing, in which a short, easily answered question is whispered in each ear, is the next appropriate step in evaluation. For people with visual or hearing impairments, it is important to provide the appropriate assistive devices (eyeglasses or hearing aids brought from home or voice amplifiers provided by the hospital), and staff may need to be instructed in the use of appliances to communicate more effectively.

Depression

Depressive symptoms in hospitalized older adults are common, prognostically important, and potentially ameliorable. Major or minor depression occurs in roughly one-third of hospitalized patients ≥65 years old but is often undiagnosed. The presence of depressive symptoms is associated with increased risk of dependence in ADLs, nursing-home placement, and shortened long-term survival, even after controlling for baseline function and the severity of acute and chronic illness.

All hospitalized older patients should be assessed for depression. Simply asking patients whether they feel down, depressed, or hopeless, or whether they have lost interest or pleasure in doing things, is a good place to start. In a systematic review of 14 studies of older medical inpatients that evaluated a depression rating scale compared with a gold standard diagnostic criteria, the Geriatric Depression Scale was found to be the only instrument that has been adequately studied. Scores of ≥5 on the GDS-15 and ≥10 the GDS-30 were associated with the best screening performance.

Psychotherapeutic interventions are safe and often effective in initial management of patients with suspected depression. Beginning pharmacotherapy during hospitalization for a medical or surgical condition may not be necessary, but follow-up shortly after discharge is critical. Those with persistently high numbers of depressive symptoms are especially at risk of functional decline and death in the year after discharge. If pharmacotherapy is started, SSRIs are often preferred, because approximately 50% of older hospitalized patients have a contraindication to tricyclic antidepressants.

Immunization

Adults ≥65 years old should be assessed at the time of hospital admission for their vaccination status and updated accordingly.

Influenza vaccine administered in the hospital and in the ambulatory setting was shown to be equally safe and immunogenic, and the complication associated with concurrent administration of influenza and pneumonia vaccines is noted to be mild in an older population.

The Advisory Committee on Immunization Practices (ACIP) recently recommended the 13-valent pneumococcal conjugate vaccine (PCV13) for routine use in those ≥65 years old based on findings from a trial involving approximately 850,000 older adults (CAPiTA). The vaccine was found to be beneficial in preventing the first episode of community-acquired pneumonia, noninvasive community acquired pneumonia, and invasive disease due to vaccine-type strains. To provide broader protection, including serotypes unique to pneumococcal polysaccharide vaccine PPSV23, ACIP recommends administering both vaccines in series. Based on immunogenicity studies, PCV13 is administered first followed by PPSV23 at least 12 months later. The sequential and time interval requirements for administering the pneumococcal vaccine series and frequent unavailability of vaccination history pose barriers to implementing a standing order system that can increase pneumococcal vaccination rates in hospitalized older adults.

Deep Venous Thrombosis (DVT) Prophylaxis

Because of diminished physiologic reserve, older adults are less able to compensate for the hemodynamic and ventilatory demands of a pulmonary embolism. Furthermore, numerous risk factors, comorbidities, and atypical presentations in older adults can lead to more challenging diagnosis of and worse outcomes from venous thromboembolic disease. Older adults are less likely to present with typical symptoms (such as chest pain, extremity discomfort, or difficulty ambulating) and are more likely to complain of dyspnea. Patients hospitalized for illness other than DVT who subsequently developed DVT were more likely to be elderly than nonelderly. Despite this, older patients receive DVT prophylaxis <50% of the time. The 2012 Guidelines from the American College of Chest Physicians recommend thromboprophylaxis with low-molecular-weight heparin, low-dose unfractionated heparin, or fondaparinux for acutely ill medical patients at high risk of venous thromboembolism. Risk can be assessed using the Padua Prediction Score, which takes into account increased age, previous venous thromboembolism, thrombophilia, cancer, heart or respiratory failure, reduced mobility, and use of hormonal medications. Renal function should be considered when deciding which antithrombotic to use and at what dosage. In patients with impaired kidney function, low-molecular-weight heparin and fondaparinux, both renally cleared agents, should be dose adjusted or completely avoided; unfractionated heparin may be preferable in these patients. Mechanical thromboprophylaxis should be used primarily for patients with high bleeding risk. Ensuring proper use and maximal adherence are key to effectiveness of mechanical prophylaxis.

Code Status Discussions

Half of all patients with cardiac arrests receiving resuscitation efforts in the United States occur in people >65 years old. Because resuscitation is an emergency procedure needed by those who at the moment of arrest are incapable of expressing treatment preference, consent is presumed and treatment administered immediately. Two scenarios are generally accepted as exceptions to this presumption: the patient's previous expression of preference that CPR be withheld and the treating physician's clinical judgment that an attempt to resuscitate would be futile.

From 2000 to 2009, rates of survival to hospital discharge of patients who had in-hospital cardiopulmonary arrests and underwent attempts at resuscitation increased from 13.7% to 22.3%. Survival to hospital discharge is better when the initial rhythm is ventricular fibrillation or pulseless ventricular tachycardia (40% in 2009) than when it is asystole or pulseless electrical activity (14% in 2009). Increasing age is associated with decreased survival to discharge and poorer outcomes. Of those >65 years old who survive to discharge, about half have clinically significant neurologic disability. Of patients with no or mild, moderate, or severe disability, or who are in a vegetative state, 27%, 39%, 58%, and 90%, respectively, died in the year after discharge.

Clinicians should solicit the wishes for resuscitation of patients who are at risk of suffering cardiac or respiratory failure. Ideally, these discussions will take place nonemergently in the clinic setting in the context of asking about the patient's general treatment preference. The strongest predictor of whether a code discussion was documented was the presence of preexisting documentation of care wishes. However, only 25% of patients have such documentation. Many states now have programs (eg, Physician Orders for Life-Sustaining Treatment [POLST]) that allow for patients with advanced illness to have their wishes for care translated by a health care provider into actionable medical orders (eg, "Do not attempt resuscitation"). In the absence of previous outpatient discussion or completed POLST forms, the patient's wishes should be determined early in the hospitalization. Subsequent discussions are necessary as the patient's condition and treatment options change. In addition, any decisions made should be periodically reevaluated. When older patients with "Do not attempt resuscitation/Do not intubate" (DNR/DNI) orders are asked about specific hypothetical situations, many would choose to have a trial of cardiac resuscitation or intubation. Fewer than half would reject these interventions under any circumstance.

Essential elements of the discussions include ensuring that the 1) patient understands his or her prognosis and the likelihood of requiring CPR; 2) patient's values and treatment goals are understood; 3) patient understands the nature of CPR and the risks, benefits, and likely outcomes; and 4) physician offers a recommendation about CPR based on the patient's prognosis and treatment goals.

Information about an individual's likelihood for surviving an in-hospital cardiac arrest (IHCA) neurologically intact or with minimal deficits is useful when making informed decisions about DNR/DNI orders. Data from 51,240 adults who suffered index IHCA was used to develop a clinical decision rule for predicting survival to discharge in good neurologic state. The mean age of individuals suffering IHCA was 65 years. Using clinical variables gathered at admission, 13 predictor variables were identified: neurologic status at admission, major trauma, acute stroke, metastatic or hematologic cancer, bacteremia, medical noncardiac diagnosis, hepatic insufficiency, admission from a skilled-nursing facility, hypotension/hypoperfusion, renal impairment, respiratory insufficiency, pneumonia, and age. The rate of survival to hospital discharge with good cerebral performance was 10.4%. The Good Outcome Following Attempted Resuscitation (GO-FAR) model identified very low to low likelihood (good neurologic outcomes in only 0.9% and 1.7%, respectively) in 28.3% of patients. This tool may provide clinicians with a more accurate survival estimate to integrate into code status discussions.

Daily Evaluation

Hospitalized older adults should be evaluated daily using a systematic approach to ensure that essential geriatric issues are not overshadowed by disease-specific or technologic concerns. For patients who are expected to recover mobility, progress toward that goal should be assessed. Time out of bed (eg, in a chair for meals) and ambulation (with assistance, if needed) should be encouraged. Progress on ADL recovery should be tracked, and patients encouraged and coached toward functional independence.

Daily physical examination should include identifying the devices attached to, or inserted in, each patient. Many of these devices can cause injury if used inappropriately, and a daily assessment of risks and benefits is wise. Central venous catheters, for example, allow for convenient blood draws and delivery of medications and parenteral nutrition, but they are also associated with infection, restricted mobility, deep venous thrombosis, and air embolism.

Special Hospital Populations

Intensive Care

Adults >65 years old account for 42%–52% of the intensive care unit (ICU) admissions and for almost 60% of total ICU days in the United States. Research is ongoing in an attempt to better understand which older patients are most likely to benefit from ICU care.

Respiratory failure is the most common reason for medical ICU admission and, because advanced age is associated with higher prevalence of chronic and acute pulmonary conditions, the number of older patients admitted to the ICU requiring mechanical ventilator support is rising. Patients with acute respiratory distress syndrome appear to have higher mortality with advancing age. Interestingly, in 3 separate studies of >1,500 patients, older patients recovered from their pulmonary physiologic abnormalities at a rate equal to that of their younger counterparts after acute lung injury; however, they required nearly twice as long to be successfully liberated from the ventilator and discharged from the ICU (SOE=A). Prolonged mechanical ventilation is likely an indicator not only of the severity of the initial illness that led to the respiratory failure but also of impairments in multiple organ systems.

Mortality in very old (>85 years) patients is 30%–70% for those with single organ failure and 80%–100% for those with multiple organ failure. Patients requiring renal replacement therapy have an extremely poor prognosis. Approximately 40% of older adults are alive 3 months after an ICU stay. Severe sepsis (defined as sepsis with acute organ dysfunction) increases the odds of developing cognitive deterioration and new ADL dependence in older survivors, and the deterioration in cognition and function after sepsis persists up to 8 years later.

ICUs provide care at end-of-life for a significant number of decedents; 1 in 5 Americans who die receive ICU services before death. Establishing goals of care in older critically ill patients is of paramount importance. In caring for critically ill patients, it may become apparent to the patient, family, and clinician that further intervention would not likely be of substantial benefit, depending on the individual patient's goals, values, and hopes. Many older patients with life-limiting illness are most concerned about maintaining function (as opposed to prolonging physiologic life) when weighing the burdens and potential outcomes of treatment options.

Defining *futility* is often difficult. The American Medical Association recommends a standardized "fair process" rather than a strict definition of futility. This approach consists of deliberation and negotiation between all parties, steps to secure alternatives in the setting of irreconcilable differences, and a final step of closure when all alternatives have been exhausted. As much as possible, clinicians should base futility decisions on factors such as clinical efficacy of treatment, likelihood of mortality, and subsequent quality-of-life considerations rather than on chronologic age alone. The limitation of life support before death is a common practice in ICUs, occurring in ~20% of ventilated older adults. The top 4 reasons for ventilator withdrawal are 1) clinicians' perception that the patient did not want life support, 2) clinicians' prediction that ICU survival was <10%, 3) clinicians' prediction that future cognitive

Table 18.3—Emergency Department Validated Risk-Screening Tools

Tool	Cut-off	Performance (Sensitivity, Specificity)	Outcomes Measured
Score Hospitalier d'Evaluation du Risque de Perte d'Autonomie (SHERPA)	≥3.5/11.5	85%, 45%	Functional decline, hospitalization, death at 3 months
Runciman test	≥2/8	86%, 38%	Emergency department readmission at 28 days
Rowland test	≥4/7	85%, 28%	Emergency department readmission at 14 days
Triage Risk Stratification Tool (TRST)	≥2/6	64%, 63%	Emergency department readmission and institutionalization at 30 days
Identification of Seniors at Risk (ISAR)	≥2/6	72%, 58%	Death, institutionalization, functional decline at 6 months

Data from: Graf CE, Zekry D, Giannelli S, et al. Efficiency and applicability of CGA in the ED: a systematic review. *Aging Clin Exp Res.* 2011;23:244–254.

function would be severely impaired, and 4) the ongoing need for an inotrope or vasopressor. Given the well-described difficulty of clinicians to accurately prognosticate beyond hours of impending death, important decisions regarding use of life-prolonging technology in older critically ill patients should be made with humility and must incorporate the patient's goals of care when known.

Emergency Department

The emergency department (ED) is an important treatment site for acute illness and injury in older adults and is frequently a path of entry to hospital care. Older adult patients made up 15% of all ED visits in the United States in 2009–2010. The annual average visit rate was 511 per 1,000 persons >65 years old and increased with age. Treatment of injury and unintentional falls accounts for 29% of ED encounters. About one-third of ED visits resulted in hospital admission, and the rate increased with age.

Older adults account for a disproportionate number of ED visits. They are more likely to be transported to the ED by ambulance and are 2.5–4.6 times more likely to be hospitalized. They use more staff time and resources because of longer ED stays and are more likely, when admitted, to require a critical care bed. ED diagnoses tend to be less accurate despite greater use of diagnostic tests and procedures.

After discharge from the ED, older adults are at greater risk of future hospitalization, repeat ED visits, functional decline, and mortality. In an analysis of 172,927 older adults discharged from Quebec EDs to the community, over the next 30 days, 1% died, 5% returned to the ED and were admitted, 16% returned to the ED but were not admitted, and 29% were prescribed a potentially inappropriate medication.

Although changes in functional capacity have been inconsistently defined, approximately 10%–45% of older adults decline in functional ability during the 3 months after an ED visit.

Commonly identified risk factors for adverse outcomes are baseline functional dependence, advanced age, recent hospitalization or ED visit, lack of social support, and living alone.

Impaired cognition is common in older adult ED patients and is a risk factor for poor outcomes. Of 297 ED patients >70 years old seen in an urban teaching hospital, 26% had evidence of mental status impairment, 16% had cognitive impairment without delirium, and 10% had delirium. A small minority of cases had any documentation by the physician of mental status impairment. This is concerning, because undetected delirium is associated with higher 6-month mortality compared with when there was no delirium or when delirium was detected.

Given the prevalence of geriatric syndromes in the ED and their association with poor outcomes, older adults, particularly the highest-risk patients, would benefit from comprehensive geriatric assessment (CGA) and targeted interventions in the ED. However, a survey of ED chief physicians and head nurses revealed that systematic screening, use of standardized cognitive and functional assessment tools, discharge planning protocol, geriatric staffing resource, and linkages with community providers were available in only a minority of EDs.

The rapid pace of the ED poses a barrier to systematic performance of CGA; therefore, simplified geriatric-specific screening tools have been developed to more efficiently identify at-risk individuals discharged from the ED. Five nurse-administered screening tools have been validated in the ED: Score Hospitalier d'Evaluation du Risque de Perte d'Autonomie (SHERPA), Runciman, Rowland, Triage Risk Stratification Tool (TRST), and Identification of Seniors at Risk (ISAR). For a summary of characteristics of screening tools, see Table 18.3.

Since 2008, geriatric EDs are increasingly being developed in hospitals across the United States, although no standard criteria currently define a geriatric ED. A survey of representatives of 24 existing and 6 planned geriatric EDs in 2013 revealed significant variation in the services offered, environmental modifications, and outcomes measured. Eighty percent served 5,000–20,000 older patients annually. The most frequently reported physical changes made were in beds, lighting, flooring, visual/hearing aids, corridor safety, and sound level. Selection of patients for treatment in the geriatric ED was based mostly on an age cutoff of 65 years and acuity of illness; only 17% used a risk screening tool for this purpose. Specialized training of geriatric ED staff was reported by 80% of respondents. Common protocols implemented addressed falls prevention (including gait assessment), medication evaluation, delirium management, and urinary catheter use. Frequently reported targeted interventions were coordination of community resource services (home aids, durable medical equipment), pharmacology review, discharge planning, communication with the primary care physician, and referral to clinical services (skilled-nursing facility, physical therapy, primary care providers, geriatric clinics). The most frequently measured outcomes were hospital admissions, patient satisfaction, hospital readmissions, and ED visits.

After ED discharge, CGA and targeted interventions delivered by an interprofessional team can improve important outcomes. For example, such interventions have been shown to reduce 30-day elective and emergency hospital admissions and 6-month functional decline.

MODELS OF CARE FOR OLDER HOSPITALIZED PATIENTS

Three systematic approaches have been demonstrated in controlled trials to improve hospital care of older adults. These approaches involve comprehensive multicomponent interventions, 2 of which were implemented on designated medical units.

Geriatric Evaluation and Management Units

Geriatric evaluation and management (GEM) units for older adults who have stabilized during an acute hospitalization were developed and pioneered in Veterans Affairs medical centers. These units incorporate CGA (including screening for geriatric syndromes, and assessment for and treatment of functional, cognitive, affective, and nutritional problems) with interprofessional team-based care. In a multicenter randomized trial, ADL function and physical performance improved for veterans assigned to GEM units relative to those who received usual hospital care (SOE=A). Some measures of health-related quality of life were also superior for patients treated on GEM units. These units did not affect mortality and were cost neutral after consideration of costs of both initial hospitalization and care after discharge.

Acute Care for Elders

Acute Care for Elders (ACE), adopted in many acute care hospitals, involves a system of care designed to help acutely ill older patients to maintain or achieve independence in ADLs and IADLs. ACE programs adopt a proactive, "prehabilitative" approach, comprising 4 components:

- A prepared environment to promote mobility and orientation (eg, carpeting, raised toilet seats, low beds, clocks, calendars, and pictures)

- Interprofessional, team-based, patient-centered care with nursing-initiated protocols for independent self-care, nutrition, sleep hygiene, skin care, mood, and cognition

- Early planning to go home, with social work intervention to mobilize family and other resources at home

- Medication review to promote optimal prescribing

This approach resulted in greater independence in ADLs at discharge, less frequent discharge to a nursing home, and somewhat shorter and less expensive hospitalization (SOE=A). In addition, ACE was associated with substantial differences in the satisfaction of patients, family members, physicians, and nurses but with only modest differences in ADL function (SOE=A). These findings demonstrate that ACE is a proven approach to improve outcomes and reduce hospital costs for acutely ill older general medical patients, but the effects of ACE on patient outcomes are likely sensitive to factors that depend on the function of the interprofessional team.

Hospital Elder Life Program

The Hospital Elder Life Program (HELP) involves a multicomponent intervention to prevent delirium in hospitalized older patients. The intervention consists of protocols to manage 6 risk factors for delirium: cognitive impairment, sleep deprivation, immobility, visual impairment, hearing impairment, and dehydration. Older patients receiving this intervention are not segregated on a special hospital ward or unit. The program makes extensive use of hospital volunteers. In one prospective controlled study, incidence of delirium was reduced by one-third, from 15.0% to 9.9% (SOE=A). Severity and duration of delirium episodes appeared not to be affected by HELP. The intervention was also associated with significantly improved cognitive function among patients with cognitive impairment at admission and with a reduced rate of use of sleep medications among all patients. A trend toward improvement was also seen in other risk factors, including immobility, visual impairment, and hearing impairment.

Surgical Co-Management

Increasingly, hospitalized surgical patients are being co-managed by surgeons and hospitalists or geriatricians. One of the more well-studied models in geriatrics is the co-management of hip fracture patients by orthopedic surgeons and geriatricians. Successful models have demonstrated reduced lengths of stay, complication, readmission, mortality rates, and cost. Key components of this model include standardized protocols and order sets, frequent communication between the surgeon and geriatrician, early discharge planning, and clear delineation of responsibilities.

Nurses Improving Care of Health System Elders (NICHE)

NICHE is a national program of the Hartford Institute for Geriatric Nursing at New York University College of Nursing, the goal of which is to improve the care of hospitalized older patients through change programs and nursing protocols.

The Geriatric Resource Nurse (GRN) Model is the foundation of the NICHE program and is based on the belief that primary nurses are most knowledgeable about the daily patterns and needs of the older adults in their units. After receiving specialized education in nursing care of older adults, the GRN receives ongoing mentorship and clinical support from an advanced practice nurse through clinical rounds and structured learning activities. GRNs serve as the unit's resource on geriatric best practices, engage in quality and research initiatives, and educate other staff regarding geriatric care.

Initially field tested in 4 hospital sites, NICHE has since grown into a national hospital network for sharing lessons and collaborating in development of inpatient geriatric nursing-care resources. After implementing the NICHE GRN model, hospitals have reported improved clinical outcomes, enhanced nurse knowledge and perceptions of quality, and increased compliance with protocol application. See www.nicheprogram.org for additional information.

ALTERNATIVES TO HOSPITAL CARE

It is often assumed that older adults would prefer to be treated for acute illness at home rather than in the hospital whenever possible. The safety and feasibility of this approach for some acutely ill older adults who would otherwise be hospitalized has been demonstrated. This approach, sometimes called the *home hospital*, requires intensive resources for medical and nursing care at home that are not yet widely available.

Older adults' preferences for care at home rather than in the hospital vary widely. In a study of community-dwelling older adults, virtually all preferred care in the site that would provide the higher probability of survival. When home care and hospital care provide equivalent probabilities of survival, roughly half preferred care in each site, with those preferring home care more likely to be white, better educated, living with a spouse, deeply religious, and dependent in ≥2 ADLs. The major difference perceived by older adults between home care and hospital care was feeling safer in the hospital than at home.

Studies suggest that hospital-at-home care can provide safe, economical, and efficacious care for some older adults with selected medical conditions, eg, heart failure, community-acquired pneumonia, cellulitis, COPD (SOE=A). Common features of the home-hospital models are the provision of care by an interprofessional team, availability of 24-hour coverage (including physician coverage), and a safe home environment. In one trial, patients with dementia in the intervention group had fewer problems with sleep, feeding, and aggression. Fewer patients were prescribed antipsychotics. There were no beneficial effects in functional ability. Patients receiving care in a home hospital were more satisfied with their care than those admitted to hospital.

HOSPITAL COMPARE

Hospital Compare is a CMS quality initiative that mandates reporting of hospital compliance with selected process measures and outcomes of patients treated for acute myocardial infarction (AMI), heart failure, or pneumonia. In April 2005, CMS began reporting hospital's performance on the Hospital Compare website. Publicly reported outcomes include risk-standardized 30-day mortality and, in 2013, risk-standardized unplanned readmission. Hospital Compare was designed to accomplish 2 goals: to guide patients who seek nonemergent care with relative performance among different hospitals and to spur hospital quality improvement. CMS aims to raise the performance level of as many hospitals as possible to the level set by the highest-performing hospitals.

Between 2004 and 2006, all process measures improved, particularly in baseline low-performing hospitals, whereas most high-performing hospitals maintained performance level. Concurrently, there were improvements in risk-adjusted outcomes only for AMI. Across all hospitals, a 10-point increase in performance was associated with declines in AMI-associated mortality rate of 0.6%, in length of stay of −0.19 days, and in readmission rate of 0.5%. Changes in outcomes for heart failure and pneumonia were smaller and less consistent. To date, the effect of reporting 30-day risk-adjusted mortality rates for pneumonia, heart failure, and AMI seems to have been negligible.

Health Compare started reporting hospital mortality performance in 2007, rating hospitals as better, worse, or no different than national average. Very few hospitals were rated as differing from average, which may have partly explained why this study found no evidence that patients shifted to higher-performing hospitals. Patient's access to higher-quality hospitals may also be constrained by other factors such as the distance to the nearest high-performing hospital, selective contracts between hospitals and insurers, and hospital crowding.

In sum, public reporting of process and outcome measures seems to be associated with significant improvement in process measures and minimal changes in mortality.

READMISSION

Readmission is costly and often considered to be a quality-of-care indicator. Although one-fifth of Medicare beneficiaries discharged from the hospital from 2003 to 2004 were readmitted within 30 days, rehospitalizations are only modestly related to age. There is significant geographic variability in readmission rates; the difference between the 5 states with the highest and lowest rates is 45%. The cost to Medicare of unplanned readmissions in 2004 U.S. dollars was estimated at $17.4 billion.

The U.S. Patient Protection and Affordable Care Act (ACA) has targeted several initiatives at reducing readmission rates. The common theme running through these strategies is incentivized coordination of care across transitions. Reducing readmissions is also a goal of public reporting through Hospital Compare. Since 2013, hospitals with high Risk-Standardized-Readmission Rates (RSRR) are penalized through reductions in Medicare reimbursement.

All-cause 30-day readmission rate between 2007 and 2011 remained stable at 19% but decreased to 18.4% in 2012, translating to 70,000 fewer readmissions. In 2009, CMS began reporting hospital-specific 30-day RSRR for 3 conditions: AMI, heart failure, and pneumonia. The RSRR trend for Medicare fee-for-service and older Veterans Affairs beneficiaries discharged with one of these diagnoses from July 2009 to June 2012 showed a decline of 9%–15%.

The diagnosis at readmission frequently differs from the index admission diagnosis. From 2007 to 2009, 30-day readmissions for the same condition of Medicare fee-for-service patients occurred in only 35% of heart failure, 10% of AMI, and 22% of pneumonia admissions. Two-thirds of readmissions occurred within 15 days of discharge. No association was identified between readmission diagnoses or timing of readmission and age, sex, or race.

CHOOSING WISELY® RECOMMENDATIONS

Eating and Feeding

- Do not recommend percutaneous feeding tubes in patients with advanced dementia; instead offer oral assisted feeding.

- Avoid using prescription appetite stimulants or high-calorie supplements to treat anorexia or cachexia in older adults; instead, optimize social supports, provide feeding assistance and clarify patient goals and expectations.

Delirium

- Avoid physical restraints to manage behavioral symptoms of hospitalized older adults with delirium.

- Do not use benzodiazepines or other sedative-hypnotics in older adults as first choice for insomnia, agitation, or delirium.

REFERENCES

- Chan PS, Nallamothu BK, Krumholz HM, et al. Long-term outcomes in elderly survivors of in-hospital cardiac arrest. *N Engl J Med*. 2013;368(11):1019–1026.

    Predictors of long-term survival of older survivors of in-hospital cardiac arrest were examined by identifying 6,972 patients ≥65 years old from the Get with the Guidelines® Resuscitation Registry and linking patient-level data with Medicare files. The patients were discharged from the hospital after an in-hospital cardiac arrest between 2000 and 2008; 58% were alive 1 year after discharge. The risk-adjusted 1-year survival rate was lower in older survivors (64% in the 65–74 year group compared with 50% in those ≥85 years old). The 1-year survival rate was also negatively correlated with severity of neurologic disability (73% in survivors who had minimal or no neurologic disability at discharge versus 10% in those who were discharged in a comatose state).

- Feldblum I, German L, Castel H, et al. Individualized nutritional intervention during and after hospitalization: the Nutrition Intervention Study Clinical Trial. *J Am Geriatr Soc*. 2011;59(1):10–17.

    In this study, 259 nutritionally at-risk older hospitalized patients were randomized to nutritional treatment in the hospital plus 3 home dietitian visits (intervention group), one in-hospital visit with the dietitian, or standard care (latter two were combined into the control group). At 6 months, 9.7% of the intervention group had serum albumin <3.5 g/dL versus 22.9% in the control group (*P*=.03), and mortality was lower in the intervention group, 3.8% versus 11.6% (*P*=.046).

- Graf CE, Zekry D, Giannelli S, et al. Efficiency and applicability of comprehensive geriatric assessment in the emergency department: a systematic review. *Aging Clin Exp Res.* 2011;23(4):244–254.

    This systematic review looked at the evidence for comprehensive geriatric assessment (CGA) in improving outcomes of older adults discharged from the emergency department, summarized the validation of 5 simplified screening tools for identifying high-risk older adults discharged from the emergency department and proposed a 2-step algorithm (identifying high-risk patients followed by CGA). Of 8 studies, 5 showed that CGA linked with geriatric interventions resulted in reduced functional decline. Of the 5 screening tools, only the triage risk screening tool and identification of seniors at risk (ISAR) had been studied in a 2-step approach. The authors recommended using ISAR at a cut-off of 2/6 as a better predictor of adverse outcomes.

- Kahn SR, Lim W, Dunn AS, et al. Prevention of VTE in nonsurgical patients: Antithrombotic Therapy and Prevention of Thrombosis, 9th ed: American College of Chest Physicians Evidence-Based Clinical Practice Guidelines. *Chest.* 2012;141(2 Suppl):e195S–226S.

    This guideline addresses the use of venous thromboembolism (VTE) prophylaxis in hospitalized medical patients, outpatients with cancer, immobilized adults, long-distance travelers, and those with asymptomatic thrombophilia. The authors provide recommendations on risk assessment for VTE and bleeding complications and suggest treatment for patients in different risk categories.

- Mehta KM, Pierluissi E, Boscardin J, et al. A clinical index to stratify hospitalized older adults according to risk for new-onset disability. *J Am Geriatr Soc.* 2011;59(7):1206–1216.

    A clinical tool for predicting new-onset disability at hospital discharge in previously independent patients >70 years old was developed and validated using data from 2 prospective studies. Seven independent risk factors known on admission were identified and weighted using logistic regression: age (80–89, 1 point; ≥90, 2 points), dependence in ≥3 IADLs at baseline (2 points), impaired mobility at baseline (unable to run, 1 point; unable to climb stairs, 2 points), dependence in ADLs at admission (2 or 3 ADLs, 1 point; 4 or 5 ADLs, 3 points), acute stroke or metastatic cancer (2 points), severe cognitive impairment (1 point), and albumin <3 g/dL (2 points). New-onset disability occurred in 6%, 13%, 18%, 34%, 35%, 45%, 50%, and 87% of participants with 0, 1, 2, 3, 4, 5, 6, and 7 or more points, respectively, in the derivation cohort. The risk score also predicted ($P<.001$) disability severity, nursing-home placement, and long-term survival.

Margarita Sotelo, MD
Edgar Pierluissi, MD

CHAPTER 19—TRANSITIONS OF CARE

KEY POINTS

- Older adults undergoing care transitions have increased risk of experiencing suboptimal care and adverse events.

- Clinicians play an important role in implementing effective solutions to improve care during transitions, which requires a team-based approach to coordinate care.

- Successful care transitions can result in more effective implementation of care plans, reduced adverse events, faster restoration of older adults' functioning, and improved satisfaction among patients, caregivers, and health care providers.

THE TREACHERY OF SUBOPTIMAL CARE TRANSITIONS

A care transition is defined as the movement of a patient from one set of providers, level of care, or health care setting to another. Other terms for care transitions include "handoffs," "handovers," or "transfers." Figure 19.1 depicts typical care transitions that older adults experience within the health care environment. Some transitions are *within* the hospital setting, such as the transition from the intensive care unit to the floor, while others are *across* health care settings, such as the transition from the hospital to a skilled-nursing facility. Although care transitions are generally well intended, eg, to provide a higher level of care for an older adult who is clinically deteriorating, care transitions are a time when older adults are vulnerable to receiving suboptimal or potentially unsafe care.

Care transitions are common, complicated, and costly. Almost 40% of older adults experience two or more care transitions within 30 days of hospital discharge. A national study of Medicare beneficiaries found that about 78% of older adults stay in place over the course of a year, while 22% experience care transitions of some kind. About half of these transitions involved a single hospitalization followed by return to the original residence, but the other half involved a complex sequence of other transitions. Few predominant transition patterns were apparent; most patterns were unique, which makes predicting (and accommodating) the traffic flow of patient transfers difficult. This has profound implications for organizations or individuals involved in care provision. The heterogeneity of transition patterns of older adults challenges approaches to improving care transitions, because it is onerous and inefficient to plan for all possible care patterns when many apply to a small number of individuals.

Suboptimal care transitions that result in hospital readmission can be costly. One in five older adults discharged from the hospital are rehospitalized within 30 days, and one in three are rehospitalized within 90 days. The cost of unplanned rehospitalizations to the Medicare program is estimated at $15 billion annually. Beyond their economic implications, suboptimal care transitions

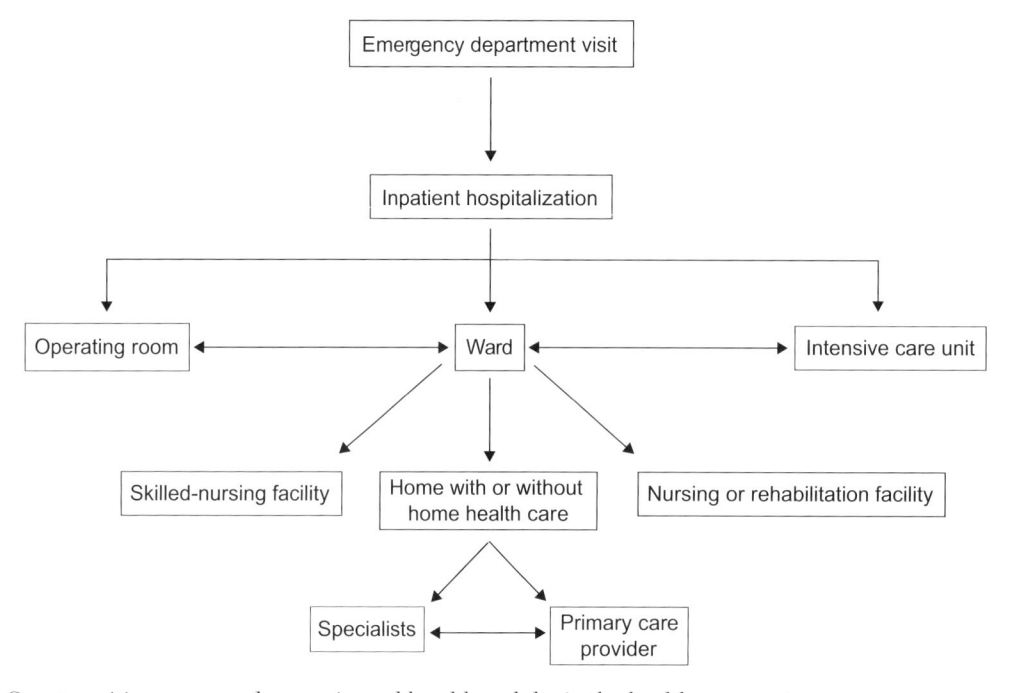

Figure 19.1—Care transitions commonly experienced by older adults in the health care environment

increase the risk of adverse events resulting from poor care coordination among providers and health care entities.

Suboptimal care transitions across care settings can pose a significant threat to patient safety. Common transitions-related hazards include medication errors, and inaccurate or incomplete information transfer. Indeed, almost half of all medication errors occur during admission or discharge, ie, care transitions to and from the acute hospital setting. Inaccurate or incomplete information is a common problem during care transitions with significant implications for patient safety, including delayed diagnosis, duplicative medical services, and reduced provider and patient satisfaction. Lack of availability of discharge summaries during follow-up clinician visits is common and can lead to duplicate testing and preventable hospital readmission.

Although suboptimal care transitions adversely affect patients of all ages, for several reasons, older adults are at particularly increased risk of safety problems. Age is a strong predictor of use of hospital services, and older adults have a 4-fold higher risk of hospitalization than the general population. Older adults also have higher rates of iatrogenic complications, greater frequency of admission through the emergency department, and longer lengths of stay than their younger counterparts. Further, older adults are more vulnerable to the hazards of hospitalization: functional decline, delirium, adverse drug events, pressure ulcers, bowel and bladder dysfunction, malnutrition, and dehydration. Because of these hazards, older adults are more likely to experience complications and therefore to require complex care after discharge. Older adults also have a greater prevalence of functional deficits and cognitive impairments at baseline, and some have limited health literacy; these can further challenge their ability to participate in the care-transitions process and to understand discharge and self-care instructions. The following are important patient- and system-level risk factors for experiencing a suboptimal care transition:

Patient-Level Risk Factors

- Limited education (less than high school)
- Unmet functional need (no help with at least one deficit in an activity of daily living)
- Limited self-management ability, eg, identifying when medical care is needed
- Worse self-rating of health
- Living alone
- Transition to home with home-care services
- Prior hospitalization
- Long hospital length of stay
- Low income or Medicaid eligible, including homelessness
- Older age
- Five or more comorbidities
- Specific diagnoses: depression, heart disease, diabetes mellitus, cancer, substance abuse

System-Level Risk Factors

- Communities with high hospital admission rate
- Lack of discharge education
- Insufficient communication across care settings
- Failure in implementation of plan of care (durable medical equipment, home health care, follow-up appointments, medications, tests)

BARRIERS TO SAFE TRANSITIONS

Improving care transitions for older adults, especially between hospital and home, is an attractive target for improving health care quality and reducing medical and liability expenditures. Older adults are among the highest users of health care services and account for the largest amount of government health spending. Interventions to improve care transitions are a high priority under the Affordable Care Act of 2010, which attempts to realign financial incentives to improve care transitions and reduce hospital readmission rates. Care transitions programs are now expected to be implemented in many health care systems. In addition, there are medicolegal liability concerns related to suboptimal care transitions. Hospital medicine and primary care physicians share the risk of liability during care transitions. Hospital medicine physicians have a duty to the patient upon discharge to assure care until the care transition is complete, including follow-up of pending tests, incidental findings, and medical treatments started in the hospital. The primary care provider has a duty to the patient to obtain hospital records if not received and ensure proper follow-up once the care transition is complete.

Several barriers exist to executing safe care transitions. Common ones include the following:

- Diverse older adult and caregiver transitional care needs depending on illness, social situation, and type of transition
- Lack of provider education and feedback on execution of care transitions, including preparation of timely and effective discharge summaries and understanding the capabilities of different types of postacute care settings

- Difficulty communicating with colleagues at the previous or next site of care
- Lack of time or financial resources (Transitional care activities that involve care coordination are largely not billable in the current American reimbursement system.)

STRATEGIES TO IMPROVE TRANSITIONAL CARE, AND OUTCOMES OF SPECIFIC CARE MODELS

Transitional care entails a broad range of time-limited services designed to ensure the coordination and continuity of health care as patients transfer between different locations or different levels of care. Transitional care contains elements of care coordination, discharge planning, and disease or case management. Many successful interventions designed to improve transitional care share common features, such as assigning a care transitions coach, guide, or navigator to monitor the older adult during care transitions. Cost-effective transitional care is focused on the highly vulnerable and chronically ill population and includes the following components:

- Accurate and timely transfer of information to the next set of providers
- Empowerment of the older adult to assert his or her own preferences
- Comprehensive assessments of older adult and caregiver needs
- Comprehensive medication review and management
- Logistical arrangements related to executing the care transition
- Education to prepare both older adults and caregivers for what to expect at the next site of care
- Support for self-management of medical conditions
- Coordination among medical and community resources
- Follow up and support after discharge

Targeted interventions, both before and after discharge—including home-health services, older adult and caregiver empowerment, and comprehensive discharge planning—may improve transitional care and avert early readmission and other adverse outcomes. For example, although it is labor-intensive, meticulous discharge planning can maximize the probability that older adults maintain the clinical and functional benefits achieved by hospitalization, as well as reduce the risk of early readmission and use of emergency services. Discharge planning ideally begins at hospital admission, with a projection of medical, nursing, rehabilitative, and functional support required by the older adult at the time of discharge.

Specific Care Models to Improve Transitional Care

Transitions from Hospital to Home

Transitions-of-care programs for home care after hospitalization using directed discharge planning and follow-up protocols have shown promise in reducing early repeat hospitalizations. The Care Transitions Intervention is a patient-centered self-management program coordinated by a health coach that has reduced repeat hospitalizations. The Re-Engineered Discharge (RED) intervention, in which a nurse discharge advocate and a clinical pharmacist work together to coordinate hospital discharge, educate patients, and reconcile medication, was found to decrease emergency department and hospital utilization within 30 days of discharge. The Transitional Care Model uses an advanced-practice nurse to assist with the transition of frail and complex older adults; this model was found to reduce readmissions, lengthen the time between discharge and readmission, and decrease the costs of providing health care.

One systematic review evaluating the effectiveness of hospital-initiated care transition strategies found that a "bridging" strategy, incorporating pre- and post-discharge interventions with a dedicated transitions provider, reduced readmission or emergency department visit rates. There was insufficient evidence to reach conclusions on the effectiveness of specific strategies that were components of these interventions. Another systematic review assessing the efficacy of transitional care interventions to reduce readmission and mortality for adults hospitalized with heart failure found home-visiting programs and multidisciplinary heart failure clinics reduced all-cause readmission and mortality. Structured telephone support interventions were also found to reduce heart failure–specific mortality but not all-cause readmissions.

Other Transitions

Some models exist for transitions other than hospital to home. Guided Care is an outpatient-based interprofessional team model of care led by a specially trained registered nurse in partnership with primary care providers and caregivers to support a practice's most complex patients. A major goal of the program is to refine transitions between sites of care. It also operates by assessing the patient and primary caregiver at home, creating an evidence-based care plan for providers and an action plan for patients and caregivers, promoting patient self-management, monthly monitoring of patients' conditions, coordinating efforts of care providers in all settings, educating and supporting family caregivers, and facilitating access to community resources. Guided Care patients tended to use less home health services, but there was no difference in hospital, emergency department, and skilled-nursing facility services or 30-day readmission rates compared with usual care patients.

The Interventions to Reduce Acute Care Transfers (INTERACT) model is a nursing home quality improvement intervention providing tools and strategies to assist nursing home staff in the early identification, assessment, and communication regarding changes in resident status. The improved communication and hand-offs between hospital and nursing home appears to prevent avoidable rehospitalizations. The Discharge of Elderly from the Emergency Department (DEED) program uses comprehensive geriatric assessment (CGA) performed by a nurse for patients ≥75 years old who are discharged from the emergency department (ED) to home. Based on the CGA findings, an interprofessional team develops a care plan, in coordination with the patient, caregivers, primary care providers, and community resources, and follows the patient for 4 weeks, including home visits. In a randomized controlled trial, the DEED II study demonstrated a significantly reduced rate of hospitalization within the first 30 days and reduced rate of ED admission for 18 months after the index ED visit. Intervention patients also experienced a significantly longer time to the first repeat ED visit.

Table 19.1 provides a brief summary of selected interventions, with their key components and demonstrated outcomes.

Policy Approaches

The common themes from transitional care models are the basis of many of the new models of care encouraged by the CMS. Increased emphasis is placed on patient-specific goals, quality, safety, and the avoidance of cost shifting to other components of the health care system. Given the high risk of problems during care transitions, the Federal government has implemented programs to improve care transitions nationally. The Community-based Care Transitions Program (CCTP) was created by Section 3026 of the Affordable Care Act and was launched in 2011. Designed to allow for testing of care models, the goals of the CCTP are to improve transitions of Medicare beneficiaries from the inpatient hospital setting to other care settings, to improve quality of care, to reduce readmissions for high-risk beneficiaries, and to document measurable savings to the Medicare program. Results from early implementation of the CCTP in intervention communities found that, compared with those in uninvolved communities, all-cause 30-day rehospitalization and all-cause hospitalization declined.

In addition to the CCTP, CMS also announced new payment codes in 2013 that incentivize ambulatory care providers to participate in transitional care management. Providers can bill under these codes for transitional care management services they perform to assist with transitions of care in the first 30 days of discharge from an inpatient hospital setting.

DISCHARGE DESTINATIONS AND CARE VENUES

The choice of discharge destination reflects a match between the needs of a given older adult and the services available at each setting. The array of possible settings includes home with family support, home with home-health care, custodial care (such as assisted living or "nursing home"), skilled-nursing facilities, acute rehabilitation hospitals, long-term acute care, and inpatient hospice. Home-health care works well for older adults requiring only intermittent skilled services (nursing, physical therapy, or speech therapy), and older adults with one of these needs may also receive assistance (under Medicare) from occupational therapy, medical social work, or home-health aides. Medicare requires that older adults receiving home-health care be homebound. Under Medicare, older adults appropriate for skilled-nursing facilities must also have a need for a skilled service, such as a requirement for intravenous therapy, artificial nutrition and hydration, complex wound care, ostomy care, or rehabilitation. Medicare covers all or part of skilled-nursing care for up to 100 days after a qualifying hospital stay, but coverage stops earlier if an older adult's treatment goals are met or if the older adult "plateaus" and no longer demonstrates improvement. Older adults with substantial rehabilitation needs (more than just physical therapy, occupational therapy, or speech therapy) and considerable rehabilitation potential may be appropriate for transfer to an acute rehabilitation unit, but many older adults are deemed ineligible because of an inability to participate in 3 hours per day of intense therapy. Long-term acute care, also known as "chronic hospitalization," is appropriate for the rare hospital patient who requires prolonged, hospital-level care. Long-term acute care facilities provide care for patients requiring long-term mechanical ventilation, multiple intravenous medications, parenteral nutrition, or complex wound care, along with a need for frequent clinician monitoring.

THE DISCHARGE MEDICATION REGIMEN

A critical activity near the time of hospital discharge is the preparation of the discharge medication list. This list should include an indication for each medication, stop dates (eg, for antibiotics) or tapering schedules (eg, for systemic corticosteroids) as appropriate, and clear behavioral triggers for as-needed psychiatric medications. Medications added during the hospital stay (such as analgesics, proton-pump inhibitors, or laxatives with as-needed orders) can be tapered and discontinued at this time. Finally, the discharge regimen should be formally reconciled with the preadmission regimen. Reconciliation results in clear documentation of which medications on the discharge list are new (relative to the preadmission regimen), which of the preadmission medications have been stopped, and which dosages of continued medications have been changed.

COMMUNICATING WITH PATIENT, CAREGIVERS, AND RECEIVING TEAM

The following items should be communicated to older adults (or their caregivers) who are being discharged directly home: follow-up appointments, warning symptoms or signs to watch for with instructions on whom to contact, clinical disciplines (eg, nursing, physical therapy) contracted for provision of services in the home, and the reconciled medication list. Older adults being discharged to other care venues should be oriented with respect to the nature of the new institution, the identity of a new attending physician (if known), and the expected frequency of provider visits. Tools are available to assist older adults and caregivers with assessing care preferences, clarifying discharge instructions, reconciling medication inaccuracies, and facilitating communication across care sites at discharge (eg, see www.caretransitions.org [accessed Jan 2016]). If the provider at the receiving institution differs from the hospital clinician, then clear and prompt communication is essential. Some items of information (such as critical but pending study results, nuances of goals of care, or family dynamics) call for direct communication between sending and receiving clinicians. Otherwise, a brief and prompt discharge summary containing the following will suffice: summary of hospital course with care provided and results of important tests; a list of problems and diagnoses; baseline physical functional status; baseline cognitive status; physical and cognitive status at discharge; reconciled medication list; allergies; tests results still outstanding; follow-up appointments; and information related to goals, preferences, and advance directives.

THREE STEPS TO IMPROVE CARE TRANSITIONS

Creating a strategy to improve care transitions consists of three essential steps. The first step is setting expectations for both the sending and receiving provider teams. The National Transitions of Care Coalition recommends shifting from the concept of "discharge" to that of "transfer with continuous management." The following are some questions to assist the transferring team with completing this step:

- Starting with the information available on the day of admission, what needs will this older adult have after transfer?
- What are the older adult's and caregiver's preferences about the transfer plan?
- How will this older adult care for himself or herself after transfer?
- What other clinicians need to evaluate the older adult to formulate an effective care plan?
- Once the transfer plan is set, do the older adult and caregiver understand the purpose of the transfer and what to expect at the next site of care?
- Has the next site of care received, understood, and clarified discrepancies about the care plan?

The second step to creating a strategy to improve care transitions involves tailoring communication strategies to the type of information being communicated and to the type of care transition. Written communication (electronic or paper) is best for information that must be a part of the medical record or used as a reference by the older adult, caregiver, or clinical provider. Written communication can be used for information transfer of discharge summaries, notification of patient admission or discharge, and other nonurgent issues. Verbal communication (phone or in person) is best for situations of urgency or uncertainty, new diagnoses of serious illnesses, difficult social situations, and when preparing patients for their next care transition. Communication strategies vary based on specific resources and institutional arrangements. The following are some questions to assist with completing this step:

- Based on this older adult's current episode of illness, what is the most relevant information to communicate to the next site of care?
- How quickly does this information need to be communicated?
- What is the best form of communication for this situation?
- Does the information also need to be given directly to the older adult and caregiver?

Table 19.1—Care Transitions: Major Interventions, Key Components, and Outcomes

Intervention	Goal of Intervention	Key Components			Demonstrated Outcome Improvements
		Pre-discharge intervention	Post-discharge intervention	Interventions bridging the transition	
Care Transitions Intervention (www.caretransitions.org/)	Minimize rehospitalization of older patients with complex care needs	N/A	Follow-up telephone call Home visit	Transition coach Patient-centered discharge instructions	Reduction in readmissions Improvement in care transition quality score
Re-Engineered Discharge ("Project RED") (www.bu.edu/fammed/projectred/)	Minimize rehospitalization of diverse inpatient populations	Patient education Discharge planning Medication reconciliation	Timely communication with primary care provider Follow-up telephone call	Patient-centered discharge instructions	Reduction in ED and hospital utilization within 30 days
Transitional Care Model (www.transitionalcare.info/)	Minimize rehospitalization of older patients with complex care needs	Patient education Discharge planning	Follow-up telephone call Post-discharge hotline	Transition coach Patient-centered discharge instructions	Reduced readmissions, increased time between discharge and readmission, decreased cost of providing health care
Better Outcomes by Optimizing Safe Transitions (BOOST) (www.hospitalmedicine.org/Web/Quality_Innovation/Implementation_Toolkits/Project_BOOST/Web/Quality_Innovation/Implementation_Toolkit/Boost/Overview.aspx)	Minimize rehospitalization of patients at high risk of readmission	Approach not stated; rather, each site receives a mentor to develop its own strategies based on local needs assessment and existing best practices			Reduction in 30 day readmission
Guided Care (www.guidedcare.org/)	Managing complex older adults in ambulatory care or home care, and through transitions	Patient education Discharge planning Medication reconciliation	Timely communication with primary care provider Timely clinic follow-up Follow-up telephone call Post-discharge hotline Home visit	Transition coach Patient-centered discharge instructions Provider continuity	Tended to use less home health services Reduced costly health care utilization in integrated health care systems
Interventions to Reduce Acute Care Transfers (INTERACT) (http://interact2.net/)	Minimize rehospitalization of nursing-home residents	Not applicable	Timely staff communication of change in clinical status Evidence-based clinical care pathways triggered by changes in clinical status Advance care planning		Reduction in readmissions
Discharge of Elderly from the Emergency Department (DEED) (www.ncbi.nlm.nih.gov/pubmed/10408663)	Reducing risk of older adults' return to the ED	Comprehensive geriatric assessment	Timely communication with primary care provider Home visit Formulation of care plan by interprofessional team Transition patient to use community services		Reduced rate of hospitalization within the first 30 days Reduced rate of ED admission for 18-months after index ED visit Longer time to the first repeat ED visit Maintained greater degree of physical and mental function
Geriatric Resources for Assessment and Care of Elders (GRACE) (http://graceteamcare.indiana.edu/case-for-grace.html)	Reducing ED visits, hospital admissions, and nursing-home admissions for frail older adults with complex needs	Not applicable	Home-based care management by nurse practitioner and social worker Collaborations with primary care provider and geriatric interprofessional team Care protocols for geriatric conditions		Improved patient-centered care transitions, reduced hospital readmissions and nursing-home placement

NOTE: ED=emergency department; above websites accessed Jan 2016.

The third step to creating a strategy to improve care transitions focuses on specific processes or outcomes as targets for improvement, using established quality improvement methods. It is important to begin by choosing one or two measures to focus on to track progress, and then expand further once initial goals are achieved. Examples of measures that can be targets for improvement include the following:

- Communication with primary care provider before older adult's transfer
- Medication reconciliation at the time of transfer
- Older adults, caregiver's, or receiving clinician's satisfaction with quality of care transition
- Timeliness of arrival of transfer summaries
- Inclusion of various components in transfer summaries, eg, documentation of cognitive and functional status
- Ease of scheduling of follow-up appointments
- Frequency of health care usage after transfer
- Table 19.1 gives examples of practical strategies drawn from the literature to consider for specific transitional care challenges.

REFERENCES

- Brock J, Mitchell J, Irby K, et al. Association between quality improvement for care transitions in communities and rehospitalizations among Medicare beneficiaries. *JAMA*. 2013;309(4):381–391.

    This paper describes the results of a quality improvement project designed by CMS to determine whether implementation of improved care transitions processes would reduce rehospitalizations in defined geographic communities. Medicare Quality Improvement Organizations facilitated evidence-based improvement activities by community organizing, providing technical assistance, and monitoring of participation, implementation processes, and outcomes. All-cause 30-day rehospitalization rates declined among Medicare fee-for-service intervention beneficiaries, compared to those in uninvolved communities.

- Feltner C, Jones C, Cene C, et al. Transitional care interventions to prevent readmissions for persons with heart failure. *Ann Intern Med*. 2014;160(11):774–784.

    This systematic review sought to assess the efficacy, comparative effectiveness, and harms of transitional care interventions to reduce readmission and mortality rates for adults hospitalized with heart failure. The investigators found home-visiting programs and multidisciplinary heart failure clinics reduced all-cause readmission and mortality; structured telephone support reduced heart failure–specific readmission and mortality.

- Hansen LO, Young RS, Hinami K, et al. Interventions to reduce 30-day rehospitalization: a systematic review. *Ann Intern Med*. 2011;155(8):520–528.

    In this systematic review, the authors describe interventions and outcomes in studies designed to reduce rates of rehospitalization within 30 days of discharge. They developed a taxonomy in which interventions were categorized into three domains: predischarge interventions (eg, patient education and medication reconciliation), postdischarge interventions (eg, follow-up telephone calls or home visits), and bridging interventions (eg, transition coaches, physician continuity across venues). Observational designs predominated in the included studies, and significant heterogeneity precluded a meta-analytic approach. A discrete intervention or discharge bundle that reliably reduced rehospitalization rates was not identified.

- Jencks SF, Williams MV, Coleman EA. Rehospitalizations among patients in the Medicare fee-for-service program. *N Engl J Med*. 2009;360(14):1418–1428.

    A landmark article provides a review of rehospitalizations in the Medicare population. Medicare claims data were analyzed to describe patterns of rehospitalizations and the relation of rehospitalization to demographic characteristics. Almost one-fifth of almost 12 million Medicare beneficiaries who had been discharged from a hospital were rehospitalized within 30 days, and 34% were rehospitalized within 90 days. For half of the patients who were rehospitalized within 30 days after a medical discharge to the community, there was no bill for a visit to a physician's office between the time of discharge and rehospitalization. The cost to Medicare of unplanned rehospitalizations in 2004 was $17.4 billion.

- National Transitions of Care Coalition (www.ntocc.org)

    This website is a rich resource that contains a compendium of literature about care transitions and includes downloadable practical tools for health care educators, health care providers, caregivers, and older adults to safely manage care transitions.

- Naylor MD, Aiken LH, Kurtzman ET, et al. The care plan: the importance of transitional care in achieving health reform. *Health Aff (Millwood)*. 2011;30(4):746–754.

    In this systematic review of 21 randomized clinical trials of transitional care interventions targeting chronically ill adults, researchers identified 9 interventions that demonstrated positive effects on measures related to hospital readmissions. Most of the interventions led to reductions in readmissions through at least 30 days after discharge. Many of the successful interventions shared similar features, such as assigning a nurse as the clinical manager or leader of care and including in-person home visits to discharged patients. Several strategies are recommended to guide the implementation of transitional care under health care reform.

- Rennke S, Nguyen OK, Shoeb MH, et al. Hospital-initiated transitional care interventions as a patient safety strategy: a systematic review. *Ann Intern Med*. 2013;158:433–440.

    This systematic review addressed the effectiveness of hospital-initiated care transition strategies aimed at preventing clinical adverse events, emergency department visits, and readmissions after discharge in general medical patients. The study found a "bridging" strategy (incorporating both predischarge and postdischarge interventions) with a dedicated transition provider reduced readmission or emergency department visit rates in 10 studies, but the overall strength of evidence for this strategy was low. Because of scant evidence, no conclusions could be reached on methods to prevent postdischarge adverse events. Most studies did not report intervention context, implementation, or cost. The authors concluded that strategies hospitals should implement to improve patient safety at hospital discharge remain unclear.

Alicia I. Arbaje, MD, MPH

CHAPTER 20—REHABILITATION

KEY POINTS

- The World Health Organization conceptual model of functioning and disability provides a useful framework for geriatric rehabilitation by taking into account the complex interactions of body functions and structures, health conditions, individual activities and participation in life situations, and environmental and personal factors.

- As rehabilitation treatments require active patient participation and long-term self-management, the patient and family are core members of the rehabilitation team.

- Factors that influence recovery after a hip fracture include prior mobility and functional status, comorbid conditions, cognitive status, and social support.

- Optimal rehabilitation outcomes depend on comprehensive assessment of the patient, coordinated interprofessional team management, multifaceted interventions, and access to appropriate and high-quality care.

Rehabilitation is a critical component of geriatric health care because of the high incidence of disabling conditions in the older adult population. Although these conditions drastically influence quality of life, they often improve with treatment. Chronic disease almost always underlies disability in older adults; for example, stroke occurs most often in people with other vascular diseases, and hip fractures occur most often in people with osteoporosis and gait disorders. Disability also worsens in progressive chronic diseases (eg, osteoarthritis, Parkinson disease, or amyotrophic lateral sclerosis) or in the context of deconditioning from inactivity during acute illness. To provide the best functional recovery possible, those providing geriatric rehabilitation must do the following:

- Use systematic approaches to assess the causes of disability
- Be familiar with the advantages and disadvantages of all potential sites of care
- Understand the role of interprofessional teams and care plans
- Adapt care to comorbidities and disabilities
- Be familiar with the basic requirements for rehabilitation of common geriatric conditions

CONCEPTUAL MODEL FOR GERIATRIC REHABILITATION

Geriatric rehabilitation services can be organized around a conceptual model of disability for assessing the status and needs of the patient, matching treatments with specific conditions, and evaluating rehabilitation outcomes. The World Health Organization (WHO) *International Classification of Functioning, Disability, and Health* (ICF) provides a useful framework for measuring health and disability. For an ICF guide and a discussion of the ICF model of disability, see the WHO website (www.who.int/classifications/icf/en/ [accessed Jan 2016]). The ICF has two main domains: "health conditions" and "contextual factors." Disability and functioning are viewed as outcomes of interactions between health conditions (diseases, disorders, injuries) and contextual factors, which includes both environmental and personal. Environmental factors range from a person's most immediate environment, like furniture in the room, to the more general environment, such as access to public transportation. Personal factors include a person's age, race, gender, educational background, personality, fitness, and lifestyle.

In the WHO model, interventions can be designed to modify a person's impairments, limitations in activities, and restrictions in participation. For example, a treatment plan can be developed to improve a person's muscle strength (impairment level), but the significance of this intervention is a result of its effect on his or her physical mobility (activity) and ultimately his or her ability to return to social or physical roles (participation). The effects of gains in strength and physical mobility on participation can be modified by the person's motivation or social support. For example, if patients improve in strength and balance but their family and friends continue to "do everything for them" and do not encourage independent function, they may remain dependent. The physical environment is another powerful modifier. Even the person who achieves improved function cannot return to prior work or household roles if physical barriers to access in the community are not removed or adapted by means such as ramps or modified bathrooms. In summary, the interaction of disease and disability is particularly complex in older adults; the ICF model is useful for structuring their comprehensive rehabilitation care.

SITES OF REHABILITATION CARE

Rehabilitation services are available through Medicare Part A on a time-limited basis. These services are

Table 20.1—Rehabilitation Sites of Care and Level of Care Requirements

Rehabilitation Sites	Level of Care Requirements	Expected Intensity of Services	Payment Source
Inpatient			
Freestanding rehabilitation hospital or rehabilitation unit attached to acute hospital	24-hour availability of a physician with training or experience in rehabilitation 24-hour nursing care Relatively intense level of rehabilitation services Interprofessional team to deliver coordinated program of care as evidenced by team conferences at least every 2 weeks Reasonable expectation of improvement	An interprofessional team approach is required and in most cases, this calls for 3 hours of therapy 5 days/week of at least two therapies; this can include physical, occupational, or speech therapy in any combination.	Medicare Part A Days 1–60: full coverage Days 61–90: partial coverage but daily co-payment >90 days: daily co-payment for up to 60 lifetime reserve days More than lifetime reserve days: no coverage
Medicare skilled-nursing facility	Physician supervision, with access 24 hours/day on emergency basis 24-hour nursing care Less intense therapy needs Interprofessional team coordination ideally will occur Maintenance of function without progress can be goal of care	Daily therapy (5 days/week) 1 hour/day or more, as tolerated by patient; ADL assistance and/or skilled-nursing care	Medicare Part A Days 1–20: full coverage Days 21–100: partial coverage but per day co-payment >100 days: no coverage
Outpatient			
Home health	Face-to-face physician visit within 90 days to establish need and order; physician certifies need every 60 days Skilled need required for homebound patient, including either intermittent skilled nursing, physical, occupational, or speech therapy	Intermittent nursing or therapy provided in home; can be no more than 7 days/week or 8 hours/day; patient must have support system to meet needs of living at home	Medicare Part A
Clinic (hospital-based or independent)	Physician orders Skilled need required; rehabilitation services to include physical, occupational, or speech therapy and reviews plan periodically	Intermittent physical, occupational, or speech therapy provided; patient must be able to get to therapy visits	Medicare Part B There are annual caps on coverage, but these can be waived if medically necessary.

SOURCE: www.cms.hhs.gov (accessed Jan 2016)

offered in both inpatient and community-based sites. Inpatient care may be provided in rehabilitation centers (freestanding hospitals or units attached to acute hospitals) or nursing facilities (Medicare skilled-nursing facilities). To receive Medicare coverage for an inpatient rehabilitation stay in either type of facility, a patient must have a hospital stay of at least 3 consecutive midnights for a related illness or injury. Typically reimbursed through Medicare Part B, outpatient rehabilitation services can be provided in hospital-based or independent clinics, in day hospital settings, or in the home. The patient's eligibility, the particular services provided, and costs vary across sites of care. The balance of advantages and disadvantages for the individual patient is an important factor for the clinician to consider in recommending a site for rehabilitation care. For a summary of the sites of rehabilitation, Medicare requirements and payment sources, and the expected intensity of the rehabilitation services, see Table 20.1.

Sites of Care: Coverage and Services

Medicare Part A covers intensive inpatient rehabilitation for patients who have complex needs requiring an interprofessional team approach, including multiple therapies. In most cases, this calls for a minimum of 3 hours of rehabilitation therapy services per day at least 5 days per week or 15 hours per week. Potential patients undergo a preadmission screen to evaluate their condition, need for services, and determine prior level of function. A Medicare-certified inpatient rehabilitation hospital program must demonstrate that at least a certain percentage of patients have at least 1 of 13 conditions: stroke, spinal cord injury, congenital deformity, amputation, major multiple trauma, hip fracture, brain injury, neurologic disorders (eg, multiple sclerosis, Parkinson disease), burns, three arthritis conditions for which appropriate aggressive and sustained outpatient therapy has failed, joint replacement for both knees or hips when the surgery immediately precedes admission, a BMI >50 kg/m², or age >85 years. Patients must have close medical supervision by a physician with specialized training or experience in rehabilitation, have 24-hour rehabilitation nursing care, and be managed by an interprofessional team of skilled nurses and therapists. Medicare prospective reimbursement is now based on case-mix groups using the Functional Independence Measure (Table 20.2).

The Medicare-approved skilled-nursing facility must provide 24-hour nursing care. Dietary, pharmaceutical, dental, and medical social services are also available. Physicians must supervise patient care and can visit the patient infrequently, but they must be available 24 hours per day on an emergency basis. Therapy services are available, and ideally interprofessional coordination will occur. In this setting, maintenance of function without progress may be the goal of care. A recent legal decision (Jimmo v. Sebelius, 2013) clarifies that the skilled services may include those interventions to prevent or slow further deterioration.

Medicare provides home-health benefits to patients who require nursing care or therapy services on an intermittent or part-time basis, defined as <7 days per week or <8 hours per day for all required services. Patients must also be homebound, defined as either not recommended based on a medical condition or requiring considerable effort to leave home. Patients can leave home for medical treatments or for short, infrequent nonmedical reasons, including attendance at religious services. Home-health services must be prescribed and recertified every 60 days by a physician. Initial certification for home health requires a documented face-to-face visit by the physician, or nonphysician practitioner within 90 days before the start of home-health care or within 30 days after the start of care. There is no prior hospitalization requirement or limit on the number of visits a person may receive. Medicare provides care in 60-day episodes. Home-health services provide skilled nursing and home-health aides, therapy services, medical social services, and supplies. Provision of part-time or intermittent home-health aide services require concomitant skilled-nursing or therapy visits.

The escalating expenditures for Medicare's post-acute care benefits from $2.5 billion in 1986 to more than $30 billion in 1996 led to the Balanced Budget Act (BBA) of 1997, which mandated prospective payment systems rather than fee-for-service reimbursement. In skilled-nursing facilities, the BBA mandated the implementation of a per diem prospective payment system covering all costs (routine, ancillary, and capital) related to the services provided to patients under Part A of the Medicare program. Per diem payments for each admission are case-mix adjusted by use of a resident classification system (RUG IV) that is based on data from patient assessments (the Minimum Data Set 3.0) and relative weights developed from staff time data. Home-health care reimbursement is also under a prospective payment system. Payment rates are based on relevant data from patient assessments conducted by clinicians using the Outcome and Assessment Information Set (OASIS). The OASIS was originally developed to assess quality of care outcomes in home health. The OASIS is lengthy, encompassing sociodemographic, environmental, support system, health status, and functional status attributes; it is required for reimbursement by Medicare for home-health services. For each 60-day episode of care, national payment rates vary, depending on the intensity of care required. Home-health agencies receive less than the full 60-day episode rate if they provide only a minimal number of visits (<4) to beneficiaries.

Less intensive rehabilitation services, including physical, occupational, and speech therapies, are available through independent and hospital-based clinics. To assist in Medicare reform, new legislation now requires a claims-based system to collect data on the provision of outpatient therapy services to Medicare B beneficiaries. Functional information on the beneficiary is reported using non-payable G-codes and complexity/severity modifiers. The functional data on mobility, self-care, and cognition must be collected using an outcomes assessment such as the Activity Measure for Post Acute Care (Table 20.2).

Sites of Care and Outcomes

The effect of site of care on rehabilitation outcomes is not well established. A study of outcomes among patients with stroke and hip fracture examined rates of discharge to home and recovery of function that were based on use of inpatient or nursing rehabilitation services. When controlling for case-mix differences, the researchers found that stroke but not hip fracture patients were more likely to be discharged home and to recover activities of daily living (ADLs) if treated in an inpatient rehabilitation setting (SOE=B). In another cohort study, patients admitted for hip fracture to inpatient facilities had better 12-week functional outcomes than did patients undergoing rehabilitation at skilled-nursing facilities (SOE=B). This type of observational study is vulnerable to bias, despite adjusting the analyses, because the prognosis for recovery may influence discharge site; patients with a poor prognosis are more likely to go to the nursing home, whereas those with a better prognosis go to inpatient or home-health settings. Nevertheless, site of care may be an important factor in recovery.

Each site of care has advantages and disadvantages from the patient's perspective. Inpatient care is the most intense but may not be endurable for frail older patients, because it usually requires 3 hours per day of active (and fatiguing) therapy. Skilled nursing offers

Table 20.2—Functional Status and Disease-Specific Assessment Instruments

Instrument	Purpose/Description
Functional Independence Measure (FIM) (www.rehabmeasures.org/Lists/RehabMeasures/DispForm.aspx?ID=889)	■ Measures assistance required for self-care, transfers, locomotion, sphincter control, social cognition, and communication. ■ An 18-item ordinal scale with scores ranging from 0 (total assist) to 7 (complete independence); the possible total score ranges from 18 (the lowest) to 126 (highest), obtained by adding points for each item.
Barthel ADL Index (www.rehabmeasures.org/Lists/RehabMeasures/DispForm.aspx?ID=916)	■ Used to establish degree of independence with regard to ADLs. ■ A 10-item ordinal scale; scores vary depending on the item in question. Bathing and grooming are scored either 0 (dependent/needs help) or 5 (independent); scores for feeding, dressing, bowels, bladder, toilet use, and stairs range from 0 (dependent/unable) to 10 (independent); scores for transfers and mobility on level surfaces range for 0 (unable) to 15 (independent); the possible total score ranges for 0 (the lowest) to 100 (the highest), obtained by adding points for each item.
Activity Measure for Post Acute Care (AM-PAC) (www.rehabmeasures.org/Lists/RehabMeasures/DispForm.aspx?ID=978)	■ Measures patient's activity limitations in the domains of cognition, self-care, and mobility. ■ Various versions available, including a computer-adapted test; inpatient short form includes 5–8 items per domain and outpatient short form consists of 15–18 items per domain.
Stroke Impact Scale (www.rehabmeasures.org/Lists/RehabMeasures/DispForm.aspx?ID=934)	■ An 8-domain, 59-item scale that measures the aspects of stroke recovery important to patients and caregivers, as well as stroke experts. ■ Includes measures of physical domain such as strength, mobility, ADLs, and hand function, as well as the domains of memory, emotion, communication, and social participation.
Harris Hip Questionnaire (www.orthopaedicscore.com/scorepages/harris_hip_score.html)	■ Asks questions regarding pain and function, including ambulation distance, presence of a limp, ability with tasks such as public transportation or stairs, and need for an assistive device. ■ Hip deformity and range of hip motion are also included.

NOTE: Above websites accessed Jan 2016.

24-hour care for those who cannot care for themselves or do not have a full-time caregiver. Outpatient services have clear advantages and disadvantages. Patients often prefer to return to their own homes but may not have the care support they need. Participation in day hospitals or outpatient clinics requires transportation, which can be costly and time consuming.

In summary, clinicians should be familiar with the services provided in a wide range of rehabilitation settings and with the advantages and disadvantages of each. The clinician is responsible for recommending the best match between patient needs and program services. However, under certain insurance plans, decisions about location of services can be heavily influenced by costs. More systematic evaluation of rehabilitation outcomes that is based on the structures and processes of care offered by various settings is essential for more rational use of rehabilitation programs. CMS is currently monitoring the quality of patient care using information from patient assessments.

TEAMS AND ROLES

A team approach is necessary to meet the complex rehabilitation needs of older adults. The interprofessional rehabilitation team often includes nursing, physical therapy, occupational therapy, speech language therapy, social work, psychology, nutrition services, prosthetics/orthotics, nurse practitioner, physician assistant, and physician. All health professionals who work with older adults should have a basic understanding of the roles and functions of various team members (Table 20.3). Each health care professional evaluates the patient, identifies goals, and then provides discipline-specific interventions to address the patient's issues. The patient's health-related outcome is the sum of the effort of each discipline.

Multidisciplinary teamwork can be inefficient and result in duplication of services and gaps in care of the older patient. The interdisciplinary or interprofessional team is the recommended approach to providing holistic and coordinated care for the older adult. Patient-centered care is efficient and effective. Health care professionals complete comprehensive evaluations on the patient; however, the patient goals and the intervention plan are determined by the entire team, including the patient and his or her family. The patient and family are core members of the rehabilitation team, and their expectations and preferences must be integrated into the care plan. In collaboration, the team members should pool their skills, experience, and knowledge to work toward the patient's goals to achieve the best outcome. Because coordinating care is the function of the interprofessional care team, team members must be able to define roles, share tasks, and collaborate within and outside the team. Team

Table 20.3—Roles of Core Health Care Providers on Rehabilitation Team

Provider	Primary Role on Rehabilitation Team
Nurse, clinical nurse specialist	Provides ongoing assessment of signs and symptoms of illness, medical conditions, and affect Provides patient and family education Evaluates self-care skills
Physical therapist	Assesses joint range of motion and muscle strength Assesses gait and mobility Provides appropriate assistive devices Instructs in exercise training to increase range of motion, strength, endurance, balance, coordination, and gait Treats with physical modalities (heat, cold, ultrasound, massage, electrical stimulation) Assesses environmental barriers in planned discharge environment
Occupational therapist	Assesses ADL and IADL abilities Screens visual perception and cognition Provides home assessment Provides self-care skills training; makes recommendations and provides training in use of assistive technology Fabricates splints and treats upper extremity deficits
Speech therapist	Assesses all aspects of communication Assesses swallowing disorders Treats communication deficits Recommends changes in diet and positioning to treat dysphagia
Social worker	Evaluates family and home-care factors Assesses psychosocial factors Provides counseling
Case manager	Assists patient and their family in coordinating services to meet recovery needs and transition toward discharge home
Dietitian	Assesses nutritional status Recommends dietary changes to maximize nutrition
Prosthetist	Makes and fits prosthetic limbs
Orthotist	Makes and fits braces and other devices to align and/or support limbs
Physician	Certifies rehabilitation need Supervises patient treatment Treats medical comorbidities Provides education
Physician assistant, nurse practitioner	Contributes to postadmission assessment Supervises patient treatment Treats medical comorbidities Provides education

building and continual efforts to improve team function are important issues for geriatric rehabilitation service providers to achieve positive patient outcomes.

The primary goal of the rehabilitation team is to ensure that patients receive comprehensive assessments and appropriate interventions for the disabling illness and associated comorbid conditions, as well as for the specific impairments and environmental factors that can affect activities and participation. The team must collaborate to establish common goals and a cohesive treatment plan to meet the needs of older adults.

IMPACT OF COMORBID CONDITIONS

In older patients, comorbid diseases and conditions can interrupt or delay treatment and often require the care plan to be modified. Many of the illnesses that can interfere with rehabilitation of older adults are predictable and potentially preventable. A systematic approach to assessment, prevention, and management of comorbid conditions can improve the patient's chance of receiving maximal benefit from rehabilitation services.

Older adults with reduced mobility are at high risk of skin breakdown, which can interfere with recovery and require extensive treatment. Immobility or altered weight bearing can precipitate pressure ulcers that heal poorly. Clinicians should monitor pressure and weight-bearing areas and be prepared to modify footwear, wheelchairs, and bedding as needed. Because thromboembolic events are also common with reduced mobility, their prevention should be a routine part of care. Length of time for prophylaxis and medication recommendations varies depending on the medical condition.

Incontinence is prevalent among older adults; causes include detrusor overactivity, obstruction, neurogenic bladder, immobility, and cognitive deficits. Indwelling catheters increase the risk of infection and are rarely appropriate in the nonacute setting. A structured approach to the assessment and treatment of bladder problems should be a basic component of any rehabilitation service.

The risk of pneumonia is increased by inactivity and disordered swallowing, as well as by underlying lung disease. The prevention of aspiration pneumonia involves difficult tradeoffs. Awareness of aspiration has been markedly increased by routine radiologic screening, but the clinical relevance of modest aspiration detected radiologically is unknown. Conservative measures such as changing food consistency with liquid thickeners and cohesive food substances and elevating head position while eating can help alleviate the problem. Sometimes aspiration risk is addressed by discontinuing all oral feeding and placing an enteral feeding tube. This approach eliminates the fundamental human pleasure of eating and may not be successful, because oral secretions or refluxed gastric contents can still be aspirated. Bleeding in the upper GI tract can occur during rehabilitation as a consequence of stress or medications and may not be preceded by typical symptoms.

Anemia is common in older adults and has been associated with adverse outcomes, including functional impairment, decreased muscle strength, and poorer quality of life. Although there is some evidence for improved exercise tolerance in older adults with end-stage kidney disease, definitive studies are lacking. Mental functioning is critical for rehabilitation, which requires the ability to follow commands and to learn. Because older adults who have been acutely ill are at increased risk of delirium, clinicians should assess mental status and screen for easily reversible causes in older rehabilitation patients. Depression is endemic in newly disabled individuals and can manifest as low motivation; formal screens for depression and early intervention are essential. Seizures can develop after stroke, and spasticity can develop during stroke recovery. Interventions for spasticity such as physical therapy or muscle relaxants have offered only modest benefit (SOE=B). Studies have shown botulinum toxin to be effective in decreasing muscle tone and increasing range of motion (SOE=A). However, these improvements have not consistently translated into improved function (SOE=B).

Certain comorbid conditions common in older adults, including diabetes mellitus, heart disease, peripheral vascular disease, musculoskeletal disorders, sensory impairments, and dementia, require ongoing adaptations in rehabilitation. Activity level is a powerful factor in glucose metabolism; diabetic patients are therefore likely to experience changes in glucose levels and medication requirements during rehabilitation. Increased caloric intake during recovery can also affect medication needs. Therapy personnel should know how to assess diabetic control, use a glucometer, and intervene for hypoglycemia. Most abnormal gaits increase the energy requirements of walking; an abnormal gait in a patient with coronary artery disease can cause coronary symptoms to worsen. Patients with poor cardiac output may have extreme exercise limitations. Medication adjustments for heart diseases may be necessary but can cause adverse events of their own, such as orthostatic hypotension. Patients with one vascular disease often have others; peripheral vascular disease is common, often associated with insensitive or painful feet and a high risk of skin breakdown. Treatment of painful peripheral neuropathy can foster increased activity and avoid pressure ulcers. Musculoskeletal status should be monitored to avoid overuse syndromes involving increased demand on vulnerable joints. For those with vision or hearing impairment, corrections must be provided and teaching approaches adapted accordingly. In patients with dementia, rehabilitation progress is still possible, but carryover may be decreased and the need for supervision and cueing may be increased.

Rehabilitation Approaches and Interventions

The primary goals of rehabilitation treatment are restitution of function, compensation for and adaptation to functional losses, and prevention of secondary complications. Ultimately, rehabilitation should maximize the person's potential for participation in social, leisure, or work roles. Many strategies can be used to achieve these goals. Restitution of physical function usually depends on therapeutic exercises to improve flexibility, muscle strength, motor control, and cardiovascular endurance. Exercise has been shown to improve strength, endurance, and balance in well-defined populations of disabled older adults (SOE=A). In stroke, speech and language therapy can be used to treat aphasia. Cognitive rehabilitation might improve alertness and attention. However, research evidence is insufficient to demonstrate that speech and language therapy, or cognitive rehabilitation, improve functional deficits.

Massage, heat, cold, and ultrasound are used to decrease pain and muscle spasm. These and other pain management strategies can contribute to increased function and tolerance for further rehabilitation. There is little research evidence supporting objective benefits from these therapies, but patients commonly report symptomatic relief.

Equipment for mobility, dressing and bathroom assistance, orthotic and prosthetic devices, and splints all can augment or replace the function of impaired body parts and thereby reduce limitations in activities and participation. For example, an ankle-foot orthosis can compensate for foot drop and improve safety and speed of walking. A wheelchair can provide mobility for community activities.

Repeated practice of task-specific activities such as bed mobility, transfers, and walking can improve functional mobility. Arm function improves with specific functional training activities, such as grasping, reaching, and fine manipulations. Balance training may improve balance and reduce the risk of falls. Older adults can benefit from retraining in instrumental activities of daily living (IADLs), such as cooking, managing finances, or driving a car.

Contextual factors, both environmental and personal, should be addressed to minimize restrictions on a person's activities and participation. For example, motivation can be addressed by collaborative goal setting, patient and family education, detection and management of depression, and use of support groups. Environmental modifications, such as grab bars and raised toilet seats in the bathroom or curb cutouts on public streets, can promote independent functioning.

To maintain function and enhance health status after rehabilitation, patients and families should assume responsibility for long-term self-management. Rehabilitation goals include a program to prevent worsening disability, including reintegration into social programs such as senior center programs, and health and wellness programs.

COMPREHENSIVE ASSESSMENT

Comprehensive assessment of rehabilitation patients is necessary for appropriate clinical management and evaluation of outcomes. The treatment plan should be guided by results of the initial assessment. The primary components of any assessment include patient demographics, social support, place of residence before illness, medical comorbidities, severity of current illness, and the patient's prior functional status. The rehabilitation stay is an ideal time for medication review and reconciliation, as patients transition from the hospital to the rehabilitation setting and ultimately to the community.

Impairments such as deficits in range of motion and flexibility, strength, sensory functions, balance, cognition, and depression should always be assessed. In conditions such as stroke, swallowing and language function should be evaluated. The patient's functional status is assessed with standardized measures of ADLs (eg, the Barthel ADL Index [Table 20.2]) and measures of IADLs. The patient's participation or quality of life is assessed with generic measures such as the SF-36 Health Survey (available at www.sf-36.org [accessed Jan 2016]) or disease-specific measures such as the Stroke Impact Scale or Harris Hip Questionnaire (Table 20.2).

STROKE

Stroke is a major cause of mortality and morbidity in the United States, particularly among adults ≥55 years old. Acute stroke occurs in >700,000 people each year, and 80% or more are likely to survive, many with residual neurologic difficulties. Stroke-related deficits are severe in approximately one-third of the survivors. Many patients with mild and moderate stroke become independent in ADLs, but other more complex dimensions of health status may still be affected. As stroke survival continues to increase, the need for comprehensive stroke rehabilitation will rise. Rehabilitation programs must address a broad range of stroke-related disabilities, including those in basic ADLs and IADLs, and participation and integration into health and wellness programs.

Goals of Rehabilitation

The overall goals of rehabilitation for older stroke patients include regaining function, compensating for or adapting to functional losses, and preventing secondary complications. Specific objectives include the following:

- Preventing or recognizing and managing comorbid illness and medical complications

- Assessing each patient comprehensively, using standardized assessments

- Matching the patient's needs to the program capabilities

- Training the patient to maximize independence in ADLs and IADLs

- Facilitating the patient's and family's psychosocial coping and adaptation

- Preventing recurrent stroke and other vascular conditions such as myocardial infarction

- Assisting the patient in reintegrating into the community

Rehabilitation for older adults with stroke is complex because of the variability of causes, symptoms, severity, and recovery. Stroke patients present with varying symptoms, depending on the site and size of the brain lesions. The most common type of neurologic deficit is hemiparesis, but other deficits can include sensory impairment, aphasia, dysarthria, cognitive impairment, motor incoordination, hemianopsia, visual-perceptual deficits, depression, dysphagia, and bowel and bladder incontinence. The degree of initial recovery and the time needed to reach maximal recovery is affected by the number of deficits. For example, individuals who have hemiparesis, hemianopsia, and sensory deficits are less likely to ambulate independently and require a longer time to regain skills than do those with only hemiparesis.

Stroke patients usually experience some degree of recovery. This recovery is most dramatic in the first 30 days but may continue more gradually for months. Stroke severity, which is based on degree of neurologic impairment and size of infarct on CT or MRI, is probably the most important factor to affect short and long-term outcomes. In the Framingham study, improvement in motor function and self-care slowed 3 months after stroke but continued at a reduced pace throughout the first year. In a study of locomotor training after stroke, participants demonstrated functional improvements up to 1 year later, even when training was begun 6 months after the stroke had occurred (SOE=B). Language and visual-spatial function was recovered over 12 months, but cognitive function improved during only the first 3 months.

Approach to Management

Guidelines for rehabilitation after stroke have been updated by a team sponsored by the Department of Veterans Affairs and the Department of Defense (available at www.healthquality.va.gov/Management_of_Stroke_Rehabilitation.asp [accessed Jan 2016]). The guidelines offer algorithms for initial assessment and rehabilitation referral, followed by management in inpatient or community settings. The guidelines emphasize that clinical outcomes are better when patients with acute stroke are treated in a setting that provides coordinated, interdisciplinary stroke-related evaluation and services (SOE=A). Studies have confirmed that adherence to guidelines promotes better outcomes. Coordinated care reduces 1-year mortality, improves functional independence, and increases satisfaction with care (SOE=A). Stroke severity should be systematically assessed, using the NIH Stroke Scale (www.strokecenter.org/wp-content/uploads/2011/08/NIH_Stroke_Scale.pdf [accessed Jan 2016]).

Benefits of rehabilitation after stroke are not restricted to any particular subgroup of patients. Studies have found that racial/ethnic minorities may be more likely to receive rehabilitation and to have longer lengths of stay (SOE=B). In one study, urban-dwelling black stroke patients were more likely to be discharged to an inpatient rehabilitation facility, possibly because of the greater number and severity of stroke cases in this population. Non-Hispanic whites who undergo rehabilitation for a stroke tend to be older, and less likely to have had a hemorrhagic stroke or have Medicaid. In a large, national, retrospective study, non-Hispanic white patients had higher functional status ratings at admission and discharge than patients in the minority groups. Despite this, whites were discharged home less frequently than blacks, Hispanics, or other minority groups (SOE=B).

In general, therapy should be started early, but later supplementary interventions can also be beneficial. The A Very Early Rehabilitation Trial (AVERT Phase 2) study showed that mobilization within the first 24 hours after stroke and at regular intervals thereafter was safe, with patients in the intervention group being more likely to be discharged home. There are several philosophical approaches to physical rehabilitation after strokes that are based on neurophysiologic, motor learning, or orthopedic principles. In a Cochrane review, a mixed approach was significantly more effective than no treatment or placebo (sham treatment) control for improving functional independence (standardized mean difference 0.78; confidence intervals 95%, 0.58–0.97), and this effect persisted beyond the intervention period. There is no convincing evidence that any one specific technique is superior to another.

Constraint-induced movement therapy discourages use of the unaffected extremity and encourages active use of the hemiparetic extremity, with a goal of improved motor recovery. In a systematic review, constraint-induced movement therapy produced statistically significant and clinically relevant improvements in arm motor function that persisted for at least 1 year (SOE=A). Treadmill walking with partial body-weight support using a harness connected to an overhead system can improve gait velocity and walking endurance significantly. Although this method did not increase the chances of walking independently compared with other physiotherapy interventions, the improvements in walking endurance were sustained among those patients who could walk at the beginning of therapy. There is evidence that mirror therapy improves recovery of arm function (SOE=B). This therapy uses visual imagery by encouraging the patient to exercise both extremities symmetrically while viewing the reflection of only the unaffected limb in a mirror. It is thought that the patient experiences proprioceptive input to the affected side through the visual input. Newer therapeutic interventions for regaining motor function are in development, including use of robotics to provide high-intensity repetitive and task-specific treatments. One systematic review found improvements in ADLs, and arm function but not arm muscle strength using robot-assisted training. The use of virtual reality for upper limb rehabilitation has also been evaluated in a systematic review that included 5 randomized controlled trials. Results showed improved motor impairment but no significant differences in motor function between the control and intervention groups (SOE=A).

Speech and language therapy are often provided for stroke patients with aphasia. However, there is no universally accepted treatment. Although a Cochrane report states that the evidence does not support a finding of either clear effect or lack of effect, the Veterans Affairs guidelines support "good" evidence for follow-up evaluation and treatment by a speech language professional for long-term residual communication difficulties. Dysphagia (or swallowing disorders) is common after stroke, affecting up to 30% of patients. The most commonly used test to diagnose dysphagia is videofluoroscopy, which allows speech therapy professionals to observe and analyze the swallowing process and to assess for aspiration. Patients who aspirate are treated using rehabilitation exercises, changes in food consistency, and changes in posture to reduce the likelihood of aspiration. Transcranial magnetic stimulation to improve muscle function has shown promise. The guidelines also support "good" evidence for cognitive retraining for attention or visual-spatial perceptual deficits and compensatory training for short-term memory deficits. The same guidelines find "good" evidence for medication treatment for depression and emotional lability. In several studies, depression was a consistent factor adversely influencing rehabilitation outcomes. Spasticity can develop gradually after stroke and can inhibit function and interfere with hygiene. Most interventions, including surgery and medications like baclofen, have been disappointing.

Patients who have had a stroke are at high risk of recurrence: up to 7%–10% annually. The rehabilitation phase is an appropriate time to ensure that assessment and treatment for stroke prevention has occurred. Assessments for significant carotid stenosis and for atrial fibrillation should be completed. Indications for carotid endarterectomy and anticoagulation with warfarin, dabigatran, or rivaroxaban should be reviewed. Antiplatelet medications such as aspirin alone or in combination with extended-release dipyridamole or clopidogrel should be considered in many patients. Treatment with ACE inhibitors[OL] and statins[OL] has also demonstrated reduced risk of stroke. Other risk factors to be targeted for preventing stroke recurrence include hypertension and smoking (SOE=A).

In summary, the evidence for specific interventions for stroke rehabilitation is weak. The collective benefits of well-organized interprofessional care, including secondary prevention, are well established.

HIP FRACTURE

Epidemiology and Surgical Care

Each year in the United States, about 300,000 older adults fracture a hip, with >90% of these fractures being the result of a fall. The risk of fracture is higher in women, whites, nursing-home residents, and in people with dementia. Mortality is about 5% during the initial hospitalization but nears 25% in the year after fracture. About 75% of survivors return to their prior level of function, but their overall mobility is more limited; up to half still require an assistive device. About half of patients will have an initial decline requiring transient long-term care, and about 25% will still be in long-term care 1 year later.

Medical management includes interventions to relieve pain and restore bone alignment to allow fracture healing and prepare the older adult to return to their prior level of functioning. For medically stable patients, surgical repair is recommended 24–72 hours after fracture. This early repair has been associated with a reduction in 1-year mortality, as well as with a lower incidence of complications such as pressure ulcers and delirium. For medically unstable patients, delaying surgery is warranted to allow sufficient improvement to tolerate the procedure. The surgical approach is determined by the location of the fracture, the presence or absence of displacement, and the prefracture mobility. One-third of hip fractures occur at the femoral neck, and the other two-thirds are intertrochanteric, occurring lateral to the femoral neck. Prefracture mobility is used as a guide to determine the goal of surgical treatment and to allow the risks and benefits of each surgical procedure to be considered. There is evidence that comanagement by geriatricians and orthopedic surgeons can result in improved outcomes, including lower than predicted length of stay, low complication rates, low mortality, and reduced cost. To be successful, comanagement must be interdisciplinary with shared decision making, equal responsibility for the patient, and daily communication.

Femoral neck fractures, which include subcapital, transcervical, and basilar fracture locations, are more common in older adults, particularly women. A femoral neck fracture without any displacement and intact blood supply can be surgically corrected with simple screws. However, femoral neck fractures with any degree of displacement and/or poor circulation are at increased risk of nonunion or avascular necrosis and therefore are usually treated with a prosthetic femoral head (hemiarthroplasty). Patients with significant underlying bony acetabular disease and a displaced femoral neck fracture may benefit from complete hip arthroplasty. Patients are usually allowed to bear weight immediately after repair of a femoral neck fracture, regardless of type of surgical procedure. However, those undergoing a total hip arthroplasty are required to adhere to total hip precautions.

For intertrochanteric fractures, the treatment of choice is open reduction and internal fixation with a compression screw or similar device. Displaced or comminuted intertrochanteric fractures commonly remain unstable, even after surgical fixation; therefore, full weight bearing is often not allowed for up to

6 weeks or until the stability of the fracture is assured. Factors that influence recovery should be assessed, including prior mobility and functional status, comorbid conditions, cognitive status, social support, type of injury, and repair and pain status. Mobility performance can be systematically assessed with numerous instruments, including the Harris Hip Questionnaire, which was developed specifically for hip fracture (Table 20.2).

Rehabilitation

Rehabilitation after hip fracture includes pain management, mobilization, and prevention of complications, such as delirium and thromboembolic events. The most important factors influencing recovery appear to be how soon mobilization is started and how frequently therapy is provided. Delay in mobilization is often driven by surgical recommendation, with proper healing of the fracture taking precedence over mobility. Partial weight bearing is difficult for many older adults to achieve. Prolonged inactivity is clearly associated with poorer functional outcomes, and early weight bearing is associated with low rates of surgical failure (SOE=A). Accelerated rehabilitation with rapid mobilization, coordinated planning, early discharge, and community follow-up has been associated with a 17% reduction in costs and no detriment to rates of recovery (SOE=B). Intensity of service clearly affects outcome, because those who receive physical therapy more than once a day during initial rehabilitation are more likely to be discharged directly to home than those who receive physical therapy once a day or less (SOE=A).

Prevention of Recurrence

Older adults who have had a hip fracture often have other comorbidities, such as osteoporosis and balance problems, that place them at risk of additional fractures resulting from falls. Efforts to diagnose and treat osteoporosis, improve balance, and reduce injury risk are a key part of treatment planning during rehabilitation. The use of hip protectors for fracture prevention in older adults has been extensively studied with mostly negative results.

TOTAL HIP AND KNEE ARTHROPLASTY

Cause and Surgical Care

In the United States, joint arthroplasty is the most common elective surgical procedure performed; approximately 400,000 are done annually. The primary indications for joint replacement are progressive pain and limitation of mobility despite conservative care. Plain radiographs are the usual method for determining the severity of joint damage at both the hip and knee. Loss of cartilage is shown by joint-space narrowing, and often osteophyte formation is also present. The most common diagnosis associated with the need for hip and knee joint replacement is osteoarthrosis, followed by rheumatoid arthritis.

The long-term results of joint replacement have generally been excellent and include significant pain relief, increased motion, and improved function. Continued success rates in the 90% range are seen 10–15 years after joint replacement. The most common reason for failure of the hip or knee replacement is loosening of the implant. Joint infection is another major concern, affecting 0.2%–1.1% of total hip and 1%–2% of total knee replacements. Deep infections often necessitate removal of the implant and long-term treatment with antibiotics until there is no sign of infection, followed by ultimate replacement with a new implant.

There are various types of hip prostheses and surgical approaches for the total hip arthroplasty; the prosthetic and approach used are determined by the surgeon and based on the condition of the joint and integrity of the bone. Depending on the approach used, the patient must adhere to certain hip precautions, ie, prevention of specific movements by the affected leg for approximately 6 weeks to ensure healing and prevent dislocation. When the anterolateral surgical approach is used, the patient must avoid external rotation, adduction, and extension of the operated leg. When the posterolateral approach is used, the patient should not internally rotate or adduct the leg and not flex the hip beyond 90 degrees. Many surgeons use a minimally invasive technique for total hip arthroplasty that involves 2-inch incisions (versus the traditional 10-inch) and no detachment of muscle. Because tissue trauma is less, recovery is often quicker.

Various types of prosthetic knees are also available and, like hip prostheses, the type used depends on the joint damage. Typically, patients can begin bearing weight on the operated leg by the first day or two after surgery. However, rotation or torsion at the knee should be avoided for up to 3 months. Surgeons have also applied the concept of minimal incisions to the total knee replacement surgery and with significantly more success, including achieving greater knee flexion. This surgery, in experienced hands, decreases blood loss and length of stay (SOE=A).

Management

Anticoagulation to prevent thromboembolism and good pain control are the major goals during the immediate postoperative period for both hip and knee arthroplasty. Patients who have undergone a major orthopedic procedure such as total hip or knee arthroplasty are at particularly high risk of both symptomatic and asymptomatic venous thromboembolism. Current guidelines for prevention of venous thromboembolism after total hip arthroplasty recommend a minimum of 10–14 days of antithrombotic prophylaxis (SOE=A). Pain in the initial postoperative period is often controlled with opioids administered orally, intravenously, or by patient-controlled analgesia pumps. For both hip and knee arthroplasty, early mobilization is the standard of care, and weight bearing often begins on the first postoperative day. Patients at low risk can often be discharged from the acute care hospital within 5 days. For those at high risk, defined as being >70 years old or having two or more comorbid conditions, early inpatient rehabilitation improves functional outcomes and decreases total length of stay (SOE=B). Age alone should not be used as a criterion for eligibility for joint replacement—excellent results can be achieved even in patients >80 years old who are in good health with stable chronic conditions. In a large retrospective study of patients receiving inpatient medical rehabilitation after hip arthroplasty, non-Hispanic whites and women had the greatest functional improvement from admission to discharge. Asians had the lowest mean change in function scores. Being of nonwhite ethnicity and being male were associated with higher odds of being discharged to home (SOE=B).

Rehabilitation

To decrease the risk of dislocation after total hip arthroplasty, rehabilitation patients are taught to complete their daily activities while adhering to hip precautions through the use of adaptive equipment and assistive devices. To prevent excessive hip flexion during toileting, a raised toilet seat is recommended for the first few months after surgery. If the patient uses a tub/shower combination at home, a tub bench is beneficial for safety in entering and exiting while maintaining hip precautions. Rehabilitation focuses on strengthening especially the abductors, which are weakened by the surgical approach, as well as on progressive range-of-motion and gait training. After total knee replacement, recovery of range of motion is the key to return of function and is often aided by use of a continuous passive-motion (CPM) machine. Based on a systematic review, early postoperative CPM decreased the need for postoperative manipulation and, combined with physical therapy, increased active range of motion and shortened the length of stay. Postoperative swelling is common and interferes with regaining motion. However, thigh-high compression stockings, CPM, and possibly cryotherapy can be used to manage swelling.

AMPUTATION

Epidemiology

Approximately 75,000 people undergo leg amputation each year in the United States. Most of these people have systemic vascular disease, with or without diabetes mellitus. Those with diabetes often have other end-organ disease, such as blindness, chronic kidney disease, and peripheral neuropathy. Mortality in this group approaches 50% at 2 years and 70% at 5 years. For up to one-fifth of patients, amputation of the other leg is needed within the first 2 years after the initial amputation. Most dysvascular amputees have such a burden of comorbid disease that the prosthesis is largely used for limited mobility, such as transfers and ambulation within the home.

The level of amputation and surgical approach depends on the status of the extremity; the surgery may be to remove devitalized tissue or may include reconstruction of the residual limb or stump. Common amputation levels include above or below the knee, as well as hip disarticulations.

Assessment

Key factors to assess include the patient's prior functional status, stability of comorbid conditions, cognition, and arm use, as well as the condition of the stump and the other leg. Successful prosthetic ambulation is associated with independent prior ambulation, ability to bear weight on the contralateral leg, stable medical status, and ability to follow directions. Blindness and chronic kidney disease do not necessarily preclude rehabilitation.

Rehabilitation

Rehabilitation starts in the preoperative stage, when the patient begins with strength and flexibility exercises and is educated about the recovery process, including prosthetic preparation and training. Amputation surgery generally aims to preserve the knee, because the energy requirement for walking is much lower for the below-the-knee amputee than for the above-the-knee amputee. This decision must be weighed against risks of poor wound healing with more distal amputation.

Postoperative rehabilitation includes efforts at early mobilization, prevention of contractures, wound healing, edema control, shaping of the stump, and psychosocial support. Patients are educated on maintaining intact skin integrity through wound care, compression wrapping, desensitization, and skin inspection to prepare the residual limb for the prosthesis. Poor wound healing delays rehabilitation in about 25% of cases. Prostheses vary in weight, socket type, style of foot, and suspensions. The older amputee benefits from a prosthesis that is lightweight, stable, and easy to use. Prosthetic rehabilitation involves progressive ambulation, education about prosthesis and stump care, and stump injury monitoring.

Lastly, phantom limb pain is common after amputation, with an estimated incidence of 60%–80%; pain management influences progress with rehabilitation. Treatment remains difficult, and clear evidence-based guidelines are lacking. Because tricyclic antidepressants[OL] and sodium channel blockers such as carbamazepine[OL] are generally effective for neuropathic pain, they are often used for phantom pain despite the lack of well-controlled trials (SOE=B). Anticonvulsants, specifically gabapentin, have been effective in several randomized controlled trials but not in others (SOE=B). A number of other medication regimens, using such agents as opioids[OL] and anesthetic blocks[OL], have also had success in small trials. Although previous controlled trials using memantine showed little success, a more recent double-blinded placebo-controlled trial using memantine in the 4 weeks immediately after amputation showed a significant decrease in phantom limb pain. Thus, memantine may be useful if used shortly after amputation but not for established, chronic phantom limb pain (SOE=B).

CARDIAC REHABILITATION

Cardiac rehabilitation (CR) programs typically include an individualized, medically supervised exercise program combined with an interdisciplinary focus on psychosocial, nutritional, and heart disease risk factor reductions. CR programs have been shown to improve exercise capacity, physical function, and quality of life, and to reduce mortality. In a study of more than 600,000 Medicare beneficiaries who had been hospitalized for coronary conditions or revascularization procedures and were eligible for cardiac rehabilitation, 1- to 5-year mortality rates were reduced for those who attended rehabilitation (21%) compared to those who did not (34%) (*P*<.001). In addition, a dose effect was demonstrated with better attendance being correlated with better outcomes (SOE=B). CR is effective in reducing symptoms of anxiety. In one study of 104 younger (<55 years) and 260 older (>70 years) adults with coronary heart disease, the prevalence of anxiety fell by 61% in the young adults and by 32% in the older ones after formal CR. Unfortunately, <30% of eligible patients are referred to CR and only 40%–60% actually complete the prescribed course of treatment. There are a number of barriers to utilization of CR, including low physician referral and lack of personal resources, making attendance difficult. Low rates of referral by primary care physicians has been attributed to lack of familiarity with CR site locations, lack of standardized referral forms, and inconvenience. Medicare provides for up to 36 sessions after myocardial infarction, percutaneous revascularization, heart valve, or coronary artery bypass surgery. At this time, heart failure is not a covered condition.

PULMONARY REHABILITATION

Pulmonary rehabilitation (PR) has been defined as "a comprehensive intervention based on a thorough patient assessment followed by patient-tailored therapies which include, but are not limited to, exercise training, education, and behavior change, designed to improve the physical and emotional condition of people with chronic respiratory disease and to promote the long-term adherence to health-enhancing behaviors." PR is most successful when delivered by an interprofessional team. Traditionally, PR has been provided to stable patients with moderate to severe chronic obstructive pulmonary disease (COPD). However, more recent studies have shown that rehabilitation in the peri-exacerbation period can reduce hospital admissions. PR has also been shown to be as effective with equivalent benefits in patients with non-COPD respiratory disease. There is little guidance regarding who should be referred for PR. However, a practical approach that has been suggested is to refer any patient with functional status limitations or persistent respiratory symptoms despite otherwise optimal therapy.

The main aim of endurance exercise training is to improve aerobic capacity and thereby enhance ability to perform activities of daily living. This improvement is attributed, in part, to reduced ventilatory requirements for a given task and improved peak aerobic capacity. In addition, there is evidence of improvements in lower limb muscles, specifically increases in muscle fiber capillarization and mitochondrial density and oxidative capacity of muscle fibers. There is strong evidence for improvements in health-related quality of life and reductions in fatigue and dyspnea with PR (SOE=A). The effect on mortality is less robust. One systematic review found in the control group, 29 of 100 people had mortality over 107 weeks compared with 10 of 100 in the active treatment group. Thus, the number needed to treat for benefit was 6 (95% CI 5–30) over 107 weeks. Treadmill walking and stationary cycle ergometry are the most common forms of exercise in PR and have been shown to improve exercise performance and muscle function (SOE=A). In addition, a number of other types of exercise training have also been explored and may be beneficial, although the evidence is less robust. These include ground walking exercise, Nordic walking exercise training, resistance exercise, aquatic exercise, and tai chi.

Table 20.4—Commonly Prescribed Mobility Aids

Assistive Device	Characteristics	Prescribed Conditions
Straight cane	Provide unilateral support Assist with balance and proprioception Reduce weight bearing on opposite leg	Osteoarthritis of knee or hip Peripheral neuropathy
Quad cane	Provides unilateral support More stable than straight cane Allows greater weight bearing on device	Stroke with hemiparesis
Stationary "pick-up" walker	Provides bilateral support Must be lifted and advanced, requiring strength and coordination Very stable and allows non-weight bearing movement	Hip fracture in which non-weight bearing needed Unilateral amputation, before prosthesis
Two-wheeled walker	Less stable than stationary walker but easier to advance Allows for smoother, faster gait	Deconditioning Parkinson disease Total joint replacement
Rollator (four-wheeled walker with seat and brakes)	Less stable but allows for smoother, faster gait Requires more coordination and safety awareness (because of brakes) Good for outside walking because of large wheels Has seat for resting	Cardiopulmonary disease Peripheral neuropathy with balance difficulty
Manual wheelchair	Requires use of arms and some cardiopulmonary endurance Often used in nursing homes and by caregivers for ease of patient mobility Easy to transport	Nonambulatory patient with cognitive impairment Low-level spinal cord injury
Power wheelchair	Allows community mobility for those with limited ambulatory ability Controls do not require intact upper extremities Need cognitive ability to operate safely May need home modifications	Neurologic diseases (eg, high-level spinal cord injury, multiple sclerosis, amyotrophic lateral sclerosis) Multiple limb amputations
Scooter	Similar benefits to power wheelchair, except need to operate with upper extremities May be more acceptable to patient than power wheelchair	Cardiopulmonary disease

MOBILITY AIDS, ORTHOTICS, ADAPTIVE METHODS, AND ENVIRONMENTAL MODIFICATIONS

Assistive devices, orthotics, adaptive methods, and environmental modifications are effective for maximizing function in older adults with disabilities. Many of the items considered durable medical equipment are 80% reimbursed for Medicare B beneficiaries with a physician prescription. It is important to identify the underlying causes of disability before prescribing a device or modification, because medical or surgical treatment for individual diseases and impairments may be more effective or may enhance the usefulness of these approaches.

An estimated 6.8 million Americans use assistive technology devices to enhance mobility. Unfortunately, many older adults who might benefit from the use of mobility aids do not or will not use them. There may be racial/ethnic influences in willingness to use mobility aids. Focus group studies with community-dwelling older adults of white, non-Hispanic black, and Hispanic backgrounds showed that for all groups, perceived benefits of mobility devices in maintaining independence and control produced positive attitudes. However, the association of use of mobility aids with aging and physical decline contributed to stigmatizing attitudes. Black and Hispanic participants expressed apprehension about using unsafe or inappropriate secondhand equipment, heightened concerns about mobility-aid users becoming the subject of negative biases, and a preference for fashionable mobility aids. Hispanic participants expressed a preference for human assistance. Participants of all groups perceived clinicians as influencing their decision to use mobility aids.

Mobility Aids

Canes typically support 15%–20% of the body weight and are used in the hand contralateral to the affected knee or hip. A straight cane has a single tip, while a quad cane has four tips. As the number of tips increases, the degree of support also increases, but the cane becomes heavier and more awkward to use. The handle of the cane may be curved or have a pistol grip; the pistol grip offers more support. Canes can be made of a variety of materials, but most are made of wood or lightweight aluminum. The length of the cane is important for stability. Some canes are adjustable, but wooden canes must be cut to size. One of two methods can be used to evaluate the proper cane length: measuring the distance from the distal wrist crease to the ground when the patient is standing erect, and measuring the distance from the greater trochanter to the ground. Straight canes are often prescribed for patients with a single joint problem, such as osteoarthritis of the knee. The cane decreases the weight bearing through the joint, thereby decreasing pain and improving ambulation. A cane can also be helpful for patients with decreased lower extremity proprioception. Proprioceptors in the hand relay vital information to the brain about where the cane and the ground are in relation to the person. Quad canes are used when a patient requires a more stable platform on which to bear weight, such as after a stroke with resultant hemiparesis. When using a quad cane, it is important that all four tips are placed on the ground simultaneously, to assure the cane is stable before weight bearing (Table 20.4).

Crutches, axillary or forearm, are usually used to provide bilateral support. Axillary crutches are seldom recommended for older adults because greater arm strength and coordination are required for use. In addition, there is a risk of brachial plexus injury if the crutches are used incorrectly. Forearm crutches are more functional because a cuff secures the crutch on the patient's arm, allowing use of the hand to manipulate objects. A single crutch can be used instead of a cane if additional unilateral support is needed.

A walker is prescribed when a cane does not offer sufficient stability. A walker can completely support one leg but cannot support full body weight. Walker types include pick-up and wheeled walkers. Walkers should be adjusted so that the user maintains an erect posture and is not required to lean forward to reach the walker. The pick-up walker is lifted and moved forward by the user, who then advances before lifting the walker again; the result is a slow, staggering gait. It requires strength to repeatedly pick up the walker and cognitive ability to learn the necessary coordination. It may be the mobility device of choice when offloading one limb and maximal stability is preferred, such as after a hip fracture in a patient with a tenuous fixation in which non-weight bearing is needed to allow the bone to heal. A wheeled walker allows for a smoother, coordinated, and faster gait and takes advantage of compensated gait patterns; it is more likely to be correctly used by those with cognitive impairment. The most commonly used type is the two-wheeled walker, which brakes automatically with increased downward pressure. Patients with Parkinson disease often do well with a wheeled walker because once they start walking, they do not have to stop and start as is required with a pick-up walker. The two-wheeled walker is also easier to stop, because patients need only to lean on the device to engage the brakes.

A "rollator" is a four-wheeled walker with hand brakes, which can be locked when the patient is transferring. This type also has a platform seat for resting and a basket for carrying objects. Because of the use of the hand brakes, the rollator requires greater skill and safety awareness. It is preferred for outdoor use, because the wheels are larger and move easier over sidewalks and slightly rough terrain. The rollator is often prescribed for patients with cardiac or pulmonary conditions and deconditioning. The ability to lean on the device increases the distance patients can travel because it decreases energy expenditure, and patients can sit to rest when fatigued.

Patients who cannot safely use or who are unable to ambulate with an assistive device require a wheelchair. A wheelchair must be fitted according to the patient's body build, weight, disability, and prognosis. Incorrect fit can result in poor posture, joint deformity, reduced mobility, pressure ulcers, circulatory compromise, and discomfort. The Rehabilitation Engineering and Assistive Technology Society of North America Wheelchair Service Guide provide detailed information for determining the most appropriate wheelchair for the patient (www.resna.org/dotAsset/22485.pdf [accessed Jan 2016]). Several factors are associated with use of a prescribed wheelchair, including age, gender, health, characteristics of the device (eg, type, size), and environmental facilitators and barriers. Often the prescribed devices do not meet the needs of the older adult. In one study, 61% of the older adults reported having difficulty with manual wheelchair propulsion. Important considerations in the evaluation for a wheelchair are cognitive status and functional ability to use the device. Manual wheelchairs are frequently used in the nursing-home setting to allow ease of mobility, either through self- or staff propulsion. The most significant factor associated with manual wheelchair use was not living at home.

The demand for power mobility devices has increased substantially in recent years, and accounts for 66% of the Medicare expenses for mobility-related devices. CMS provides a checklist for physician prescribing of power mobility devices (www.cms.gov/Outreach-and-Education/Medicare-Learning-Network-MLN/MLNMattersArticles/downloads/SE1112.pdf [accessed Jan 2016]) Motorized wheelchairs can be used by mentally alert individuals with bilateral arm weakness or other neurologic disorders that limit arm use. Power wheelchairs can be controlled using a joystick or an alternative control device like a sip-and-puff switch or head control. Examples of patients who might do well with a power wheelchair include those with spinal cord injuries, multiple sclerosis, or amyotrophic lateral sclerosis. Motorized scooters offer less trunk support than motorized wheelchairs but are more acceptable to some people. Patients are more likely to use scooters rather than power wheelchairs if they have a primary diagnosis of cardiovascular and pulmonary disease and if they are living at home. Motorized scooters and wheelchairs increase patients' mobility, but there is a risk of deconditioning because patients might otherwise push a wheelchair or ambulate. The use of a wheelchair commonly requires home modifications, including ramps and widened doorways. Cars may need to be adapted with lifts.

Orthotics, Adaptive Methods, and Environmental Modifications

Orthotics are exoskeletons designed to assist, resist, align, and stimulate function. Orthotics are named by the use of letters for each joint that the device involves in its structure. Thus, an AFO is an ankle and foot orthotic device used to support weak calf or pretibial muscles (eg, for a stroke patient with leg weakness). It is important to obtain a physical or occupational therapy evaluation early in the hospitalization to assess for equipment needs, including mobility aids and adaptive equipment. This assessment is critical to providing older adults with the correct equipment to maximize their independent function.

Adaptations to facilitate dressing may be necessary for older adults with problems such as range of motion loss, decreased strength, incoordination, and limited endurance. Clothing that is easy to clean and tops that fit easily over the head or fasten in the front and allow for freedom of movement are helpful. Hook-and-loop tape is usually easier to use than buttons and can be sewn on to replace buttons and zippers. When buttons are necessary, if they are sewn on with elastic thread, the need to manipulate them can be eliminated. Putting on shoes and socks is particularly difficult for older adults with decreased agility. Longer, looser socks (eg, tubular socks) are easier to put on. For patients who find that reaching the feet to put on socks and shoes is a problem, a sock aid and long-handled shoehorn may be useful. Elastic shoelaces eliminate the need for tying and untying.

Environmental modifications can have a major impact on the older adult's ability to function independently or with minimal assistance at home (SOE=A). A variety of assistive devices, such as reachers, door knob extenders, and plug pullers, can reduce the difficulty of performing daily tasks and have a significant impact on a person's quality of life.

The bathroom is a common place for falls. Any older adult with impaired balance or leg weakness should have grab bars installed near the toilet and tub or shower. Raised toilet seats and bathtub benches are available to assist those with leg weakness, poor balance, or limited endurance. These are also useful for older adults with arthritis of the hips or knees, because they reduce biomechanical stress on the joint. Long-handled bath brushes, hand-held shower heads, and "soap on a rope" can be helpful for older adults with arm weakness or other impairment.

REFERENCES

- Fleury AM, Salih SA, Peel NM. Rehabilitation of the older vascular amputee: a review of the literature. *Geriatr Gerontol Int.* 2013;13(2):264–273.

  This review presents an overview of predictive factors for successful prosthetic rehabilitation outcomes in older adults after amputation secondary to a vascular condition. Premorbid functioning and mobility is a solid predictor of success. Comorbidities, such as cardiac and pulmonary diseases, as well as ischemia in the remaining leg, make it physically difficult for older adults to participate in gait training. Similarly, cognitive impairments are contraindicated to learning to use a prosthetic. Multidisciplinary teams can often identify successful users.

- Jette AM. Toward a common language of disablement. *J Gerontol A Biol Sci Med Sci.* 2009;64(11):1165–1168.

  This paper reviews selected contemporary disablement models leading to the current World Health Organization International Classification of Functioning, Disability, and Health framework. The concepts and terminology inherent to each model are described, and evidence is provided for the importance of a common language among rehabilitation providers.

- Langhorne P, Bernhardt J, Kwakkel G. Stroke rehabilitation. *Lancet.* 2011;377(9778):1693–1702.

  This review focuses on the evidence underlying stroke rehabilitation, including principles of rehabilitation practice, systems of care, and specific interventions. Randomized trials and systematic reviews of the effects of rehabilitation interventions for stroke-related impairment and disability are emphasized.

- Latham NK, Harris BA, Bean JF, et al. Effect of a home-based exercise program on functional recovery following rehabilitation after hip fracture. *JAMA.* 2014;311(7):700–708.

  The aim of this randomized controlled trial was to determine whether a comprehensive 3 times per week, 6-month home exercise program with only minimal therapist contact improved the physical functioning of community-dwelling older adults after discharge from rehabilitation services for a hip fracture. Results showed a significant improvement in functional mobility at 6 months; this increase remained at the 6-month follow up, indicating that home programs are beneficial.

- Menezes AR, Lavie CJ, Milani RV, et al. Cardiac rehabilitation in the United States. *Prog Cardiovasc Dis.* 2014;57(2):152–159.

  This review describes the benefits of cardiac rehabilitation, as well as factors that affect referral and participation in these programs.

Kathleen T. Foley, PhD, OTR/L
Cynthia J. Brown, MD, MSPH, AGSF

CHAPTER 21—NURSING-HOME CARE

KEY POINTS

- Currently, there are 15,663 nursing homes with 1.7 million beds, 1.4 million residents, and 2.4 million discharges each year.

- The Omnibus Budget Reconciliation Act of 1987 requires a periodic comprehensive assessment of all nursing-home residents, sets minimum staffing requirements, and fosters residents' rights by limiting the use of restraints and psychoactive medications.

- The care of nursing-home residents has become more complex over the past several years, commensurate with an increasing level of medical acuity in an environment constrained by limited resources.

Nursing homes have evolved dramatically over the past several years, responding to a variety of government and market-driven forces. The almshouse, common at the turn of the 20th century, has been transformed into a highly regulated institution for people who often have severe physical and mental disabilities. Nursing homes, more than ever, present the clinician with a set of unique and complex care issues, many of which are best understood in the context of population needs, government policy, and reimbursement and staffing patterns.

THE NURSING-HOME POPULATION

Currently, more than 1.4 million Americans live in nursing homes. Relatively speaking, this is a small portion of Americans who are >65 years old (2.8%); 15% of nursing-home residents are <65 years old. The typical nursing-home resident is a white, unmarried (usually widowed) woman >85 years old with limited social supports. Most people admitted to nursing homes are older adults, with an average age at of 82.6 years. In recent years (1999–2008), the numbers of Hispanic, Asian, and black Americans living in nursing homes have increased by 55%, 54%, and 11% respectively. Although some of this increase is explained by increasing numbers of these populations in American demographics, the rate of increase of minority populations in nursing homes has exceeded changing population demographics, suggesting that nursing-home use is increasing by these populations. It has been speculated that disparities in access to community-based long-term care services may mediate this differential use, but more study is needed. Some cultural groups, particularly Hispanic and Asian Americans may be reluctant to consider nursing-home placement because of concerns about the lack of staff on all shifts who speak the same language as their relative, as well as the perception that the nursing home will not be able to serve familiar foods or follow other cultural traditions of their loved one. Older adults with intellectual and/or developmental disabilities constitute another unique population that is requiring increasing nursing-home care as their older parent-caregivers are lost. These individuals often require specialized care that many nursing homes have difficulty providing.

Functional disability is prevalent in nursing-home residents. More than half of long-stay nursing-home residents require supervision or hands-on assistance from another person in 5 ADLs (ie, eating, dressing, bathing, transferring, and toileting). Cumulative disability is high, with >80% of nursing-home residents requiring assistance in ≥3 ADLs. Many residents are dependent on assistance for eating (57%), more than a third require a mechanically altered diet consistency (32.5%), and 5% receive tube feedings. Difficulty with bladder or bowel control, or both, is reported in >60% of long-stay nursing-home residents. Hearing and visual impairments are also common, with each affecting approximately one-third of nursing-home residents. Not surprisingly, most residents have communication problems, with frequent difficulty both in being understood and understanding others. In 2000, <18% of nursing-home residents ambulated independently; the number of nursing-home residents able to independently ambulate has diminished steadily since that time. Currently, few residents (9.4%) walk without assistance or supervision, and most (60.6%) can be described as "chairfast," reflecting reliance on a chair for mobility, and an inability to take steps without extensive or constant weight-bearing support. For selected demographic and functional characteristics of older adults who live in nursing homes, see Table 21.1.

Today's population in the nursing home is sicker than the nursing-home population of the past. Over two-thirds of long-stay residents in skilled-nursing facilities have multiple medical conditions. More than 1 in 20 nursing-home residents have pressure ulcers. Nearly 40% of older adults in the nursing home are diagnosed with heart failure or ischemic heart disease. Diabetes and stroke are reported in 22% and 26% of new nursing-home admissions, respectively. COPD, hypertension, arthritis, and hip fractures are also prevalent health conditions among nursing-home residents. Moderate to severe cognitive impairment is seen in 63% of older adults residing in nursing homes, making dementia the most commonly occurring condition in nursing homes.

The prevalence of cognitive impairment is reflected in the fact that about 80% of nursing-home residents are felt by nursing home staff to be impaired in their ability to make daily decisions, and two-thirds have orientation difficulties or memory problems, or both. Depression is diagnosed in 20%–25% of residents. In 39% of nursing-home residents >65 years old, both medical and psychiatric conditions have been diagnosed, reflecting a 60% increase from 1999 data in prevalence of comorbid physical and mental diagnoses in this population. Additionally, behavioral issues, such as verbal and social inappropriateness, wandering, and resistance to care, are seen in one-third of nursing-home residents.

NURSING-HOME AVAILABILITY

According to CMS data, there are currently 15,663 nursing homes in the United States with 1,707,817 beds and 2.4 million discharges (ie, to home, hospital, or secondary to death). Of these facilities, 69% are proprietary (ie, for profit), with voluntary nonprofit (25%) and government nursing homes (5.8%) accounting for the remainder. Nursing-home care is provided to eligible veterans in 134 Veteran's Administration Community Living Centers. The Veteran's Administration also recognizes 140 State Veterans Homes, which are owned, operated, and funded by all 50 states and Puerto Rico to provide long-term care services to veterans. In some states, nonveteran spouses and parents may also be eligible for care in a State Veterans Home. Nationally, nursing homes operate an average of 108 beds, but facility size varies greatly by state. More than 80% of homes have 50–199 beds; only a minority (6.1%) has >200 beds. Associations between facility size and quality of care have been explored, and suggest that smaller facilities may provide higher quality of care on average than larger facilities. Although the current evidence also suggests a relationship between nurse staffing levels and quality, this relationship is complex and may be mediated in part by proprietary status. A little more than half of all nursing homes are part of a chain. Nursing homes vary with respect to what ancillary services are available. Many facilities offer on-site mobile radiography services; however, challenges exist in obtaining optimal quality of images. Similarly, many nursing homes provide infusion service, but results of studies have been variable with respect to the impact of the availability of the infusion service on resident hospitalization.

Most admissions to nursing facilities come from acute hospitals, followed by private residences and other nursing homes. Not surprisingly, assisted-living facilities are becoming a greater source of older adults admitted to nursing facilities, accounting for 7.9% of total admissions. Assisted-living facilities do not operate under the oversight of a single national regulatory or licensure agency. In general, assisted-living facilities have greater heterogeneity than nursing homes in services offered and are most commonly paid for with out-of-pocket funds.

By age 65, a person's lifetime risk of nursing-home admission is high, estimated at 46%. The risk of nursing-home admission rises steeply with age. While 7.4% of those ≥75 years old reside in nursing homes, this figure approaches 16% for those ≥85 years old. Barring breakthroughs in the treatment of dementia, the number of people ≥65 years old using nursing homes will double by the year 2030. Interestingly, the occupancy rates in nursing homes nationally have declined over the past several years and now stand at 80%. This decline has generally been attributed to the availability of other long-term care options, such as assisted living, but there are likely other causal social and financial variables that have yet to be identified. The availability and use of home-care services for Medicare-eligible patients have not been found to consistently reduce nursing-home admissions.

Postacute care is increasingly being offered in nursing-home settings, a response to the higher-care needs of older adults in conjunction with shorter hospital stays and the presence of a Medicare payment stream. Although the types of postacute services and programs vary significantly from one locale to another (eg, dialysis, orthopedic, ventilator, postoperative, rehabilitative, wound care), they remain distinct from the standard nursing-home services by integrating the features of acute medical, long-term care nursing, and rehabilitative settings. The challenge in postacute care is that of accommodating patients with varying degrees of disease severity, functional dependence, and comorbidities. Some limited studies suggest that, for selected patient populations, postacute care in the nursing home has outcomes equal to or better than those of postacute care in acute hospitals. Definitions as to what constitutes postacute care, however, vary widely, as do regulatory standards, which make comparison studies difficult.

On any given day, residents with a length of stay of <3 months comprise about 20% of the total nursing-home population. Conversely, long-stay residents, whose length of stay is ≥90 days after admission, account for 80% of the nursing-home population. Among all nursing-home residents, about 25% have a length of stay >3 years. This diversity in nursing-home stays is reflected in a mean length of stay for those admitted to a nursing home of 835 days, with a median length of stay of only 463 days. Historically, increases in the number of residents with shorter lengths of stay coincided with increased Medicare funding of postacute care in nursing homes.

This continuum spanning subacute and long-term care in nursing homes contributes to the development of two populations of residents. Many short-stay residents are admitted for rehabilitation, targeting restoration of the functional ability and endurance that will allow them to return to community-based living settings. Others enter nursing homes for terminal care. In contrast, many of those who ultimately become long-stay residents present to nursing homes for the ongoing supportive care of progressive, chronic illnesses. Interestingly, improvement in function among long-stay nursing-home residents is quite common, further reflecting the heterogeneity of the nursing-home population. The role of the nursing home in the continuum of health care is expected to become more important as health care systems adapt to the need to provide high-quality, accountable care to the expanding population of older adults and disabled adults.

NURSING-HOME FINANCING

Across all payers, nursing-home expenditures total more than $140 billion dollars. In 2012, the national average daily rate for a private room in a nursing home was $248, or $90,520 annually. Public health programs primarily finance this cost; Medicaid and Medicare account for 64% and 14% of nursing-home care payments, respectively. With the high annual costs, those paying for nursing-home care out-of-pocket often deplete their personal funds and turn to public funding. Although purchase of long-term care insurance has been increasing, these policies generally pay for only a small fraction of nursing-home care. Medicare funding for nursing-home costs is available for certain limited conditions for beneficiaries who require skilled-nursing or rehabilitation services. In general, to be covered, beneficiaries must receive services from a Medicare-certified skilled-nursing home after a qualifying hospital stay. A qualifying hospital stay is a hospital stay of at least 3 days before entering a nursing home. Some groups have argued for elimination of this requirement for a 3-day qualifying hospital stay on the basis that it limits accessibility to appropriate levels of care for patients, increases cost, and unnecessarily exposes patients to hazards of hospitalization.

Medicare covers only those skilled-nursing facility services rendered to help a beneficiary recover from an acute illness or injury. Medicare pays for skilled care in full for the first 20 days in a skilled-nursing facility. For days 21–100, a co-payment from the resident is required for skilled-nursing facility services; beyond 100 days, Medicare does not cover skilled-nursing facility care.

As part of the Balanced Budget Act of 1997, Medicare payments to nursing homes are based on an individual's functional needs and potential for rehabilitation. This prospective payment system, also called PPS, requires careful documentation of functional gains, particularly by rehabilitation therapists. Although the PPS has not conclusively limited access to skilled-nursing care for Medicare beneficiaries, it has forced nursing homes to be more diligent with regard to their admission policies. Not unexpectedly, physical, occupational, and speech therapies are commonly prescribed in the nursing home, with half of all patients admitted to nursing homes receiving at least 90 minutes of these rehabilitation services, according to one study. The PPS requires nursing-home staff to carefully document gains in function to ensure reimbursement. A recent legal decision (Jimmo v. Sebelius, 2013) clarifies that the skilled services may include those interventions to prevent or slow further deterioration.

Supplemental increases in reimbursement are made to offset costs of caring for those with HIV/AIDS. Despite the high cost of nursing-home care, resources remain constrained. In general, psychiatric conditions are undervalued with respect to reimbursement in long-term care. Residents with active psychiatric illness often require increased care and staff time, but mechanisms do not exist for increased reimbursement for those efforts. Shortages of psychiatric specialists trained in nursing-home care, combined with relatively low reimbursement rates for care in nursing homes, add to the challenge of providing optimal mental health care in this setting.

STAFFING PATTERNS

Resident care and evaluation in the nursing home largely depend on nurses and nursing assistants. Nursing facilities are required to provide nurse staffing sufficient to provide the care outlined in its care plans. According to federal guidelines, every nursing home must have the following on staff: a licensed nurse who acts as charge nurse on each shift; a registered nurse who is on duty at least 8 consecutive hours, 7 days a week; and a registered nurse who is designated as the director of nursing. Studies have confirmed the correlation between the provision of quality care to total nursing hours and the ratio of professional nurses (ie, registered nurses) to nonprofessional nursing staff. A 2001 Institute of Medicine report recommended increasing nurse staffing levels to enhance the quality of nursing-home care, spurring Congress to debate the merits of mandatory minimal staffing ratios. Although recommendations for minimal and optimal staffing at nursing facilities have been made by CMS based on links to quality of care, current federal regulations do not mandate specific nurse-to-resident staffing ratios. The total direct care staffing averages 4.04 hours per

Table 21.1—Activities of Daily Living (ADL) Functional Characteristics of Nursing-Home Population (%), 2013

ADL	Independent	Limitations Present	Level of Dependence	
			Assistance of 1 or 2 People	Dependent
Bathing	3.76	96.24	63.45	32.79
Dressing	8.54	91.45	70.67	20.78
Toileting	12.65	87.36	63.25	24.11
Transferring	15.45	84.55	63.38	21.17
Eating	42.96	57.04	43.77	13.27

SOURCE: Data from Cowles CM. *Nursing Home Statistical Yearbook*, 2013. Cowles Research Group; 2014.

Table 21.2—Quality Measures for Nursing Homes Based on the Minimum Data Set and Publicly Reported by CMS

For Long-Stay Residents
  Percent assessed and given, appropriately, the seasonal influenza vaccination
  Percent assessed and given, appropriately, the pneumococcal vaccination
  Percent whose need for help with daily activities has increased
  Percent who self-report moderate to severe pain
  Percent who were physically restrained
  Percent who have depressive symptoms
  Percent who have/had a catheter inserted and left in their bladder
  Percent with a urinary tract infection
  Percent who lose too much weight
  Percent who experience one or more falls with major injury
  Percent who received an antipsychotic medication

For Long-Stay Low-Risk Residents
  Percent who lose control of their bowels or bladder

For Long-Stay High-Risk Residents
  Percent who have pressure ulcers

For Short-Stay Residents
  Percent assessed and given, appropriately, the seasonal influenza vaccination
  Percent assessed and given, appropriately, the pneumococcal vaccination
  Percent who newly received an antipsychotic medication
  Percent who self-report moderate to severe pain
  Percent with pressure ulcers that are new or worsened

SOURCE: Adapted from Department of Health and Human Services, Medicare. *Nursing Home Compare*. www.medicare.gov/NHcompare/ (accessed Jan 2016).

resident day (HPRD), or roughly 242 minutes per resident per day but varies significantly both within and between states. Nursing assistants contribute most direct staff time, at 2.5 HPRD. Licensed nurses and registered nurses contribute 0.85 and 0.77 HPRD, respectively. Physical and occupational therapy staff hours per resident day have increased to 0.190 and 0.159 HPRD, respectively, commensurate with increasing medical acuity and a rise in the proportion of skilled-nursing facility days. However, HPRD has remained flat for licensed nurses and nursing assistants providing direct care. It has been estimated that 9 of 10 nursing homes are inadequately staffed, and nearly $8 billion dollars would be needed to bring staffing to adequate levels.

Recruiting and retaining staff, particularly nursing assistants who constitute the bulk of the nursing-home workforce, also continues to be difficult. Turnover rates of approximately 50% for direct care staff of nursing facilities, including 50% of nurse assistants and registered nurses and 35% of licensed practical nurses, have been reported. Stability of staff has been associated with better quality of care. Turnover rates have been associated with increased rates of hospitalization for nursing-home residents and have been linked to the organizational culture within the nursing facility.

Staffing issues are also pertinent to physicians practicing in nursing homes. Many physicians avoid nursing-home practice because of perceptions of excessive regulations, paperwork, limited reimbursement, and aversion to the long-term care environment. Although older data suggest that the typical nursing-home physician is a primary care internist or family physician who devotes ≤2 hours per week to nursing-home care, a recent trend of more physicians who dedicate their practice to nursing-home medicine has been described, although national data do not yet

Table 21.3—Roles and Responsibilities of the Nursing Facility Medical Director

Physician Leadership
- Help the facility ensure that patients have appropriate physician and health care provider coverage and services
- Help the facility develop a process for reviewing physician and health care provider credentials
- Provide guidance for physician performance expectations
- Help the facility ensure that a system is in place for monitoring the performance of health care providers
- Facilitate feedback to physicians and other health care providers on performance and practices

Patient Care—Clinical Leadership
- Participate in administrative decision making and development of policies and procedures related to patient care
- Help develop, approve, and implement specific clinical practices for the facility to incorporate into its care-related policies and procedures, including areas required by laws and regulations
- Develop procedures and guidance for staff regarding contacting practitioners, including information gathering and presentation, change in condition assessment, and when to contact the medical director
- Review, consider, and/or act on consultant recommendations, as appropriate, that affect the facility's resident care policies and procedures or the care of an individual resident
- Review, respond to, and participate in federal, state, local, and other external surveys and inspections
- Help review policies and procedures regarding adequate protection of patients' rights, advance care planning, and other ethical issues

Quality of Care
- Help the facility establish systems and methods for reviewing the quality and appropriateness of clinical care and other health-related services and provide appropriate feedback
- Participate in the facility's quality improvement process
- Advise on infection control issues and approve specific infection control policies to be incorporated into facility policies and procedures
- Help the facility provide a safe and caring environment
- Help promote employee health and safety
- Assist in development and implementation of employee health policies and programs

Education, Information, and Communication
- Promote a learning culture within the facility by educating, informing, and communicating
- Provide information to help the facility provide care consistent with current standards of practice
- Help the facility develop medical information and communication systems with staff, patients, and families and others
- Represent the facility to the professional and lay community on medical and patient care issues
- Maintain knowledge of the changing social, regulatory, political, and economic factors that affect medical and health services of long-term care patients
- Help establish appropriate relationships with other health care organizations

SOURCE: Adapted with permission from American Medical Directors Association. *Medical Director Roles and Responsibilities*. Copyright 2006. www.amda.com/about/roles.cfm (accessed Jan 2016).

---

exist. In this vein and taking a lead from the recent hospitalist practice movement in acute care hospitals, formal creation of postacute and long-term care specialists has been proposed, a concept that has been put into practice in the Netherlands. Closed-staff models are thought to deliver a higher intensity and quality of care in part because of the integration of the physician into the nursing-home facility culture, which ultimately improves interdisciplinary communication and treatment. Emerging evidence suggests that quality of clinical outcomes and hospitalization rates for nursing-home residents may be lower in facilities that employ a limited number of committed physicians (SOE=B). In one study, physicians who spent >85% of their total practice time in nursing homes had a 50% lower rate of potentially preventable hospitalizations than those physicians devoting ≤5% of their practice to nursing-home care. In another study, the quality of prescribing in the nursing home was positively correlated with enhanced nurse-physician communication and with regular interprofessional team discussions.

Historically, a paucity of credible role models for physicians in training also contributed to a lack of interest and involvement in long-term care issues. However, use of the nursing home as an academic training site can offer important exposure to this practice opportunity and professional role models and may help to stimulate interest among trainees. The American Medical Director's Association has recently developed a set of 26 competencies specific to attending physicians practicing in the postacute and long-term care setting (Table 21.5). These competencies will serve

Table 21.4—Brief Summary of Selected Medicare and Medicaid Requirements for Long-Term Care Facilities

Tag Number	Subject	Regulation	Guideline
F309	Quality of care	CFR 483.25	Each resident must receive and the facility must provide the necessary care and services to attain or maintain the highest practicable physical, mental, and psychological well-being, in accordance with the comprehensive assessment and plan of care. "Highest practicable" is defined as the highest level of functioning and well-being possible, limited only by the individual's presenting functional status and potential for improvement or reduced rate of functional decline.
F319-320	Quality of care: mental and psychosocial functioning	CFR 483.25(f)	Based on the comprehensive assessment of a resident, a facility must ensure that a resident who displays mental or psychosocial adjustment difficulty receives appropriate treatment and services to correct the assessed problem and a resident whose assessment did not display a pattern of decreased social interaction and/or withdrawn, angry, or depressive behaviors, unless that residents' clinical condition demonstrates that such a pattern is unavoidable.
F329-331	Medications, appropriate and unnecessary	CFR 483.25(I)(1)	Residents' medications regimens must be free of unnecessary drugs. These are defined as "those given without indication, at excessive doses, for excessive duration, without adequate monitoring, or in setting of significant adverse reaction."
F385-386	Physician services	CFR 483.40	It is the attending physician's responsibility to participate in the resident's assessment and care planning, monitoring changes in the resident's medical status and providing consultation or treatment when called by the facility. At scheduled visits, the physician must review the total plan of care; write, sign, and date a progress note; and sign and date all orders.
F501	Medical director, required duties	CFR 483.75(i)	Each facility must designate a physician to serve as medical director. The medical director is responsible for implementation of resident-care policies and the coordination of care in the facility.

SOURCE: Adapted with permission from the American Medical Directors Association. *Synopsis of Federal Regulations in the Nursing Facility.* Copyright 2010.

to frame a formal curriculum and possibly lead to future certification. Research is planned that will examine the link between these new competencies and relevant clinical outcomes.

FACTORS ASSOCIATED WITH NURSING-HOME PLACEMENT

Although there is a significant chance of being admitted to a nursing home with increasing age, other factors, such as low income, poor family supports (especially lack of spouse and children), and low social activity have been associated with institutionalization (SOE=B). Cognitive and functional impairments have also predicted nursing-home placement. Interestingly, for patients with dementia, education and caregiver support have been shown to delay the need for nursing-home placement for up to 1 year (SOE=B). The range of long-term care services that are now available (ie, skilled nursing, home care, assisted living) further increases the complexity of placement decisions. The use of formal (ie, paid-for) community services does not necessarily reduce the likelihood of nursing-home placement for patients with severe disabilities.

THE INTERFACE OF ACUTE AND LONG-TERM CARE

Approximately 1 in 5 Medicare beneficiaries are discharged from hospitals to a skilled-nursing facility. The number of hospital discharges to nursing homes and long-term care settings increased 35% between 1997 and 2008. Conversely, nursing-home residents have high rates and frequently use emergency department and acute hospital care. Nursing-home residents account for >2.2 million emergency department visits annually in the United States, or 1.6 emergency department visits for every nursing-home resident. The Office of the Inspector General reported that in 2011, one-quarter of Medicare nursing-home residents experienced hospitalizations at a cost of $14.3 billion. Although most nursing-home residents who were hospitalized were hospitalized once (63.8%), many experienced multiple transfers with 20% having two transfers, 7% three transfers, and 5% four or more transfers. Hospital admissions from nursing homes cost a third more than the average Medicare hospital admission. The most frequent causes of hospital admission by nursing-home residents include septicemia, pneumonia, and congestive heart failure.

Unfortunately, the transitions between acute and long-term care settings are often complicated by suboptimal information transfer. Illegible or nonexistent transfer summaries; omission of prescribed medications; and the lack of documentation of advanced directives, psychosocial information, and behavioral issues are but a few of the information gaps commonly reported. In 2006, almost one-fourth of Medicare beneficiaries (23.5%) discharged from the hospital to the skilled-nursing facility were readmitted to the acute hospital within 30 days at a cost to Medicare of $4.34 billion dollars. Five conditions account for most (78%) of these rehospitalizations: congestive heart failure, respiratory infection, urinary tract infection, sepsis, and electrolyte imbalances.

A better understanding of contributing factors and best practices to target reduction in the high rates of hospital admission and readmission by nursing-home residents are needed. Health care financing reform, including bundled payments as part of accountable care partnerships, have drawn additional attention to this issue. Several recent quality initiatives have focused on early identification of change in condition in the nursing home, as well as improved transition of care to and from the nursing home. One example is the "Interventions to Reduce Acute Care Transfers" program, also known as INTERACT (http://interact2.net/ [accessed Jan 2016]). INTERACT is a quality improvement project developed with the support of CMS to improve the early identification, assessment, documentation, and communication about changes in the status of residents of skilled-nursing facilities, with the goal of reducing the frequency of transfers from the nursing home to the acute hospital. The INTERACT II intervention, which includes communication tools, clinical care paths, and advanced care planning tools, has resulted in a 17% reduction in acute-hospital admissions in a group of community-based nursing homes.

QUALITY ISSUES AND LEGISLATION INFLUENCING CARE IN THE NURSING HOME

In 1983, a published Institute of Medicine report documented significant deficiencies in the care of nursing-home residents and influenced the passage of the Omnibus Budget Reconciliation Act (OBRA) in 1987. As the first major revision of nursing-home legislation in over 20 years and the first detailed source of clinical expectations for nursing-home care, OBRA has had significant impacts on medical care in nursing homes. OBRA set new, higher standards for quality of care provided in nursing facilities certified for reimbursement under Medicare and Medicaid (which includes most skilled-nursing facilities) by CMS. CMS pays Medicare claims and interprets legislation into written regulations for skilled-nursing facilities. CMS interprets federal statutes and also writes regulations for Medicaid that are administered by each state's Medicaid program. Federal regulations, including those pertaining to long-term care, are compiled in the *Code of Federal Regulations*. Each federal regulation is given a tag number, often called "F-tags." To qualify for federal reimbursement under Medicare and Medicaid, facilities must comply with these CMS regulations. OBRA regulations targeted many residents' rights issues, including setting limits on restraint use and regulating use of psychoactive medications. In the years since OBRA was instituted, the use of restraints in nursing homes has decreased significantly, registered nurse staffing has increased, and training requirements for certified nursing assistants have been established. Assisted-living facilities do not operate under such all-inclusive mandates, which some believe contribute to the significant variability of care practices and quality of care in that setting.

OBRA also mandates comprehensive periodic assessments of all nursing-home residents. This is accomplished by the Minimum Data Set (MDS), which surveys a host of clinical issues thought to directly relate to the quality of resident care and thus considered pertinent to effective care planning. A resident's medical regimen must be consistent with the assessment compiled in the MDS. CMS also uses the MDS for individual facilities to compile nursing-facility quality measures data, which are reported publicly on the CMS website (www.medicare.gov/NHcompare/Home.asp) (accessed Jan 2016). Measures include outcomes data such as prevalence of pain, pressure ulcers, weight loss, and depression, as well as rates of vaccination, restraint use, and urinary tract infection. Although publication of these measures is intended to offer a way to compare facilities, it has been criticized for lack of standardization of data to account for the substantial variability in disability and medical acuity between different facilities. For quality measures of nursing homes that are publicly reported by CMS, see Table 21.2. The MDS was updated to version 3.0 by CMS in 2010 and resulted in changes in the publicly reported quality measures. Included in the measures of nursing-home quality publicly reported by CMS is the 5-star quality rating for nursing homes. This rating was developed to help consumers, families, and caregivers make comparisons about nursing homes and areas of strength or concern. The 5-star rating is based on three sources of data: the facility's health inspection survey results, staffing levels, and quality measures. Beginning in 2015, nursing-home ratings will also take into account the percentage of a facility's residents who are prescribed antipsychotic drugs. Further, staffing levels will be reported quarterly rather than annually and use a system that allows verification with payroll data. The focus on antipsychotic medication is consistent with a recent Office of Inspector General report that highlighted the inappropriate use of certain drug classes in nursing home-residents.

Pay-for-performance (P4P) programs in nursing homes have been conducted over the past several years but have met with limited success. In a Medicaid-sponsored P4P of 8 states spanning 8 years, the total number of nursing-home deficiencies increased, while there was an inconsistent change in quality measures. The CMS sponsored Nursing Home Value Based Purchasing Demonstration (NHVBP) involved 3 states and was conducted between 2009–2012. Performance was based on nurse staffing, MDS-derived quality outcomes, survey deficiencies, and potentially avoidable hospitalization rates. Overall, quality was unchanged by the NHVBP demonstration.

Adherence to regulations is assessed by mandatory site visit surveys. These surveys are mandated every 15 months but occur on average every 12 months. During traditional nursing home surveys, facility procedures and records are reviewed, and quality of care and quality of life for residents are observed. CMS recently began national implementation of the Quality Indicator Survey process (QIS) during regulatory survey. QIS is a computer-assisted, two-staged long-term survey process used to systematically review nursing-home requirements and objectively investigate any triggered regulatory areas. In the QIS, a sample of residents, developed from census, admission, and MDS data, is created and used to strategically perform interviews, observations, and chart reviews that calculate indicators of quality of care and quality of life in that facility. Those areas, as well as a group of standard facility-level tasks, are then assessed in an in-depth fashion.

Failure to meet regulatory standards for care is cited in a "deficiency." Penalties imposed for deficiencies depend on the nature and severity of the deficiency and can range from implementation of a corrective action plan to monetary fines, limits on facility admissions, or even facility closure. Each deficiency is rated according to a standard matrix of scope and severity. Severity refers to the level of harm to the resident or residents involved from no harm with minimal potential for harm to immediate jeopardy to health or safety. Scope of a deficiency may be isolated, a pattern, or widespread in nature. Scope and severity scores follow an alphabetical pattern from least severity "A" to greatest severity "L." Inspections can also occur at any time in between mandated surveys as a result of a complaint received by the state. In 2012, the mean number of deficiencies received by nursing homes during regulatory visits was 5.9, with 11.2% of these deficiencies relating to actual harm or immediate jeopardy of residents.

OBRA mandates that each individual in a nursing facility receive and be provided the necessary care and services to achieve and maintain "the highest practicable physical, medical, and psychological well-being" that can be obtained. The facility must ensure that the resident optimally improves or deteriorates only within the limits of that resident's right to refuse treatments and within the influence of their illnesses and normal aging. When a resident declines (or does not improve), a survey team may investigate whether the decline was avoidable. A decline may be determined unavoidable if the resident has been given a careful and thorough assessment, which directs the resident's care plan. The interventions included in the care plan should be evaluated and revised as necessary. Documentation of a resident's reasonable prognosis and the risks versus reasonable expected benefits of treatments has an important role in care planning in the nursing home, particularly given current regulatory and liability influences.

OBRA requires that a state agency must screen and preapprove the admission of individuals with intellectual disability or serious mental illness to a nursing facility (F285). This screening is done to ensure that the facility can provide appropriate programs and services to meet the individual's needs. Residents readmitted to a nursing facility from a hospital, or those admitted from a hospital with an anticipated stay of <30 days who require treatment at the nursing facility for the same problem for which they were hospitalized, are exempt from screening.

The quality of physician practice in the nursing home is, in many ways, determined by the medical director. CMS requires that every skilled-nursing facility designate a licensed physician to serve as medical director (F501). The United States is the only country in the world that requires a nursing home medical director. The medical director has many roles (Table 21.3) that differ from the roles of the attending physician and include coordination of medical care that meets current standards for care in the nursing home. Integral to the medical director's role is providing guidance in development and implementation of resident-care policies. The medical director must ensure compliance with all relevant state and federal guidelines and work with the nursing-home administrator and director of nursing to foster effective team care and continuing staff education. The medical director of a nursing home works closely with all disciplines and must be constantly aware of the unique interplay between laws, regulations, organization, and delivery of medical care. Certification for medical directors (CMD) after completion of a formal course is offered through the American Medical

Table 21.5—Competencies for Attending Physicians in Post-Acute and Long-Term Care Medicine

Foundation
- Addresses conflicts that may arise in the provision of clinical care by applying principles of ethical decision-making.
- Provides and supports care consistent with (but not based exclusively on) legal and regulatory requirements.
- Interacts with staff, patients, and families effectively by using appropriate strategies to address sensory, language, health literacy, cognitive, and other limitations.
- Demonstrates communication skills that foster positive interpersonal relationships with residents, their families, and members of the interdisciplinary team (IDT).
- Exhibits professional, respectful, and culturally sensitive behavior toward residents, their families, and members of the IDT.
- Addresses patient/resident care needs, visits, phone calls, and documentation in an appropriate and timely fashion.

Medical Care Delivery Process
- Manages the care of all postacute patients/long-term care residents by consistently and effectively applying the medical care delivery process, including recognition, problem definition, diagnosis, goal identification, intervention, and monitoring of progress.
- Develops, in collaboration with the IDT, a person-centered, evidence-based medical care plan that strives to optimize quality of life and function within the limits of an individual's medical condition, prognosis, and wishes.
- Estimates prognosis based on a comprehensive patient/resident evaluation and available prognostic tools, and discusses the conclusions with the patient/resident, his or her family (when appropriate), and staff.
- Identifies circumstances in which palliative and/or end-of-life care (eg, hospice) may benefit the patient/resident and family.
- Develops and oversees, in collaboration with the IDT, an effective palliative care plan for patients/residents with pain, other significant acute or chronic symptoms, or who are at the end of life.

Systems
- Provides care that uses resources prudently and minimizes unnecessary discomfort and disruption for patients/residents (eg, limited nonessential vital signs and blood glucose checks).
- Can identify rationale for and uses of key patient/resident databases (eg, the Minimum Data Set [MDS]) in care planning, facility reimbursement, and monitoring of quality.
- Guides determinations of appropriate levels of care for patients/residents, including identification of those who could benefit from a different level of care. Performs functions and tasks that support safe transitions of care.
- Works effectively with other members of the IDT, including the medical director, in providing care based on understanding and valuing the general roles, responsibilities, and levels of knowledge and training for those of various disciplines.
- Informs patients/residents and their families of their health care options and potential impact on personal finances by incorporating knowledge of payment models relevant to the postacute and long-term care setting.

Medical Knowledge
- Identifies, evaluates, and addresses significant symptoms associated with change of condition, based on knowledge of diagnosis in individuals with multiple comorbidities and risk factors.
- Formulates a pertinent and adequate differential diagnosis for all medical signs and symptoms, recognizing atypical presentation of disease, for postacute patients and long-term care residents.
- Identifies and develops a person-centered medical treatment plan for diseases and geriatric syndromes commonly found in postacute patients and long-term care residents.
- Identifies interventions to minimize risk factors and optimize patient/resident safety (eg, prescribes antibiotics and antipsychotics prudently, assesses the risks and benefits of initiation or continuation of use of physical restraints, urinary catheters, and venous access catheters).
- Manages pain effectively and without causing undue treatment complications.
- Prescribes and adjusts medications prudently, consistent with identified indications and known risks and warnings.

Personal QAPI
- Develops a continuous professional development plan focused on postacute and long-term care medicine, using relevant opportunities from professional organizations (American Medical Directors Association, American Geriatrics Society, American Academy of Family Physicians, American College of Physicians, Society of Hospital Medicine, American Academy of Hospice and Palliative Medicine), licensing requirements (state, national, province), and maintenance of certification programs.
- Utilizes data (eg, Physician Quality Reporting System indicators, MDS data, patient satisfaction) to improve care of their patients/residents.
- Strives to improve personal practice and patient/resident results by evaluating patient/resident adverse events and outcomes (eg, falls, medication errors, health care–acquired infections, dehydration, rehospitalization).

SOURCE: Adapted with permission from American Medical Directors Association. Competencies for Post-Acute and Long-Term Care Medicine Setting of Care: SNF/NF. Available at www.amda.com/strategic-initiatives/AMDA_Physician_Competencies.pdf (accessed Jan 2016).

Directors Association. Over 3,000 physicians have the "CMD" designation. Presence of certified medical directors has been found to be an independent predictor of quality in U.S. nursing homes (SOE=B).

Additional regulations require medication review at regular intervals and that each resident's medication regimen includes no unnecessary drugs. Clinical documentation must demonstrate the indication for all drugs, especially psychoactive medications. Unnecessary medications are those given without indication, at excessive dosages, for excessive duration, without adequate monitoring, or when there has been a significant adverse event. Residents without a history of antipsychotic drug use should not be treated with antipsychotic medication unless the drug is required to treat a specific diagnosed condition (eg, schizophrenia, Huntington disease, psychosis) that is documented in the medical record. For those residents receiving psychoactive medications, gradual dosage reductions and behavioral interventions are mandated unless a clinical contraindication exists and is documented in the medical record. In 2012, CMS convened "The National Partnership to Improve Dementia Care in Nursing Homes." This initiative joined efforts of federal and state partners, nursing homes and other providers, advocacy groups, and caregivers to improve the quality of care for adults with dementia, including a specific target of appropriate care and use of antipsychotic medications for nursing-home patients. As of the second quarter of 2014, the national prevalence of antipsychotic medication use among long-stay residents had reduced by more than 18%. CMS anticipates a 30% reduction in the unnecessary use of antipsychotics by the end of 2016.

A thorough evaluation of medication regimens, done monthly by a pharmacist, is also required. This monthly medication review is intended to minimize adverse events and unnecessary medication use and to ensure proper medication monitoring. A facility must ensure that the medication error rate is <5% and that no significant medication errors occur. No errors should occur that cause a resident discomfort or jeopardize his or her health and safety. Care in assisted-living facilities does not have the same regulations that guide care in nursing homes. For a brief summary of selected regulations influencing medical and psychiatric care in skilled-nursing facilities, see Table 21.4.

The 2010 Affordable Care Act included a provision that will require all 16,000 nursing homes in the nation certified by CMS to establish Quality Assurance and Performance Improvement (QAPI) programs in the near future. Adding performance improvement to the traditional quality assurance required in nursing homes significantly expands the level and scope of facility activities not only to correct defects but also to be proactive in preventing problems and optimizing performance throughout all levels of the organization. A number of tools have are available to assist nursing homes in their preparation for QAPI planning and implementation, including CMS technical assistance and resources for QAPI and quality improvement organizations.

MEDICAL CARE ISSUES

The care of nursing-home residents has become more complex over the past several years, commensurate with an increasing level of medical acuity in an environment continually constrained by lack of adequate resources. Comprehensive, ongoing assessment within an interdisciplinary framework works to restore function, when possible, and to enhance quality of life.

Clinical challenges abound in the nursing home, created, in part, by the atypical and subtle presentation of illness so characteristic of residents with profound physical and psychologic frailty. In addition, limited access to biotechnology, frequent dependence on nonphysicians such as nurses and nurse assistants for resident evaluation, and the high prevalence of cognitive impairment in a setting of intense regulatory oversight all complicate the medical decision-making process. Families of nursing-home residents often remain an integral part of the overall care plan and may require specific educational and psychosocial supports. Ethical and legal concerns are also very common, particularly those regarding end-of-life, feeding, hydration, and resident rights issues. Finally, the heterogeneity among nursing-home residents demands an individualized, thoughtful, and reasoned approach to each individual.

Problems in nursing homes that commonly require unique diagnostic and treatment strategies include infections, falls, malnutrition, dehydration, incontinence, behavioral disturbances, the use of multiple medications, and prevention and screening. For example, determining the risks and benefits of tube feedings for frail nursing-home residents must be predicated not only on underlying illness but also on the resident's and family's value system, the resources available in the nursing facility, and staff acceptance of the intervention. Given that the evidence for and against enteral feeding in nursing-home residents is controversial (ie, benefits are not well established), therapy must be individualized. Many of the problems commonly encountered in the nursing home result when multiple comorbidities interact with a host of environmental factors, all of which may be only partially remediable. Unfortunately, expectations of family, as well as regulations, often do not account for these complexities and commonly engender "risk-averse" behavior that may be counter to autonomy and optimal quality of life.

Over the last 40 years, many have advocated for culture change in nursing-home care from institutional, provider-centered models to person-centered models that are driven by choice and self-determination of older adults and their caregivers. Transformed nursing-home culture includes resident direction of activities; homelike atmosphere; close relationships between staff, residents, and families; empowered staff members who are trained to respond to residents' needs; and collaborative decision making with residents about care. Several culture-change initiatives, including the Eden Alternative, the Wellspring Model, and the Green House Model, have been described. The Eden Alternative focused on development of collaborative partnerships between caregivers and older adults and development of a human habitat with continued contact with plants, animals, and children. Wellspring developed learning collaborative alliances between nursing homes to share management, training, and data systems with the goal of implementing interdisciplinary best-care practices through empowerment of frontline workers. In the Green House Model, 6 to 10 older adults reside in small noninstitutional homes set in residential neighborhoods. Care in these homes is provided by empowered direct-care staff that accomplishes all care and meal preparation. Close relationships between staff and residents are developed in each of the models. Evidence to date suggests these models improve resident quality of life and employee satisfaction, while preserving or improving quality of care; however, additional research regarding the benefits and costs of culture change is needed.

Physician Practice in the Nursing Home

Physicians have traditionally had limited involvement in nursing homes. Perceptions of excessive regulations, paperwork, and limited reimbursement are further disincentives to nursing-home practice. In reality, the medical care of nursing-home residents is challenging and fulfilling, requiring excellent clinical skills as well as sensitivity to a variety of ethical, legal, and interdisciplinary issues. Medical interventions, whether curative, preventive, or palliative, demand an individualized approach that recognizes the complex interplay among resident, family, and staff needs. Further, the evidence on which to base treatment may be nonexistent.

The comorbidity present in most nursing-home residents commonly creates the need for multiple drug therapies, with attendant risk of complications. The prevalence of nursing-home residents who were prescribed ≥9 medications was reported as a quality measure for nursing facilities for many years, with 32% of all nursing-home residents falling into this group. With revisions to the MDS, this is no longer included in the regulated quality measures, in part reflecting that the use of multiple medications by nursing-home residents with prevalent comorbid illnesses cannot always be avoided. In fact, on average, nursing-home residents are prescribed 7 or 8 medications. The most common health conditions found in the nursing home for those ≥65 years old are dementia, heart disease, hypertension, arthritis, and stroke. The approaches to these and other illnesses have evolved dramatically and complicate treatment decisions when cost-effectiveness is increasingly considered a desirable goal. Clear documentation of the rationale for a given medication or intervention is the best way to protect against potential scrutiny; frequent discussion with the facility's consultant pharmacist is also helpful.

Physicians who schedule and structure their visits to the nursing home will benefit from the resultant efficiencies and will be more fully integrated into the health care team. Nurse practitioners and physician assistants have become increasingly involved in the primary care of nursing-home residents. Studies suggest that nurse practitioners and physician assistants who act in concert with the primary care physician as a coordinated team provide more intensive care to nursing-home residents and may decrease hospitalization rates while maintaining cost neutrality (SOE=A). For information regarding physician responsibilities, see Table 21.5 and the website of the American Medical Directors Association (www.amda.com).

Responsibilities encompass ongoing comprehensive assessment and coordination of care to ensure resident autonomy and safety as well as optimal physical and psychosocial function. Regulations mandate that the initial comprehensive visit for the purpose of certifying that a newly admitted nursing-home resident requires a skilled level of care be done by a physician. During this visit, physicians performs a thorough assessment, develops a plan of care, and writes appropriate orders for the nursing-home resident. Nurse practitioners may perform initial history and physical examination visits for long-term care residents who do not require a skilled level of care. Regulations mandate that nursing-home residents be seen for subsequent face-to-face medical visits every 30 days for the first 90 days after admission and then at least every 60 days thereafter. For these subsequent visits, a visit by a nonphysician provider may be substituted for every other physician visit. Additional medical visits should take place if acute medical needs or changes in condition develop. Medicare allows for physician reimbursement for evaluation and management activities for both nursing home regulatory visits and medically necessary visits to provide acute care. Availability of on-site medical providers can improve timeliness of acute medical care and decrease hospitalization rates.

Opportunities to improve medical care in nursing homes exist. Several studies have documented misdiagnoses, inappropriate interventions, and poor preventive care practices in nursing homes. Intensive research is underway to understand the processes necessary to integrate validated care guidelines into nursing homes in an effort to improve quality of care. The Office of Inspector General reported that 22% of Medicare beneficiaries experienced at least one harmful adverse event during a postacute nursing home stay. Over half (59%) of the adverse events were clearly or likely preventable and resulted in $2.8 billion spent on hospital readmissions for corrective treatment. The Office of Inspector General recommendations to reduce resident harm included strategies to develop more effective safety cultures, like those that have been used in hospitals.

Vaccination rates for eligible chronic-care nursing-home residents vary. Nationally, current vaccination rates in nursing homes are 94% for both influenza and pneumococcal vaccines. Vaccination programs for long-term care employees have also been taken as a primary prevention strategy for influenza in nursing facilities. Vaccination of employees is thought to decrease the influenza incidence in residents through decreased entry of influenza virus into facilities and decreased resident-to-resident transmission through staff. Unfortunately, health care worker vaccination rates are generally suboptimal. Although brief educational programs have been associated with increased acceptance of vaccines, improved understanding of individual and operational barriers to and facilitators of optimal immunization is needed.

Strategies have been developed that may enhance the quality of care in nursing homes. The commonly used special-care units, although conceptually attractive, have not consistently been shown to enhance quality of care apart from the involvement of individual professionals. Specific consultation services in the nursing home, however, may improve care practices and condition-specific resident outcomes, such as reduction of falls (SOE=A). In addition, an interactive educational program for physicians and nursing staff may improve practice, as has been demonstrated in programs to promote appropriate psychoactive drug use (SOE=B). Clinical practice guidelines for the care of nursing-home residents have been developed by the American Medical Directors Association (www.amda.com/) and the American Geriatrics Society (www.americangeriatrics.org).

Understanding each nursing-home resident's preference for care in the context of his or her underlying value system will undoubtedly improve overall quality.

According to the CDC, 65% of nursing-home residents have at least one advance care directive on record. Living wills and do-not-resuscitate orders are the most common advance directives, in place for 18% and 56%, respectively, of all nursing-home residents. Nursing-home residents >65 years old are more likely to have advance directives than their younger counterparts. White nursing-home residents are more likely than black nursing-home residents to have a living will (20% versus 6%) and do-not-resuscitate orders (61% versus 28%). This disparity in advance directives highlights the need for long-term care research that contributes to development of culturally sensitive approaches to advance care determination in the nursing home.

Durable power of attorney for health care documentation is present for 26% of nursing-home residents at admission and for 39% after 1 year of residence. Less than 5% of nursing-home residents have "do-not-hospitalize" orders, which document that the resident is not to be hospitalized even after developing a condition that is generally treated in the hospital. Although ongoing discussion of care preferences appears to be present in the nursing home, there likely remain ongoing opportunities for improved understanding of nursing-home resident preferences for care. A recent study found almost one-third of older adults receive care in a skilled-nursing facility in the last 6 months of life under the Medicare post-hospitalization benefit, and 1 in 11 older adults will die while enrolled in the skilled-nursing facility benefit. Although use of formal hospice programs to augment end-of-life care for long-term residents in nursing homes has increased in recent years, many have called for the provision of additional palliative care services to care for the diverse population receiving care in nursing-home settings. When ethical dilemmas arise in nursing-home care, institutional ethics committees can provide important guidance. The multidisciplinary nature of these committees ensures a spectrum of opinion and insight critical for nursing-home residents.

REFERENCES

- Coon JT, Abbott R, Rogers M, et al. Interventions to reduce inappropriate prescribing of antipsychotic medications in people with dementia resident in care homes: a systematic review. *J Am Med Dir Assoc*. 2014;15(10):706–718.

    Antipsychotic medications have often been used in the nursing-home setting to manage behavioral and psychological symptoms of dementia. Given studies demonstrating increased morbidity and mortality associated with this practice, a call has been made to decrease inappropriate prescribing of antipsychotics in those with dementia. This review systematically assesses the effectiveness of interventions in care homes, including educational, in-service, medication review, and multicomponent programs.

- Grabowski DC, O'Malley AJ, Afendulis CC, et al. Culture change and nursing home quality of care. *Gerontologist*. 2014;54 Suppl 1:S35–45.

    An important development in nursing-home care in recent decades has been the concept of "culture change." Improved quality of life has been emphasized in culture change; however, this study is the first to evaluate the impact on quality of care when transforming nursing homes from health care institutions to person-centered homes offering long-term care services. Culture change adopters were found to have less survey deficiencies, but no significant difference in MDS quality indicators.

- Katz PR, Wayne M, Evans J, et al. Examining the rationale and processes behind the development of AMDA's competencies for post-acute and long-term care medicine. *Annals of Long-Term Care: Clinical Care and Aging*. 2014;22(11):36–39.

    As the complexity of clinical care in nursing home settings increases, the association between physician care and quality in skilled-nursing homes is gaining interest. This article describes AMDA – The Society for Post-Acute and Long-Term Care Medicine's efforts to develop and define physician competencies necessary for attending physicians in nursing homes. These competencies offer objective metrics with the hope that physicians are adequately prepared to provide effective, high-quality care.

- Ouslander JG, Lamb G, Tappen R, et al. Interventions to reduce hospitalizations from nursing homes: evaluation of the INTERACT II collaborative quality improvement project. *J Am Geriatr Soc*. 2011;59(4):745–753.

    This study evaluates the INTERACT, a multisite quality improvement program designed to improve the early identification, assessment, documentation, and communication about changes in condition of residents in skilled-nursing facilities with the goal of reducing avoidable transfers to the acute hospital. Nursing homes highly engaged in the program had a 24% reduction in hospital admissions. Since this publication, the INTERACT program has been adopted by many nursing facilities in an effort to improve resident care.

- Tolson D, Rolland Y, Katz PR, et al. An international survey of nursing homes. *J Am Med Dir Assoc*. 2013;4(7):459–462.

    A variety of models of nursing-home care exist. This international survey of nursing-home care identifies frequent use of social or nursing-home models with engagement of advanced practice nurses.

- Zimmerman S, Anderson WL, Brode S, et al. Systematic review: effective characteristics of nursing homes and other residential long-term care settings for people with dementia. *J Am Geriatr Soc*. 2013;61(8):1399–1409.

    This study compares the health and psychosocial outcomes of those with dementia and their informal caregivers in nursing home and other long-term residential care settings to identify characteristics associated with the most effective care. Although additional research is sorely needed in this arena, evidence supports the use of pleasant sensory stimulation in reducing agitation for those with dementia.

Suzanne M. Gillespie, MD, RD, CMD, FACP
Paul R. Katz, MD, CMD, AGSF

CHAPTER 22—COMMUNITY-BASED CARE

KEY POINTS

- Home care will play an increasingly important role as health care reform continues, helping to keep people living in their homes longer.

- Community-based services that do not require a change of residence may often be used as an alternative to hospitalization or institutionalization. The availability of such services vary strongly depending on location, financial reimbursements, and state policies.

- Health care providers should be familiar with the types of community-based care services available in their own communities to help advise patients and their families about care options.

HOME CARE

Home care organizations include home health care agencies, home care aide organizations, and hospices. Some of these organizations are Medicare certified, which allows providers to bill Medicare for reimbursement. Agencies that are not Medicare certified cannot be reimbursed through Medicare.

Approximately 12 million people received home care in 2009 at a cost of $72 billion dollars. For a large number of these people, home care has the potential to improve their quality of life and avoid unnecessary hospitalization or institutionalization.

Under a cost-based reimbursement system, home care grew rapidly in the 1980s and 1990s. This growth coincided with the initiation of the prospective payment system (diagnostic-related groups [DRGs]) for hospitals, which resulted in patients being discharged sooner from hospitals and an increased need for home services. New technologies created the possibility of providing therapies in the home that were previously available only in hospitals or nursing homes. Because of an increase in costs, Congress placed limits of Medicare spending as mandated in the Balanced Budget Act of 1997, which led to development of a prospective payment system (PPS) for home services. By the end of 2001, the number of Medicare-certified home care agencies had declined by 30.4%, many as a result of financial pressures. However, with implementation of a PPS, the financial stability has allowed growth of Medicare-certified agencies to well over 10,000 agencies nationally. The Outcome and Assessment Information Set (OASIS) is a tool that classifies patients into home health–related groups (HHRGs). The OASIS instrument is completed by the home care agency and tracks several domains of the patient's functional status and medical needs. Like the DRGs, the HHRGs provide the basis for agency reimbursement and are based on severity of the patient's illness, disabilities, and nursing needs. They include a payment adjustment based on location in the United States. The instrument is also intended to provide a means of uniformly measuring quality of care across all home care agencies. Although there are 10 HHRGs, comorbid conditions are considered in the ultimate reimbursement. The OASIS assessment and the International Classification of Disease (ICD) codes must be accurate to ensure that reimbursement matches the needs of the patient being served. Like other sectors of the health care system, home care agencies are charged with developing cost-effective, high-quality care despite diminishing reimbursement.

Medicare coverage of home health services require that a patient meets the criteria for being homebound and have a need for a skilled service provided by a licensed nurse or rehabilitation professional. To be considered homebound, a patient's condition makes leaving home a "considerable and taxing effort." For example, leaving home may require extensive assistance such as using a wheelchair or walker, needing special transportation, or getting help from another person. The patient may still be able to leave the home for nonmedical reasons as long as these occurrences are "infrequent and short in duration" such as for attending a religious service or special family event.

Home care services paid under Medicare must be provided by a Medicare-certified home health agency. To compare quality measures of agencies, one may use the Home Health Compare tool available at Medicare.gov (www.medicare.gov/homehealthcompare).

The Primary Provider's Role in Home Care

Home care often requires an interprofessional team that is generally composed of nurses, rehabilitation professionals (speech, physical, occupational, and respiratory), social workers, personal care aides, home medical equipment suppliers, and informal caregivers. Physicians certify and recertify the plan of care and the need for individual therapy services for Medicare-covered home health services. Billing codes and requirements for these services may be found at www.cms.gov/Medicare/Medicare-Fee-for-Service-Payment/HomeHealthPPS/coding_billing.html (accessed Jan 2016). The documentation requirements for billing allow activities over multiple days in a month to be combined. Reimbursement can vary in different parts of the country by as much as 20% based on a Medicare adjustment called "Geographical Practices Cost Indices."

Nurse practitioners cannot certify home care services under Medicare, but they are authorized by law to provide both primary care and registered nurse services in the home. Reimbursement for these services depends on the type of care provided. If the nurse practitioner provides a service described by a Current Procedural Terminology (CPT) code made necessary by an ICD diagnosis to a homebound patient, then it is billable to Medicare Part B as a medical service. It does not require a physician's order and could be billed directly using the nurse practitioner's provider number. Nursing services provided by the nurse practitioner are billable under Medicare Part A, in which case the nurse is working as an employee of a certified home care agency that would bill for these services using the agency's Medicare provider number.

House calls can add an important dimension to the primary provider's knowledge of the patient's circumstances, function, and environment. Home evaluation can identify additional problems not readily apparent in office-based assessment. House calls have the additional benefit of reducing the burden for patients who have difficulty getting transportation. Section 3024 of the Affordable Care Act created the Independence at Home Demonstration, which is taking place for 3 years beginning in 2012. Under this demonstration project, 10,000 home-limited Medicare beneficiaries with multiple chronic conditions are provided longitudinal primary care and care coordination services by teams of provider groups headed by physicians or nurse practitioners. Care coordination is comprehensive, involving both social service and medical needs. If participant groups meet the savings target of 5%, they will be eligible for varying levels of shared savings to help finance the incremental costs of the program.

Medical care in the home may be provided as part of an ongoing office-based program, as an extension of hospitalization through a postacute care program, or as a free-standing entity. Regardless of the method chosen, the organization of the home care program must be well conceived to maximize effectiveness and efficiency and to remain financially solvent. Current regulations allow house calls to be provided by physicians, nurse practitioners, and physician assistants. Their services are often delivered as part of those of an interprofessional team.

For house calls to be financially feasible for clinicians, thorough documentation is key to receiving reimbursement. There are no specific restrictions on the number of visits, as long as sufficient justification for evaluation, management, and medical necessity is included in the progress notes. As is the case with other outpatient visits, the provider must identify historical data, physical examination findings, diagnostic test results, and an assessment that reflects an active diagnosis. Evaluations of the patient's function, caregiver issues, and the medical plan of care are also critical elements of the documentation. There are specific CPT codes for house calls and domiciliary care. When visits are prolonged, time codes can sometimes be used to justify an enhanced reimbursement.

Patient Assessment

Homebound patients generally have significant functional impairment. Comprehensive geriatric assessment is particularly valuable in this setting to establish a baseline, monitor the course of illness, and evaluate the effects of intervention. However, assessment in the home has some important differences from office-based assessment.

During a home visit, the patient's daily environment can be assessed for safety in the context of the patient's unique needs. Performance-based functional assessment can focus on the practical aspects of performing ADLs by directly observing bathing, dressing, and transferring. Challenges and safety issues can be identified, and the assessor can evaluate the caregiver's abilities to support the patient's needs. The caregiver's needs for counseling, training, support, and education can also be identified and addressed.

Environmental modifications can be recommended to improve function. For example, modifications of the bathtub, a hand-held shower, a shower seat, grab bars, and a bedside commode can improve the patient's quality of life and functioning. Barriers to wheelchairs and walkers (eg, door sills) can be identified and removed. Chair lifts and outdoor ramps can help patients circumvent stairs. Occupational therapy consultation can be particularly useful in identifying other personal care needs and assistive devices for performing ADLs such as dressing, eating, and housekeeping chores. Numerous home safety checklists are available online to help a reviewer assess the home. Additional technological additions to improve home safety, including personal emergency response systems (in which a person pushes a button for emergency assistance), can help aid the homebound patient.

Limitations of Home Care

Most older adults would prefer to remain in their own home, but certain situations arise that make institutional care a more appropriate choice than in-home care. For example, caregivers in the home may not be available or able to safely or adequately meet the needs of the patient. Unstable medical conditions that require frequent laboratory testing, respiratory interventions,

IV medications, or very frequent dressing changing, may make institutional care a better choice than home care. Additionally, the features of the home setting may make mobility and completion of ADLs unsafe. Another consideration is the substantial cost of home care beyond what is covered by a patient's insurance. Out-of-pocket expenses for additional services may be prohibitive, making a nursing facility a more feasible option for patients and their families.

Liability and Legal Issues

As in other areas in the practice of medicine, clinicians are potentially liable for adverse outcomes in home care. It is important to maintain accurate and thorough documentation of the patient's needs, conditions, assessments, and care plans. Clinicians must also ensure that the patient meets the defined criteria for being home bound. Inaccurate certificates of medical necessity for home care could lead to charges of Medicare fraud. All home care forms should be carefully reviewed before they are signed.

When providing home care, a provider must be sensitive to potential conflicts of interest. Federal legislation prohibits physicians from receiving financial benefit, compensation, or rebate for referring a patient to a home care provider. Further, physicians may not refer patients to home care companies in which the physician or the physician's family has a substantial financial interest. Legal advice should be sought by providers for any question of a potential conflict of interest.

Ethics and Decisions about Institutionalization

Two ethical themes commonly arise in home care. The first is the balance between patient autonomy and maintaining safety. The second involves issues surrounding mistreatment and neglect of older adults.

Respect for patient autonomy often dictates that the patient remain in the home as a result of the patient's (or surrogate decision maker's) choice. An assessment of the patient's capacity for decision making should be conducted if in question. Conflict arises when a patient's medical care or safety cannot be adequately maintained in the home, yet the patient insists on remaining in the home. It is difficult to balance respect for patient autonomy with prevention of medical neglect. In some situations when the patient has a terminal prognosis, a hospice referral can help provide additional services in the home and supports for both the patient and family. In cases when there is a neglectful or abusive situation, local Adult Protective Services should be notified.

COMMUNITY-BASED SERVICES NOT REQUIRING A CHANGE IN RESIDENCE

Adult Day Care

Adult day care is a community-based option that provides a wide range of social and support services in a congregate setting. Adult day care has become increasingly common. Providers of adult day care may offer a variety of services, ranging from simple nonskilled custodial care to more advanced skilled services. The availability of a registered nurse allows for onsite health services, clinical assessment and monitoring, and assistance with medication management. Adult day care is also used commonly for patients with dementia who need supervision and assistance with their ADLs while the primary caregiver is at work or tending to other responsibilities. Adult day care may be used on a regular basis or temporarily as a form of respite for the primary caregiver. In general, custodial adult day care is not covered by Medicare, although some costs may be covered by Medicaid or other insurers.

Day Hospitals

Day hospitals provide a broad range of skilled nursing care services, including parenteral antibiotic treatment, chemotherapy, and intensive rehabilitation. They may also be referred to as partial hospitalization programs. Most programs are housed in chronic care hospitals or rehabilitation centers. This arrangement allows for the provider to take advantage of in-house professional expertise and resources, while allowing the patient to return to his or her home or alternative living site after day treatments are complete. Services are covered under Medicare, with similar requirements to those surrounding home health care.

Day hospitals are most often used for 2 groups of patients: those needing multidisciplinary rehabilitation and those with psychiatric illnesses. A systematic review of day hospital care found no significant differences between day hospitals and alternative sources of care with respect to death, disability, or use of health services. Among those receiving care in a day hospital, there was a trend toward less functional decline and less hospital and institutional care.

The Program of All-inclusive Care for the Elderly (PACE)

PACE is a capitated model of care that provides comprehensive care services to frail, community-dwelling older adults by a single organization. The program provides all inpatient, outpatient, and long-term care services to frail older adults. Participants in the PACE program must be age ≥55 years old to meet state-defined requirements regarding their need for a nursing home level of care. Most will also qualify for Medicaid and Medicare; pooling funds from Medicaid and Medicare allows for comprehensive care to be planned and coordinated by the PACE interprofessional team. Without Medicaid and Medicare coverage, out-of-pocket expenses are high. Few private insurance programs provide a PACE program as part of their policies. The average PACE enrollee is 80 years old and has an average of 8 medical conditions and 3 ADL limitations. Half of PACE participants have dementia. As of 2015, there are 114 PACE programs operating in 32 states.

The goal of the PACE program is to keep the participant in the community for as long as is medically, socially, and financially feasible. The system, designed to be seamless, uses an interprofessional team of health care providers who know the patients and their caregivers well. The team provides care across the spectrum of hospital, home, alternative living situations, and institutional care. The team consists of a physician (often a geriatrician), nurse practitioner or physician assistant, clinic and home health nurses, social workers, physical, occupational, and speech therapists, pharmacists, dieticians, and transportation workers. The hub of care is the PACE center, which provides adult day health care. Other care and services may include, but are not limited to, respite care, transportation, prescription drug coverage, audiology, dentistry, optometry, and podiatry. Hospital and nursing home care may remain an option when necessary. The interprofessional team aims to provide assistance for the complex social needs as well as the medical needs of the participant.

The National PACE Association (NPA) studies and disseminates information on who PACE serves and the experience of individuals enrolled in PACE. NPA leads the effort to determine how the model should evolve in response to the rapid changes in the health care system.

In 1997, legislation was passed that changed the status of PACE from a demonstration program to a permanent provider under Medicare. PACE is an optional program under state Medicaid. There are more than 3 million dually eligible and nursing home–certifiable older adults in the United States that might benefit from PACE, but only a small fraction have enrolled. The growth of PACE has been slower than expected. Barriers to growth have included large start-up costs, insufficient supply of physicians, and the reluctance of patients to leave their primary care physician. NPA and CMS are evaluating modifications to the PACE model that would allow for community physician involvement as primary care providers (rather than using a PACE-paid, staff health maintenance organization model). This change in the model may result in more significant growth of PACE, because it could allow patients to keep their primary care physicians.

Managed Long-Term Care Programs

Managed long-term care programs are state-developed systems that aim to streamline the delivery of long-term services to people with chronic illnesses or disability who wish to stay in their homes and communities. These services, such as home care or adult day care, are provided through managed long-term care plans. These programs often include patients with Medicare and Medicaid and those who are eligible for both ("dually eligible"). Some of these programs have been referred to as "PACE without walls" and provide funding to test new models of care that build on the successful PACE model. States are partnering with entities such as home care agencies, nursing homes, hospitals, and integrated delivery systems to develop these programs. These programs provide financing through various capitated per member, per month payments. The aim of the managed long-term care programs is to provide safe and cost-effective care.

Home Hospital

The home hospital focuses on providing more complex care at home to older adults who would have been hospitalized for an acute care need. Patients receiving home-hospital care have access to nurses and physicians on a regular basis and for episodic care through an on-call system that allows problems to be addressed promptly. Such programs have been successfully implemented in nations with single-payer health systems. Studies conducted outside of the United States suggest that care is comparable for selected patients and that patient satisfaction is higher. The Veterans Administration Program at Home is a research-based home-hospital program run by physicians and nurses with the goal of preventing hospitalization or reducing the length of hospital stays. This program has demonstrated that complications such as falls and confusion are lower for patients in the home-hospital program than those who remain in hospital.

In-Home Technology

A wide array of technologies have been developed that can assist patients with ADLs and provide valuable information to caregivers. Devices such as personal emergency response systems, usually worn on the wrist or around the neck, can alert care providers that help is needed. Newer technologies can provide help in administering and tracking medications, monitoring

Table 22.1—Levels of Care

Adult day care	Structured day programs for older and disabled individuals permitting family caregivers time to pursue personal and employment opportunities while still maintaining affected individuals in the home setting.
Respite care	Temporary in-home assistance or placement in an alternative care setting of a disabled individual, usually for a period of days to weeks to allow a rest period for family caregivers. The patient is eventually returned to the home setting.
Assisted living	Residence that provides a variety of services designated to facilitate continued residence in the community for older and disabled persons. Assistance may include meals, administration of medication, homemaker services, transportation, health reminders, and personal care.
Board and care	Residence for infirm individuals who are able to ambulate or self-propel in a wheelchair. Meals, personal care, medicine administration, and group living environment are provided.
Nursing home/ long-term care	May provide custodial care for individuals whose functional disabilities or illnesses preclude a lower level of care. Some patients may also have skilled nursing needs, such as wound management, acute rehabilitation, and intravenous antibiotics.

and transmitting vital signs, and connecting patients to care providers through audio and visual telemedicine screens. Homes can be equipped with fully automated systems to adjust heating and lighting, to allow doors to be opened and closed with remote devices and to monitor activity throughout the home. Home robotics are under development that assist in ADLs or IADLs, including meal preparation and service. Computers and smartphones can also be used to connect patients through social networks to combat isolation and loneliness. The rapid development and interconnectivity of these tools will likely become increasingly important in the safe and efficacious delivery of home care services.

Telemedicine

Telemedicine is a rapidly growing modality of providing in-home health care services. Telemedicine can improve access to medical services that may not be readily available otherwise, such as in rural communities. A wide variety of technology and services are broadly included in the telemedicine category. Commonly used technologies include videoconferencing connections, usually through a web-connected camera or tablet computer, allowing a clinician to speak with and observe a patient to conduct a "virtual home visit." More advanced models use trained technicians on-site with a patient and incorporate higher resolution cameras and additional equipment (eg, stethoscope and otoscope attachments), while the off-site clinician can conduct a clinical assessment remotely. Some telemedicine services also include clinical monitoring (telehealth), mobile laboratory/phlebotomy, radiography, and home-nursing components, and as such begin to resemble a hospital-at-home type service. Telemedicine psychiatric services, including longitudinal medication management and treatment of depression, have been successfully implemented across many areas of the country. Current obstacles to the wider implementation of telemedicine include unclear or variable regulations across states (including licensing requirements across state lines), as well as marked variation in reimbursement for such services. A number of health care companies and insurers are now adopting telemedicine services as supplemental benefits, which can include urgent care visits and other medical consultations with health care providers. These services have varying levels of insurance coverage, copayment, and out-of-pocket costs to patients.

COMMUNITY-BASED SERVICES REQUIRING A CHANGE OF RESIDENCE

See Table 22.1.

Senior Villages and Senior Cohousing

Senior villages and cohousing are intentional communities where residents tend to be more independent, healthy, and active than in other forms of senior housing. These are typically not associated with provision of medical supervision or health care services.

Assisted-Living Facilities

Assisted-living facilities continue to grow in number as the U.S. population ages. They may be categorized or marketed under different titles (such as personal care homes, residential care homes, domiciliary care, and sheltered care) and are housing increasingly frail and medically complex individuals. The average length of stay for persons in an assisted-living facility is 2 years, and the most common reason for discharge is the need for nursing home care.

Assisted-living residences are characterized by some level of coordination or provision of personal care services, social activities, health-related services, and supervision in a home-like atmosphere that maximizes autonomy and privacy. Additional individual services may be provided at additional cost to the resident.

Table 22.2—Examples of Skilled Versus Nonskilled Nursing Needs

Skilled	Nonskilled
Acute rehabilitation	Dementia
Complex wound care	Functional dependency
Intravenous antibiotics	Incontinence
Titrating oxygen and insulin requirements	Lack of a caregiver

Assisted-living facilities may provide private or shared rooms or apartments. They may provide housekeeping, meals, and assistance with ADLs. Facilities vary with regard to whether they will accept residents with cognitive impairment or dementia. Many assisted-living facilities do not have a registered nurse on staff. State licensing requirements vary in terms of medication administration by facility personnel. Depending on the requirements, medication administration and management can be directed by staff with varying levels of training requirements or licensure.

In states where regulations do not require skilled care (see Table 22.2) in assisted-living facilities, home health skilled care is often provided as an external or independent service to the individual patient at the facility. In this context, the boundary between assisted-living and skilled-nursing facilities often becomes blurred.

Costs for assisted-living residences vary greatly, depending on the size of the unit, services provided, and location. Assisted living is covered in a growing number of long-term care insurance policies, but only a small minority of older Americans possess long-term insurance. Assisted living is not covered by Medicare, but certain services are paid under Supplementary Security Income and Social Services Block Grant programs. Some states reimburse or plan to reimburse for assisted-living services through Medicaid. In addition, states have the option to pay for certain assisted-living services under their Medicaid plans or to petition the Department of Health and Human Services for a waiver.

Group Homes

Group homes (including domiciliary care, single room occupancy residences, board-and-care homes, and some congregate living arrangements) are houses or apartments in which 2 or more unrelated people live together. Group homes vary in types of residents they serve, such as those with chronic mental illness or dementia. Residents share common living spaces but have their own bedrooms. Advantages of this arrangement include a lower cost of living and peer socialization. Independence and functional status are supported through the interdependence and relationships of the residents, although staff are present and assist residents to varying degrees. Resident-to-staff ratios may be higher than in other supported-living environments. Most group homes are run as for-profit businesses, and some states require licensing.

Adult Foster Care

Foster care homes generally provide room, board, and some assistance with ADLs by the sponsoring family or by paid caregivers, who customarily live on the premises. Perhaps the longest experience with adult foster care is in the state of Oregon, where it is used as an alternative to long-term care and institutionalization. Adult foster care has the advantages of maintaining frail older adults in a more home-like environment. Regulations for foster care vary by state, and some states require licensing. Some states provide coverage of adult foster care through their Medicaid programs.

Sheltered Housing

Sheltered housing is funded though the Older Americans Act and is offered as an option for housing subsidized through Section 8, Housing and Urban Development programs for seniors and disabled residents. Often, these arrangements are sheltered homes offering personal care assistance, housekeeping services, and meals. Programs may be supplemented by social work services and activities coordinators. Charges to clients are based on a sliding scale, which may cost up to 30% of income.

Continuing Care Retirement Communities

Continuing care retirement communities (CCRC) possess a variety of living options with the expectation that a resident will transition to those offering additional supports as needed over time. Such communities may include houses, condominiums, apartments, assisted living, home care, and skilled-nursing home care. Three financial models are common in such communities: the all-inclusive model, which provides total health care coverage, including long-term care; fee-for-service models, which match payments to the level of care; and the modified coverage model, which covers long-term care to a predetermined maximum. CCRCs often require an entry fee that may or may not be refundable, plus a variable monthly fee to pay for rent and supportive services. Funding for care in such communities is largely private (out-of-pocket or one-time investment), although some facilities have Medicare- or Medicaid-funded beds for skilled care.

REFERENCES

- Medicaid.gov Community-Based Long-Term Services & Supports. www.medicaid.gov/affordablecareact/provisions/community-based-long-term-services-and-supports.html (accessed Jan 2016).

    This website highlights a number of program and funding improvements authorized under the Affordable Care Act to help ensure that people can receive long-term care services and supports in their home or community.

- National PACE Association. www.npaonline.org/website/article.asp?id=4&title=Homepage (accessed Jan 2016).

    This website describes the PACE model, enumerates federal regulations, and provides a toolkit for states incorporating PACE into integrated care initiatives.

- The National Hospice and Home Care Survey 2007. Centers for Disease Control and Prevention (www.cdc.gov/nchs/nhhcs.htm) (accessed Jan 2016).

    This website provides extensive information about home care, utilization patterns, and surveys of workers and patients.

- The National Association for Home Care and Hospice (www.nahc.org) (accessed Jan 2016).

    This website has comprehensive information about the various forms of home care. It explains funding mechanisms, eligibility criteria for different patient populations, and the range of services offered.

Kristen Thornton, MD, FAAFP, AGSF, CWSP

Thomas V. Caprio, MD, MPH, MSHPE, FACP, CMD, HMDC, AGSF

CHAPTER 23—OUTPATIENT CARE SYSTEMS

KEY POINTS

- Outpatient interventions that improve the quality and outcomes of care of older adults include personalized care that is provided by a team in accordance with best practice, coordination among all providers and settings of care, consideration of the resources and environment of older adults, and inclusion of older adults as active partners in their care.

- For optimal cost-effectiveness, outpatient programs need to be targeted to patients identified in advance who are likely to be active participants in an intervention that is known to better meet their specific clinical needs.

- Broad dissemination of effective models of outpatient care for older adults may be aided by payment reform (eg, patient-centered medical homes and accountable care organizations) and initiatives to expand the geriatrics workforce.

Traditional outpatient care in the United States does not deliver the recommended standard of care to older adults for preventive services, chronic disease management, and geriatric syndromes. In addition, traditional approaches are associated with racial and ethnic disparities in preventive and chronic care. Realizing that a more proactive, patient-centered, and population-based approach is needed to improve the overall quality of geriatric care, several innovative outpatient care systems have been developed over the past two decades. This chapter describes new system approaches supported by evidence from clinical trials that demonstrated improved processes or outcomes of care, or both. Some new approaches integrate geriatrics into primary care, whereas others involve geriatric specialty care. Current methods for targeting these approaches to those older adults who are most likely to benefit are also reviewed.

A variety of new models of primary care aimed at improving the quality and outcomes of care for older adults have been studied and share many concepts with the new patient-centered medical home (PCMH) model of practice. In 2007, four primary care organizations—the American Academy of Pediatrics, the American College of Physicians, the American Association of Family Physicians, and the American Osteopathic Association—agreed on a set of Joint Principles of the PCMH (www.medicalhomeinfo.org/downloads/pdfs/JointStatement.pdf) (Table 23.1). The PCMH model builds on a strong evidence base showing that higher-quality care and lower costs can be achieved through greater emphasis on primary care.

The accountable care organization (ACO) is another model for delivery-system reform and is synergistic with the PCMH model. An ACO aims to manage the full continuum of care and to be accountable for the overall quality of care and costs for a defined population. An ACO is a provider-led organization and may take on many forms, including large integrated delivery systems, physician-hospital organizations, and independent practice associations. ACOs typically receive fee-for-service payment and if specified quality performance metrics are met, share in any cost savings achieved relative to a risk-adjusted projected spending target for their patient population. ACOs need a strong primary care foundation to succeed and, in turn, can provide important infrastructure beyond the primary care practice to facilitate the full realization of the PCMH model. Payment reform such as that proposed for PCMH and ACOs may offer a means for implementing the new system approaches to outpatient geriatric care discussed below.

GERIATRICS IN PRIMARY CARE

Enhanced Primary Care

Guided Care was designed to improve the quality of life and efficiency of resource use for older adults with multiple morbidities. Consistent with the PCMH approach, Guided Care aims to enhance primary care by infusing the operating principles of 7 chronic care innovations: disease management, self-management, case management, lifestyle modification, transitional care, caregiver education and support, and geriatric evaluation and management. A specially trained registered nurse works with assigned primary care physicians (PCPs) and office staff to provide the intervention to a panel of the practice's older patients at highest risk of requiring abundant health care services. Preliminary results from a multisite randomized controlled trial of Guided Care demonstrated improved quality of chronic care as measured by patient ratings, reduced family caregiver strain, increased patient and clinician satisfaction with care, and a trend toward less use of expensive health services in the first 8 months. Final trial results concluded that Guided Care reduced the use of home health care but had little effect on the use of other health services at 32 months. Interestingly, in the same trial and among the subgroup of Kaiser-Permanente patients, Guided Care reduced skilled-nursing facility admissions and days and also showed

Table 23.1—Joint Principles of the Patient-Centered Medical Home

- Each patient has an ongoing relationship with a personal physician.
- A physician-directed medical practice includes a team of individuals who collectively take responsibility for care.
- The practice adopts a "whole-person orientation" and provides or arranges for all the patient's health care needs.
- Care is coordinated across all elements of the complex health care system.
- Physicians engage in continuous quality improvement, and patients participate in decision making.
- Access to care is enhanced.
- Payment recognizes the added value provided to patients who have a patient-centered medical home (eg, via enhanced fee-for-service, care management fee, and/or shared savings).

a trend toward reduced hospital admissions and emergency department visits.

The Geriatric Resources for Assessment and Care of Elders (GRACE) model of primary care, now referred to as GRACE Team Care™, also includes each of the PCMH principles and could be described as an intensive "medical home" or complex care management program for high-risk older patients. GRACE provides patients with home-based comprehensive geriatric assessment and long-term care management by a nurse practitioner and social worker (GRACE support team) who collaborate with the office-based PCP and a geriatrics interprofessional team, including a geriatrician, pharmacist, and mental health liaison. Individualized care planning during weekly team meetings is guided by 12 care protocols for common geriatric conditions (eg, "difficulty walking/falls," "cognitive impairment," and "depression"). Three protocols are used in all patients: "medication management," "health maintenance," and "advance care planning." The nurse practitioner and social worker (employees of the primary care practice) review and prioritize the care plan with the patient's PCP, assure the plan is consistent with the patient's goals and preferences, and then implement it in collaboration with the PCP. The GRACE support team provides ongoing home-based care management, including coordination and continuity of care among all health care professionals and sites of care, facilitated by an electronic medical record and Web-based care management tracking system.

The GRACE model was developed specifically to improve the quality of care of a mixed-race population of seniors who are poor (many dually eligible for Medicare and Medicaid), have multiple comorbid conditions, and receive primary care in community-based health centers affiliated with an urban safety net healthcare system. Low-income seniors enrolled in a randomized controlled trial of the GRACE intervention, compared with usual care, received better quality of care for the geriatric conditions (eg, falls and depression) and general health processes (eg, preventive care and advance directives) targeted, had improvements in health-related quality-of-life measures, and made fewer emergency department visits over 2 years. In addition, hospital admissions were significantly reduced in the second year among GRACE patients identified at baseline as being at high risk of future hospitalization (SOE=A). Cost analysis of the GRACE intervention revealed that in the high-risk group, increases in chronic and preventive care costs were offset by reductions in acute care costs such that the intervention was cost neutral in the first 2 years. Two-year costs were higher in the low-risk group. The intervention reduced costs in the high-risk group during the post-intervention, or third, year because of continued lower hospital costs for GRACE patients than for those who received usual care.

Replication of the GRACE model has been successful in Medicare managed-care and Veterans Administration health care settings and demonstrated consistent improvements in quality of care and reductions in hospital utilization (http://graceteamcare.indiana.edu [accessed Jan 2016]). The GRACE model has been applied within a home visitation program, as a care transition intervention, and as a model for integrated medical and social services in seniors enrolled in the Medicaid Home and Community-Based Services waiver. Other successful models of enhanced primary care demonstrating reduced acute care utilization have also involved an interprofessional team that provides ongoing care management (usually including home visitation) in support of and integrated with the PCP (SOE=A).

The CareMore model was developed by a for-profit, privately held corporation in southern California to provide intensive management for the approximately 15% frail and chronically ill Medicare Advantage program members who accounted for 70% of medical costs. Although rigorous evaluations have not been reported in the peer-reviewed literature CareMore has demonstrated excellent performance on quality, utilization, cost, and patient satisfaction compared with the overall Medicare population. CareMore's risk-adjusted total per capita health spending has been reported as 15% below the national Medicare average. Patients enrolled in the CareMore model are assessed for chronic diseases and geriatric conditions and are managed by an outpatient care center team consisting of a nurse practitioner, nurse care manager, and medical assistant care extenders. CareMore hospitalists, termed "extensivists," provide inpatient care and postdischarge follow-up care in the Care Centers and in skilled-nursing facilities and conduct home visits as needed. CareMore makes intensive use of condition-specific protocols, team-based chronic disease care management programs, and a home monitoring technology system to transmit blood pressures, weights, and blood sugars to nurse care managers. Patients with their own PCP have their care co-managed between the CareMore teams and the PCP. The PCP's role includes the diagnosis and treatment of undifferentiated illnesses, diseases not covered under condition-specific protocols, and acute problems that do not require hospitalization.

Disease Management

Disease management programs focus health care delivery around a single disease with the goal of optimizing patient care for that condition. The most effective disease management programs are those that are integrated with the patient's primary care or specialty physician, or both. Heart failure and depression interventions are examples of disease management programs that lead to better outcomes in older adults and that are potentially cost saving. One notable heart failure program that was nurse-directed and multidisciplinary (geriatrician, cardiologist, nurse, dietitian, and social worker) reduced readmission rates and costs in hospitalized older adults with heart failure (SOE=A). Key components included comprehensive education of the patient and family, a prescribed diet, social-service consultation and planning for an early discharge, medication review, and intensive follow-up.

In the disease management program for late-life depression called Improving Mood—Promoting Access to Collaborative Treatment (IMPACT), patients had access to a depression care manager (a specially trained nurse or psychologist), supervised by a psychiatrist and a primary care liaison physician, who offered education, care management, and support of antidepressant drug therapy prescribed by the patient's PCP or a brief psychotherapy for depression. In a large multicenter clinical trial, depressed patients who received the IMPACT intervention were more likely than patients who received usual care to be given guideline-concordant depression care and to recover from depression (SOE=A).

A collaborative care model developed for older adults with Alzheimer disease has demonstrated improvements in the quality of care and in behavioral and psychological symptoms of dementia among primary-care patients (SOE=A). In this program, known as the Aging Brain Care Medical Home, an advanced practice nurse supported by an interprofessional team (psychologist, neuropsychologist, geriatrician, and geriatric psychiatrist) served as the care manager working with the patient's family caregiver and PCP. The team used standard protocols to initiate treatment and to identify, monitor, and treat behavioral and psychological symptoms of dementia with an emphasis on nonpharmacologic approaches to management.

Outpatient Consultation

Comprehensive geriatric assessment (CGA) is a process intended to determine a patient's medical, psychosocial, and functional capabilities and limitations, with the goal of developing an overall plan for treatment and long-term follow-up. Because CGA typically requires highly trained teams of geriatricians, geriatric nurse clinicians, physical and occupational therapists, geriatric psychiatrists, and social workers, it is expensive and time consuming. Success generally requires the geriatric team to take over the direct care of the patient. An extended period of intensive team involvement with ongoing care is essential to ensure the efficacy of the intervention. When the geriatric team assumes a purely consultative role (ie, without a role in implementing the recommendations), CGA is unlikely to be successful in improving patient outcomes (SOE=A). However, CGA coupled with an intervention designed to improve PCP and patient adherence to recommendations has demonstrated improved outcomes. In a randomized controlled trial, CGA coupled with adherence strategies was associated with less decline in physical functioning, less fatigue, and better social functioning among community-dwelling older adults with at least one of four conditions (functional impairment, falls, urinary incontinence, or depressive symptoms [SOE=A]). In this care model, patients undergo an in-depth, standardized assessment from a social worker, a geriatrics nurse practitioner/geriatrician team, and a physical therapist (when indicated by falls or impaired mobility), after which the evaluation team holds a short interdisciplinary case conference to form its recommendations for care. The adherence intervention includes the geriatrician contacting the patient's PCP to convey the recommendations and also sending a letter describing the recommendations, a copy of the dictated consultation, and full-text references specific to the patient's conditions. In addition, the patient receives a written list of recommendations at the time of the CGA and is subsequently mailed a copy of the dictated consultation and list of recommendations, as well as a "How to Talk to Your Doctor" booklet. Approximately 2 weeks later, a health educator telephones the patient to review the team's recommendations and to help prepare the patient for discussion of the proposed recommendations with the PCP.

A more intensive outpatient consultation model is short-term geriatric evaluation and management (GEM). In GEM, a geriatrics interprofessional team diagnoses *and treats* problems, including adjusting medications, providing counseling and health education, and making referrals to other health professionals and community services. In addition, monitoring and coordination of care between visits is provided through regular telephone calls. In one trial, community-dwelling adults ≥70 years old and found to be at high risk of hospital admission by mailed screening questionnaire underwent CGA followed by interdisciplinary primary care by the GEM team (geriatrician, geriatrics nurse practitioner, nurse, and social worker) for an average of 6 months before being discharged and returned to the care of their original PCP. This GEM model prevented functional decline, improved patients' satisfaction with their health care, and lessened caregiver burden. Other trials of GEM have shown similar positive results (SOE=A). However, fully implementing the above GEM model was more expensive than usual care. Other GEM trials have produced varying results on costs, with some costing more than usual care, some costing the same, and some costing less.

Forms of CGA may also be attempted in the home setting. Accumulating evidence suggests that preventive home visitation programs, based on CGA with extended follow-up of patients at lower risk of death, can reduce functional decline and nursing-home placement (SOE=A).

GERIATRIC SPECIALTY CARE

Senior Health Clinic

The senior health clinic (SHC) care model is a specialized ambulatory clinical service center for older adults providing primary care using an interprofessional team approach to developing and implementing a plan of care. All SHC providers have competency in geriatrics, and care is provided and/or coordinated throughout the continuum of care, including hospital, skilled-nursing facility, assisted living, and home care. Team members work with patients, families, and caregivers, and link patients with needed community-based services and information. The chronic care model offers an organized framework to provide the comprehensive resources and processes needed to deliver evidence-based primary care within an integrated health care system that supports the interactions between the informed, activated (ie, engaged) patient and a prepared, proactive team. Patients new to the SHC are screened for risk status, and a comprehensive geriatric-focused evaluation is completed.

The core interprofessional clinical practice team consists of a geriatrician, nurse practitioner, and social worker. An extended team may include other professionals, such as a pharmacist, physical therapist, dietitian, and home-health nurse. Provider teams share a common medical record and meet at least weekly to review complex care plans and discuss new or anticipated patient issues. When SHC patients are admitted to the hospital or skilled-nursing facility, care is delivered directly and/or coordinated by providers from the SHC.

Studies in community settings and Veterans Affairs medical centers have demonstrated that geriatric patients cared for in the SHC model have improved mental health status and better maintained health-related quality of life over time than patients in traditional care (SOE=A). Financially, SHCs may be a cost center when viewed in isolation, but these clinics are more likely revenue generators when viewed from the perspective of an integrated health system because of the associated "downstream" fee-for-service revenues generated from hospital inpatient, hospital outpatient, and professional fees (SOE=B). There exist financially viable private practice groups who provide this type of care in a fee-for-service environment; however, broad uptake of the SHC model is limited by health system administrators who consider the clinic in isolation as a cost center, and by the limited number of specialty-trained geriatrics health care professionals available to staff such clinics. However, under a capitated/risk sharing environment or one of the newer payment models (PCMH or ACO), the SHC model has the potential to thrive by focusing on high-risk Medicare Beneficiaries and delivering higher-quality care at lower costs from reduced need for expensive services such as emergency department visits and hospitalizations.

Program of All-inclusive Care for the Elderly (PACE)

PACE is a capitated model of care that provides comprehensive care services to frail community-dwelling older adults by a single organization. The program provides all inpatient, outpatient, and long-term care services to its enrolled population. Participants in the PACE program must be ≥55 years old and meet state-defined requirements regarding their need for a nursing-home level of care. Most will also qualify for Medicaid and Medicare; pooling funds from Medicare and Medicaid allows for comprehensive care to be planned and coordinated by the PACE interprofessional team. Without Medicaid and Medicare coverage, out-of-pocket expenses are high. Few private insurance plans provide a PACE benefit as part of their policies. The average PACE enrollee is 80 years old and has an average of 8 medical conditions and 3 ADL limitations; half of PACE participants have dementia.

The goal of the PACE program is to keep the participant in the community for as long as is medically, socially, and financially feasible. The system, designed to be seamless, uses an interprofessional team of health care providers who know the patients and caregivers well and who provide care across the spectrum of hospital, home, alternative living situations, and institutional care. This team includes a physician (often a geriatrician), nurse practitioner, clinic and home-health nurses, social workers, physical therapist, pharmacist, dietician, and transportation workers. The hub of care is the PACE center, which provides adult day health care. Other care includes respite, transportation, medication coverage, rehabilitation (including maintenance physical and occupational therapy), hearing aids, eyeglasses, and a variety of other benefits. The program, at the discretion of the interprofessional team, has the flexibility to pay for nonmedical costs in unusual circumstances (eg, paying a person's electric or gas bill). Care by the interprofessional team provides for the complex social needs as well as the medical needs of the participant. PACE has been described as one of the few truly integrated systems of care in the United States. Although the effectiveness of PACE has not been directly tested by a randomized controlled trial, research has shown that PACE provides high-quality care, albeit with significant site-to-site variation (SOE=B).

In 1997, legislation was passed that changed the status of PACE from a demonstration program to a permanent provider under Medicare. PACE is an optional program under state Medicaid. There are more than 3 million dually eligible and nursing home–certifiable older adults in the United States who might benefit from PACE, but only a small fraction have enrolled. The growth of PACE has been slower than expected. Barriers to growth have included large start-up costs, insufficient supply of physicians, and reluctance of patients to leave their primary care physician. The National PACE Association and CMS are evaluating modifications to the PACE model that would allow for community physician involvement as primary care providers (rather than using a PACE-paid, staff health-maintenance organization model). This change in the model may result in more significant growth of PACE.

PATIENT SELECTION FOR OUTPATIENT INTERVENTIONS

Programs described above have been developed to better address the multiple health care needs of older adults with chronic conditions and in response to rising costs. For these interventions to be successful and cost effective, they must target patient populations whose clinical needs are addressed by the intervention, or who are at risk of high health care expenditures in the future, or both. Ideally, identifying individuals in advance who are also likely to participate in the intervention program is also desirable. Patient selection for intensive outpatient interventions is one of the major challenges facing health care organizations that serve older adults.

Three complementary approaches have been used to identify high-risk older adults: referral by clinicians, screening by mail or telephone, and analysis of administrative data (predictive modeling). The ideal system for identifying high-risk individuals would rely on multiple sources of information. Clinicians in primary care settings are perhaps well-positioned to identify some high-risk older adults, especially when provided with objective criteria on which to base referral. However, they may lack the time, skills, and incentives to do so. Surveys can be administered systematically by mail or telephone to a defined population of older adults. The Probability of Repeated Admission Questionnaire (Pra) has been used extensively in managed-care settings to identify high-risk older adults upon enrollment. A risk score is calculated based on age, sex, perceived health, availability of an informal caregiver, heart disease, diabetes, and frequency of physician visits and hospitalizations. A score above a certain threshold indicates that the member is at high risk of hospital admission and use of other health-related services during the coming year. The Pra has been found to be valid in many different populations of community-dwelling older adults, including Medicaid, fee-for-service, and managed-care patients (SOE=B). Because of the associated expenses and limited survey response rates, an administrative proxy has been developed as a close substitute to the Pra.

The Vulnerable Elders Survey-13 (VES-13), another risk screening instrument, is a 13-item questionnaire that produces a vulnerability score from 0 to 10 based on age, self-reported health, physical function (ability to stoop, crouch, kneel, walk modest distances, etc), and self-care function (selected basic and instrumental ADLs). Patients with a VES-13 score of ≥3 are at four times the risk of functional decline or death over the next 2 years, compared with those whose scores are <3, and are therefore defined as vulnerable (SOE=B).

Finally, predictive modeling approaches use administrative data for identifying high-risk older adults and are usually proprietary (and therefore not described in the peer-reviewed literature). They typically analyze health insurance enrollment records and claims data, producing predictions based on age, gender, diagnoses, prior use of health services and associated costs, and pharmacy data.

REFERENCES

- Boult C, Wieland GD. Comprehensive primary care for older patients with multiple chronic conditions: "Nobody rushes you through". *JAMA*. 2010;304(17):1936–1943.

    This is a review of articles published between 1999 and 2010 reporting results of studies about the effects of U.S. models of comprehensive primary care for older patients with multiple chronic conditions. Articles were selected that compared an intervention group with an equivalent concurrent control group to evaluate the effect on quality of health care, quality of life or functional status, and the use or cost of health services. Three comprehensive models of primary care were identified as having the greatest potential to improve quality of care and quality of life for older patients with complex health care needs, while reducing or at least not increasing the costs of their health care: the GRACE model, Guided Care, and PACE. Details are given as to what these models have in common and how they differ.

- Brown RS, Peikes D, Peterson G, et al. Six features of Medicare coordinated care demonstration programs that cut hospital admissions of high-risk patients. *Health Aff.* 2012;31(6):1156–1166.

    Using data from the Centers for Medicare and Medicaid Services' Medicare Coordinated Care Demonstration and focusing on effects on subgroups of patients at high-risk of hospitalization over the 6-year study period, authors identified six approaches present in programs that reduced hospitalizations. As practiced by program care coordinators, these approaches were 1) frequent in-person meetings with patients, 2) in-person meetings with physicians, 3) serving as a communications hub for physicians, 4) providing evidence-based patient education, 5) emphasizing medication management, and 6) delivering proactive transitional care. Including these design features in future care coordination programs should increase the likelihood of success in reducing hospitalizations in high-risk patients.

- Callahan CM, Boustani MA, Weiner M, et al. Implementing dementia care models in primary care settings: The Aging Brain Care Medical Home. *Aging Ment Health.* 2011;15(1):5–12.

    This article describes the experience of the authors in implementing a primary care–based dementia and depression care program. Findings from prior randomized controlled trials provided the rationale and basic components for implementing the new memory care program. Care for patients with dementia or depression, or both, is facilitated through a care manager working in collaboration with a primary care clinician and supported by specialists in a memory care clinic as well as by information technology resources. The process by which system-level barriers were overcome to implement the program is described.

- Counsell SR, Callahan CM, Clark DO, et al. Geriatric care management for low-income seniors: a randomized controlled trial. *JAMA.* 2007;298(22):2623–2633.

    This landmark study describes the Geriatric Resources for Assessment and Care of Elders (GRACE) model. In this controlled clinical trial, 951 low-incomes seniors (≥65 years old) with primary care physicians established in community-based health centers were randomized to either GRACE or usual care. The GRACE intervention entailed 2 years of home-based care management in which a nurse practitioner and a social worker collaborated with the primary care physician and an interdisciplinary team to provide care, using protocols for 12 common conditions. Compared with patients in usual care, patients in the intervention arm demonstrated significant improvements in general health, mental health, social functioning, and vitality. The two groups did not differ in physical functioning (ADLs) or mortality. A predefined, high-risk group was found to have reduced acute care utilization with the GRACE model.

- GRACE Training and Resource Center (http://graceteamcare.indiana.edu [accessed Jan 2016]).

    This website provides additional information on GRACE Team Care™ including news and publications, and training and technical assistance tools and resources for organizations and healthcare systems that would like to implement the GRACE model.

- Hong CS, Siegel AL, Ferris TG. Caring for high-need, high cost patients: what makes for a successful care management program? New York: The Commonwealth Fund; 2014.

    This study compares the operational approaches of 18 successful complex care management programs to identify best practice to improve care and thereby control costs. Effective programs had several characteristics in common: adopted a tailored approach to local contexts and target population, considered care coordination as a key role, focused on building trusting relationships with patients and PCPs, matched team composition and interventions to patient needs, and used technology to facilitate care management.

- NCQA Programs for Patient-Centered Medical Home Recognition and Accountable Care Organization Accreditation (www.ncqa.org/Programs.aspx [accessed Jan 2016]).

    NCQA standards and specific criteria for PCMH Recognition and ACO Accreditation are available on this website. Extensive PCMH and ACO program information and resources are also provided.

- Nelson KM, Helfrich C, Sun H, et al. Implementation of the patient-centered medical home in the Veterans Health Administration: Associations with patient satisfaction, quality of care, staff burnout, and hospital and emergency department use. *JAMA Intern Med.* 2014;174(8):1350–1358.

    The Veterans Health Administration implemented across the entire system a PCMH-type model in 2010 called the Patient Aligned Care Team (PACT) focusing on team-based care, improved access, and care management. This study reports on the results of a large-scale implementation of PACT in primary care clinics (mean patient age 64 years). Investigators found that the more effective a clinic site was at PACT implementation, the higher the level of patient satisfaction and the lower the level of staff burnout. In addition, a greater extent of PACT implementation correlated with significant reductions in emergency department visits and hospital admissions.

Steven R. Counsell, MD, AGSF

CHAPTER 24—FRAILTY

KEY POINTS

- Frailty occurs in 7%–10% of community-dwelling older adults.

- Frailty is a clinical syndrome of dysregulation of energetics and multiple physiologic systems. Its definable clinical manifestations become apparent when physiologic dysregulation reaches a critical threshold. It has recognizable causes associated with altered physiology and underlying alterations in mitochondrial, genetic, and molecular processes, particularly those affecting the body's energy production and utilization.

- The validated frailty syndrome is manifested when 3 or more of 5 phenotypic components are present: weakness, slowed walking speed, low physical activity, low energy or exhaustion, and weight loss. Consistent with the clinical definition of a syndrome, the whole is greater than the sum of the parts, and the clinical presentation signifies the presence of advanced pathophysiology.

- Frail patients are at high risk of adverse clinical outcomes, including falls, fractures, hospitalization, worsened outcomes from chemotherapy or surgery, hemodialysis, disability and dependency, and mortality. They may be candidates for palliative care.

- Stressors such as hospitalization, surgery, illness, or environmental extremes are less tolerated by frail older adults.

- Frailty develops along a continuum of severity. This spectrum probably ranges from a latent phase of vulnerability that is not clinically apparent in the absence of stressors; to early stages of weakness, slowed gait, or low physical activity that may be most responsive to intervention; to an end-stage with high risk of short-term mortality.

- The most effective preventive approaches appear to be maintaining muscle mass and strength (through walking and resistance exercise) and consuming a Mediterranean diet. Dietary protein supplementation also appears to be beneficial. Consistent with theory regarding the wide-ranging dysregulation underlying frailty, interventions that optimize multiple physiologic systems, such as exercise, are most likely to be effective for prevention or amelioration.

EVIDENCE-BASED FINDINGS

Frailty as a Core Clinical Concept

The care of frail older adults is a central focus of geriatrics. Frail older adults are a subset of the older population at high risk from stressors such as extremes of heat and cold, acute infection or injury, or hospitalization or surgery. In the face of such stressors, frail older adults are more likely to experience delayed recovery from illness, to fall, to develop greater functional impairment (including becoming disabled or dependent), and/or to die. As a group, frail older adults are at high risk of needing hospitalization, and they risk worse outcomes, including dependency, once hospitalized.

Frailty is clinically observed to be a chronic, progressive condition with a spectrum of severity. The most severely frail older adults appear to be in an irreversible, pre-death phase with high risk of mortality over 6–12 months. Earlier phases may be responsive to treatment, which may prevent or ameliorate the clinical manifestations of frailty. The late phase appears to be an indication for palliative care.

Frailty may, in some individuals, result from intrinsic aging processes, ie, *primary frailty*. It also appears that the same phenotype and vulnerability is associated with the end stages of several chronic diseases associated with inflammation and wasting, such as cancer, heart failure, COPD, and HIV/AIDS, in which case the condition is termed *secondary frailty*. The similarity of presentation between primary and secondary frailty suggests that, clinically, frailty is a physiologic entity unto itself that can be triggered by disparate causes and, ultimately, represents a final common pathway resulting from these causes. In this sense, it resembles the sepsis syndrome, another recognizable constellation of symptoms and signs arising from a variety of external insults, although frailty develops over years instead of days.

Frailty and Associated Vulnerability: Clinical Implications of Frailty

Frailty is associated with heightened vulnerability to adverse outcomes, and this vulnerability may most likely become manifest in the face of stressors. All frailty theories suggest that, regardless of the causes, frail older adults have decreased reserves to compensate for, or recover from, stressors. Aggregate loss of physiologic function is the process thought to increase the risk of and underlie the vulnerability to adverse outcomes. An emerging research agenda is focused on developing approaches that can identify older adults with this vulnerable physiologic status before frailty becomes clinically apparent.

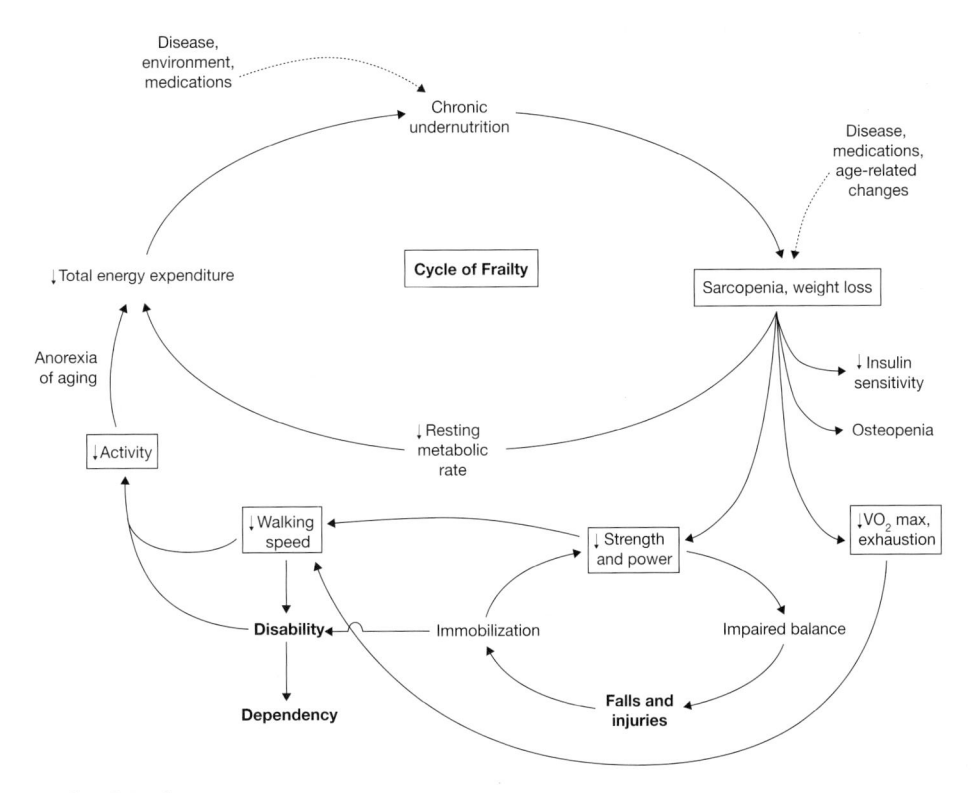

Figure 24.1—The Cycle of Frailty

SOURCE: Fried LP, Tangen CM, Walston J, et al. Frailty in older adults: evidence for a phenotype. *J Gerontol A Biol Sci Med Sci*. 2001;56(3):M146–156.

Frailty as a Clinical Syndrome

Beyond the consensus that frailty is a physiologic state of heighted vulnerability, current definitions place frail older adults into two major categories. One definition identifies frailty as the physiologic vulnerability resulting from accumulation of a number of likely unrelated diseases, impairments, and other health conditions in an individual. This state of multimorbidity is associated with increased risk of both mortality and disability; the number of conditions predicts this vulnerability. In this approach, a large number of prevalent conditions marks an individual as frail.

The second definition of frailty (the so-called *phenotypic* construct used in this chapter) is that it is a distinct physiologic process resulting from dysregulation of multiple systems; many of these systems interact with each other, and resulting impairments and compromised resilience result in an observable clinical phenotype. The aggregate impact of too many dysregulated systems is a decreased ability to maintain homeostasis in the face of stressors, resulting in vulnerability to adverse outcomes. These two definitions and measures of frailty identify populations that overlap to a modest degree (SOE=A).

A phenotype has been developed and validated that links all aspects identified as clinical presentations of frailty (strength, balance, motor processing, nutrition, endurance, physical activity, mobility; note that cognition is excluded), based on the hypothesis that the clinical presentation of frailty results from a vicious cycle of dysregulated energetics, leading to the following:

- Decreased muscle mass, or sarcopenia, with resulting loss of strength
- Slowed motor performance (such as walking speed)
- Decreased physical activity
- Worsened exercise tolerance (or low energy or fatigue or exhaustion)
- Inadequate nutritional intake (even when physical activity is low)

The latter three result in further sarcopenia and, when nutritional intake is inadequate, weight loss as well (Figure 24.1). Identifying the presence of multiple manifestations (defined as ≥3 of the list above) provides specificity in formally defining an individual as frail (Table 24.1). Research has shown this construct is consistent with the definition of a clinical syndrome, and that it is chronic and progressive, with early stages generally predicting progression to more severe frailty. Progression is not inexorable, however, because some afflicted individuals may show improvement. Early stages of frailty are likely most amenable to intervention. The first manifestations of frailty tend to be weakness, slowed walking speed, and/or decreased physical activity.

Table 24.1—Criteria that Define Frailty[a]

Characteristic	Criteria for Frailty[b]
Weight loss	Lost >10 pounds unintentionally last year
Exhaustion	Felt last week that "everything I did was an effort" or "I could not get going"
Slowness	Time to walk 15 feet (cutoff depends on sex and height)
Low activity level	Expends <270 kcal/ week (calculated from activity scale incorporating episodes of walking, household chores, yard work, etc)
Weakness	Grip strength measured using hand dynamometer (cutoff depends on sex and BMI)

[a] Syndrome present when ≥3 characteristics identified
[b] For specific measures and details for determining frailty criteria, see Fried LP, Tangen CM, Walston J, et al. Frailty in older adults: evidence for a phenotype. *J Gerontol Med Sci.* 2001;56A:M146–M156.

Observations to date support the concept of frailty as a clinical syndrome, the manifestations of which become apparent when physiologic dysregulation reaches a critical threshold. It has recognizable causes at the level of both altered physiology and potentially altered genetic, cellular, and molecular processes, conceptually illustrated in Figure 24.2.

Frailty is distinct from disability, a common outcome of frailty, and therefore a commonly coinciding condition. However, disability can occur without frailty, as in the case of a vigorous young man who, after a motorcycle accident, uses an electric wheelchair.

Many patients present for medical attention without the full syndromic definition of frailty, and clinicians caring for older adults should be adept at constructing a differential diagnosis for such individuals. The differential diagnosis of malnutrition and undesired weight loss is extensive and includes conditions that can be grouped into three broad categories. The medical category includes endocrine disorders (eg, uncontrolled diabetes mellitus), end-stage organ failure, malignancy, chronic infections (eg, osteomyelitis or lung abscess), polymyalgia rheumatica/giant cell arteritis, oral cavity disorders, and a number of GI problems (eg, diseases of the pharynx or esophagus, malabsorption syndromes, intestinal angina, gastroparesis). The psychosocial category includes depression; social stressors; difficulty obtaining, affording, or preparing food; and occult alcoholism. Finally, medications, when used for prolonged periods, can lead to unexpected weight loss, and review of the regimen (looking for NSAIDs, antibiotics, digoxin, and others) is often rewarding.

The differential diagnosis of isolated fatigue is similarly extensive and overlaps with that of weight loss. Additional causes to consider include anemia, adrenocortical insufficiency, various neurologic conditions (see weakness, below), sleep disorders, anxiety, and deconditioning.

Causes of isolated global weakness commonly arise in the nervous system (eg, amyotrophic lateral sclerosis, myasthenia gravis, Lambert-Eaton syndrome, cervical myelopathy, Parkinson disease, autonomic failure) but also include myopathies (inflammatory, endocrine, and others) and electrolyte derangements (particularly involving potassium and phosphate).

EVIDENCE AS TO CAUSE

Primary Frailty

Sarcopenia, or loss of lean body mass, is a central component of frailty and a key predictor of the other clinical manifestations. Predictors of loss of muscle mass and strength with aging include decreased anabolic factors such as testosterone and IGF-1, diminished physical activity, reduced nutritional intake (including protein, energy, vitamin D and other micronutrients), and older age itself.

Although the fundamental underlying cause of frailty is still unknown, the intermediate process appears to entail the dysregulation of a critical number of physiologic systems. In addition to sarcopenia, systemic abnormalities include a pro-inflammatory state (indicated by increased IL-6 and C-reactive protein), decreased immune function, anemia, glucose intolerance, increased insulin resistance, low levels of DHEA-S and IGF-1, increased cortisol, low testosterone, decreased heart rate variability, and nutritional derangements (low levels of certain vitamins and carotenoids, reduced intake of protein and energy). The number of abnormal systems is a stronger predictor of frailty than dysfunction in any one system, and there is evidence that abnormal systems synergistically interact to increase frailty risk. There is no evidence to date that intervention on any one system modifies frailty risk.

In frail older adults, dysfunction in a physiologic system may not be apparent at rest but is unmasked by a stressor. For example, in a resting state, levels of blood glucose and insulin may be in normal ranges but after a glucose tolerance test, levels are increased and return to baseline is delayed in those who are frail compared with those who are not.

Secondary Frailty

A variety of primary diseases independently predict development of the frailty phenotype, potentially through inflammation and/or their effect on cardiopulmonary

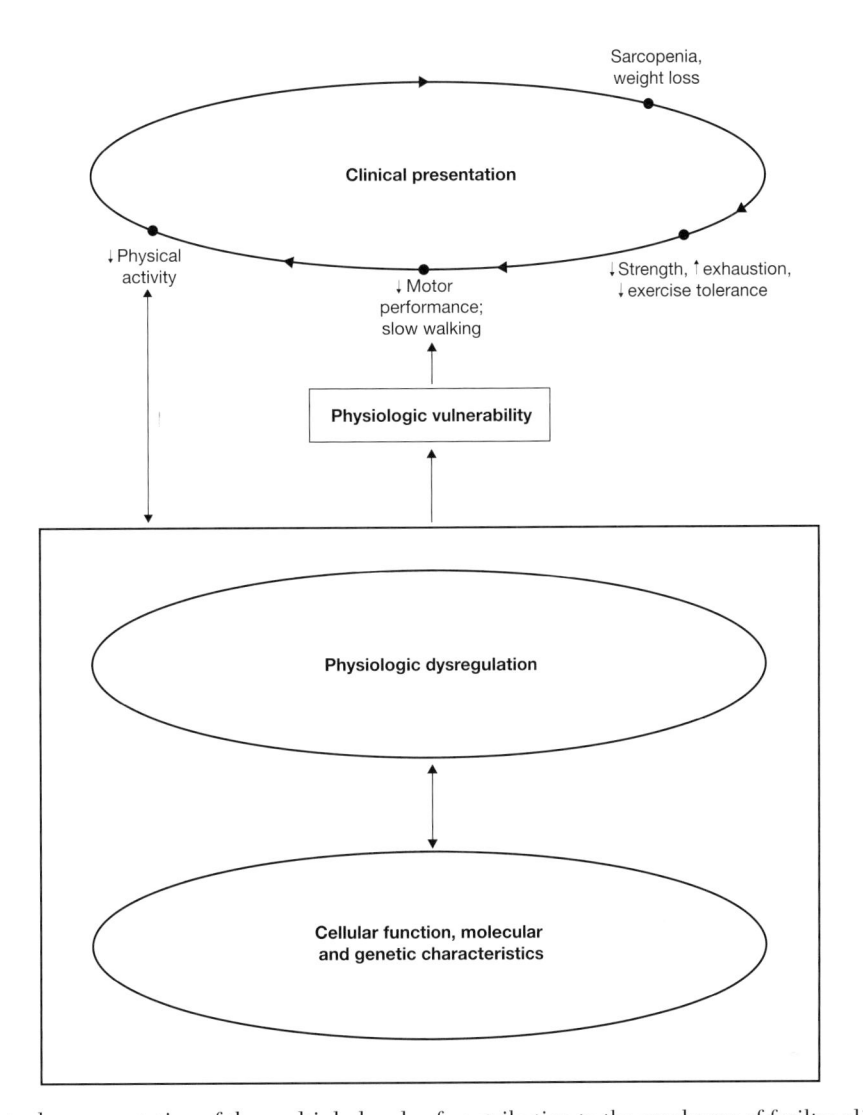

Figure 24.2—Conceptual representation of the multiple levels of contribution to the syndrome of frailty: clinical phenotype, physiologic and biologic causes, and resulting vulnerability in the face of stressors

function and inactivity. Such diseases include immune disorders (eg, HIV/AIDS), heart failure, COPD, and chronic infections (eg, cytomegalovirus, tuberculosis). Data on HIV-positive men indicate that HIV infection, even in the absence of clinical AIDS, is associated with rates of a frailty-like presentation that would be found in HIV-negative men who are 10 years older. Additionally, frailty in association with HIV/AIDS predicts a lower response to therapy and a worse prognosis than HIV infection alone. Similarly, there is early evidence that frailty is a risk factor for intolerance of some cancer chemotherapies and worse outcomes after kidney transplantation.

ASSESSMENT OF FRAILTY

Although the benefits of screening for frailty have not been conclusively demonstrated, an international consensus conference has recommended that adults at least 70 years old be screened for the condition. The presence of frailty can be determined by use of several established methods. The approach chosen may differ depending on the setting and goal. In the clinical setting, assessing older adults for frailty (Table 24.1) is appropriate to identify those at risk of adverse outcomes and to gauge the severity of risks, find those who may benefit from prevention or treatment, track change in status over time, or determine eligibility for palliative care for those at end stage.

Frailty can be assessed in several different ways:

- For frailty as a clinical syndrome with a distinct phenotypic presentation, determining the number of criteria present (out of 5) offers a standardized approach to diagnosis and stage of severity (Table 24.1).

- Some rapid screening/assessment tests have been developed and validated, such as the interview-based FRAIL scale. These may be sensitive in clinical settings but should be followed up using more specific evaluations for the syndrome of frailty.

- For frailty as a clinical composite or "gestalt", an instrument providing a clinical global impression of change in frailty has been validated. Called the Clinical Global Impression of Change in Physical Frailty (CGIC-PF), it draws on clinical judgment and incorporates intrinsic domains (mobility, balance, strength, endurance, nutrition, neuromotor performance) as well as outcome/consequence domains (medical complexity, healthcare utilization, appearance, self-perceived health, activities of daily living, emotional status, and social status).

- Walking speed has been shown to predict mortality and mobility disability. It, along with grip strength, is an early manifestation of frailty, and can serve as a marker in screening (SOE=A).

- The cumulative number of symptoms, signs, illnesses, and disabilities present is useful to characterize aggregate morbidity burden, and those present can be combined into an index of accumulated deficits, which predicts risk of mortality, presumably due to multisystem dysregulation.

PREVAILING MANAGEMENT STRATEGIES

Comprehensive geriatric assessment and management is a clinical care model designed to optimize outcomes for frail older adults, particularly preservation of their independence. This team-based, multidisciplinary approach has been shown to produce positive effects on polypharmacy, falls, functional status, nursing-home admission, and mortality. The assessment should include accurate screening for frailty, including assessment of gait speed, combined with ongoing, expert geriatric care. The focus of care should be 1) to exclude any modifiable precipitating causes of frailty, particularly those that are treatable or environmental; 2) to improve the clinical manifestations of frailty, especially low physical activity, strength, exercise tolerance, and nutrition; and 3) to minimize the consequences of the vulnerability of frail older adults, by directing attention to environmental risks, extent of social support, falls prevention, and the risks from stressors such as acute illness or injury, hospitalization, or surgery. Frail adults subject to such stressors should be provided support for a potentially prolonged recovery. Resistance, or strengthening, exercise, with added nutritional support, particularly protein-calorie supplementation, appears to be a key management approach for frailty and for its prevention. This can be supplemented by walking for exercise and balance training.

The approach that many older adults use to adapt to age-related psychosocial losses and behaviors can also be applied to challenges in physical health and frailty. In the face of diminished resources or reserves, older adults must carefully choose their goals, focus on optimizing the abilities needed to reach their goals, and then compensate for any diminished competencies by increased reliance on other functions or by resort to replacement. Such compensations could include services such a "meals on wheels" or supportive residential environments that offer personal care or meals if needed. Clinical management needs to include such approaches for care of frail older adults, as well as more standard medical approaches, as described above. Further, implementing systematic approaches to decrease the stress of environments such as hospitals, surgical centers, and rehabilitation facilities may be effective as well. For severe frailty, palliative care or hospice may be appropriate, depending on severity and patient preferences.

POTENTIAL APPROACHES FOR PREVENTION OF FRAILTY

Points of Vulnerability and Precipitants

Exposure to any of a variety of stressors appears to put frail older adults at risk of adverse outcomes and may precipitate clinically apparent frailty in those already at risk. Immobility is one key precipitant, causing frailty to develop or worsen, as well as accelerating the onset of adverse outcomes such as dependency. This holds regardless of whether immobility results from pain, illness, or in the context of hospitalization or surgery. Depression may be another precipitant, given its association with decreased activity, energy, and nutritional intake, as well as with inflammation and social isolation. (Depression also appears to be an outcome of frailty as well as a precipitant.) Overall, attention should be paid to minimizing these precipitants or the stress associated with them, through systematic screening, case finding, and quality improvement approaches. Evidence supporting the benefit of such efforts in the context of frailty is limited.

Potential Pharmacologic Treatments

It has not been demonstrated that replacing deficiencies of any one hormone or repleting defects in other systems as a sole intervention can prevent or ameliorate frailty. Theoretically, this is understandable, given that the number of deficits in multiple physiologic systems most strongly predicts frailty, rather than the presence of any one deficit alone. This suggests that improving only one system (eg, immune, hormonal, musculoskeletal) may not be clinically effective, and future effective drug treatments will likely be those that target multiple systems simultaneously. The prototype of such approaches, along with comprehensive geriatric assessment and management, has been shown to decrease polypharmacy and related adverse medication events in frail older adults (SOE=A).

Behavioral Approaches to Prevention or Treatment

Maintaining physical activity and muscle mass is critical in older adults at risk of frailty. Evidence is substantial that resistance, or strengthening, exercise is effective in increasing muscle mass, strength, and walking speed in frail older adults, such as nursing-home residents (SOE=A). Other forms of exercise, including stretching, Tai Chi, and aerobic exercise, are also helpful. Prevention of immobility is critical. Overall, exercise has proven beneficial physiologic effects on sarcopenia, inflammation, and other systems associated with frailty, making maintenance of physical activity as well as strength a cornerstone of prevention, "prehabilitation," and treatment. Importantly, randomized controlled trials of exercise interventions have demonstrated increased gait speed and reduced functional limitations. It remains to be determined if they can prevent or ameliorate frailty and disability.

Consumption of a Mediterranean diet has been shown to lower the risk of becoming frail over 6 years in community-dwelling adults ≥65 years old. More broadly, attention to preventing nutritional inadequacy is important, including supplementation of protein, calories, and micronutrients. In many studies, nutritional supplementation appears to be effective only when added to exercise.

FRAILTY AND FAILURE TO THRIVE

A clinical concept that is an antecedent of current conceptualizations of frailty is that of failure to thrive. In geriatrics, this was historically used as a blanket diagnosis at admission to a hospital or long-term care setting, in the context of an older patient with a range of severe symptoms, including fatigue, poor nutritional intake, weight loss, social withdrawal, and/or decline in cognitive and physical function, often in a state of functional collapse, and without an apparent cause. It was commonly thought that depression was a key component as well. This diagnosis was observed to be associated with poor response to treatment or rehabilitation, increased rates of pressure sores, infection, diminished cell-mediated immunity, and high surgical and short-term mortality rates. Some experts have argued that the term should be abandoned because it does not assist thoughtful evaluation, while others have expressed concern that the application of a term initially used for delayed development in children appeared pejorative when applied to older adults. Nevertheless, there may well be conceptual overlap between the concept of failure to thrive and very severe, or end-stage, frailty.

FRAILTY AND PALLIATIVE CARE

Frailty predicts functional decline and onset and progression of dependency at the end of life. Severe frailty, with a score of 4–5 using a syndromic definition (Table 24.1), and metabolic abnormalities of low cholesterol and albumin predict particularly high short-term mortality rates in frail older adults (SOE=B); these characteristics can be considered to mark a pre-death phase of severe frailty. Clinical case series document a poor response to treatment in those with end-stage frailty, and the adoption of palliative approaches for such patients may be appropriate.

REFERENCES

- Fried LP, Tangen CM, Walston J, et al. Frailty in older adults: evidence for a phenotype. *J Gerontol A Biol Sci Med Sci*. 2001;56(3):M146–156.

    This research operationalizes and validates a phenotype for frailty in older adults, utilizing the study population in the Cardiovascular Health Study. Frailty was defined as a clinical syndrome in which 3 or more of the following criteria were present: unintentional weight loss (10 lbs in past year), self-reported exhaustion, weakness (grip strength), slow walking speed, and low physical activity. The number of manifestations present are related to the severity of frailty, with 3 or more of 5 manifestations characterized as frail, 1 or 2 as prefrail or intermediate, and 0 as nonfrail or robust. This phenotype is consistent with energy dysregulation and predictive of disability, falls, hospitalization, and mortality. This study provides a potential standardized definition for frailty in community-dwelling older adults and offers concurrent and predictive validity for the definition as a distinct clinical syndrome.

- Cesari M, Vellas B, Hsu F-C, et al. A physical activity intervention to treat the frailty syndrome in older persons—Results From the LIFE-P Study. *J Gerontol A Biol Sci Med Sci*. 2015;70(2):216–222.

    This article reports results from exploratory analyses of the LIFE pilot study, a randomized controlled trial enrolling 424 people (mean age 77 years) with a sedentary lifestyle and risk of mobility disability. Participants were randomly allocated to a 12-month physical activity intervention or a successful aging education group. At 12 months follow-up, those in the physical activity group had a 10% frailty prevalence compared with 19% prevalence in the successful aging group. Regular physical activity may reduce frailty in individuals at high risk of disability.

- Talegawkar SA, Bandinelli S, Bandeen-Roche K, et al. A higher adherence to a Mediterranean-style diet is inversely associated with the development of frailty in community-dwelling elderly men and women. *J Nutr.* 2012;142(12):2161–2166.

> This article reports analyses of InChianti longitudinal cohort study over 6-year follow-up. Results show that higher adherence to a Mediterranean-style diet was associated with 70% lower odds of developing frailty compared with those with lower adherence score.

- Theou O, Stathokostas L, Roland KP, et al. The effectiveness of exercise interventions for the management of frailty: A systematic review. *J Aging Res.* 2011 Apr 4;2011:569194.

> In this systematic review of randomized controlled trials in which exercise interventions were used in the management of frail patients, there was insufficient evidence to recommend a particular regimen. However, superior outcomes arose from programs that had multiple components, lasted at least 5 months, and consisted of 30- to 45-minute sessions conducted 3 times a week.

Linda P. Fried, MD, MPH, AGSF

CHAPTER 25—VISUAL LOSS AND EYE CONDITIONS

KEY POINTS

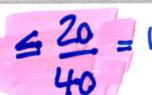

- Visual loss, defined as visual acuity less than 20/40, increases exponentially with age such that 20%–30% of the population ≥75 years old is affected. Blindness, defined as visual acuity of 20/200 or worse, affects 2% of the population ≥75 years old. Those ≥65 years old make up 12% of the total U.S. population but 50% of the blind population.

- Cataracts and refractive error are common; both are correctable, and correction improves quality of life.

- Age-related macular degeneration (ARMD) is common; the wet form, the major complication of ARMD leading to blindness, is treatable with a series of intravitreal antiangiogenesis injections. Antioxidant multivitamins can slow progression to the wet form.

- Glaucoma is common, and increased intraocular pressure is no longer required to meet diagnostic criteria. Screening for glaucoma should be done every 1–2 years after age 50 and more often in high-risk individuals.

- Control of blood glucose and blood pressure in type 2 diabetes reduces retinopathy. Glycemic and blood pressure control needs to be sustained to achieve significant benefit. Intravitreal antiangiogenic injections and laser therapy are the mainstay treatments for complications of diabetic retinopathy.

Visual loss has considerable impact on the medical system and older age groups. Chronic eye conditions are one of the most common reasons for office visits to the physician among those ≥65 years old. Of all office visits by older adults, 14% are to ophthalmologists, one of the highest rates of all specialty visits. Falls and car crashes, each associated with visual loss in older adults, consume considerable medical resources. Moreover, visual loss has been linked to a significant deterioration in the quality of life and activities of daily living of older adults.

The American Academy of Ophthalmology recommends a comprehensive eye examination every 1–2 years for adults ≥65 years old. Prophylactic and therapeutic ocular management can effectively alter the course of various conditions causing visual loss. About one-third of all new cases of blindness can be avoided with effective use of available ophthalmologic services.

COMMON EYE CONDITIONS IN OLDER ADULTS

Many changes common with aging involve the eyes and surrounding structures (Table 25.1). Consequences of these changes range from cosmetic concerns to discomfort and disease predisposition. Lid abnormalities are a common problem for older adults. Because of the gradual loss of elasticity and tensile strength that develops with age, secondary degenerative changes can develop. Blepharochalasis (drooping of the brow) and blepharoptosis (drooping of the eyelid) can cause cosmetic deformity and, if severe, can cause visual loss. Lid ectropion or entropion (ie, eversion and inversion of the lid margins, respectively) can disrupt the ocular surface and cause discomfort. These conditions can be addressed by various surgical procedures. Ocular lubricant ointments (those without antibiotics) can be recommended to minimize discomfort from exposure of the globe. Older adults can also develop squamous cell and basal cell carcinomas of the eyelids. Ulcerations or chronic irritation, especially if associated with loss of eyelashes, should be evaluated by an ophthalmologist. In addition, older adults frequently develop nasolacrimal tear duct obstruction that prevents tears from exiting into the nose, which causes chronic epiphora leading to blurry vision. Patients can be offered surgery if the epiphora is highly symptomatic.

Older adults with eye complaints frequently first seek care from their primary care provider. Common complaints include red eye, ocular swelling or discomfort, blurred or sudden loss of vision, diplopia, and floaters (Table 25.2). "Has your vision changed?" is a key question that helps determine whether a patient can be treated by the primary care provider as opposed to needing a referral to the ophthalmologist. A decrease in vision can indicate a serious condition. For this reason, it is vitally important to check visual acuity in each eye separately with the patient's current corrective aid (eg, eyeglasses) in place for any eye complaint.

Significant vision loss can also be indicated by the presence of a relative afferent pupillary defect, which can be assessed using a "swinging flashlight test." While in a dark room, the patient is asked to stare into the distance. A bright flashlight is then placed in front of one eye to check the pupillary light reflex; the other eye should also constrict because of the consensual light reflex. The flashlight is then quickly swung over to the second eye. If this eye dilates, there is an afferent pupillary defect (ie, the second eye is not detecting the light as the first eye detects it).

Table 25.1—Common Aging Changes of the Eye and Consequences

Change	Finding	Functional Consequence
Eyelids		
Laxity of eyelid tendons	Entropion (turning in of lid)	Eyelashes rub and irritate eye, chronic tearing, drying of eye; ptosis blocks visual axis, particularly when looking down to read
	Ectropion (turning out of lid)	
	Ptosis (drooping of lid)	
Atrophy of periorbital fat	Sunken eyes	
Tear ducts		
Stenosis of nasolacrimal duct	Chronic tearing	Blurred vision
Reduced production of tears	Reduced tears	Dry eye, irritation
Cornea		
Lipid deposition in cornea	Arcus senilis (white ring in peripheral cornea)	Cosmetic
Sclera		
Calcium deposition among scleral fibers	Ovoid zone of grayish translucency on sclera	Cosmetic, sometimes confused for a pigment tumor
Subconjunctival deposition of fat	Yellowish appearance of sclera	Cosmetic
Lens		
Lens thickening	Anterior chamber shallowing	Predisposes to an acute attack of angle-closure glaucoma
Changes in lens proteins	Cataracts	Blurred vision
Pupils		
Unknown etiology	Pupil size shrinks	Difficulty in dim light, glare
Intraocular drainage		
Thickening of basement membranes in trabecular meshwork	Increased intraocular pressure	Glaucoma
Vitreous		
Liquefaction	Posterior vitreous detachment	Floaters and retinal tears
Retina		
Decreased phagocytotic activity of cells	Accumulation of drusen	Macular degeneration

For serious eye conditions that require immediate attention from an ophthalmologist, see Table 25.3. All of the listed conditions are usually associated with a decrease in vision that can be profound but masked by good vision in the other eye. The symptoms of a retinal detachment include new floaters in one eye along with photopsias (the perception of flashes of light), distorted peripheral vision, or decreased vision. Ocular pain and hyperemia do not accompany a retinal detachment; the only signs a primary care provider may detect are a relative afferent pupillary defect, decreased vision, or a monocular visual field deficit. Signs and symptoms of acute angle-closure glaucoma include an injected eye with fixed, dilated pupil and cloudy cornea; the patient is often in severe pain, nauseous, and vomiting. In ischemic optic neuropathy, vision in one eye is lost suddenly, usually in the upper or lower hemifield (this can be detected on visual field testing by confrontation). Giant cell arteritis must be excluded quickly in patients with ischemic optic neuropathy to prevent bilateral blindness. Diplopia and central retinal artery occlusion can also be the result of giant cell arteritis. Bacterial keratitis usually presents with pain and a corneal infiltrate. Scleritis is frequently associated with significant autoimmune disease; symptoms include boring pain, decreased vision, and a red eye. Posterior uveitis presents with decreased vision and floaters.

RED EYE

Red eye is an extremely common eye complaint, the cause of which may be benign or malignant (Table 25.4). Hyperemia of the eye can accompany any inflammation or infection. Causes of red eye that require referral include corneal ulcers, which are usually accompanied by a visible white infiltrate on the cornea, anterior and posterior uveitis, herpes simplex and herpes zoster ophthalmicus, scleritis, angle-closure glaucoma, ocular surface tumors, and postoperative infections. The reason for referral is to prevent permanent vision loss, which can be the end point of any of these conditions. Although it is sometimes difficult to differentiate one cause from another without a slit lamp ophthalmologic examination, signs and symptoms that should prompt referral are decreased vision, severe pain, photophobia, recent intraocular surgery, or even distant surgery (especially if glaucoma surgery).

Relatively benign causes of red eye include blepharitis or inflammation of the Meibomian glands in the eyelids, dry eye, allergic conjunctivitis, corneal exposure due to lid malposition, viral conjunctivitis, and subconjunctival hemorrhages. Blepharitis and dry eye often present together because blepharitis affects the integrity of the tear film, which then evaporates more readily. Tears serve several important functions,

Table 25.2—Symptoms and Treatment of Most Common Eye Diseases of Older Adults

Condition	Comments	Signs and Symptoms	Treatment	Prevention
Cataracts	*Reversible* cause of blindness	Decreased vision; cause refractive shifts, reduced visual acuity, reduced contrast sensitivity, glare, monocular diplopia/ghosting *[handwritten: glare = blending]*	Change eyeglasses to match changing refractive error. Surgical cataract extraction when eyeglasses no longer improve vision: extremely successful in improving vision in those without other ocular pathology; can also be helpful in those with other ocular pathology.	Smoking cessation, healthy diet with fruits and vegetables, decrease alcohol intake, sunglasses, manage other disease
Age-related macular degeneration	Most common cause of *irreversible* blindness			Smoking cessation, healthy diet with fruits, vegetables, and fish, manage other diseases, regular eye examinations
Dry form		Slow onset, vision loss not severe, usually asymptomatic	To decrease rate of conversion to wet form: vitamin supplements (vitamins C, E, zinc, lutein, zeoxanthine)	
Wet form		Sudden onset of vision loss or distortion of vision; central vision loss can be severe, peripheral vision maintained	Intravitreal injections of vascular endothelial growth factor inhibitors and laser	
Glaucoma	Second leading cause of *irreversible* blindness	Peripheral vision loss first, but in advanced stages all vision can be lost; early glaucoma typically asymptomatic		Treat high eye pressure, healthy diet, regular eye examinations
Open angle		Typically asymptomatic until advanced; may note contrast sensitivity loss or night vision problems in earlier stages	Lowering of intraocular pressure with medications, laser trabeculoplasty, and/or incisional surgery	
Narrow angle	Drug warnings apply to this type of glaucoma. Avoid medications that can dilate the pupil (anticholinergic and sympathomimetic drugs, ie, those used for bladder problems, decongestants, and some antidepressant drugs)	Acute: painful, red eye, decreased vision, nausea, vomiting, headache	Acute: pilocarpine 2% ophthalmic solution (2 drops in affected eye), acetazolamide 250 mg IV or po, if tolerated, and immediate laser treatment needed; may require continued medical and/or surgical treatment	
		Chronic: usually asymptomatic until vision loss advanced or central vision affected	Chronic: lowering of intraocular pressure with medications, laser, and/or incisional surgery	
Diabetic retinopathy	Vision loss is caused by macular edema and ischemia, vitreous hemorrhage, and retinal detachments.	Decreased/blurred vision, sudden loss of vision, floaters	Laser treatment and intravitreal injections; tight control of blood glucose and blood pressure	Manage blood glucose and blood pressure, healthy diet, exercise, regular eye examinations

including corneal lubrication, debris clearance, and immune protection. Tear production decreases with age, and older adults are prone to develop keratitis sicca, characterized by redness, foreign body sensation, and reflex tearing. Patients may complain of severe eye discomfort and blurred vision, which usually improves with blinking or eye rubbing because these two maneuvers spread the remaining tear film over the cornea. Dry eye can be especially problematic in older women, in whom hormonal changes are thought to play a role. Keratitis sicca can also be associated with autoimmune disease; conditions such as Sjögren syndrome should be excluded. Management of dry eye includes tear replacement with artificial tears during the day (preservative-free tears if being used more than four times daily) and a lubricant ointment at bedtime. Topical cyclosporine A (0.2%) eye drops can be used for more severe cases of dry eye to combat the underlying ocular inflammation that affects tear production; however, caution is warranted in patients with a history of ocular herpetic infections. If there is a severe tear deficiency, an ophthalmologist can place punctal plugs to retain what tears are made. Treatment for accompanying blepharitis includes lid hygiene, consisting of gentle scrubbing of the lash bases with nontearing baby shampoo twice daily and applying topical antibiotic ointment to the eyelids nightly. Oral doxycycline can also be a useful adjunct, especially when blepharitis is associated with acne rosacea. If symptoms continue despite these conservative measures, referral is warranted.

Subconjunctival hemorrhages are very common and, despite being benign, elicit worried responses from patients. Many patients are on a blood thinner, and minor trauma such as eye rubbing, which usually is not recalled by the patient, can cause a small blood vessel to tear and bleed. Artificial tears are recommended for comfort until the hemorrhage clears. If the patient is on warfarin, checking an INR, if not done recently, may be prudent.

Herpes zoster ophthalmicus, or shingles, is a painful reactivation of varicella zoster virus that not uncommonly affects older adults. Dermatomal distribution of weeping vesicles affecting the ophthalmic branch of the trigeminal nerve is the classic presentation. Ocular involvement can be signaled by lesions on the tip of the nose (Hutchinson sign) and can include dendritic keratopathy or uveitis. Oral antiviral therapy can shorten the course of disease. Trifluridine eye drops are indicated for herpes simplex dendriform corneal ulcers (not for herpes zoster). Postherpetic neuralgia can be quite debilitating; systemic medications (narcotics, tricyclic antidepressants[OL], gabapentin, pregabalin) can reduce pain; less often, topical agents such as capsaicin and lidocaine patches can be tried (these should not be used near the eye—capsaicin can be extremely irritating to the eye, and lidocaine can anesthetize the eye, placing the patient at risk of eye injury while the eye is numb).

Viral conjunctivitis (or pink eye) is associated with severe tearing, mucous discharge, and matting of the eyelids, especially in the morning. Symptoms include eye irritation and blurred vision. Viral conjunctivitis is distinguished from bacterial conjunctivitis by history and, because it is highly contagious, patients frequently report either an upper respiratory tract infection or recent contact with someone suffering from a red eye. Viral conjunctivitis is treated conservatively with warm compresses and artificial tears; topical antibiotics are not indicated. If it is accompanied by severely reduced vision, the patient should be referred for an ophthalmologic examination, because corneal infiltrates can (rarely) develop, requiring steroid eye drops. Viral conjunctivitis is extremely contagious (by contact), and patient education is necessary to limit spread of the infection to the other eye or to contacts (including office staff).

Allergic conjunctivitis is a common benign condition; its hallmark is ocular pruritus. Patients should be advised to avoid known precipitants (eg, pet dander or cosmetics). Management of allergic conjunctivitis includes cool compresses, systemic antihistamines, topical antihistamines or decongestants, and ophthalmic corticosteroids for limited periods of time. Allergic conjunctivitis can also be an adverse event of some topical glaucoma medications. Usually, the conjunctivitis is accompanied by dermatitis of the eyelids. This problem should prompt referral to the ophthalmologist treating the glaucoma.

OPHTHALMIC CORTICOSTEROIDS

The use of ophthalmic corticosteroids merits comment. Ophthalmic steroid drops or ointment can have serious potential adverse events, including risks of ocular hypertension and glaucoma development (which can be asymptomatic for a long period of time), secondary infections, cataract formation, and corneal thinning if used in undiagnosed infections. Because of these risks, the prescription of ophthalmic corticosteroids is best limited to practitioners with the tools to monitor for these adverse events. The risk of adverse events increases greatly with prolonged steroid use (months to years); therefore, prescriptions for any steroid-containing eye medication should never be refilled without ophthalmic evaluation. Ocular hypertension that can lead to glaucoma can develop within 2–3 weeks with daily use of topical steroids in susceptible individuals (those with glaucoma, either diagnosed or undiagnosed, or with a family history of glaucoma). Low-potency steroids given for 7–10 days will not be problematic for the vast majority of patients, but patients and caregivers should be warned of the risks of prolonged and unmonitored use of steroids in and around the eyes.

REFRACTIVE ERROR AND CATARACTS

The leading causes of visual loss worldwide are refractive error and cataracts, for which eyeglasses and surgical cataract extraction, respectively, are mainstays of treatment. Despite the considerable successes of these therapeutic options, many populations do not receive adequate treatment for these problems.

Refractive error can be categorized as emmetropia (neutral refraction), ametropia, or presbyopia. Three forms of ametropia exist: myopia (nearsightedness), hyperopia (farsightedness), and astigmatism (distorted vision). Typically, older adults have increasing hyperopia, unless a cataract is present, which can induce a myopic shift. Although contact lens wear and laser refractive surgery are available for myopic and hyperopic refractive errors, these forms of refractive treatment are not favored by older people. Corneal refractive surgery, such as LASIK, is not the best remedy for refractive problems in older adults who usually have some degree of cataracts. Removal of the cataract and replacement with an artificial intraocular lens, the power of which can be chosen to eliminate refractive error, is a better option in older adults. Toric intraocular lenses can correct astigmatism, and multifocal lenses can decrease the need for eyeglasses after surgery. After the age of approximately 40, emmetropic individuals begin to develop progressive presbyopia, loss of ability to focus on near objects that is caused by gradual hardening of the lens and decreased muscular effectiveness of the ciliary body. Reading glasses can be obtained OTC, or bifocal eyeglasses can be prescribed.

Approximately 20% of adults ≥65 years old and 50% of adults ≥75 years old have cataracts, a lens opacity that reduces vision. Cataracts are associated with decreased visual acuity that is not correctable by glasses, glare symptoms, changes in color perception, and decreased contrast sensitivity. The most important risk factor is increased age; other risk factors include decreased vitamin intake, light (ultraviolet B) exposure, smoking, alcohol use, long-term corticosteroid use, and diabetes mellitus.

Cataract extraction is one of the most successful surgeries in medicine (90% of patients achieve vision of 20/40 or better). Approximately 3 million cataract procedures are performed each year in the United States. The benefits of cataract surgery include not only improved vision but also a decreased rate of falls (SOE=B) and improved vision-related quality of life (SOE=A).

Indications for cataract surgery are a decrease in vision that affects ability to perform activities of daily living. Cataract removal may also be recommended if the cataract impairs the ophthalmologist's ability to monitor diseases of the retina. Cataract extraction is safe and can be completed in <30 min under local or topical anesthesia. The surgery involves the breakdown of the lens by ultrasound energy and its aspiration (phacoemulsification). An artificial implant (intraocular lens) is placed in the capsular bag, which is the only remnant of the native lens retained. A secondary laser procedure (capsulotomy) may be necessary to ablate subsequent capsular opacification that can develop in ≥15% of patients. As mentioned previously, 20/40 vision or better is achieved in 90% of surgeries. Reasons for not attaining that level of vision include diseases of the retina and optic nerve that limit best correctable vision.

AGE-RELATED MACULAR DEGENERATION (ARMD)

ARMD is the most common cause of irreversible blindness in older adults throughout the developed world. It is a multifactorial disease involving age-related changes and multiple genes and environmental interactions. A dysregulation of the complement cascade plays an integral role in development of disease. Mutations in a number of complement proteins appear to be involved with various forms of ARMD, including complement factor H (CFH), complement factor B (CFB), complement factor I (CFI), and complement components C2 and C3. Mutations in these factors can lead to increased inflammation and development of ARMD and complications such as atrophy and/or angiogenesis. Currently, there is no role for genetic screening as a clinical tool, because it is not yet clear how to use this information. The percentage of patients who harbor these gene mutations who will actually develop disease is unknown. Other risk factors include smoking and hypertension. Fair-skinned individuals are at greater risk of developing this disease than are black individuals, in whom pigment may serve as a protective element. Exposure to ultraviolet light is a debated risk factor. Researchers are also looking at links between ARMD and Alzheimer disease, because both are common in older adults. The two diseases share the accumulation of amyloid beta within brain plaques and drusen, respectively, which may contribute to angiogenesis.

ARMD is classified into two forms: dry and wet. The dry form is much more common and is characterized by deposits of macular drusen. Drusen, submacular yellow lipoprotein deposits composed of metabolic by-products, do not typically cause vision loss but are a marker for the wet form of ARMD, which is characterized by angiogenesis or choroidal neovascularization (CNV). The presence of larger, more numerous drusen conveys the greatest risk of development of CNV. The 2001 Age-Related Eye Disease Study (AREDS) found that the risk of CNV development could be decreased by 25% (absolute risk reduction [ARR] of 8% for progression to advanced ARMD, and 6% for loss of vision of 3 lines or more) when patients with high-risk drusen are treated with high-dose oral multivitamin therapy (SOE=A). AREDS II studied the addition of omega-3 fatty acids or lutein/zeaxanthin to the original AREDS vitamin formulation. Compared with placebo, there was no statistically significant reduction in risk for either group; however, for patients with very low levels of lutein/zeaxanthin in their diets, the supplement helped reduce their risk of advanced ARMD.

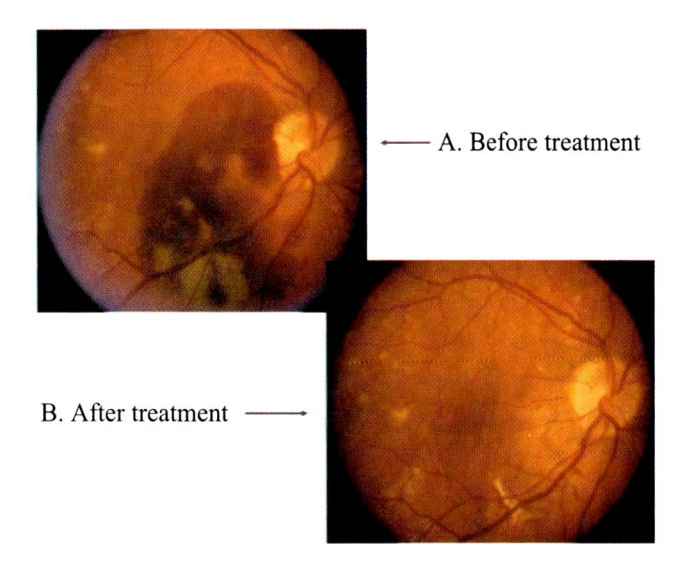

Figure 25.1—Resolution of submacular hemorrhage after intravitreal anti-VEGF therapy in patient with neovascular ARMD.

A. Fundus showing submacular hemorrhage due to choroidal neovascularization and the wet form of ARMD.

B. Resolution of the hemorrhage after a series of intravitreal anti-VEGF injections. Note the presence of macular drusen temporally and subretinal fibrosis inferiorly under the vessels.

Combination multivitamins containing lutein 10 mg, zeaxanthin 2 mg, vitamin E 400 IU, vitamin C 500 mg, and zinc 25 mg are available OTC. Supplements are recommended indefinitely or until the wet form of ARMD develops, which then necessitates other treatment. Lutein and zeaxanthin have replaced β-carotene in the original multivitamin studied, because they are naturally found in the retina and because they do not incur an increased risk of lung cancer as does β-carotene. The multivitamin supplement used in AREDS II (listed above) is not recommended for patients with less than high-risk drusen who have a very low baseline risk of progressing to wet ARMD.

Patients with the dry form of ARMD should be examined periodically by an ophthalmologist for development of early signs of CNV. CNV in wet ARMD is marked by the presence of subretinal fluid and blood that may appear as a gray-green membrane (Figure 25.1). The development of CNV is signaled by sudden vision loss or distortion of vision and requires urgent evaluation, because untreated CNV can lead to severe central vision loss. The natural history of CNV is progressive subfoveal growth and leakage with eventual fibrotic scarring and central blindness.

Angiogenesis inhibition has proved to be a major breakthrough in the treatment of CNV. Various inhibitors of vascular endothelial growth factor (VEGF) have been approved by the FDA for treatment of wet ARMD. Ranibizumab is a fragment antibody that exhibits broad-spectrum inhibition of VEGF. In a multicenter, prospective randomized clinical trial, visual acuity improved by approximately 2 lines in patients with CNV treated with ranibizumab compared with those given sham treatments (ARR=33%, number needed to treat [NNT] =3 [SOE=A]). Serial intravitreal injections of ranibizumab are now the gold standard of care for all subtypes of wet ARMD (according to data from the pivotal ANCHOR and MARINA trials). Ranibizumab is costly (approximately $2,000 per vial), and one vial is needed per eye. The manufacturer has recommended an injection every month for 2 years (approximately $48,000). However, most clinicians are giving a monthly injection for 3–4 months per eye, monitoring, and reinjecting as needed when neovascularization recurs. Injections may be necessary indefinitely. Bevacizumab is another VEGF inhibitor related to the ranibizumab molecule that has shown promise as being equally efficacious and is significantly less expensive than ranibizumab; however, it must be compounded by an accredited pharmacy for intraocular use. In 2012, the Comparison of AMD Treatments Trial (CATT) sponsored by the National Institutes of Health published 2-year results from a 2-year multicenter randomized controlled trial comparing ranibizumab and bevacizumab, either monthly or as needed, for wet ARMD in which the primary outcome measure was visual improvement. Visual improvement was not significantly different for either group. Two international trials had similar findings. In CATT, the as-needed bevacizumab group fared the poorest (SOE=A). Anatomically, monthly ranibizumab injections were most effective in resolving macular edema but were also associated with increased rates of macular atrophy. Serious adverse events (primarily hospitalizations) occurred at a 24% rate for patients receiving bevacizumab and a 19% rate for patients receiving ranibizumab. However, the number of deaths, heart attacks, and strokes were low and similar for both drugs during the study.

A third medication approved by the FDA called aflibercept (or VEGF Trap-Eye) is a fusion protein that has greater binding affinity of VEGF-A than ranibizumab and bevacizumab. In addition to binding all forms of VEGF-A, it binds placental growth factor. The advantage of aflibercept is a longer duration of action and, therefore, less frequent injections. Injected every 2 months after a loading dose of 3 monthly injections, it has been found to be equal in efficacy to ranibizumab.

Although the great majority (90%) of AMD patients with blindness develop complications due to the neovascular or wet form, a small proportion of patients (10%) develop blindness due to geographic atrophy of the macula. No therapies exist for this form of ARMD, although recent interest has been shown with an intravitreal injected antibody directed against the alternate complement pathway in an effort to down-regulate inflammation.

DIABETIC RETINOPATHY

Duration of disease, control of blood glucose, and control of blood pressure are the most important variables in the development and progression of diabetic retinopathy. After 10 years, 70% of those with type 2 diabetes have some form of retinopathy, and nearly 10% show proliferative disease. The Diabetic Control and Complications Trial demonstrated that tight control of blood glucose in individuals with type 1 diabetes resulted in a long-lasting decrease in the rate of development and progression of diabetic retinopathy. The United Kingdom Prospective Diabetes Study (UKPDS) validated these results in an older population with type 2 diabetes. Tight blood glucose control was shown to decrease the need for the studies' primary outcome measures (ie, the need for laser) and the level of retinopathy; therefore, it was indirectly shown to influence and benefit vision, although some authors have questioned this surrogate measure. For example, a patient with poor control of blood glucose is more likely to progress to preproliferative and proliferative levels of retinopathy and need surgery, which is more likely to result in poor vision. The benefit of tight glucose control reduced the need for laser therapy within 3–4 years in the groups with no baseline retinopathy and within 2–3 years in the groups with mild to moderate baseline retinopathy; however, most other studies and guidelines indicate that 7–8 years of tight control are needed to show microvascular benefits. However, tight control of blood pressure (≤130/80 mmHg) is an important factor in decreasing microvascular complications, and becomes evident within 2–3 years.

More recent data from the ACCORD, ADVANCE, and VADT studies have raised the question of whether intensive glycemic control is of enough benefit to outweigh the risks of hypoglycemia. The ACCORD study was stopped early because of excessive mortality in the intensive control group (relative risk increase 20%, absolute risk increase 1.0%, number needed to harm 100) and showed no significant benefit for macro- or microvascular disease in a group of patients of average age 62 years old and with longstanding diabetes. The ADVANCE study showed reductions in microvascular disease (relative risk reduction [RRR]=14%, ARR=1.5%, NNT=66.6); however, the significant benefits were in reductions of albuminuria rather than retinopathy. In contrast to the ACCORD study, a follow-up of UKPDS found evidence of a "legacy effect," of benefits of intensive control early in the course of the disease. In a group of patients followed for 10 years after the end of the trial, intensive control during the trial reduced microvascular disease (RRR=25%, ARR=0.37%, NNT=270 in the group treated with sulfonylureas plus insulin; RRR=7%, ARR=0.1%, NNT=1,000 in the group treated with metformin), even though patients had not maintained the low target hemoglobin A_{1c} levels. The results of these studies prompted significant controversy in both the lay press and the medical literature, and led the American Diabetes Association, the American Heart Association, and the American College of Cardiology to issue a revised position statement in 2009 about the value of intensive control in type 2 diabetes mellitus. In this statement, the recommended hemoglobin A_{1c} target remains 7.5%–7.9%; however, it notes that targets should be individualized and that patients with limited remaining life expectancy, those with longstanding diabetes mellitus, and those with preexisting vascular disease are less likely to benefit from intensive control (see Item 3 at: www.americangeriatrics.org/health_care_professionals/clinical_practice/clinical_guidelines_recommendations/choosingwisely). Many, and probably most, geriatric patients fall into the latter categories; thus, the benefits of intensive control need to be very carefully weighed against the potential for harm. The risk of hypoglycemia is significantly greater in those who are frail, demented, or otherwise unable to comply with medical regimens and merit particular attention.

Other systemic risk factors, including kidney function and serum cholesterol, can also influence the course of diabetic retinopathy and should be optimized. ACE inhibitors decrease progressive nephropathy in diabetic patients and may have similar benefits on the retina.

Patients with type 2 diabetes require baseline ophthalmologic screening at diagnosis of systemic disease and annually thereafter. Subsequent follow-up depends on the grade of retinopathy. Nonproliferative diabetic retinopathy, the earliest stage of retinopathy, can first be manifested by retinal microaneurysms. Intraretinal hemorrhages and exudates, with or without associated macular edema, can ensue. Progressive ischemia characterized by increasing hemorrhages, venous caliber changes or intraretinal microvascular abnormalities or both, and capillary nonperfusion on fluorescein angiography characterize the preproliferative stage of diabetic retinopathy. About 40% of patients with preproliferative retinopathy develop proliferative diabetic retinopathy within 1–2 years, characterized by neovascularization or new blood vessel growth of the retina or disc, or both.

Visual loss in patients with diabetes can occur as a result of macular nonperfusion or macular edema. In 1985, the Early Treatment Diabetic Retinopathy Study demonstrated the benefit of focal or grid laser photocoagulation in stabilizing and improving vision

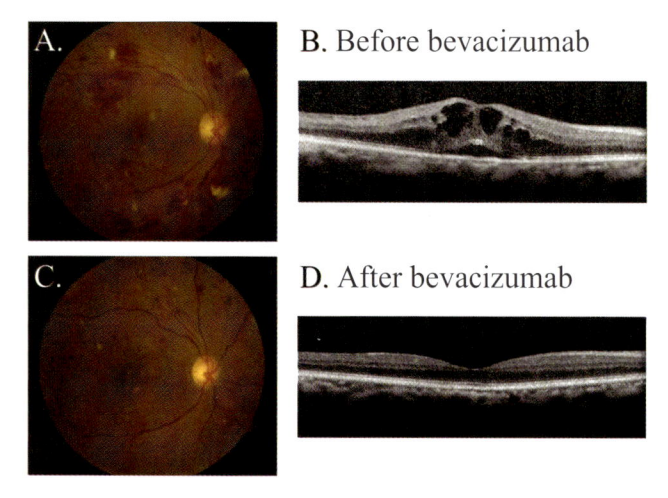

Figure 25.2—Severe nonproliferative diabetic retinopathy with macular edema before and after anti-VEGF therapy.

A. Fundus showing multiple retinal hemorrhages and cotton wool spots in a diabetic patient with severe nonproliferative diabetic retinopathy.
B. Optical coherence tomography of the same eye showing diabetic cystoid macular edema.
C. Marked improvement of the retinal hemorrhages and cotton wool spots after intravitreal anti-VEGF therapy.
D. Complete resolution of diabetic cystoid macular edema after intravitreal anti-VEGF therapy.

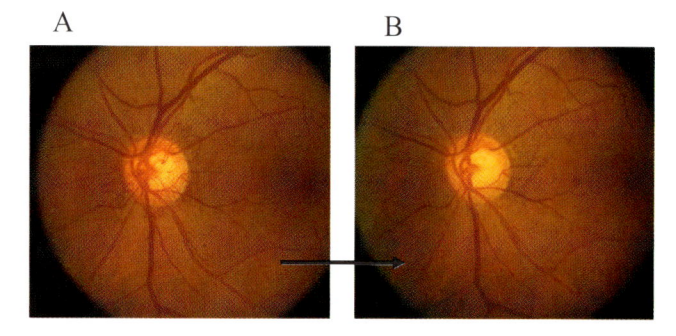

Figure 25.3—Resolution of severe neovascularization of the disc after intravitreal anti-VEGF therapy in proliferative diabetic retinopathy.

A. Fundus showing florid neovascularization of the disc.
B. Complete resolution of neovascularization of the disc after intravitreal anti-VEGF therapy.

in diabetic patients with clinically significant macular edema (Figure 25.2). More recently in 2013, the Study of Ranibizumab Injection in Subjects with Clinically Significant Macular Edema with Central Involvement Secondary to Diabetes Mellitus (RIDE and RISE trials) established anti-VEGF injections as the gold standard treatment for diabetic macular edema. Compared with laser therapy, monthly intravitreal injections of ranibizumab were associated with significantly greater visual gains and greater anatomic reduction of macular edema and also reduced the rate of progression of retinopathy and even reversed the grade of retinopathy. Intravitreal injection of a slow-releasing steroid (dexamethasone) implant has also been FDA approved for treatment of diabetic macular edema. Steroid injection should be used with caution because it increases risk of cataracts and glaucoma.

Neovascularization (Figure 25.3) and proliferative diabetic retinopathy is the most important cause of severe vision loss or blindness in diabetic patients because of vitreous hemorrhage or tractional retinal detachment. Proliferative diabetic retinopathy is amenable to treatment by panretinal laser photocoagulation to inhibit the growth stimulus for neovascularization. In the Diabetic Retinopathy Study, incidence of severe visual loss in patients treated with panretinal photocoagulation was 11%, but the incidence in those who did not receive laser during a 2-year follow-up was 26% (ARR=15%, NNT=6–7). Intravitreal anti-VEGF injections are also used in proliferative retinopathy to expedite regression of neovascularization. Pars plana vitrectomy, membrane peeling, and endolaser are surgical methods of addressing nonclearing vitreous hemorrhage or tractional macular detachment.

GLAUCOMA

Glaucoma is the second most common cause of irreversible blindness worldwide and in the United States the most common cause of blindness in black Americans. It affects more than 2.25 million Americans ≥40 years old and results in >3 million office visits each year. The financial burden is considerable because of the prevalence and chronicity of glaucoma and the debilitation that results.

The definition of glaucoma has evolved considerably, and it is now defined as characteristic optic nerve head damage and visual field loss. Increased intraocular pressure (IOP) is no longer considered an absolute criterion, although it is a very important risk factor. There are many different types of glaucoma, of which primary open-angle glaucoma (POAG) is the most common. Adults >50 years old should be screened for glaucoma every 1–2 years. Older adults with a family history of glaucoma, black ethnicity, or other risk factors may need more frequent screening.

POAG is a chronic disease most commonly affecting older adults. The "clogged" drain of the eye impairs passage of aqueous humor out of the angle. Slow aqueous drainage leads to chronically increased IOPs. This is in contrast to acute angle-closure glaucoma, in which the eye's drain is suddenly blocked off, IOP increases precipitously, and the patient has considerable redness and pain with acute vision loss. Pain may be so severe as to cause headache, nausea, and vomiting. Emergent ophthalmologic referral is required to reverse the angle closure and decrease the IOP through the use of aqueous

Table 25.3—Common Signs and Symptoms of Eye Conditions Requiring Immediate Referral to an Ophthalmologist

Condition	Symptoms and Signs
Retinal detachment	Flashes, floaters, decreased vision
Acute angle-closure glaucoma	Eye pain or headache, ocular hyperemia, dilated pupil, decreased vision, nausea, vomiting
Ischemic optic neuropathy	Sudden painless loss of vision (complete or partial) in one eye
Central artery occlusion or giant cell arteritis	Sudden painless loss of vision in one eye; if from giant cell arteritis, then review of symptoms may reveal accompanying jaw claudication, headache, transient diplopia, etc
Bacterial keratitis	Decreased vision, eye redness, pain, discharge
Scleritis	Eye redness, pain, decreased vision
Posterior uveitis	Floaters, decreased vision
Corneal ulcers	Eye redness, pain, decreased vision, corneal infiltrate
Uveitis	Photophobia, eye redness, decreased vision
Herpes zoster ophthalmicus	Eye redness, pain, burning, rash, decreased vision, light sensitivity

Table 25.4—Treatment of Eye Conditions Commonly Seen by Primary Care Providers

Condition	Treatment and/or Cause
Red eye	
Subconjunctival hemorrhage	Supportive treatment with artificial tears
Dry eye	Artificial tears, cyclosporine 0.2% eye drops
Blepharitis	Lid scrubs, ophthalmic antibiotic ointment qhs, oral doxycycline
Lid malposition/exposure	Ocular lubricant, refer for surgical repair
Allergic conjunctivitis	Cold compresses, allergen avoidance, topical/systemic antihistamines
Viral conjunctivitis	Supportive treatment with artificial tears; refer to ophthalmologist if vision significantly affected
Chalazion	Warm compresses, may refer for excision
Herpes simplex keratitis	Trifluridine eye drops, refer to ophthalmologist
Herpes zoster ophthalmicus	Tear drops, refer to ophthalmologist immediately
Angle-closure glaucoma	Pilocarpine 2% ophthalmic solution, refer to ophthalmologist immediately
Floaters, flashes	Refer to ophthalmologist immediately; may be retinal detachment or vitreous hemorrhage
Sudden decrease in vision	Refer to ophthalmologist immediately; may be secondary to a number of vision-threatening problems
Diplopia	
Monocular	Refractive error, cataract
Binocular	Microvascular infarct to cranial nerve, giant cell arteritis, compressive tumor

suppressants, miotics, and laser iridotomy. Conversely, the increase in IOP in POAG is slow and much less severe. Individuals with POAG are asymptomatic and can suffer substantial field loss before consulting an ophthalmologist, which underscores the importance of regular ophthalmologic screening of older adults.

Development of POAG is most likely multifactorial and polygenic. Initial pedigrees demonstrated linkage to the 1q locus. Subsequent investigations have more precisely defined the GLC1A gene that encodes for myocilin, the trabecular meshwork-induced glucocorticoid response protein. Several other chromosomal loci, including those mapped to chromosomes 2, 3, 7, and 10, are also associated with development of glaucoma.

The management of POAG is approached by the ophthalmologist in a stepwise manner. A variety of IOP-lowering medications, both local and systemic, are available. Mechanisms of action include decreased aqueous production or increased aqueous outflow. Various eye drop formulations are available, and all have some adverse effects (Table 25.5). In the face of visual field progression despite maximal medications, intolerance to medications, or inability to comply with eye drop administration (eg, because of problems such as rheumatoid arthritis or dementia), laser trabeculoplasty (application of laser energy to the trabecular meshwork) can be effective in lowering IOP in approximately 50% of patients for 3–5 years after treatment. Intraocular surgery involves the creation of a fistula or filtration site to allow an alternative route of aqueous egress (trabeculectomy). Adjunctive antimetabolite use with 5-fluorouracil[OL] or mitomycin-C[OL] has increased the success of this procedure in those patients at high risk of surgical failure because of fibrosis and scarring of the filtration site. Alternative surgeries for glaucoma include drainage devices or aqueous shunts. These devices made of silicone shunt fluid from the anterior chamber to the subconjunctival space. Cryotherapy or laser procedures to destroy the ciliary body

Table 25.5—Adverse Events of Selected Eye Drops for Glaucoma

Class	Adverse Events
Aqueous suppressants	
α-Agonists (eg, brimonidine)	Allergic dermatoconjunctivitis, dry mouth/nose, mental status changes occasionally
β-Blockers (eg, timolol)	Bradycardia, dyspnea, asthma, heart failure exacerbations, impotence, exercise intolerance, hypoglycemia masking
Carbonic anhydrase inhibitors (eg, dorzolamide)	Blurry vision, stinging, bad taste in mouth, allergic dermatoconjunctivitis
Aqueous outflow facilitators	
Epinephrine (eg, dipivefrin)	Palpitations, angina, cystoid macular edema
Miotics (eg, pilocarpine)	Brow ache, blurriness, detached retina, small pupils
Prostaglandins (eg, latanoprost)	Hyperemia, increased length and thickness and darkness of eyelashes, increased iris and eyelid pigmentation, orbital fat atrophy, cystoid macular edema, exacerbation of herpetic eye disease

(cyclocryoablation or cyclophotocoagulation) can be used when the prognosis for vision in the eye is poor.

The strength of evidence is high in support of treating ocular hypertension to prevent the onset of glaucoma and of treating prevalent glaucoma to slow down progression of disease. Based on a meta-analysis of the literature, 12 ocular hypertensive patients need to be treated to prevent 1 patient from developing visual field defects or optic nerve changes consistent with glaucoma (SOE=A). From a meta-analysis of literature on treatment of established glaucoma patients, the NNT to prevent 1 glaucoma patient from progressive vision damage within 5 years of treatment is 7. The ARR is 14.2%.

ANTERIOR ISCHEMIC OPTIC NEUROPATHY

Anterior ischemic optic neuropathy (Figure 25.4) can result in acute vision or field loss. Microvascular occlusion of the blood supply to the optic nerve can be attributed to atherosclerotic vascular disease or inflammation in the setting of giant cell (temporal) arteritis. The nonarteritic form typically affects patients with vasculopathic risk factors such as diabetes mellitus and hypertension; the latter, the arteritic form, tends to occur in older adults with a history of myalgias, headaches, and weight loss. An increased Westergren erythrocyte sedimentation rate and a positive temporal artery biopsy are diagnostic. Systemic corticosteroid treatment is crucial to avoid visual loss in the other eye. Because of the hypotensive effects of phosphodiesterase inhibitors (eg, sildenafil), it has been speculated that they may contribute to nonarteritic ischemic neuropathy; however, causation has not been proved.

CHARLES BONNET SYNDROME

Between 10% and 13% of patients with significant visual loss (bilateral acuity worse than 20/60) experience visual hallucinations, a condition known as Charles

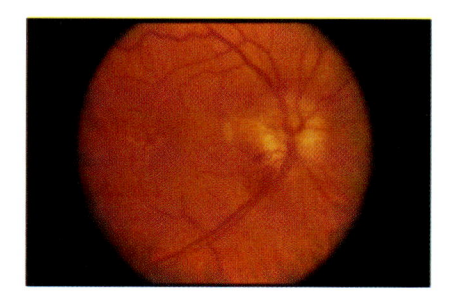

Figure 25.4—Pallid swelling of the optic nerve head in anterior ischemic optic neuropathy.

Bonnet syndrome. Hallucinations may be elementary shapes, or more commonly they are complex and highly organized with patients seeing small children, multiple animals, or a vivid scene as one would see in a movie. Patients with this syndrome have a clear sensorium and are aware that the visions are not real. It has been suggested that this syndrome is a concomitant of the phantom limb syndrome. Underlying conditions include age-related macular degeneration, glaucoma, diabetic retinopathy, and cerebral infarction. If the cause of vision loss is known and there is no homonymous visual field defect present, neuroimaging is not necessary.

The best treatment for the Charles Bonnet syndrome is education, reassurance, and support. Patients should be informed that the hallucinations are a sign of eye disease, not mental illness. An occasional patient has partial insight or loses insight and becomes very distressed by this symptom. When this distress is significant or leads to dangerous behavior, a cautious trial of low dosages of a second-generation antipsychotic medication can be considered.

LOW-VISION REHABILITATION

Despite considerable advancements in the medical treatment of ocular conditions, many patients, especially those with the wet form of ARMD, can ultimately sustain permanent visual loss. Visual training and the provision of visual aids are indispensable services for those with low vision (visual acuity <20/60).

Patients with low vision can develop useful adaptive skills with proper instruction. Eccentric viewing by ARMD patients with central macular pathology uses the principle of off-center fixation. The patient can benefit from formal training to find and use the most effective eccentric viewing points. Instruction in scanning and tracking and other skills can help the patient integrate his or her visual environment.

Various low-vision aids are available to improve the ability to see both near and far. The fine detail required for reading is the most common indication for visual aids. Improved lighting is a simple modification that can enhance visualization of print. Selection of reading material using bold, enlarged fonts and accentuated black-on-white contrast can also be helpful. Magnification also is commonly used. Various devices such as high-plus spectacles, hand-held magnifiers, stand magnifiers, and closed-circuit television can also enhance reading. Distance magnification can be achieved with the use of telescopic devices that can be hand-held for spot viewing or spectacle mounted for continual viewing. Talking devices, which are computers used to create voice synthesis such as those used at stoplights, or Braille can be especially helpful for those who have completely lost vision. Downloadable smart phone apps that can provide magnification, money recognition, and dictation functions are also available.

CHOOSING WISELY® RECOMMENDATIONS

Visual Loss and Eye Conditions

- Do not perform preoperative medical tests for eye surgery without specific indications.
- Most cases of acute conjunctivitis have a viral etiology. Do not treat viral infections with antibiotics; if diagnosis is uncertain, patients may be followed closely for resolution.
- Do not place temporary or permanent punctal plugs for mild dry eye syndrome before trying other medical treatment.

Diabetes Mellitus

- Avoid using medications to achieve hemoglobin A_{1c} <7.5% in most adults ≥65 years old; moderate control is generally better.

REFERENCES

- ACCORD Study Group; ACCORD Eye Study Group, Chew EY, Ambrosius WT, Davis MD, et al. Effects of medical therapies on retinopathy progression in type 2 diabetes. *N Engl J Med.* 2010;363(3):233–244.

    This randomized trial of 10,251 participants with type 2 diabetes showed that at 4 years both intensive glycemic control and combination therapy for dyslipidemia limited the progression of diabetic retinopathy. Intensive blood pressure control was not shown to reduce the rate of progression.

- Lindblad B, Håkansson N, Wolk A. Smoking cessation and the risk of cataract: a prospective cohort study of cataract extraction among men. *JAMA Ophthalmol.* 2014;132(3):253–257.

    In this cohort study of 44,371 men, smoking cessation significantly decreased the risk of cataract extraction. Higher intensity of smoking was associated with both greater risk of cataract extraction and longer duration of risk after smoking cessation.

- Lindsley K, Matsumura S, Hatef E, et al. Interventions for chronic blepharitis. *Cochrane Database Syst Rev.* 2012 May 16;5:CD005556.

    This article is a Cochrane review of randomized, controlled trials of interventions for chronic blepharitis, which accounts for many patient complaints of eye irritation, dry eyes, and tired eyes. Lid hygiene and topical antibiotics provide symptomatic relief, but there is no strong evidence for any treatments providing a cure for chronic blepharitis.

- Peeters A, Webers CA, Prins MH, et al Quantifying the effect of intraocular pressure reduction on the occurrence of glaucoma. *Acta Ophthalmol.* 2010;88(1):5–11.

    This article is a meta-analysis of the randomized controlled trials looking at the treatment of ocular hypertension and open-angle glaucoma.

- Ying GS, Kim BJ, Mcguire MG, et al. Sustained visual acuity loss in the comparison of age-related macular degeneration treatments trials. *JAMA Ophthalmol.* 2014;132(8):915–921.

    This study shows that sustained visual acuity loss was relatively rare after 2 years of treatment with two antivascular endothelial growth factors, one FDA-approved for the eye and another that is commonly used off-label for the eye, in the treatment of wet age-related macular degeneration.

JoAnn A. Giaconi, MD
David Sarraf, MD

CHAPTER 26—HEARING LOSS

KEY POINTS

- Hearing loss is among the most common chronic diseases among older adults: 10% of adults 65–75 years old and 25% of those >75 years old have hearing loss.

- Treatment of hearing loss and attention to communication strategies can improve quality of life for individuals who have difficulty with hearing.

- Important issues when considering hearing aids for an older adult with hearing loss are the nature and degree of hearing loss, the person's ability to manipulate the aid and adapt to its use, and the person's social support and financial resources.

Hearing loss is the fourth most common chronic disease among older adults. Hearing loss is often assumed to be benign, but it has profound effects on quality of life. The psychological effects of hearing loss include family discord, social isolation, loss of self-esteem, anger, and depression. Epidemiologic studies suggest an association between hearing loss and cognitive impairment, and between hearing loss and reduced mobility. Hearing loss can also affect an older adult's interaction with clinicians, making history taking and patient education difficult. Treatment of hearing loss and attention to communication strategies can improve quality of life for individuals with hearing loss by facilitating interaction with family, friends, and caregivers. Studies indicate that use of a hearing aid can relieve symptoms of depression that are associated with hearing loss.

NORMAL HEARING AND AGE-RELATED CHANGES IN THE AUDITORY SYSTEM

The normal ear is an efficient transducer of sound energy into nerve impulses. Sound energy is transmitted through the external ear to the tympanic membrane and the auditory ossicles. The malleus, incus, and stapes in series transmit vibrations to the oval window of the cochlea. Fluid waves within the cochlea stimulate the outer hair cells of the scala tympani. These cells stimulate the inner hair cells, which generate impulses that are sent via cochlear neurons to the cochlear nuclei and then to auditory pathways elsewhere in the brain.

Age-related changes in the auditory system can interfere with its function. The walls of the external ear canal become thin. Cerumen becomes drier and more tenacious, increasing the likelihood of cerumen impaction. The tympanic membrane becomes thicker and appears duller in older adults than in younger people. The ossicular joints undergo degenerative changes, but this generally does not interfere with sound transmission to the cochlea. Cochlear changes include loss of sensory hair cells and fibrocytes in the organ of Corti, stiffening of the basilar membrane, calcification of auditory structures, and cochlear neuronal loss. Changes in the stria vascularis include thickening of capillaries, decreased production of endolymph, and decreased Na^+/K^+-ATPase activity. These degenerative changes occur to varying degrees in different individuals. It is currently not possible to fully correlate the degree of hearing loss with histologic changes in the aging ear.

Changes in central auditory processing also occur with aging. In one study, when competing speech stimuli were presented to each ear, the right ear had a 5%–10% advantage over the left ear in younger people (the effect of right- and left-handedness was not assessed; all the participants were right-handed). In adults 80–89 years old, this difference increased to >40%. This difference may be related to a loss of efficiency of transfer of auditory information from one side of the brain to the other through the corpus callosum.

EPIDEMIOLOGY

Hearing loss can result from dysfunction of the auditory system at any point from the external ear to the brain. This loss can be described in terms of the loss of ability to hear pure tones across the range of audio frequencies important for understanding speech, but in practical terms, difficulty in understanding spoken language and perceiving environmental sounds significantly affects quality of life. The prevalence of hearing loss increases with age. Hearing loss is present in 10% of adults 65–75 years old and in 25% of those >75 years old. In nursing homes, estimates of prevalence vary from 50% to 100%, depending on the criteria used to define hearing loss.

In addition to age, male sex is a risk factor for hearing loss. Loss of hearing in the higher audio frequencies is associated with noise exposure; higher levels of education are associated with a lower prevalence of hearing loss. Black race is associated with a lower risk of age-associated hearing loss. The association of hearing loss with cardiovascular risk factors is less clear, with results differing among studies.

Hearing loss can be caused by pathology in the external ear canal, the middle ear, the inner ear, the auditory nerve, central auditory pathways, or a combination of these. For typical audiograms for common forms of hearing loss, see Figure 26.1.

Conductive hearing loss is caused by disease in the external ear, such as cerumen impaction or a foreign body in the canal, or by middle-ear pathology, such as otosclerosis, cholesteatoma, tympanic membrane perforation, or middle-ear effusion.

Sensorineural hearing loss is most often caused by cochlear disease. Noise is the most common factor in cochlear damage. Hearing loss is less common among people in quiet rural environments than among those in industrialized communities. Other causes of hearing loss include ototoxic medications, genotype, vascular disease, and rarely, occupational and environmental chemical exposures. Smokers have higher rates of hearing loss than nonsmokers. Autoimmune disease and auditory nerve tumors are rare causes of sensorineural hearing loss. Neuronal loss can affect the brain stem and cortical ascending auditory pathways. The resulting deficits in central auditory processing can affect perception of sound and the ability to understand speech. These deficits are not apparent on a simple audiogram.

PRESBYCUSIS

Most hearing loss in older adults is categorized as presbycusis (literally, "older hearing"). Presbycusis is a sensorineural, usually symmetrical hearing loss. It is usually due to cochlear pathology but may have central components. Many people with presbycusis can be helped by amplification, especially if speech discrimination is preserved.

Sensory presbycusis is attributed to a loss of sensory hair cells in the basal end of the cochlea. It results in a steeply sloping audiogram. It is often slowly progressive, beginning with the higher frequencies of 8,000 Hz, 6,000 Hz, and 4,000 Hz. It can involve the 3,000 and 2,000 Hz range, which is the higher portion of the range of frequencies in human speech (Figure 26.2). Loss of auditory acuity can begin when people are in their twenties but may not become clinically evident until later decades. People with this type of hearing loss often have trouble hearing in the presence of background noise but are able to hear adequately in quiet settings. Amplification often helps these patients, because speech discrimination is satisfactory.

Strial presbycusis results from atrophy of the stria vascularis. It typically begins between the ages of 20 and 60 years old and is characterized by mild to moderate hearing loss in most frequencies. People with strial presbycusis usually have good speech discrimination and do well with amplification.

Neural presbycusis is caused by a cochlear neuronal loss of ≥50%. Despite preserved pure-tone thresholds, which are not affected until >90% of cochlear neurons have been lost, individuals with neural presbycusis show very poor speech discrimination. Successful use of amplification is difficult for this form of presbycusis.

Cochlear conductive presbycusis is caused by changes in cochlear mechanics produced by mass or stiffness changes or spiral ligament atrophy. It has a unique audiogram, which gradually descends over at least 5 octaves with no more than a 25-dB difference between any 2 adjacent frequencies. Speech discrimination can also be impaired. Pathologically, this form is defined by the absence of histologic changes seen in the other forms of presbycusis.

Most presbycusis is probably a mixture of these forms. The shape of the audiogram and speech discrimination scores depend on the extent of injury to various components of the cochlea.

CLINICAL PRESENTATION AND HEARING LOSS DETECTION

It is common for patients with hearing loss not to bring it to medical attention. Partly because of the slowly progressive nature of hearing loss, many older adults are unaware of their hearing deficit. They may also be unaware of advances in hearing instrument technology that can help people who did not benefit from older devices. In some cases, the perceived stigma of wearing a hearing aid causes the patient to deny the problem. The hearing loss may be brought to medical attention by family members, who complain that the patient does not hear them or plays the television or radio too loudly. Clinicians may notice that the patient does not respond when spoken to by someone out of the patient's field of view, or seems to misunderstand questions. Hearing loss can also be interpreted as cognitive impairment. Caregivers and clinicians may not recognize the presence of hearing loss or may assume it is a benign component of aging.

Tinnitus, or "ringing in the ears," can be an early sign of hearing loss. Individuals with tinnitus or buzzing should be evaluated by an otolaryngologist. Medical treatment for tinnitus is often unsuccessful, but hearing aids for those with hearing loss, or the use of devices that provide background white noise, may be useful to reduce the impact of tinnitus.

Fitting hearing aids early in the course of hearing loss can help the person adjust to their use (SOE=B), and treatment can reduce psychological morbidity related to hearing loss (SOE=A). Hearing aid use may reduce the frequency of behavioral problems in older adults who have both hearing loss and dementia. However, robust evidence that treatment of hearing loss can prevent or reduce cognitive decline is lacking.

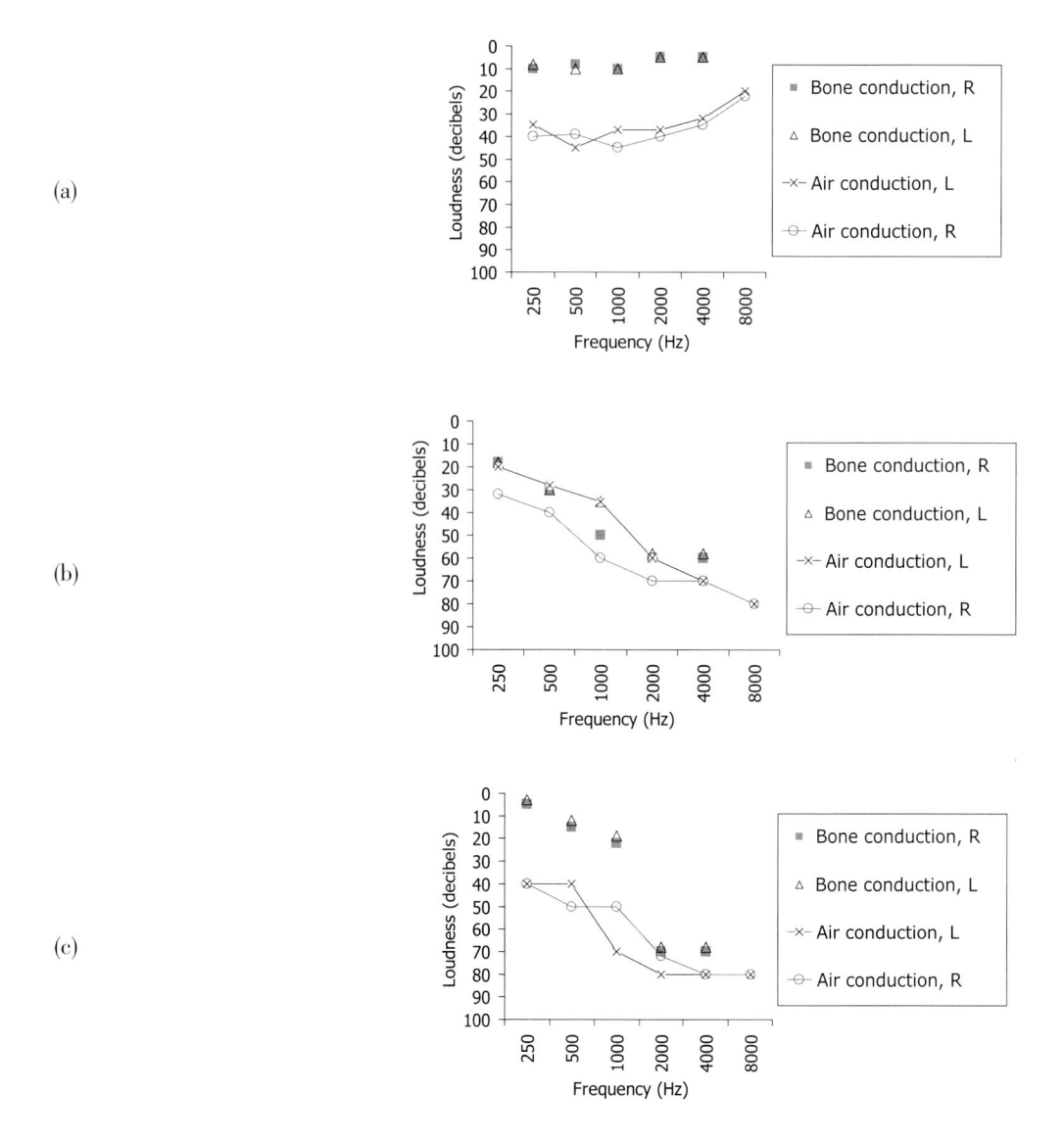

Figure 26.1—Audiograms for conductive, sensorineural, and mixed hearing loss

(a) Conductive hearing loss. Air conduction thresholds are greater than bone conduction thresholds, most likely because of middle-ear pathology.
(b) Sensorineural hearing loss. Air and bone conduction thresholds are the same, most likely because of inner-ear damage. The high-frequency pattern of this patient's hearing loss is typical of presbycusis.
(c) Mixed hearing loss. Air and bone conduction thresholds are abnormal, with the greatest difference seen for the left ear. This patient has pathology in both the middle and inner ears. Bone conduction thresholds for the left ear are measured by masking the right ear.

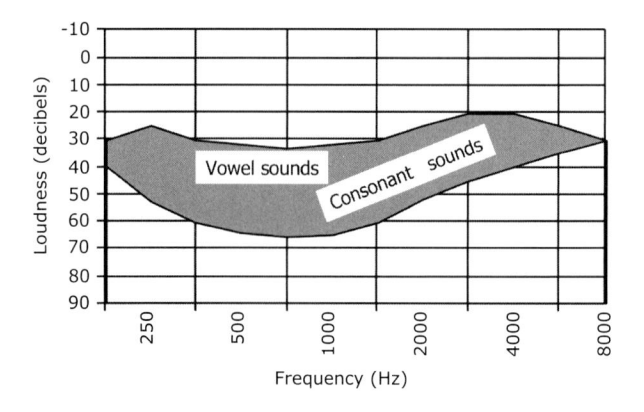

Figure 26.2—Speech range on the audiogram

Hearing loss assessments can include questionnaires, testing with speech or pure tones, or a combination. The Hearing Handicap Inventory for the Elderly–Screening Version is a 10-item questionnaire that asks about difficulty with communication in various settings. It can be useful to determine the impact that hearing loss has on a patient's daily activities. The Whisper Test, when performed from 2 feet away, was associated with a median positive LR of 5.1 (range, 2.3–7.4) and a median negative LR of 0.03 (range, 0.007–0.73) for detecting hearing loss poorer than 25 dB. A handheld otoscope with a tone generator can be used by primary care providers to assess for the presence of hearing loss at selected frequencies (0.5, 1, 2, and 4 kHz) and 2 loudness levels (25 and 40 dB hearing loss). This device should be used in a quiet environment. When set at 40 dB hearing loss, testing at 1 and 2 kHz has a sensitivity of 94% and a specificity of 82%–90% for detecting hearing loss. A similar device costs $660–$900 with accessories; the cost of using it would not be directly reimbursable by third-party payors. One app for the iPhone (uHear by Unitron, a hearing device manufacturer) uses pure-tone testing. It has high sensitivity and specificity for identifying moderate hearing loss in the office setting (SOE=B). Other apps and online hearing tests may also be helpful for identifying hearing loss. Results of hearing tests can be affected by background noise and other factors.

When a hearing loss is detected and the patient is willing and able to pay for a hearing aid, referral to an audiologist should be discussed.

EVALUATION OF SUSPECTED HEARING LOSS

The clinician should exclude causes of hearing loss that are readily treatable or that warrant referral to an otolaryngologist before signing medical clearance forms for hearing aids (see Table 26.1). The ear canals should be examined with an otoscope to exclude the presence of obstruction or effusion before referral for audiologic testing. Medications should be reviewed for their potential contribution to hearing loss. Furosemide and salicylates can cause reversible hearing loss. Other medications, such as aminoglycosides and vancomycin, can cause irreversible sensorineural hearing loss and should be used only with caution.

Cerumen impaction can cause a clinically significant hearing loss, as much as 40 dB. If the patient has a history of tympanic membrane surgery or perforation, referral to an otolaryngologist for removal of the impaction is advisable. Otherwise, cerumen can be removed by manual extraction in cooperative patients. Cerumenolytics alone, used for several days, are effective about 40% of the time in treating cerumen impaction. Alternatively, cerumenolytics or saline can be applied to soften the wax 15–30 min before irrigating the ear with warm water. If irrigation fails, using a cerumenolytic for several days may clear the impaction or soften it enough that repeat irrigation is successful. If the impaction remains, the patient should be referred to an otolaryngologist.

The otolaryngologist will further evaluate the hearing loss and identify treatable causes. An asymmetrical hearing loss demands thorough investigation. Auditory nerve tumors are rare, but tumors of the posterior pharynx can obstruct the eustachian tube, causing a middle-ear effusion with conductive hearing loss.

The audiologist will assess hearing to determine the presence and type of hearing loss. A comprehensive audiologic assessment consists of pure-tone thresholds for both air and bone conduction, speech-recognition thresholds, speech discrimination, and middle-ear function. This information, along with the medical evaluation, is used to determine appropriate treatment. Audiologists recommend and fit hearing aids and provide auditory rehabilitation. Medicare will pay for an audiologic examination if it is ordered by a physician.

TREATMENT

Some causes of hearing loss are amenable to medical or surgical treatment. Paget disease of the bone can affect the middle ear, causing conductive loss, or the inner ear, leading to sensorineural loss. Bisphosphonate therapy rarely restores hearing, although it may stabilize hearing loss (SOE=C). Otosclerosis or tympanosclerosis may be correctable with surgery (SOE=C). Otosclerosis may respond to bisphosphonate therapy (SOE=C). Sudden hearing loss may be autoimmune in nature and sometimes responds to corticosteroids (SOE=B) or immunosuppressant therapy (SOE=C). Most older adults with hearing loss are treated with communication strategies or amplification, or both. Hearing aids often improve ability to understand speech, particularly soft speech and conversational loud speech (SOE=B). Almost all hearing aids currently sold use digital sound processing to limit noise to comfortable levels and to reduce feedback, and have dual microphones for reduction of background noise. They may have automatic volume control.

Surgical treatment of sensorineural hearing loss may include implantation of prosthetic devices (see bone-anchored hearing aids and cochlear implants, below).

Strategies to Enhance Communication

Individuals with hearing loss should be encouraged to let others know about their hearing loss and to suggest

Table 26.1—Indications for Medical Evaluation of Hearing Loss

- Unilateral hearing loss with sudden or recent onset (within the last 90 days)*
- Acute or chronic dizziness
- Air-bone gap ≥15 dB at 500, 1000, and 2000 Hz*
- Visible congenital or traumatic ear deformity*
- Pain or discomfort in the ear
- Active drainage from the ear within the previous 90 days
- Visible deformity of the outer ear
- Cerumen impaction or foreign body in the ear canal
- Cerumen impaction with history of tympanic membrane surgery or perforation*

*Indication for referral to an otolaryngologist

Table 26.2—Strategies to Improve Communication with People Who Have Hearing Loss

- Ask the listener what is the best way to communicate with him or her.
- Obtain the listener's attention before speaking.
- Eliminate background noise as much as possible.
- Be sure the listener can see the speaker's lips:
    - Speak face-to-face in the same room.
    - Do not obscure the lips with hands or other objects.
    - Make certain that light shines directly on the speaker's face, not from behind the speaker.
- Speak slowly and clearly, but avoid shouting.
- Speak toward the better ear, if applicable.
- Change phrasing if the listener does not understand at first.
- Spell words out, use gestures, or write them down.
- Have the listener repeat back what he or she heard.

strategies that will help them communicate more easily (Table 26.2). In addition to using these strategies, clinicians should provide options for patients with hearing loss, such as sign language interpreters, the use of writing materials (eg, pen and paper, dry-erase board, or computer screen), or assistive devices. Office and hospital staff should be alerted to a patient's hearing loss. Background noise from the environment can interfere with hearing and should be reduced as much as possible.

Lipreading can be a useful adjunct to listening, but it requires thoughtfulness on the part of the speaker. When speaking to a person with hearing loss who lip-reads, it is important to face him or her and to obtain the person's attention before speaking; a gentle touch on the hand or arm will usually suffice. Each word should be spoken clearly and distinctly. Shouting not only distorts lip movements so they are harder to read but also can make the speaker sound angry even when not. It is best to speak in complete sentences; single words are hard to lip-read because the listener often needs cues from context to identify meaning. It is helpful to make certain the person knows the topic of conversation. The language used should be appropriate for the listener's educational level. Unlike deaf persons who have usually had hearing loss all or most of their lives, most older adults with hearing loss do not know sign language. Sometimes, amplification and lipreading are not enough. Gestures can aid communication even with cognitively impaired individuals.

For patients with hearing loss, it can also be helpful to write words down. For those with both hearing loss and visual impairment, large printing with a marker pen or a laptop computer screen with magnified print may be necessary. These patients may benefit from correction of the visual problem, if possible (eg, cataract removal or use of eyeglasses). In any case, providing written instructions generally improves understanding and retention of important information.

The clinician should be alert to misunderstandings, which are common. If a reply does not make sense, repeating the idea of what was said using different words can help, as can asking the patient to express what he or she heard.

Assistive Listening Devices

For some people with hearing loss, a personal amplifier may be more useful than hearing aids. These pocket-sized devices are considerably less expensive than hearing aids and are harder to misplace. Headphones stay on the head better than earbuds and provide sound to both ears. The volume and microphone placement of the amplifier should be adjusted to find the best combination for a given user. At least one or two of these devices should be available in every health care

Table 26.3—Effects and Rehabilitation of Hearing Loss, by Degree of Loss

Degree of Loss	Hearing Loss (dB)	Sounds Difficult to Hear	Effect on Communication	Amplification or Other Assistance Needed
Mild	25–40	Whisper	Difficulty understanding soft speech or normal speech in presence of background noise	Hearing aid needed in specific situations
Moderate	41–55	Conversational speech	Difficulty understanding any but loud speech	Frequent need for hearing aid
Severe	56–80	Shouting, vacuum cleaner	Can understand only amplified speech	Amplification needed for all communication
Profound	≥81	Hair dryer, heavy traffic, telephone ringer	Difficulty understanding amplified speech; may miss telephone calls	May need to supplement hearing aid with lipreading, assistive listening devices, sign language

SOURCE: Data in part from *A Report on Hearing Aids: User Perspectives and Concerns*. Washington, DC: American Association of Retired Persons; 1993:2.

facility; these devices are not personalized and so can be used by different people.

Adaptive equipment can facilitate telephone use. State agencies may provide amplified telephones, vibrating and flashing ringer alert devices, and text telephones (TTY) or captioned telephones to people with hearing loss. This equipment can also be purchased from retailers of assistive devices. Text telephones can be contacted through telecommunications relay services by dialing 711, then the number. A communications assistant transcribes the caller's voice into text that is displayed for the listener. Captioned telephones and Web-based captioning services allow the user to hear the caller's voice and then to read a transcription of the caller's voice during the call.

Many other assistive devices are available. Television listening devices can spare others from overly loud volume levels. FM loop systems can be used for groups of people with FM receivers or telecoil switches in their hearing aids. Wireless FM transmitters and receivers are also available for indoor or outdoor use. Infrared group-listening devices are primarily useful indoors. Vibrating and flashing devices such as alarm clocks and timers, smoke alarms, doorbell alerts, and motion sensors can improve quality of life and safety for people with hearing loss. These items can be purchased through the agencies mentioned above, or from catalog retailers of assistive listening devices.

Electronic communication such as text messaging and e-mail can be helpful for patients and caregivers with hearing loss. However, measures to protect patient confidentiality must be considered if using these mediums.

Hearing Aids

Hearing aids are the most common form of amplification. Many factors need to be considered in deciding whether to fit an individual with a hearing aid. In addition to the nature and degree of hearing loss (Table 26.3), the person's motivation and ability to adapt to use of the aid and to physically manipulate the aid (Table 26.4), the degree of his or her social support, and his or her ability to afford the aid (Table 26.5) must be considered. Although hearing aids can be purchased from numerous sources, including over the Internet, working with an audiologist or other individual who has master's level training in audiology is advisable because of his or her expertise in hearing-aid fitting and adjustment.

Not everyone benefits from a hearing aid. The pattern of sensorineural damage can be such that speech discrimination is poor even with amplification. Some individuals are unable to tolerate the presence of the hearing aid in the ear. It is important to be sure that the aid can be returned during an initial trial period, usually 30 days, without having to pay the full cost of the aid. It is equally important not to give up on the aid too soon, because the audiologist often can adjust it to improve comfort and sound quality. The audiologist should provide counseling for optimal use of the aid. In general, two hearing aids are more beneficial than one. The first aid provides the most gain; the second one helps with speech discrimination and with localizing the source of sounds. However, the presence of asymmetrical hearing loss or significant difficulty in understanding competing speech stimuli may mean that use of a single hearing aid is more appropriate.

Many different styles of hearing aids are available (Table 26.4). Behind-the-ear aids hang behind the ear and are connected directly to an earmold. The earmold is usually custom made to fit each ear. Some behind-the-ear aids can be connected to assistive listening devices via a "boot," which fits over the end of the aid to provide direct audio input. Some newer models of hearing aids can be used with Bluetooth devices, including mobile telephones, remote microphones, and computers. Body aids are worn on the belt or in a pocket or harness, and they are connected to a custom-made earmold by a wire. These are rarely used. All-in-the-ear aids and canal aids usually have cases that are custom fit to the user. The smaller hearing aids may have remote controls.

Table 26.4—Advantages and Disadvantages of Styles of Hearing Aids

Style	Degree of Hearing Loss	Advantages	Disadvantages
CIC	Mild to moderate	Almost invisible Less occlusion of ear canal allows more natural sound Easier to use with headphones and telephone	Dexterity may be a problem. Small size may limit available features. May cost more than canal or in-the-ear aids Shorter battery life
Canal	Mild to moderate	More cosmetic than larger aids Telecoil available in some models May be able to use with headphones	Dexterity may be a problem. Small size may limit available features.
In the ear	Mild to severe	Ease of handling Comfortable fit Available options: telecoil, directional microphone More power than CIC or canal aid	More conspicuous than CIC or canal aid May be difficult to use with headphones
Behind the ear	Mild to profound	Greatest power Available options: telecoil, direct audio input, directional microphone Earmold can be changed separately	More conspicuous May be more difficult to insert than in-the-ear aids Difficult to use with headphones
Body aid	Severe to profound	Greatest separation of microphone from receiver reduces feedback	Most conspicuous Body-level microphone is subject to noise from clothing. Microphone is on chest or at waist, but speech is usually directed at ear level.
Bone conduction aid	Mild to severe	Bypasses middle ear; used if ear canal is unable to tolerate aid or earmold, or for unilateral hearing loss	Receiver of traditional aid causes pressure on the scalp, which can be uncomfortable; does not correct sensorineural loss. Being replaced by bone-anchored hearing aids

NOTE: CC = completely in the canal

Selection of aid style for each individual depends on the degree of hearing loss, available features, and the person's dexterity and motivation.

The telecoil is an induction coupling coil that can be built into the hearing aid. It detects the magnetic field produced by telephones that are compatible with hearing aids. The telecoil is used to listen to the telephone with less distraction from noise in the same room. It can also be used with many assistive listening devices. The amount of coupling, and therefore the volume of the signal, depends on the angle of the telecoil with respect to the magnetic field. Users may need to experiment to find the right angle. Strongly magnetic devices such as computer monitors often produce interference, which also depends on the angle and the distance of the telecoil from the device. These drawbacks aside, the telecoil is a useful feature and can be added to hearing aids at relatively low cost. Individuals with moderate to severe hearing loss should be encouraged to consider purchasing an aid with a telecoil.

Analogue hearing aids were the first type available but are rarely sold now. Digital technology has allowed improved sound quality, reduced size, and increased ability to customize the amplification of the aid to the needs of the user. Programmable aids are adjusted for each individual while he or she is wearing the aid. Often, 2 or more programs are available within a single aid. Using a computer, the audiologist makes adjustments to gain, response in different frequency ranges, and loudness balance for each program. One program may be most useful in the presence of background noise, whereas another works better in a quiet environment, and a third works with a telecoil. Patients with Ménière disease can have their aids reprogrammed to accommodate fluctuating hearing loss. Many hearing aids automatically adjust the volume to increase amplification of soft sounds while avoiding uncomfortable loudness, reducing the need for the user to manipulate the aid. This can be helpful for first-time users, although experienced users may require time to adjust to this feature. Hearing aids may have an automatic telecoil feature that switches to the telecoil program when a hearing-aid compatible telephone is brought close to the ear. Background noise is a significant problem for hearing-aid users. Traditional hearing aids amplify sound indiscriminately, so that background noise, eg, papers rustling or water running, can be very distracting. For new hearing-aid users, this problem can be addressed by having the audiologist gradually increase the gain of the hearing aid as the listener adjusts to being able to hear environmental sounds over the course of weeks. However, background noise in the presence of speech is a problem even for experienced hearing-aid users. The use of multiple microphones in

Table 26.5—Approximate Costs of Assistive Listening Devices and Hearing Aids

Type of Technology	Cost	Comments
Assistive listening devices (eg, personal amplifiers, telephone amplifiers, television listening devices)	$100 and up	Useful for specific situations (see text for details)
Hearing aids		
	One aid/two aids	
Digital, economy	$1,200/$2,200	Economy aids process signals more slowly and have fewer programs. Telecoils are available on request. Background noise suppression may be switched on manually. Economy aids may be very appropriate for persons with a quiet lifestyle.
Digital, value	$1,500/$2,800	Multiple programs, telecoil
Digital, mid-range	$2,100/$4,000	Multiple programs, telecoil, Bluetooth input
Digital, premium	$2,800/$5,400	Multiple features available, including multiple programs, telecoil, Bluetooth input, and more rapid signal processing

NOTE: Assistive listening devices and hearing aids are not covered by Medicare. Features of hearing aids in a given price range vary by manufacturer.

the hearing aid, combined with digital signal processing, can decrease the effects of background noise. This can significantly improve the user's ability to understand speech and increase satisfaction with the aid. Most hearing aids now include noise reduction and feedback suppression.

Unfortunately, the cost of hearing aids is often a significant barrier to their use and can affect the purchaser's choice of features (Table 26.5). The cost of a hearing aid ranges from $1,200 to $3,000 per device, or $2,200 to $5,400 for a pair. The features available in a given price range vary by manufacturer. Typically the cost of the aid includes follow-up visits to the hearing-aid dispenser through the life of the aid, although some audiologists may unbundle the follow-up visits from the original fitting and purchase. Hearing aids can be expected to last 3–5 years, although with care, aids may last longer. Although hearing aids are covered by Medicaid in most states, the amount of reimbursement often does not cover aids with advanced features. Hearing aids are not covered by Medicare or by private health insurance in many states, except in rare circumstances. Federal programs such as the Department of Veterans Affairs may pay for hearing aids, depending on the recipient's eligibility for services. Some charitable organizations assist in providing hearing aids to low-income persons.

Caring for Hearing Aids

Hearing aids should be stored with the battery compartment door open; this may be the only way to turn the hearing aid off. They should be wiped with a dry cloth daily (earmolds of behind-the-ear aids should be cleaned according to manufacturer's instructions). Wax may plug the sound outlet of a hearing aid, and the manufacturer's instructions should be consulted before trying to clean it.

Patients may need assistance to insert the hearing aid. First, it should be noted whether the hearing aid goes into the right ear (the aid may be marked with red) or the left ear (marked with blue). The battery door faces the outside of the ear. If there is a vent or a removal string, these are usually at the bottom. The following instructions apply to all except behind-the-ear aids:

The aid should first be turned on to be sure it is working. If so, a high-pitched squeal or vibration (feedback) should be heard; if no noise is heard when the volume is set at maximum, the battery should be replaced. The hearing aid should be oriented right side up, with the canal portion of the aid or earmold facing toward the canal. The wide, flat portion of an in-the-ear aid or earmold should be posterior. This part of the aid may need to be rotated so that it fits into the external ear, and the helix lifted gently to ease this part in. If there is feedback, the aid may be gently pushed to seat it more firmly into the ear. Turning the volume down may also reduce feedback.

Patients with dementia may remove and dispose of the aid. To reduce this risk, it can be helpful to order a loop attached to the hearing aid case; a piece of fishing line can be attached to the loop and the other end of the line pinned to the patient's clothing to catch the aid when the patient removes it. In long-term care institutions, a system for collecting the aids each night and placing them in the patients' ears each morning may facilitate use of the aids, while reducing the number that are lost.

Bone-Anchored Hearing Aids (BAHA)

People with unilateral hearing loss, inability to tolerate an earmold or hearing aid in the canal, or conductive/mixed hearing loss may be treated with a BAHA. A BAHA has a small post that is surgically implanted in the mastoid bone, which connects to a speech processor that converts sound into vibrations. The vibrations are transmitted through the post in the skull to the inner

Table 26.6—Characteristics of Older Candidates for Cochlear Implants

- Severe to profound sensorineural hearing loss in both ears
- Functional auditory nerve
- Short duration of severe hearing loss
- Good speech, language, and communication skills
- Not benefiting enough from other kinds of hearing aids
- No medical contraindication to surgery (eg, active infection, inability to tolerate general anesthesia)
- Realistic expectations about results
- Appropriate support services available for aural rehabilitation after cochlear implant
- Adequate motivation and cognition to participate in aural rehabilitation

ear, bypassing the middle ear. BAHAs are replacing bone conduction aids.

Cochlear Implants

For patients with severe to profound hearing loss who gain little or no benefit from hearing aids yet who are motivated to participate in the hearing world, cochlear implants can provide useful hearing (Table 26.6). A cochlear implant is an electronic device that bypasses the function of damaged or absent cochlear hair cells by providing electrical stimulation to cochlear nerve fibers. A receiver-stimulator and an intracochlear electrode array are surgically implanted. A headset is worn behind the ear. The headset microphone transmits signals to the speech processor, which filters and digitizes the sound into coded signals. The coded signals are sent to the cochlear implant, which then stimulates auditory nerve fibers in the cochlea. Nerve signals are then sent through the auditory system to the brain. Patients must be able to tolerate general anesthesia and to participate in extensive pre-implant testing and post-implant training. Meningitis is a rare complication of cochlear implants.

The cochlear implant procedure is covered by most Medicare carriers and insurance companies, although prior authorization is generally required. In general, outcomes of cochlear implantation in adults ≥65 years old have been comparable to those of younger adults, with many patients obtaining excellent results by both audiologic and quality-of-life measures. Cochlear implants do not restore normal hearing, but users can sense environmental sounds and are able to understand speech more easily. Many can use a telephone, and some can even enjoy music.

REFERENCES

- Lin FR, Yaffe K, Xia J, et al; Health ABC Study Group. Hearing loss and cognitive decline in older adults. *JAMA Intern Med.* 2013;173(4):293–299.

    Nearly 2,000 adults 70–79 years old were followed for up to 12 years to evaluate whether hearing loss is associated with accelerated cognitive decline. Baseline hearing loss appeared to be independently associated with accelerated cognitive decline and incident cognitive impairment in older adults.

- McKee M. Caring for older patients who have significant hearing loss. *Am Fam Physician.* 2013;87(5):360–366.

    A case scenario illustrates issues related to end-of-life care and long-term care facility placement for individuals with significant hearing loss. Socialization, communication during cognitive testing, and advance care planning are all affected by hearing loss. Treatment strategies are presented, although in many localities the availability of long-term care facilities specializing in care of those with severe hearing loss is limited.

- Pacala JT, Yuch B. Hearing deficits in the older patient: "I didn't notice anything". *JAMA.* 2012;307(11):1185–1194.

    This article incorporates progressive case disclosure as it reviews hearing loss demographics, detection and evaluation, and management including amplification. The case effectively illustrates the patient and family centered view on the impact, importance, and management challenges of this common condition.

- Szudek J, Ostevik A, Dziegielewski P, et al. Can uHear Me Now? Validation of an iPod-Based Hearing Loss Screening Test. *J Otolaryngol Head Neck Surgery.* 2012;41(S1):S78–S84.

    An iPod-based application used in an otology clinic and a sound booth was compared with standard audiogram done by the same audiologist on 100 adult patients. The app was a reasonable screening test to exclude moderate hearing loss (pure tone average > 40 dB) but slightly overestimated the degree of hearing loss.

- Weinstein BE, Taylor B. *Hearing Healthcare Toolkit for Use in Primary and Geriatric Care.* Unitron 2014. Request a link for downloading the kit at: http://unitron.com/content/unitron/us/en/professional/build-your-practice/hearing-healthcare-toolkit-hhcp.html#form-2 (accessed Jan 2016).

    This toolkit is a PDF file that includes information about the demographics and impact of hearing loss in the older population, a screening protocol and recommendations for evaluation of a person with hearing loss, communication techniques and aids, and intervention options for hearing loss. Some smart phone apps that turn the device into an amplifier are listed. The toolkit includes several annotated references to articles about hearing loss.

Priscilla F. Bade, MD, FACP, CMD

CHAPTER 27—DIZZINESS

KEY POINTS

- The classification of dizziness into vertigo, presyncope, dysequilibrium, mixed, or others may be useful in guiding patient evaluation; however, precise classification is often difficult, and multiple causes of the same symptoms are common.
- Dizziness is associated with increased fear of falling, functional disability, and depressive symptoms.
- Multiple factors can contribute to chronic dizziness.
- Expensive tests like electronystagmography, rotational chair testing, posturography, and neuroimaging, such as CT or MRI, are not often needed in the evaluation of dizziness.
- Multifactorial interventions can help in ameliorating chronic dizziness.

Dizziness ranks among the most common symptoms presented by older adults to primary health care providers. The various and often nonspecific terms—light-headedness, giddiness, wooziness, vertigo, spinning, floating, and imbalance—that patients typically use to describe dizziness add to the diagnostic and management challenge. Dizziness that continues >1–2 months is considered chronic. The prevalence of dizziness in adults ≥65 years old ranges from 4% to 30%. The wide prevalence range is related to differences in age, symptoms, and sample population among the various studies. The prevalence of dizziness is lower between the age of 65 and 69 years and increases as people get older. Dizziness is more common in women than in men.

Acute dizziness, which is independent of age, usually results from a disorder of one system. The causes, evaluation, and interventions are similar to those of chronic dizziness. The most common causes of acute dizziness are acute vestibular neuritis, cerebrovascular ischemia, and cardiovascular disorders resulting in hypotension. The approach to management in older adults is similar to that in younger patients.

Chronic dizziness is much more common in older adults, has a larger variety of contributing causes, and requires additional skill and patience to evaluate and manage successfully. This chapter focuses on chronic dizziness in older adults, which is commonly associated with increasing fear of falling, depressive symptoms, fall risk, and general functional disability.

CLASSIFICATION

Dizziness has been classified into 4 types of sensations: vertigo, presyncope, dysequilibrium, and other. A fifth type—mixed—results from a combination of two or more of the above and is the most common type of dizziness reported by older adults (Table 27.1).

Vertigo

Vertigo is an often episodic spinning or rotational sensation; objective vertigo ("the room is spinning") versus subjective vertigo ("I am spinning") results from disturbances in the vestibular system. The most common causes of vertigo are benign paroxysmal positional vertigo (BPPV) and Ménière disease. BPPV, an inner ear disorder, is characterized by sudden onset, seconds-long bouts of vertigo precipitated by certain changes in head position (rolling over in bed, gazing up or down). BPPV probably results from changes in endolymphatic pressure during head movements, resulting from dislodged otoconia in the semicircular canal. Ménière disease, an idiopathic inner ear disorder, is characterized by episodic vertigo, tinnitus, fluctuating hearing loss, and a sensation of fullness in the inner ear. Other causes of vertigo include idiopathic recurrent vestibulopathy and central vestibular lesions such as cerebrovascular disease and acoustic neuroma. Absence of spinning sensation does not exclude vestibular diseases, because patients with vestibular problems can describe dizziness as an imbalance, dysequilibrium, or other sensation. Patients with cervical dizziness secondary to cervical arthritis can also present with vertigo.

Presyncope

Presyncope, a feeling of faintness or lightheadedness, usually results from a cardiovascular problem causing brain hypoperfusion through postural hypotension. There is no specific definition of postural hypotension in older adults, but it is commonly defined as a drop in systolic arterial blood pressure of at least 20 mmHg and/or a drop in diastolic blood pressure of 10 mmHg after standing up from a supine position. However, older adults commonly describe dizziness on standing from a supine position without any orthostatic changes in blood pressure. Another common condition, postprandial hypotension, is defined as a decrease in systolic blood pressure of ≥20 mmHg in a sitting or standing posture within 1–2 hours of eating a meal.

Dysequilibrium

Dysequilibrium, a feeling of imbalance or unsteadiness on standing or walking, usually results from visual or proprioceptive system abnormalities, with or without vestibular system involvement. Common contributing conditions include vision problems (eg, refractory

Table 27.1—Classification of Dizziness

Type	Common Causes or Coexisting Conditions	Diagnostic Features	Treatment
Vertigo	Benign paroxysmal positional vertigo	History of episodic vertigo; rotational nystagmus; Dix-Hallpike maneuver confirms diagnosis	Epley maneuver is treatment of choice
	Meniere disease	Episodic vertigo lasting for a few hours; tinnitus; fluctuating hearing loss; sensation of fullness in ears; audiogram reveals sensorineural hearing loss (at low more than high frequencies)	Salt restriction, diuretics; vestibular suppressants may be helpful during acute attacks; in severe cases, may need surgical interventions, including endolymphatic decompression, vestibular nerve resection, and labyrinthectomy
	Ototoxic medications, eg, aminoglycosides, diuretics, NSAIDs	Presence of nystagmus, bedside vestibular function tests (eg, head thrust test can be abnormal)	Discontinue, substitute, or reduce dosage of offending medication
Presyncope	Cerebral ischemia secondary to orthostatic hypotension, cardiac causes, dehydration, medications, vasovagal attack, autonomic dysfunction secondary to diabetes, parkinsonism	Near fainting/lightheadedness when getting up from lying down or sitting position; orthostatic changes in blood pressure; investigations relevant to predisposing diseases	Treatment of specific cause, eg, proper hydration; dosage adjustment or removal of offending medications; slow rising from sitting or lying down position; graduated support stockings; physical therapy and/or occupational therapy; medications (eg, fludrocortisone, midodrine) as needed
	Postprandial hypotension	Near fainting/lightheadedness when getting up from lying down or sitting position; orthostatic hypotension usually within 45–60 min of eating	Frequent small meals; avoid exertion after meals; slow rising from sitting position; avoid antihypertensive drugs with or near meal time
Dysequilibrium	Vertebrobasilar ischemia and/or cerebellar infarcts/ hemorrhages	History of dizziness usually associated with slurred speech; visual changes; one-sided weakness and/or gait ataxia; truncal ataxia; CT or MRI or magnetic resonance angiography scan may be helpful	Low-dose aspirin, clopidogrel, or extended-release dipyridamole/ aspirin; rehabilitation
	Cerebellopontine angle tumor, eg, acoustic neuroma	History of vertigo or dysequilibrium, unilateral hearing loss, tinnitus; audiometry reveals sensorineural hearing loss more for higher frequencies; MRI is diagnostic	Surgery
	Parkinson disease	Bradykinesia; muscular rigidity; tremor; orthostatic hypotension	Drug therapy; rehabilitation therapy
	Peripheral neuropathy secondary to diabetes; vitamin B_{12} deficiency; idiopathic, etc	Decreased vibration or position sense; gait abnormality; hyperglycemia; low vitamin B_{12} level	Treatment of the underlying disease
	Cervical spine degenerative arthritis, spondylosis	Limitation of range of motion of neck; decreased vibratory or joint position sense; signs of radiculopathy or myelopathy; cervical spine radiologic abnormalities	Cervical or vestibular rehabilitation; cervical collar; surgery if needed
Other	Anxiety, depression, or psychosomatic disorders	Usually continual nonspecific dizziness; fatigue; poor appetite; sleep problems; somatic complaints; positive results on anxiety or depression screening scales	Psychotherapy and/or antidepressant therapy
Mixed	Medications: antianxiety drugs, antidepressants, anticonvulsants, antipsychotics, antihypertensives, anticholinergics	History of fatigue; dizziness often vague and can be continual, postural, or associated with confusion	Discontinue, substitute, or reduce dosage of offending medication
	Combination of any of the above causes	Combination of any of the above features	Multifactorial intervention

errors, cataract, macular degeneration), musculoskeletal disorders (eg, arthritis, muscle weakness, deconditioning after prolonged illness), proprioceptive disorders (eg, neuropathies), and gait disorders (eg, cerebrovascular stroke, Parkinson disease, cerebellar disorders).

Other Forms of Dizziness

Other forms of dizziness include a vague feeling other than vertigo, presyncope, or dysequilibrium. The patient may describe "floating," "lightheadedness," "wooziness," "spaciness," "whirling," or other nonspecific sensations. Patients with psychogenic dizziness commonly report anxiety or depressive symptoms. The psychiatric symptoms can primarily cause or contribute to the dizziness complaint in older adults.

Mixed Dizziness

Mixed dizziness, a combination of two or more of the above types, is the most common type of dizziness reported by older adults. It most likely results from combinations of diseases affecting the vestibular, CNS, visual, or proprioceptive systems. Systemic disorders like anemia, heart failure, diabetes mellitus, and hypothyroidism can contribute to instability or dizziness by affecting the sensory, central, or effector components. Although less commonly reported, carotid sinus hypersensitivity or carotid sinus syndrome can also cause dizziness. Patients with dementia often get fixated on being dizzy or unsteady.

Many medications can contribute to chronic dizziness through various mechanisms. Important classes of medications to consider in the dizziness evaluation include anxiolytics, antidepressants, antihistaminics, antihypertensives, aminoglycosides, anticholinergics, antipsychotics, and NSAIDs.

Research data indicate that chronic dizziness often has a multifactorial etiology. Chronic dizziness is associated with risk factors such as angina, myocardial infarction, stroke, arthritis, diabetes, syncope, anxiety, depressive symptoms, impaired hearing, and the use of medications in several classes. In a study of a large community sample and in another study in which patients attended a geriatric clinic, the complaint of chronic dizziness was associated with factors such as anxiety, depressive symptoms, postural hypotension, use of ≥5 medications, and impaired gait and balance (SOE=B). Complaints of chronic dizziness were more common in patients who had >5 of these risk factors than in those having <2 of these risk factors. Similar to delirium and falls, chronic dizziness can be thought of as a geriatric syndrome that prompts a multifactorial assessment and intervention strategy, which is likely more effective at alleviating symptoms than a standard disease-oriented approach.

EVALUATION

The evaluation of dizziness is challenging, and diagnostic evaluation can be extensive. Patients present with vague sensations, which generate a broad differential diagnosis. An expansive evaluation can often be avoided by taking a more detailed history and conducting a more directed physical examination.

History

The clinical history begins with helping patients to describe their symptoms as precisely as possible, which is potentially daunting for those with multiple sensations. Patients should be encouraged to use their own words to distill the symptoms into specific sensations such as spinning, imbalance or unsteadiness, or fainting. Documenting the frequency and duration of dizziness, and whether changing head position exacerbates the dizziness, is important. Establishing whether symptoms peak at any specific time of day, such as after meals or first thing in the morning, is also useful. Patients should be asked about associated symptoms such as hearing loss, ear fullness, diplopia, dysarthria, and tinnitus. Patients with Meniere disease complain of recurrent dizziness associated with ear fullness and/or tinnitus along with fluctuating hearing loss. Patients with acoustic neuroma complain of hearing loss and tinnitus but not of ear fullness. Patients with Meniere disease, CNS diseases, and BPPV complain of recurrent dizziness, whereas patients with psychogenic and central dizziness usually complain of continual dizziness. Inquiring about precipitating factors such as after eating meals (postprandial hypotension), looking down or rolling over in bed (vestibular conditions), or standing from supine position (orthostatic hypotension) can suggest interventions, as well as corroborate timing of symptoms. Any evaluation must include a critical review of medications, including OTC medications. It is also important to elicit the impact on the patient's quality of life.

Physical Examination

The physical examination should begin with measurements of orthostatic changes in blood pressure. Nystagmus should be evaluated; horizontal or rotatory nystagmus usually indicates a peripheral vestibular lesion, whereas vertical nystagmus is seen in central lesions. Hearing and vision tests should be done, and the cranial nerves examined if vertebrobasilar ischemia or infarction is suspected. The Timed Up and Go test can be performed to look for gait and balance problems.

The following provocative tests of the vestibular system can be done at the bedside:

Dix-Hallpike maneuver: This is a useful test for diagnosis of BPPV. Ask the patient to sit on the

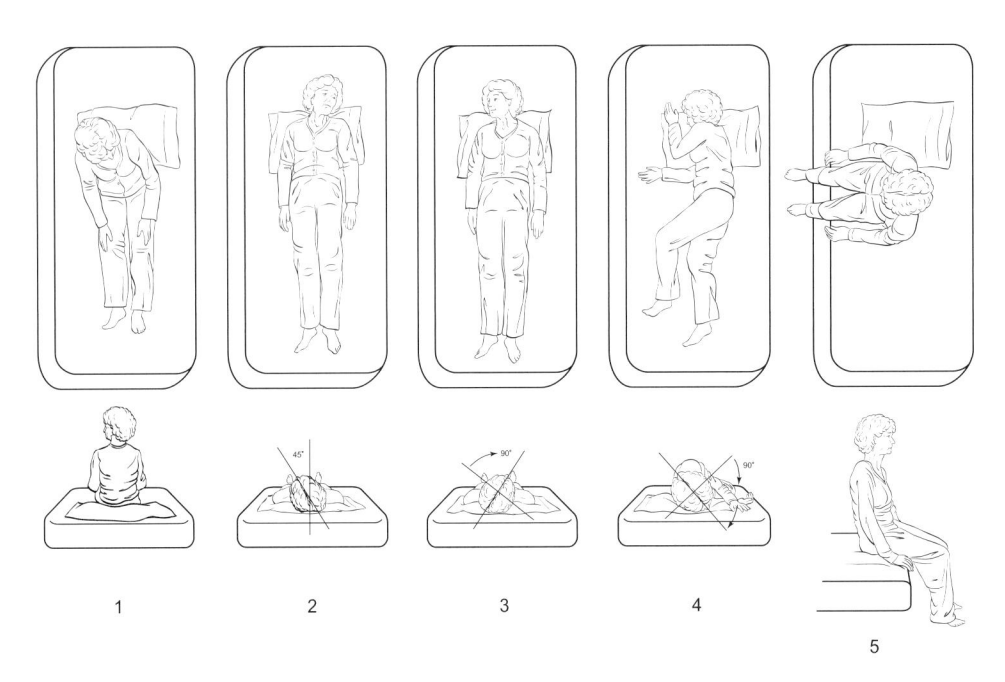

Figure 27.1 —Self-treatment of benign paroxysmal positional vertigo using Epley maneuver.

Perform the maneuver 3 times a day until free of positional vertigo for 24 hours. Use the positions shown here when the right ear is affected. Reverse all positions (left instead of right) when the left ear is affected. The affected ear is the ear that when turned downward during the Dix-Hallpike maneuver triggers vertigo or nystagmus, or both.

Each maneuver consists of the following steps (numbered to match the illustration):
1. Sit on the bed with a pillow far enough behind you to be under your shoulders when you lie back. Turn your head 45 degrees to the left.
2. Holding your head in the turned position, lie back quickly so that your shoulders are supported on the pillow and your head is reclined on the bed. Hold this position for 30 sec.
3. Remain supine on the bed and turn your head 90 degrees to the right. Hold this position for 30 sec.
4. Turn your head and body another 90 degrees to the right; you should now be looking down at the bed. Hold this position for 30 sec.
S5. it up, facing to the right.

SOURCE: Data from Radtke A, Neuhauser H, von Brevern M, et al. A modified Epley's procedure for self-treatment of benign paroxysmal positional vertigo. *Neurology.* 1999;53(6):1358–1360.

examination table with the head rotated 30–45 degrees to one side. Instruct the patient to fix his or her vision on the examiner's forehead. The examiner holds the patient's head firmly in the same position, and moves the patient from a seated to a supine position with the head hanging below the edge of the table and the chin pointing slightly upward. The examiner notes the direction, latency, and duration of the nystagmus, if present. The diagnostic criteria for BPPV include 1) paroxysmal vertigo along with a rotatory nystagmus, 2) latency for 1–2 sec between the completion of the maneuver and the onset of vertigo and nystagmus, and 3) fatigability (decrease in the intensity of the vertigo and nystagmus with repeated testing).

Head-thrust test: Ask the patient to fixate on the examiner's nose. The examiner then rotates the head rapidly about 10 degrees to the left or right. In patients with a vestibular deficit, the eyes move away from the target along with the head, followed by a corrective saccade back to the target, whereas normal eyes remain fixed on the target without a saccade.

Fukuda stepping test: Draw a circle on the floor, and ask the patient to stand in the center. Blindfold the patient and ask him or her to take a few steps forward as if walking on a straight line with outstretched arms. The examiner notes the patient's body sway as the patient takes the steps. In a unilateral vestibular lesion or acoustic neuroma, the patient's body will sway by >30 degrees toward the affected side.

Diagnostic Testing

A small battery of laboratory tests, including hematocrit, glucose, electrolytes, BUN, vitamin B_{12}, folic acid, and thyrotropin, should be performed on all patients with chronic dizziness. An ECG should be done if a cardiac cause is suspected, and a Holter and event monitor only if suspicion of arrhythmia is strong. Tilt-table testing should be done only for select patients with postural hypotension or syncope. Audiometry assists in the evaluation of patients with tinnitus or hearing loss and helps differentiate between acoustic neuroma and Meniere disease.

Suspected vestibular disorders can be evaluated with vestibular function tests such as electronystagmography, and rotational testing. Electronystagmography helps in detecting unilateral vestibular dysfunction, whereas rotational chair testing helps in identifying bilateral vestibular loss. These tests should be used selectively, based on initial assessment.

Likewise, neuroimaging is not needed in all patients with dizziness. MRI provides better resolution than CT for posterior fossa lesions. However, in a community-based study of adults ≥65 years old, the similar prevalence of MRI abnormalities in the dizzy and nondizzy group led to the conclusion that routine MRI will not identify a specific cause of dizziness in most patients (SOE=B).

MANAGEMENT

Medical therapy of acute dizziness depends on its cause, and patients with chronic dizziness, especially older adults, can have multiple comorbid conditions or impairments. Given the multifactorial nature of dizziness, it has been suggested that dizziness may be a geriatric syndrome. Therefore, a multifaceted approach to interventions can help treat chronic dizziness and reduce the impact on day-to-day functioning. Treatment of coincident symptoms from depression, anxiety, hearing loss, and vision loss can help reduce the disability arising from dizziness. Dizziness from medication responds to dosage adjustment or to withdrawal of the offending medication.

Vestibular suppressants, including antihistamines (eg, meclizine), provide effective symptomatic relief of vertigo but generally do not provide benefit in management of chronic dizziness or dysequilibrium. In general, meclizine should be used with caution because of its anticholinergic properties and potential adverse events in older adults. Long-term use should be avoided, because it suppresses central and vestibular adaptation and can thus eventually worsen or exacerbate dizziness.

Vestibular rehabilitation therapy (VRT) can help suppress symptoms in patients with peripheral and central vestibular causes of dizziness. VRT includes different exercises such as vestibulo-ocular reflex adaptation exercises and habituation exercises. Vestibulo-ocular reflex adaptation exercises help the CNS to adapt to a change or loss in input of the vestibular system. Habituation exercises include a combination of exercises designed to provoke dizziness; the movements are repeated until they can no longer be tolerated. Initially, the exercises can worsen the dizziness, but over time (weeks to months) movement-related dizziness improves, likely because of central adaptation. VRT has been shown to improve dizziness as well as quality of life (SOE=B).

The canalith repositioning procedure, introduced by Semont as well as Epley, can provide quick relief for those patients with BPPV (Figure 27.1). Other repositioning procedures include Li's maneuvers, which consist of 3 different sets of movements developed to manage BPPV of posterior, anterior, and horizontal semicircular canals.

A small subset of patients require surgical intervention. Surgical excision remains the treatment of choice for cerebellopontine angle tumors. Surgery should be reserved for disabling unilateral peripheral disease that is unresponsive to medical therapy. Surgical procedures are ablative or nonablative. Surgeons select ablative procedures, including transmastoid labyrinthectomy and partial vestibular neurectomy, for uncontrolled Meniere disease. Nonablative procedures, such as posterior canal occlusion, provide benefit to those patients whose BPPV remains refractory to repeated attempts of canalith repositioning procedures.

REFERENCES

- Alrwaily M, Whitney SL. Vestibular rehabilitation of older adults with dizziness. *Otolaryngol Clin North Am.* 2011;44(2):473–496.

    This excellent review article discusses the role of vestibular rehabilitation therapy in older adults with vestibular dysfunction. It describes evidence-based effect of vestibular rehabilitation on various vestibular disorders responsible for dizziness in older adults.

- Bruintjes TD, Companjen J, van der Zaag-Loonen HJ, et al. A randomised sham-controlled trial to assess the long-term effect of the Epley manoeuvre for treatment of posterior canal benign paroxysmal positional vertigo. *Clin Otolaryngol.* 2014;39(1):39–44.

    This randomized, controlled, double-blinded trial examined 44 patients with at least one month of posterior canal benign paroxysmal positional vertigo (BPPV). Patients were randomly assigned to receive the Epley maneuver or a sham head movement procedure and followed up to 1 year. The Epley maneuver group had a treatment success rate of 20/22 patients (91%), whereas the sham procedure group had a positive effect in 10/22 patients (46%). The authors concluded that the Epley maneuver provided long-term symptom resolution in patients with posterior canal BPPV.

- Navi BB, Kamel H, Shah MP, et al. Rate and predictors of serious neurologic causes of dizziness in the emergency department. *Mayo Clin Proc.* 2012;87(11):1080–1088.

    In this retrospective review of 907 patients presented to the emergency department of a tertiary care center with dizziness, vertigo, or imbalance, 49 (5%) patients had a serious neurologic diagnosis. The authors concluded that most cases of acute dizziness or vertigo in the emergency department are due to benign conditions. Clinical suspicion should be high for serious neurologic causes if patients are older, report imbalance, or have focal neurologic deficits.

- Tarnutzer AA, Berkowitz AL, Karen A et al. Does my dizzy patient have a stroke? A systematic review of bedside diagnosis in acute vestibular syndrome. *CMAJ.* 2011;183(9):E571–592.

    This is a systematic review of predictors of bedside diagnosis in 10 studies describing a total of 392 patients presenting with acute vestibular syndrome in the emergency department.

Aman Nanda, MD, AGSF, CMD

CHAPTER 28—SYNCOPE

KEY POINTS

- The incidence of syncope increases with age.

- In older adults, the cause of syncope is often multifactorial. In nearly one in five cases, the cause of syncope is not determined, but the prognosis is generally favorable.

- Although many diagnostic procedures are available to search for the cause of syncope, most are expensive and have a low yield unless findings from the history or physical examination suggest a particular cause.

- Bradycardia is the single most common cardiac cause of syncope in older adults.

- Treatment of syncope often requires addressing multiple potential causes in geriatric patients, including polypharmacy, frailty, orthostasis, bradycardia, and tachyarrhythmias.

Syncope is a symptom complex composed of a sudden and transient loss of consciousness resulting from a temporary interruption of global cerebral perfusion. It is a common reason for evaluation in both outpatient clinics and emergency departments, and for hospital admission. Annually it accounts for approximately 3% of emergency department visits and 2%–6% of hospital admissions. Incidence of syncope increases with age; incidence doubles in those ≥70 years old, and the rate among those ≥80 years old is three to four times that seen among younger people. Approximately 80% of patients hospitalized for syncope are ≥65 years old.

Syncope is a clinically important condition that is challenging to evaluate. Its potential causes range from those that are benign and self-limiting to those that are life threatening. In older adults, the cause of syncope can often be multifactorial, adding to the diagnostic difficulty. Additionally, limited recall of details surrounding the event may make it difficult to determine whether syncope truly occurred. Because syncope encompasses a wide range of potential causes (Table 28.1), its diagnostic evaluation can be complex and expensive.

NATURAL HISTORY: DIAGNOSIS AND PROGNOSIS

Causes of syncope in older adults are often multifactorial. Decreases in cardiac output or peripheral vascular resistance, or both, resulting in decreased systemic blood pressure and cerebral perfusion are common mechanisms of syncope. In addition, adverse effects of drugs must be considered during evaluation of syncope in older adults. Thus, the common causes of syncope in older adults are:

- Neurally mediated

- Cardiac rhythm disturbances

- Decreased intravascular volume due to blood loss or dehydration

- Alterations in the peripheral vasculature due to arterial vasodilation or increased venous pooling

- Medication related

Localized atherosclerotic diseases, such as vertebral basilar insufficiency and subclavian steal, can result in syncope without alteration in systemic blood pressure. These causes are uncommon.

Epileptic seizure, a common cause of transient loss of consciousness, is no longer categorized as a cause of syncope, because seizure is not mediated by a decrease in cerebral perfusion. Nevertheless, differentiation of seizure from syncope as a cause of transient loss of consciousness is clinically relevant, because both conditions are common and have overlapping clinical features in the older population. For clinical characteristics differentiating cardiac syncope due to arrhythmia, vasovagal syncope, and seizure, see Table 28.2.

The prognosis of syncope depends on the underlying cause. Patients with syncope from cardiac causes have the worst prognosis; their 1-year mortality is 18%–33%, with deaths chiefly due to underlying disease, not syncope. Patients with syncope due to noncardiac causes have a 1-year mortality of approximately 6%. Neurally mediated or vasovagal syncope, which has a benign prognosis in the young, was once thought to be an unusual cause of syncope in older adults. However, reports from syncope evaluation centers have found vasovagal mechanisms as the cause of syncope in approximately 30%–50% of patients >65 years old (SOE=A). It has not been established that vasovagal syncope in older adults has the same benign prognosis as it does in younger individuals, because there has been some suggestion that vasovagal syncope in older adults is often associated with comorbid illness that can increase overall mortality (SOE=B). In approximately 10%–20% of syncopal patients, no cause can be found. The prognosis for these patients is no worse or better than that of the general population (SOE=C).

Table 28.1—Common Causes of Syncope (and Frequency) in Older Adults

Reduced cardiac output
  Cardiac
    Rhythm disturbances: tachyarrhythmias, bradyarrhythmias, blocks, chronotropic incompetence (11%)
    Structural heart diseases: aortic stenosis, hypertrophic cardiomyopathy (2%–4%)
    Coronary artery disease (2%–5%)
  Reduced intravascular volume
    Bleeding (4%)
    Dehydration (16%–20%)
  Pulmonary
    Massive pulmonary embolism (<1%)
Altered peripheral vascular resistance
  Functional autonomic reflexes
    Vasovagal (21%–31%)
    Carotid sinus syndrome (carotid sinus hypersensitivity may be present in up to 39%)
    Situational: swallowing, micturition, defecation, postprandial hypotension (likely under-recognized)
  Structural autonomic insufficiency
    Primary conditions: pure autonomic failure, multiple system atrophy, Parkinson disease (2%–4%)
    Secondary conditions: diabetes mellitus, spinal cord lesions, uremia (2%–4%)
Drugs causing reduced cardiac output or altered peripheral resistance (6%)

Table 28.2—Distinguishing Characteristics of Seizure and Syncope Due to Arrhythmia and Vasovagal Syncope[a]

Phase	Sign/Symptom	Seizure	Cardiac Syncope Due to Arrhythmia	Vasovagal Syncope
Before	Position	Any	Any	**Upright; aborted by lying flat**
	Warning/prodrome	None	**<5 seconds**	**Seconds to minutes**
	Precipitant	Usually absent	Absent	**Present**
	Palpitations	Absent	Sometimes	Absent
	Nausea/diaphoresis	Rare	Absent	**Common**
	Visual changes	None	None	**Common**
During	Tone	**Rigid**	Flaccid	Motionless, relaxed
	Pulse	**Rapid**	Absent or faint	Slow, faint
	Color	Pale or normal	Blue, ashen	Pale
	Incontinence	**Common**	Rare	Very rare
	Eye findings	**Tonic eye deviation**	Variable pupils	Dilated, reactive pupils
	Oral frothing	**Common**	Absent	Absent
After	Type of recovery	Slow, incomplete	**Rapid, complete**	Fatigue common
	Mental status	**Disorientation**	No retrograde amnesia	No retrograde amnesia
	Nausea/diaphoresis	Rare	Absent	**Common**
	Focal neurologic findings	**Common**	Absent	Absent

[a] Characteristics most distinctive in determining the cause of syncope are highlighted in bold.

PATHOPHYSIOLOGY

The integrity of a number of control mechanisms is crucial for maintaining adequate perfusion of the brain and cerebral oxygen delivery after sudden changes in blood pressure. These mechanisms include carotid and aortic baroreceptors, sympathetic renal stimulation of the renin-angiotensin system, and arteriolar autoregulation.

In aging, many of these reflex mechanisms are less responsive. For example, the arterial baroreceptor reflex and cardiac response to β-adrenergic stimulation (cardiac acceleration and increased contractility) decrease with advancing age. In addition, comorbid conditions such as diabetes mellitus and Parkinson disease affect postural reflexes. Medications such as α-blockers, β-blockers, calcium channel blockers, ACE inhibitors, and tricyclic antidepressants can also impair postural reflexes. Because the ability to increase heart rate in response to sympathetic stimulation is decreased in older adults, maintaining blood volume and vasoconstriction become more important in maintaining postural blood pressure. Thus, older adults can be particularly sensitive to the effects of dehydration, diuretics, and vasodilator medications. These three factors—age-related decline in adaptive reflexes, comorbid conditions, and medications—are all likely to have a role in older patients presenting with syncope, and can be addressed by increasing caution with postural change, physical counter-pressure maneuvers (eg, leg crossing) and compression stockings to increase venous return, adequate hydration, and simplification of the patient's medication regimen to eliminate excessive medications.

EVALUATION

History

An accurate recall of the syncopal event is frequently inadequate because of the high prevalence of cognitive dysfunction in the older population. The medical history, if possible, should be obtained from a witness to the event. This history, in combination with a physical examination, plays a key role in the initial evaluation. It is important to establish whether the patient suffered a true syncopal event, as opposed to dizziness (dysequilibrium) or falls. Falls are common in older adults (estimated annual incidence up to 30% in ambulatory community-dwelling older adults); it is important to differentiate accidental falls from syncope causing falls. Key elements to obtain from the history are:

- Was there a precipitant? Could the patient's activities around the time of the event have triggered it? Such activities include eating, urinating, coughing, using medication, and experiencing emotional stress. Syncope occurring while sitting or supine suggests a profound hemodynamic disturbance and should raise a concern about a significant cardiac arrhythmia. Syncope occurring during physical exertion should raise the possibility of myocardial ischemia or aortic stenosis. A history of syncope after turning motions of the head should raise the possibility of carotid sinus hypersensitivity.

- Were there prodromal symptoms before the event? Chest pain, palpitations, or shortness of breath suggests a cardiac or pulmonary cause. Diaphoresis, presyncope, and GI symptoms, such as nausea or vomiting, can be associated with vasovagal syncope. Sudden onset of syncope with <5 sec of warning is characteristic of syncope due to a cardiac arrhythmia and should be evaluated as such. However, in older adults, vasovagal syncope can present with short or no prodrome because of inability to precisely recall the event. Thus, if the initial evaluation for arrhythmia in an older adult with syncope without a prodrome is unrevealing, a vasovagal mechanism should also be considered.

- What medications are being used? It is important to establish how medications were taken with relationship to meals and other activities, and whether the medication regimen was recently changed. Specifics about dosage times should be obtained. Many antiarrhythmic medications and other commonly used medications can increase the propensity for ventricular arrhythmias by prolonging the QT interval (for a full current list, see www.qtdrugs.org).

Table 28.3—Evaluation of Guidelines in Syncope Study (EGSYS) Score: Predictors of Cardiac Syncope

Variable	Score[a]
Palpitations preceding syncope	4
Heart disease or abnormal ECG	3
Syncope during effort	3
Syncope while supine	2
Precipitating or predisposing factors, or both[b]	–1
Autonomic prodromes (nausea/vomiting)	–1

[a] Scores ≥3 are associated with higher rates of cardiac syncope and higher mortality.
[b] Warm or crowded place, prolonged orthostasis, fear, pain, or emotional distress

SOURCE: Data from Del Rosso A, Ungar A, Maggi R, et al. Clinical predictors of cardiac syncope at initial evaluation in patients referred urgently to a general hospital: the EGSYS score. *Heart*. 2008;94(12):1620–1626.

- What did witnesses observe? They should be queried about the duration of the event and the appearance of the patient during the event. Patients with cardiac causes of syncope are generally flaccid in tone and motionless while unconscious, unless the event lasts for >15 sec, when myoclonic jerks and truncal extension can be seen. In contrast, increased body motion, tone, and head turning to one side with loss of consciousness are more common with seizure activity.

- Are there significant comorbid conditions? A history of coronary artery disease or its associated symptoms is particularly important. Approximately 5% of myocardial infarctions present as syncope. Sustained ventricular tachycardia resulting in syncope is most common in patients with prior myocardial infarction. Patients with diabetes mellitus are at increased risk of coronary atherosclerosis, as well as autonomic dysfunction predisposing to syncope.

For a summary of the characteristics of three common causes of loss of consciousness, see Table 28.2. A scoring system has been useful in distinguishing cardiac from noncardiac syncope (Table 28.3). The probability of cardiac syncope increases with higher scores; notably, scores ≥3 are associated with 95% sensitivity and 61% specificity. Mortality was 17%–21% in those with a score ≥3, and 2%–3% in those with a score <3 after 600 days of follow-up (SOE=B).

Physical Examination

A physical examination should focus on elements raised by the history. Blood pressure should be measured in both arms, as well as with postural changes. The pulse should

Table 28.4—Diagnostic Evaluation of Older Adults with Syncope

Evaluation	Finding	Comments
Orthostatic vital signs	Systolic blood pressure drop of >20 mmHg on standing	Maintain adequate hydration. Consider reducing antihypertensive therapy. Repeat measurements to identify situations that precipitate orthostasis (eg, postprandial hypotension).
Gait evaluation	Gait unsteadiness	Increased risk of falls
	Failure of heart rate to increase	Chronotropic incompetence preventing appropriate increase in heart rate
Carotid sinus massage	Reproducible symptoms	Contraindicated in patients with carotid bruits, recent stroke. Patients with transient asystole and carotid sinus syncope may benefit from pacemaker placement.
Laboratory testing	Hyperglycemia Electrolyte disturbance Anemia Occult heme in feces Increased creatinine	Correctable pathophysiologic states that either precipitate syncope or result in a state of altered consciousness that can be confused with syncope
Resting ECG	Arrhythmias, Q waves, prolonged QT_c	Increased likelihood of cardiac causes of syncope, including arrhythmias
Echocardiogram	Aortic stenosis, left ventricular outflow tract obstruction	Treatable causes of cardiac syncope are identified.
Ambulatory (24-hour) blood pressure monitor	Diurnal variation in blood pressure	Can identify patterns in variation in blood pressure, in particular, supine hypertension and postprandial hypotension
Holter monitor	Arrhythmias Chronotropic incompetence	Likelihood of identifying cause of syncope is low.
Implantable loop recorder	Arrhythmias	Ultimately demonstrates whether or not infrequent syncope is arrhythmic in origin
Head-up tilt table testing	Reproduces vasovagal syncope	Adequate usefulness in older adults Reproduces vasovagal syncope
Electrophysiologic study	Inducible ventricular tachyarrhythmias	Limited utility
Validated depression assessment	Syncope is more common in depressed patients	Identification of another treatable risk factor for syncope
Autonomic neurologic testing	Autonomic nervous system dysfunction	Diagnoses primary syndromes of autonomic dysfunction and demonstrates extent of dysfunction with targets for therapeutic intervention.
Electroencephalogram	Epileptiform activity	Diagnostic for seizure

Note: Not every test is required; the history and physical examination are used to determine appropriate testing. In all patients, an assessment of orthostatic vital signs, gait, laboratory tests, and ECG are reasonable.

be taken with the patient in both supine and standing positions. Blood pressure with the patient in the standing position should be obtained after 1 min and 3 min of standing. Although any definition of postural hypotension is arbitrary, a decrease in systolic blood pressure of >20 mmHg is the definition used most frequently (SOE=C).

The character of the carotid pulse should also be assessed for the delayed upstroke and low volume characteristic of significant aortic stenosis. The presence of a carotid bruit, a history of cerebrovascular disease, and recent myocardial infarction are relative contraindications to carotid sinus massage. Even in the absence of contraindications, carotid sinus massage should be performed only under continuous ECG monitoring (to detect induced sinus pauses, atrioventricular [AV] block, or other arrhythmias) in a setting where resuscitation equipment is available.

Physical examination of the patient with syncope should include cardiac examination for evidence of murmurs characteristic of valvular abnormalities or extra heart sounds suggestive of cardiomyopathy. Fecal examination for occult blood and neurologic examination for focal deficits are also important.

Diagnostic Testing

Several clinical characteristics and diagnostic approaches are particularly important for evaluation of syncope in older adults (Table 28.4).

Electrocardiogram (ECG)

An ECG is indicated for all patients presenting with syncope. Although an ECG establishes a diagnosis in only 5% of those with syncope, approximately 50% have an abnormal ECG. Abnormalities on an ECG can provide clues for further cardiovascular evaluation; a normal ECG is associated with a more favorable prognosis. Key features to assess on an ECG include evidence of acute or remote myocardial infarction. Conduction abnormalities, especially block in the AV node or in the His Purkinje system, and preexcitation, such as Wolff-Parkinson-White, can be detected as well. A prolonged QT interval can predispose to ventricular arrhythmias, including torsade de pointes.

Ambulatory Electrocardiographic Monitoring

An ambulatory ECG recording can establish or exclude many causes of syncope if the patient experiences syncopal or presyncopal symptoms during the recording. Unfortunately, the occurrence of symptoms during ambulatory ECG monitoring is relatively infrequent in most patients with syncope that remains unexplained after a history, physical examination, and ECG. On average, studies examining the diagnostic yield of ambulatory ECG monitoring report an arrhythmia correlating with symptoms in approximately 4% of patients. In another 15% of patients studied, an arrhythmia was excluded by the presence of symptoms during the recording but without evidence of an arrhythmia; in approximately 14% of patients, arrhythmias were found to be present but without concomitant symptoms (SOE=B). These patients can represent a diagnostic dilemma. However, certain arrhythmias, even asymptomatic ones, such as nonsustained ventricular tachycardia, second- and third-degree AV block, and sinus pauses >3 sec, are rare in people without heart disease. Their presence, even if asymptomatic, in a patient with a history of syncope indicates the need for further evaluation.

Ambulatory external Holter monitoring devices are usually used for 24–48 hours. Because symptoms do not recur in most patients during the monitoring period, the positive diagnostic yield of Holter for syncope evaluation is low, approximately 1%–2% in unselected populations. External loop recorders have a loop memory that continuously records rhythm in single or multiple leads. When activated by the patient, typically after a symptom has occurred, 5–15 min of pre- and post-activation ECG is stored and can be retrieved for analysis. Patients are typically given the external loop recorder for 1 month. The diagnostic yield can be up to 25% in selected patients. The external loop recorder is less useful when recurrence of syncope is infrequent.

Implantable Loop Recorders

Implantable loop recorders (ILRs) are implanted subcutaneously in the prepectoral region under local anesthesia with a battery life of up to 36 months. A smaller injectable device (volume of 1 cc) is now available. These devices have a solid-state loop memory that stores ECG recordings, when activated either by the patient or a bystander, usually after a syncopal episode or are automatically activated in the case of occurrence of predefined arrhythmias. Some of these devices have remote (at home) telemetry capable of transmitting the signals in real time. Studies have shown that symptom–electrocardiogram correlation ranges between 35% and 88%. Additional studies have shown that implantation of an ILR early during the evaluation was more likely to provide a diagnosis than the conventional strategy (52% vs 20%). Current guidelines recommend that use of an ILR should be considered early in patients when an arrhythmic cause of syncope is suspected but not sufficiently proved (SOE=B).

Echocardiography and Exercise Stress Testing

In the absence of features suggestive of heart disease by history, physical examination, or ECG, two-dimensional echocardiography has a low yield (SOE=C). It is most useful in confirming a specific diagnosis suspected by other assessment. Occult coronary artery disease is also prevalent among older adults, and stress testing is often used for screening. In some patients, particularly those in whom the history, physical examination, or ECG suggest structural cardiac abnormalities and ischemia, it is efficient to perform stress echocardiography as a single procedure.

Tilt-Table Testing

Head-up tilt-table testing results in pooling of blood in the legs and, in susceptible individuals, can trigger syncope mediated by neurocardiogenic mechanisms or to confirm postural hypotension. Tilt-table testing is useful for patients suspected of having vasovagal syncope and those with unexplained syncope who are not suspected of having a cardiac cause. Responses to tilt testing performed for evaluation of syncope tend to differ by age among adults without significant structural heart disease. Those ≥65 years old tend to have far higher rates of symptoms due to pure vasodilatation without significant change in heart rate than individuals ≤35 years old. In contrast, individuals ≤35 years old tend to have more profound cardioinhibitory responses, characterized by profound bradycardia or asystole induced by tilt testing, than those ≥65 years old. The different patterns of responses induced by tilt studies between younger and older adults suggest that different mechanisms for neurocardiogenic syncope predominate at different ages. Exaggerated autonomic response is common in younger people, whereas attenuated autonomic responses become predominant with advancing age.

Electrophysiologic Study (EPS)

The diagnostic efficacy of EPS to determine the cause of syncope greatly depends on patient selection and the degree of suspicion of an arrhythmic substrate for syncope. The development of effective noninvasive methods, ie, prolonged rhythm monitoring, has decreased the importance of EPS as a diagnostic test. Nevertheless, this test is still useful for diagnosis in suspected intermittent bradycardia, tachyarrhythmia, or in patients with bundle-branch block (suggestive of impending high-grade AV block). EPS is not recommended for patients with normal ECGs or without a history of heart disease or symptoms of palpitations.

Neurologic Testing

Extensive neurologic testing is generally not required in syncope evaluation. Neurologic testing, including imaging of the head by CT or MRI and electroencephalographic recording, is appropriate in situations when focal neurologic signs or symptoms are present or when the history suggests seizure during the evaluation of loss of consciousness. Also, neuroimaging may be required to evaluate trauma that occurred during the loss of consciousness. Autonomic evaluation should be considered when symptoms and signs of autonomic insufficiency are present.

Is Hospital Admission Required?

Syncope is a frequent reason for emergency department visits, and older patients are frequently hospitalized for evaluation because they are presumed to be higher risk. However, patients with no risk factors for adverse events (Table 28.5) were found to have no significant increase in adverse events regardless of age. A specialized syncope observational unit in the hospital setting has been shown to reduce hospital admission and expedite the diagnosis of potential causes of syncope.

TREATMENT

The goals of treatment for syncope, particularly in older adults, are to improve quality of life and prevent physical injuries. Effectiveness of therapy depends on whether a cause of syncope can be clearly established.

Polypharmacy is increasingly identified as a risk of syncope because of the actual number of medications and risk of interaction and adverse effects, and potentially because of the number of comorbid conditions requiring complex pharmacotherapy. Before any new medication is added, the medication list must be reviewed for potential culprits (in particular, α-antagonists, clonidine, vasodilators, and excessive diuretics). Timing of medication administration should also be reviewed, and shifting antihypertensive medications to evening administration may reduce daytime orthostatic symptoms.

Table 28.5—Risk Factors for Adverse Prognosis in Syncope

Symptoms	Chest pain
	Shortness of breath
	Palpitations or rapid heart beat
	GI bleeding
Cardiac history	Coronary artery disease
	Heart failure
	Hypertrophic cardiomyopathy
	Pacemaker or defibrillator
	Antiarrhythmic medications
	Ventricular tachycardia or ventricular fibrillation
Syncope characteristics	Syncope during exercise
	>1 episode within 6 months
Family history	First-degree relative with sudden death, hypertrophic cardiomyopathy, Brugada syndrome, or long QT syndrome
Physical examination	Tachypnea
	Hypoxia (O_2 saturation <90%)
	Sinus heart rate <50 beats/min or >100 beats/min
	Systolic blood pressure <90 mmHg
	Heart murmur
	Volume depletion
	Neurologic deficits
ECG abnormalities	Q waves
	Ischemic ST segment or T wave changes
	Ventricular or supraventricular arrhythmias, including rapid atrial fibrillation
	Second- or third-degree AV block
	Corrected QT interval >500 ms
Laboratory abnormalities	Hematocrit <30%
	Occult blood in feces

Note: Patients with no risk factors for adverse prognosis can likely be safely dismissed from the emergency department without hospitalization.
SOURCE: Data from Grossman SA, Chiu D, Lipsitz L, et al. Can elderly patients without risk factors be discharged home when presenting to the emergency department with syncope? *Arch Gerontol Geriatr*. 2014;58:110–114.

Reflex Syncope and Postural Hypotension

Nonpharmacologic measures with physical counter-pressure maneuvers such as leg crossing, arm tensing, hand grip, and buttock clenching are able to induce a significant blood pressure increase during the phase of impending reflex syncope so that the patient can avoid or delay losing consciousness in most cases (SOE=B). These measures in conjunction with conventional therapies have been shown to reduce the recurrence by 39% (SOE=A). However, effectiveness of these physical counter-pressure maneuvers in older adults has not been confirmed. Compression stockings and abdominal binders can be helpful in some patients with postural hypotension. Smaller and frequent meals can be effective in patients with postprandial hypotension.

Medical Management

The baroreceptor reflex plays a key role in blood pressure hemostasis. Drugs that mimic sympathetic activity such as α-agonists, including midodrine, have been used to increase vasoconstriction. Midodrine is a useful addition to the nonpharmacologic approaches in patients with persistent postural hypotension. However, use of an α-agonist is limited by supine hypertension, particularly in older adults with decreased vascular compliance. The use of an α-agonist for treatment of orthostatic hypotension requires careful titration of the drug dosage and close monitoring of blood pressure response and symptoms.

In studies that assessed the effects of pyridostigmine, an acetylcholinesterase inhibitor, on facilitating transmission of impulses from the cholinergic neurons across the synaptic cleft, both standing blood pressure and peripheral resistance were significantly increased, while orthostatic blood pressure was attenuated. Supine blood pressure increased modestly in some patients but overall was not significantly affected. Common adverse events include abdominal cramps with diarrhea from increased peristalsis and urinary urgency (SOE=C). The use of pyridostigmine in syncopal patients with orthostatic hypotension and autonomic failure should be closely supervised. Because there are limited data on the efficacy and safety of pyridostigmine in older adults, caution is advised when initiating administration, because the adverse effects may not be tolerated well.

Volume expansion with added salt (liberalize diet) or fludrocortisone, or both, to increase renal sodium retention and intravascular volume can be effective in patients with persistent postural hypotension (SOE=C).

Additional and less frequently used treatments, alone or in combination, include desmopressin in patients with nocturnal polyuria, selective serotonin-reuptake inhibitors in patients with depression, octeotride in postprandial hypotension, erythropoietin in anemia, and use of walking sticks.

Role of Pacemakers

Beyond the discontinuation of culprit medications, pharmacologic treatment has little place in the long-term treatment of bradycardia associated with syncope. Atropine or isoproterenol is indicated only in emergencies and temporary situations before cardiac pacing can be introduced. The mainstay of treatment for sinus node dysfunction or high-grade AV block is a pacemaker. Permanent pacing is clearly indicated when syncope or near syncope is correlated with bradycardia, regardless of the site of block. Although the recommendation to avoid pacemaker placement but rather discontinue medications causing bradycardia in patients taking them makes sense, often these medications are treatment for a significant cardiac condition (ie, β-blockers) or dementia (acetylcholinesterase inhibitors). Acetylcholinesterase inhibitors are associated with a significant risk of bradycardia, and bradycardic patients have a significant risk of syncope. Although recommendations for when it is appropriate or necessary to discontinue acetylcholinesterase inhibitors are needed, the risk of these medications in patients with bradycardia may outweigh the benefits. Pacemaker therapy is not recommended in patients with unexplained syncope or falls without documentation of bradycardia.

The role of pacemaker therapy in patients with reflex syncope remains to be defined. In older adults with recurrent syncope of a vasovagal nature, pacemaker placement should be considered when a cardioinhibitory response is documented during monitoring. Pacemaker therapy is effective in preventing recurrent syncope in patients with carotid sinus syndrome.

CHOOSING WISELY® RECOMMENDATIONS

Syncope

- Do not perform imaging of the carotid arteries for simple syncope without other neurologic symptoms.

- In the evaluation of simple syncope and a normal neurologic examination, do not obtain brain imaging studies (CT or MRI).

REFERENCES

- Grossman SA, Chiu D, Lipsitz L, et al. Can elderly patients without risk factors be discharged home when presenting to the emergency department with syncope? *Arch Gerontol Geriatr.* 2014;58(1):110–114.

  This prospective study demonstrated no significant difference in future adverse events for older adults without risk factors for an adverse prognosis than for younger patients. The authors conclude that such patients with no risk factors can be safely discharged from the emergency department despite advanced age.

- Kim DH, Brown RT, Ding EL, et al. Dementia medications and risk of falls, syncope, and related adverse events: meta-analysis of randomized controlled trials. *J Am Geriatr Soc.* 2011;59(6):1019–1031.

  This thorough meta-analysis of published and unpublished trials includes recent observational studies that have described associations between cholinesterase inhibitors and syncope, bradycardia, pacemaker insertion, and hip fractures. The authors concluded that cholinesterase inhibitors increase the risk of syncope with no effect on accidental injury in patients with cognitive impairment.

- Pirozzi G, Ferro G, Langellotto A, et al. Syncope in the elderly: an update. *J Clin Gerontol Geriatr.* 2013;4:69–74.

    This review highlights the common multifactorial contributors to syncope in older patients and the importance of a comprehensive geriatric assessment in every older patient with syncope.

- Ruwald MH, Hansen ML, Lamberts M, et al. Comparison of incidence, predictors, and the impact of co-morbidity and polypharmacy on the risk of recurrent syncope in patients <85 versus ≥85 years of age. *Am J Cardiol.* 2013;112(10):1610–1615.

    In a retrospective study of patients with syncope, factors that contributed the most to syncope in patients ≥85 years old included an increased incidence of aortic valvular stenosis, atrioventricular conduction block, atrial fibrillation, heart failure, renal insufficiency, COPD, and polypharmacy. In particular, medications known to cause orthostasis were commonly taken by patients before their syncopal event, with 40% of the patients ≥85 years old on at least 3 medications known to cause orthostasis. The number of orthostatic medications also predicted syncope recurrence.

- Shen WK, Traub SJ, Decker WW. Syncope management unit: evolution of the concept and practice implementation. *Prog Cardiovasc Dis.* 2013;55(4):382–389.

    This is a detailed review on the evolving concept and implementation of a specialized syncope observational unit in the hospital or emergency department setting to improve clinical outcomes among patients presenting with syncope. This syncope unit practice is especially relevant to the older population to expedite the diagnosis and risk stratification for prognosis.

- Task Force for the Diagnosis and Management of Syncope of the European Society of Cardiology (ESC); European Heart Rhythm Association (EHRA); Heart Failure Association (HFA); Heart Rhythm Society (HRS). Guidelines for the diagnosis and management of syncope (version 2009). *Eur Heart J.* 2009;30(21):2631–2671.

    This detailed guideline and recommendations for the approach and management of patients with syncope is based on available evidence. This includes the most recent update on indications for the use of electrophysiologic study, ambulatory monitoring preferences, and pacemaker implantation in the select populations.

J. William Schleifer, MD
Win-Kuang Shen, MD

CHAPTER 29—NUTRITION AND WEIGHT

KEY POINTS

- Aging is associated with changes in body composition such that well-standardized nutrient requirements for younger or middle-aged adults cannot be generalized to older adults.

- The Mini-Nutritional Assessment–Short Form is a brief and simple instrument useful for nutritional screening in geriatric patients.

- Identification of the presence of undernutrition or obesity can be facilitated by determining a person's BMI.

- Lean body mass (muscle mass) is inversely associated with mortality risk in older adults.

- Many medications cause anorexia or can reduce nutrient availability in older adults.

- Therapeutic diets should be avoided unless their clinical value is certain; appetite stimulants have not been demonstrated to improve long-term survival and may cause serious adverse effects.

- Cultural competence extends to understanding the many factors influencing nutrition and health behaviors in the increasingly heterogeneous population of older adults.

Malnutrition in older adults spans the spectrum from under- to overnutrition. Nutritional problems accompany many chronic disease processes of older adults. Moreover, age-related changes in physiology, metabolism, and function can alter the older adult's nutritional requirements. Better understanding among clinicians of the aging process and of nutritional screening, assessment, and interventions could potentially improve the health and independence of older adults.

AGE-RELATED CHANGES

Body Composition

Aging is associated with notable changes in body composition. Bone mass, lean mass, and water content all decrease, while fat mass generally increases. The volume of distribution of many medications changes as a result of these shifts in body composition, and creatinine-based determinations can overestimate renal clearance in older adults. The increase in total body fat is commonly accompanied by greater intra-abdominal fat stores. The consequence of these changes in body composition is that well-standardized nutrient requirements for younger or middle-aged adults cannot be generalized to older adults. The aging process also affects organ functions, although the degree of change observed is highly variable among individuals. Decline in organ functions can affect nutritional assessment and intervention.

Energy Requirements

The reduced basal metabolic rate in older adults reflects loss of lean body mass, including muscle mass. The resting energy expenditure is the principal contributor to total energy expenditure; energy expenditure in relation to physical activity is the most variable component. The Harris-Benedict or similar equations can be used to predict basal energy expenditure. In any determination of energy needs for older adults, care must be taken to avoid overfeeding while still meeting basal requirements.

Macronutrient Needs

MyPlate (www.choosemyplate.gov [accessed Jan 2016]), a modified food guide pyramid for older adults based on the 2010 U.S. Department of Agriculture food guidelines, is a USDA initiative with helpful, culturally sensitive advice; it is replacing the formerly used Food Pyramid. This pictorial recommendation depicts easy-to-understand examples to balance energy, avoid oversized food and meal portions, encourage lower-fat dairy and low-sodium food choices, and make half the plate fruits and vegetables and half of all grains whole grain.

The Food and Nutrition Board of the Institute of Medicine of the National Academies (formerly National Academy of Sciences) has released macronutrient guidelines that recommend a prudent diet, with 20%–35% of energy as fat, and reduced intakes of cholesterol, saturated fatty acids, and trans-fatty acids. Carbohydrates should constitute 45%–65% of total energy; complex carbohydrates are the preferred fiber source. More specifically, the recommended daily fiber intake for those ≥60 years old is 30 g for men and 21 g for women. Protein intake is recommended at 0.8 g/kg/day at approximately 10%–35% of total energy. With stress or injury, protein requirements are typically estimated at 1.5 g/kg/d, but underlying renal or hepatic insufficiency may warrant protein restriction (SOE=C).

Micronutrient Needs

Revisions of the dietary reference intakes, defined as the general term for a set of reference values used to plan and assess the nutrient intakes of healthy people, include recommended dietary allowances (RDAs),

Table 29.1—Recommended Dietary Intakes of Micronutrients for Adults ≥71 Years Old

Nutrient	Recommended Daily Allowance	
	For Men	For Women
Calcium	1,000 mg	1,000 mg
Magnesium	350 mg	265 mg
Vitamin D	10 mcg	10 mcg
Thiamine	1.0 mg	0.9 mg
Riboflavin	1.1 mg	0.9 mg
Niacin	12 mg	11 mg
Vitamin B_6	1.4 mg	1.3 mg
Folate	320 mcg	320 mcg
Vitamin B_{12}	2.0 mcg	2.0 mcg
Pantothenic acid	5 mg*	5 mg*
Vitamin A	625 mcg	500 mcg
Vitamin K	90 mcg*	90 mcg*
Iron	6 mg	5 mg
Zinc	9.4 mg	6.8 mg
Vitamin C	75 mg	60 mg
α-Tocopherol	12 mg	12 mg
Selenium	45 mcg	45 mcg
Potassium	4,700 mg*	4,700 mg*

*Adequate intake, not recommended dietary allowance.

SOURCES: Data from Standing Committee on the Scientific Evaluation of Dietary Reference Intakes, Food and Nutrition Board, Institute of Medicine, *Dietary Reference Intakes for Calcium, Phosphorus, Magnesium, Vitamin D, and Fluoride*. Washington, DC: National Academy Press; 1997; Standing Committee on the Scientific Evaluation of Dietary Reference Intakes, Institute of Medicine, *Dietary Reference Intakes for Thiamin, Riboflavin, Niacin, Vitamin B6, Folate, Vitamin B12, Pantothenic Acid, Biotin, and Choline*. Washington, DC: National Academy Press; 1998; Standing Committee on the Scientific Evaluation of Dietary Reference Intakes, Food and Nutrition Board, *Dietary Reference Intakes for Vitamin C, Vitamin E, Selenium, and Beta Carotene, and Other Carotenoids*. Washington, DC: National Academy Press; 2000; Standing Committee on the Scientific Evaluation of Dietary Reference Intakes, Food and Nutrition Board, *Dietary Reference Intakes for Vitamin A, Vitamin K, Arsenic, Boron, Chromium, Copper, Iodine, Iron, Manganese, Molybdenum, Nickel, Silicon, Vanadium, and Zinc*. Washington, DC: National Academy Press; 2001; Standing Committee on the Scientific Evaluation of Dietary Reference Intakes, Institute of Medicine, *Dietary Reference Intakes for Water, Potassium, Sodium, Chloride, and Sulfate*. Washington, DC: National Academy Press; 2004; *Dietary Reference Intakes for Calcium and Vitamin D* (2011). Available at www.nap.edu (accessed Jan 2016).

the average daily nutrient intake level estimated to meet the requirements of 97%–98% of the healthy individuals in a group, with more specific guidelines for older adults. For RDAs for the group ≥71 years old, see Table 29.1. The Food and Nutrition Board has also updated the RDAs with population-weighted estimated average requirements, defined as the average daily nutrient intake level estimated to meet the requirements of half of the healthy individuals in a group, based on updated census data. This information may be helpful for individualized recommendations to avoid over-nutrification http://books.nap.edu/openbook.php?record_id=11537&page=R1 (accessed Jan 2016).

Fluid Needs

Dehydration is the most common fluid or electrolyte disturbance in older adults. Normal aging is associated with a decreased perception of thirst, impaired response to changes in serum osmolality, and reduced ability to concentrate urine after fluid deprivation. A decline in fluid intake can also result from disease states that reduce mental or physical ability to recognize or express thirst, or that result in decreased access to water. In general, fluid needs of older adults can be met with 30 mL/kg/d or 1 mL/kcal ingested. Fluid needs may increase during episodes of fever or infection, as well as with diuretic or laxative therapy. Common signs of dehydration are decreased urine output, confusion, constipation, and mucosal dryness, although none of these signs is sensitive or specific.

NUTRITION SCREENING AND ASSESSMENT

Anthropometrics

Anthropometric measurements are often used for assessing nutritional status of older adults. An unintended weight loss of 10 pounds in the preceding 6 months is a useful indicator of morbidity; this degree of weight loss is predictive of functional limitations, health care charges, and the need for hospitalization (SOE=B). The Minimum Data Set (MDS-3) used by Medicare-certified nursing homes defines significant weight loss as ≥5% of body weight in the past month or ≥10% in the past 6 months. BMI, calculated by weight in kg/(height in meters)^2, is a useful measure of body size and indirect measure of body fat that does not require use of a reference table of ideal weights. For National Institutes of Health guidelines regarding body size classification based on BMI, see www.cdc.gov/healthy-weight/assessing/bmi/adult_bmi/index.html (accessed Jan 2016). The risk threshold for low BMI is set at 18.5 but should be interpreted in the context of the individual's lifelong weight history. Other anthropometric tools include skin-fold and circumference measurements, but these have had limited practical application because of the difficulty of achieving acceptable reliability among those taking the measurements.

Nutritional Intake

Generally, inadequate nutritional intake has been defined as average or usual intake of servings of food groups, nutrients, or energy below a threshold level of the RDI. Poor intake is often an indication of illness. The limited reliability of accurately assessing dietary intake measures is well known, so thresholds of 25%–50% below the RDI have generally been selected as an indicator of inadequate intake. In one study, energy intake (<50% of calculated maintenance energy requirements) was reduced in 21% of the population of hospitalized older adults. This subset of patients had higher rates of in-hospital mortality and 90-day mortality than did those with energy intakes above the threshold. Surveys of nutritional status conducted among long-term institutionalized older adults suggest that 5%–18% of nursing-home residents have energy intakes below their recommended average energy requirements. However, evidence is generally lacking to support any benefits of nutritional supplementation in this population (SOE=B).

Energy intakes of men and women 65–98 years old have been estimated in a nationwide food consumption survey; 37%–40% of the men and women studied had energy intakes lower than two-thirds of the RDIs, and many participants reported skipping at least one meal every day. However, estimated intakes obtained from consumption surveys may be unreliable, because some studies suggest that older adults under-report energy intakes by 20%–30%.

Problems with obtaining food commonly contribute to inadequate nutritional intakes among older adults. It is important to ascertain whether limitations in resources, transportation, or functionality may limit access to food or the ability to prepare and/or consume food.

Laboratory Tests: Albumin, Prealbumin, Cholesterol

Serum albumin has been recognized as a risk indicator for morbidity and mortality. Hypoalbuminemia lacks specificity and sensitivity as an indicator of malnutrition; however, it can be associated with injury, disease, or inflammatory conditions. As a negative acute-phase reactant, albumin is subject to cytokine-mediated decline in synthesis and to increased degradation and transcapillary leakage. Longitudinal studies of serum albumin levels suggest a modest decline with aging that may be independent of disease. The prognostic value of hypoalbuminemia may be largely because of its use as a proxy measure for injury, disease, or inflammation. In the community setting, hypoalbuminemia has been associated with functional limitations, sarcopenia, increased health care use, and mortality (SOE=B). In the hospital setting, hypoalbuminemia has been associated with increased length of stay, complications, readmissions, and mortality (SOE=B).

Serum prealbumin is another protein marker of nutritional status with clinical significance. Prealbumin has a considerably shorter half-life (48 hours) than albumin (18–20 days) and may more adequately reflect short-term changes in protein status. In the absence of an inflammatory state, prealbumin appears to have limitations similar to those of albumin as a diagnostic tool for nutritional status assessment. In the presence of inflammation, neither albumin nor prealbumin are accurate predictors of malnutrition. However, prealbumin can be used to assess the effectiveness of nutritional interventions or as an indicator of recovery (SOE=B). Because of a shorter half-life and a smaller serum pool than albumin, prealbumin can be used to detect small changes in nutritional status over a shorter time period if inflammation is not present. Serum cholesterol concentration has also been linked to nutritional status. Low cholesterol levels (<160 mg/dL) are often detected in individuals with serious underlying disease such as malignancy. Poor clinical outcomes have been reported among hospitalized and institutionalized older adults with hypocholesterolemia. In a study of community-dwelling older adults, nutrient intakes were not different in those in the lowest quartile of serum cholesterol levels from other quartiles. It appears likely that acquired hypocholesterolemia is a nonspecific feature of poor health status that is independent of nutrient and/or energy intakes, and that it may be a marker of pro-inflammatory conditions. Of interest is the observation that community-dwelling older adults with both hypoalbuminemia and hypocholesterolemia have higher rates of mortality and adverse functional outcomes than those with hypoalbuminemia or hypocholesterolemia alone (SOE=B).

Drug-Nutrient Interactions

Medications can modify the nutrient needs and metabolism of older adults. Certain medications, such as digoxin and phenytoin, even at therapeutic levels, can cause anorexia in older adults. Additional agents that have anorexia as a major potential adverse effect include SSRIs, calcium channel blockers (eg, dihydropyridines), H_2-receptor antagonists, proton-pump inhibitors, narcotic and nonsteroidal analgesics, furosemide, potassium supplements, ipratropium bromide, and theophylline. Many medications are known to interfere with taste and smell, and others can reduce the availability of specific nutrients (Table 29.2). Some medications can reduce intake by causing inattention, dysphagia, dysgeusia, or xerostomia. Medications that precipitate constipation can also reduce appetite.

Multi-Item Tools for Nutrition Screening

The nutritional status of older adults can be influenced by a variety of factors (Table 29.3). The lack of single assessment measures that are valid indicators of comprehensive nutritional status has prompted the development of multi-item tools. Older adults in acute- or chronic-care facilities have been extensively studied to identify indicators and predictors of nutritional status. In contrast, substantially fewer studies have been conducted in community-dwelling adults. Nutritional screening tools for older adults have been widely disseminated. Their effectiveness remains to be demonstrated and, more specifically, whether these tools can identify undernourished individuals whose problems are amenable to intervention.

The Nutrition Screening Initiative (a collaborative effort of the American Dietetic Association, the American Academy of Family Practitioners, and the National Council on Aging, Inc.) developed three interdisciplinary tools to screen for nutrition risk and help evaluate the nutritional status of older adults. The DETERMINE checklist (http://nutritionandaging.fiu.edu/downloads/NSI_checklist.pdf [accessed Jan 2016]) was created to raise public awareness about the importance of nutrition to the health of older adults. This self-report questionnaire is composed of 10 items and is intended to identify risk but not to diagnose malnutrition. The Level I screen, intended for use by health care professionals, incorporates additional assessment items regarding dietary habits, functional status, living environment, and weight change, as well as measures of height and weight. The Level II screen, for use by more highly trained medical and nutrition professionals and suggested for use in the diagnosis of malnutrition, contains all the items from Level I with additional biochemical and anthropometric measures, as well as a more detailed evaluation of depression and mental status.

The Mini-Nutritional Assessment tool was developed to evaluate the risk of malnutrition among frail older adults and to identify those who may benefit from early intervention (SOE=B). This assessment tool requires administration by a trained professional and consists of 18 items, including questions about BMI, mid-arm and calf circumferences, weight loss, living environment, medication use, dietary habits, clinical global assessment, and self-perception of health and nutrition status. A shortened screening version that contains only 6 items, the short form Mini-Nutritional Assessment, is also available (www.mna-elderly.com [accessed Jan 2016]). Another nutritional assessment tool, the Simplified Nutrition Assessment Questionnaire can be answered by patients through the mail or while sitting in a waiting room; it has a sensitivity and specificity of 88.2% and 83.5% for identifying those at risk of weight loss (www.slu.edu/readstory/newslink/6349 [accessed Jan 2016]).

Table 29.2—Drug-Nutrient Interactions

Drug	Reduced Nutrient Availability
Alcohol	Zinc, vitamins A, B_1, B_2, B_6, B_{12}, folate
Antacids	Vitamin B_{12}, folate, iron
Antibiotics, broad-spectrum	Vitamin K
Colchicine	Vitamin B_{12}
Digoxin	Zinc
Diuretics	Zinc, magnesium, vitamin B_6, potassium, copper
Isoniazid	Vitamin B_6, niacin
Levodopa	Vitamin B_6
Laxatives	Calcium, vitamins A, B_2, B_{12}, D, E, K
Lipid-binding resins	Vitamins A, D, E, K
Metformin	Vitamin B_{12}
Mineral oil	Vitamins A, D, E, K
Phenytoin	Vitamin D, folate
Salicylates	Vitamin C, folate
Trimethoprim	Folate

Table 29.3—Risk Factors for Poor Nutritional Status

Alcohol or substance abuse
Cognitive dysfunction
Decreased exercise
Depression, poor mental health
Functional limitations
Inadequate funds
Limited education
Limited mobility, transportation
Medical problems, chronic diseases
Medications
Poor dentition
Restricted diet, poor eating habits
Social isolation

NUTRITION SYNDROMES

Involuntary Weight Loss

Involuntary weight loss and low body weight can have potentially serious clinical implications. Clinically important weight loss is commonly defined as loss of 10 lbs (4.5 kg) or >5% of usual body weight over a period of 6–12 months. Weight loss >10% of body weight often represents protein-energy malnutrition, and 20% loss is associated with impaired physiologic function, including cell-mediated and humoral immunity. A BMI <17 is consistent with under-nutrition. Excess loss of lean body mass results in skeletal muscle wasting, loss of visceral protein, and associated nutrient deficiencies, and is associated with poor wound healing, infections, pressure sores, depressed functional ability, and mortality. Involuntary weight loss is present in approximately 13% of older outpatients, 25%–50% of hospitalized older adults, and >50% of nursing-home residents.

Etiologies of involuntary weight loss include approximately 50% organ related (congestive heart failure, COPD, renal failure, chronic infection and inflammatory states, GI conditions, adverse medication effects, and neurodegenerative conditions), 20% neoplastic, 20% idiopathic, including sarcopenia associated with aging, and 10% psychosocial conditions. In evaluating involuntary weight loss the following strategy is recommended: careful documentation of weights over time; detailed history including medical, dietary, and psychosocial elements; a physical examination; focused additional testing based on the history, physical, and limited standard laboratory profile; institution of treatment of underlying cause; and appropriate follow-up to assess response to management.

Nutritional therapy should include dietary education, removing dietary restrictions for chronic conditions, nutritional supplements given between meals and supervised by a dietitian, and a multivitamin/multimineral supplement to prevent micronutrient deficiencies (SOE=C). Unfortunately, the clinical benefits of full replacement nutrition are difficult to document and avoidance of severe nutritional compromise is of critical importance.

Obesity

The growing prevalence of obesity in America extends to older adults in their 60s and 70s. According to National Health and Nutrition Examination Surveys, the prevalence of obesity (BMI ≥30 kg/m^2) has climbed from 14% to 32% between 1976 and 2004. Trends were similar for all ages, both genders, and all racial or ethnic groups.

Excess body weight and modest weight gain (≥5 kg) in middle age can be associated with medical comorbidities in later life that include hypertension, diabetes mellitus, cardiovascular disease, obstructive sleep apnea, and osteoarthritis. Adverse outcomes associated with obesity include impaired functional status, increased use of health care resources, and increased mortality (SOE=B). A BMI ≥35 kg/m^2 is associated with increased risk of functional decline among older adults. Of interest, poor diet quality and micronutrient deficiencies are relatively common among obese older adults, especially obese older women living alone. However, in older individuals, higher BMI may have a protective effect with mortality rates lowest for individuals with BMIs between 27 and 29. This effect may be related to lean body mass, because muscle mass is inversely associated with mortality risk in older adults independent of fat mass and cardiovascular and metabolic risk factors. Many homebound older adults are also obese. The National Institutes of Health has suggested: "Age alone should not preclude weight loss treatment for older adults. A careful evaluation of potential risks and benefits in the individual patient should guide management." The focus must be on achieving a more healthful weight to promote improved health, function, and quality of life. A combination of prudent diet, behavior modification, and physical activity, including exercise, may be appropriate for selected patients. For frail, obese older adults, the emphasis may better be placed on preservation of strength and flexibility and maintaining weight rather than on weight reduction.

NUTRITIONAL INTERVENTIONS

Oral Nutrition and Nutritional Supplements

Preventing undernutrition is much easier than treating it. Food intake can be enhanced by catering to food preferences as much as possible and by avoiding therapeutic diets unless their clinical value is certain. Patients should be prepared for meals with appropriate hand and mouth care, and they should be comfortably situated for eating. Assistance should be provided for those who need help. Placing two or more patients together for meals can increase sociability and food intake. Foods should be of appropriate consistency, prepared with attention to color, texture, temperature, and arrangement. The use of herbs, spices, and hot foods helps to compensate for loss of the sense of taste and smell often accompanying older age and to avoid the excessive use of salt and sugar. Hard-to-open individual packages should be avoided. Adequate time should be given for leisurely meals. Title IIIC of the Older Americans Act has provided for congregate and home-delivered meals for older adults, regardless of economic status. This service is available in most parts of the country, albeit with a waiting list in many locations. Adequate access to nutritious and appetizing food should be assured for patients of various cultural backgrounds and in all settings.

Nutritional supplements containing protein and energy (calories) have been widely used in an effort to enhance caloric and nutrient intake, especially when patients eat only small amounts of food. The use of such supplements may decrease food intake, but overall nutritional intake usually increases owing to the nutrient quality and density of the supplements (SOE=C). Standard supplements contain macro- and micronutrients. Many different oral formulations are available in both liquid and solid bar forms. They can be chosen based on patient preferences, chewing ability, or product cost. Oral formulas can also be selected based on their caloric density, osmolality, protein, fiber, or lactose content. Most formulas provide 1–1.5 calories/mL, and many are lactose- and/or gluten-free. Supplementation with energy and protein produces a small but consistent weight gain in older people. Mortality may be reduced in older people who are undernourished. There may also be a beneficial effect on complications which needs to be confirmed. However, there is no evidence of improvement in functional benefit or reduction in length of hospital stay with supplements. In addition, current evidence does not support routine supplementation for older people at home or for well-nourished older patients in any setting.

Interest is also growing in the use of micronutrient supplements in health promotion to ensure adequate dietary intake of essential nutrients. Many vitamin and mineral supplements are commonly available in supermarkets and drugstores and are generally safe except for excessive intake of some such as vitamins A, D, and iron. New recommendations for older adults include higher than before intakes of calcium and vitamin D to prevent osteoporosis (SOE=B) (Table 29.1). Vitamin D deficiency occurs in 30% of individuals >70 years old and is associated with impaired calcium absorption and reduced physical activity level. Screening for vitamin D deficiency with measurement of total vitamin D levels is appropriate in older patients, because repletion is associated with improved physical performance, reduced falls, improved bone healing, and response to bisphosphonates (SOE=B). Supplements of vitamin D up to 4,000 IU (100 mcg) daily are considered safe. Folic acid, vitamins B_6, and B_{12} can lower homocysteine levels; however, evidence to date from randomized controlled trials with folic acid or vitamin B_6 supplementation is poor and has not demonstrated reduced risk of coronary artery disease or prevention of cognitive decline. Insufficient evidence also exists to determine whether immune function can be improved by protein, vitamin E, zinc, or other micronutrient supplementation (SOE=C). Whether the effects of antioxidants are beneficial is also the subject of controversy. Although it has previously been suggested that antioxidants can help in preventing age-related cataracts and macular degeneration, evidence indicates that they may have little or no effect. Although naturally occurring dietary antioxidants can reduce cardiovascular disease and mortality, supplementation with specific antioxidants, namely β-carotene, vitamin A, and vitamin E, can increase mortality in some settings (SOE=C). In addition, vitamin E supplementation has not been shown to slow progression of Alzheimer disease or prevent cardiovascular disease, but it may be associated with higher risk of hemorrhagic stroke. Further, among individuals with diabetes or vascular disease, supplementation with vitamin E can increase risk of heart failure (SOE=C).

Because approximately 60% of older adults take self-prescribed dietary supplements, it is imperative that the clinician obtain information about the patient's use of all supplements. The appropriateness and safety of each supplement should be evaluated, because patients are often unaware of potential risks and adverse events of many OTC supplements, and solid evidence in favor of these purported benefits is currently lacking.

Drug Treatment for Undernutrition Syndromes

A number of agents have been suggested to promote appetite or to serve as anabolic aids. Although some studies involving selected patient populations (eg, AIDS, certain cancers) suggest limited efficacy, there are no reports demonstrating improvement in long-term survival, and some agents may cause serious adverse effects. Appetite stimulants include mirtazapine[OL], an alpha$_2$-antagonist antidepressant that antagonizes the 5-HT$_3$ receptor, possibly stimulating appetite by that mechanism, but proof of this effect is limited. Dosing is 7.5–30 mg po at bedtime. Caution is required for dosages of 15–30 mg/d because of hepatic or renal insufficiency and more noradrenergic and serotonin effects, some of which may counteract the appetite stimulatory effects. Cyproheptadine[OL], a serotonin and histamine antagonist, can also enhance appetite (SOE=C), but there is the potential for confusion in older adults. It is given at a dose of 2–4 mg po with meals. Megestrol[OL] is a progestin that stimulates appetite and is given daily at 320–800 mg po in two equal doses. Appetite and weight usually improve with megestrol acetate; however, this weight gain is primarily fat, and clinical benefits have not been demonstrated (SOE=A). In addition, megestrol acetate in nursing-home populations can be associated with a higher risk of deep-vein thrombosis, fluid retention, edema, and exacerbation of congestive heart failure. There is a strong Beers List warning to avoid prescribing this agent. Finally, megestrol acetate taken during rehabilitation may negate the benefits of exercise on strength and function. Dronabinol^{OL}, a cannabinoid, can stimulate appetite at 2.5 mg twice daily before lunch and dinner (maximum 20 mg/d), but it is associated with somnolence and dysphoria in older adults.

Cytokine-modulating agents are experimental in the treatment of undernutrition syndromes, even though anticytokines have been breakthrough treatments for selected forms of disease-related cachexia. Approaches include anti–tumor necrosis factor, consisting of antibodies that can inhibit cytokine-mediated inflammation, and n-3 fatty acids and antioxidants, which can modulate cytokine production.

Anabolic agents include human growth hormone^{OL}, which induces preferential usage of carbohydrates and fats while preserving proteins and increasing muscle mass. However, increased muscle strength and functional capacity, depend on exercise rehabilitation. Growth hormone is contraindicated in cancer states. Hyperglycemia and fluid retention can be seen, and no studies have demonstrated significant functional benefits. Oxandrolone is an anabolic steroid that increases muscle protein synthesis; it is given at 2.5–20 mg/d po in divided doses. Anabolic agents can increase muscle mass, but questions remain concerning long-term safety and cost that currently mitigate endorsement (SOE=B). Likewise, although muscle mass has consistently improved with anabolic agents, significant improvements in strength and function, or a reduction in fractures have not been demonstrated.

CULTURALLY APPROPRIATE NUTRITIONAL CARE

Cultural factors dramatically influence health behaviors and outcomes. In the United States, minority older adult (>65 years old) populations are projected to increase from 16% of the population in 1999 to 25% by 2030. The Hispanic population is expected to increase by 328%; African Americans by 131%; and American Indians, Eskimos, Asians, and Pacific islanders by 285%. The United States will continue to be characterized as an increasingly diverse population. In addition to genetics and nutrition intake, nutritional status of older adults could be affected by socioeconomic factors, such as education and income level and environmental factors, such as proximity to stores and transportation that can affect food variety and availability. Ethnic and religious customs are 2 of many factors that influence food preferences. Cultural variation is additionally influenced by regionalism and within-culture diversity. Nutrition and aging are connected inseparably, because eating patterns affect progress of many chronic and degenerative diseases associated with aging. In turn, disease progression, health status, and ultimately quality of life may be adversely affected by a number of cultural and ethnic factors associated either directly or indirectly with nutrition and aging.

For example, many Latinos believe in disease as destiny (ie, fatalism) and often fear adverse effects of medications given to treat disease. Some patients expect the healer to cure the ailment, with difficulty comprehending the concept of chronic illness. This can greatly compromise the care of certain conditions such as diabetes. The hot and cold theory of disease traditionally held by Hispanic cultures is a continuing influence of ancient Greek and Arabic *humoral* pathology, which maintained that the four body "humors" regulated health and disease: blood, phlegm, and black and yellow bile, each characterized as warm or cold, wet or dry. Although disagreement exists within Latino populations, warm illnesses (kidney ailments, rashes, dysentery) are produced by the body, and cold illnesses (pain, paralysis, stomachache) are produced by outside influences. Warm illnesses are treated by avoiding cold foods (vegetables, dairy products, tropical fruits), and cold illnesses by avoiding warm foods (lamb, beef, grains, temperate fruits).

Multicultural nutrition counseling competencies are critical in managing nutritional health and chronic illness for diverse populations. It is important for clinicians to be aware of how cultural background and experiences and attitudes, values, and biases influence nutrition counseling and to be advised to acquire cultural knowledge and sensitivity for appropriate nutrition intervention and materials. Many culturally appropriate nutrition education materials are available in English and other languages, including My Plate for Older Adults, a USDA product also available in Spanish (http://hnrca.tufts.edu/my-plate-for-older-adults/ [accessed Jan 2016]). Oldways® (http://oldwayspt.org [accessed Jan 2016]), a nonprofit organization that promotes healthy eating based on regional diets, has developed consumer-friendly pyramids that display prudent food choices in a culturally sensitive manner. These pyramids include Mediterranean, Hispanic, Asian, African-American, and vegetarian alternatives to the USDA My Plate for Older Adults and reflect consistency with eating patterns of healthy populations around the world.

LEGAL AND ETHICAL ISSUES

In the nursing home, unacceptable weight loss, as defined by the Omnibus Budget Reconciliation Act of 1987, is any loss ≥5% in the past month or ≥10% in the past 6 months. Sections of the Minimum Data Set related to nutritional status include those assessing cognitive function, mood and behavior, physical function, health condition, oral and nutritional status, dental status, skin condition, and special treatments and procedures, including restorative care for eating and swallowing. Care Area Assessments (formerly called Resident Assessment Protocols) ensure prompt identification of problems focused on by the MDS. The MDS uses intake of <75% of food provided as the threshold to trigger nutrition assessment. Standards of care dictate the following:

- Acceptable parameters of nutritional status such as body weight and protein levels should be maintained; unless the resident's clinical condition demonstrates that this is not possible.

- A resident should receive a therapeutic diet when there is a problem.

Food and fluids should always be offered to all patients; however, the decision to start or to discontinue artificial nutrition or hydration must be considered very carefully. Competent adults may choose to forgo artificial feeding, just as they have the right to decline any invasive procedure. Some adults have advance directives executed at a time when the individual was competent that prohibit the use of feeding tubes. These should be honored unless there is compelling evidence that the individual would have changed his or her mind in the current situation. Incompetent adults without advance directives pose a greater challenge. The decision to start or to discontinue artificial feeding should be considered carefully with the surrogate, taking into account the risks and burdens of such an action, the risks and burdens of alternative actions, and the evidence to support likely benefits of the various actions. To date, evidence does not support the use of feeding tubes in patients with end-stage cancer, dementia, or COPD.

After total cessation of nutrition, depending on underlying conditions, several weeks may ensue before death, and some patients who consume very little may survive much longer. In this setting, palliative care, including emotional support, is extremely important and complex.

REFERENCES

- Buchowski MJ, Sidani MA, Powers JS. Minority Elders: Nutrition and dietary interventions. In: Whitfield KE, Baker TA, eds. *Handbook of Minority Aging*. New York: Springer Publishing; 2014.

    This review examines cultural factors on nutrition and health with detailed descriptions of Far Asian, Mediterranean, Hispanic, African American, Middle Eastern, and Eastern European influences.

- Casaer MP, Van den Berghe G. Nutrition in the acute phase of critical illness. *N Engl J Med*. 2014;370(25):1227–1236.

    This review of nutrition in acute illness examines pathophysiology of malnutrition and nutritional interventions in critically ill patients, providing current information on the limited clinical benefits of refeeding.

- ChooseMyPlate. www.choosemyplate.gov/healthy-eating-tips.html (accessed Jan 2016).

    MyPlate is a USDA initiative with helpful, culturally sensitive nutritional advice and recommendations that is replacing the food pyramid formerly used.

- Institute of Medicine of the National Academies, Food and Nutrition Board. *Dietary Reference Intakes*. www.iom.edu/Global/Topics/Food-Nutrition.aspx (accessed Jan 2016).

    This source provides up-to-date nutrient guidelines from the Food and Nutrition Board that specifically address the needs of older adults.

- Srikanthan P, Karlamangla AS. Muscle mass index as a predictor of longevity in older adults. *Am J Med*. 2014;127(6):547–553.

    This study demonstrates the survival prediction ability of relative muscle mass and the need to look beyond total body mass in assessing the health of older adults.

- Winter JE, MacInnis RJ, Wattanapenpaiboon N, et al. BMI and all-cause mortality in older adults: a meta-analysis. *Am J Clin Nutr*. 2014;99(4):875–890.

    In this review, the authors examine the complex relationship between BMI and mortality, and how this risk changes with older age.

James S. Powers, MD, AGSF
Maciej S. Buchowski, PhD

CHAPTER 30—FEEDING AND SWALLOWING

KEY POINTS

- With aging, chewing becomes less efficient, and swallowing is slowed for most healthy older adults.

- Dementia is the most common cause of oral dysphagia.

- Most healthy people aspirate regularly without any important clinical consequences.

- Aspiration pneumonitis results when gastric contents, usually sterile, are misdirected into the lungs. This condition is not treated with antibiotics.

- Aspiration pneumonia is believed to occur when contaminated oral secretions arrive in the lungs in a high enough inoculum to overcome host defenses.

- Many studies identify feeding tubes as major risk factors for aspiration of both oral and gastric contents.

- Given the absence of data linking interventions resultant from swallowing studies with clinical outcomes, the assessment of swallowing function is controversial. Performing swallowing studies in delirious patients is nonsensical.

Swallowing is an important and complex event affected by both normal aging and diseases that are common in older adults. Treatment of eating and feeding problems depends on identified cause(s) and contributing factors. Many medications contribute to feeding problems at a variety of levels.

SWALLOWING IN HEALTH AND DISEASE

Swallowing and Aging

Swallowing can be divided into 3 phases on the basis of anatomy. First is the preparatory or oral phase, which includes the complex activities of mastication and propelling the food bolus to the back of the mouth toward the pharynx. This stage is under voluntary control and requires attention, praxis, and coordination. The second or pharyngeal phase is involuntary and involves initiation of the swallow reflex with propulsion of the food bolus past the laryngeal vestibule and into the esophagus. Execution of the oral and pharyngeal phases of swallowing requires the complex coordination of 5 cranial nerves and a large number of small muscles in the head and neck, with regulation from cortical input to the medullary swallow center, all in the appropriate sequence, usually within 1 second. The third stage of swallowing is the esophageal phase, during which food is propelled down the esophagus by the action of skeletal muscle proximally and smooth muscle distally; this phase is regulated by its own intrinsic innervation.

Normal aging is associated with several changes in eating. With advanced age, taste sensation decreases but not taste discrimination (older adults may be able to distinguish sweet from salty but may need to add more salt to food to taste it sufficiently). Olfactory function declines with advancing age, further impairing taste sensation. Loss of teeth greatly reduces chewing efficiency (ie, chewing is needed for a longer period of time and with more chewing strokes to achieve the same level of food maceration), which is only partly ameliorated with dental prostheses. Sarcopenia, or age-related loss of lean muscle mass, can contribute to loss in chewing efficiency and to pharyngeal muscle weakness demonstrated on videofluoroscopic deglutition examination (VDE) of asymptomatic older adults. Whether aging alone contributes to esophageal dysmotility (so-called *presbyesophagus*) remains a subject of debate. Esophageal function is probably well preserved, except perhaps in very advanced age. In total, these changes with age result in a prolonged duration of each swallow.

Dysphagia

Dysphagia, or difficulty swallowing, can occur when a disease affects any level of swallowing function. Dysphagia is usually classified as oral, pharyngeal, or esophageal. In oral dysphagia, there is difficulty with the voluntary transfer of food from the mouth to the pharynx. This might be diagnosed, for example, when scrambled eggs are discovered in the cheeks of a demented patient shortly before lunch. The most common cause of oral dysphagia is dementia.

In pharyngeal dysphagia, there is a problem with reflexive transfer of the food bolus from the pharynx to initiate the involuntary esophageal phase of swallowing while simultaneously protecting the airway from misdirection of food. The affected person or a caregiver may notice coughing, choking, or nasal regurgitation while eating and localize the symptoms to the throat. The most common cause of pharyngeal dysphagia is stroke, but any disease that impairs the swallowing center in the brain stem or the cranial nerves involved (eg, Parkinson disease, CNS tumor), the oropharyngeal striated muscle (eg, myasthenia gravis, amyotrophic lateral sclerosis), or the local structures involved (eg, retropharyngeal abscess, tumor) can lead to pharyngeal dysphagia. Management of both oral and pharyngeal dysphagia involves treating the underlying disorder and devising an individualized, often labor-intensive, feeding program.

In esophageal dysphagia, the patient has the sensation that food has gotten "stuck" after a swallow. Dysphagia for both solids and liquids suggests an esophageal motility disorder (eg, achalasia, scleroderma), whereas progressive dysphagia for solids suggests a mechanical obstruction (eg, cancer, esophageal ring, stricture from mucosal irritation). None of these diseases is unique to the geriatric population, although older adults tend to take more medications and are therefore more likely to experience medication-induced esophagitis (which manifests initially as odynophagia, followed by dysphagia). Medications most commonly causing esophagitis in older adults are potassium, NSAIDs, oral bisphosphonates, and tetracycline-related antibiotics. Indirectly, medications that promote candidal esophagitis, such as prednisone or immunosuppressants, also contribute to esophageal dysphagia.

Aspiration

The misdirection of oral or gastric contents into the airway is termed *aspiration*. However, controversy persists over the definition of *aspiration pneumonia*. Aspiration pneumonia is believed to occur when bacteria arrive in the lungs from the pharynx in a large enough inoculum to overcome host defenses. In the case of more virulent organisms, defenses can be overwhelmed by smaller inocula, and when host defenses are weak, smaller inocula may also be problematic. Pneumococcal pneumonia arises from aspiration of *Pneumococcus* from a colonized oropharynx and is usually not considered an aspiration pneumonia, highlighting how inexactly the nomenclature is applied. Aspiration of gastric contents, or Mendelson syndrome, usually results in a chemical pneumonitis; the usefulness of antibiotics in this situation is questionable. Most often, after a period that can include fever, tachypnea, hypoxemia, and rales that last <24 hours, local host defense mechanisms clear the lung of the offending aspirate, without serious clinical effect. Many healthy individuals episodically aspirate without any important clinical consequences.

Aspiration of contaminated oral or gastric contents is not prevented by placement of a feeding tube. In fact, tube feeding is universally cited as a risk factor for major aspiration, and some patients who have never previously aspirated begin to do so after a feeding tube has been placed. A review found no evidence that tube feeding of any sort would reduce the risk of aspiration pneumonia (SOE=B). A common misconception is that jejunostomy tube feeding has lower rates of associated aspiration of gastric contents than does gastrostomy. Most studies do not demonstrate reduced aspiration with jejunostomy compared to gastrostomy (SOE=C). Whether hand feeding (personal assistance with oral intake) is safer than tube feeding is also unclear. In a single nonrandomized prospective comparison of hand feeding with tube feeding in patients with oropharyngeal aspiration, hand feeding resulted in lower rates of pneumonia. No prospective randomized trials comparing hand with tube feeding to reduce aspiration have been published. An active area of clinical research is focused on the role of substance P in swallowing and aspiration and the potential benefit of ACE inhibitors (which prevent the breakdown of substance P) in patients who aspirate. Using compensatory swallowing techniques and ensuring an upright posture during mealtimes both have some evidence of benefit in reducing aspiration associated with meals (SOE=C); whether altering food consistencies also reduces clinically meaningful aspiration is not yet established.

Assessment of Oropharyngeal Dysphagia

Several tools can be used to assess swallowing function when oropharyngeal dysphagia is suspected clinically. The most common are the full bedside evaluation (of which there are many variations), the videofluoroscopic deglutition examination (VDE; a variant of the modified barium swallow), and nasopharyngeal laryngoscopy performed by an otolaryngologist. There is considerable controversy regarding the relative efficacy of these tools.

VDE is usually performed by a speech-language pathologist who videotapes the patient swallowing barium-impregnated foods of several consistencies while maintaining various head positions. This can permit identification of the food consistency or compensatory mechanisms that minimize fluoroscopic evidence of aspiration. Depending on the results of the VDE, the therapist may recommend swallow therapy or diet modifications, or both. Swallow therapy may be compensatory (eg, turn head toward weaker side while swallowing), indirect (eg, exercises to improve the strength of the involved muscles), or direct (ie, exercises to perform while swallowing, such as swallowing multiple times per bolus). Dietary recommendations generally consist of altering bolus size or consistency of food or fluid, or of restricting foods of certain consistencies (Table 30.1). Unfortunately, there is insufficient evidence to support any clinical benefit in altering dietary consistency (SOE=D).

Data regarding the usefulness of VDE and nasopharyngeal laryngoscopy have been derived from small, historically controlled studies rather than from larger prospective randomized trials. A systematic review of studies of dysphagia secondary to stroke

Table 30.1—Characteristics of Altered Diet Consistencies

Prescribed Consistency	Description
Solids	
Regular or whole foods	Food served as it would be at a restaurant
Cut up	No pieces larger than ½" cubes
Chopped*	Food chopped into pea-sized pieces no larger than ¼" cubes
Ground*	Size/consistency of cottage cheese, moist, soft
Pureed*	Smooth, like yogurt or very thick soup
Liquids	
Unrestricted	Also known as "thin" liquids with the consistency of water
Nectar	Consistency of tomato juice (usually some thickening agent added)
Honey	Liquid can be poured but slowly (most liquids require addition of thickening agent)
Pudding	Liquids cannot be poured and must be spooned

* Avoid foods that are tough to chew (eg, nuts, seeds, bacon, meat with casing, bagels, popcorn, dried fruits) for any consistency other than regular or cut up.

published by the Agency for Healthcare Research and Quality concluded that evidence was insufficient to recommend one type of swallowing study over another and that data correlating specific findings from any type of examination with clinically meaningful outcomes are lacking (SOE=C).

FEEDING

Hand Feeding Versus Tube Feeding

When an older adult experiences difficulty eating, the two main therapeutic approaches are careful feeding by hand or tube. The first requires extraordinary patience and is labor intensive; the latter is an invasive intervention associated with its own risks. Data about either approach are limited, and randomized comparisons have not been done. The role of dietary supplements, if any, in augmenting the caloric intake of hand-fed older adults has not been clearly defined. One systematic review suggested that mortality was less with the use of oral protein and energy supplements in acutely hospitalized or community-dwelling adults >65 years old, although the quality of the studies reviewed were not optimal. Functional status does not appear to be improved with oral nutritional supplements in any of the studies evaluating this outcome.

The number of percutaneous endoscopic gastrostomy feeding tubes placed in patients ≥65 years old has grown at an astonishing rate over the past two decades. Low procedure-related complication rates are often cited; however, long-term studies reveal substantial mortality among tube-fed patients. Despite the popularity of feeding tubes, studies have not demonstrated improved survival, reduced incidence of pneumonia or other infections, improved symptoms or function, or reduced pressure ulcers with the use of feeding tubes of any type in demented patients who have eating difficulties. A 2009 Cochrane review of tube feeding in patients with advanced dementia found no decrease of a decrease in mortality (SOE=B).

Median survival after placement of a feeding tube is well under a year, but it is unknown whether this results from tube feeding or if the need for tube feeding is a marker that death is near.

Complications described with feeding tubes are numerous and include an increased risk of aspiration pneumonia, metabolic disturbances, diarrhea, and local cellulitis. Monitoring for these complications should be meticulous. In a study that used a large administrative data set, 1-year mortality was higher in 5,266 nursing-home residents with chewing or swallowing difficulties who were fed with a tube than in those who were not, even when statistically accounting for potential confounding variables (SOE=B). No prospective randomized studies comparing tube and hand feeding have been published, and information on quality-of-life outcomes is sorely needed. Patients in nursing homes fed by tube have less contact time with nursing and support staff than those who are hand fed. Although paradoxically likely a marker of poorer quality of care in a nursing home, feeding by tube is reimbursed at a higher rate than the more labor-intensive hand feeding approach. Tube feedings may interfere with absorption of some medications, eg, levodopa/carbidopa and phenytoin. Time-released medications cannot be crushed for administration through the tube.

Placement of a percutaneous endoscopic gastrostomy or jejunostomy bypasses the oropharynx and the esophagus, allowing nutrients and medications to be instilled directly into the stomach or the jejunum to be absorbed by a functioning gut. It is clear that neither gastrostomy nor jejunostomy feeding tubes reduce aspiration compared with a program of hand feeding, but no randomized trials comparing these interventions have been published. The only condition for which feeding tubes have been shown to be of clinical benefit to the patient is esophageal obstruction, such as from malignancy. For most other disease states, their use remains unproved (SOE=D). The American Geriatrics Society has issued a helpful position statement regarding the use of feeding tubes (see References).

Contraindications to gastrostomy include the inability to pass an endoscope into the stomach, uncorrectable coagulopathy, massive ascites, peritonitis, and bowel obstruction. After successful placement of a gastrostomy, the stoma is not epithelialized for up to a month but the tube may be used right away with tube feedings of commercially available canned nutritional supplements as slow gravity boluses for gastrostomy tubes over 30–60 minutes or as a continuous infusion. The feeding tube should be flushed with water before and after each feeding or at least 4 times a day in cases of continuous feedings.

Consideration of feeding tube placement requires careful examination of the data, with a focus on whether there is evidence of clinical benefit to support this invasive and potentially burdensome approach.

Approaches to Nondysphagia Feeding Problems

Not all feeding problems are related to dysphagia, and many contributing factors are quite amenable to therapy. Other approaches to consider in older adults who demonstrate eating or feeding problems are evaluating for depression, eliminating unduly restrictive diets, considering individual food preferences, considering the environment in which the person eats to improve socialization and reduce disruptive stimuli, examining the oral cavity, determining the need for personal assistance with feeding, and reducing or eliminating medications that can cause inattention, xerostomia, movement disorders, or anorexia. Small studies have documented improved clinical outcomes in nursing-home residents with the use of flavor enhancers, increased food variety, and attention to the meal ambiance.

CHOOSING WISELY® RECOMMENDATIONS

Feeding and Swallowing

- Do not recommend percutaneous feeding tubes in patients with advanced dementia; instead offer oral assisted feeding.

- Avoid using prescription appetite stimulants or high-calorie supplements for treatment of anorexia or cachexia in older adults; instead, optimize social supports, provide feeding assistance, and clarify patient goals and expectations.

REFERENCES

- American Geriatrics Society. Feeding tubes in advanced dementia position statement. *J Am Geriatr Soc.* 2014;62(8):1590–1593.

  In this state-of-the-art comprehensive review, the AGS synthesized the evidence and identified further areas that are less well understood in regards to use of feeding tubes in patients with dementia. The position of the AGS is that careful hand feeding is the preferred approach to feeding patients with dementia. When considering the more aggressive and burdensome option of a feeding tube, institutions and providers should engage patients and families in a careful discussion around preferences and goals of care.

- Sura L, Madhavan A, Carnaby G, et al. Dysphagia in the elderly; management and nutritional considerations. *Clin Interv Aging.* 2012;7:287–298.

  This well-written and comprehensive review of the causes of dysphagia focuses on the evidence behind options for evaluation and treatment of dysphagia. The authors find little evidence to support various assessment and treatment options to improve clinical outcomes. In some instances, the authors argue in favor of interventions that improve "nutritional status" even if there is no evidence of clinically meaningful benefit to patients.

- Swaminath A, Longstreth GF, Runnman EM, et al. Effect of physician education and patient counseling on inpatient nonsurgical percutaneous feeding tube placement rate, indications, and outcome. *South Med J.* 2010;103:126–130.

  This is an interesting study in which a single geriatrician and one institution were engaged in discussing feeding options with patients and families at the time of contemplating feeding tube placement during acute hospitalization. Involvement of the geriatrician in these discussions resulted in a 50% reduction in the placement of feeding tubes with no change in 30-day, 1-year, or 2-year mortality for those patients.

- Teno JM, Gozalo PL, Mitchell SL, et al. Feeding tubes and the prevention or healing of pressure ulcers. *Arch Intern Med.* 2012;14;172(9):697–701.

  The relationship between feeding tubes and pressure ulcer outcomes is controversial, and few studies have evaluated carefully their relationships. In this cohort study of nursing-home residents with advanced cognitive impairment, the Minimum Data Set was used to assess risk factors and outcomes. Placement of a feeding tube was associated with double the rate of newly developed stage 2 or higher pressure ulcers and with worse measures of healing of existing ulcers when compared to controls matched for pressure ulcer risk who did not have a feeding tube placed.

Colleen Christmas, MD, FACP

CHAPTER 31—URINARY INCONTINENCE

KEY POINTS

- The prevalence of urinary incontinence (UI) increases with age and ADL dependence, affecting 15%–30% of all adults ≥65 years old and 60%–70% of long-term care residents.

- UI in older adults can be caused or worsened by medical conditions, functional and cognitive impairment, and medications, with or without concomitant lower urinary tract dysfunction. Therefore, assessment of comorbidity, medications, and function are essential components of evaluation.

- Even in frailer older adults, UI is manageable through a stepped approach that starts with addressing comorbidity, impairments, and medications, followed by lifestyle interventions, behavioral therapy, medications, and finally minimally invasive and surgical interventions as appropriate.

UI is the involuntary leakage of any amount of urine. Even when UI is differentiated by type of leakage (eg, urge or stress), in older adults urinary leakage does not necessarily represent a specific diagnosis or pathophysiologic entity. In younger people, the etiology of UI often can be attributed after evaluation to specific pathophysiology in the lower urinary tract (LUT) and/or pelvic floor. In older adults, however, UI can be caused or worsened by comorbid conditions, medications, or functional and cognitive impairments, either alone or in combination with LUT dysfunction. Thus, UI is a classic geriatric syndrome in which multiple risk factors interact with one another and other modulating factors to produce a clinical phenotype (ie, incontinence of urine).

The most common types of UI symptoms in older adults are:

- Urge UI—leakage associated with urgency, the compelling and often sudden need to void; most common type in both men and women

- Stress UI—leakage associated with coughing, sneezing, laughing, physical activity; second most common form in women and also seen in men after radical prostatectomy

- Mixed UI—leakage occurs with both urgency and activity; common in women

- UI associated with incomplete bladder emptying—leakage occurs in the setting of an increased postvoid residual (PVR), often with symptoms of intermittent small dribbling; uncommon. The cut-off level for an increased PVR is not well established, although 200 mL is commonly used.

The coexistence of urge UI and increased PVR (in the absence of bladder outlet obstruction) in frail patients is called detrusor hyperactivity with impaired contractility (DHIC).

UI may be accompanied by other LUT symptoms (eg, frequency, nocturia [awakening to void >1 time during sleep], slowed stream, hesitancy, sense of incomplete emptying, intermittent stream). "Overactive bladder" refers to a symptom complex of urgency, with or without urge UI, often accompanied with frequency and nocturia. These symptoms are all nonspecific and can be due to a variety of LUT conditions as well as comorbid diseases.

The terms "transient UI" and "functional UI" have been used to describe UI that is caused or exacerbated by factors beyond the LUT, such as comorbid conditions, medications, and impaired mobility. However, in many cases LUT dysfunction is present as well, and thus correction of contributing factors may be insufficient to resolve UI. There is no widely accepted alternative term, although some authors suggest "UI due to potentially reversible factors."

PREVALENCE AND IMPACT

UI increases with age and affects women more than men (ratio 2:1) until age 80, after which men and women are equally affected. The prevalence is 15%–30% in community-dwelling adults ≥65 years old, and 60%–70% in long-term care settings. In most studies, overall rates of UI are higher in white women than in black, Hispanic, and Asian women, and stress UI is more common in white and Hispanic women than in black women. Racial and ethnic differences among older men are less clear. The few longitudinal studies in older women suggest annual UI incidence rates of 5%–11% in the community and 22% in long-term care, with remission rates that nearly match incidence.

UI significantly impairs quality of life, including emotional well-being, social function, and general health. Older adults with UI may maintain social activities but do so with an increased burden of coping, embarrassment, and poor self-perception. Morbidity from UI includes dermatitis and cellulitis, pressure ulcers, urinary tract infections, falls with fractures, sleep deprivation, social withdrawal, depression, and sexual dysfunction. UI is not associated with increased mortality. UI increases caregiving time and burden, which may be why it remains a significant cause of long-term care placement. Estimated annual costs related to UI in older adults total more than $26 billion.

Table 31.1—Medications That Can Cause or Worsen Urinary Incontinence

Medication	Effect on Continence
Alcohol	Frequency, urgency, sedation, delirium, immobility
α-Adrenergic agonists	Outlet obstruction (men)
α-Adrenergic blockers	Stress leakage (women)
ACE inhibitors	Associated cough worsens stress and possibly urge leakage in older adults with impaired sphincter function
Anticholinergics	Impaired emptying, retention, delirium, sedation, constipation, fecal impaction
Antipsychotics	Anticholinergic effects plus rigidity, sedation, and immobility
Calcium channel blockers	Impaired detrusor contractility and retention; dihydropyridine agents can cause pedal edema, leading to nocturnal polyuria
Cholinesterase inhibitors	Urinary frequency, potential interactions with anticholinergics
Estrogen (oral)	Worsens stress and mixed leakage in women
GABAergic agents (eg, gabapentin, pregabalin)	Sedation, dizziness, night time incontinence
Loop diuretics	Polyuria, frequency, urgency
Narcotic analgesics	Urinary retention, fecal impaction, sedation, delirium
NSAIDs	Pedal edema causing nocturnal polyuria
Sedative hypnotics	Sedation, delirium, immobility
Thiazolidinediones	Pedal edema causing nocturnal polyuria
Tricyclic antidepressants	Anticholinergic effects, sedation

RISK FACTORS AND ASSOCIATED COMORBID CONDITIONS

The evidence-based risk factors for UI in older adults include obesity (best demonstrated in young-old women), functional impairment, dementia, medications (eg, estrogen and α-blockers [in women], cholinesterase inhibitors), and environmental barriers to toilet access. The association of vaginal delivery and parity with UI attenuates with age. These data pertain primarily to white women; much less is known about UI risk factors in other racial and ethnic populations and in men (other than prostate disease and adverse effects from its treatment).

Especially in older adults, continence depends not only on LUT function but also on the ability to toilet, which requires sufficient physical function (mobility and manual dexterity), cognition, motivation, and available toilets.

Medications (Table 31.1) and medical conditions (Table 31.2) can cause or worsen UI via multiple pathways that include direct and indirect effects on LUT function, toileting, and/or urine output. For example, incontinence in people with diabetes can occur from direct neurologic effects (with detrusor overactivity [DO] being far more common than cystopathy), disease complications (eg, constipation, glycosuria, impaired ambulation from peripheral vascular disease), and complications from treatment (eg, thioglitazone- and gabapentin-associated edema causing nocturia).

Not all older adults with a comorbid condition or taking a medication that is associated with UI will develop UI, and the presence of such factors in an individual person with UI does not imply that they are causative. The best example of this is the relationship between UI and dementia. Although older adults with dementia may have impairment in central inhibitory pathways that control urgency, impaired functional status and mobility are at least as strong or stronger predictors of UI than cognitive status. Older adults with advanced dementia may remain continent if they can transfer and ambulate with minimal to moderate assistance. Furthermore, older adults with dementia may have other types of LUT dysfunction and symptoms than urge UI: one-third of nursing-home residents with UI have stress UI or bladder outlet obstructions on urodynamic testing.

PATHOPHYSIOLOGY

Age-related LUT Changes

A number of age-related physiologic changes in LUT function predispose older adults to UI. In both genders, bladder contractility decreases, uninhibited bladder contractions are more prevalent, diurnal urine output occurs later in the day, and sphincteric striated muscle attenuates, while bladder capacity decreases and PVR

Table 31.2—Comorbid Conditions That Can Cause or Worsen Urinary Incontinence

Comorbidity	Effect on Continence
Cardiovascular disease	
Arteriovascular disease	Detrusor underactivity or areflexia from ischemic myopathy or neuropathy
Congestive heart failure	Nocturnal polyuria
GI disease	Retention and overflow UI from constipation; fecal and urinary incontinence commonly coexist
Metabolic diseases	
Diabetes mellitus	DO with urge UI; detrusor underactivity due to neuropathy; osmotic diuresis; altered mental status from hyper- or hypoglycemia; retention and overflow from constipation
Hypercalcemia	Diuresis; altered mental status
Vitamin B_{12} deficiency	Impaired bladder sensation and detrusor underactivity from peripheral neuropathy
Musculoskeletal disease	Mobility impairment; DO from cervical myelopathy in rheumatoid arthritis and osteoarthritis
Neurologic conditions	
Cerebrovascular disease, stroke	DO with urge UI from damage to upper motor neurons; impaired sensation to void from interruption of subcortical pathways; impaired function and cognition
Delirium	Impaired function and cognition
Dementia	DO with urge UI from damage to upper motor neurons; impaired function and cognition
Multiple sclerosis	DO, areflexia, or sphincter dyssynergia (depending on level of spinal cord involvement)
Normal-pressure hydrocephalus	DO from compression of frontal inhibitory centers; impaired function and cognition
Parkinson disease	DO from loss of inhibitory inputs to pontine micturition center; impaired function and cognition; retention and overflow from constipation
Spinal cord injury	DO, areflexia, or sphincter dyssynergia (depending on level of injury)
Spinal stenosis	DO from damage to detrusor upper motor neurons (cervical stenosis); DO or areflexia (lumbar stenosis)
Obstructive sleep apnea	Nocturnal polyuria
Peripheral venous insufficiency	Nocturnal polyuria
Pulmonary disease	Conditions with chronic cough can worsen stress UI.
Psychiatric disease	
Affective and anxiety disorders	Decreased motivation
Alcoholism	Functional and cognitive impairment; rapid diuresis and retention in acute intoxication
Psychosis	Functional and cognitive impairment; decreased motivation

NOTE: UI = urinary incontinence; DO = detrusor overactivity

increases (both modestly and without clear clinical significance). In women, urethral closure pressure decreases, and vaginal mucosal atrophy is prevalent. Benign prostatic hyperplasia and prostate hypertrophy increase in men. Why some older adults with age-related LUT changes develop UI and others do not remains unclear; differences in LUT function and other compensatory mechanisms may play a role.

LUT Pathophysiology in UI

Specific UI symptoms and LUT pathophysiology overlap substantially. However, some general associations (with caveats) are possible:

- **Urge UI with DO (uninhibited bladder contractions):** Up to 40% of continent healthy older adults demonstrate DO on urodynamic testing, suggesting that urge UI requires not only DO but also impaired compensatory mechanisms. Research now emphasizes the roles of afferent stimulation from the bladder urothelium and impaired CNS control of urgency in DO and overactive bladder. DO may be idiopathic, age-related, secondary to lesions in cerebral and spinal inhibitory pathways, due to bladder outlet obstruction, or (less commonly) result from local bladder irritation (eg, infection, stones, tumor).

- **Stress UI and impaired urethral sphincter support and/or closure:** Stress UI can result from 1) damage to pelvic floor supports (levator ani, connective tissues), such that they fail to provide firm resistance and compress the urethra with any increase in intra-abdominal pressures; or 2) failure of the proximal urethra and its sphincter components to remain closed during bladder filling (usually due to surgical damage or severe atrophy or, in rare cases, subsacral spinal cord injury). DO can cause apparent "stress" UI when a cough triggers an uninhibited detrusor contraction. In such cases, leakage usually occurs after and not coincident with the cough, is large in volume, and difficult to stop.

Table 31.3—Causes of Nocturia

Nocturnal polyuria (nocturnal output >35% of total 24-hour output)	Late day/evening fluids, especially with caffeine or alcohol
	Pedal edema (eg, due to medications, venous stasis, heart failure)
	Heart failure
	Obstructive sleep apnea
Sleep disturbance	Medications
	Cardiac or pulmonary disease
	Pain
	Restless legs syndrome
	Depression
	Obstructive sleep apnea
	Sleep partner
Lower urinary tract	Detrusor overactivity
	Benign prostatic hyperplasia
	Impaired bladder emptying

- **Mixed UI with both DO and impaired sphincter support/function:** Mixed UI occurs when the mechanisms of urge and stress UI are both present. The contribution of the different mechanism can vary, such that some mixed UI is urge-predominant and some stress-predominant.

- **UI with impaired bladder emptying due to bladder obstruction and/or detrusor underactivity:** The most common cause of obstruction in men is prostate hyperplasia causing prostate enlargement, and in women urethral surgical scarring or a large cystocele/prolapse that kinks the urethra. Detrusor underactivity can be caused by intrinsic bladder smooth muscle damage (eg, from ischemia, scarring, fibrosis), peripheral neuropathy (diabetes mellitus, vitamin B_{12} deficiency, alcoholism), or damage to the spinal cord and spinal bladder efferent nerves by disc herniation, spinal stenosis, tumor, or degenerative neurologic disease. Neurologic diseases affecting the spinal cord (eg, multiple sclerosis, spinal cord injury) can cause detrusor underactivity and/or neurally mediated obstruction, depending on the exact level and extent of spinal cord involvement.

- **Nocturia:** This is a nonspecific symptom, even in older men, and causes other than urge UI and prostate disease should be considered (Table 31.3).

EVALUATION

Similar to other geriatric syndromes, UI requires multifactorial evaluation with a focus on comorbidity, function, and medications as contributing factors. Evaluation and management of UI in nursing-home residents is discussed separately below.

Screening

All older patients, especially women, should be asked at least yearly about UI, because 50% of affected individuals do not voluntarily report their symptoms to a health care provider.

Screening questions

- Do you have any problems with bladder control?
- Do you have problems making it to the bathroom on time?
- Do you ever leak urine?

Follow up positive screen with questions to determine the type of UI (SOE=B)

Do you leak urine most often:

- When you are performing some physical activity, such as coughing, sneezing, lifting, or exercising? (stress)
- When you have the urge or feeling that you need to empty your bladder but cannot get to the toilet fast enough? (urge)
- With both physical activity and a sense of urgency? (mixed)
- Without physical activity and without sense of urgency? (other)

History

The history should include UI onset, frequency, volume; timing and exacerbating and ameliorating factors; other LUT symptoms; and amount and types of fluid intake. Understanding any success or failure of past treatment(s) and current management (types and frequency of changing protective pads) can help direct management.

UI may be the herald symptom of neurologic disease and cancer. "Red flag" symptoms that require prompt evaluation and referral are abrupt onset of UI, pelvic pain (constant, worsened, or improved with voiding), and hematuria.

Medical conditions and their status, medications, functional status, and access to toilets should be reviewed, including their association with onset or worsening of UI. For example, was UI present before a stroke, or subsequent to any medication change? Review of systems should include fecal incontinence, which is common in older adults with UI. Ask patients (and/or caregivers) specifically about UI-associated bother and impact on quality of life, starting with simple questions (eg, "What bothers you most about your leakage?" or "How does leakage affect your daily life?"), followed by more specific probes, as appropriate, regarding impact on ADLs and IADLs, social role, emotional and interpersonal relations, sexual function and relations, self-concept, general health perception, and financial burden.

Physical Examination

The initial general examination should include cognition and functional status, if not recently assessed, and focus on presence and severity of comorbid conditions that may be associated with UI (SOE=D). Abdominal palpation is insensitive and nonspecific for bladder distention. Digital rectal examination should check for masses, fecal loading, and prostate nodules or firmness, but it cannot accurately determine prostate size. Neurologic evaluation is especially important in patients with known neurologic disease, new-onset or sudden worsening of UI, or in those with motor and sensory symptoms. Tests for integrity of the sacral cord (the origin of the pelvic and pudendal nerves innervating the LUT) are perineal sensation, anal "wink" (lightly scratch the perianal area and look for [or palpate during a DRE] anal sphincter contraction), and bulbocavernosus reflex (lightly touch the clitoris or glans and look for or palpate for anal contraction same as with anal wink). A basic pelvic examination in women should include checking for labial and vaginal lesions and marked pelvic organ prolapse (eg, large uterine prolapse, cystocele extending to or through the introitus). Uncircumcised men should be checked for phimosis, paraphimosis, and balanitis.

Depression screening is recommended because of the bidirectional association between depression and UI (SOE=B). Screening for sleep apnea should be considered in patients with nocturia associated with nocturnal polyuria (see below).

A clinical stress test can corroborate stress UI symptoms. The patient should have a full bladder and is instructed to relax the perineum and buttocks, while the examiner is positioned to observe or catch any leakage when the patient gives a single vigorous cough. Clinical stress testing is highly sensitive (most helpful when negative) but less specific (SOE=B). Sensitivity is highest when the patient is standing. It is insensitive if the patient cannot cooperate, is inhibited, or the bladder volume is low.

Additional Testing

The only recommended test for all patients is urinalysis to look for hematuria (and glycosuria in diabetic patients) (SOE=D). If a woman does not have an acute onset of UI, dysuria, fever, or other signs of urinary tract infection, then any pyuria and bacteriuria represent asymptomatic bacteriuria. Asymptomatic bacteriuria is not associated with UI and should not be treated with antibiotics.

Bladder diaries (also called frequency-volume charts) can help to determine whether urine volume contributes to UI frequency and especially nocturia (Table 31.4) and can assist in evaluation of UI frequency, timing, and circumstances. Typically, a diary entails recording the time and volume of all continent voids and UI episodes for 2–3 days, including day and evening.

PVR measurement is not routinely needed in evaluation of UI (SOE=B), because the cut-off for an "increased" PVR is not standardized, the overall prevalence of high PVR (eg, >200 mL) is low, and there is insufficient evidence that routine PVR measurement affects outcomes. Even older men with LUT symptoms and/or known prostate disease do not require routine PVR testing. PVR measurement may be considered in patients with prior urinary retention, longstanding diabetes, recurrent urinary tract infections, severe constipation, complex neurologic disease, higher than routine risk for prostate enlargement (eg, men with known increased PSA) and in women with marked pelvic organ prolapse or who have had prior surgery for UI (SOE=C). PVR can be measured in the office with ultrasonography or catheterization.

Routine urodynamic testing is not necessary or desirable; it should be considered only if the cause of UI is unclear and knowing it would change management (eg, determine whether a man with severe urge UI also has bladder outlet obstruction), or when empiric treatment has failed and the patient would consider invasive or surgical therapy. Cystometry can determine bladder proprioception, capacity, and detrusor stability. Simultaneous measurement of abdominal pressure is necessary to exclude abdominal straining and detect DHIC. Leak-point pressure, profilometry, and/or fluoroscopic monitoring are necessary to diagnose physiologic stress UI. Pressure-flow studies are required to diagnose outlet obstruction.

Table 31.4—Example Bladder Diary

Date	Time	Measured Amount of Urine (mL)	Are You Wet or Dry?	Approximate Amount of Leakage (mL)	Comments
Day 1	3:50 PM	90	Dry		
	6:05 PM	90	Dry		
	8:15 PM	120	Dry		
	10:20 PM	150	Dry		
	12:00 AM	30	Dry		
Day 2	2:15 AM	150	Dry		
	3:40 AM	120	Dry		
	5:00 AM	120	Dry		
	6:05 AM	240	Dry		Almost had accident
	8:40 AM	120	Dry		Coffee
	12:50 PM	120	Dry		
	6:00 PM	120	Dry		
	9:20 PM	210	Dry		Dribbled on way
	11:40 PM	120	Dry		
	2:00 AM	150	Dry		
	4:50 AM	180	Dry		
	6:20 AM	180	Dry		

NOTE: Bladder diary of an older woman with nocturia 4 to 5 times a night, occasional urge incontinence (less than daily), and frequency ("every 2 or 3 hours"). The diary indicates that she does not have her self-reported daytime frequency and that her nocturnal urine output (including all voids from bedtime up to and including first morning void) is 630–660 mL, or just over 50% of the 24-hour urine output on Day 2 (630 − [630 + 570]). With a functional bladder capacity of 240 mL (largest voided volume on the diary), this amount of nocturnal polyuria necessitates that she void at least twice (630 − 240) during the night. Thus, despite the presence of daytime urgency and rare urge incontinence, the cause of her nocturia is likely nocturnal polyuria. Evaluation and treatment should focus on potentially reversible causes of the polyuria.

TREATMENT AND MANAGEMENT

As with all geriatric practice, it is important to establish the goals of care for incontinence management from the patient and/or caregivers. For example, desired outcomes may range from complete continence, control sufficient to prevent large volume leakage with tolerance of small volume, to skin integrity and comfort. Patients and caregivers may have different tolerance for or perceptions of the bother, invasiveness, burden of treatment, and desired outcome of treatment.

Treatment should proceed stepwise, from correcting contributory factors and lifestyle modification, to behavioral therapy, medications, and then minimally invasive procedures and surgery as appropriate and consistent with the goals of care. Not all steps will be needed or appropriate for all patients, and some patients may want to proceed directly to specific therapy (eg, women with severe stress UI desiring surgery). Some treatments are effective for several UI symptoms (see below). Management should focus on relieving the aspect of UI that is most bothersome for the patient; eg, treatment that only decreases daytime UI episodes may not be sufficient for those most bothered by the timing of UI, nocturia, or leakage with exercise.

Geriatricians should be able to conduct an initial evaluation and begin stepped treatment for most older patients with UI. However, patients presenting with pelvic pain, hematuria, recurrent symptomatic urinary tract infections, pelvic mass, previous pelvic irradiation, prior pelvic or LUT surgery, significantly increased PVR, significant pelvic organ prolapse, or suspected fistula should be referred for specialty management, if appropriate for goals of care.

Lifestyle Modification

Weight loss significantly reduces stress incontinence in obese, young-old women (SOE=A). Other lifestyle interventions lack confirmatory evidence but may be helpful (SOE=D): avoiding extremes of fluid intake, caffeinated beverages, and alcohol; minimizing evening intake in those with nocturia; and quitting smoking (to decrease coughing) in patients with stress UI.

Behavioral Therapies

Bladder training and pelvic muscle exercises (PMEs) are effective for urge, mixed, and stress UI, and are often used in combination (SOE=A).

Bladder training uses two principles: frequent voluntary voiding to keep bladder volume low, and urgency suppression using CNS and pelvic mechanisms.

- The initial voiding frequency can be every 2 hours or based on the smallest voiding interval on bladder diary.

- To decrease or suppress a strong urge, the patient should not walk to or focus on getting to the bathroom but instead stand still or sit down, do several pelvic muscle contractions, and concentrate on making the urgency decrease by taking a deep breath and letting it out slowly, or visualizing the urgency as a wave that peaks and then falls. Once the patient feels more in control (the urgency can still be present), they should walk to the bathroom and void.

As patients progress, they can increase the time between scheduled voids by ~30-minute intervals, until they reach a comfortable level balancing voiding frequency and continence. Successful bladder training usually takes several weeks, and patients need reassurance to proceed despite any initial failure.

PMEs strengthen the muscular components of urethral support and are effective for urge, mixed, and stress UI. PMEs also are effective for prevention and treatment of UI after prostatectomy. PMEs are based on similar strategies to other muscle strength training: correct isolation of the target muscle(s), high intensity contraction, and low repetitions. Patient instruction and motivation are necessary, although simple instruction booklets alone have moderate benefit (SOE=A).

To do PMEs, the patient 1) performs an isolated pelvic muscle contraction, without contracting buttocks, abdomen, or thighs (this can be checked during a bimanual examination in women), and holds it for 6–8 seconds (initially, only shorter durations may be possible); 2) repeats the contraction 8 to 12 times (one set), relaxing the pelvis between each contraction; 3) completes 3 sets of contractions daily at least 3 to 4 times a week, and continuing for at least 15 to 20 weeks. As patients progress, they should try to increase the intensity and duration of the contraction, perform PMEs in various positions (sitting, standing, walking), and alternate fast and slower contractions. Many experts believe biofeedback can improve bladder retraining and PME teaching and outcomes, but marginal benefit is unproved. Medicare covers biofeedback for patients who do not improve after 4 weeks of conventional instruction.

Patients with moderate to severe cognitive impairment cannot participate in the behavioral therapies described above. The only behavioral treatment with proven efficacy in cognitively impaired patients is prompted voiding (SOE=B). A caregiver monitors the patient and encourages him or her to report any need to void; prompts the patient to toilet on a regular schedule during the day (usually every 2–3 hours); leads the patient to the bathroom; and gives the patient positive feedback when he or she toilets. Patients most likely to improve are able to state their name, transfer with a minimum of one assist, void ≤4 times during daytime hours, and are able to accept and follow the prompt to toilet at least 75% of the time with an initial 3-day trial. Toileting routines without prompting, such as habit training (based on a patient's usual voiding schedule without prompting) and scheduled voiding (using a set schedule) are not effective.

Medications

Medications are used to treat urge UI or urge-predominant mixed UI insufficiently responsive to behavioral therapy. There are currently no approved medications for stress UI.

Antimuscarinic agents are moderately effective for urge UI, overactive bladder, and mixed incontinence (SOE=A). They work by decreasing basal excretion of acetylcholine from the urothelium and thus increasing bladder capacity; they do not ablate uninhibited contractions. Data are conflicting whether combined antimuscarinic and behavioral therapy is better than either alone for reducing UI; the combination is significantly better for improving quality of life (SOE=A), and in stepped therapy behavioral therapy is usually continued when medications are added. Antimuscarinics are safe and effective in men with urgency and urge UI associated with benign prostatic hyperplasia who have a PVR <200 mL (SOE=A). Antimuscarinics are contraindicated for patients with narrow-angle glaucoma (not open-angle), impaired gastric emptying, and urinary retention. It is not necessary to routinely monitor PVR with antimuscarinic treatment. However, PVR should be checked if UI increases with antimuscarinic treatment, because a significant PVR reduces the functional capacity of the bladder, making voiding and UI more frequent.

There are six antimuscarinics with established efficacy (SOE=A):

- Oxybutynin (immediate release 2.5–5 mg q6–12h; extended release 5–20 mg/d; topical patch 3.9 mg/24 hr applied twice weekly to abdomen, thighs, or buttocks; and topical gel [3% gel or 10% sachet daily])

- Tolterodine (immediate release 1–2 mg q12h; extended release 2–4 mg/d)

- Trospium (immediate release 20 mg q12h or q24h; extended release 60 mg/d in am)

- Darifenacin (7.5–15 mg/d)

- Solifenacin (5–10 mg/d)

- Fesoterodine (4–8 mg/d)

Based on systematic reviews, the six antimuscarinic agents have similar efficacy in reducing urge UI frequency (best data are in women, ARR for continence 0.9–0.13, NNT 8–11; ARR for clinically important improvement 0.08–0.18, NNT 6–13) but differ in adverse events, metabolism, drug interactions, and dosing requirements. Only fesoterodine has been evaluated in a community-based population of vulnerable older adults; efficacy and tolerability were similar to those observed in trials of younger and healthy old adults (SOE=A). Comparative effectiveness trials are limited and industry supported.

Anticholinergic adverse events can limit tolerability and safety of these medications. The major concern is cognitive impairment. Although antimuscarinics as a class are associated with cognitive impairment, the risk, prevalence, type, and magnitude of cognitive changes from specific antimuscarinic UI medications in individual patients or patient groups are not clear. Short-term (4 week) use of extended-release oxybutynin (5 mg/d) did not increase delirium in frail nursing-home patients (SOE=A). A systematic review found low-moderate evidence for impairment of divided attention and reaction time, but overall the effects were inconsistent. Evidence is insufficient that one drug is "safer" for all patients, for those with mild cognitive impairment, or for those with moderate-severe dementia. What is clear is that antimuscarinics should not be combined with cholinesterase inhibitors because of lack of efficacy and risk of increased functional and possibly cognitive impairment.

Other important anticholinergic adverse effects include dry mouth with increased risk of dental caries, and constipation, with similar rates across antimuscarinics except for dosages of oxybutynin ≥10 mg/d, which is highest.

All antimuscarinics except trospium are metabolized by cytochrome P-450 pathways and can interact with drugs that induce CYP2D6 (eg, fluoxetine) or are metabolized by CYP3A4 (eg, erythromycin, ketoconazole). Fesoterodine is a prodrug that is metabolized to tolterodine by nonspecific peripheral esterases. Trospium is renally cleared and should be given once daily in patients with renal insufficiency; it should be taken on an empty stomach. Other antimuscarinics that should be considered for dose adjustment in chronic renal disease are tolterodine, fesoterodine, and solifenacin. Therefore, choice of agent for a particular patient should depend on potential adverse events to be avoided, possible drug-drug and drug-disease interactions, dosing frequency, titration range, and cost. A lack of response to one agent does not preclude response to another.

Mirabegron (25–50 mg/d) is a β_3-adrenergic agonist that stimulates detrusor relaxation and increases bladder capacity, with the same similar moderate efficacy as the antimuscarinics (SOE=A). To date, it has not been shown to have cognitive adverse effects, but it can raise blood pressure. Important drug-drug interactions can occur with digoxin, metoprolol, venlafaxine, desipramine, and dextromethorphan.

There is insufficient evidence for the efficacy of propantheline, dicyclomine, imipramine, hyoscyamine, calcium channel blockers, NSAIDs, and flavoxate. Vasopressin (DDAVP) should not be used for nocturia in older adults because of the risk of hyponatremia (SOE=A).

The serotonin–norepinephrine uptake inhibitor antidepressant duloxetine decreases stress UI but is not FDA approved for this indication. Oral estrogen, alone or in combination with progestins, increases UI (SOE=A). There is insufficient evidence whether vaginal topical estrogen improves UI (cream, vaginal tablet, or slow-release ring), but it is helpful for uncomfortable vaginal atrophy and may decrease recurrent urinary tract infections. Oral estrogen increases UI; this has not been found to be the case so far with topical vaginal estrogen.

Minimally Invasive Procedures

These procedures are used primarily for refractory urge UI. Sacral nerve neuromodulation has some effect for both urge UI refractory to drug treatment and urinary retention (idiopathic and neurogenic). The mechanism of action is unknown. The procedure involves percutaneous implantation of a trial electrode at the S3 sacral root, which is connected to an external stimulator. Patients responding to the trial have a permanent lead with a pacemaker-like energy source implanted. Posterior tibial nerve stimulation is a less invasive form of neuromodulation with a variably defined response rate of 60%–81% in small short-term trials (SOE=C).

Intravesical injection of botulinum toxin is effective for refractory urge UI (SOE=A). Optimal dosing for specific patient groups is uncertain, and patients must be willing to do self-catheterization because of the risk of urinary retention.

Pessaries may benefit women with stress and urge UI exacerbated by bladder or uterine prolapse.

Surgery

Surgery provides the highest cure rates for stress UI in women (SOE=A). The most commonly used procedures are colposuspension (Burch operation), and midurethral and bladder neck slings (synthetic mesh or autologous fascia placed transvaginally). Older women have similar improvement with midurethral slings as middle-aged women, but older women have more persistent postoperative urgency (SOE=A). Periurethral injection of a bulking agent is a short-term (≤1 year) alternative and usually requires a series of injections; previously widely used, collagen is no longer commercially produced.

Artificial sphincters are used for refractory stress UI from sphincter damage, typically after radical prostatectomy. A cuff is placed internally around the urethra, and its inflation controlled by the patient squeezing a reservoir device placed in the scrotum. They are moderately effective (SOE=B) but require manual dexterity and intact cognition; an alert bracelet should be considered, because catheter insertion through a closed artificial sphincter can cause significant damage. Revision rates can be high (up to 40%).

Supportive Care

Pads and protective garments should be chosen based on patient gender and type and volume of UI. For example, an absorbent sheath may be sufficient for a man with mild UI after prostatectomy. In some states, Medicaid may cover the cost of pads; Medicare and private insurance do not. Medical supply companies and patient advocacy groups publish illustrated catalogs to guide product selection. Because these products are often expensive, some patients may not change pads frequently enough.

EVALUATION AND MANAGEMENT OF UI IN NURSING-HOME RESIDENTS

The CMS *Guidance for Surveyors for Long Term Facilities* sets the nursing-home compliance standards, known as the F-tag 315, for evaluation and management of UI and urinary catheters. The 2006 revision of F-tag 315 changed the focus from documentation of toileting plans to an increased emphasis on screening, the process and documentation of UI assessment, and reevaluation. The Minimum Data Set requires that residents are screened for UI at admissions and quarterly, and with any change in cognition, function, or urinary tract function. F-tag 315 guidance suggests an evaluation essentially equivalent to that described above. Instead of bladder diaries, toileting patterns and UI episodes are monitored over several days. Although evaluation is largely a nursing responsibility, physician input is especially important given the F-tag 315 emphasis on physical examination, evaluation of medications and comorbidity as a cause of UI, and differential diagnosis.

Nearly all studies of UI treatment in long-term care involve behavioral therapy. Evidence is moderate that prompted voiding is effective in reducing daytime UI (SOE=B), but treatment is rarely continued long term. Interventions that combine prompted voiding with bedside exercise improve both incontinence and physical function (SOE=B). Prompted voiding should be tried in all eligible patients (able to state their name, can transfer with at most an assist by one), but continued only in those who are able to accept and follow the prompt to toilet at least 75% of the time in an initial 3-day trial (SOE=B). Long-term care residents who do not respond should be managed with "check and change." The revised F-tag 315 supports this targeted approach and the role of patient and family preferences in evaluation and treatment. Unfortunately, many nursing homes practice only scheduled toileting without prompting, which is ineffective. Quality improvement efforts focused on staff organization and systems may ultimately be necessary to reduce UI in long-term care.

The only randomized studies of antimuscarinic efficacy in nursing-home residents used oxybutynin. A 4-week randomized controlled trial found no difference between extended-release oxybutynin given at 5 mg/d and placebo. Consequently, antimuscarinics are infrequently prescribed, despite evidence that patients may prefer medications over behavioral therapy and "check and change." It is reasonable to consider an antimuscarinic trial for residents with urge UI who respond to prompted voiding but still have bothersome incontinence.

It is important to remember that up to a third of nursing-home residents with UI have an underlying bladder outlet problem (stress incontinence or bladder outlet obstruction) and may be candidates for alternative medical or surgical treatment.

CATHETERS AND CATHETER CARE

Indwelling catheters cause significant morbidity, including polymicrobial bacteriuria (universal by 30 days), febrile episodes (1 per 100 patient days), nephrolithiasis, bladder stones, epididymitis, chronic renal inflammation and pyelonephritis, and meatal damage. Condom catheters, often assumed to be less morbid than indwelling catheters, also cause bacteriuria, infection, penile cellulitis and necrosis, and even urinary retention and hydronephrosis if the condom twists or its external band is too tight. Indwelling catheters should be used only for short-term decompression of acute urinary retention, chronic retention that cannot be managed medically or surgically, protection of wounds that may be contaminated by urine, and for comfort in terminally ill or severely impaired patients who cannot tolerate garment changes and there is an informed preference for catheter management despite risks. Inappropriate and/or poorly documented indications for catheter use are a major focus in the revised F-tag 315 guidance for nursing homes. The guidance states that catheters should primarily be used for short-term decompression of acute retention but also allows for the indications above.

All patients with acute retention should have decompression with an indwelling catheter while being evaluated and treated for potentially remediable causes, such as medications that impair detrusor contractility or increase urethral tone, outlet obstruction, and constipation. Duration of catheterization before voiding trial should depend on time course for reversing underlying cause. A voiding trial without catheter should follow decompression. To do so, the catheter should be removed (never clamped), the patient adequately hydrated, and a PVR checked after the first void or bladder volume checked if there is no void after about 6 hours. Studies have not confirmed any benefit of bethanechol chloride for patients with retention (SOE=B).

Intermittent clean catheterization is an effective alternative to an indwelling catheter for willing and able patients and/or caregivers. Strict sterility is not necessary, although good hand washing and regular decontamination of the catheters is needed. Specialized stiff and smooth short catheters are available for use. Bacteriuria can be minimized by a frequency of catheterization that keeps bladder volume <400 mL. Sterile intermittent catheterization is preferred for frailer patients and those in institutionalized settings.

Bacteriuria is universal in catheterized patients and should not be treated unless there are clear symptoms of cystitis or pyelonephritis, eg fever. Routine cultures should not be done because of changing flora and difficulty in differentiating colonization from active infection. In symptomatic patients, urine for culture is best obtained by removing the old catheter and urine obtained from a newly placed catheter. Institutionalized patients with catheters should be kept in separate rooms to decrease cross-infection. Topical meatal antimicrobials, catheters with antimicrobial coating, collection bag disinfectants, and antimicrobial irrigation are not effective in preventing catheter-associated urinary tract infection. Use of antibiotics for anything other than symptomatic infection induces resistant organisms and secondary infections (such as with *Clostridium difficile*) and should not be used. Prophylactic antibiotics are recommended only in high-risk patients (eg, those with prosthetic heart valves) during short-term catheterization. For patients with chronic obstruction, suprapubic catheters may be preferable to avoid meatal and penile trauma.

Catheters do not need to be changed routinely as long as monitoring is adequate and catheter blockage does not develop. Risk factors for blockage include alkaline urine, female gender, poor mobility, calciuria, proteinuria, copious mucin, *Proteus* colonization, and bladder stones. Changing the catheter every 7–10 days may decrease blockage in such patients. If patients cannot be monitored, changing catheters every 30 days is reasonable (SOE=D). Possible causes of persistent leakage around the catheter are large Foley balloon, detrusor overactivity, bacteriuria, constipation or impaction, and improper catheter positioning. These can be addressed by trials of partial deflation of the balloon, smaller catheter, treatment of constipation, use of an anticholinergic, or treatment with pyridium.

Catheters coated with silver alloys reduce asymptomatic bacteriuria in hospitalized patients requiring short-term urethral catheterization, but their use in reducing symptomatic bacteriuria is less certain. Data are scant whether silver alloy catheters reduce asymptomatic or symptomatic bacteriuria in other settings (such as long-term care or home care) or with longer-term catheterization.

CHOOSING WISELY® RECOMMENDATIONS

Urinary Incontinence

- Do not order creatinine or upper tract imaging if only lower urinary tract symptoms.

REFERENCES

- American Medical Directors Association. Clinical Corner: Urinary Incontinence. Available at www.amda.com/tools/clinical/urinaryincontinence.cfm (accessed Jan 2016).

   This website provides a variety of useful resources on the topic of incontinence, including links to key articles, tools, and resources.

- Catheterout.org. www.catheterout.org (accessed Jan 2016).

   This is an excellent and practical website regarding prevention of catheter-associated urinary tract infections, with a focus on quality improvement. It includes tools for physician and nurse engagement, nurse-led "catheter patrols" to assess patients for catheter and initiate removal, and brochures for patients and families who request catheter use without an evidence-based medical indication. Although geared to the inpatient setting, the information and tools can be helpful in long-term care settings.

- Goode PS, Burgio KL, Richter HE. Incontinence in older women. *JAMA*. 2010;303(21):2172–2181.

   This review from the *JAMA* series "Care of the Aging Patient: From Evidence to Action" combines a case-based approach with evidence-based practice.

- Madhuvrata P, Cody JD, EllisG, et al. Which anticholinergic drug for overactive bladder symptoms in adults. *Cochrane Database Syst Rev*. 2012;1:CD005429.

   This systematic review covers nonsurgical and surgical treatment of overactive bladder and/or urge incontinence in women. Each uses slightly different objectives, methodology, and scope. The first is a report done for AHRQ Evidence-based Practice Center, and the second a recent Cochrane review comparing anticholinergics. The Cochrane Collaborative Group on Incontinence has systematic reviews with updates on a wide range of UI treatments.

- Richter HE. Surgery for stress incontinence in the older woman—some considerations. *Eur Obstet & Gynaecol*. 2010;5(1):58–60.

   Older women undergoing surgery for stress incontinence have overall similar operative risks and subjective, objective, and quality-of-life outcomes to those of younger women, although their risk for surgical re-treatment may be higher.

Catherine E. DuBeau, MD

CHAPTER 32—PRESSURE ULCERS AND WOUND CARE

KEY POINTS

- Critical components of managing pressure ulcers include wound examination, documentation, diagnosis, and understanding and implementing basic principles of wound care.

- Because of their association with the perception of quality, pressure ulcers are an important concern in regulatory, reimbursement, and risk-management arenas.

- Pressure ulcers have severe consequences, including increased length of stay, increased chance of readmission within 30 days of hospital discharge, prolonged rehabilitation, pain, disfigurement, infection, loss of limb, and death.

- Risk assessment and risk factor intervention are key to pressure ulcer prevention. It is now accepted that nonmodifiable risk factors in many patients can lead to pressure ulcers even when appropriate interventions are implemented.

- Many wounds have reduced or no chance of healing. For these wounds, palliative care principles may curtail suffering, improve quality of life, and decrease health care costs.

- Physicians are key members of the interprofessional team involved with preventing and treating pressure ulcers. Because advanced age is associated with many pressure ulcers, geriatricians have a responsibility to shape the future of care for these wounds.

Pressure ulcers are a common chronic wound in the geriatric population. Care of pressure ulcers is interdisciplinary and involves nursing, nutrition, rehabilitation, and surgical subspecialties. Pressure ulcers cause pain and are associated with a decreased quality of life, longer hospital stay, increased chance of readmission within 30 days after hospital discharge, increased chance of admission to a long-term care facility, and increased risk of death. Infectious complications include cellulitis, abscess, sepsis, pyarthrosis, and osteomyelitis. Pressure ulcers often require surgical procedures ranging from sharp debridements to myocutaneous flaps, amputations, and ostomies for fecal diversion. Care for pressure ulcers is costly, with estimates of \$3,500 to more than \$60,000 per patient, depending on stage. A vexing variety of treatments is available with few studies to prove efficacy of one over the other. The standard of care for pressure ulcers is evolving, and all primary care providers, particularly geriatricians, need to be aware of prevention strategies, documentation standards, and treatment choices. These choices include a palliative care approach, which can avoid unnecessary and futile procedures, improve quality of life, and curtail health care costs.

Pressure ulcers affect from 1.3 to 3 million adults in the United States, and their incidence and prevalence varies greatly depending on stage, setting, and how data are collected. In acute care, one study showed incidence ranging from 7% to 9% per year. Higher rates are consistently reported in older populations. Hospital prevalence rates range from 11.9% to 15.8%. In long-term care, prevalence ranges from 8.5% to 32.2%. One study reported that up to 54.7% of terminally ill nursing-home residents have pressure ulcers. The increase in pressure ulcer prevalence that occurred in the 20th century was largely a result of modern public health measures and advances in medical technology that resulted in longer life expectancy and greater numbers of people living with multiple chronic illnesses.

Pressure ulcers are a designated quality measure in hospitals, long-term care, and home-care settings. As a result of their association with quality of care, pressure ulcers have become a major risk management issue. Pressure ulcer data for skilled nursing facilities is currently published by CMS on the Nursing Home Compare website, but as yet there is no federal mandate for publication of pressure ulcer statistics for hospitals and home care. In addition, pressure ulcers have been spotlighted in value-based purchasing and pay-for-performance initiatives. For example, in 2008 the CMS introduced a policy to decline payment to hospitals for certain hospital-acquired conditions that include stage III or IV pressure ulcers. These factors have resulted in an evolving standard of care that designates physicians as key players. Many hospitals and long-term care facilities require physician orders for wound care products, dressings, and devices to obtain Medicare reimbursement. Because pressure ulcers are an identified geriatric syndrome, geriatrics providers with proper training can play a pivotal role in improving quality of care for this condition.

It has become increasingly recognized that many pressure ulcers are unavoidable. Patients at severe risk with immobility and multiple chronic conditions can develop pressure ulcers even when standards of care for prevention are met. A pressure ulcer is therefore not necessarily indicative of poor quality care but rather may be a marker for disease severity or impending death. An expert panel (SCALE Panel 2009) assembled consensus statements about skin changes at life's end that support the concept of unavoidable pressure ulcers in patients who are actively dying. An extensive literature review and consensus study summarizing factors that lead to unavoidable pressure ulcers was published in 2014. A key concept for understanding unavoidable pressure ulcers is the nonmodifiable risk factor for which effective interventions cannot be implemented. NPUAP defines an unavoidable pressure ulcer as one that develops despite the provider having 1) evaluated the individual's clinical condition and pressure ulcer risk factors; 2) defined and implemented interventions consistent with individual needs, goals, and recognized standards of practice; and 3) monitored and evaluated the impact of the interventions, revising the approaches as appropriate.

Chronic Wound Healing

Normal wound healing is a complex but orderly sequence of biologic events that includes hemostasis, inflammation, proliferation, and remodeling. Neutrophils are involved in the inflammatory phase, phagocytizing debris and microorganisms and providing a first line of defense. Macrophages play an important role in phagocytosis, debriding damaged tissue with proteases, creating granulation tissue, laying down extracellular matrix, and secreting chemotactic and growth factors. Granulation tissue consists of new blood vessels, fibroblasts, endothelial cells, myofibroblasts, and extracellular matrix. Fibroblasts produce collagen that increases the strength of the wound, plus other critical substances such as elastin, fibronectin, glycosaminoglycans, and proteases. Myofibroblasts, descended from fibroblasts, assist in contraction. Keratinocytes are the main cells responsible for epithelialization, the process of migrating across a bed of granulation tissue. Because of the disruption in normal anatomy and disorganization of new collagen, the tensile strength of a healed wound is only 50%–80% of that of undamaged skin.

Pressure ulcers are one of a diverse group of lesions classified as chronic wounds (see Table 32.1). Chronic wounds share in common prolonged healing time and interference with normal wound healing that renders them stalled in the inflammatory and proliferative phases. The surface of a chronic wound often harbors an "antihealing environment" with elements that include biofilm, exudate that contains pro-inflammatory cytokines such as matrix metalloproteases and tumor necrosis factor alpha (TNF-α), and lack of pro-regenerative agents such as transforming growth factor (TGF-β),

Table 32.1—The Spectrum of Chronic Wounds

- Pressure ulcers
- Arterial ulcers, or wounds from peripheral arterial disease
- Venous insufficiency ulcers
- Diabetic or neuropathic ulcers
- Nonhealing surgical wounds
- Wounds from malignancy
- Wounds from autoimmune source or vasculitis
- Wounds from trauma and burns (including skin tears, lacerations, and self-induced)

platelet-derived growth factor, and vascular endothelial growth factor.

Conditions leading to chronic wounds include repetitive trauma, decreased vascular perfusion, poor nutrition, poor oxygenation from anemia, diabetes or pulmonary disease, edema that interferes with nutrient delivery, pharmacologic barriers such as corticosteroids and immunosuppressants, incontinence, and biofilms. A biofilm is a community of microorganisms that secretes a mucilaginous extracellular coating that protects them from antibiotics and inhibits healing. These factors have greater impact on older adults, because they add to the processes of aging that include reduced fibroblasts, macrophages and mast cells, loss of extracellular matrix components such as collagen and glycosaminoglycans, decreased amount and morphology of elastin, altered surface pH, reduced sebum secretion with decreased pilosebaceous units, and flattening of the dermal-epidermal junction.

Pressure Ulcer Definition and Classification

A pressure ulcer is defined as a localized injury to the skin and/or underlying tissue, usually over a bony prominence, that results from pressure or from pressure in combination with shear. The current staging system defined by NPUAP is used only for pressure ulcers (see Table 32.2 and Figures 32.1–32.4). Staging of pressure ulcers is determined by visible depth. If the base of the wound cannot be seen, the wound is determined as "unstageable" (Figure 32.5). A wound is designated "deep tissue injury" (DTI) when the skin is intact and a purple bruise-like area is present in an area subjected to pressure (Figure 32.6). A DTI can dissipate leaving intact skin, or it can evolve into a wound of varying severity. Stage I and DTI can be difficult to assess in persons with dark skin, and examinations should be performed with adequate lighting and include palpation for detection of induration or warmth.

The heel, the second most common site for pressure ulcers after the sacrum, has unique anatomic features

Table 32.2—NPUAP Staging Criteria for Pressure Ulcers

Stage I **Nonblanchable erythema**	Intact skin with nonblanchable redness of a localized area, usually over a bony prominence. Darkly pigmented skin may not have visible blanching; its color may differ from the surrounding area. The area may be painful, firm, soft, or warmer or cooler than adjacent tissue. May be difficult to detect in those with dark skin tones. May indicate "at risk" patients.
Stage II **Partial thickness**	Partial-thickness loss of dermis presenting as a shallow open ulcer with a red pink wound bed, without slough. May also present as an intact or open/ruptured blister filled with serum or serosanguineous fluid. Presents as a shiny or dry shallow ulcer without slough or bruising (the latter indicates deep-tissue injury). This category should not be used to describe skin tears, tape burns, incontinence-associated dermatitis, maceration, or excoriation.
Stage III **Full-thickness tissue loss**	Full-thickness tissue loss; subcutaneous fat may be visible but bone, tendon, or muscle are not exposed/visible or directly palpable. Slough may be present but does not obscure the depth of tissue loss. May include undermining and tunneling. The depth of a Stage III pressure ulcer varies by anatomical location. The bridge of the nose, ear, occiput, and malleolus do not have (adipose) subcutaneous tissue, and Stage III ulcers can be shallow. In contrast, areas of significant adiposity can develop extremely deep Stage III pressure ulcers.
Stage IV **Full-thickness tissue loss**	Full-thickness tissue loss with exposed/visible bone, tendon, or muscle that is directly palpable. Slough or eschar may be present. Often includes undermining and tunneling. The depth of a Stage IV pressure ulcer varies by anatomical location. The bridge of the nose, ear, occiput, and malleolus do not have (adipose) subcutaneous tissue, and these ulcers can be shallow. Stage IV ulcers can extend into muscle and/or supporting structures (eg, fascia, tendon or joint capsule) making osteomyelitis or osteitis likely to develop.
Unstageable/unclassified **Full-thickness skin** **or tissue loss, depth** **unknown**	Full-thickness tissue loss in which actual depth of the ulcer is completely obscured by slough (yellow, tan, gray, green, or brown) and/or eschar (tan, brown, or black) in the wound bed. Until enough slough and/or eschar are removed to expose the base of the wound, the true depth cannot be determined; but it will be either a Stage III or IV. Stable (dry, adherent, intact without erythema or fluctuance) eschar on the heels serves as "the body's natural (biological) cover" and should not be removed.
Suspected deep tissue **injury, depth unknown**	Purple or maroon localized area of discolored intact skin or blood-filled blister due to damage of underlying soft tissue from pressure and/or shear. May be preceded by tissue that is painful, firm, mushy, boggy, and warmer or cooler than adjacent tissue. May be difficult to detect in those with dark skin tones. Evolution may include a thin blister over a dark wound bed. The wound may further evolve and become covered by thin eschar. Evolution may be rapid, exposing additional layers of tissue even with optimal treatment.

© National Pressure Ulcer Advisory Panel, 2014
SOURCE: Adapted with permission from the National Pressure Ulcer Advisory Panel, 2014 (www.npuap.org [accessed Jan 2016]).

that warrant special consideration when evaluating an ulcer. These include thick skin, very little subcutaneous tissue and muscle, and vascular perfusion delivered around the large calcaneus bone that underlies the rear portion of the foot. The foot is also susceptible to circulatory impairment because of atheromatous disease of the leg, microvascular disease from diabetes mellitus, and decreased sensation from peripheral neuropathy of any etiology. Pressure ulcers of the heels often present as blisters. A clear blister over a bony prominence is considered a stage II pressure ulcer, whereas a blood-filled blister is considered DTI.

PRESSURE ULCER ASSESSMENT AND DOCUMENTATION

Pressure ulcers must be detected early, because these wounds can usually heal quickly if discovered in early stages and treated properly. Alternatively, wounds can deteriorate quickly, particularly in patients with severe immobility in conjunction with multisystemic disease. As a result, timely examination and documentation is an important component of management. Consistent and complete documentation is required for coding and reimbursement, public reporting, risk management, and accurate transmittal of information as patients traverse the health care continuum. Providers should take the time to perform the examination rather than rely on others for the information. Proper wound evaluation can be time consuming, particularly in patients with multiple wounds. It often involves obtaining assistance with lifting or turning an immobile patient who may be in pain, and removing and replacing dressings. However, timely and thorough examination is mandatory for all patients with pressure ulcers and will bring dividends in accurate documentation and improved decision making.

Wound documentation includes diagnosis, stage, location, length, width, depth, presence of odor and/or drainage, presence of undermining and tunneling, as well as characteristics of the wound bed, margins, and surrounding skin. Supplemental information can include warmth, capillary refill, and presence of

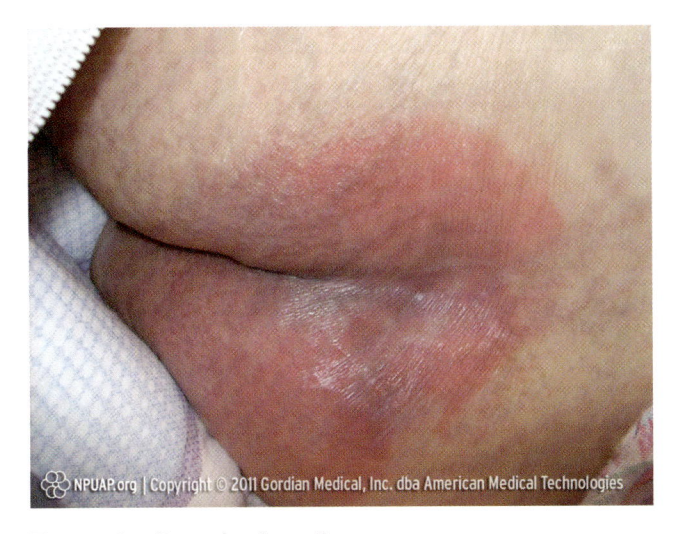

Figure 1—Buttocks, Stage I

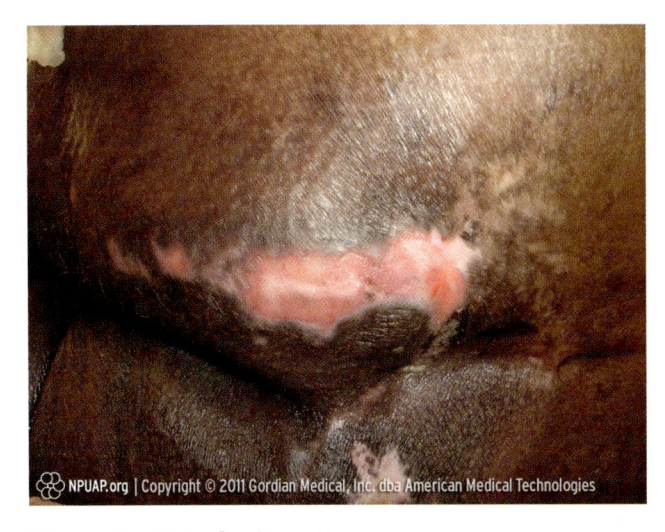

Figure 2—Buttocks, Stage II

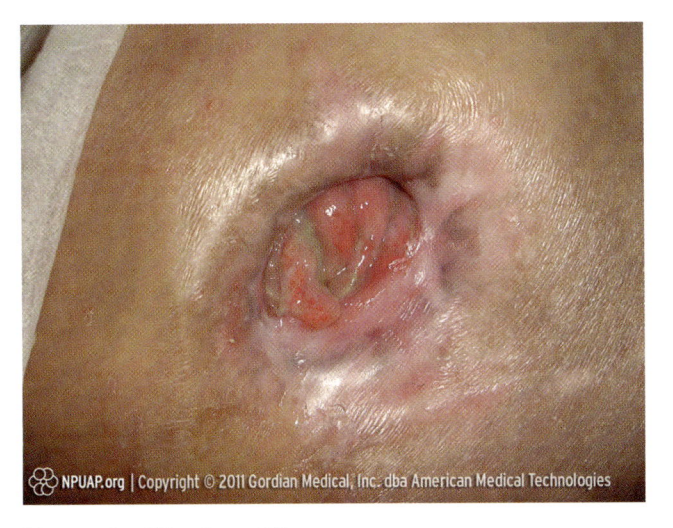

Figure 3—Hip, Stage III

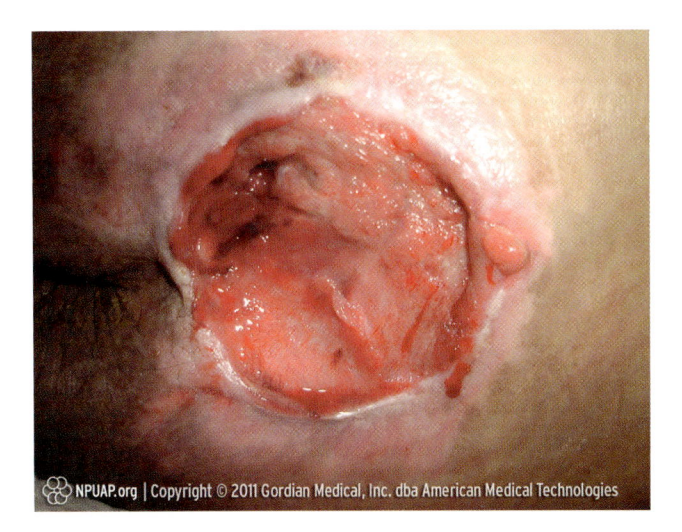

Figure 4—Sacrum, Stage IV

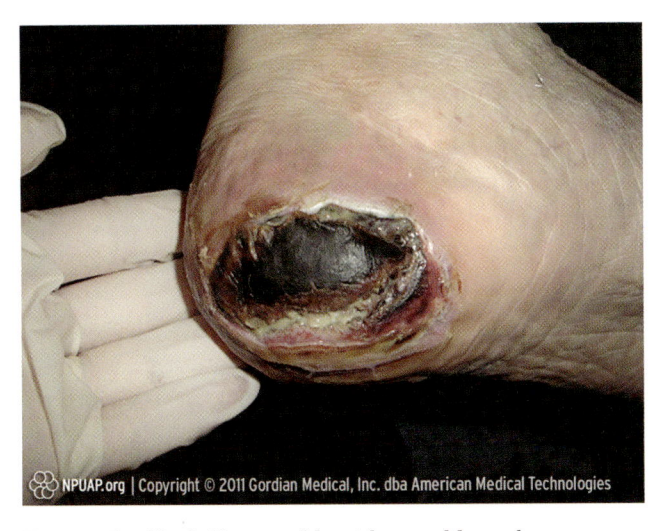

Figure 5—Heel, Unstageable with unstable eschar

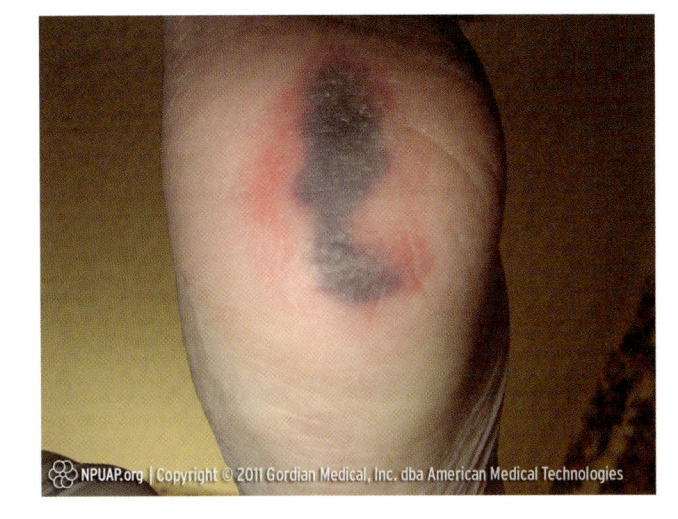

Figure 6—Heel, Deep Tissue Injury

Chapter 32: Pressure Ulcers and Wound Care

Table 32.3—Risk Factors for Pressure Ulceration and Their Associated Causes

Intrinsic Risk Factors	Associated Causes
Dermatitis	Radiotherapy (radiation dermatitis), yeast infection, moisture-associated skin damage, incontinence-associated dermatitis
Edema	Hypoalbuminemia, renal disease, heart failure, venous insufficiency
Hypoperfusion	Anemia, atherosclerotic vascular disease, hypoxia, heart failure, hypotension, shock, peripheral vasoconstriction with pressor agents
Immobility	Neurologic disease, musculoskeletal illness, pain
Long-term corticosteroid use	COPD, rheumatologic illness, etc
Circulatory impairment	Diabetes mellitus, vasculitis, atherosclerotic disease, smoking, post-thrombotic syndrome
Nutritional compromise	Failure to thrive, depression, inflammation, terminal cancer, cachexia of congestive heart failure
Extrinsic Risk Factors	
Friction	Sliding in bed, rubbing against sheets or clothing
Immobility	Physical restraints, multiple life-support modalities, sedatives
Medical devices	Tubing, orthopedic devices, face mask, trach collar, etc
Moisture	Incontinence, sweat, wound exudate
Pressure	Immobility, medical device, operative table
Shear forces	Changes in position, sitting up in bed

pulses, edema, anasarca, and lymphedema. Measurement is an important component of wound assessment, particularly for determining the effectiveness of clinical interventions. Measurement involves head-to-toe length, width, and depth and should be both consistent and accurate. The simplest method uses a centimeter ruler to measure length and width, and a cotton-tipped swab to measure depth, tunneling, and undermining. Wound clinics and skilled-nursing facilities usually have structured documentation sheets with entry points for diagnosis, length, width, and depth, along with diagrams to designate location and undermining, as well as treatment in progress and response to treatment. If such structured documents are unavailable, it is advisable to describe the wound with as much detail as possible in narrative form.

Documentation of wound progression is an important component of management and should be ongoing, systematic, and consistent. Wounds should be formally assessed at least weekly, with descriptors that include measurements, nature of the wound bed and periwound area, pressure redistribution modalities, treatments in progress, and response to healing. Some authorities recommend a validated healing scale such as the Pressure Sore Status Tool or the Pressure Ulcer Scale for Healing. No single standard exists that mandates the type and extent of information to include in a wound assessment, but the more descriptors the better. Patients with pressure ulcers frequently undergo transitions between locations within the health care continuum, and wounds should be thoroughly documented on both admission and discharge from hospitals and long-term care facilities. Similarly, initial home care visits should include thorough skin inspection. Reverse staging is not a recognized standard, because it does not accurately characterize the anatomic and physiologic process that occurs during healing.

Photographs can be valuable adjuncts to wound documentation; however, their implementation in a medical record must be consistent and within a formal policy and procedure guideline. Photographs must be of reasonable quality and accompanied by a label within the visual field that contains a patient identifier (name, initials, or medical record number), location of the wound, and date. Haphazard use of photographs or poor photographic technique can create discontinuities in documentation with risk-management implications. Providers who use personal cell phones to take photographs are committing potential HIPAA violations.

PRESSURE ULCER PREVENTION

The standard of care for pressure ulcer prevention includes risk assessment followed by appropriate pressure redistribution interventions if the patient is deemed at risk.

Risk Assessment

There are many recognized risk factors for pressure ulcers, and several validated instruments are available that quantify risk. The most widely used tool is the Braden Scale (www.in.gov/isdh/files/Braden_Scale.pdf) that combines sensory perception, moisture, activity, mobility, and friction and shear. This scale has been validated in home, skilled-nursing facilities, and hospital settings but not in ICUs. However, other studies have noted that risk assessment tools can be weak predictors of which patients are more likely to develop pressure ulcers (SOE=B). Current scales also do not contain information related to organ system failure or physiologic factors such as hypoxia and hypotension, which may also engender increased pressure ulcer risk. Therefore, clinical judgment should be relied on to determine "at risk" status in addition to the formalized risk assessment scale.

Risk factors for pressure ulcers can be classified as either extrinsic, intrinsic, or both (see Table 32.3). Immobility is a major risk factor that results from causes that are both external and internal to the patient. Nutritional compromise is a known risk factor for pressure ulcers, and patients >75 years old with malnutrition and weight loss are 3.8 times more likely to develop pressure ulcers.

Medical devices are increasingly recognized as causes of pressure ulceration. These include external devices such as tubing and orthopedic splints, casts, limb immobilizers, abdominal binders, and CPAP masks. Care plans for patients with external orthopedic devices should always include periodic skin assessment. Pressure ulcers can develop over internally placed medical devices such as implantable neurostimulators and pain-control pumps that create new pressure points under the skin.

Skin assessment is an important component of prevention and should be done at least once per day for patients considered at risk in any setting. Areas of skin exposed to chronic moisture, over bony prominences, or under medical devices require special attention to detect early signs of impairment. Inspection of skin over bony prominences and under medical devices should be a routine part of the physician assessment, particularly on admission to hospital or nursing home. Routine nursing care should include skin assessment, and skin should be cleansed with efforts to minimize both dryness and excessive moisture.

Moisture-associated skin damage (MASD) that occurs from perspiration, urine, diarrhea, fistulas, or wound exudate increases susceptibility to pressure ulcers, and is a common occurrence in patients with constant loose stools from tube feeding or *Clostridium difficile* colitis. MASD involves more than simple maceration of skin, and contributors include mechanical factors such as friction, chemical irritants, and microbes, including bacteria and fungi (Figure 32.7). Strategies to avoid or treat MASD include moisture barrier creams, absorbable undergarments, continence care, and fecal and urinary diversion devices. Fungal infections require early diagnosis, because they can lead to impaired skin integrity if untreated. The diagnosis of fungal infection is sometimes missed because of the similarity in appearance to MASD, but close inspection of the border of redness and inflammation can reveal telltale satellite lesions characteristic of *Candida albicans*.

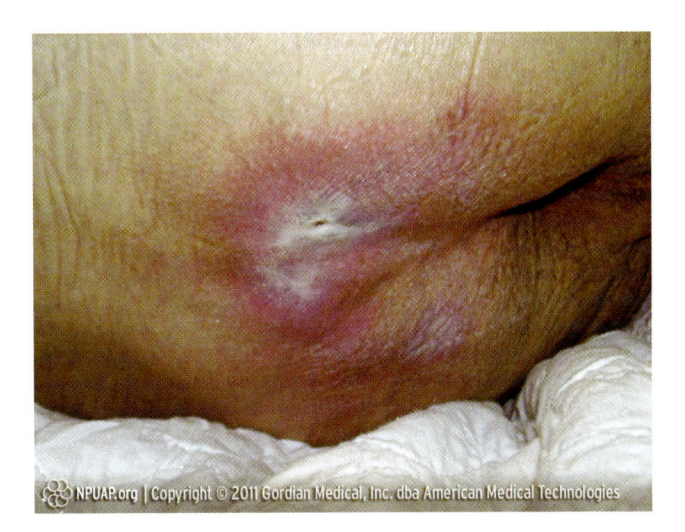

Figure 7—Sacrum with moisture-associated skin damage (MASD)

Prevention Strategies

There are many strategies for minimizing pressure, friction, and shear. Positioning devices such as pillows and foam wedges can help keep pressure off bony prominences, and lifting devices and draw sheets can minimize friction. Shear is a mechanical force that occurs when skin is pulled parallel to the body and is commonly caused by sitting up in bed. Backrest elevation of 30–45 degrees is associated with reduced risk of ventilator-associated pneumonia and aspiration related to tube feeding; however, sustained backrest elevation of >30 degrees is associated with increased pressure and shear to the lower back and buttocks. There is no current consensus as to how to balance the risks of pressure ulceration with minimizing the risks of ventilator-associated pneumonia and aspiration.

The industry standard for turning and positioning is every 2 hours, but there is minimal research to support this schedule (SOE=C). In addition, this standard was developed before the advent of advanced mattress and continence care technology. Research challenges the need for every-2-hour repositioning for patients using high-density foam mattresses (SOE=B). Patients who sit for long periods of time in chairs should be assessed for proper posture and alignment and provided with pressure relief schedules and cushioning. Strategies for preventing heel wounds include local skin care, cushioning, and lifting the heels off the mattress by placing a pillow under the legs when supine, also called "floating the heels" (SOE=B).

NPUAP defines "support surface" as a specialized device designed for management of tissue loads, microclimate, and/or other therapeutic needs. Pressure redistribution surfaces are a type of durable medical equipment categorized into 3 groups by CMS. Group 1 support surfaces are nonpowered devices made of gel, foam, or water that are designed to replace a standard hospital or home mattress, or as an overlay placed on top of the mattress. Group 2 support surfaces are designed to replace the standard hospital or home mattress or as mattress overlays, and include alternating-pressure air mattresses and pressure-reducing air mattresses of the low air loss type. This group includes both powered and nonpowered devices. Low air loss technology is a support surface that provides a flow of air for managing skin microclimate, including heat and humidity. Group 3 support surfaces are complete bed systems using air-fluidized technology using pressurized silicone-coated beads that promote a flotation environment. Other advanced features of the specialized bed include pulsations for pulmonary toilet, multizoned surfaces, and lateral rotation. There is little evidence to guide surface choices other than the general principal that persons at risk require offloading of pressure points and pressure redistribution devices when immobile.

The terms "static" and "dynamic" are also commonly applied to support surfaces, where the latter refers to powered devices. There is some evidence that a more advanced static mattress or overlay is associated with lower risk of pressure ulcers than a standard hospital mattress; however, there are little data to support the effectiveness of one type of powered device over another (SOE=C). Given the lack of evidence on efficacy of prevention devices, choices are generally made on the basis of ease of use, nursing preference, cost, availability, and reimbursement.

PRINCIPLES OF PRESSURE ULCER TREATMENT

A holistic, patient-centered approach to pressure ulcer treatment involves assessing the overall health status of the patient, addressing psychosocial needs, treating underlying comorbidities, assessing and correcting causes of tissue damage, and assessing and monitoring the wound. It is essential to understand the patient's functional and cognitive status, home environment, family support, and other factors such as the presence of depression. Wound assessment entails examination and description as discussed above, along with proper documentation. If the wound is an alteration in skin or tissue integrity over a bony prominence, it is most likely a pressure ulcer and staged in accordance with NPUAP criteria. Local malignancy must be considered in any chronic wound with consideration of biopsy, and all wounds should be assessed for infection (discussed below). Elements of pressure ulcer treatment involve offloading and pressure redistribution strategies, removing debris and necrotic tissue, and addressing moisture balance. Finally the clinician must address pain, acknowledge advance directives, and be able to recognize wounds appropriate for a palliative approach and alter the plan accordingly.

Laboratory tests provide important information regarding the patient's health and ability to heal. Anemia contributes to decreased oxygen delivery to vulnerable or healing tissue. Nutritional status as reflected in serum albumin and prealbumin levels can impair wound healing, but these laboratory tests are unreliable in the presence of inflammation. Increases in WBC count, erythrocyte sedimentation rate, or C-reactive protein may indicate ongoing infection or inflammation. The clinician must be aware of endocrinopathies such as hypothyroidism and poorly controlled diabetes mellitus. For wounds of the lower extremity, tests such as ankle-brachial index (ABI), pulse volume recording, and Doppler ultrasound can assist in evaluating arterial supply. ABI loses diagnostic value when arteries are noncompressible due to advanced atherosclerotic disease.

Numerous wound products are available, and the lack of controlled clinical trials and reliable measures of efficacy can make choosing an appropriate treatment bewildering. The lack of research is partially attributable to the FDA classification of most wound care products as medical devices, as opposed to pharmaceuticals, which exempts manufacturers from the requirement to demonstrate efficacy. With little evidence-based support for individual treatments, choices are often made based on product availability, insurance coverage, personal preference, cost considerations, expert opinion, and intrinsic rationale for product type. Table 32.4 presents some commonly used treatment modalities along with rationale for each.

Wound bed preparation has emerged as a useful tool to conceptually organize the array of wound products in a manner that achieves maximal benefit for chronic wounds such as pressure ulcers. Wound bed preparation focuses on critical components of management, including moisture and exudate, bacterial balance, and debridement. The foundation of this concept is an orderly approach to accelerate endogenous healing and facilitate the effectiveness of therapeutic measures. The goal is to reestablish the balance of growth factors, cytokines, proteases, and their natural inhibitors as found in acute wounds, thereby stimulating the healing process.

Moisture balance is an important component of wound healing, because a moist environment promotes autolytic debridement and encourages matrix formation. Alternatively, excess moisture inhibits wound healing through maceration that impairs both the wound bed and periwound area. Several products promote moist wound healing such as hydrocolloids, hydrogels, and other biocclusives. The exudate of chronic wounds contains

Table 32.4—Common Wound Treatment Modalities

Type	Content	Rationale	Best Use
Gauze	Cotton, polyester, or other fabrics	Versatile, can be absorptive or protective, primary or secondary dressing	Secondary dressing, wet to moist, or wet to dry, or as a protective to the wound and surrounding skin. *Note:* wet to dry is not recommended.
Hydrocolloid	Adhesive pad with moisture-activated, gel-forming material; gelatin and pectin	Moisture retention	Superficial, clean pressure ulcers with no necrosis or infection
Semipermeable films	Transparent polymer with acrylic adhesive	Moisture retention	Superficial, clean pressure ulcers with no necrosis or infection
Hydrogel	Water in a delivery vehicle such as glycerin or cross-linked polymer sheets	Promote moist wound healing and autolytic debridement	Dry wounds; wounds with some necrosis
Foam	Polyurethane with or without adhesive borders	Absorb exudate, cushioning, secondary dressing	Control exudate, protect the wound
Alginate	Seaweed derivative; can be in different forms, including sheet or rope, and combined with other materials such as silver or charcoal	Absorptive dressing	Control of exudate
Collagen	Animal-derived collagen formulated into gel, powder, paste, or sheet	Deactivates matrix metalloproteases that inhibit wound healing	Partial- or full-thickness wounds with minimal necrosis
Silver-containing dressings	Silver can be impregnated into multiple types of dressings	Silver has broad-spectrum antimicrobial activity	Wounds requiring control of bacterial balance
Enzymatic debriding agent	Enzyme in a petrolatum vehicle	Selected degradation of denatured collagen	Wounds with necrosis and slough
Cadexomer iodine dressing	Iodophor in a polysaccharide polymer	Absorbent, antimicrobial	Wounds with slough, infected wounds
Silicone dressings	Inert silicone polymer; sometimes has pores that allow passage of exudate	Contact layer that can be removed without causing trauma to wound or surrounding skin	When a nonadherent dressing is required, protects the wound and surrounding skin
Activated charcoal	Combined with silver or other vehicles	Control odor	Palliative wounds with odor
Honey	Medicinal grade honey can be used as a gel or impregnated into other dressing types	Antimicrobial properties, anti-inflammatory	Autolytic debriding agent on noninfected wounds
Topical antiseptics	Includes hydrogen peroxide, Dakin's solution (hypochlorite), povidone-iodine	Reduce bacterial burden of wounds	Can be cytotoxic to healing wounds; for limited use in heavily contaminated or nonhealable wounds
Petrolatum-impregnated gauze	Woven mesh; medical petrolatum and 3% bismuth tribromophenate	Bacteriostatic, nonadherent, retains moisture	Use with larger wounds with minimal necrosis and slough

heightened proteolytic activity, matrix metalloproteases, and macromolecules that inhibit growth factors, and products such as foams, hydrofibers, and alginates provide absorptive capabilities. Collagen-containing products inactivate harmful cytokines and factors that inhibit healing.

Bacterial balance in the wound bed is facilitated by cleansing, topical antibiotics, disinfectants, and debridement. Debridement removes necrotic tissue and bacteria, providing a clean surface that promotes healing. Debridement can be achieved by several ways, and selection should be individualized in accordance with goals of care and degree of necrosis. Autolytic debridement uses moisture retentive topical dressings to take advantage of endogenous enzymes present in the wound, whereas enzymatic debridement uses a commercially produced enzyme to digest debris and dead tissue. Mechanical debridement methods include hydrotherapy (whirlpool), irrigation (pulsed lavage), and scraping the wound base and periwound area with a blunt instrument. Wet-to-dry or wet-to-moist gauze dressings are discouraged because of their nonselective nature in removing both debris and healthy granulation tissue.

Management of eschar depends on whether the tissue is stable or unstable. The term stable eschar is used to describe leathery or dry tissue, whereas unstable describes tissue that is undergoing a softening process caused by bacteria or developing infection. Sharp or excisional debridement includes the use of scalpel, curette, or scissors, and requires written informed consent regardless of the location of care delivery. Other methods of debridement are available using ultrasonic or laser technology. Sharp debridement is best handled by an experienced clinician. Options for sharp debridement include scoring of the eschar with application of topical enzymatic debriding agents and use of curette, scalpel, or scissors to remove eschar. Depending on the extent of the eschar, considerations include local or general anesthesia. Timing of debridement is a matter of clinical judgment as to whether the eschar is stable or unstable, and serial debridements are often needed. Pain management and control of bleeding are important components of mechanical and sharp debridement. Some clinicians advocate maggot debridement therapy, also called biological or larval therapy, which involves application of sterilized larvae of the *Lucilia sericata* fly directly in the wound. The fly larvae digest bacteria, secrete proteinases that degrade necrotic tissue, and stimulate granulation.

Many adjunctive therapies are available for wound care, including electrical stimulation, therapeutic ultrasound, light therapy, negative-pressure wound therapy (NPWT), hyperbaric oxygen, and others (SOE=C). Of these, NPWT has had greatest market penetration and popularity with wound specialists.

NPWT is the application of suction to a wound bed to facilitate healing. The wound is packed with foam and sealed with adhesive membrane, and a vacuum device delivers controlled negative pressure while collecting exudate and debris into a collection chamber or absorptive pad. Since its introduction in the 1980s, NPWT has become a multimillion dollar industry despite the limited evidence in controlled clinical trials for efficacy. NPWT is marketed for all types of wounds, including open abdominal incisions, dehisced surgical wounds, burns, preparation for skin grafts, traumatic wounds, venous stasis ulcers, diabetic foot ulcers, and pressure ulcers.

The mechanism by which NPWT promotes healing is not known but may include removal of excess fluid, improved circulation, reduced bacterial load, and the mechanical effect of negative pressure. The FDA has issued a safety communication regarding complications of NPWT, including pain, retention of foreign bodies from the dressing, bleeding, infection, death, and complications stemming from power outages. NPWT should not be used over necrotic or infected wounds and is not a substitute for good nursing care with keeping a wound clean. Patients should be carefully selected for NPWT and educated regarding use and risks of the device. NPWT initiation should be cautiously considered in a wound that is not expected to heal; and if no observable improvement is seen after 2 weeks, NPWT should be discontinued.

Most experts agree that nutrition is an important component of pressure ulcer management. Carbohydrates and fats supply energy to cells, and protein is used in anabolic repair, whereas many vitamins and trace elements are essential for healing. Nutritional recommendations should be individualized in response to clinical conditions and goals of care. In general, the caloric requirement for wound healing is 30–35 Kcal/kg/day (SOE=B). Protein is required for wound healing, but the exact amount is not established. The current recommendation for protein is 1–1.5 g/kg/day, but more may be required depending on clinical condition. When determining nutritional needs, it is important to consider other factors such as preexisting protein-calorie nutrition and comorbidities. In the absence of documented deficiencies, vitamin and mineral supplements are not useful for wound healing (SOE=B).

Caution is advised when delegating wound care decisions to consultants, particularly with regard to procedures and ancillary treatment such as NPWT. Long-term care facilities that outsource wound care must ensure that treatment decisions remain part of the interprofessional team approach. Many types of providers practice wound care, including general surgeons; plastic and vascular surgeons; emergency physicians; dermatologists; physicians from nonsurgical specialties; podiatrists; advanced practice nurses; wound, ostomy, and continence nurses (WOCNs); physician assistants; and physical therapists. Wound care practitioners may not have had training in geriatrics or palliative care and may lack knowledge or skill with decision making in light of advance directives and end-of-life issues. The wound care consultant should be integrated into an overall and reasonable plan, particularly for patients in whom palliative principles apply. Wound care takes teamwork and communication, and weaknesses in the system have adverse consequences in terms of unnecessary procedures, pain, increased health care costs, risk-management, and quality of patient-centered care.

INFECTIOUS ASPECTS OF PRESSURE ULCERS

All chronic wounds are contaminated or colonized with bacteria but may not be infected. Contamination and/or colonization of a wound will not elicit host reaction and does not interfere with healing. Critical colonization is synonymous with biofilm and refers to polymicrobial communities of bacteria and fungi on the wound surface that delay wound healing but do not precipitate an inflammatory response. Localized infection or cellulitis occurs when microorganisms replicate and produce large enough numbers to elicit host response and cause injury. Local infectious complications of pressure ulcers include cellulitis, abscess, osteomyelitis and pyarthrosis. Pressure ulcers can be the starting point for necrotizing fasciitis, a rapidly progressive infection that spreads along fascial planes within subcutaneous tissue. Systemic infections resulting from pressure ulcers include sepsis and hematogenous seeding of distant structures causing further problems such as endocarditis, infected prosthetic joints, and bacterial meningitis.

Identification and treatment of infection are critical to healing a pressure ulcer; however, there is little consensus on definition of wound infection in a chronic wound. Signs and symptoms include fever, increased drainage, pain, warmth, edema, erythema, slough, odor, cessation of healing, or worsening of the wound. Many of these may not be present in older patients, people with diabetes, or patients with malnutrition or immunocompromise. Diagnosis is based on clinical evaluation of local and systemic symptoms in concert with laboratory studies. Increased WBC count may be found when the infection is acute but is an unreliable indicator of chronic infection.

Because all wound surfaces are contaminated, swab cultures are best reserved for wounds with purulent drainage in the setting of high suspicion for infection. One reliable technique involves rotating a swab over a 1-cm² area with enough pressure to express fluid from the wound (SOE=B). Tissue biopsy culture method includes removing a piece of the wound with scalpel or curette, but this is painful and unavailable in many settings.

Treatment of infected wounds involves managing underlying conditions, including diabetes, anemia, poor nutritional status, cardiopulmonary disease, and any cause of edema. All wounds should be protected from contamination with urine and feces. Wound cleansers include water, saline, commercial cleansers, and irrigation devices, but these do not remove deeper bacteria. Bioburden can be managed by removing devitalized tissue with debridement, which can be autolytic, enzymatic, mechanical, or surgical. Antiseptics such as povidone-iodine, betadine, peroxide, and Dakin's solution are generally discouraged because they harm living tissue but can be useful in heavily contaminated wounds when used in limited fashion.

Table 32.5—Palliative Care of Wounds: The Mnemonic "SPECIAL"

S	= Stabilize the wound
P	= Prevent new wounds
E	= Eliminate odor
C	= Control pain
I	= Infection prophylaxis
A	= Absorbent wound dressings
L	= Lessen or reduce dressing changes

SOURCE: Alvarez OM, Kalinski C, Nusbaum J, et al. Incorporating wound healing strategies to improve palliation (symptom management) in patients with chronic wounds. *J Pall Med*. 2007;10(5):1161–1189e.

Wound infections can be treated locally, systemically, or both depending on the clinical situation. Local treatments include dressings containing antimicrobial compounds such as gentian violet, methylene blue, silver, and cadexomer iodine. Topical antibiotics include mupiricin, neomycin, polymixin B, and bacitracin. Multiple topical antifungals are available, including the imidazole, triazole, and thiazole compounds. Systemic treatment depends on the suspected organisms and clinical setting, and bone infection requires 6 weeks of intravenous therapy. Aggressive treatment and hospitalization should be guided by goals of care and advance directives in conjunction with education of the patient and family.

PALLIATIVE CARE FOR CHRONIC WOUNDS

Pressure ulcers are the most common wound type at the end of life, followed by vascular wounds. A palliative approach can reduce suffering, improve quality of life, and decrease health care costs by eliminating expensive and/or painful procedures and treatments. Palliative care for chronic wounds should be considered when it becomes clear that there is little or no realistic chance of healing within the patient's lifetime, and when the burdens of operative procedures or advanced treatment options outweigh the benefits. The decision to designate a wound as palliative arises when the wound is unresponsive to therapy and the process of achieving healing is inconsistent with overall goals of care. Some wounds that are designated as palliative can show signs of healing, but this should not alter the palliative plan. Because of the difficulty of studying this population, evidence-based guidelines are limited and the strength of evidence for existing guidelines is generally level C. For a mnemonic that summarizes the palliative care approach to wounds, see Table 32.5.

Factors leading to designating a wound as palliative include unmodifiable risk factors or medical conditions such as poor nutrition, inadequate perfusion, multisystem organ failure, immunocompromise, irreversible anasarca, or a terminal prognosis that prevents the normal healing process. For example, there might be little benefit from serial sharp debridement, skin grafts, endovascular procedure, or flap rotation in patients with severe malnutrition who choose to forego or are otherwise not candidates for tube feeding, patients with terminal diseases such as end-stage dementia or metastatic cancer, or patients with anasarca from hypoalbuminemia or advanced congestive heart failure. NPWT, hyperbaric oxygen, and other ancillary treatments are generally used when the goal is healing. The decision to consider a palliative approach is made in consultation with the patient, family, and wound specialist with honest and open dialogue regarding prognosis for healing and the burdens, benefits, adverse effects, and potential complications of more aggressive cure-oriented procedures.

A palliative approach to wounds involves counseling and emotional support for the patient and family, preventing further skin deterioration and infection, promoting comfort, and optimizing pain management and other symptoms such as odor and bleeding. The timing of dressings and repositioning can be modified to decrease pain associated with physical manipulation of the patient and the wound. Topical pain treatments include viscous lidocaine gel and dressings that deliver locally applied ibuprofen and opiates. An FDA advisory warns that topical skin-numbing products may have cardiopulmonary adverse effects when absorbed into the bloodstream, so caution is advised. Wound odor can be minimized with charcoal- or chlorophyll-containing dressings, or metronidazole gel[OL]. Dressings such as alginates and absorptive foam can manage excess drainage and protect the periwound areas from MASD.

REFERENCES

- Bergstrom N, Horn SD, Rapp MP, et al. Turning for ulcer reduction: a multisite randomized clinical trial in nursing homes. *J Am Geriatr Soc*. 2013;61(10):1705–1713.

    This multisite, randomized clinical trial examined optimal repositioning frequency of nursing-home residents at risk of pressure ulcers when cared for on high-density foam mattresses. Residents studied were at moderate or high risk as measured by the Braden Scale. No significant differences were found in the incidence of pressure ulcers between residents turned at intervals of 2, 3, or 4 hours. However, residents at very high risk of pressure ulcers (ie, Braden Scale <10) were not included in this study.

- Chou R, Dana T, Bougatson C, et al. Pressure ulcer risk assessment and prevention: a systemic comparative effectiveness review. *Ann Intern Med*. 2013;159(1):28–39.

    This paper reviews the clinical utility of pressure ulcer risk assessment instruments and the comparative effectiveness of preventive interventions in patients at high risk. The authors selected both randomized trials and observational studies on the effects of risk assessment and randomized trials of preventive interventions. Only one good-quality trial showed no advantage of a formalized pressure ulcer risk assessment instrument over a less standardized risk assessment based on nurses' clinical judgment. In high-risk populations, limited effectiveness was found for low air loss and alternating air mattresses, with no clear differences from advanced static support surfaces. Advanced static support surfaces were more effective than standard mattresses in preventing ulcers in high-risk populations.

- Edsberg LE, Langemo D, Baharestani MM, et al. Unavoidable pressure injury: state of the science and consensus outcomes. *Wound Ostomy Continence Nurs*. 2014;41(4):313–334.

    This paper summarizes the evidence for unavoidability and gives results of the 2014 consensus conference on the topic. Numerous references are cited for conditions contributing to unavoidable pressure ulcers, including impaired tissue oxygenation, cardiopulmonary dysfunction, hypovolemia, sepsis, anasarca, peripheral vascular disease, multiorgan dysfunction, critical illness, and issues related to end of life. Extrinsic risk factors are also addressed such as head-of-bed elevation, hip fracture, hospital length of stay, medical devices, and behavioral factors.

- National Pressure Ulcer Advisory Panel. Prevention and Treatment of Pressure Ulcers: Clinical Practice Guideline. Washington, DC: NPUAP; 2014.

    This guideline is the result of a collaborative effort among the National Pressure Ulcer Advisory Panel (NPUAP), European Pressure Ulcer Advisory Panel (EPUAP), and Pan Pacific Pressure Injury Alliance (PPPIA). A comprehensive literature review was conducted on pressure ulcer prevention and treatment. A rigorous scientific methodology was used to appraise available research and make evidence-based recommendations for the prevention and treatment of pressure ulcers. It includes numerous recommendations for prevention, assessment, monitoring of healing, and treatment.

- Pieper B, ed, with the National Pressure Ulcer Advisory Panel. *Pressure Ulcers: Prevalence, Incidence, and Implications for the Future*. Washington, DC: NPUAP; 2012.

    This monograph is a compendium of pressure ulcer epidemiology studies in the United States and internationally. The literature sources draw from an 11-year period (January 2000 to November 2011) and include data from various clinical settings and special populations with attention to special topics such as public policy and staff education.

- Sibbald RG, Krasner DL, Jutz J, et al. SCALE: Skin Changes at Life's End: Final Consensus Statement. *Adv Skin Wound Care*. 2010;23(5):237–238.

    This document presents ten consensus statements (reached using an international modified Delphi process). Physiologic changes that occur as a result of the dying process may affect the skin and soft tissues and may manifest as observable changes in skin color, turgor, or integrity, or as subjective symptoms such as localized pain. These changes can be unavoidable and may occur with application of appropriate interventions that meet the standard of care. Skin changes at life's end are a reflection of compromised skin that include reduced soft-tissue perfusion, decreased tolerance to external insults, and impaired removal of metabolic wastes.

- Smith ME, Totten A, Hickam DH, et al. Pressure ulcer treatment strategies: a systematic comparative effectiveness review. *Ann Intern Med*. 2013;159(1):39–50.

    This paper summarized evidence comparing the effectiveness and safety of treatments for adults with pressure ulcers. Literature from January 1985 to October 2012 was reviewed, looking at randomized trials and comparative observational studies for treatments, as well as noncomparative intervention series (n>50) for surgical interventions. Investigators found moderate strength evidence that air-fluidized beds, protein-containing nutritional supplements, radiant heat dressings, and electrical stimulation improved healing of pressure ulcers. Low-strength evidence showed that alternating pressure surfaces, hydrocolloid dressings, platelet-derived growth factor, and light therapy improved healing of pressure ulcers. Application of results was limited by study quality, heterogeneity in methods and outcomes, and inadequate duration to assess complete wound healing.

- Woo KY, Krasner DL, Kennedy B, et al. Palliative wound care management strategies for palliative patients and their circles of care. *Adv Skin Wound Care*. 2015;28(3):130–140.

    This paper sets forth palliative care principles for wounds, summarizing key concepts and strategies for palliative wound care and the importance of an interprofessional team approach. Issues of patient preferences, symptom management, and local wound care are discussed.

Jeffrey M. Levine, MD, AGSF, CWSP

CHAPTER 33—GAIT IMPAIRMENT

KEY POINTS

- Gait disorders are common in older adults and are a predictor of functional decline.

- The cause of gait impairment in older adults is usually multifactorial; therefore, a full assessment must include consideration of a number of different causes, as determined from a detailed physical examination and a functional performance evaluation.

- Various interventions, ranging from medical to surgical to exercise, can reduce the degree of impairment, although some residual impairment is often present.

Gait disorders are commonly associated with falls and disability in older adults. This chapter reviews the epidemiology of gait impairments, comorbidities that contribute to these disorders, and office-based clinical assessments and interventions to reduce their functional impact.

EPIDEMIOLOGY

Limitations in walking increase with age. At least 20% of noninstitutionalized older adults admit to difficulty with walking or require the assistance of another person or special equipment to walk. In some samples of noninstitutionalized older adults ≥85 years old, the prevalence of walking limitations can be over 50%. Age-related gait changes such as slowed speed are most apparent after age 75 or 80, but most gait disorders appear in connection with underlying diseases, particularly as disease severity increases. For example, advanced age (>85 years old); three or more chronic conditions at baseline; and the occurrence of stroke, hip fracture, or cancer predict catastrophic loss of walking ability (SOE=B).

Determining that a gait is disordered is difficult, because there are no clearly accepted general standards of normal gait for older adults. Some believe that slowed gait speed suggests a disorder; others believe that deviations in smoothness, symmetry, and synchrony of movement patterns suggest a disorder. Regardless, a slowed and aesthetically abnormal gait can in fact provide the older adult with a safe, independent gait pattern. Attributing a gait disorder to one specific disease in older adults is particularly difficult, because similar gait abnormalities are common to many diseases.

Longitudinal observational studies suggest that certain gait-related mobility disorders progress with age and that this progression is associated with morbidity and mortality. Community-dwelling older adults with gait disorders, particularly neurologically abnormal gaits, are at higher risk of institutionalization and death (SOE=B).

CONDITIONS THAT CONTRIBUTE TO GAIT IMPAIRMENT

Impaired gait may not be an inevitable consequence of aging but rather a reflection of the increased prevalence and severity of age-associated diseases. These diseases, both neurologic and non-neurologic, are the major contributors to impaired gait. (For a glossary of gait abnormalities, see Table 33.1.)

Patients in primary care report that pain, stiffness, dizziness, numbness, weakness, and sensations of abnormal movement are the most common causes of their walking difficulties. The most common conditions seen in primary care that are thought to contribute to gait disorders are degenerative joint disease, acquired musculoskeletal deformities, intermittent claudication, impairments after orthopedic surgery and stroke, and postural hypotension. Usually, more than one contributing condition is found. In a group of community-dwelling adults >88 years old, joint pain was by far the most common contributor, followed by multiple causes such as stroke and visual loss. Factors such as dementia and fear of falling also contribute to gait disorders. The disorders found in a neurologic referral population include frontal gait disorders (usually related to normal-pressure hydrocephalus [NPH] and cerebrovascular processes), sensory disorders (also involving vestibular and visual function), myelopathy, previously undiagnosed Parkinson disease or parkinsonian syndromes, and cerebellar disease. Known conditions causing severe gait impairment, such as hemiplegia and severe hip or knee disease, are commonly not mentioned in these neurologic referral populations. Thus, many gait disorders, particularly those that are classical and discrete (eg, those related to stroke and osteoarthritis) and those that are mild or may relate to irreversible disease (eg, vascular dementia), are presumably diagnosed in primary care and treated without a referral to a neurologist. Other less common contributors to gait disorders include metabolic disorders (related to renal or hepatic disease), CNS tumors or subdural hematoma, depression, and psychotropic medications. Case reports also document reversible gait disorders due to clinically overt hypo- or hyperthyroidism and B_{12} and folate deficiency.

Table 33.1—Glossary of Gait Abnormalities

Term	Description
Antalgic gait	Pain-induced limp with shortened stance phase of gait on painful side
Circumduction	Outward swing of leg in semicircle from the hip
Equinovarus	Excessive plantar flexion and inversion of the ankle
Festination	Acceleration of gait
Foot drop	Loss of ankle dorsiflexion secondary to weakness of ankle dorsiflexors
Foot slap	Early, frequent audible foot–floor contact with steppage gait compensation
Freezing of gait	Sudden, short duration diminution or cessation of walking usually associated with shift in attention or movement circumstance or direction
Genu recurvatum	Hyperextension of knee
Propulsion	Tendency to fall forward
Retropulsion	Tendency to fall backward
Scissoring	Hip adduction such that the knees cross in front of each other with each step
Steppage gait	Exaggerated hip flexion, knee flexion, and foot lifting, usually accompanied by foot drop
Trendelenburg gait	Shift of the trunk over the affected hip, which drops because of hip abductor weakness
Turn en bloc	Moving the whole body while turning

Factors associated with slowed gait speed are also considered contributors to gait disorders. These factors are commonly disease associated (eg, cardiopulmonary or musculoskeletal disease) and include decreased leg strength, vision, aerobic function, standing balance, and physical activity, as well as joint impairment, previous falls, and fear of falling. Longitudinal data suggest that multiple organ system changes contribute to age-related changes in gait speed, but no single system is primarily associated with this decline. Combining factors can result in an effect greater than the sum of the single impairments (as when combining balance and strength impairments). Furthermore, the effect of improved strength and aerobic capacity on gait speed may be nonlinear; that is, for very impaired individuals, small improvements in strength or aerobic capacity yield relatively larger gains in gait speed, whereas these small improvements yield little gait speed change in healthy older adults.

Although older adults can maintain a relatively normal gait pattern well into their 80s, some slowing occurs, and decreased stride length thus becomes a common feature in descriptions of gait disorders of older adults. Some authors have proposed the emergence of an age-related gait disorder without accompanying clinical abnormalities, ie, essential "senile" gait disorder. This gait pattern is described as broad-based with small steps, diminished arm swing, stooped posture, decreased flexion of the hips and knees, uncertainty and stiffness in turning, occasional difficulty initiating steps, and a tendency toward falling. These and other nonspecific findings (eg, the inability to perform tandem gait) are similar to gait patterns found in a number of other diseases, and yet the clinical abnormalities are insufficient to make a specific diagnosis. This "disorder" may be a precursor to an as-yet-undiagnosed disease (eg, related to subtle extrapyramidal symptoms) and is likely to be a manifestation of concurrent, progressive cognitive impairment (eg, Alzheimer disease or vascular dementia). Thus, "senile" gait disorder may reflect a number of potential diseases and is generally not useful in labeling gait disorders in older adults.

Subclinical as well as clinically evident cerebrovascular disease is increasingly recognized as a major contributor to causes of gait disorders (SOE=B). Individuals without a dementia diagnosis and with clinically abnormal gait (particularly unsteady, frontal, or hemiparetic gait) followed for approximately 7 years were found to be at higher risk of developing non-Alzheimer, particularly vascular, dementia. Of note, those with abnormal gait at baseline may not have met criteria for dementia but already had abnormalities in neuropsychologic function, such as in visual-perceptual processing and language skills. Gait disorders with no apparent cause (also termed "idiopathic" or "senile" gait disorder) are associated with a higher mortality rate, primarily from cardiovascular causes (SOE=B). These cardiovascular causes are likely linked to concomitant, possibly undetected, cerebrovascular disease.

ASSESSMENT

Gait disorders can be assessed and categorized according to the sensorimotor levels that are affected (Tables 33.1 and 33.2).

Disorders that are the result of pathology of the low sensorimotor level can be divided into peripheral sensory and peripheral motor dysfunction, including myopathic or neuropathic disorders that cause weakness and musculoskeletal diseases. These disorders are generally distal to the CNS. With peripheral sensory impairment, unsteady and tentative gait is commonly caused by vestibular disorders, peripheral neuropathy, posterior column (proprioceptive) deficits, or visual impairment. With peripheral motor impairment, a number of classical gait patterns emerge. Examples of

Table 33.2—Abnormalities of Gait and Associated Findings, by Sensorimotor Level

Sensorimotor Level: Type of Impairment	Condition or Disease	Clinical/Physical Findings	Gait Abnormalities[a]
Low: peripheral sensory dysfunction	Peripheral neuropathy, proprioceptive deficits	Loss of touch sense, loss of position sense	Possible steppage gait; wide-based, unsteady, uncoordinated, especially without visual input; may lift feet high and slap on ground to increase sensory feedback
	Vestibular disorders	Dysequilibrium, abnormal Romberg	Weaving ("drunken"), falling to one side
	Visual impairment	Visual loss	Tentative, uncertain, uncoordinated
Low: peripheral motor dysfunction	Painful or deforming conditions	Pain and decreased motion of hip, knee, or spine; signs of arthritis; thoracic kyphosis; decreased lumbar lordosis; stooped posture	Antalgic gait with shortened stance phase on affected side, Trendelenburg gait, buckling of painful limb with weight bearing
	Focal myopathic, neuropathic weakness	Proximal muscle weakness, distal muscle weakness, exaggerated lumbar lordosis (secondary to pelvic girdle weakness)	Trendelenburg gait, waddling gait, steppage gait with foot drop or foot slap
Middle: postural and locomotor impairment	Cerebellar ataxia	Poor trunk control, incoordination or other cerebellar signs	Wide-based with increased trunk sway, irregular stepping, staggering, especially on turns
	Parkinsonism	Rigidity, bradykinesia, tremor, stooped posture	Small shuffling steps, hesitation, festination, propulsion, retropulsion, turning en bloc, absent arm swing, freezing of gait
	Hemiplegia or hemiparesis	Arm and leg weakness, spasticity, equinovarus, genu recurvatum	Leg circumduction, loss of arm swing, foot drag or scrape
	Paraplegia or paraparesis	Leg weakness, spasticity	Bilateral leg circumduction, scraping feet, possibly also scissoring
High: cognitive and white matter disorders	Frontal lobe disease, dementia, normal-pressure hydrocephalus	Cognitive impairment, weakness and spasticity, urinary incontinence	Range of findings may include difficulty initiating gait, freezing, leg apraxia, and shuffling gait similar to that seen in Parkinson disease but with wider base, upright posture, preservation of arm swing
	Dementia (Alzheimer disease, vascular)	Mid- to late-stage dementia, may have fear of falling	Cautious gait with normal to widened base, shortened stride, decreased speed, en bloc turns

[a] For descriptions of gait abnormalities, see Table 33.1.

these patterns include Trendelenburg gait (ie, weight shifts over the weak hip, which drops because of hip abductor weakness), antalgic gait (weight bearing is avoided and stance shortens on one side because of pain), and foot drop (due to ankle dorsiflexor weakness and characterized by a frequently audible foot-floor contact with steppage gait compensation, ie, excessive hip flexion). These gait impairments are the result of body segment and joint deformities, pain, and focal myopathic and neuropathic weakness. In general, if the gait disorder is limited to this low sensorimotor level (ie, the CNS is intact), the person can adapt well to the gait disorder, compensating with an assistive device or learning to negotiate the environment safely.

At the middle sensorimotor level, the execution of centrally selected postural and locomotor responses is faulty, and the sensory and motor modulation of gait is disrupted. Gait may be initiated normally, but stepping patterns are abnormal. Diseases causing spasticity (eg, those related to myelopathy, B_{12} deficiency, and stroke), parkinsonism (idiopathic as well as medication induced), and cerebellar disease (eg, alcohol induced) are examples of those that cause this type of impairment. Gait abnormalities appear when the spasticity is sufficient to cause leg circumduction and fixed deformities (eg, equinovarus), when the Parkinson disease produces shuffling steps and reduced arm swing, and when the cerebellar ataxia increases trunk sway sufficiently to require a broad base of gait support. Recent attention has focused on the pathophysiology, diagnosis, and therapy of freezing of gait, found commonly in parkinsonian syndromes.

At the high or central level, gait impairments become more nonspecific. Lesions in the frontal lobe account for most gait abnormalities at this level. The severity of the frontal-related disorders runs a spectrum from difficulty with initiation of gait to frontal dysequilibrium, in which unsupported stance is not possible. Cerebrovascular insults to the cortex, as well as to the basal ganglia and their interconnections, may contribute to difficulty with initiation of gait and to apraxia.

Dementia and depression are also thought to contribute to an abnormal gait at the high or central level. With increasing severity of the dementia, particularly in patients with Alzheimer disease, frontal-related symptoms also increase. Gait impairments in this category have been given a number of overlapping descriptions, including *gait apraxia*, *marche a petits pas*, and *arteriosclerotic parkinsonism*.

More than one disease or impairment is likely to contribute to a gait disorder; one example is the long-standing diabetic patient with peripheral neuropathy and a recent stroke who is now very fearful of falling. Certain disorders can actually involve multiple parts of the nervous system, such as Parkinson disease affecting cortical and subcortical structures. Drug and metabolic causes (eg, from sedatives, tranquilizers, and anticonvulsants) can involve both central and peripheral nervous systems (eg, phenothiazines can cause central sedation and extrapyramidal effects).

History and Physical Examination

A careful medical history can help elucidate the multiple factors contributing to gait impairments in older adults. A brief systemic evaluation for evidence of subacute metabolic disease (eg, thyroid disorders), acute cardiopulmonary disorders (eg, myocardial infarction), or other acute illness (eg, sepsis) is warranted because an acute gait disorder may be the presenting feature of acute systemic decompensation in older adults. The physical examination should include an attempt to identify motion-related factors, eg, by provoking both vestibular and orthostatic responses. A focused examination, based on symptoms, should include the Dix-Hallpike test to test for vestibular dysfunction, postural blood pressure measurements to exclude orthostatic hypotension, and vision screening at least for acuity. In addition, the neck, spine, extremities, and feet should be evaluated for pain, deformities, and limitations in range of motion, particularly regarding subtle hip or knee contractures. Leg-length discrepancies such as can occur with a hip prosthesis and either as an antecedent or subsequent to lower back pain can be measured simply as the distance from the anterior superior iliac spine to the medial malleolus. A formal neurologic assessment is critical and should include assessment of strength and tone, sensation (including proprioception), coordination (including cerebellar function), station, and gait. The Romberg test screens for simple postural control and whether the proprioceptive and vestibular systems are functional. Some investigators have proposed that one-legged stance time <5 seconds is a risk factor for injurious falls, although even relatively healthy adults ≥70 years old can have difficulty with one-legged stance. Given the importance of cognition as a risk factor, assessing cognitive function is also indicated.

Laboratory and Imaging Assessments

Depending on the history and physical examination, further laboratory and diagnostic imaging evaluation may be warranted. A CBC, serum chemistries, and other metabolic studies may be useful when systemic disease is suspected. Head or spine imaging, including radiography, CT, or MRI, are not indicated unless history and physical examination identifies neurologic abnormalities, either preceding or of recent onset, that are related to the gait disorder. However, cerebral white matter changes, often considered to be vascular (termed *leukoaraiosis*), have been increasingly associated with nonspecific gait disorders (SOE=B). Periventricular high signal measurements on MRI as well as increased ventricular volume, even in apparently healthy older adults, are associated with gait slowing. White-matter hyperintensities, white matter atrophy, and ventricular enlargements on structural MRI correlate with longitudinal changes in balance and gait, and the periventricular frontal and occipitoparietal regions appear to be most affected. Functional MRI generally supports these structural MRI findings, and diffusion tensor imaging techniques show that small vessel disease, even in normal-appearing white matter, can affect gait. Age-specific guidelines for and the sensitivity, specificity, and cost-effectiveness of these evaluations remain to be determined.

Performance-Based Functional Assessment

Higher technology assessments providing laboratory-based kinematic and kinetic analyses have not been applied widely in clinical assessments of balance and gait disorders in older adults. Most recent tools include timing devices and instrumented gait mats. Advancing beyond simple accelerometers, wearable sensors for gait analysis now commonly include an inertial measurement unit that comprises a 3-axis accelerometer and gyroscope, with or without a magnetometer, typically to measure motion of the trunk and shank. Although most of these assessments are conducted in healthy older adults, clinical outcomes assessed thus far include the identification of movement disorders and the assessment of surgical outcomes.

Comfortable gait speed and related endurance measures (such as the 6-minute walk) are powerful predictors of a number of important outcomes, such as falls, disability, hospitalization, institutionalization, and mortality (SOE=B). Another endurance measure, the 400-meter walk, has been increasingly used in research settings and considered a marker of major mobility disability that was responsive to a physical activity intervention. Gait speed is faster in individuals who are taller, who have a lower disease burden, and who are more active and less functionally disabled. Usual gait speed is frequently tested from a standing start over a distance of 4 meters. Although speeds between 0.6 and 0.8 m/s are associated with poor outcomes, a speed of 0.6 m/s has been proposed as the cut point for dismobility, given the rapid rise in disability and poor health outcomes below this speed. As expected, in clinical settings, gait speed is slowest in the acute hospital versus in subacute or outpatient settings (0.46, 0.53, and 0.74 m/s respectively, in a recent review). Speeds of >1.0 m/s and perhaps 1.2 m/s are associated with better functional outcomes and increased life expectancy. Several studies have found age- and disease-associated deficits in the ability to walk and perform a simultaneous cognitive task ("dual tasking," such as talking while walking), and also linked these deficits with increased fall risk (SOE=B), and include gait speed changes as well as gait variability. However, dual task changes in gait speed as well as variability may be equivalent to single task changes in discriminating fallers from non-fallers even when considering those who walk more slowly or who are cognitively impaired. The dual task effect may thus be most clinically useful in very high-risk groups who require extensive attentional resources to maintain safe gait. Although slower gait speed can predict decreased cognition in healthy older adults, the opposite is true as well, namely that decreased cognitive function, in multiple domains including executive function, is associated with slower speed.

A number of timed and semiquantitative balance and gait scales have been proposed as a means to detect and quantify abnormalities and to direct interventions. Fall risk, for example, can be increased with more abnormal gait and balance scale scores, such as with the Berg Balance Scale or the Performance-Oriented Mobility Assessment. Perhaps the simplest battery in the clinical setting is the Timed Up and Go (TUG), a timed sequence of rising from a chair, walking 3 meters, turning, and returning to sit in the chair. One study suggests a TUG score of ≥14 seconds as an indicator of fall risk. Other investigators have found limitations in TUG in the presence of cognitive impairment and difficulty in completing the test because of immobility, safety concerns, or refusal. Another functional approach that can be useful clinically is the Functional Ambulation Classification scale, which rates the use of assistive devices, the degree of human assistance (either manual or verbal), the distance the person can walk, and the types of surfaces the person can negotiate.

INTERVENTIONS TO REDUCE GAIT DISORDERS

Even if a condition can be diagnosed on evaluation, many conditions causing a gait disorder are, at best, only partially treatable. The patient is often left with at least some residual disability. However, other functional outcomes such as reduction in weight-bearing pain may be equally important in justifying treatment. Functional improvement becomes the treatment goal. Comorbidity, disease severity, and overall health status tend to strongly influence treatment outcome.

Achievement of premorbid gait patterns may be unrealistic, but improvement in measures such as gait speed is reasonable as long as gait remains safe. Recent studies have estimated the extent to which a change in gait performance, such as usual gait speed, is clinically meaningful. For example, in cohorts that include mobility-impaired individuals, estimates range from 0.05 m/s to 0.10 m/s for small and substantial change, respectively. Exercise interventions in more physically impaired older adults may have lower meaningful differences (eg, 0.07 m/s in one review). However, using a cut-off of even 0.10 m/s may not coincide with perceived change in mobility in certain patient populations, such as in patients with a previous hip fracture. The most striking changes in gait speed occur with strength or combined training (including aerobic exercise), especially with higher intensity or dosage. Innovative motor control–oriented, task-specific training in subclinically gait-impaired older adults may show more effect than standard treadmill walking training. Task-specific training may also improve dual-task performance, but the same training in impaired populations may also improve single-task performance.

Many of the older reports dealing with treatment and rehabilitation of gait disorders in older adults are retrospective chart reviews and case studies. Gait disorders presumably secondary to B_{12} or folate deficiency, thyroid disease, knee osteoarthritis, and Parkinson disease improve with medical therapy.

In meta-analyses of controlled interventions in osteoarthritis, largely in the knee, strength, flexibility, and aerobic exercise, particularly with a single goal (eg, quadriceps strengthening) and when provided at least 3 times per week, show at least moderate effects (Standardized Mean Difference = 0.63 [SOE=A]) in improving overall function, although not specifically in gait. These effects in the hip and knee may be sustained up to 6 months but may be comparable to medical (nonsteroidal) therapy or an active (sham) control.

Regarding neurologic disorders, key outcomes in reviews of controlled studies in stroke patients include the ability to walk independently as well as gait speed. Treadmill training may improve gait speed and walking endurance but not walking independence (SOE=A); patients receiving electromechanical and robotic assistance, particularly those in the first 3 months after stroke and who are unable to walk, are more likely to walk independently (SOE=A); outcomes for other methodologies such as magnetic stimulation, transcranial direct stimulation, and virtual reality are less clear. In a growing number of studies in patients with Parkinson disease, physical therapy to include complementary treatments (including treadmill training, visual and auditory cueing, and dance) yields short-term gains in functional mobility and in gait speed (SOE=B), with speed improvements compared with controls ranging from 0.06 to 0.34 m/s.

Modest improvement and residual disability are also the result of surgical treatment for compressive cervical myelopathy, lumbar stenosis, and NPH. Few controlled prospective studies and no well-controlled randomized studies address the outcome of surgical versus nonsurgical treatment for these 3 conditions. A number of problems plague the available series: outcomes such as pain and walking disability are not reported separately, the source of the outcome rating is not clearly identified or blinded, the criteria for classifying outcomes differ, the outcomes may be subjective and subject to interpretation, the follow-up intervals are variable, the participants who are reported in follow-up may be a highly select group, the selection factors for conservative versus surgical treatment between studies differ or are unspecified, and there is publication bias (only positive results are published). Many of the surgical series include all ages, although the mean age is usually >60 years old. A few studies document equivalent surgical outcomes with conservative, nonsurgical treatment.

With regard to lumbar stenosis procedures, many older adults have reduced pain after laminectomies and lumbar fusion surgery, although they have continued residual disability and if there is improvement in walking ability, the improvement may wane long term (SOE=B). Nonoperative treatment (with a variety of interventions, including oral anti-inflammatory medications, heating modalities, exercise, mobilizations, and epidural injections) can also result in modest improvements such as in walking tolerance (SOE=B). A randomized trial found that physical therapy yielded similar effects to those of surgical decompression (no gait data shown). However, methodologic differences, such as a large percentage of physical therapy patients crossing over to surgery, undermine the outcome, and similar to results of other studies, long-term benefits of surgery diminish after 24 months. Part of the problem in determining long-term gait outcomes of surgery for lumbar stenosis is other comorbidity, such as cardiovascular or musculoskeletal disease, that influences mobility. Regarding cervical stenosis, studies involving postoperative gait outcomes in older adults are limited, but in one nonrandomized study, walking speed improved significantly in most of the postcervical myelopathy decompression patients whose mean age was 60 years old (SOE=B).

A recent review of prospective, nonrandomized studies of patients with NPH suggests short-term gait improvement after shunt placement (60%–90%) but long-term maintenance of the improvement can drop to as low as 33%. Factors contributing to a better outcome include early diagnosis, gait disturbance as the predominant complaint, and a positive response to cerebrospinal fluid dynamic tests. Complication rates can be as high as 30%–40%, and the most important negative predictor of shunt response is comorbidity.

Outcomes for hip and knee replacement surgery for osteoarthritis are better, although some of the same study methodologic problems exist. Multidisciplinary rehabilitation (versus more limited rehabilitation) after hip or knee replacement results in improved global functioning beyond walking measures (SOE=A). Other advances include "total body preoperative exercise" ie, "prehabilitation," which may have positive effects on length of stay and possibly postoperative function, as noted in a review that included primarily orthopedic surgeries. Despite rehabilitation after joint replacement, some residual weakness, stiffness, and slowed/altered gait and balance may remain. Simple function may be maintained after knee replacement, such as maintaining the ability to safely clear an obstacle, but usually at the expense of additional compensation by the ipsilateral hip and foot. Other than pain relief, sizable gains in gait speed and joint motion occur, although residual walking disability continues for a number of reasons, including residual pathology on the operated side and symptoms on the nonoperated side. Controlled trials of specific exercise programs offered at least 2 months after total knee replacement (such as aquatic or general exercise) generally show retention of strength but varying retention of walking speed gains at 1-year follow-up. In patients undergoing total hip replacement for osteoarthritis versus patients with osteoarthritis who received medical therapy, self-reported walking-related function at 6 months was improved (SOE=B). Nevertheless, in a review of hip replacements, reduction in strength output continues compared with controls and the nonoperated hip, with reductions in walking speed at long term (eg, 2 year) follow-up.

Finally, the use of orthoses and other mobility aids can help reduce gait disorders (SOE=C). Although there are few data supporting their use, lifts (either internal or external) to correct for limb length inequality can be used in a conservative, gradually progressive manner. Other ankle braces, shoe inserts, shoe body and sole modifications, and their subsequent adjustments are part of standard care for foot and ankle weakness, deformities, and pain but are beyond the scope of this chapter. In general, well-fitting walking shoes with low heels, relatively thin firm soles, and if feasible, high, fixed heel collar support are recommended to maximize balance and improve gait. Mobility aids such as canes and walkers reduce load on a painful joint and increase stability. Note that light touch of any firm surface like walls or "furniture surfing" provide feedback and assist with balance.

REFERENCES

- Brach JS, Van Swearingen JM, Perera S, et al. Motor learning versus standard walking exercise in older adults with subclinical gait dysfunction: a randomized clinical trial. *J Am Geriatr Soc*. 2013;61(11):1879–1886.

    In older adults with subclinical gait dysfunction, innovative motor learning exercise, consisting of goal-oriented stepping and walking to promote timing and coordination, improved some parameters of mobility performance more than standard exercise.

- Callisaya ML, Beare R, Phan TG, et al. Brain structural change and gait decline: a longitudinal population-based study. *J Am Geriatr Soc*. 2013;61(7):1074–1079.

    Longitudinal data demonstrate the relative contributions of brain atrophy and white-matter lesion progression to gait decline in older adults. Effect modification according to age and infarcts suggests a contribution of reduced physiological and brain reserve.

- Cummings SR, Studenski S, Ferrucci L. A diagnosis of dismobility–giving mobility clinical visibility. A mobility working group recommendation. *JAMA*. 2014;311(20):2061–2062.

    This short article further refines the importance of gait speed and key clinical cutpoints for usual gait speed, arguing for a diagnosis of dysmobility at 0.6 m/s.

- Montero-Odasso M, Verghese J, Beauchet O, et al. Gait and cognition: a complementary approach to understanding brain function and the risk of falling. *J Am Geriatr Soc*. 2012;60(11):2127–2136.

    This review highlights quantifiable alterations in gait in older adults that are associated with falls, dementia, and disability. In addition, early disturbances in cognitive processes such as attention, executive function, and working memory are associated with slower gait and gait instability during single- and dual-task testing, and these cognitive disturbances assist in the prediction of future mobility loss, falls, and progression to dementia.

- Studenski S, Perera S, Patel K, et al. Gait speed and survival in older adults. *JAMA*. 2011;305(1):50–58.

    Based on analysis of 9 cohort studies, usual gait speed predicted survival as well as a number of other key clinical predictors, such as age and chronic disease.

Neil B. Alexander, MD

CHAPTER 34—FALLS

KEY POINTS

- A fall is one of the most common events threatening the independence of older adults. Complications resulting from falls are the leading cause of death from injury in adults ≥65 years old.

- The causes of a fall often involve a complex interaction among factors intrinsic to the individual (age-related declines, chronic disease, medications), challenges to postural control (environment, changing position, routine activities), and mediating factors (risk-taking behaviors, situational hazards, acute illness).

- For patients presenting with a fall, important components of the history include the activity of the patient at the time of the fall, the occurrence of prodromal symptoms (lightheadedness, imbalance, and dizziness), and the location of the fall. Older adults with a single fall should be evaluated for gait and balance.

- For older adults with two or more falls in the past 12 months or with gait or balance abnormalities, a multifactorial falls risk assessment should be pursued.

- Interventions shown to be effective in reducing falls include medication review, exercise programs that include muscle strengthening and balance training, vitamin D supplementation, use of appropriate footwear, and multifactorial interventions including home hazards assessment for those at high risk of falls.

A fall is one of the most common events threatening the independence of older adults. A fall is considered to have occurred when a person comes to rest inadvertently on the ground or lower level. Most of the literature on falls in older adults does not include falls associated with loss of consciousness (eg, syncope, seizure) or with overwhelming trauma, because most falls are not associated with syncope or trauma.

PREVALENCE AND MORBIDITY

According to a CDC report, one of three adults ≥65 years old reports falling in the previous year. The incidence of falls is more frequent with advancing age and among nursing-home residents, such that one-half of individuals >80 years old or nursing-home residents will fall each year. Among those with a history of a fall in the previous year, the annual incidence of falls is close to 60%. Almost one-third of those who fall need medical attention related to the fall or need to restrict their activities for at least 1 day as a result of the fall. Most falls result in minor soft-tissue injury, whereas 5%–10% of falls result in fracture or a more serious soft-tissue injury or head trauma. Women and nursing-home residents are more likely to experience a nonfatal fall-related injury than men. Even among those who do not experience physical injury, falls are associated with subsequent declines in functional status, greater likelihood of nursing-home placement, increased use of medical services, and development of a fear of falling. Of those older adults who fall, only half are able to get up without help, thus experiencing the "long lie." Long lies are associated with lasting declines in functional status. Fall-related injuries are not a common cause of death in older adults; however, complications resulting from falls are the leading cause of death from injury in adults ≥65 years old. The death rate attributable to falls increases with age, with white men ≥85 years old having the highest death rate (>180 deaths per 100,000 population).

The true cost of falls in healthcare dollars is difficult to ascertain. Because many falls result in injury, use of emergency department facilities among those who fall is common. In 2009, 2.2 million nonfatal falls were treated in emergency rooms, with 26% of these visits resulting in hospitalization. Thus, the direct cost of medical visits for falls and services/therapies for fall-related injuries is substantial. Indirect costs from fall-related injuries, such as hip fractures, can also be considerable.

CAUSES

Falls, incontinence, delirium, and other geriatric syndromes result from the accumulated effects of multiple impairments. In older adults, falls rarely have a single cause. Rather, there is often a complex interaction among factors intrinsic to the individual (age-related declines, chronic disease, medications), challenges to postural control (environment, changing positions, routine activities), and mediating factors (risk-taking behaviors, acute illness, or situational hazards, such as unfamiliar staff or high patient-to-staff ratios in hospitals and long term care facilities).

In multiple prospective cohort studies, several risk factors have been consistently associated with falls, including older age, cognitive impairment, female gender, past history of a fall, leg or gait problems, foot disorders, balance problems, hypovitaminosis D, psychotropic medication use, pain, Parkinson disease, stroke, and arthritis (SOE=B). These studies differed significantly in the types of risk factors evaluated, the types of population studied (eg, past fall history was sometimes an entry criterion), and the outcome (one fall, two or more falls, rate of falls, injurious falls). The differences in risk factors found across the studies highlight the multifactorial nature of falls and suggest that there may also be unique mediating factors surrounding falls that were not accounted for. In general, the risk of falling increases with the number of risk factors, although as many as 10% of falls occur in individuals with no identifiable risk factor for falls. Also, risk factors for indoor and outdoor falls differ: indoor falls tend to occur among older, frail adults with mobility disorders, whereas outdoor falls occur in younger, healthier persons.

Successful prevention of falls begins with knowledge of the age-related changes that increase the risk of falls. With aging, there are declines in the visual, proprioceptive, and vestibular systems. For example, visual changes with aging include reduced visual acuity, depth perception, contrast sensitivity, and dark adaptation. The proprioceptive system loses sensitivity in the legs. The vestibular system has a loss of labyrinthine hair cells, vestibular ganglion cells, and nerve fibers.

Despite these age-related changes in sensory systems, quantifying the age-related changes in postural control that are independent of disease is difficult. When postural stability is tested in young and old people with no apparent musculoskeletal or neurologic impairment, there are measurable age-related differences in sway with perturbations of stance, such as changing the support surface, changing body position, changing the visual input, or moving the support surface horizontally or rotationally. This occurs because these perturbations of stance stress the redundancy of the sensory systems in their ability to maintain postural control. This is borne out by the observation that gait speed deteriorates when individuals are presented with a dual task ("walking while talking"). In addition, there may be other age-related changes in the CNS that affect postural control, including the loss of neurons and dendrites, and the depletion of neurotransmitters, such as dopamine, within the basal ganglia.

Some of the most striking postural control differences between young and old people relate to the order or grouping of muscle activation patterns: in response to perturbations of the support surface, older adults tend to activate the proximal muscles, such as the quadriceps, before the more distal muscles, such as the tibialis anterior. This strategy may not be an efficient way to maintain postural stability. Similarly, in older adults, there may be greater co-contraction of antagonistic muscles, and the onset of the muscle activation and associated joint torque may be delayed. Finally, the ability to recover balance after a postural disturbance may be compromised by an age-related decline in the ability to rapidly develop joint torque by using muscles of the leg. All these mechanisms potentially impair maintenance of upright posture.

Another important physiologic contributor to the maintenance of upright posture is regulation of systemic blood pressure. With advancing age, baroreflex sensitivity declines, which manifests as an inability to increase heart rate in response to common stresses (such as changing posture, eating a meal, or suffering an acute illness) and results in subsequent hypotension. Because many older adults have a resting cerebral perfusion that is compromised by vascular disease, even slight reductions in blood pressure can result in cerebral ischemic symptoms and subsequent falls. Finally, with aging, the amount of total body water is reduced, which places older adults at increased risk of dehydration with acute illness, diuretic use, or hot weather. Because basal and stimulated renin and aldosterone levels progressively decrease with aging, dehydrating stresses can lead to orthostatic hypotension and falls.

A number of age-related chronic conditions deserve special mention because of their association with fall risk. Parkinson disease increases the risk of falls through several mechanisms, including the rigidity of leg musculature, the inability to correct sway trajectory because of the slowness in beginning movement, hypotensive effects of medication, and in some cases, cognitive impairment. Strokes can result in an increased risk of falls secondary to visuospatial defects, impaired peripheral sensation, cerebellar dysfunction, muscle weakness, and residual dizziness. Knee osteoarthritis can affect mobility, the ability to step over objects and maneuver, and the tendency to avoid complete weight bearing on a painful joint, which may also increase the risk of falls. Chronic pain has been associated with an increased risk of falls possibly due to changes in gait and muscle strength or because pain can act as a cognitive distractor.

One of the most modifiable risk factors for falls that has been repeatedly demonstrated in observational studies is medication use. Individual classes of psychotropic medications, such as the benzodiazepines, other sedatives, antidepressants, and antipsychotic medications, have been associated with an increased risk of falls and hip fracture. There appears to be no difference in the risk of falling with the use of older antidepressants or antipsychotics compared with the newer SSRIs or second-generation antipsychotics. Similarly, there is no protection with respect to risk of falls and fracture by choosing one of the newer, nonbenzodiazepine hypnotics ("Z-drugs") to treat insomnia versus using a benzodiazepine. As might be expected, the risk of falls increases in older adults taking more than one psychotropic medication, and among older adults taking more than 3 or 4 medications of any type.

Other classes of medications affect falls risk as well. Antihypertensive medications increase the risk of injurious falls. It is not clear that any individual class of antihypertensive mediations is preferable with respect to falls risk. Meta-analyses have demonstrated an increased risk of falls among those taking digoxin, diuretics, type 1A antiarrhythmic agents, and NSAIDs. Acetylcholinesterase inhibitors, which are used to treat dementia, have been associated with an increased risk of syncope. Diabetic medications can also be associated with falls risk during periods of hypoglycemia.

Older adults may be particularly vulnerable to falls in the days to weeks after a new medication is started or the dosage of an existing medication is increased. An increased risk of falling has been observed after a new prescription or dosage increase of a non-SSRI antidepressant, benzodiazepine, antihypertensive, or diuretic medication. Older adults are more vulnerable to hip fractures after a new prescription for a non-benzodiazepine hypnotic, diuretic, or antihypertensive medication. Providers should alert older patients and their caregivers to the increased risk of falls after a new prescription of these medications in an effort to avoid injury.

The relative importance of environmental and mediating factors on the risk of falling has not been well quantified. Most intervention studies have focused on improving the risk-factor profile of the individual or have combined individual interventions with environmental manipulation, making it difficult to isolate the contributions of the environmental factors. Nevertheless, attention to safety hazards in the home environment appears to be worthwhile in those at high risk of falls.

CLINICAL GUIDELINES

For older adults presenting with a fall, or with two or more falls in the past 12 months or with gait or balance abnormalities, a multifactorial falls risk assessment should be pursued.

For older adults who have no history of falling, providers should still ask about falls and use traditional geriatric assessment to target major risk factors. For a summary of the recommendations of the expert panel on falls prevention assembled by the American Geriatrics Society (AGS) and the British Geriatrics Society (BGS), see www.americangeriatrics.org.

DIAGNOSTIC APPROACH

History and Physical Examination

Many falls never come to clinical attention for a variety of reasons: the patient may never mention the event, there is no injury at the time of the fall, the clinician may neglect to ask the patient about a history of falls, or the patient or clinician may make the invalid assumption that falls are an inevitable part of the aging process. The treatment of injuries resulting from falls commonly fails to include an investigation of the cause of the fall.

In the clinical evaluation of noninstitutionalized older adults who are not being seen specifically as the result of a fall, it is still important to include an assessment of fall risk in the history and physical examination. (For an overview of falls assessment and management in all older adults, see Figure 34.1.) The most important point in the history is asking whether there has been a previous fall, because this is a strong risk factor for future falls. Older adults presenting with a single fall should be evaluated for gait and balance problems. Older adults with two or more falls in the past 12 months or with gait or balance abnormalities should undergo a multifactorial falls risk assessment; evaluation of recurrent indoor falls is most likely to uncover multiple risk factors.

For patients presenting with a fall, important components of the history include the activity at the time of the fall, the occurrence of prodromal symptoms (lightheadedness, imbalance, dizziness), and the location and time of the fall. Loss of consciousness is associated with injurious falls and should raise important considerations, such as orthostatic hypotension or cardiac or neurologic disease.

Information on previous falls should be collected to identify patterns that may help determine strategies to reduce future falls. A complete medication history should focus on newly added medications or recent dosage changes, as well as the use of antihypertensives, diuretics, and psychotropic medications because of their association with falls and their common use in older adults.

In addition to inquiring about the circumstances surrounding the fall, the clinician should attempt to identify any potential contributing environmental factors. Information on lighting, floor coverings, door thresholds, railings, and furniture can add important clues. Footwear can also be an important factor. In one small study that evaluated the effect of various shoe types on balance in older men, shoes with thin, hard soles produced the best results, even though they were perceived as less comfortable than thick, soft, mid-soled shoes, such as running shoes. In another nested case control study of men and women, athletic shoes

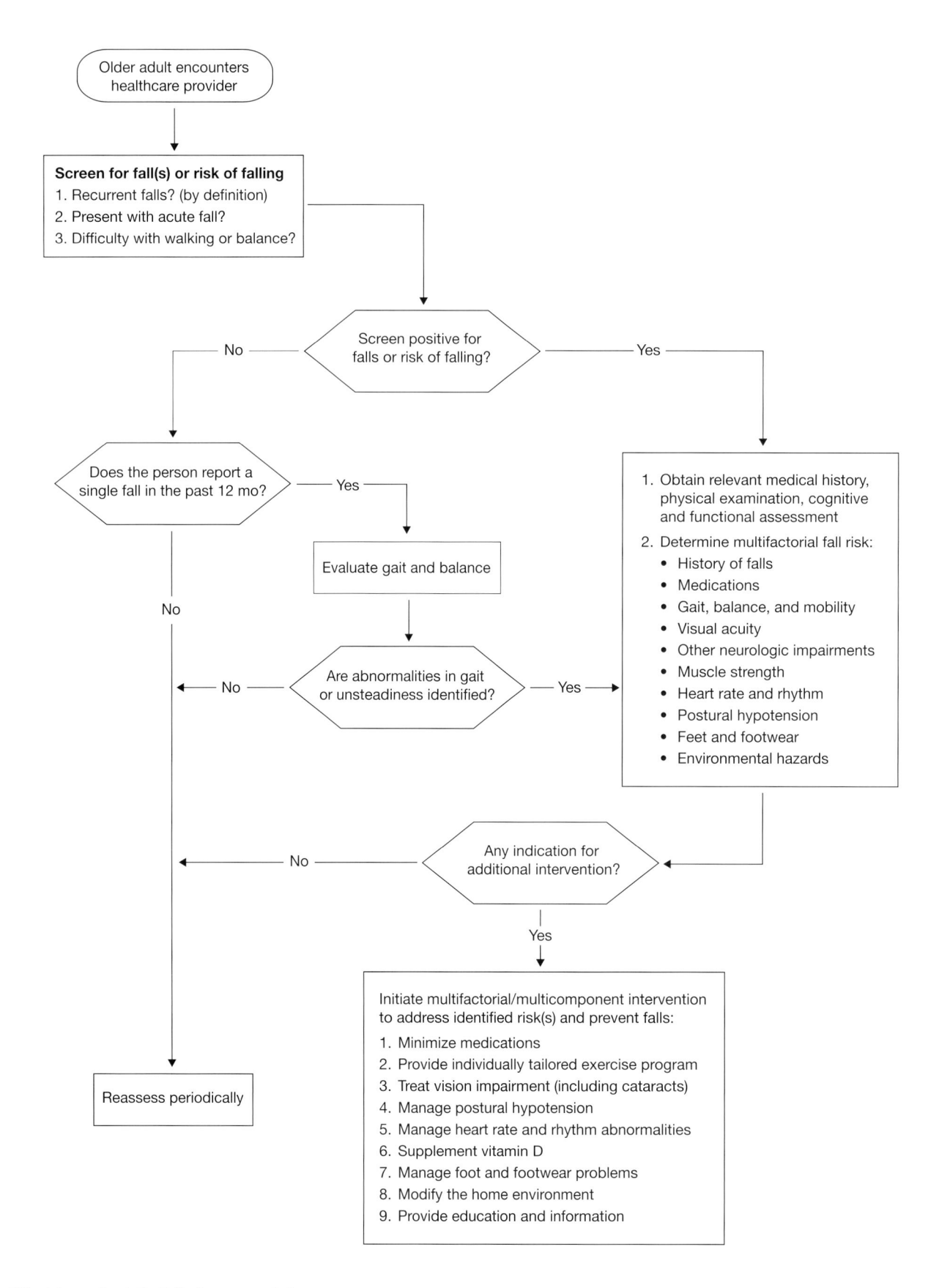

```
Older adult encounters healthcare provider
         │
         ▼
Screen for fall(s) or risk of falling
1. Recurrent falls? (by definition)
2. Present with acute fall?
3. Difficulty with walking or balance?
         │
         ▼
Screen positive for falls or risk of falling?
   ─ No ──→                                   ─ Yes ──→
         │                                            │
         ▼                                            ▼
Does the person report a single fall in the past 12 mo?   1. Obtain relevant medical history, physical examination, cognitive and functional assessment
   ─ Yes ──→ Evaluate gait and balance                   2. Determine multifactorial fall risk:
         │                 │                                 • History of falls
         No                ▼                                 • Medications
         │        Are abnormalities in gait                  • Gait, balance, and mobility
         │        or unsteadiness identified?                • Visual acuity
         │           ─ No ──→   ─ Yes ──→                    • Other neurologic impairments
         │                                                   • Muscle strength
         │                                                   • Heart rate and rhythm
         │                                                   • Postural hypotension
         │                                                   • Feet and footwear
         │                                                   • Environmental hazards
         │
         │                        ▼
         │             Any indication for additional intervention?
         │                ─ No ──→       ─ Yes ──→
         ▼                                    │
Reassess periodically                         ▼
                                   Initiate multifactorial/multicomponent intervention
                                   to address identified risk(s) and prevent falls:
                                   1. Minimize medications
                                   2. Provide individually tailored exercise program
                                   3. Treat vision impairment (including cataracts)
                                   4. Manage postural hypotension
                                   5. Manage heart rate and rhythm abnormalities
                                   6. Supplement vitamin D
                                   7. Manage foot and footwear problems
                                   8. Modify the home environment
                                   9. Provide education and information
```

Editorial note: "periodically" refers to every 1-2 years

Figure 34.1—Prevention of Falls in Older Adults Living in the Community

SOURCE: American Geriatrics Society and British Geriatrics Society. *Clinical Practice Guideline for the Prevention of Falls in Older Persons*. New York: American Geriatrics Society; 2010.

were associated with the lowest risk of falls, and shoes with increased heel height and decreased surface area between the sole and the floor were associated with a higher risk of falls.

When performing a physical examination on an older adult with a fall, the provider should focus on risk factors, including gait assessment. Probably the most important part of the physical examination is an assessment of integrated musculoskeletal function, which can be accomplished by performing one or more of the following tests of postural stability. The functional reach test is a practical way to test the integrated neuromuscular base of support and has predictive validity for falls in older men. This test is performed with a leveled yardstick secured to a wall at the height of the acromion. The person being tested assumes a comfortable stance without shoes or socks and stands so that his or her shoulders are perpendicular to the yardstick. He or she makes a fist and extends the arm forward as far as possible along the wall without taking a step or losing balance. The total reach is measured along the yardstick and recorded. Inability to reach ≥6 inches is cause for concern and merits further evaluation. Another useful test of integrated strength and balance is the Up and Go test, which can be performed with or without timing. It consists of observation of an individual standing up from a chair without using the arms to push against the chair, walking across a room (about 3 meters), turning around, walking back, and sitting down without using the arms. This test can grade muscle weakness, balance problems, and gait abnormalities using a scale of 1–5, with 5 indicating severe abnormalities. This test may be timed, with failure to complete the test within 15 seconds suggesting an increased risk of falls. A third test of integrated musculoskeletal function is the Berg Balance Test. This test includes 14 items of balance, including timed tandem stance, semitandem stance, and the ability of a person to retrieve an object from the floor. Berg scores <40 have been associated with an increased risk of falls. Lastly, the Performance-Oriented Mobility Assessment (POMA) tests balance and gait through a number of items, including ability to sit and stand from an armless chair, ability to maintain standing balance when pulled by an examiner, and ability to walk normally and maneuver obstacles. POMA scores are considered abnormal if there is a 1-point deduction from two or more items, or if there is a 2-point deduction from a single item.

A number of screening tools for risk of falls have been developed for use in the acute hospital setting, including the Morse Fall Scale and the St. Thomas's Risk Assessment Tool (STRATIFY). The Morse Fall Scale, one of the more commonly used scales, comprises 6 items: history of falling in the past 3 months, presence of any secondary diagnosis, use of an ambulatory aid, receipt of intravenous therapy, abnormal gait, and impaired mental status. Scores range from 0 to 125, with higher numbers indicating a greater risk of falls. A cutpoint of >45 is often used to identify patients at high risk of falls.

Although these screening tools perform relatively well in predicting falls, a systematic review and meta-analysis of prospective studies suggests that they are comparable with nursing clinical judgment when predicting falls in the hospital setting. Screening tools are likely to be even less useful in the nursing-home setting, where most residents have multiple risk factors for falls. For this reason, all nursing-home residents should be considered at high risk of falls, prompting a consideration of modifiable, individual risk factors.

Laboratory and Diagnostic Tests

There is no standard diagnostic evaluation of a person with a history of falls or a high risk of falling. Laboratory tests for hemoglobin, BUN, creatinine, or glucose concentrations can help to exclude anemia, dehydration, or hyperglycemia with hyperosmolar dehydration as the cause of falling. There is no proven value of routinely performing Holter monitoring of individuals who have fallen. Because data demonstrate that carotid sinus hypersensitivity contributes to falls and even hip fracture, some have advocated performing carotid sinus massage with continuous heart rate and phasic blood pressure measurement in older adults with unexplained falls. Similarly, the decision to perform echocardiography, brain imaging, or radiographic studies of the spine should be driven by the findings of the history and physical examination. Echocardiography should be reserved for those with cardiac conditions believed to contribute to the maintenance of blood flow to the brain. Spine radiographs or MRI can be useful in patients with gait disorders, abnormalities on neurologic examination, leg spasticity, or hyperreflexia to exclude cervical spondylosis or lumbar stenosis as a cause of falls.

TREATMENT AND PREVENTION

The evaluation and management of falls in older adults may differ according to the clinical setting. For example, in the home, the fall may be reported by the patient or family, or in response to clinician query. In the hospital or nursing home, staff may directly witness a fall, or find the patient on the floor. For evidence-based approaches to the management of falls, see Table 34.1.

Multiple studies of preventive interventions have been conducted, including programs to improve strength or balance, educational programs, optimization of medications, and environmental modifications in

Table 34.1—Evidence-Based Interventions for Lowering Fall Risk by Site of Care

Home	Hospital	Nursing Home
Muscle strengthening or balance training prescribed by clinician (SOE=A) Tai Chi (SOE=B) Home-hazard assessment prescribed for those with history of falls (SOE=A) Multidisciplinary, multifactorial health and environmental risk-factor screening or intervention for: (SOE=A) ■ unselected community-dwelling older adults ■ older adults with a history of falling ■ older adults selected because of known risk factors Withdrawal of psychotropic medications (SOE=B) Vitamin D supplementation at ≥800 IU/d in persons with vitamin D deficiency (SOE=A) First cataract surgery, when indicated (SOE=B)	Many risk assessments have reasonable sensitivity and specificity to be of potential value in targeting high-risk patients. Multifactorial interventions that target an individual's greatest risk factors for falls, including a plan that uses health information technology, has been effective in reducing falls (SOE=B).	No proven interventions have been reported other than vitamin D supplementation. Reasonable to assume all nursing-home residents are at high risk of falls and to target resident's most important individual risk factors, using an interprofessional team (SOE=C). Vitamin D supplementation at ≥1,000 IU/d for residents independent in transfers at risk of falls (SOE=A) Exercise programs may reduce risk of falls (SOE=C).

NOTE: MDS = minimum data set

homes or institutions. Some interventions have targeted single risk factors; others have attempted to address multiple factors by either targeting patient-specific risk factors (multifactorial intervention) or by offering the interventions to an entire population (multicomponent intervention).

A Cochrane collaboration systematic review of interventions to reduce the incidence of falling in older adults has been performed. Because of the large numbers of fall intervention trials and because interventions may be more effective in certain settings, systematic reviews of fall prevention interventions were divided into two groups: those among community-dwelling adults and those among institutionalized adults. The 2012 update of the Cochrane systematic review of fall interventions among community-dwelling adults included 159 individual trials. The results of this review demonstrated that the following falls prevention interventions are likely to be beneficial in the community setting: medication review; home hazards assessment by health care professionals in older adults at high risk of falling; Tai Chi; multiple-component interventions (strength, balance, or gait training) or home-based exercises; vitamin D supplementation in patients with vitamin D deficiency; an antislip shoe device to be worn in icy conditions; pacemaker placement in patients with carotid sinus hypersensitivity; first cataract surgery; and multifactorial, multidisciplinary interventions.

In 2011, the AGS and the BGS updated clinical practice guidelines for the prevention of falls in older adults. These guidelines advocate for interventions tailored to major falls risk factors, coupled with an appropriate exercise program. All older adults in the community at risk of falling should be offered an exercise program incorporating balance, gait, and strength training. Flexibility and endurance training should also be offered but not as sole components of the program. Interventions should include an education component tailored to the individual's cognitive ability and language. The interventions most commonly identified and that are considered to be efficacious in preventing falls in community dwellers include the following:

- **Modify the home environment:** When included as part of a multifactorial intervention, home environment assessments with environmental modification performed by a health care professional reduced the risk of falling among older adults who have fallen or are at high risk of falling because of visual impairment (2 trials; 491 participants; relative risk [RR] 0.56; CI 95%, 0.42–0.76) (SOE=A). Home environment assessment and intervention performed by a health care professional should be included in a multifactorial assessment and intervention for older adults who have fallen or who have risk factors for falling.

- **Discontinue or minimize psychoactive medications:** In one study of 93 community-dwelling adults, a gradual taper of psychotropic medications was associated with a decreased rate of falls (relative hazard 0.34; CI 95%, 0.16–0.74) (SOE=B).

- **Discontinue or minimize other medications:** A prescribing modification program for primary care physicians that included a medication review checklist, education and feedback from a pharmacist, and financial incentives significantly reduced the risk of falling (1 cluster randomized trial; 20 providers and 849 participants; RR 0.61; 95% 0.41–0.91) (SOE=B). There was no effect of medication reviews led by pharmacy on the risk of falls (2 trials; 445 participants; RR 1.03; CI 95%, 0.81–1.31). Multifactorial interventions that have been successful in preventing falls often include a review of medications.

- **Manage postural hypotension:** The sensation of dizziness is strongly associated with an increased risk of falls; thus, assessment and treatment of postural hypotension should be included as components of multifactorial interventions to prevent falls in older adults Achieving better control of systolic blood pressure has been associated with a decrease in postural changes in blood pressure. It is unclear whether this might also translate into a decreased risk of falls. Although no trial to date has addressed whether a single intervention to reduce orthostasis results in decreased falls, multifactorial interventions that include fluid optimization, medication review and reduction, and behavioral changes have shown a modest effect in reducing the risk of falls among community-dwelling adults (SOE=C).

- **Manage foot problems and footwear:** One trial comparing multifaceted podiatry intervention including foot and ankle exercises with standard care in people with disabling foot pain significantly reduced the rate of falls (305 participants; relative attributable risk (RAR) 0.64; CI 95%, 0.45-0.91) but not the risk of falls (SOE=B). Footwear associated with higher heels and decreased surface area has been associated with an increased risk of falls (SOE=C). Clinicians should advise their patients to use walking shoes with high contact surface area. In older adults with disabling foot pain, falls may be reduced by a multifaceted intervention, including customized insoles, attention to shoe wear, foot and ankle exercises, and falls prevention education.

- **Prescribe exercise, particularly balance, strength, and gait training:** The 2012 Cochrane review of fall interventions included 59 trials that tested the efficacy of exercise as an isolated intervention to prevent falls in the community setting. Exercise classes incorporating more than one type of exercise (eg, gait training, balance, strengthening) were effective in reducing the risk of falls (22 trials; 5,333 participants; RR 0.85; CI 95%, 0.76–0.96) (SOE=A). Multiple-component home-based exercise was also effective in reducing the risk of falls (6 trials; 714 participants; RR 0.78; CI 95%, 0.64–0.94). In a separate meta-analysis, home-based and group exercises reduced the rate of injurious falls in community dwellers (10 trials; 2,922 participants; RAR 0.63; CI 95%, 0.51–0.77) (SOE=A). Tai Chi, which combines both strengthening and balance measures, is effective in reducing the risk of falls among community-dwelling adults (6 trials; 1,625 participants; RR 0.71; CI 95%, 0.57–0.87) (SOE=A). The AGS/BGS recommendations state "Exercise programs should consider the functional status and comorbidities of the older person, and they should be prescribed by qualified health professionals or fitness instructors, whenever possible. The exercise program should include regular review, progression and adjustment of the exercise prescription as appropriate."

- **Supplement vitamin D:** A Cochrane meta-analysis concluded that vitamin D supplementation did not reduce the risk of falls among community dwellers overall (13 trials; 26,747 participants; RR 0.96; CI 95%, 0.89–1.03), but it did reduce the risk of falls in community dwellers with a low vitamin D level at baseline (4 trials; 804 participants; RR 0.70, CI 95%, 0.56–0.87) (SOE=A). The effectiveness of vitamin D supplementation on falls appears to be dose dependent.

- **Treat vision impairment:** There is insufficient evidence to recommend for or against the inclusion of vision interventions within multifactorial fall prevention interventions. However, first cataract surgery results in a decreased rate of falls (1 trial; 306 participants; RR 0.66; CI 95%, 0.45–0.95) (SOE=B). Second cataract surgery showed no benefit in reducing the rate of falls or number of fallers. Although routine eye screening with correction of visual defects is considered good medical practice, one trial with an intervention to treat vision problems resulted in a significant increase in the risk of falls (616 participants; RR 1.54; CI 95%, 1.24–1.91). In another trial of 597 participants, regular wearers of multifocal glasses who routinely participated in outdoor activities experienced a reduced rate of falls when given single lens glasses (SOE=B). However, there was a significant increase in outside falls in intervention group participants who infrequently participated in outside activity. The AGS/BGS recommends cautioning older adults with multifocal lenses to be more attentive to falling while walking, particularly on stairs (SOE=C).

- **Manage heart rate and rhythm abnormalities:** One trial demonstrated a reduction in the rate of falls among older adults with carotid sinus hypersensitivity treated with a pacemaker (175 participants; weighted mean difference −5.20; CI 95%, −9.40 to −1.00) (SOE=B). In contrast, a small randomized cross-over trial of 34 participants with carotid sinus hypersensitivity and a history of falls found no benefit in preventing falls when their pacemaker was switched to the on mode as compared to the off mode (RR of falling when pacemaker was off: 0.82, CI 95%, 0.62–1.10) (SOE=B)

Table 34.2—Preventing Falls: Selected Risk Factors and Suggested Interventions

Factors	Suggested Interventions
General Risk	Offer exercise program to include combination of resistance (strength) training, gait, balance, and coordination training: ■ medical assessment before starting ■ tailor to individual capabilities ■ initiate with caution in those with limited mobility not accustomed to physical activity ■ prescribed by qualified health care provider ■ regular review and progression Education and information, cognitive-behavioral intervention to decrease fear of falling and activity avoidance Recommend daily supplementation of vitamin D_3 (1,000 IU). After supplementation, vitamin D levels may be appropriate for select patients at risk of vitamin D deficiency with the goal of achieving a 25-hydroxy vitamin D level of 30 ng/mL.
Medication-Related Factors	
Use of benzodiazepines, sedative-hypnotics, antidepressants, antipsychotics, and antihypertensive medications	Consider whether medication is really needed. If medication is needed, reduce dosage as possible. Address sleep problems with nonpharmacologic interventions. Educate regarding appropriate use of medications and monitoring for adverse events.
Recent change in dosage or number of prescription medications, *or* use of ≥4 prescription medications, *or* use of other medications associated with fall risk	Review medication profile and reduce number and dosage of all medications, as possible. Counsel patients at risk of falls with new prescription or dosage increase. Monitor response to medication changes.
Mobility-Related Factors	
Presence of environmental hazards (eg, improper bed height, cluttered walking surfaces, lack of railings, poor lighting)	Improve lighting, especially at night. Remove floor hazards (eg, loose carpeting in home or carpeted flooring in nursing home). Replace existing furniture with safer furniture (eg, correct height, more stable). Install support structures, especially in bathroom (eg, railings, grab bars, elevated toilet seats). Use nonslip bath mats.
Impaired gait, balance, or transfer skills	Refer to physical therapy for comprehensive evaluation, rehabilitation, and training in use of assistive devices. Provide gait training. Prescribe balance and strengthening exercises. If able to perform tandem stance, refer for Tai Chi, dance, or yoga. Provide training in transfer skills. Prescribe appropriate assistive devices. Recommend appropriate footwear (eg, good fit, nonslip, low heel height, large surface contact area).
Impaired leg or arm strength or range of motion, or proprioception	Strengthening exercises (eg, use of resistive rubber bands, putty) Resistance training 2–3 times/week to 10 repetitions with full range of motion, then increase resistance Tai Chi Refer to physical therapy or occupational therapy
Medical Factors	
Parkinson disease, osteoarthritis, depressive symptoms, impaired cognition, carotid sinus hypersensitivity, other conditions associated with increased falls	Optimize medical therapy. Monitor for disease progression and impact on mobility and impairments. Determine need for assistive devices. Use bedside commode if frequent nighttime urination. Cardiac pacing in patients with carotid sinus hypersensitivity who experience falls due to syncope
Postural hypotension: drop in systolic blood pressure ≥20 mmHg (or ≥20%) with or without symptoms, within 3 min of rising from lying to standing	Review medications potentially contributing and adjust dosing or switch to less hypotensive agents; avoid vasodilators and diuretics if possible. Educate on activities to decrease effect (eg, slow rising, ankle pumps, hand clenching, elevation of head of bed) and to slow rising from recumbent or seated position, grab bars by toilet and bath. Prescribe pressure stockings (eg, Jobst). Optimize hydration. Liberalize salt intake, if appropriate. Recommend caffeinated coffee (1 cup) or caffeine 100 mg with meals for postprandial hypotension. Consider medication to increase blood pressure (if hypertension, heart failure, and hypokalemia not serious): midodrine 2.5–10 mg given 3 times/day 4 hr apart fludrocortisone 0.1 mg q8–24h
Visual impairment	Cataract extraction (first but not second cataract removal) Increase awareness and vigilance when wearing multifocal lenses while walking, particularly up stairs.

SOURCE: Adapted with permission from Reuben DB, Herr KA, Pacala JT, et al. *Geriatrics At Your Fingertips*, 17th ed. New York: American Geriatrics Society; 2015:121–122.

Additionally, several multifactorial interventions in which participants received more than one intervention targeting their major risk factors were effective in reducing the rate of falls (19 trials; 9,503 participants; RR 0.76; CI 95%, 0.67–0.86) (SOE=A). Because these trials were conducted in different populations and used different interventions, it is unclear which combinations of interventions are the most effective.

The health professional or team conducting the fall risk assessment should directly implement interventions or assure that the interventions are carried out by other qualified health care professionals. It is also reasonable to educate cognitively intact older adults at risk of falls on home hazards, proper footwear choices, and the importance of regular exercise. In one trial of 1,206 hospitalized older adults, intensive falls education as provided by a physiotherapist in combination with written and video materials on falls reduced the risk of falls as compared with usual care in cognitively intact persons (RR 0.51; CI 95%, 0.28–0.94) (SOE=B). However, results from a meta-analysis do not demonstrate that education reduces falls risk or fall-related injuries (4 trials; 2,555 participants; RR 0.88; CI 95%, 0.75–1.03). Thus, education alone should not be provided as a single intervention to prevent falls.

A number of interventions have not been effective for fall prevention, including group-delivered exercise interventions (SOE=B), nutritional supplementation (SOE=C), isolated modification of home hazards (SOE=B), cognitive-behavioral approach (SOE=B), and hormone therapy (SOE=C). Fall prevention programs in nursing-home settings have been largely unsuccessful to date. Multifactorial interventions were successful in reducing falls in the hospital setting and, when delivered by an interprofessional team, were marginally successful in reducing falls in the nursing-home setting. Among 8 trials of exercise in the acute hospital and rehabilitation settings, there was no clear effect of exercise on the risk of falls (1,887 participants; RR 1.07; CI 95%, 0.94–1.23). However, in subgroup analyses, it appeared that exercise may be beneficial in reducing falls risk in the nursing-home setting, whereas it may increase the risk of falls in the acute hospital setting (SOE=C). A multicenter randomized controlled trial of more than 10,000 acutely hospitalized adults found that a fall prevention tool kit using individual patient characteristics as ascertained from health information technology reduced the absolute rate of falls by 1.16 falls/1,000 bed days (CI 95%, 0.17–2.16). Vitamin D supplementation has been demonstrated in the nursing-home setting to reduce the rate of falls (5 trials; 4,603 participants; RAR 0.63; CI 95%, 0.46–0.86) but not the risk of falling (6 trials; 5,186 participants; RR 0.99; CI 95%, 0.90–1.08) (SOE=A).

The AGS/BGS makes the following recommendations regarding interventions to prevent falls in the nursing-home setting: Multifactorial/multicomponent interventions should be considered in long-term care to reduce falls. Exercise programs should be considered to reduce falls in older adults living in long-term care settings with caution regarding risk of injury in frail persons. Vitamin D supplements of at least 800 IU/day should be provided to older adults residing in long-term care settings with proven or suspected vitamin D insufficiency or who have abnormal gait and balance and are otherwise at risk of falls. Limited data exist on falls prevention in the assisted-living setting. These individuals often resemble nursing-home residents, and thus, it is reasonable to approach falls prevention in the assisted-living setting using a similar multidomain approach.

A practical approach for clinicians who are treating older adults, including nursing-home residents, at risk for falls targets risk factors in three major domains: medications, mobility, and medical conditions (Table 34.2).

Hip Protectors

Although hip protectors have been advocated as a means to reduce fracture risk in those at risk of falls, meta-analyses of studies that randomized individual patients within an institution or among older adults living at home have not shown a significant reduction in hip fractures. However, adherence to the use of hip protectors was low in these studies, which many argue could explain the lack of efficacy. In prior studies that found a benefit with hip protectors, groups of patients were randomly assigned to an intervention based on setting (eg, by ward in a nursing home). These studies were potentially susceptible to bias because unintended "co-interventions" can occur when whole units or facilities participate in trials and are allocated to use hip protectors. A multi-institutional study in which individual nursing-home residents were randomized for use of a right- or left-sided hip protector found no reduction in fractures on the protected hip (SOE=B).

REFERENCES

- American Geriatrics Society and British Geriatrics Society. Summary of the Updated American Geriatrics Society/British Geriatrics Society clinical practice guideline for prevention of falls in older persons. *J Am Geriatr Soc*. 2011;59(1):148–157. http://geriatricscareonline.org/ProductAbstract/updated-american-geriatrics-societybritish-geriatrics-society-clinical-practice-guideline-for-prevention-of-falls-in-older-persons-and-recommendations/CL014 (accessed Jan 2016).

  The aim of this publication is to guide clinicians in assessing fall risk and managing older adults at risk of falling or who have fallen. A review of the literature was performed to allow recommendations to be evidence based, whenever possible. Grades, based on the quality of the evidence and potential effect of the intervention, are provided for each recommendation. The recommendations cover the following areas: approach to assessing older adults without a recent fall; approach to assessing older adults with one or more falls, or who report recurrent falls or abnormalities of gait or balance; multifactorial interventions for managing falls by older adults in various settings; and single interventions for managing falls by older adults.

- American Geriatrics Society. Recommendations abstracted from the American Geriatrics Society consensus statement on vitamin D for prevention of falls and their consequences. *J Amer Geriatr Soc.* 2014;62(1):147–152.

    This work group concluded that older adults at risk of falls should receive a total of 4,000 IU of vitamin D daily from sunlight, food, and supplement use in an effort to prevent injurious falls. The minimum target serum 25 hydroxyvitamin D level for older adults is 30 ng/mL. However, it is not necessary for providers to measure 25-hydroxy vitamin D concentrations in older adults in the absence of underlying conditions that increase the risk of hypercalcemia or in whom there are concerns of malabsorption of vitamin D.

- Cameron ID, Gillespie LD, Robertson MC, et al. Interventions for preventing falls in older people in care facilities and hospitals. *Cochrane Database Syst Rev.* 2012 Dec 12;12:CD005465.

    Multifactorial interventions were successful in reducing falls in the hospital setting and, when delivered by a multidisciplinary team, were marginally successful in reducing falls in the nursing-home setting. Exercise may be effective in reducing falls in the subacute hospital setting, but its effectiveness in preventing falls in the long-term care setting is unclear. Vitamin D reduced the rate of falls in long-term care facilities.

- Gillespie L, Robertson M, Gillespie W, et al. Interventions for preventing falls in older people living in the community. *Cochrane Database Syst Rev. Cochrane Database Syst Rev.* 2012 Sep 12:9:CD007146.

    The results of this systematic review of falls prevention demonstrated which interventions are likely to be beneficial in the community setting: medication review; home hazards assessment by health care professionals in older adults at high risk of falling; Tai Chi; multiple-component (strength, balance, or gait training) group or home-based exercises; vitamin D supplementation in patients with vitamin D deficiency; an antislip shoe device to be worn in icy conditions; pacemaker placement in patients with carotid sinus hypersensitivity; first cataract surgery; and multifactorial, multidisciplinary interventions.

- Gillespie WJ, Gillespie LD, Parker MJ. Hip protectors for preventing hip fractures in older people. *Cochrane Database Syst Rev.* 2010;10:CD001255.

    Thirteen trials of hip protectors in the nursing home and three trials in the community were included in this analysis. After excluding five studies at high risk of bias because of cluster randomization, there was no effect of hip protectors on the risk of hip fracture (pooled RR 0.93; CI 95%, 0.74–1.18) among community dwellers. Adherence to use of hip protectors in these studies was generally low.

Sarah D. Berry, MD, MPH
Douglas P. Kiel, MD, MPH

CHAPTER 35—OSTEOPOROSIS

KEY POINTS

- Osteoporosis is a common metabolic bone disorder affecting older adults that is preventable and treatable. The resultant fractures can lead to chronic pain, decreased mobility, loss of independence and function, and increased mortality.

- Bone mineral density (BMD) measurement establishes the diagnosis of osteoporosis (T-score ≤–2.5). Osteoporosis can also be defined clinically in at-risk persons who sustain a fragility or low-trauma fracture.

- Secondary osteoporosis should be excluded in men and women with osteoporosis. Common causes of secondary osteoporosis include glucocorticoid use, hyperparathyroidism, hypogonadism, hyperthyroidism, hypercalciuria, and vitamin D deficiency.

- Screening for osteoporosis is recommended for all postmenopausal women ≥65 years old and men ≥50 years old with risk factors for osteoporosis. FRAX is a free online clinical tool that estimates the 10-year probability of osteoporotic fracture based on a patient's clinical risk factors and femoral neck BMD.

- Prevention of osteoporosis includes adequate calcium and vitamin D intake, weight-bearing exercise, and reduction of known risk factors for osteoporosis.

- Bisphosphonates are first-line pharmacologic therapy for osteoporosis. Consideration of denosumab and teriparatide as effective therapies for osteoporosis is also warranted.

Osteoporosis, the most common metabolic bone disease, is a major cause of morbidity, loss of independence, and mortality in older adults. It is a systemic skeletal disorder defined by decreased bone strength and increased risk of fracture. Bone strength is determined by both BMD and bone quality. In osteoporosis, bone density is decreased through reduced bone mass and increased loss of bone tissue while bone quality and strength are impaired by disrupted skeletal microarchitecture, accelerated skeletal turnover, altered bone mineralization, and other factors. Osteoporosis can be categorized as primary (age-related) or secondary (result of other diseases or medications). Prevention of fractures is the main goal of any prevention and treatment program.

The World Health Organization (WHO) defines osteoporosis by a BMD measurement that is less than or equal to 2.5 standard deviations below the young normal adult reference (T-score ≤–2.5). For WHO classifications of BMD measurements, see Table 35.1. BMD measurement at the spine, hip, or forearm is achieved through dual energy x-ray absorptiometry (DEXA). The basis for the WHO-defined BMD criteria is from analysis of fracture data in postmenopausal white women, with fracture risk increasing exponentially below the –2.5 T-score cut point. However, most fractures occur in patients with T-scores above this cut point. Therefore, osteoporosis can also be diagnosed clinically in at-risk individuals who sustain a fragility or low-trauma fracture, which is defined as any nonpathologic fracture that occurs from a fall from standing height or less. Specific standards for definitions of osteoporosis have not been established for men or for racial and ethnic groups other than whites, although conventional practice applies similar standards universally.

EPIDEMIOLOGY AND IMPACT

In 2010, the National Osteoporosis Foundation estimates that approximately 10.2 million Americans had osteoporosis by bone density criteria and another 43.4 million adults ≥50 years old with low bone density were at increased risk of fracture. Osteoporosis affects people of all ethnic backgrounds. Although less prevalent than in the estimated 7.7 million white and Asian adults, osteoporosis is found in 600,000 Mexican Americans and 500,000 non-Hispanic blacks ≥50 years old.

Osteoporosis is the most important cause of fracture in older adults. In 2005, osteoporosis caused >2 million fractures in the United States; this number is expected to rise to >3 million by the year 2025. One in two postmenopausal women and up to one in five men >50 years old will have an osteoporotic-related fracture in their remaining lifetime. Increased mortality is related primarily to hip fractures, although vertebral fractures have also been associated with increased mortality, generally from associated comorbidities. An estimated 20% greater mortality occurs in older adults in the year after hip fracture with the rate of death in men nearly double that of women (SOE=B). In a recent meta-analysis, the excess mortality risk persists for at least 10 years after the hip-fracture event. Hip fractures are also associated with 2.5-fold increased risk of future fractures. Hip fracture rates in black Americans, Japanese Americans, Hispanics, and Native Americans occur at lower frequencies than in white Americans, with the rate of hip fractures in Mexican Americans higher relative to that in other Hispanic groups.

Table 35.1—WHO Bone Mineral Density (BMD) Definitions

Classification	BMD	T-score
Normal	Within one SD[a] of reference mean[b]	≥–1.0
Osteopenia (low bone mass)	More than 1 but less than 2.5 SD below reference mean	Between –1.0 and –2.5
Osteoporosis	2.5 or more SD below reference mean	≤–2.5
Established osteoporosis	Below 2.5 SD of reference mean in the presence of one or more fragility fractures	<–2.5

[a] Standard deviation
[b] For young, normal adult

Osteoporotic fractures can lead to permanent declines in functional status, independence, and quality of life. In patients who were previously ambulatory, only approximately 40% regain their previous level of functioning after hip fracture and 20% require long-term nursing-home care. Pain, kyphosis, height loss, and other changes in body habitus can develop from vertebral fractures. Patients may be unable to bathe, dress, or walk independently. The economic costs associated with osteoporotic-related fractures are substantial. In 2005, the total direct health care costs were estimated at $19 billion. By 2025, this number is expected to rise to $25.3 billion. Thus, because the social and economic costs associated with osteoporotic fractures in older adults are substantial, reduction of this burden is widely seen as a health care policy imperative.

BONE REMODELING AND BONE LOSS IN AGING

Bone is a dynamic tissue that undergoes active remodeling (also called bone turnover), a coupled process of bone resorption followed by bone formation throughout adult life. Bone remodeling maintains both skeletal strength through repair of microfractures and systemic calcium homeostasis. Local signals bring osteoclasts to specific areas of bone where resorption is initiated and resorption cavities are formed. Once osteoclasts move to the area, osteoblasts are recruited to the resorption lacunae and lay down osteoid, which is subsequently mineralized into new, mature bone. Under steady state conditions, bone resorption and formation is equally balanced. However, after menopause in women and with aging in both sexes, the remodeling cycle becomes unbalanced, with bone resorption exceeding bone formation, resulting in net bone loss. Menopause and estrogen deficiency are associated with an increase in the rate of remodeling, which can also lead to loss of bone tissue and disrupted bone architecture.

Osteoblast activity decreases with aging in both men and women, compounding the bone loss that results from increased resorption seen with aging and menopause. Growth factors, such as transforming growth factor β and insulin-like growth factor 1, can be impaired with estrogen deficiency or with aging, resulting in decreased osteoblast function.

Bone mass changes over the life span of an individual. In women, bone mass increases rapidly from puberty until approximately the mid-20s to mid-30s, when bone mass peaks. Peak bone mass appears to be 75%–80% genetically determined. Other contributing factors include physical activity, nutrition, and endocrine status, as well as comorbid disease processes. Once women reach peak bone mass, bone loss occurs very slowly until the onset of menopause. After menopause, the rate of bone loss is accelerated for 8–10 years. Bone loss continues in later life, albeit at a slower rate of 1%–2% per year; however, some older women may lose bone density at a higher rate. Data suggest that reducing bone loss and skeletal turnover at any time will decrease fracture risk.

Although studies thus far have focused mostly on women, it is well documented that men also lose bone with age. It is estimated that men 30–90 years old lose approximately 1% per year in the radius and spine; some men with risk factors lose as much as 6% per year (SOE=B). The pattern of bone loss differs between men and women: men lose bone mass due to trabecular thinning, while women have a decrease in total number of trabeculae. Preservation of trabeculae may in part explain the lower lifetime risk of fracture in men. Both men and women predominantly lose the inner, spongy cancellous bone, which is concentrated in the vertebral spine. Cortical bone accounts for 45%–75% of the mechanical resistance to compression of the vertebral spine, and men actually gain cortical bone with age through periosteal bone deposition. The cross-sectional area of the vertebrae of men increases by 15%–20% through adulthood, increasing maximal load levels until the age of 75 years. Subsequently, bone strength seems to be reversed by thinning of the cortical ring by age 75, the age at which men begin to present with vertebral fractures from osteoporosis. Although bone loss at the hip has not been extensively studied in men, in cross-sectional analyses, healthy 90-year-old men have a 40% lower femoral neck BMD than 20-year-olds.

PATHOGENESIS

The pathogenesis of osteoporosis in men and women is complex, encompassing factors that affect the level of peak bone mass, the rate of bone resorption, and the rate of bone formation. Peak bone mass seems to be 75%-80% genetically determined. A number of candidate genes that may be important to osteoporosis are currently being studied, including the vitamin D receptor, estrogen receptor, transforming growth factor, interleukin-6, interleukin-1 receptor 2, type I collagen genes, and collagenases. However, it is clear from studies to date that osteoporosis in the vast majority of individuals is in part a polygenic disorder.

Estrogen Deficiency in Women

After menopause, the natural decline of estrogen levels is associated with risk of osteoporosis, with fracture risk inversely related to estrogen levels (SOE=A). Increased resorption appears to be the major factor for bone loss in estrogen deficiency. More recent evidence also suggests a role of estrogen deficiency in reducing bone formation, although both markers of bone resorption and formation are increased after menopause.

Estrogen has both direct and indirect effects on osteoclasts, the cells that are responsible for bone resorption and bone loss. It can act on cells of the osteoblastic lineage to decrease the expression of human receptor activator of nuclear factor kappa-B ligand (RANKL), the major cytokine that promotes the development and facilitates the differentiation of osteoclasts to mature forms. Estrogen deficiency also decreases production of osteoprogerin, a soluble receptor that neutralizes the effect of RANKL. It can also have direct effects on cells of hematopoietic lineage, including osteoclast precursors, mature osteoclasts, and lymphocytes.

Calcium and Vitamin D Deficiency and Secondary Hyperparathyroidism

A major mechanism by which older men and women continue to lose bone is likely related to calcium deficiency, which results in secondary hyperparathyroidism. Decreased dietary calcium intake, impaired intestinal absorption of calcium due to disease or aging itself, and vitamin D deficiency can all lead to calcium deficiency and secondary hyperparathyroidism. Older black Americans are at particular risk of vitamin D deficiency as they age.

Aging skin and decreased exposure to sunlight reduce the conversion of 7-dehydrocholesterol to cholecalciferol (vitamin D_3) by ultraviolet light, causing vitamin D deficiency and reduced calcium absorption. The hormonally active form of vitamin D is $1,25(OH)_2D_3$, or calcitriol. It is necessary for optimal intestinal absorption of calcium and phosphorus, and also exerts a tonic inhibitory effect on parathyroid hormone (PTH) synthesis. Vitamin D deficiency not only contributes to accelerated bone loss and increasing fragility but also appears to promote muscle weakness that can increase the risk of falls.

PTH is a potent stimulator of bone resorption when chronically increased. As a result of decreased serum concentrations of calcium, PTH increases, which leads to increased bone resorption. In one study, older women (mean age 79 years) hospitalized with a hip fracture had lower 25(OH)D levels and bone formation, and higher PTH and bone resorption than women in the control group (mean age 77 years). Further, data from the Study of Osteoporotic Fractures indicate that women with low fractional absorption of calcium are at increased risk of hip fracture. Trials involving older adults at high risk of calcium and vitamin D deficiency show that supplementation of both can reverse secondary hyperparathyroidism (SOE=A); increase bone mass (SOE=B); and decrease bone resorption (SOE=A), fracture rates (SOE=B), and possibly the frequency of falling (SOE=C).

Hormonal Influences in Men

Hypogonadism is an important risk factor for osteoporosis in men. Androgens are important determinants of peak bone mass in young men and fall gradually as men age. Although total testosterone levels remain relatively stable because of an increase in sex-hormone binding globulin levels, a decline in free or bioavailable testosterone levels at a rate of approximately 1% per year has been demonstrated in observational studies. Bioavailable testosterone levels are below the normal reference range of young adult men in approximately half of men >70 years old.

Several studies have demonstrated that late-onset hypogonadism can also play a role in osteoporosis in men. Although it is evident that severe hypogonadism in men (eg, due to pituitary tumors or androgen-deprivation treatment) can cause osteoporosis, the effect of moderate decreases in testosterone levels in aging men on rates of bone loss is uncertain. In one study, >60% of men presenting with hip fracture had low testosterone levels compared with about 20% of those in the control group. In several studies in which men with low-normal testosterone levels received supplemental testosterone, femoral bone density increased in the testosterone group and leg muscle strength increased in some but not all.

Evidence for a pivotal role of estradiol in bone metabolism in men has been demonstrated in several studies. Estradiol in older men has been positively associated with BMD, and a threshold bioavailable estradiol level of 40 pmol/L (11 pg/mL) has been identified at which bone loss at the lumbar spine and femoral neck is increased below this value.

z-Score = pt's age

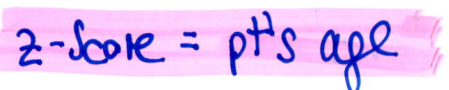

Table 35.2—Risk Factors for Osteoporosis

- Age (postmenopausal in women, >70 years in men)
- Female sex
- Low body weight (BMI <20 kg/m^2)
- 10% decrease in weight (from usual adult body weight)
- Physical inactivity
- Glucocorticoids
- Previous fragility fracture as adult
- White or Asian race
- Current smoking
- Low dietary calcium
- Alcohol intake ≥3 drinks a day

Table 35.3—Modifications to Reduce Risk of Osteoporosis

Exercise	Encourage regular, weight-bearing exercise at least 5 times per week for 30 min
Nutrition	Encourage adequate intake of calcium (1,200 mg/d in divided doses) and vitamin D_3 (800–1000 IU/d)
Smoking	Encourage smoking cessation
Alcohol consumption	Avoid excessive intake
Medications that can increase risk of osteoporosis—use with caution	Glucocorticoids Anticonvulsants Cancer chemotherapeutic agents Long-term heparin Excess thyroid hormone replacement Gonadotropin releasing-hormone agonists (used for prostate cancer) Aromatase inhibitors (used for breast cancer)

Table 35.4—Common Causes of Secondary Osteoporosis

- Male hypogonadism
- Vitamin D insufficiency
- Idiopathic hypercalciuria
- Malabsorption (often celiac disease)
- Multiple myeloma
- Glucocorticoids
- Hyperthyroidism
- Primary hyperparathyroidism
- Solid organ transplantation

DIAGNOSIS AND PREDICTION OF FRACTURE

Osteoporosis is a preventable disease; however, because bone loss is silent, it is often not diagnosed until a fracture occurs. The National Osteoporosis Foundation recommends clinical assessment of osteoporosis risk factors for all postmenopausal women and men ≥50 years old. The diagnosis of osteoporosis should be considered in any older adult with a fracture. BMD measurement is used to establish the diagnosis of osteoporosis in those at high risk clinically but without a prior fragility fracture.

Risk Factors

Clinical evaluation begins with a thorough history to uncover risk factors that may lead to increased bone fragility. Risk factors for osteoporosis and osteoporotic fracture have been identified (Table 35.2) and can be used to determine who should be placed on preventive or therapeutic regimens. Obtaining a thorough history of fracture and the setting in which the fracture occurred is important. Vertebral fractures directly reflect bone fragility and are strong predictors of future fractures. The WHO has developed a specific set of risk factors as part of its 10-year fracture risk model (FRAX) (www.shef.ac.uk/FRAX [accessed Jan 2016]). These factors are associated with an increased risk of fracture independent of BMD. For a list of modifiable risk factors for osteoporosis, see Table 35.3; all of these risk factors should be addressed as part of the routine care of older adults.

Secondary Causes

The diagnosis of idiopathic or primary osteoporosis is made by BMD measurement before fracture or by incident fracture. Exclusion of other diseases that can present with fracture or low bone mass is important in evaluating women and men with osteoporosis, because different or additional interventions may be required. For the major secondary causes of osteoporosis, see Table 35.4. Certain laboratory tests should be considered for all older adults who present with acute fracture or with a diagnosis of osteoporosis by BMD measurement (Table 35.5). Idiopathic hypercalciuria, found in approximately 10% of the general population, is an important secondary cause of osteoporosis. It is diagnosed by a 24-hour urinary calcium excretion >4 mg/kg and can be treated with a thiazide-type diuretic. Primary hyperparathyroidism is a cause of secondary osteoporosis in women with an incidence in older women as high as 1:500. A previous observational study has suggested preservation of BMD in women who undergo parathyroidectomy. The most commonly reported secondary causes of osteoporosis in men include hypogonadism and excessive alcohol use. Androgen-deprivation therapy with gonadotropin-releasing hormone (GnRH) agonists to treat prostate cancer reduces BMD from 3% to 7% per year and increases the risk and rates of fracture. Men are more likely to have a secondary cause of osteoporosis than women, with up to 50% of men having a secondary cause identified based on clinical and laboratory evaluations.

Glucocorticoid use is the most common drug-induced cause of osteoporosis in both men and women.

An estimated 2.5% of people 70–79 years old take an oral glucocorticoid. Glucocorticoid-induced osteoporosis is caused by an early increase in bone resorption and turnover; with prolonged exposure, osteoblastogenesis is reduced, resulting in low bone turnover and decreased bone formation. Fracture risk is greatest in the first 3–6 months of therapy because of rapid bone loss in the hip and spine. Increased fracture risk may be present at daily dosages as low as 2.5–7.5 mg/d. The risk of fracture increases with increasing glucocorticoid dosages and duration, partially independent of BMD. Stopping glucocorticoids is associated with a decrease in fracture risk, although it is unclear if it ever returns to the preexposure level. Although inhaled corticosteroids have not been as well studied, high doses of high-potency inhaled steroids can also result in bone loss. The best strategy for older adults who require long-term glucocorticoid therapy is to maximize bone health by a variety of interventions, including using the lowest possible dosage of glucocorticoids, ensuring adequate intake of calcium and vitamin D, serial monitoring of BMD, and starting prescription osteoporosis therapy (see treatment, below). Other medications that adversely affect BMD include aromatase inhibitors, excess thyroid supplementation, anticonvulsants, methotrexate, calcineurin inhibitors, and heparin. More recent studies have also implicated a negative skeletal effect of SSRIs, antiretroviral agents, and proton-pump inhibitors.

Physical Examination

The physical examination is directed toward detecting signs of fracture as well as potential secondary causes. Key elements include height, weight, posture, mobility, nutritional status, and overall build. Vertebral fractures are suggested by thoracic kyphosis, although this finding is not diagnostic. Wall-to-occiput distance >0 cm and rib-pelvis distance ≤2 fingerbreadths are findings that suggest occult spinal fracture. Height loss >4 cm in women and >6 cm in men from peak young adult height or prospective height loss of 2 cm in women and 3 cm in men is also suggestive of previous vertebral fracture.

Bone Density Measurement

BMD measurement establishes the diagnosis of osteoporosis and is the best predictor of fracture risk. As BMD decreases, the risk of fracture increases exponentially. The relative risk of fracture is 10 times greater in women whose BMD is in the lowest quartile than in women whose BMD is in the highest quartile (SOE=A).

Bone density of the hip, spine, wrist, or calcaneus can be measured by a variety of techniques. The preferred method of BMD measurement is central DEXA, which measures BMD of the proximal femur and lumbar spine. Femoral neck BMD is the best predictor of hip and other osteoporotic fractures. Other methods of measuring BMD include quantitative CT, ultrasonography of the calcaneus, single radiographic absorptiometry of the calcaneus, peripheral DEXA, and radiographic absorptiometry. These methods are not currently recommended in the United States, although they are used globally.

BMD is expressed in grams of mineral per square cm scanned (g/cm²). The Z-score is the relationship between the patient's BMD to the expected BMD for the patient's age and sex, while the T-score compares it to "young normal" adults of the same sex. The lowest T-score from the lumbar spine, femoral neck, or total proximal femur is used to make the overall diagnosis. Forearm BMD from the distal 1/3 radius can be used for diagnosis, specifically if that from the hip or spine cannot be interpreted, the patient has a history of hyperparathyroidism, or weight is >300 pounds (thus precluding measurement of the other sites). Osteoporosis is defined as 2.5 or more standard deviations below the young adult mean (ie, T-score ≤–2.5). For every standard deviation below the young adult mean (or a 1-unit decrease in T-score), fracture risk at the spine and hip approximately doubles. For example, if a woman has a T-score of –2, her risk of fracture is four times that of a woman with normal bone density for her age (controlled for height and weight).

The U.S. Preventive Services Task Force (USPSTF) recommends BMD testing for all women ≥65 years old, regardless of risk-factor status. Women <65 years old should be screened if their 10-year fracture risk is equal to or greater than that of a 65-year-old white woman without additional risk factors (SOE=B). There is insufficient evidence to recommend screening in men according to the USPSTF (SOE=C). For indications for BMD testing, see Table 35.6. The National Osteoporosis Foundation recommends screening all men ≥70 years old regardless of risk factors (SOE=C). DEXA is also recommended in men 50–69 years old with diseases or medications known to increase risk of osteoporosis and in those with a history of fracture after age 50.

Table 35.5—Recommended Initial Laboratory Testing in Those with Osteoporosis

- Fasting comprehensive metabolic panel (including albumin and alkaline phosphatase)
- Serum phosphorus
- 25(OH)D concentration
- Serum parathyroid hormone
- Thyrotropin
- 24-hour urine collection for calcium and creatinine
- CBC
- Serum testosterone

Table 35.6—U.S. Preventive Services Task Force Guidelines: Indications for Osteoporosis Screening

Women	▪ ≥65 years old without previous known fractures or secondary causes of osteoporosis ▪ <65 years old whose 10-year fracture risk is equal to or greater than that of a 65-year-old white woman without any additional risk factors (according to FRAX-US, 10-year fracture risk is 9.3% for a 65-year-old white woman without any additional risk factors for osteoporosis)
Men	Not currently recommended in those without known previous fracture or secondary causes of osteoporosis

Although data relating BMD to fracture risk are derived from studies of women, data also suggest that similar associations may be valid for men. Men tend to fracture at a higher BMD than women, but like women most fractures occur in men with a T-score greater than −2.5. There are limited data to determine the frequency of screening or the age to stop screening for osteoporosis. In the Study of Osteoporotic Fractures, no additional benefit was achieved from repeat BMD testing at an interval of 15 years for healthy, older postmenopausal women. Post-hoc analyses of the Framingham Osteoporosis study suggest no benefit of a screening interval <4 years in older men and women (mean age 75).

Interpretation of BMD involves evaluating the quality of the DEXA as well as the T-scores. Several considerations are important when evaluating BMD of the spine over time. BMD of lumbar vertebrae L1–L4 should be measured when making a decision about therapy. Vertebral, arterial, or lymph node calcification as well as any scoliosis can falsely increase BMD of the anterior-posterior spine DEXA. Thus, a woman with osteoporosis of the spine can have a DEXA T-score that is higher than −2.5. Usually, these changes can be seen on the DEXA report if the picture of the scan is included in the report. Proximal femoral neck BMD is preferred because it is more likely to be free of osteoarthritic changes and is most associated with fracture risk. Proximal femur is based on the lower measure of the total hip or femoral neck. Another important issue of DEXA testing is measurement variability. It is critical to scan a patient on the same DEXA machine, given that unaccountable inter-machine differences can substantially impair the ability to detect statistically different changes in BMD over time. In addition, patient positioning should be consistent on repeated measurements. The International Society of Clinical Densitometry offers guidelines and standardized training courses for technicians and clinicians acquiring and interpreting the results.

FRAX

The WHO fracture risk assessment tool (FRAX) has been the most widely adopted method to incorporate clinical risk factors and BMD. FRAX is a free online clinical tool (www.shef.ac.uk/FRAX [accessed Jan 2016]) that estimates the 10-year probability of fracture at the hip or major osteoporotic fracture (hip, spine, proximal humerus, or distal forearm). It is used for both women and men from different geographic settings. The data used to calculate this risk includes femoral neck BMD; patient's age, sex, height, and weight; 7 clinical risk factors (previous fracture, parental history of fracture, current smoking, glucocorticoid use, rheumatoid arthritis, secondary osteoporosis, alcohol consumption of ≥3 drinks per day); and the brand of DEXA scanner used. FRAX was developed through the WHO after analyzing 12 population-based cohorts of nearly 60,000 men and women with approximately 250,000 person-years of observation; this data was then externally validated in another 11 cohorts comprising 230,000 men and women with >1.2 million person-years of observation. It is most useful for patients who have a low hip BMD, because fracture risk may be underestimated if BMD is low at the spine but relatively preserved at the hip. It has not been validated in patients who have or are currently taking medications for osteoporosis or for individuals <40 years old or >90 years old. Currently in the United States, FRAX limits its algorithm to four ethnicities (white, black, Hispanic, and Asian).

Vertebral Fracture Assessment

Vertebral fracture assessment (VFA) is a technology used for diagnosis of vertebral fractures that can be performed as part of a routine DEXA measurement. Vertebral fractures are highly associated with future fracture risk and morbidity (SOE=A), but they are often not clinically apparent and can be present in patients with T-scores greater than −2.5. In addition, under-reporting of radiographic vertebral fractures by radiologists is well established. Treatment of patients with vertebral fractures, including those with T-scores greater than −2.5, reduces further fracture risk (SOE=A). For diagnosing vertebral fractures, VFA has lower resolution than CT and spine radiographs but has the advantage of less radiation, lower cost, convenience (at time of BMD), and comparable sensitivity and specificity to spine radiographs. VFA can therefore be a useful adjunct to BMD testing, particularly when results can influence clinical decision making. Risk stratification of patients at risk of fracture, who otherwise might not be considered for pharmacologic therapy, is an important benefit of this technology. The

International Society of Clinical Densitometry (www.iscd.org [accessed Jan 2016]) published a position statement in 2007 on indications for VFA.

The following are suggested indications for VFA:

- When results will influence clinical decision making (eg, regarding beginning medical therapy for bone loss)
- Documented height loss >2 cm or historical height loss >4 cm in postmenopausal women with osteopenia, or >3 cm or historical height loss >6 cm in men with osteopenia
- Long-term glucocorticoid use (≥5 mg of prednisone or equivalent for ≥3 months)
- History or findings suggestive of vertebral fracture not previously documented

Biochemical Markers of Bone Turnover

Serum and urine biochemical markers can estimate the rate of bone turnover (remodeling) and provide additional information to assist the clinician. A number of markers have been developed that reflect collagen breakdown (or bone resorption) and bone formation (proteins secreted from osteoblasts). Several markers have been associated with increased risk of hip fracture, decreased bone density, and bone loss in older adults. Markers of bone resorption and formation decrease in response to antiresorptive treatment. Two markers of bone resorption, deoxypyridinoline cross-links and cross-linked N-telopeptides of type I collagen, and one formation marker, bone alkaline phosphatase, can be used clinically to provide an early assessment of treatment efficacy. A decrease in the level of these markers from baseline after 3–6 months of therapy may indicate a therapeutic response. However, the use of markers in clinical practice is controversial because of the substantial overlap of marker values in women with different bone densities or rates of bone loss. Few studies have investigated the magnitude of decrease of a biochemical marker necessary to prevent bone loss or, more importantly, fracture. Therefore, routine measurement is not recommended.

PREVENTION AND TREATMENT

Whom To Treat

Treatment should be offered to all postmenopausal women and men ≥50 years old who meet the criteria for osteoporosis by DEXA or have a history of hip, vertebral, or prior fragility fracture. However, some individuals may be at high risk despite not meeting the BMD criteria for osteoporosis or having a fracture by history. The National Osteoporosis Foundation recommends considering treatment in patients with a 10-year probability of hip fracture ≥3% or major osteoporotic fracture ≥20%, as calculated by FRAX-US algorithm. The National Osteoporosis Guidelines Group (NOGG) recommends calculating the 10-year probability of major osteoporotic fracture using FRAX. This probability as well as the patient's age can be manually input into the NOGG website (www.shef.ac.uk/NOGG) to provide additional guidance to clinicians on the benefit of BMD testing and/or treatment. In patients whom treatment is being considered, secondary causes should be evaluated and excluded as appropriate. All patients should have adequate calcium and vitamin D supplementation, engage in regular weight-bearing exercise, avoid excessive alcohol intake and all tobacco products, and receive falls prevention counseling.

The Role of Exercise

Weight-bearing and muscle strengthening exercises are an important component of osteoporosis treatment and prevention, although exercise alone is not adequate to prevent the rapid bone loss associated with estrogen deficiency in early menopause. Regular exercise is positively associated with BMD, and starting an exercise program even late in life can help to preserve BMD (SOE=A). The effectiveness of high-intensity strength training in maintaining femoral neck BMD as well as in improving muscle mass, strength, and balance in postmenopausal women has been demonstrated, supporting the use of resistance training in helping to maintain BMD and to reduce the risk of falls (SOE=B).

Marked decrease in physical activity or immobilization results in a decline in bone mass; accordingly, it is important to encourage older adults to be as active as possible. Weight-bearing exercise, such as walking, can be recommended for all adults. Older adults should be encouraged to start slowly and to gradually increase both the number of days as well as the time spent walking each day.

Calcium and Vitamin D

Current recommendations for calcium intake to maintain a positive calcium balance for postmenopausal women >50 years old is elemental calcium at 1,200 mg/d. For men 51–70 years old, the recommendation is 1,000 mg/d and after age 70 years, 1,200 mg/d. The upper intake level for all groups is 2,000 mg/d. The average dietary intake of calcium for postmenopausal women in the United States is 500–700 mg/d; thus, most require some form of additional dairy or calcium supplementation to ensure adequate intake. For information on the amount of calcium in selected foods, see Table 35.7. Common calcium supplements are carbonate or citrate, and absorption of either supplement is best in dosages

Table 35.7—Calcium-Containing Foods

Food	Serving Size	Calcium (mg) per serving
Dairy Products		
Milk	1 cup	290–300
Yogurt	1 cup	240–400
Swiss cheese	1 ounce (1 slice)	250–270
American cheese	1 ounce (1 slice)	165–200
Ice cream	½ cup	90–100
Cottage cheese	½ cup	80–100
Parmesan cheese	1 tablespoon	70
Powdered nonfat milk	1 teaspoon	50
Other		
Sardines in oil with bones	3 ounces	370
Calcium-fortified orange juice	1 cup	300
Canned salmon with bones	3 ounces	170–210
Broccoli	1 cup	160–180
Tofu (soybean curd)	4 ounces	145–155
Turnip greens	½ cup, cooked	100–125
Kale	½ cup, cooked	90–100
Cornbread	2 ½-inch square	80–90
Egg	1 medium	55
Other fortified foods (eg, bread, cereal, fruit juices)	1 serving	Varies; read label

≤600 mg at a time. Calcium citrate can be absorbed efficiently without food, whereas calcium carbonate is best absorbed with food. Calcium carbonate may cause adverse effects such as bloating and constipation more commonly than calcium citrate. Recent studies have suggested an increased cardiovascular risk with calcium supplementation; however, no definitive association has been proved, and these adverse events were not seen with high calcium dietary intake.

The recommended requirement of vitamin D is 600 IU/d for women and men 51–70 years old, and 800 IU/d for women and men >70 years old. The upper intake level for all groups is 4,000 IU/d. Dietary sources of vitamin D include liver, egg yolks, saltwater fish, and vitamin D–fortified food. Many patients may require higher levels of supplementation to achieve serum 25(OH)D concentrations of ≥30 ng/mL (75 nmol/L).

Fracture risk is decreased with the combination of calcium and vitamin D (SOE=A). However, recent studies, primarily involving postmenopausal women, have questioned the benefit of routine supplementation in the absence of risk factors for osteoporosis and an adequate dietary intake of calcium and vitamin D. Vitamin D supplementation alone has not been shown to be beneficial in osteoporosis prevention in community-dwelling older adults (SOE=A). The greatest benefit for dual supplementation is in homebound or institutionalized older adults who often have low calcium intake and vitamin D deficiency.

Pharmacologic Options

For dosing and special considerations for medications used to prevent and treat osteoporosis, see Table 35.8. Combination therapy is not currently recommended.

Bisphosphonates

Bisphosphonates decrease bone resorption and bone remodeling, which leads to stabilization or an increase in BMD. The oral bisphosphonates alendronate and risedronate are approved for osteoporosis prevention in postmenopausal women and as treatment in both men and women. Both medications increase BMD and decrease fractures at the spine and hip in postmenopausal women with osteoporosis (SOE=A). Ibandronate, which can be taken orally on a monthly basis or intravenously every 3 months, is approved for osteoporosis prevention and treatment in postmenopausal women. Ibandronate has shown efficacy in preventing vertebral fractures only (SOE=A). These medications can be given weekly (alendronate, risedronate) or monthly (risedronate, ibandronate). In post-hoc analyses of the Fracture Intervention Trials, alendronate decreased the relative risk of hip, symptomatic vertebral, and wrist fractures in postmenopausal women up to age 85. Risedronate has been shown to decrease the relative risk of new vertebral fractures in women >80 years old with osteoporosis. Alendronate and risedronate are also approved to treat glucocorticoid-induced osteoporosis.

Zoledronic acid is an IV bisphosphonate approved for osteoporosis prevention and treatment in postmenopausal women and for patients after osteoporotic hip fracture. It is also indicated as treatment for osteoporosis in men and for prevention of osteoporosis in men and women who are expected to receive ≥12 months of glucocorticoid therapy. In the HORIZON studies, which were randomized clinical trials involving 8,000 postmenopausal women and >2,100 patients who were 3 months after surgical hip-fracture repair, zoledronic acid increased BMD at the spine and hip and decreased vertebral, spine, and nonvertebral fractures (SOE=A). Zoledronic acid has also been proven to reduce all-cause mortality when given to patients after surgical hip-fracture repair (SOE=A). Post-hoc analyses have shown a risk reduction for new clinical fracture in women ≥75 years old with treatment.

The major adverse events of oral bisphosphonates are GI symptoms, which can include abdominal pain, dyspepsia, esophagitis, nausea, vomiting, and diarrhea. Musculoskeletal pain can also rarely occur. Esophagitis,

Table 35.8—Prescription Medications Used to Prevent and Treat Osteoporosis

Medication	Dosage	Special Considerations	Observed Beneficial Treatment Outcomes[a]
Bisphosphonates (should not be used if CrCl <30 mL/min)			
Alendronate	70 mg/wk; 35 mg/wk for prevention	Adherence to dosing instructions required; used in men and women to prevent glucocorticoid-induced osteoporosis	Vertebral fracture: ARR=7.1%, NNT=14 over 3 years Hip fracture: ARR=1.1%, NNT=91 over 3 years
Risedronate	35 mg/wk or 150 mg/mo	Adherence to dosing instructions required	Vertebral fracture: ARR=5%, NNT=20 over 3 years Nonvertebral fracture: ARR=4%, NNT=25 over 3 years
Ibandronate	150 mg/mo or 3 mg IV every 3 mo (treatment only)	Adherence to dosing instructions required	Vertebral fracture: ARR=4.9%, NNT=20 over 3 years
Zoledronic acid	5 mg/year IV; 5 mg every 2 years for prevention	Adherence to dosing instructions required	Morphometric vertebral fracture: ARR=7.6%, NNT=13 over 3 years Clinical vertebral fracture: ARR=2.1%, NNT=48 over 3 years All nonvertebral fractures: ARR=2.7%, NNT=37 over 3 years Hip fracture: ARR=1.1%, NNT=91 over 3 years
Selective estrogen-receptor modulator			
Raloxifene	60 mg/d	Also approved for breast cancer prevention	Vertebral fracture: ARR=3.5%, NNT=29 over 3 years
Estrogen	See text	Not recommended as first-line choice	See text
Parathyroid hormone			
Teriparatide	20 mcg/d SC	For use in patients who cannot tolerate other approved treatments for osteoporosis	Vertebral fracture: ARR=9%, NNT=11 over 21 months Nonvertebral fracture: ARR=3%, NNT=33 over 21 months
RANKL inhibitor			
Denosumab	60 mg SC every 6 months	For treatment of postmenopausal women at high risk of fractures	New vertebral fractures: ARR=4.9% Nonvertebral fractures: ARR=1.5%

[a] Patient populations were not comparable across studies, so direct comparisons of absolute risk reduction (ARR) and number needed to treat (NNT) may not be valid.

particularly erosive esophagitis, is seen most commonly in patients who do not take the medication properly, including not remaining upright for 30 minutes after administration. The absorption of oral bisphosphonates is very poor; thus, it is extremely important for patients to follow the specific and detailed instructions for taking them. Zoledronic acid has been associated with an acute-phase response (fever, myalgias, arthralgias, and headache) as soon as 6 hours and lasting up to 72 hours after infusion. Timing of bisphosphonate administration after fracture has been controversial given concerns that these drugs may interfere with bone healing in animal models. However, several studies show no detectable delay in fracture repair via external callus formation.

Bisphosphonate use is rarely associated with osteonecrosis of the jaw, a necrotic area of bone more commonly found in the mandible than the maxilla. The preponderance of cases has been reported in patients receiving parenteral bisphosphonates for malignant bone disorders such as myeloma who have undergone dental procedures such as tooth extraction. There are rare reports of patients contracting osteonecrosis of the jaw on long-term conventional oral bisphosphonates for osteoporosis. Osteonecrosis of the jaw is also a reported possible effect of denosumab. There is also concern that long-term use of bisphosphonates could be associated with atypical fractures, such as subtrochanteric and diaphyseal femur fractures. Cohort studies have shown an increased risk of subtrochanteric and femoral shaft fractures with ≥5 years of bisphosphonate use as well as a drug-dose effect. However, secondary analyses of randomized trials have not found an association. Overall, the absolute risk of osteonecrosis of the jaw and atypical femoral fractures is very low and is outweighed by the benefits of bisphosphonate use in the vast majority of patients.

Patients taking bisphosphonates are encouraged to report new groin or thigh pain to their health care providers. When such pain is reported, radiographs of both femurs should be obtained, which can identify those who may be at risk of these atypical fractures. Further studies such as MRI or whole-body scan may be warranted in certain circumstances given the low sensitivity of plain radiographs in detecting stress fractures. Evidence is conflicting for an association between bisphosphonates and esophageal cancer. No clear association with atrial fibrillation and bisphosphonates exists.

The optimal duration of treatment with bisphosphonates is unclear; however, the effects of bisphosphonates may extend for months to years after treatment is stopped. In the FLEX study, patients who took alendronate for 10 years had less decline in their BMD at the hip and spine than those who stopped the drug after 5 years. Risk of clinical (symptomatic) vertebral fractures, but not total fractures or hip fractures, was higher in those who stopped alendronate after 5 years (SOE=A). This data suggest that alendronate can be discontinued after 5 years of treatment in patients at low risk of future fracture (eg, no new fractures on therapy, T-score greater than −2.5, and T-score that has increased while on therapy). The American Association of Clinical Endocrinologists guidelines recommend a "drug holiday" of 1–2 years. After 10 years of therapy, those at highest risk of fracture should be offered a drug holiday with consideration of possible interval treatment with another agent. After 3 years of therapy with risedronate, no change in fracture risk was seen after a 1-year drug holiday, although BMD did significantly decline. Ibandronate and zoledronic acid have been proved safe and effective for up to 3 years of treatment. In the long-term care population, expert opinion recommends discontinuation of bisphosphonates when a person is no longer ambulatory or has a remaining life expectancy of <2 years. An FDA review of the clinical studies that explored the long-term benefit of bisphosphonates concluded that patients at low risk of fracture may be good candidates to discontinue treatment after 3–5 years, while those at increased risk may continue to benefit from continued bisphosphonate treatment. However, further research is needed to better understand an individual's risk of fracture after stopping bisphosphonate therapy and when and whether to resume therapy in the future.

Selective Estrogen-Receptor Modulators

The selective estrogen-receptor modulators act as estrogen agonists in bone and heart but as estrogen antagonists in breast and uterine tissue. These medications have the potential to prevent osteoporosis or cardiovascular disease without increased risk of breast or uterine cancer. Several studies have reported that tamoxifen, an agent used to treat breast cancer, has beneficial effects on bone, but because of stimulatory effects on the uterus, it is not indicated for osteoporosis treatment or prevention.

Raloxifene is approved for treatment and prevention of osteoporosis in postmenopausal women. Efficacy has not been proved beyond 4 years of treatment, although long-term beneficial effects on bone and reduction of breast cancer risk have been demonstrated with treatment up to 8 years. Comparison of raloxifene with placebo in postmenopausal women with osteoporosis found that raloxifene decreases bone turnover, maintains BMD, and reduces incident vertebral fractures (SOE=A). However, raloxifene has not been shown to decrease nonvertebral fractures, and it significantly increases the risk of venous thromboembolism and fatal stroke (SOE=A). Additional adverse events with raloxifene include flu-like symptoms, hot flushes, leg cramps, and peripheral edema.

Another important finding with raloxifene was reduced risk of breast cancer in women who participated in the Multiple Outcomes of Raloxifene Trial, with a relative risk of developing breast cancer in women receiving raloxifene of 0.24 (95% CI, 0.13–0.44). Raloxifene is approved for prevention of breast cancer.

Calcitonin

Calcitonin, which inhibits bone resorption, is available as a subcutaneous injection and as a nasal spray for treatment of postmenopausal osteoporosis in women. The nasal spray is more widely used. Although there are no direct comparisons, calcitonin appears to be less effective than other antiresorptive drugs. Compared with placebo, calcitonin modestly improves spine BMD and reduces vertebral fractures but has not been demonstrated to reduce hip or other nonvertebral fractures (SOE=B). There is some evidence that calcitonin produces an analgesic effect in some women with painful vertebral compression fractures, particularly in its subcutaneous injectable form (SOE=C). Safety and efficacy data are available for up to 5 years of treatment. In 2013, the FDA recommended against the use of calcitonin to treat osteoporosis in postmenopausal women because of a potential increased risk of cancer.

Estrogen

Estrogen replacement therapy is an option for osteoporosis prevention (approved by the FDA; indication as a treatment withdrawn); however, it is not recommended as a first-line choice. Multiple studies have demonstrated that postmenopausal estrogen use prevents bone loss at the hip and spine when begun within 10 years of menopause (SOE=A). Decreased incident vertebral fractures were seen in a small study of postmenopausal women using a transdermal estradiol preparation. In the Women's Health Initiative (WHI) trial,

>16,000 postmenopausal women with and without low BMD were randomized to receive estrogen plus progesterone versus placebo. After a mean of 5.2 years of follow-up, hormone therapy reduced hip fracture (relative risk reduction [RRR]=34%, absolute risk reduction [ARR]=0.25%, NNT=403), vertebral fracture (RRR=34%, ARR=0.26%, NNT=386), and colon cancer (RRR=37%, ARR=0.30%, NNT=336). However, hormone therapy also increased the risk of breast cancer (relative risk increase [RRI]=26%, absolute risk increase [ARI]=0.42%, number needed to harm [NNH]=238), heart disease (RRI=29%, ARI=0.42%, NNH=235), stroke (RRI=41%, ARI=0.44%, NNH=227), and venous thromboembolism (RRI=111%, ARI=0.95%, NNH=105). Given the WHI findings, recent USPSTF guidelines advise against the routine use of estrogen plus progesterone for prevention of chronic conditions in postmenopausal women. The estrogen-only arm of the WHI was also stopped a year ahead of schedule and demonstrated an increased risk of stroke but not of coronary heart disease or breast cancer; estrogen alone also decreased hip fracture risk. Previously, hormone therapy was recommended for prevention of osteoporosis; however, given the results of the WHI and the availability of other effective medications for osteoporosis prevention and treatment, the FDA changed its indication for estrogen and estrogen-progestin products: "When these products are being prescribed solely for the prevention of postmenopausal osteoporosis, approved non-estrogen treatments should be carefully considered. Estrogens and combined estrogen-progestin products should only be considered for women with significant risk of osteoporosis that outweighs the risks of the drug."

Other data suggest that lower-than-usual doses of estrogen, when given with adequate calcium and vitamin D, are effective in reducing bone turnover and bone loss in older women. In a randomized controlled study, women treated with conjugated equine estrogen at 0.3 mg/d plus medroxyprogesterone acetate at 2.5 mg/d gained spine and hip BMD, whereas women treated with placebo showed no change. In another study, 17β-estradiol at 0.25 mg/d increased BMD at all sites and decreased bone turnover in older women versus placebo, with minimal adverse events. The effect of lower-dose estrogen on fracture incidence and other health outcomes is unknown.

Parathyroid Hormone

Recombinant 1-34 human PTH (teriparatide) is the only anabolic agent approved for treatment of osteoporosis in men and women. PTH increases both bone formation and resorption. Because formation is increased before resorption, the resultant "anabolic window" appears to result in increased bone mass, trabecular connectivity, and mechanical strength when PTH is administered in a daily pulsatile manner. This is in contrast to the chronic increases of PTH seen in primary hyperparathyroidism, which lead to increased resorption, bone loss, and osteoporosis.

Recombinant 1-34 human PTH increases spine and hip BMD in osteoporotic men and women, and reduces vertebral and nonvertebral fractures in postmenopausal women (SOE=A). In men with primary or hypogonadal osteoporosis, PTH also has been shown to increase BMD at all sites, although BMD declines when the drug is stopped. Studies have shown that using PTH for 2 years followed by bisphosphonate therapy maintains the BMD gains afforded by PTH, although the impact of this strategy on fracture risk is not known.

Teriparatide, which is given subcutaneously on a daily basis, is approved for men and women who are at risk of osteoporotic fracture and unable to tolerate or take other approved agents. It is also the preferred treatment of glucocorticoid-induced osteoporosis. It is typically reserved for those with severe osteoporosis and a higher prevalent fracture burden, although cost and parenteral administration have limited its use. Teriparatide increased the incidence of osteosarcoma in rats in drug development trials; therefore, it has a "black box" warning and is contraindicated in patients with Paget disease or who have a history of skeletal irradiation, and in all others who are at higher baseline risk of osteosarcoma. Because teriparatide may make patients feel fatigued, some clinicians suggest giving it before bedtime.

RANKL Inhibitor

Denosumab is a human monoclonal antibody that binds and neutralizes RANKL, a critical mediator of bone resorption by cells of osteoclast lineage. Specifically, denosumab inhibits RANKL, which decreases bone turnover and increases BMD. It is FDA approved for postmenopausal women at high risk of fracture or in whom other therapies for osteoporosis have failed or who are otherwise intolerant of other medications. In the FREEDOM clinical trial, postmenopausal women were randomized to treatment with denosumab every 6 months for 36 months or placebo (all patients received calcium and vitamin D supplementation). Those who received denosumab had a reduced risk of vertebral, nonvertebral, and hip fractures than those who received supplements alone. Planned subgroup analyses demonstrated a reduction in vertebral fractures that persisted in women ≥75 years old. The most statistically significant adverse events associated with denosumab were eczema and serious infections.

Investigational Agents

Strontium ranelate is an anabolic agent that increases bone formation and decreases bone resorption in animals. In a randomized, placebo-controlled study in postmenopausal women with osteoporosis (at least one vertebral fracture plus lumbar spine T-score less than or equal to −2.5) at baseline, strontium ranelate increased BMD and decreased the incidence of vertebral fractures at the highest dosage tested (2 g/d). At this dosage, bone alkaline phosphatase increased, and urinary excretion of N-telopeptides of type I collagen decreased. Strontium ranelate is approved in a number of European countries but not in the United States. Other osteoporosis treatments under study include additional bisphosphonates; cathespin K inhibitors (odanacatib) and *src* kinase inhibitors (saractinib), which impair osteoclast activity; calcium receptor antagonists (calcilytic), which pulse endogenous PTH secretion; and sclerostin antibody, which enhances osteoblast function.

Monitoring

Patients receiving treatment for osteoporosis commonly undergo serial BMD measurements at least every 2 years to assess effectiveness, an interval that is currently covered by Medicare. This interval is not a universal recommendation, and there is not sufficient evidence to date to support modifying treatment based on BMD response. Serial BMD measurement is generally used to identify patients who are losing BMD and thus may not be adhering to treatment, who have an underlying secondary cause of bone loss that is undermining therapy, or in whom the prescribed osteoporosis treatment is failing. Compliance with treatment, especially with oral bisphosphonates, should be questioned at each visit. Patients on bisphosphonates who experience GI adverse events are 50% more likely to discontinue their medication; poor compliance is associated with increased risk of fractures (SOE=A).

VERTEBRAL FRACTURE MANAGEMENT

Vertebral compression fractures are often asymptomatic and diagnosed incidentally by spinal radiographs. They most commonly occur in the thoracolumbar transition zone or midthoracic region. In affected individuals, height may decrease, kyphosis may increase, or clothes may no longer fit properly over time. Many older adults have chronic back pain caused by changes in the spine that develop with degenerative osteoarthritis or vertebral compression; distinguishing the source of the pain can be difficult. On a practical level, pain should be treated if it interferes with ADLs and quality of life, regardless of cause. However, identifying vertebral fractures is important so that future fractures can be prevented.

In the case of symptomatic vertebral compression fractures, adequate pain control is essential. The pain usually lasts 2–4 weeks and can be quite debilitating. In addition to medication, physical therapy is an important part of osteoporosis treatment programs to manage acute and chronic pain and to provide patient education. A physical therapist can provide postural exercises, alternative interventions for pain reduction, and information on changes in body mechanics that can help prevent future falls. Back braces may also help to decrease pain and disability after a fracture. Support groups for patients with osteoporosis can also be helpful.

Vertebroplasty and Kyphoplasty

Vertebroplasty and kyphoplasty are surgical approaches for management of painful vertebral compression fractures. In 2009, two randomized trials of vertebroplasty were published that involved 280 patients with painful vertebral fractures. No significant differences in pain reduction were seen between the vertebroplasty and placebo (sham procedure) groups at 1–6 months of follow-up (SOE=A). Currently, the American Academy of Orthopedic Surgeons recommends against vertebroplasty (SOE=A).

CHOOSING WISELY® RECOMMENDATIONS

Osteoporosis

- Do not routinely repeat BMD more than once every 2 years.

REFERENCES

- Berry SD, Samelson EJ, Pencina MJ, et al. Repeat bone mineral density screening and prediction of hip and major osteoporotic fracture. *JAMA*. 2013;310(12):1256–1262.

    This study sought to determine if changes in BMD after 4 years provides additional fracture risk assessment beyond the initial BMD. Using a population-based cohort study design, the authors analyzed femoral neck BMD measurements and the risk of hip or major osteoporotic fracture after a second BMD measurement in 310 men and 492 women from the Framingham Osteoporosis Study (mean age 75). BMD change of the femoral neck over an average of 4 years was independently associated with hip and major osteoporotic fracture. The second BMD measurement, however, only reclassified a small percentage of patients as high risk, thus putting into question the common screening interval of 2 years.

- Brown JP, Morin S, Leslie W et al. Bisphosphonates for treatment of osteoporosis: expected benefits, potential harms, and drug holidays. *Can Fam Physician*. 2014;60(4):324–333.

    This article reviews the role of bisphosphonates for treatment of osteoporosis. It includes a discussion of potential adverse effects, including osteonecrosis of the jaw and atypical fractures, as well as guidance for patients who may be eligible for drug holidays.

- Ensrud KE, Schousboe JT. Vertebral fractures. *N Engl J Med.* 2011;364(17):1634–1642.

    This article reviews vertebral fractures, a common sign of osteoporosis in older adults. Recommendations for evaluation and diagnosis are described, along with treatment strategies, including pain management, rehabilitation, vertebroplasty, and pharmacologic therapy. Guidelines from professional societies are provided as well as the authors' expert opinion.

- Gourlay ML, Fine JP, Preisser JS et al. Bone-density testing interval and transition to osteoporosis in older women. *N Engl J Med.* 2012;366:225–233.

    Using the Study of Osteoporotic Fractures data, the authors sought to determine the optimal intervals between BMD tests, as defined by the time for 10% of women to make the transition to osteoporosis before having a hip or clinical vertebral fracture. This group of nearly 5,000 postmenopausal women was divided into 4 subgroups based on baseline testing: normal BMD and mild, moderate, and advanced osteopenia. Results included an estimated BMD testing interval of 16.8 years (95% CI, 11.5–24.6) for normal BMD, 17.3 years (95% CI, 13.9–21.5) for mild osteopenia, 4.7 years (95% CI, 4.2–5.2) for moderate osteopenia, and 1.1 years (95% CI, 1.0–1.3) for advanced osteopenia.

- Park-Wyllie LY, Mamdani MM, Juurlink DN, et al. Bisphosphonate use and risk of subtrochanteric or femoral shaft fractures in older women. *JAMA.* 2011;305(8):783–789.

    This study investigated whether prolonged bisphosphonate use is associated with increased risk of subtrochanteric or femoral shaft fractures in the absence of trauma. Using a population-based, nested case-control study design, the authors examined women ≥68 years old in Ontario who were treated with a bisphosphonate between April 1, 2002 and March 31, 2008. Medication use was determined using the Ontario Public Drug Program database, while hospitalizations were obtained from the Canadian Institute for Health Information Discharge Abstract database. Cases were defined as women hospitalized with a subtrochanteric or femoral shaft fracture. Each case was matched with 5 controls. In total, 716 women experienced such fractures after initiation of bisphosphonate therapy. Treatment with bisphosphonate therapy for ≥5 years was associated with an increased risk of subtrochanteric or femoral shaft fractures (adjusted odds ratio 2.74 [1.25–6.02]). Of the 52,595 women treated with a bisphosphonate for at least 5 years, a subtrochanteric or femoral shaft fracture occurred in 71 (0.13%) during the subsequent year and in 117 (0.22%) within 2 years. These results suggest that despite an increased risk of subtrochanteric or femoral shaft fractures with prolonged bisphosphonate use, such fractures remain a rare event.

Loren M. Wilkerson, MD
Kenneth W. Lyles, MD, AGSF

CHAPTER 36—DEMENTIA

KEY POINTS

- Alzheimer disease, vascular dementia, and dementia with Lewy bodies are the most common forms of degenerative dementias seen in late life.

- Cholinesterase inhibitors and N-methyl-D-aspartate antagonists can be modestly helpful in delaying decline of the cognitive symptoms of Alzheimer dementia.

- Behavioral symptoms can occur with any type of dementia and tend to respond best to a combination of psychosocial and environmental modifications as well as to medication management of symptoms.

With the institution of criteria in the *Diagnostic and Statistical Manual of Mental Disorders, Fifth Edition (DSM-5)* for mild and moderate neurocognitive disorder (NCD), dementia has evolved to describe in general several disorders that cause significant decline in one or more areas of cognitive functioning, severe enough to result in functional decline. The *DSM-5* differentiates mild versus moderate NCD with regard to impairment in instrumental activities of daily living (IADLs) versus activities of daily living (ADLs), respectively. More details of this diagnostic categorization will be discussed later in the chapter. For the purposes of maintaining consistency with the clinical identification of these disorders in current practice, the term "dementia" will be used when referencing the various disorders.

Of those who suffer from dementia, most have Alzheimer disease (AD), which affects an estimated 5 million people in the United States. The pain and anguish of dementia also afflicts millions more caregivers and relatives, who must cope with the patient's progressive and irreversible decline in cognition, functioning, and behavior. Both caregivers and patients can misinterpret the initial symptoms of dementia as normal age-related cognitive losses; clinicians as well may not recognize early signs or can misdiagnose them. However, dementia and aging are not synonymous. As people age, they usually experience such memory changes as slowing in information processing, but these kinds of changes are minimal and do not affect function. By contrast, dementia is progressive and disabling and is not an inherent aspect of aging.

Diagnostic and treatment advances have benefited many patients. Early and accurate diagnosis of dementia and its cause can minimize use of costly medical resources and give patients and their relatives time to anticipate future medical, financial, and legal needs (SOE=B). Sustained reversal of the progressive cognitive decline of dementia is not currently possible, but psychosocial and pharmacologic treatments can improve such associated conditions as depression, psychosis, and agitation, and enhance quality of life.

EPIDEMIOLOGY AND SOCIETAL IMPACT

Dementia is typically a disease of later life, generally beginning after 65 years of age. AD is the most common type of dementia, accounting for approximately two-thirds of all cases and affecting 6%–8% of those ≥65 years old. The disease prevalence doubles every 5 years after age 60; an estimated 45% or more of those who are ≥85 years old have AD. Vascular dementia is thought to cause an estimated 15%–20% of cases and often coexists with AD pathology, ie, so-called "mixed dementia." In recent years, dementia associated with Lewy bodies has received increased attention and is now thought to be the second most common cause of dementia. Frontotemporal dementia is also a more recent diagnostic category of dementia and represents a smaller percentage of cases, with a younger age of onset than seen in other dementias. Neurodegenerative diseases such as Huntington disease, Parkinson disease, or other causes such as head injury and alcoholism account for other dementia syndromes.

Dementia has a major impact on society. According to the World Report on Alzheimer's 2010, total costs for dementia were $604 billion annually, which were attributable to the direct costs of medical care, direct costs of social care, and informal care. Medicare, Medicaid, and private insurance pay much of the direct cost, but families caring for patients with dementia bear the greatest burden of expense. In 2013, the Alzheimer's Association reported family caregivers provided an estimated 17.7 billion hours of care, estimated to cost more than $220.2 billion dollars in the United States alone.

The financial costs of dementia are only one aspect of the total burden. The emotional toll is immense for both patients and their families. Nearly half of primary caregivers of patients with dementia experience psychologic distress, particularly depression, and have more physical health issues. An accurate economic assessment of the problem underestimates the true cost of the disease to society unless the quality of life of both patients and caregivers is included in the analysis.

ETIOLOGY

Research into the pathophysiologic mechanisms of dementia has rapidly evolved over the last several decades. For each type of dementia, a putative protein or set of proteins has been implicated in the cause and progression of the neurodegenerative process. Whether it is the amyloid plaques/oligomers or tau neurofibrillary tangles (or both) associated with AD; the tau or ubiquitin proteins of frontotemporal dementia, or the cytoplasmic α-synuclein inclusion bodies of Lewy body dementia and Parkinson dementia, it is the accumulation of these proteins or protein aggregates within the brain that appears to set off a cascade of events that directly affect neuronal function and ultimately cell death in a disease-specific pattern. Efforts continue to better understand the genetics and environmental influences on these mechanisms, which appear to be well underway, possibly even up to 30 years, before any pathology is clinically identifiable. Therefore, current research is focusing on determining how best to analyze these pathologic processes in their earliest and most insidious stages, possibly providing us with the tools to intervene early or to prevent dementia altogether.

RISK FACTORS AND PREVENTION

The two greatest risk factors for AD are age and family history. Studies that account for death from other causes suggest that by 90 years of age, nearly half of those with first-degree relatives (eg, parents, siblings) with AD develop the disease themselves. Rare forms of familial AD are caused by mutations in one of three genes—amyloid precursor protein (APP), presenilin 1 (PS1), or presenilin 2 (PS2)—and account for approximately 1% of individuals with AD. These individuals usually have a pattern of illness in the family called autosomal dominant, which describes many family members, who are closely related to each other, with AD before age 60. Most commonly, AD begins late in life, and for many such late-onset cases, the apolipoprotein E gene (APOE) on chromosome 19 influences risk. The APOE gene has three alleles: epsilon (ε) 2, 3, and 4. Epsilon 4 (ε4) is the risk-conferring allele; it does not cause AD directly. Epsilon 2 (ε2) is considered a protective allele, and epsilon 3 (ε3) is neutral. Individuals with two APOE ε4 alleles have increased lifetime risk, as compared to those in the general population. Those carrying one APOE ε4 allele are still at increased risk. The APOE ε4 allele increases risk by decreasing age of onset in a dose-related fashion; every ε4 allele decreases age of onset by about 9 years. The ε3 allele is the most frequently occurring allele among whites. About 25% of whites carry one APOE ε4 allele. The APOE ε4 allele is less common in black Americans than in white Americans. Using APOE genotyping as a prognostic test for asymptomatic older adults is not currently recommended. Merely a risk factor, the ε4 allele cannot accurately predict whether or not a person will develop AD. It is unclear whether or not APOE genotyping increases diagnostic confidence for AD if an individual already has dementia. Genome-wide association studies have identified genes in addition to APOE that confer risk of AD. These additional risk genes include triggering receptor expressed on myeloid cells 2 (TREM2), bridging integrator 1 (BIN1), ATP-binding cassette subfamily A member 7 (ABCA7), clusterin (CLU), and phosphatidylinositol-binding clathrin assembly protein (PICALM). Genetic testing is not clinically available for these genes. Other types of dementia have genetic etiologies. Huntington disease is caused by mutations in the Huntington gene. A proportion of frontotemporal dementia with or without amyotrophic lateral sclerosis is also genetic in origin, and may be caused by mutations in select genes. Any evaluation should include a thorough family history and referral to a genetics counselor if indicated.

Other established risk factors include a history of head trauma, cardiovascular disease and its risk factors (hyperlipidemia, smoking, diabetes, and hypertension), depression, diminished physical activity, and possibly fewer years of formal education. Head trauma is thought to disrupt neuronal synapses and predispose to b-amyloid formation. Cardiovascular risk factors are thought to increase risk by predisposing individuals to impairment in cognition through ischemic mechanisms, although there is newer evidence linking some vascular risk factors to Alzheimer pathology. Physical activity may be protective, because it decreases other cardiovascular and inflammatory factors and increases plasticity and neurogenesis. Research suggests that more years of formal education can delay the onset of dementia, which may represent a confounding variable of socioeconomic status or a factor that truly provides protection by supplying a cognitive "reserve." Emerging risk factors that need further study include diet, sleep quality, and obesity.

Prevention of dementia, especially AD, is an active area of research. Drugs associated with reduced risk in epidemiologic studies include NSAIDs[OL], statins[OL], Ginkgo biloba, insulin, and possibly antioxidants. Several of these have been studied in randomized clinical trials, but to date, none has been shown to be effective. Research in healthy older adults shows a possible protective effect of physical and intellectual activity on the risk of cognitive decline (SOE=B). Preliminary trials have yielded promising results, particularly in those with mild cognitive impairment, but large-scale, longitudinal studies are still needed. The onset of dementia can also be delayed by adequate

Table 36.1—Protective Factors and Risk Factors for Alzheimer Disease

Protective Factors	Risk Factors
Definite	
None identified	Age
	Family history
	APOE4 allele
	Down syndrome
Possible	
NSAID use	Head trauma
Antioxidant use	Fewer years of formal education
Intellectual activity	History of depression
Physical activity	Cardiovascular risk factors (hypertension, hypercholesterolemia, diabetes, obesity)
Statin use	

treatment of hypertension (SOE=B). Several randomized controlled trials are beginning to test multicomponent interventions that target several of these risk factors together. Recent reviews suggest that even a 25% reduction in 7 modifiable risk factors, including diabetes, hypertension, obesity, depression, physical inactivity, smoking, and education/cognitive inactivity, could prevent up to 3 million cases worldwide. For both risk and protective factors for dementia, see Table 36.1.

ASSESSMENT AND DIFFERENTIAL DIAGNOSIS

Most cases of dementia can be diagnosed on the basis of a general medical and psychiatric evaluation. It is important for primary care providers to be alert to the early symptoms, because dementia is often undetected until severe symptoms or an adverse event, such as behavioral disturbances, flags its presence. Subjective complaints are significant, and, if a patient or family member expresses concerns about cognitive decline, a mental status assessment and probably a dementia evaluation are indicated. Subtle signs of cognitive change can include displaying behavioral changes, missing deadlines or having other problems at work, increasing difficulty managing complex tasks such as finances, or giving up a hobby or interest that may have become too challenging. Several consensus guidelines are now available for the clinical diagnosis and treatment of most types of dementia.

The informant interview and office-based clinical assessment are the most important diagnostic tools for dementia. Both the patient and a reliable informant should be interviewed to determine the patient's current condition, medical and medication history, patterns of substance use, and living arrangements. Determination of onset and nature of symptoms can help differentiate clinical syndromes. Useful informant-based instruments, such as the Functional Activities Questionnaire, can help determine whether lapses in memory or language use have occurred and assess the patient's ability to learn and retain new information, handle complex tasks, and demonstrate sound judgment. Any changes are best determined by comparing present with previous performance, because functional decline and multiple cognitive deficits support the diagnosis.

Cognitive performance is influenced by number of years of formal education. Affected patients with more years of education may have normal cognitive test scores, whereas patients with less education may have low scores and no decline in function. This must be considered, especially in patients with more subtle deficits or subjective complaints. In addition, in tests that are most sensitive to language performance, cultural differences can lead to an over-interpretation of dementia in minority patients. One way to improve the accuracy of assessment is to perform serial evaluations (using a medical interpreter if needed), which allow determination of decline in an individual that is consistent with a neurodegenerative process. In addition, measuring changes in everyday memory function by evaluating a person's performance of ADLs, either by direct observation or obtaining information from a reliable informant may be helpful. A comprehensive physical examination should include a neurologic and mental status evaluation. Brief quantified screening tests of cognitive function, such as the Folstein Mini–Mental State Examination, the Mini-Cog Assessment Instrument for Dementia, the St. Louis University Mental Status, or the Montreal Cognitive Assessment (see Table 36.2), can be useful, particularly if they demonstrate change over a 6-month or 1-year follow-up period, and can provide a practical approach to acquiring a quantitative baseline against which to compare future assessments. These tests are generally useful for screening and monitoring change. However, full neuropsychologic testing may be necessary when the presentation is atypical or if results are confounded by a high level of education or subtle changes. Cognitive and functional assessments should be conducted in the patient's native language, if at all possible. (In the face of cognitive decline, dementia patients commonly retain the greatest fluency in their native language.)

A routine laboratory evaluation, generally including a CBC, serum sodium and calcium concentrations, BUN/creatinine, fasting glucose rapid plasma reagin test, thyrotropin, and vitamin B_{12} concentration, is recommended. Optional tests, based on clinical examination and clinical suspicion, include liver function tests, serum folic acid, serum homocysteine and methylmalonic acid concentrations, urinalysis, urine toxicology, CSF analysis, and HIV testing. In addition, the history or physical examination may

Table 36.2—Screening Instruments for the Evaluation of Cognition

Instrument Name	Items Scoring	Domains Assessed	Available (accessed Jan 2016)
Mini-Cog	2 items Score = 5	Visuospatial, executive function, recall	http://geriatrics.uthscsa.edu/tools/MINICog.pdf
St. Louis University Mental Status (SLUMS) Examination	11 items Score = 30	Orientation, recall, calculation, naming, attention, executive function	http://medschool.slu.edu/agingsuccessfully/pdfsurveys/slumsexam_05.pdf
Montreal Cognitive Assessment (MoCA)	12 items Score = 30	Orientation, recall, attention, naming, repetition, verbal fluency, abstraction, executive function, visuospatial	www.mocatest.org
Folstein Mini–Mental Status Examination (MMSE)	19 items Score = 30	Orientation, registration, attention, recall, naming, repetition, 3-step command, language, visuospatial	www.minimental.com (for purchase)
Functional Activities Questionnaire	10 items Score = 30	Informant based, executive functioning, activities of daily living, attention, concentration, memory, home safety	www.healthcare.uiowa.edu/familymedicine/fpinfo/Docs/functional-activities-assessment-tool.pdf

indicate the need for other tests, such as an ECG or a chest radiograph, or a neurology consultation.

Brain imaging studies may be especially useful in the following situations:

- Onset occurs at an age <65 years old.
- Symptoms begin suddenly or progress rapidly.
- There is evidence of focal or asymmetrical neurologic deficits.
- The clinical picture suggests normal-pressure hydrocephalus (eg, onset has occurred within 1 year, gait disorder or unexplained incontinence is present).
- There is a history of a recent fall or other head trauma.

In general, a noncontrast CT head scan is adequate to exclude intracranial bleeding, space-occupying lesions, and hydrocephalus. If vascular dementia is suspected, MRI is often performed but not recommended. If performed, white-matter changes revealed by T2-weighted MRI images should not be overinterpreted. Functional brain imaging studies such as positron emission tomography (PET) may be useful when the diagnosis remains uncertain. Functional analysis with FDG-PET can reveal the characteristic parietal and temporal deficits in AD or the widespread irregular deficits in vascular dementia. More recent advances in PET imaging focus on the molecular underpinnings of AD, ie, β-amyloid. Although the FDA has approved PET scanning with florbetapir, which binds brain amyloid, few insurers provide payment, and guidelines from the National Institute on Aging and Alzheimer's Association still recommend limited use by specialists. CSF analysis has gained interest in helping detect AD early, but analysis of β-amyloid and phosphorylated-tau is available only from limited laboratories and interpretation remains challenging. At this stage, these biomarkers provide only marginal additive value over clinical diagnosis and should be used by specialists in atypical presentations.

In general, the diagnosis of dementia is a clinical one, and laboratory assessment and imaging are used to identify uncommon treatable causes and common treatable comorbid conditions and, when used in the setting of specialty care clinics, can help further differentiate atypical presentations.

DIFFERENTIATING TYPES OF DEMENTIAS OR NEUROCOGNITIVE DISORDERS

For the purpose of inclusion, the *DSM-5* subsumed all dementing illnesses into the subheading of mild NCD and major NCD with the identified etiologic source of illness still being defined as a dementia when appropriate. A diagnosis of mild NCD indicates a measurable decline in one or more cognitive domains causing the individual to use compensatory strategies in their management of IADLs. In major NCD, an individual must exhibit a measurable decline in one or more cognitive domains to a degree impairing his or her ability to manage IADLs or ADLs independently. The *DSM-5* has also added specifiers with respect to behavioral disturbances (with or without), the degree of severity in major NCDs (mild, moderate, or severe), and lastly a specifier of possible versus probable when designating a specific dementia, ie, dementia with Lewy bodies versus AD. Diagnosis requires further investigation into identifying the cause of the dementia by mapping the chronology of symptoms along with the pattern and extent of deficits. A general discussion of the most common dementias is provided below; for an overview of diagnostic features, see Table 36.3.

Cognition in aging is now understood to be a continuum, ranging from the mild changes of normal aging

Table 36.3—Diagnostic Features and Treatment of Dementia Syndromes

Syndrome	Onset	Cognitive Domains, Symptoms	Motor Symptoms	Progression	Imaging	Pharmacologic Treatment of Cognition
Mild cognitive impairment	Gradual	Primarily memory	Rare	Unknown, 12% per year proceed to Alzheimer disease	Possible global atrophy, small hippocampal volumes	Cholinesterase inhibitors (ChIs) possibly protective for 18 months (SOE=B) in subset of high-risk patients
Alzheimer disease	Gradual	Memory, language, visuospatial	Rare early, apraxia later	Gradual (over 8–10 years)	Possible global atrophy, small hippocampal volumes	ChI for mild to severe (SOE=A); memantine for moderate to severe stages
Vascular dementia	May be sudden or stepwise	Depends on location of ischemia	Correlates with ischemia	Gradual or stepwise with further ischemia	Cortical or subcortical changes on MRI	Consider ChI for memory deficit only (SOE=C); risk factor modifiers
Lewy body dementia	Gradual	Memory, visuospatial, hallucinations, fluctuating symptoms	Parkinsonism	Gradual but faster than Alzheimer disease	Possible global atrophy	ChI (SOE=B); ± carbidopa/levodopa for movement
Frontotemporal dementia	Gradual; age <60 years	Executive, disinhibition, apathy, language, ± memory	None	Gradual but faster than Alzheimer disease	Atrophy in frontal and temporal lobes	Not recommended per current evidence

to the significant impairments that define dementia. Although studies are not conclusive, it appears that normal aging involves some mild decline in memory, usually requiring more effort and time to recall new information. However, this decline does not impair functioning; new learning is slower but still occurs and is usually well compensated with lists, calendars, and other memory supports.

As our attention shifts to earlier signs of cognitive decline, mild NCD allows for greater clarification around the diagnosis of mild cognitive impairment (MCI), which was assigned to individuals who have a subjective complaint of cognitive decline in at least one domain (complex attention, executive function, learning and memory, language, perceptual-motor or social cognition) to a degree that is noticeable and measurable, but not to a degree that causes impairment in independent living. Using the "probable" versus "possible" criteria for each dementia subtype further enhances ability to define and predict outcomes and prognosis. For example, the institution of MCI as a diagnostic entity allowed for identification and possible early treatment of individuals who may convert to AD (9.4–14.3/1,000 person-years). For individuals with MCI whose single domain of impairment is memory (amnestic MCI versus nonamnestic MCI), the rate of conversion to AD is predictably higher but not wholly predictive of AD or other dementias. Nearly half of individuals with amnestic MCI maintain a stable degree of impairment or return to a state of normal cognition over 3–5 years. Although there are no currently accepted criteria, the National Institute on Aging and Alzheimer's Association have designated "preclinical AD" in expectation of developing a set of biomarkers to assess for presence of preclinical brain changes that have yet to manifest as clinical signs and symptoms of cognitive impairment.

Alzheimer Disease

Clinically, AD is characterized by gradual onset and progressive decline in cognitive functioning; motor and sensory functions are spared until middle and late stages. Memory impairment is often a core symptom of any dementia, but in AD it is typically *the* core feature present in the earliest stages. Typically, AD patients demonstrate difficulty learning and retaining new information. In later disease stages, their ability to learn and retrieve information is compromised even more, and patients are unable to access older, more distant memories. Aphasia, apraxia, disorientation, visuospatial dysfunction, impaired judgment, and executive dysfunction are also often present. Neurologic examination is usually nonfocal. The "probability" of AD is amplified by the presence of a genetic marker, ie, APOE4, in addition to the clear evidence of decline in memory and learning.

Vascular Dementia

Vascular dementia refers to cognitive deficits most often associated with vascular damage in the brain, either micro or macro in nature. It is sometimes associated with focal neurologic deficits that accompany cognitive loss, and the cognitive and neurologic impairments should correlate anatomically with the areas of ischemia, although the often diffuse nature of vascular disease may make this correlation difficult to identify. This is especially true in the case of small-vessel ischemic disease, which can be found in up to 50% of the cases of vascular dementia. Small-vessel ischemic disease involves white-matter damage and subcortical vessel damage, which in contrast to large-vessel disease, can present with more subtle neurologic signs, ie, pronator drift, gait instability, slowing of motor performance, and/or a neuropsychologic profile consistent with a dysexecutive syndrome of slow information processing and inattention. These changes are often seen as focal or diffuse white-matter changes on MRI (T2-weighted hyperintensities) and, as a function of volume, are often associated with worsening cognitive function. Parsing the differences between AD and vascular dementia can be challenging, especially given the relatively high rate of "mixed" etiology found in AD. The temporal association of cardiovascular events, genetic predispositions, and/or neuroimaging data increase the probability of a diagnosis of vascular dementia.

Dementia (or NCD) with Lewy Bodies

For a diagnosis of dementia with Lewy bodies, both dementia and at least one of the following core features must be present: recurrent and detailed visual hallucinations, parkinsonian signs, and fluctuating changes in alertness or attention. Additional suggestive features may include autonomic dysfunction, sleep disorder, severe neuroleptic sensitivity, and psychiatric misidentification syndromes. The diagnosis may overlap with AD and the dementia associated with Parkinson disease but having at least 2 core features raises the probability of dementia with Lewy bodies. Poor visuospatial abilities are also often out of proportion to other cognitive deficits. If Parkinson disease has been diagnosed or has been present for ≥1 year before cognitive symptoms are seen, the diagnosis is more consistent with Parkinson disease dementia. If parkinsonian symptoms are present at the same time as cognitive symptoms, a diagnosis of dementia with Lewy bodies should be considered.

Frontotemporal Dementia

Frontotemporal dementia is a disease often seen in patients with onset of cognitive symptoms at a younger age; these patients present most often with executive and language dysfunction and significant behavioral changes. These behaviors include disinhibition and hyperorality, and they often have had a profound effect on the patient's social functioning. Memory deficits are often not as pronounced in these patients in the early stages as they are in patients with other dementias. The language impairment in frontotemporal dementia may be detected in neuropsychologic tests such as the Boston Naming Test and may progress even early in the course of illness much faster than other cognitive domains. It is important to recognize the difference between frontotemporal dementia and AD with "frontal" symptoms. The latter refers to social disinhibition and behavioral impulsivity that can be seen with AD. In these patients, the behavioral problems occur much later in the course of illness, after a cognitive problem is already clearly evident. In contrast, patients with frontotemporal dementia display social disinhibition before prominent memory decline. The probability of frontotemporal dementia is increased by the presence of a known genetic marker and/or evidence of disproportionate frontal and/or temporal lobe involvement from neuroimaging.

Differentiating Delirium and Depression

Recognition of dementia can be complicated by the presence of either delirium or depression. Delirium has been defined as an acquired impairment of attention, alertness, or perception. Delirium and dementia are in some ways similar; both are characterized by global cognitive impairment. Delirium can be distinguished by acute onset, cognitive fluctuations throughout the course of a day, impaired consciousness and attention, fluctuating levels of alertness, and altered sleep cycles. In hospitalized patients, delirium and dementia often occur together. The presence of dementia increases the risk of delirium and accounts in part for the high rate of delirium in older patients. A delirium episode in an older adult, therefore, should alert the clinician to search for dementia once the delirium clears.

Symptoms of depression and dementia often overlap, presenting additional diagnostic challenges. Patients with primary dementia commonly experience symptoms of depression, and such patients may minimize cognitive losses. By contrast, patients with primary depression can demonstrate decreased motivation during the cognitive examination and express cognitive complaints that exceed objectively measured deficits. Moreover, patients with primary depression usually have intact language and motor skills, whereas patients with primary dementia may show impairment in these domains. As many as half of older adults who present with severe depression and signs of cognitive loss become progressively demented within 5 years.

Common to all types of dementia, cognitive impairment eventually has a profound effect on the patient's daily life. Difficulties in planning meals, managing finances or medications, using a telephone, and driving without getting lost are not uncommon. Such functional impairments may first alert others that a problem is emerging. Numerous functions are maintained in patients with dementia of mild to moderate severity, including such ADLs as eating, bathing, and grooming, and the behaviors of many patients remain socially appropriate during the early disease stages.

Behavior and mood changes eventually become commonplace, including personality changes, apathy, irritability, anxiety, or depression. During the middle and late stages of the disease, delusions, hallucinations, aggression, resistance to care, and wandering may develop. These behaviors are extremely troubling to caregivers and often result in family distress and long-term care placement. Although the course of dementia is variable, the progression of dementia often follows a sequential clinical and functional pattern of decline (Table 36.4).

TREATMENT AND MANAGEMENT

The primary treatment goals for patients with dementia are to enhance quality of life and maximize functional performance by improving or stabilizing cognition, mood, and behavior. Both pharmacologic and non-pharmacologic treatments are available, and the latter should be emphasized. However, research has shown only modest effects on cognition, and providers should educate patients and caregivers to have realistic expectations. Patients with dementia often develop significant behavioral symptoms that are a challenge to both family members and professional caregivers. Any acute change requires an evaluation for undiagnosed medical problems, pain, depression, infection, metabolic disturbance, or delirium. Other factors that can contribute to behavioral symptoms include interpersonal or emotional issues. Addressing such issues, treating underlying medical conditions, providing reassurance, and attending to the possible need for changes in the patient's environment can reduce agitation. The use of pharmacologic treatments for behavioral problems is recommended only after nonpharmacologic ones prove ineffective, or when there is an emergent need such as extreme patient distress or risk of physical violence.

Nonpharmacologic Treatment

Cognitive Rehabilitation

Reality orientation, memory retraining, and cognitive training have all been proposed as possible techniques to perhaps improve cognitive function. A 2013 Cochrane review of cognitive training found no indication of significant benefit in patients with dementia (SOE=B). Studies in this review were limited primarily by poor design and inadequate outcome measures. Given that new learning is a skill lost very early in the course of AD, an overemphasis on quizzing or retraining may lead to anxiety and self-depreciation. In general, a preferred approach is to provide support to accommodate for lost skills.

Supportive Therapy

Emotion-oriented psychotherapy, such as "pleasant events" and "reminiscence" therapy, and stimulation-oriented treatment, including art and other expressive recreational or social therapies, such as exercise or dance, are examples of psychosocial treatments that can minimize depressive symptoms and reduce behavioral symptoms. These interventions can be provided by professionals or informal caregivers who have been specifically trained. Support groups can provide meaningful support and education for both patients and caregivers. Early-onset dementia groups are especially helpful for patients with mild deficits and insight. Research has begun to demonstrate benefits of caregiver education and support in reducing behavioral symptoms and improving quality of life among patients and caregivers with dementia (SOE=C).

Other Therapies

There are some data supporting physical exercise as having effects on functional performance, cognitive function, and behavioral symptoms. A recent Cochrane review reported evidence on ADL performance and cognition, as well as promising data on caregiver burden associated with exercise programs. Physical activity should be encouraged as part of the treatment plan for any patient with dementia. Early research also suggests a role for occupational therapy in providing caregiver education strategies and environmental modification.

Regular Appointments

One approach to ensuring optimal health care for patients with dementia is to schedule regular patient surveillance and health maintenance visits every 3–6 months. During such visits, the clinician should address and treat comorbid conditions, evaluate ongoing medications, and consider initiating medication-free periods. In addition, it is useful to check for sleep and behavioral disturbances and to provide guidance on proper sleep hygiene. Caregiver well-being should also be regularly assessed.

Family and Caregiver Education and Support

Research has demonstrated that caring for an individual with dementia is more difficult and more stressful than caring for someone with normal cognition. Working closely with family members and caregivers will help

Table 36.4—The General Progression of Dementia

Stage 1: No cognitive impairment

Unimpaired individuals experience no memory problems, and none is evident to a health care professional during a medical interview.

Stage 2: Very mild cognitive decline

Individuals at this stage feel as if they have memory lapses, especially in forgetting familiar words or names or the location of keys, eyeglasses, or other everyday objects. However, these problems are not evident during a medical examination or apparent to friends, family, or coworkers.

Stage 3: Mild cognitive decline

Early-stage Alzheimer disease can be diagnosed in some, but not all, individuals with these symptoms.

Friends, family, or coworkers begin to notice deficiencies. Problems with memory or concentration may be measurable in clinical testing or discernible during a detailed medical interview. Common difficulties include the following:

- Word- or name-finding problems noticeable to family or close associates
- Decreased ability to remember names when introduced to new people
- Performance issues in social or work settings noticeable to family, friends, or coworkers
- Reading a passage and retaining little material
- Losing or misplacing a valuable object
- Decline in ability to plan or organize

Stage 4: Moderate cognitive decline (mild or early-stage Alzheimer disease)

At this stage, a careful medical interview detects clear-cut deficiencies in the following areas:

- Decreased knowledge of recent occasions or current events
- Impaired ability to perform challenging mental arithmetic, eg, to count backward from 100 by 7s
- Decreased ability to perform complex tasks, such as marketing, planning dinner for guests, or paying bills and managing finances
- Reduced memory of personal history

The affected individual may seem subdued and withdrawn, especially in socially or mentally challenging situations.

Stage 5: Moderately severe cognitive decline (moderate or mid-stage Alzheimer disease)

Major gaps in memory and deficits in cognitive function emerge. Some assistance with day-to-day activities becomes essential. At this stage, individuals may:

- Be unable during a medical interview to recall such important information as their current address, their telephone number, or the name of the college or high school from which they graduated
- Become confused about where they are or about the date, day of the week, or season
- Have trouble with less challenging mental arithmetic, eg, counting backward from 40 by 4s or from 20 by 2s
- Need help choosing proper clothing for the season or occasion
- Usually retain substantial knowledge about themselves and know their own name and the names of their spouse or children
- Usually require no assistance with eating or using the toilet

Stage 6: Severe cognitive decline (moderately severe or mid-stage Alzheimer disease)

Memory difficulties continue to worsen, significant personality changes may emerge, and affected individuals need extensive help with customary daily activities. At this stage, individuals may:

- Lose most awareness of recent experiences, events, and surroundings
- Recollect their personal history imperfectly, although they generally recall their name
- Occasionally forget the name of their spouse or primary caregiver but generally can distinguish familiar from unfamiliar faces
- Need help getting dressed properly; without supervision, may make errors such as putting pajamas over daytime clothes or shoes on wrong feet
- Experience disruption of their normal sleep-wake cycle
- Need help with handling details of toileting (flushing toilet, wiping, and disposing of tissue properly)
- Have increasing episodes of urinary or fecal incontinence
- Experience significant personality changes and behavioral symptoms, including suspiciousness and delusions (eg, believing that their caregiver is an impostor); hallucinations (seeing or hearing things that are not really there); or compulsive, repetitive behaviors such as hand wringing or tissue shredding
- Tend to wander and become lost

Stage 7: Very severe cognitive decline (severe or late-stage Alzheimer disease)

This is the final stage of the disease when individuals lose the ability to respond to their environment, to speak, and ultimately to control movement.

- Frequently lose the ability for recognizable speech, although words or phrases may occasionally be uttered
- Need help with eating and toileting, and there is general urinary incontinence
- Lose the ability to walk without assistance, then the ability to sit without support, smile, and to hold up head; reflexes become abnormal, muscles grow rigid, and swallowing is impaired

SOURCE: Excerpted from www.alz.org/AboutAD/Stages.asp and reproduced with permission of the Alzheimer's Association. © 2011 Alzheimer's Association. All rights reserved. This is an official publication of the Alzheimer's Association but may be distributed by unaffiliated organizations and individuals. Such distribution does not constitute an endorsement of these parties or their activities by the Alzheimer's Association.

establish a therapeutic alliance. Education of family and caregivers about diagnosis, clinical course, treatment options, and management strategies is critical. Recent research has focused on developing a framework to analyze behaviors and develop individualized strategies for use by caregivers. Several of these studies have demonstrated efficacy on reducing caregiver burden, especially around behavioral symptoms, and include programs such as COPE, REACH, and the Savvy Caregiver. These programs provide information about community resources as well as strategies for managing challenging behavioral symptoms and can allow families to cope more effectively, reduce institutionalization, and improve quality of life. A recent Cochrane review of these studies suggested potential beneficial effects but was unable to prove efficacy.

Relatives are often helpful sources of information about cognitive and behavioral changes, and generally they take the primary responsibility for implementing and monitoring treatment. Often, they are also responsible for medical and legal assistance. However, early identification of dementia can allow the affected individual to participate in treatment decisions and future planning. Subjects to pursue with family include medical and legal advance directives (also called advance care plans in some contexts). It is often best for a trusted relative to co-sign important financial transactions and attend to paying bills.

Community programs such as enrollment in adult daycare centers or respite programs can provide support to family caregivers, allowing the individual with dementia to remain at home longer. Patients also benefit from these programs through opportunities for socialization and structured activities. Although most care for dementia patients is provided in the home, many patients with dementia need admission to a long-term care facility at some point. Discussion about long-term care placement options should be started early rather than late, to provide the individual or family members time to complete arrangements and begin to adjust emotionally. Palliative care teams may be consulted to assist in developing goals of care around symptom management and may provide support in planning for this very unpredictable prognosis. Hospice can be an alternative for end-stage dementia patients who wish to remain at home and have comfort as the goal for care. Caregivers often express concern about their own memory lapses, which should be addressed with counseling or neuropsychologic assessment. Caregiver distress is often reduced with participation in support groups, which may relieve common feelings of anger, frustration, and guilt. Respite care is another community resource that offers caregivers relief. Caregiver support interventions involving individual and family counseling combined with regular participation in support groups have demonstrated improvement in caregiver well-being and delay in time to nursing-home placement. Use of support groups and counseling services by family caregivers has also been associated with a delay in nursing-home placement of ≥1 year (SOE=B).

Environmental Modification

Patients with dementia can be extremely sensitive to their environment; in general, a moderate level of stimulation is best. When they experience overstimulation, confusion or agitation can increase, whereas too little stimulation can cause boredom and withdrawal. As deficits change over time, this balance must be re-evaluated and activities adjusted regularly. Familiar surroundings maximize existing cognitive functions, and predictability through daily routines is often reassuring. Other helpful orientation and memory measures in early stages include conspicuous displays of clocks, calendars, and to-do lists. Links to the outside world through newspapers, radio, and television can benefit some mildly impaired patients. Adaptive strategies for more impaired individuals can involve providing visual clues to assist patients (eg, picture of a toilet for the bathroom, or of food for the dining room) or to distract patients from exposure to unsafe situations (eg, STOP sign on door, covering elevator buttons). Attention to a simple and compassionate communication style can reduce behavioral symptoms in the patient and burden for the caregiver. Strategies such as using simple sentences, phrasing commands in a positive fashion, avoiding slang and pronouns, and speaking in a calm tone of voice can enhance communication.

Attention to Safety

In early stages, safety concerns may be minimal, because the person with dementia is still able to make appropriate judgments about safety. However, the need for supervision usually increases as the disease progresses and the person becomes more forgetful and is no longer able to anticipate or avoid dangerous situations. Interventions should balance allowing as much independence as possible while ensuring safety, focusing initially on environmental strategies. Door locks or electronic guards prevent wandering, and many families benefit from registering with Safe Return through the Alzheimer's Association (www.alz.org). Patient name tags and medical-alert bracelets can assist in locating lost patients. Emerging technologies include watches and other devices that incorporate a global positioning system to monitor the individual's location.

Cognitive impairment affects driving skills, and the visuospatial and planning disabilities of even mildly demented patients can make them unsafe drivers. Discussions about driving are best started early in treatment.

In California and some other states, physicians must report patients with dementia to the health department, which forwards the information to the motor vehicle department for further assessment. Patients with advanced dementia definitely should not drive, but clinicians disagree about whether mildly demented patients should drive. Referral for an independent driving assessment is recommended if there is any concern regarding safety. Certainly, when a patient has a history of traffic accidents or significant spatial and executive dysfunction, driving abilities should be carefully scrutinized.

Pharmacologic Treatment

General Issues

Several factors should be considered when prescribing medications for older adults with dementia. Patients in the older age groups vary in their response, so treatments need to be individualized. In addition, age is associated with decreased renal clearance and hepatic metabolism. Older patients often take several medications simultaneously, so drug interactions and adverse events are likely. Medications with anticholinergic effects are a particular problem for patients with dementia, because they can worsen cognitive impairment and lead to delirium. Another group of problem medications that can worsen cognition include those causing CNS sedation. Any nonessential medications with CNS adverse events should be considered carefully. The best strategy, in light of such factors, is to start with low dosages and increase dosing gradually ("start low and go slow"). The goal is to identify the lowest effective dosage, thus minimizing adverse events while avoiding subtherapeutic dosing. Before starting any treatment, a thorough medical examination should be conducted to identify and treat any underlying medical conditions that might impair cognition.

Cholinesterase Inhibitors (ChIs)

The primary medications available for stabilizing cognitive function in AD are ChIs. Currently, three ChIs are approved by the FDA: donepezil, rivastigmine, and galantamine. By slowing the breakdown of the neurotransmitter acetylcholine, these medications are thought to facilitate memory function because of the association of acetylcholine and memory.

In clinical trials, these medications demonstrate a modest delay in cognitive decline compared with placebo in patients with AD. Onset of behavioral problems and decline in ADLs is modestly delayed compared with treatment with placebo (SOE=A). In a Cochrane review of 10 randomized, double-blind, placebo-controlled trials, treatment for 6 months improved cognitive function on average −2.7 points (95% confidence interval, −3.0 to −2.3, P <.00001) on the 70-point Alzheimer's Disease Assessment Scale-Cognitive Subscale; there was also small improvement on measures of ADLs and behavior. Over the last decade, a large body of evidence has grown to support the modest clinical benefits of cholinesterase inhibitors in AD for short- and long-term treatment not only with respect to outcomes on cognitive performance but also with slight reductions in volumetric loss within the hippocampus, suggesting a somewhat neuroprotective effect. With the increase in focus on identifying a prodromal phase of AD, several clinical trials, including a few randomized double-blind, placebo-controlled trials, have sought to determine the efficacy of ChIs in MCI in preventing/delaying onset of AD, but to date no study has achieved its endpoint. However, some of the subanalysis suggests a positive response within specific populations toward prevention of progression to AD (ie, APOE ε4 allele).

Results of studies of patients with dementing disorders other than AD are also becoming available. Widespread treatment in vascular dementia was not recommended in a meta-analysis because of the limited cognitive benefit and lack of sufficient data (SOE=B). Some studies suggest that ChIs may be helpful in managing attention and behavioral disturbances (eg, hallucinations) associated with dementia with Lewy bodies (SOE=B), and one ChI, rivastigmine, is approved by the FDA for mild to moderate dementia in Parkinson disease. There appears to be no role for ChIs in treating frontotemporal dementia, and in fact, evidence suggests they may worsen agitation (SOE=B). Because effects are modest in all disorders, patients and families should be counseled to have realistic expectations, and discontinuation of medication should be considered after a reasonable time period if decline continues at the rate expected without treatment. Clinical evaluation after 6 months of therapy is suggested. In the case of long-term therapy with initial positive responses to treatment but continued advancement of cognitive decline, the question of discontinuation effect on cognition ultimately arises. If cognitive decline persists despite maximal treatment with ChIs, the clinician should discuss the risks and benefits of therapy with the patient and caregivers. Tapering the medication over time may be considered. Abrupt discontinuation is not recommended.

All three ChIs can be dosed once daily, either in oral form (donepezil and galantamine) or as a 24-hour patch (rivastigmine). Dosing adjustments should follow a slow titration curve to maximize the tolerable dosage while avoiding adverse events, such as nausea, diarrhea, insomnia, headaches, dizziness, orthostasis, and nightmares. However, a lower initial dosage and/or an even slower titration curve can help further mitigate adverse events if they occur, especially GI adverse events. Increasing the dosage of donepezil to the recently approved dosage of 23 mg/d or rivastigmine patch to 13.3 mg/24 hours may offer some benefit in severe dementia but is unlikely to affect overall global functioning and should only be used with caution given the observed increase in adverse events (SOE=A). The most serious adverse event associated with ChIs is bradycardia. Because of limited direct comparisons, there is currently no evidence for any difference in efficacy among the ChIs.

Memantine

Memantine, an N-methyl-d-aspartate antagonist, has been used worldwide for many years. It is thought to have neuroprotective effects by reducing glutamate-mediated excitotoxicity. Clinical trials in the United States support the efficacy of memantine in moderate to severe stages of AD (SOE=A). A Cochrane review of two 6-month studies showed modest beneficial effects on cognition, ADLs, and behavior. Memantine is approved by the FDA for treatment of moderate to severe AD. Research has not supported use in earlier stages of AD, and trials have yet to establish efficacy in other dementias. A Cochrane review and a meta-analysis of memantine in vascular dementia found limited effect on cognition and no evidence to recommend widespread use (SOE=A). The recommended dosage of memantine in management of Alzheimer-type dementia starts at 5 mg/d po, which may then be increased on a weekly basis in 5-mg increments to a target dosage of 20 mg/d dosed as 10 mg q12h after a 4-week titration period. For the extended-release formulation, the starting dosage of 7 mg/d can be increased to the maximal dosage of 28 mg/d over 3 weeks. The most common adverse events are constipation, dizziness, and headache. Memantine has been used safely as a single agent and in conjunction with ChIs for moderate to severe AD (SOE=B).

Other Cognitive Enhancers

Ongoing studies are assessing a variety of other agents in AD, including antioxidants and *Ginkgo biloba* extract. In a trial including >300 patients with moderately severe AD, treatment with vitamin E (α-tocopherol) or the selective monoamine oxidase B inhibitor selegiline (approved for treatment of Parkinson disease) lowered rates of functional decline but was not associated with evidence of cognitive improvement. However, this study involved patients with moderate to severe dementia, so effects on cognition earlier in the illness remain unknown. Results from a randomized, placebo-controlled trial of vitamin E and donepezil in MCI showed some short-term benefit from donepezil in delaying conversion to AD but no effect of vitamin E.

Although a 2005 meta-analysis posited an increased risk of all-cause mortality in individuals with chronic illness taking vitamin E at >400 IU/d, the TEAM-AD VA Cooperative Randomized Trial conducted from 2007–2013 not only demonstrated the safe use of vitamin E at dosages >2,000 IU/d in individuals taking a ChI with mild to moderately severe AD but also demonstrated a significant slowing of functional decline over 4 years as well as significantly lowering caregiver burden. Thus, the clinical efficacy and safety of vitamin E has yet to be fully established.

Extract from the leaf of the *Ginkgo* tree has been promoted primarily in Europe for peripheral vascular disease as well as for "cerebral insufficiency." Other studies in Europe and the United States have explored its use in AD. However, a recent large, multicenter, randomized, double-blind, placebo-controlled trial in normal individuals and individuals with MCI did not show any slowing of cognitive decline in either population over a median follow-up of 6.1 years.

Nutrient-based interventions have failed to show any consistent, clinical benefit in improving cognition or function. Trials of antioxidants, B vitamins, omega 3 fatty acids, and medium-chain triglycerides have all been negative. The results may be confounded by the heterogeneity of the compounds and stage of illness, but further research is needed before recommending their routine use in treatment.

Many patients also use OTC preparations for cognitive enhancement. A complete review of medications should always include questions about use of OTC medications.

Disease-Modifying Therapies—Immunotherapy

Attempts at active or passive immunization directed at key putative proteins central in the neurodegenerative process and thus slowing or reversing the disease process continues to show promise. To date, however, no trials have produced a deliverable product because of either excessive inflammatory responses, ie, meningoencephalitis, or simply a lack of efficacy. Efforts are under way to refine these techniques by reducing the inflammatory response and targeting high-risk individuals at preclinical stages so as to attenuate the downstream effects of early amyloid deposition.

Antidepressants

Antidepressant drug treatment is generally considered for AD patients with depressive symptoms, including depressed mood, appetite loss, insomnia, fatigue, irritability, and agitation. Anecdotal evidence exists that SSRIs can be helpful in managing the disinhibitions and compulsive behaviors associated with frontotemporal dementia. However, patients with dementia are at risk of falls, and the use of SSRIs and SNRIs can possibly exacerbate these risks, especially those with greater anticholinergic tone (eg, paroxetine).

Psychoactive Medications

Behavioral and psychologic symptoms of dementia such as paranoia, agitation, and irritability are best managed by nonpharmacologic strategies, such as reducing overstimulation, distraction, redirection, and physical activity. However, when medications are required, target symptoms should be identified and therapy selected accordingly. There is some limited evidence that first- and second-generation antipsychotics help control these symptoms, but recent trials have revealed that all antipsychotics increase the risk of "all-cause" mortality in the setting of dementia (SOE=A). Therefore, these medications must be used cautiously to manage delusions, hallucinations, and paranoia as well as some of the irritability associated with dementia. To help mitigate these risks, frequent attempts to taper off each medication should be undertaken (SOE=A). Medications such as carbamazapine[OL] and valproic acid[OL] are possible alternatives for managing irritability and agitation, but again both have limited evidence for effectiveness in dementia and can also be associated with increased mortality risk (SOE=B). The use of benzodiazepines and medications with anticholinergic effects should be avoided. Finally, antidepressants with sedating effects such as mirtazapine and trazodone can be considered in management of insomnia.

Other Resources

Most primary care providers successfully treat and manage most patients with dementia, but referral to a specialist is sometimes necessary, especially for diagnosis. When the presentation or history is atypical or complex, particularly when the onset begins before age 60, consultation with a specialist in treating dementia patients (eg, geriatric psychiatrist, neurologist) can be useful. Geriatric specialists with psychology or psychiatry training can assist with behavioral management, particularly when patients are agitated, psychotic, or violent. They are also helpful when patients are suicidal or suffer from a major depressive disorder or when individual or family therapy is indicated for patients or caregivers.

A neurologist can be helpful for patients with parkinsonism, focal neurologic signs, unusually rapid progression, or abnormal neuroimaging findings. Neuropsychologic consultation can clarify diagnostically complex cases, and clinical psychologists can provide psychotherapy, especially for caregivers. Social workers can provide counseling and contact with community resources. Physical therapists can provide guidance on physical and group activity, and occupational therapists can assess the patient's functional level and suggest approaches to maximize functioning. Nurses can make management suggestions and guide behavior management, feeding, and other care issues. Pharmacists can perform medication reviews to minimize adverse drug events and can assist caregivers with practical advice on the administration of medications to demented patients. Wills, conservatorships, estate planning, and other legal matters are best addressed with the assistance of an attorney. Because most dementias are progressive, patients with early dementia should be offered an opportunity to plan for future incapacity and illness.

Community support can be informal, in which neighbors or friends help out, or formal, through home-care or family service agencies, the aging or mental health networks, or adult daycare centers. Available specialized services include adult daycare and respite care, home-health agencies that can provide skilled nursing, help lines of the Alzheimer's Association, and outreach services offered by Area Agencies on Aging and Councils on Aging, which are mandated and funded under the federal Older Americans Act. Food services for the homebound are available from Meals-on-Wheels, and many senior citizens' centers, church and community groups, and hospitals offer transportation options.

CHOOSING WISELY® RECOMMENDATIONS

Dementia

- Do not prescribe cholinesterase inhibitors for dementia without periodic assessment for perceived cognitive benefits and adverse GI effects.

REFERENCES

- Barnes DE, Yaffe, K. The projected effect of risk factor reduction on Alzheimer's disease prevalence. *Lancet Neurol.* 2011;10(9):819–828.

    This review summarizes the evidence regarding 7 potentially modifiable risk factors for Alzheimer disease (AD): diabetes, midlife hypertension, midlife obesity, smoking, depression, cognitive inactivity or low educational attainment, and physical inactivity. Additionally, the effect of risk factor reduction on AD prevalence was projected by calculating population-attributable risks (the percent of cases attributable to a given factor) and the number of AD cases that might be prevented by risk-factor reductions of 10% and 25% worldwide and in the United States. Together, up to half of AD cases worldwide (17.2 million) and in the United States (2.9 million) are potentially attributable to these factors. A 10%–25% reduction in all 7 risk factors could potentially prevent as many as 1.1–3 million AD cases worldwide and 184,000–492,000 cases in the United States.

- Dysken MW, Sano M, Asthana S, et al. Effect of vitamin E and memantine on functional decline in Alzheimer disease. The TEAM AD Cooperative Randomized Trial. *JAMA*. 2014;311(1):33–44.

    This large, randomized, controlled trial was directed at testing the efficacy of alpha tocopherol (vitamin E) and memantine alone or in combination in reducing the primary outcome of decline in Alzheimer disease (AD) in the Alzheimer's Disease Cooperative Study/Activities of Daily Living [ADCS-ADL]) Inventory, a measure of functional ability, in mild to moderate AD. What is notable about this trial is the significant reduction in functional decline (19%; $P =.03$) observed in the vitamin E–alone treatment arm. Moreover, the study did not find any significant increase in mortality associated with use of vitamin E at 2,000 IU/d, which runs counter to a large meta-analysis of vitamin E conducted in 2005, suggesting an increase risk of all-cause mortality at dosages >400 IU/d. Thus, further investigation into the use of vitamin E in delaying functional decline in AD is warranted, especially given the possibility of a more favorable risk profile.

- Kales HC, Gitlin LN, Lyketsos CG, et al. Management of neuropsychiatric symptoms of dementia in clinical settings: recommendations from a multidisciplinary expert panel. *J Am Geriatr Soc*. 2014;62(4):762–769.

    This article reports on the recommendations of a multidisciplinary expert panel to define critical elements of care for neuropsychiatric symptoms in clinical and research settings and how best to integrate nonpharmacologic and pharmacologic approaches. It includes discussion of a framework for assessing and managing these symptoms.

- McKhann GM, Knopman DS, Chertkow H, et al. The diagnosis of dementia due to Alzheimer's disease: Recommendations from the National Institute on Aging-Alzheimer's Association workgroups on diagnostic guidelines for Alzheimer's disease. *Alzheimers Dement*. 2011;7(3):263–269.

    The National Institute on Aging and the Alzheimer's Association charged a workgroup with the task of revising the 1984 criteria for Alzheimer's disease (AD) dementia. The workgroup sought to ensure that the revised criteria would be flexible enough to be used both by general health care providers without access to neuropsychological testing, advanced imaging, and cerebrospinal fluid measures, and by specialized investigators involved in research or in clinical trial studies who would have these tools available. This article presents criteria for all-cause dementia and for AD dementia.

- Swaminathan A, Jicha G. Nutrition and prevention of Alzheimer's dementia. *Front Aging Neurosci*. 2014;6(282):1–13.

    This review focuses on several key nutritional compounds and dietary modifications that have been studied in people, and further discusses the rationale underlying their potential use for prevention and treatment of AD.

Alexander W. Threlfall, MD, MA
Cynthia Barton, RN, MSN

CHAPTER 37—BEHAVIORAL DISTURBANCES IN DEMENTIA

Key Points

- Behavioral disturbances in dementia require evaluation of the specific symptoms, including the comfort of the patient, medical comorbidities, the environment of care, the needs of the caregiver, and the degree of distress of all those involved in the life of the demented adult.

- Delirium secondary to an underlying condition such as dehydration, urinary tract infection, or medication toxicity is a common cause of abrupt behavioral disturbances in patients with dementia.

- Nonpharmacologic interventions must be considered the first-line choice for all behavioral disturbances in dementia. These include caregiver education and support, patient-centered use of music, physical activity, support for activities of daily living, and cognitive stimulation programs.

- Pharmacologic treatment of behavioral disturbances in dementia is of limited efficacy and should be used only after environmental and nonpharmacologic interventions have been implemented.

- Increased mortality has been identified with the use of both first-generation antipsychotic agents such as haloperidol and perphenazine, as well as second-generation antipsychotic agents such as risperidone and olanzapine. All antipsychotic agents carry an FDA warning regarding increased all-cause mortality in patients with dementia.

- Despite these FDA warnings, antipsychotic medications may be needed for treatment of distressing delusions and hallucinations, and antidepressants may be helpful if symptoms of depression are evident. There is limited evidence for considering mood stabilizers for symptoms such as impulsivity and aggression in patients who have a significant behavioral disturbance.

Most dementias are associated with a range of behavioral and psychologic disturbances, with as many as 80%–90% of patients developing at least one distressing symptom over the course of their illness. The development of behavioral disturbances or psychotic symptoms in dementia often precipitates early nursing-home placement and causes significant caregiver burden and distress. These disturbances are potentially treatable, and it is vital that they are anticipated and recognized early. As these symptoms emerge, it is essential to perform a thorough evaluation of contributing factors, identify the target symptoms for treatment, and implement appropriate interventions for the patient and caregiver.

The *Diagnostic and Statistical Manual of Mental Disorders, Fifth Edition (DSM-5)* uses the term *neurocognitive disorders* to classify conditions of acquired cognitive loss but retains the term *dementia* for clinical and practical uses. ICD-10 continues to use the term dementia in its classifications.

Research that compares different treatment strategies for the behavioral and psychologic symptoms of dementia is growing in response to the great need for evidence-based treatment guidelines. Some conclusions can be drawn from randomized controlled trials evaluating medications for the treatment of depression and psychosis, but these results are limited by marginal efficacy and FDA warnings regarding increased mortality among patients with dementia who are treated with antipsychotic agents. Interventions using behavioral treatment modalities have also been studied, with more robust outcomes in the ability to delay the need for nursing-home placement (SOE=A) and to improve quality of life among patients and caregivers (SOE=B). These studies have allowed for recommendations in many areas; however, many aspects of treatment must still draw on case reports and clinical experience.

Clinical Features

Behavioral and psychologic symptoms are a common feature of all dementias. These include anxiety, apathy, depression, sleep disturbance, resistance to care, appetite changes, elation, irritability, disinhibition, wandering, hoarding, verbal disruptions, physical aggression, delusions, and hallucinations. Discrete psychiatric symptoms may develop that take on a variety of characteristics resembling mental disorders such as depression or mania; however, the course and features are more difficult to predict, and treatments are less reliably effective than when these disorders occur in younger adults without dementia. Depressive symptoms are common and often manifest as sadness, tearfulness, or a lack of interest in previously enjoyable activities. This depressive syndrome can also include a loss of interest in self-care, eating, or interacting with peers.

A propensity for irritability and impulsivity can also occur. If these features become progressive, overt hostility or violence may ensue, and patients may be characterized as "agitated," reflecting a loss of the ability to modulate their behavior in a socially acceptable way. These behaviors may include verbal outbursts, physical aggression, resistance to bathing or other care needs, and restless motor activity such as pacing or rocking. Among the behavioral complications of dementia, the most severe disruptions in caregiving occur when patients develop physical behaviors such as hitting, scratching, or pushing, or when they develop paranoid delusions that lead to hostility and altercations with caregivers. This type of overlap across symptoms, in which some are associated with a well-described psychiatric disorder but others such as wandering and hoarding are considered atypical, often creates a significant challenge in diagnostic labeling. In this situation, the nonspecific term *agitation* is commonly used to describe the patient, but it is too broad and nonspecific to be clinically useful and may best be accompanied by additional description as to whether the problem is accompanied by irritability, vocal or physical aggression, or motor disturbances. Assessment of disruptive behavior must include a careful description of the nature of the symptom, when it occurs, where it develops, and if any precipitants or antecedents are identified. Treatment cannot be provided without adequate assessment of the behavioral disturbance.

In many cases, behavioral disruption can occur concomitantly with evidence of paranoia or delusional thinking, such as a fixed false belief that caregivers have stolen possessions or money, or are plotting against the patient. When delusions occur, the patient is then characterized as suffering from "psychotic" symptoms. Sensory experiences without stimuli such as hallucinations are another type of psychotic symptom that can accompany episodes of agitated behavior. Depending on the degree of communication deficits in a given patient, the ability to discern the presence of psychosis is variable, and in many cases disruptive behaviors can occur without clear evidence as to whether delusions or other psychoses may be precipitating the disturbance. Antipsychotic medications are commonly used in management of disruptive behaviors, with the presumption that disturbed perceptions may be the underlying problem. There is little evidence to support this presumption, and there is increasing concern over the lack of efficacy of antipsychotic agents for nonspecific symptoms of disruptive behavior, in addition to risks of adverse events and mortality related to these medications in dementia.

Occasionally, a behavioral syndrome occurs that includes features of hyperactivity, mood lability, disinhibition, and grandiose beliefs that resemble a manic episode associated with bipolar affective disorder. The features of this "manic-like" syndrome are described below, and much like other mood symptoms in dementia, the features in older adults are similar but less predictable than those seen in younger adults; treatment strategies are also more challenging. One key feature of the manic-like syndromes seen in dementia patients is the tendency to develop additional symptoms outside the typical course of a bipolar manic episode, such as resistance to care, stubbornness, wandering, and hoarding behaviors, as well as a significant degree of fluctuation in symptoms over the course of a single day.

The complaints from family caregivers and professional caregivers in a nursing home or assisted-living facility often arise from behavioral complications occurring during care that involved a resistance to bathing, dressing, feeding, or other routines. Environmental precipitants such as excessive stimuli or a change in the environment (eg, a new roommate, frequent changes in staff and caregivers) can induce behavioral problems. The presenting complaint may relate to internal cues such as pain, hunger, thirst, or other needs that the patient is not able to express. Family members may feel more overwhelmed than professional caregivers and may consequently attribute more overall distress to these episodes. Overt resistance to care is most often seen in later stages of dementia, but behavioral problems can also be a first sign of an incipient cognitive decline in earlier stages. Neuropsychiatric symptoms such as apathy, poor self-care, or paranoia may be the first indication of dementia before cognitive decline is recognized, such that an evaluation for dementia in any older adult who presents with new behavioral or emotional symptoms may reveal a previously undetected dementia syndrome.

ASSESSMENT AND DIFFERENTIAL DIAGNOSIS

Comprehensive assessment includes a history from both the patient and an informant or other source. The information should include a clear description of the behavior: temporal onset, course, associated circumstances, and its relationship to key environmental factors such as caregiver status and recent stressors. The problem behaviors and symptoms should then be considered in the context of the patient's family and personal, social, and medical history.

Rating scales are available for the behavioral and psychologic symptoms of dementia. Some of these include the Cohen-Mansfield Agitation Inventory (CMAI), the Neuropsychiatric Inventory (NPI), and the Behavioral Pathology in Alzheimer Disease Rating Scale (BEHAVE-AD). These allow the clinician to note and quantify the symptoms based on a caregiver interview.

A differential diagnosis of the disturbance should proceed based on findings of a comprehensive geriatric evaluation. The first step is to decide whether the disturbance is a symptom of a new condition, of a preexisting medical problem, or of an adverse drug event. Disturbances that are new, acute in onset, or evolving rapidly are most often due to a medical condition or medication toxicity. An isolated behavioral disturbance in a demented patient can be the *sole* presenting symptom for many acute conditions such as pneumonia, urinary tract infection, acute pain, angina, constipation, or poorly controlled diabetes mellitus. Additionally, the need to satisfy basic physical needs, such as hunger, sleepiness, thirst, boredom, or fatigue, which the patient cannot adequately communicate, can precipitate a behavioral disturbance. Medication intolerance toxicity due to new or existing medications might also present as solely behavioral symptoms. Treatment or stabilization of the medical or physical cause is often sufficient to resolve the disturbance. Older adults with dementia may require several weeks longer to recover from routine medical problems than those who are cognitively intact.

The second step is to consider whether the behavioral disturbance is related to an environmental precipitant. These include disruptions in routine, time change (eg, with daylight savings time or travel across time zones), changes in the caregiving environment, new caregivers, a new roommate, or a life stressor (eg, death of a spouse or family member). Other common environmental precipitants include overstimulation (eg, too much noise, crowded rooms, close contact with too many people, too much time spent out of the familiar environment), understimulation (eg, relative absence of people, spending much time alone, use of television as a companion), and the disruptive behavior of other patients. For many disturbances, correcting an environmental precipitant or removing the stressor commonly improves the symptoms.

Another consideration is whether the disturbance results from stress in the patient-caregiver relationship. Caring for dementia patients is difficult and requires a degree of perseverance of which most caregivers are capable if proper guidance and support is provided. Inexperienced caregivers, domineering caregivers, or caregivers who themselves are impaired by medical or psychiatric disturbances can exacerbate or cause a behavioral disturbance. Caregiver burden can be a problem both in community settings and in nursing homes. Assessing the level of stress and burden on the caregiver is an important part of the evaluation of behavioral disturbances. Interventions to improve the patient-caregiver relationship and to provide caregiver education and support are a vital part of treatment of behavioral disturbances in dementia. Providing resources to caregivers such as referral to support groups and respite services is often very helpful.

After medical, environmental, and caregiving causes are excluded, it is often concluded that the behavioral problem is a manifestation of the dementia and may not be amenable to a pharmacologic intervention. Such disturbances that are closely linked to the dementia syndrome take on the form of a catastrophic reaction. A catastrophic reaction is an acute behavioral, physical, or verbal reaction to environmental stressors that results from an inability to make routine adjustments in daily life. The reaction might include anger, emotional lability, or aggression when patients are confronted with a deficit, such as the inability to find a word, or confusion about where they are or what they are supposed to do. Catastrophic reactions are best treated by identifying and avoiding their precipitants, by providing structured routines and activities, and by recognizing early signs of the impending catastrophic reaction so that the patient can be distracted and supported before reacting.

If the disturbance is not related to an identifiable cause or environmental precipitant, it may be a consequence of the brain deterioration that occurs during the course of dementia. Disturbances with a more insidious onset or that are persistent are more likely to be symptoms of the underlying disease. Epidemiologic and clinical studies suggest that such disturbances fall into three groups: mood symptoms, psychosis, and specific behavior problems that occur without significant specific psychiatric symptoms. The overlap in the symptoms of these groups can make treatment choices difficult. One approach is to decide whether the predominant symptom of a polysymptomatic disturbance is psychosis (delusions or hallucinations), mood symptoms (dysphoria, sadness, irritability, lability), aggression, or behavioral disruption, and then direct treatment toward the most distressing feature.

Behavioral disturbances can occur in all types of dementias, including Alzheimer type, vascular, and mixed. Frontotemporal dementia (ie, Pick disease) is a less common type of dementia often associated with prominent disinhibition, compulsive behaviors, and social impairment due to more advanced frontal lobe degeneration. In severe cases, a syndrome of hyperphagia, hyperactivity, and hypersexuality can occur that is related to bilateral temporal lobe atrophy. Another dementia associated with prominent psychiatric symptoms and behavioral disturbances is dementia with Lewy bodies. This form of dementia may be more common than previously thought. It is characterized by cognitive deterioration and parkinsonian features with prominent psychosis characterized by visual hallucinations. Affected older adults often suffer from distressing hallucinations and a fluctuating clinical course. These patients are extremely sensitive to

Table 37.1—Behavioral Interventions for Dementia Care

- Evaluate and treat underlying medical conditions.
- Correct sensory deficits; replace poorly fitting hearing aids, eyeglasses, and dentures.
- Remove offending medications, particularly anticholinergic agents.
- Keep the environment comfortable, calm, and homelike with use of familiar possessions.
- Provide regular daily activities and structure; refer patient to adult daycare programs, if needed.
- Assess for new medical problems.
- Attend to patient's sleep and eating patterns; offer regular snacks and finger foods.
- Install safety measures to prevent accidents.
- Ensure that the caregiver has adequate respite.
- Educate caregivers about practical aspects of dementia care and about behavioral disturbances.
- Teach caregivers the skills of caregiving: communication skills, avoiding confrontational behavior management, techniques of support for activities of daily living, activities for dementia care.
- Simplify bathing and dressing with use of adaptive clothing and assistive devices if needed; offer toileting frequently, and anticipate incontinence as dementia progresses.
- Provide access to experienced professionals and community resources.
- Refer family and patient to local Alzheimer's Association.
- Consult with caregiving professionals, such as geriatric case managers.

the extrapyramidal adverse events of antipsychotic medications (eg, muscle rigidity and tremor) and often cannot tolerate even low dosages of second-generation antipsychotic medications.

TREATMENT APPROACH

The treatment of the psychiatric and behavioral disturbances in dementia is complex and may require several interventions as part of a comprehensive plan of care. Specialists should be consulted in refractory cases. In general, treatment begins with appropriate environmental and caregiver interventions. Caregiver education and support interventions have been useful in reducing distress and delaying the need for nursing home placement (SOE=A). Nonpharmacologic interventions should always be used as a first-line treatment in the management of disruptive, aggressive, or agitated behavior. For a list of key behavioral interventions that might ameliorate behavioral symptoms in patients with dementia, see Table 37.1. Having a daily routine and introducing meaningful activities is vital. Behavioral disturbances in patients with dementia may decrease with the use of music, particularly during meals and bathing, and with light physical exercise or walking (SOE=B). Massage, pet therapy, white noise, videotapes of family, and cognitive stimulation programs may also be helpful. If the disturbances persist despite best efforts, pharmacologic interventions for specific target symptoms are often necessary.

TREATMENTS FOR SPECIFIC DISTURBANCES

The core of treatment is identifying any possible underlying cause of the behavior change, recognizing that multiple causes may exist. Managing pain, dehydration, hunger, and thirst is paramount. The possibilities of positional discomforts or nausea secondary to medication effects should be considered, because these are common possible culprits. Environmental modifications can improve patient orientation. Good lighting, one-on-one attention, supportive care, and attention to personal needs and wants are also important aspects of treatment. If there is sleep-wake cycle disturbance, efforts should be made to stabilize the sleep cycle by maintaining a consistent routine, using bright lights, or prescribing short-term use of medications.

Mood Disturbances

In dementia patients experiencing mood symptoms, measures similar to those used in other behavior disturbances should be implemented, ie, the environment should be optimized by reducing adversive stimuli, and physical health should be assessed comprehensively. Recreational programs and activity therapies have shown positive results in improving mood in depressive symptoms in dementia. Criteria for the diagnosis of depression in Alzheimer dementia have been proposed that note common features of irritability and social isolation or withdrawal. The waxing and waning course of mood symptoms in dementia is attributed to the cognitive loss and reduced communication skills related to the dementia. In patients with depression that lasts ≥2 weeks and that results in significant distress, a trial of an antidepressant medication should be strongly considered. Similarly, if depressive symptoms last >2 months after behavioral interventions have been implemented, treatment with antidepressant medications is warranted.

First-line agents are the SSRIs, preferred for their favorable adverse-event profiles. Studies of depression in patients with dementia have demonstrated the efficacy of sertraline and citalopram versus placebo (SOE=B), but other studies using the same medications as well as paroxetine and fluoxetine have been inconclusive.

Table 37.2—Medications to Treat Depressive Features of Behavioral Disturbances in Dementia

Medication	Dosage (mg/d)	Uses	Precautions
Selective serotonin reuptake inhibitors (SSRIs)			
Citalopram	10–20	Depression, anxiety[OL]	GI upset, nausea, insomnia (common among all SSRIs), risk of QT_c prolongation with doses >20 mg
Escitalopram	5–20	Depression, anxiety	
Fluoxetine	10–40	Depression, anxiety	Long half-life, greater inhibition of the cytochrome P-450 system
Paroxetine	10–40	Depression, anxiety	Greater inhibition of cytochrome P-450 system, some anticholinergic effects
Sertraline	25–100	Depression, anxiety	
Vilazodone	10–40	Depression, anxiety	Take with food, dosage adjustment required in severe hepatic impairment, reduce dose to 20 mg if given with CYP3A4 inhibitors
Vortioxetine	5–10	Depression	Nausea, dizziness, fewer sexual adverse events than other SSRIs
Serotonin norepinephrine reuptake inhibitors (SNRIs)			
Desvenlafaxine	25–50	Depression, fibromyalgia	Nausea, hypertension, dry mouth, headaches, dizziness
Duloxetine	20–60	Depression, diabetic neuropathy	Nausea, dry mouth, dizziness, hypertension
Mirtazapine	7.5–30	Useful for depression with insomnia and weight loss	Sedation, hypotension, potential for neutropenia
Venlafaxine	25–150	Useful in severe depression, anxiety	Hypertension may be a problem, insomnia
Tricyclic antidepressants (TCAs)			
Desipramine	10–100	Useful in severe depression, anxiety; high degree of efficacy	Anticholinergic effects, hypotension, sedation, cardiac arrhythmias (conduction delays)
Nortriptyline	10–75	High efficacy for depression if adverse events are tolerable; therapeutic range 50–150 ng/mL	Anticholinergic effects, hypotension, sedation, cardiac arrhythmias (conduction delays), caution in patients with glaucoma
Other			
Buproprion	75–225	More activating, lack of cardiac effects	Irritability, insomnia
Gabapentin	100–300	Anxiety[OL], insomnia[OL]	Sedation, falls, hypotension
Trazodone	25–150	When sedation is desirable	Sedation, falls, hypotension

For the antidepressants most commonly used to treat depressive symptoms in dementia, see Table 37.2. The FDA warns that there is a dose-dependent risk of QT prolongation with citalopram and advises that for patients >60 years old the maximum dose should be 20 mg/d.

The treatment of depression in dementia requires persistence. If a first agent has failed after administration of an adequate therapeutic dose for 8–12 weeks, an alternative agent should be tried. Venlafaxine, bupropion, mirtazapine, and the tricyclic agents desipramine and nortriptyline might be considered. Tricyclics should be avoided if a bundle-branch block or other significant cardiac conduction disturbance is present. For patients who have a partial response to an antidepressant, augmentation strategies might be considered. The addition of a stimulant such as methylphenidate[OL] (2.5–10 mg/d) may be helpful in some cases (SOE=C), but there is some risk of increasing psychotic symptoms if the patient tends to be suspicious or delusional. Also, the addition of stimulants such as methylphenidate to augment bupropion should be avoided, because bupropion already has stimulant effects. If the patient does not improve, the agents should be discontinued. If a patient continues to be significantly depressed after several antidepressant trials and is in danger because of serious weight loss or suicidal ideas, electroconvulsive therapy might be considered. This is the most efficacious and rapidly effective treatment for severe major depression and has a favorable safety profile even in mild dementia (SOE=B).

Table 37.3—Mood Stabilizers for Behavioral Disturbances in Dementia with Manic-like Features

Medication	Geriatric Dosage	Adverse Events	Comments
Carbamazepine[OL,a,b]	200–1,000 mg/d (therapeutic level 4–12 mcg/mL)	Nausea, fatigue, ataxia, blurred vision, hyponatremia	Poor tolerability in older adults; monitor CBC, liver function tests, electrolytes every 2 weeks for first 2 months, then every 3 months
Lamotrigine[OL,b]	25–200 mg/d	Skin rash, rare cases of Stevens-Johnson syndrome, dizziness, sedation, neutropenia, anemia	Increased adverse events and interactions when used with divalproex, slow-dose titration required
Lithium[OL,a,b]	150–1,000 mg/d (therapeutic level 0.5–0.8 mEq/L)	Nausea, vomiting, tremor, confusion, leukocytosis	Poor tolerability in older adults; toxicity at low serum concentrations; monitor thyroid and renal function
Divalproex sodium[OL,a,b]	250–2,000 mg/d (therapeutic level 50–100 mcg/mL)	Nausea, GI upset, ataxia, sedation, hyponatremia	Monitor CBC, platelets, liver function tests at baseline and every 6 months; better tolerated than other mood stabilizers in older adults

[a] Approved by FDA for treatment of bipolar disorder
[b] 2009 FDA warning regarding increase in suicidal thoughts and behaviors among all populations treated with anticonvulsant agents, including those used as mood stabilizers

Common adverse effects of antidepressants include sedation, insomnia, GI upset, falls, and for tricyclic agents cardiac adverse events. The serotoninergic-norepinephrine reuptake inhibitors venlafaxine, duloxetine, and desvenlafaxine may cause dose-related hypertension. Patients should be monitored for development of serotonin syndrome, a potentially fatal result of multiple or high-dose agents that increase availability of serotonin.

Manic-like Behavioral Syndromes

Occasionally, mood syndromes may develop in dementia patients that are characterized by pressured speech, disinhibition, elevated or irritable mood, intrusiveness, hyperactivity, impulsivity, and reduced sleep. These syndromes frequently bear a resemblance to the manic episodes seen in the context of bipolar affective disorder in younger adults, although they are generally considered to be secondary to the dementing disorder. The important distinction in the dementia patient is the frequent co-occurrence with confusional states and a tendency to have more of a fluctuating mood, ie, the patient's mood may be irritable or hostile as opposed to euphoric. The appearance of hypersexual behaviors may be seen in this clinical presentation, although sexual disinhibition frequently occurs with dementia as a consequence of reduced frontal-executive functioning and may not necessarily be part of a manic syndrome.

Treatment of manic-like states, emotional lability, disinhibition, or irritability typically begins with the use of mood-stabilizing agents such as divalproex sodium[OL] (Table 37.3). The sustained-release preparation divalproex sodium is commonly recommended (SOE=C). In dementia patients, a typical starting dosage of divalproex is 125 mg q12h. The dosage should be titrated upward slowly while the patient is monitored for sedation, ataxia, and falls. Serum concentrations in the range of 50–100 mcg/mL have been shown to be effective, but individual variability in dosage and response is great. Because of the potential adverse effects on the liver and thrombocytopenia, transaminase levels and a CBC with platelets should be done before therapy is started, rechecked with each dosage increase, and repeated at least every 6 months while the patient remains on the medication. Alternatives to divalproex sodium are carbamazepine[OL], lamotrigine[OL], or lithium[OL]. Carbamazepine starting at 100 mg q12h (with monitoring of liver enzymes and CBC) is an acceptable alternative for manic-like states, mood lability, or irritability in dementia. Leukopenia is of concern with carbamazepine, and monitoring the CBC with every dosage increase and at least every 3 months while the patient remains on the medication is needed. Lamotrigine is approved by the FDA for treatment of mania, but no trials have been conducted in older adults. Lithium is valuable as a mood stabilizer, but its use may be a problem in older adults because of enhanced sensitivity to adverse events. Increased lithium concentrations may occur in the context of reduced renal function and dehydration, resulting in ataxia, tremor, GI distress, and confusion.

Delusions and Hallucinations

Delusions (fixed false beliefs) or hallucinations (sensory experiences without stimuli), whether occurring independently or in association with mood syndromes, typically require specific pharmacologic treatment if

Table 37.4—Antipsychotic Medications for Treatment of Psychosis (Hallucinations and Delusions) in Dementia

Medication	Dosage (mg/d)	Adverse Events[a]	Formulations	Comments
Aripiprazole[OL]	2–20	Mild sedation, mild hypotension	Tablet, rapidly dissolving tablet, IM injection, liquid concentrate	Give in AM
Asenapine[OL]	5–10	Sedation	Sublingual tablet	Only sublingual use
Clozapine[OL]	12.5–200	Sedation, hypotension, anticholinergic effects, agranulocytosis	Tablet, rapidly dissolving tablet	Weekly CBCs required; poorly tolerated by older adults; reserved for treatment of refractory cases
Haloperidol[OL]	0.5–3	Extrapyramidal symptoms, sedation	Tablet, liquid, IM injection, long-acting injection	First-generation agent
Iloperidone[OL]	1–12	Sedation, orthostatic hypotension	Tablet	Dosage reduction with use of CYP3A4 and CYP2D6 inhibitors
Lurasidone[OL]	40–80	Sedation	Tablet	Do not exceed 40 mg/d with CYP3A4 inhibitors
Olanzapine[OL]	2.5–15	Sedation, falls, gait disturbance	Tablet, rapidly dissolving tablet, IM injection	Weight gain, hyperglycemia
Paliperidone[OL]	1.5–12	Sedation, fatigue, GI upset, extrapyramidal symptoms	Sustained-release tablet, depot IM long-acting injection	Dosage reduction in renal impairment
Perphenazine[OL]	2–12	Extrapyramidal symptoms, sedation	Tablet	First-generation agent
Quetiapine[OL]	25–200	Sedation, hypotension	Tablet, sustained-released tablet	Ophthalmologic examination recommended every 6 months
Risperidone[OL]	0.5–2	Sedation, hypotension, extrapyramidal symptoms with dosages >1 mg/d	Tablet, rapidly dissolving tablet, depot IM long-acting injection, liquid concentrate	
Ziprasidone[OL]	40–160	Higher risk of QT_c prolongation	Capsule, IM injection	Warning about increased QT_c prolongation; little published information on use in older adults

[a] All listed medications have warnings about hyperglycemia, cerebrovascular events, and increase in all-cause mortality in patients with dementia.

the patient is disturbed by these experiences, or if the experiences lead to disruptions in the patient's environment that cannot otherwise be controlled. Clinical criteria for the diagnosis of Alzheimer dementia with psychosis specifies that the presence of delusions or hallucinations occur for at least 1 month, at least intermittently, and must cause distress for the patient. A sample of antipsychotic drugs is listed in Table 37.4, along with dosing information. The second-generation agents risperidone[OL], olanzapine[OL], quetiapine[OL], andaripiprazole[OL] are used more commonly than first-generation agents such as haloperidol[OL]. The first-generation agents are more likely to cause extrapyramidal adverse events, such as parkinsonism and tardive dyskinesia. Sedation, hypotension, and falls are common adverse events with all antipsychotic agents.

As these medications are more widely used, differences in adverse-event profiles are emerging. The FDA has required that warnings regarding diabetes mellitus, hyperglycemia, ketoacidosis, and hyperosmolar states be included as a risk of therapy with all second-generation antipsychotic agents. Quetiapine is the most sedating of the second-generation agents. Clozapine[OL], the first of the second-generation agents to be introduced, is difficult to use because of the need for weekly CBC monitoring, adverse events of sedation and orthostatic hypotension, and risk of agranulocytosis. Clozapine is still helpful in a small group of patients with psychosis associated with Parkinson dementia or dementia with Lewy bodies who are unable to tolerate the extrapyramidal adverse events of other agents; quetiapine can also be used in this situation. Clinicians must be prepared to monitor for the emergence of adverse effects among all patients treated with antipsychotic agents and to counsel caregivers regarding the possible adverse effects of these medications before treatment is started.

Table 37.5—Behavioral Management of Insomnia

- Establish a stable routine for going to bed and awakening.
- Advise and educate caregivers regarding the natural fragmented sleep patterns associated with dementia.
- Optimize sleep environment (attention to noise, light, temperature).
- Increase daytime activity, use of regular light exercise and exposure to natural sunlight.
- Reduce or eliminate caffeine, nicotine, alcohol.
- Reduce evening fluid consumption to minimize nocturia.
- Give activating medications (eg, steroids) early in the day.
- Control nighttime pain.
- Limit daytime napping to periods of 20–30 min.
- Use relaxation, stress management, breathing techniques to promote natural sleep.
- Provide a safe environment for the patient to stay awake if unable to sleep.

An increased risk of cerebrovascular events in patients with dementia was identified with use of second-generation agents in 2002. All such agents, including risperidone, olanzapine, aripiprazole, quetiapine, clozapine, ziprasidone, and paliperidone must carry this warning. It should be noted that most cerebrovascular events were not fatal.

In 2005, the FDA required that the manufacturers of aripiprazole[OL], olanzapine[OL], quetiapine[OL], risperidone[OL], clozapine[OL], and ziprasidone[OL], and all additional second-generation antipsychotic agents add a "black box" warning to their labeling describing an increased risk of mortality that was observed in 17 placebo-controlled studies (SOE=A). In these studies, the rate of death for patients with dementia was approximately 1.6–1.7 times that of placebo. In most cases, the cause of death appeared to be heart related or from infections (eg, pneumonia). All new second-generation agents, including rapid-release clozapine and paliperidone, must carry this warning. Based on two observational studies, in 2008, the FDA required that all first-generation antipsychotic agents also have a "black box" warning regarding an increase in all-cause mortality among patients with dementia who are treated with these agents (SOE=B). The mechanism of action of the increase in mortality is not understood, and the FDA has stated that it is not indicating that clinicians should never use these agents to treat patients with dementia and psychosis. It is strongly suggested that clinicians discuss the risks and benefits of treatment with these agents with families and caregivers before starting therapy. More information on these warnings is available at www.fda.gov/.

Although antipsychotic agents have demonstrated efficacy in large controlled trials in the treatment of dementia with psychosis and aggression, overall positive effects have been relatively modest (SOE=B). Controlled studies of geriatric patients have had very high placebo responses. Although 45%–55% of patients improved on antipsychotic medications, the response to placebo ranged from 30% to 50% across studies. Studies of several antipsychotic agents show that risperidone and aripiprazole may be more effective than placebo for symptoms such as anger, aggression, and paranoid ideation when used for ≤12 weeks (SOE=B). However, use of antipsychotic agents did not appear to improve functional status, care needs, or quality of life. Antipsychotic agents clearly play an important role in the treatment of delusions, hallucinations, and aggression in dementia, but they must be part of a comprehensive treatment plan that includes frequent dosage evaluation, monitoring of adverse effects, and time-limited treatment.

There is some evidence that cholinomimetic agents such as donepezil or galantamine may reduce the onset of psychosis and behavioral disturbances of Alzheimer disease. Studies comparing these agents with placebo in patients with mild to moderate Alzheimer disease have suggested that they may reduce the rate of emergence of behavioral disturbances and psychosis (SOE=B). One area in which cholinesterase inhibitors may be likely to improve psychosis is in the case of dementia with Lewy bodies. Reduced visual hallucinations have been reported with cholinesterase inhibitor treatment (SOE=C). Galantamine[OL] in dosages of 16–24 mg/d may be useful in the treatment of patients with Lewy body dementia, who are uniquely sensitive to the extrapyramidal adverse events of antipsychotic agents. More recent studies including patients with Alzheimer dementia and behavioral disturbances failed to demonstrate that agents such as donepezil or memantine were effective in reducing behavioral and psychologic disturbances once the symptoms were present. Benzodiazepines are generally avoided due to concerns about causing disinhibition with increased agitation in older and demented patients.

Disturbances of Sleep

Treatment of insomnia and sleep-wake cycle disturbance should begin with improvement of sleep hygiene (Table 37.5). This consists of efforts to get the patient to go to sleep later every day, around 10:00 or 11:00 pm, while keeping the environment calm, comfortable, and conducive to sleep, into the next morning. If the sleep disturbance is associated with depression, suspiciousness, or delusions, those conditions should be treated.

For primary sleep disturbances when good sleep hygiene and increasing daytime activity level are not successful, trazodone[OL] (25–50 mg at bedtime) or mirtazapine^OL (7.5–15 mg at bedtime) might be used (SOE=D). Gabapentin is increasingly used because of its sedative properties for insomnia and anxiety (SOE=D). Benzodiazepines or antihistamines, such as diphenhydramine, should be avoided, because they carry a high risk of falls, hip fractures, disinhibition, and cognitive disturbance when prescribed for patients with dementia.

Zolpidem^OL and zaleplon^OL are short-acting nonbenzodiazepine sedative hypnotics that may be helpful for sleep disturbances in older adults, although there have been no controlled trials for their use in sleep disturbances secondary to dementia. Zolpidem has been studied in older patients without dementia and appears to be effective in improving sleep onset, although it does not improve sleep duration because of its short half-life. The recommended dose of zolpidem in older adults is 5 mg, because an increased risk of adverse events appears to be dose related. Zaleplon has also been studied in older patients and appears to have similar properties. Melatonin is commonly available OTC and found to be helpful in some older adults. It has a relatively benign adverse-event profile (SOE=C).

Inappropriate Sexual Behavior

Inappropriate sexual behavior includes exposing oneself, touching, or grabbing in a sexual aggressive manner. It is imperative to exclude treatable causes such as underlying urinary tract infections or other general medical conditions. Simple solutions like changes in bedding, providing adaptive clothing, following a toileting schedule, and providing comfort measures may reduce the incidence of inappropriate sexual behaviors. If this occurs in association with another recognizable syndrome such as a mania-like state, treatment of the specific syndrome, such as with mood stabilizers, should be undertaken. SSRIs have also been used for behavioral issues in patients with dementia.

In men with dementia who are dangerously hypersexual or aggressive, clinical case reports have suggested that a trial of an antiandrogen might be attempted to reduce the sexual drive (SOE=D). Patients have been tried on oral progesterone^OL starting at 5 mg/d. The dosage should be adjusted to suppress serum testosterone well below normal. If the patient responds well behaviorally, 10 mg of depot intramuscular progesterone may be given weekly to maintain reduced sexual drive. An alternative treatment to reduce sexual drive is leuprolide acetate^OL (5–10 mg IM every month), also an antiandrogen. The use of antipsychotic medications is often adopted clinically, given the seriousness of hypersexual behaviors in institutionalized settings such as nursing homes; however, there are no controlled studies supporting this use. Presumably, these medications may enhance the cognitive focus of the individual's perceptions by reducing any psychotic thinking that may in some way be contributing to hypersexual behavior. Studies of nonpharmacologic interventions are needed for this problem.

Intermittent Aggression or Agitation

When disruptive behavior occurs intermittently or episodically, such as once per week or less, behavioral interventions focusing on identifying the antecedents of the behavior and avoiding the triggers are often most useful. Behavior modification using positive reinforcement of desirable behavior has been shown to be helpful, and it also helps encourage the caregiver to focus on times when behavior is not a problem. Caregiver education and support, music therapy, and physical activity appear to show promise in reducing behavioral disturbances (SOE=B). Reminiscence, validation therapy, and environmental modifications (ie, of light, sound, and space) may all help promote positive behavior. Distraction techniques, activity therapies, and aromatherapy also show promise in reducing troublesome behaviors (SOE=C).

The combination agent dextromethorphan-quidine is being studied for the treatment of generalized agitation. Early studies show promise but are limited.

Physical restraint in any form should be avoided if at all possible. If restraining measures are necessary, careful supportive care should be provided to the patient. Over time, it is usually possible to reduce or eliminate the amount of restraint.

CHOOSING WISELY® RECOMMENDATIONS

Behavioral Disturbances in Dementia

- Do not use antipsychotics as first choice to treat behavioral and psychological symptoms of dementia.

REFERENCES

- Bardell A, Lau T, Fedoroff JP. Inappropriate sexual behavior in a geriatric population. *Int Psychogeriatr.* 2011;23(7):1182–1188.

    Inappropriate sexual behavior is an uncommon but vexing problem among older patients. This includes such things as public masturbation and excessive or inappropriate sexual comments to health care staff or others (eg, in nursing homes). Patients exhibiting inappropriate sexual behavior typically suffer from neurodegenerative diseases or stroke involving the frontal lobes. Although many strategies have been tried (eg, behavior modification, β-blockers), often without success, second-generation antipsychotics are sometimes effective and medroxyprogesterone is more often effective.

- Berman K, Brodaty H, Withall A, et al. Pharmacological treatment of apathy in dementia. *Am J Geriatr Psychiatry.* 2012;20(2):104–121.

    This article identifies the clinical syndrome of apathy in dementia and reviews the available literature on treatment. Apathy was found to be nearly universal among patients with dementia. There is limited evidence for the efficacy of most psychopharmacologic agents for the treatment of apathy in dementia. The best results were found for cholinesterase inhibitors, with limited efficacy for memantine. Very modest effects were found for the use of stimulants, calcium channel blockers, and antipsychotics, with adverse effects limiting treatment. No evidence was found in the literature to support the use of antidepressant or anticonvulsant agents for treatment of apathy in dementia. Unfortunately, psychosocial interventions were not of sufficient quality to be reviewed.

- Brodaty H, Arasaratnam C. Meta-analysis of nonpharmacological interventions for neuropsychiatric symptoms of dementia. *Am J Psychiatry.* 2012;169(9):946–953.

    Nonpharmacological interventions delivered by family caregivers have the potential to reduce the frequency and severity of behavioral and psychological symptoms of dementia, with effect sizes at least equaling those of pharmacotherapy, as well as to reduce caregivers' adverse reactions.

- Kales HC, Kim HM, Zivin K, et al. Risk of mortality among individual antipsychotics in patients with dementia. *Am J Psychiatry.* 2012;169(1):71–79.

    This large, retrospective cohort study of older outpatients in the Department of Veterans Affairs included those treated with haloperidol, risperidone, olanzapine, quetiapine, and valproic acid. All agents were identified as having some increase in risk of mortality, although the time frame (30 days for haloperidol and 120 days for second-generation agents) was variable. Valproic acid and its derivatives may carry a small risk as well. This study indicates that the need for treatment should be carefully identified, and the risks and benefits discussed with patients and caregivers.

- Livingston G, Kelly L, Lewis-Holmes E, et al. A systematic review of the clinical effectiveness and cost-effectiveness of sensory, psychological and behavioral interventions for managing agitation in older adults with dementia. *Health Technol Assess.* 2014;18(39):1–226.

    This review concluded that person-centered care, communication skills and dementia care mapping (all with supervision), sensory therapy activities, and structured music therapies reduce agitation in care-home dementia residents.

- Nelson JC, Devanand DP. A systematic review and meta-analysis of placebo-controlled antidepressant studies in people with depression and dementia. *J Am Geriatr Soc.* 2011;59(4):577–585.

    The evidence for the efficacy of antidepressant treatment of patients with dementia and depression is suggestive but weak based on this meta-analysis of 7 placebo-controlled trials. Studies were limited by confounding factors, including comorbid medical conditions, severity of dementia, and heterogeneity of the samples. Antidepressant therapy may be beneficial in some populations of patients with dementia.

- Small G, Bullock R. Defining optimal treatment with cholinesterase inhibitors in Alzheimer's disease. *Alzheimers Dement.* 2011;7(2):177–184.

    Cholinesterase inhibitors became available for the treatment of dementia in 1992. Optimal strategies to identify who may benefit most from the use of these agents is still perplexing to many clinicians. These agents may delay the need for institutional placement and, in some patients, may slow the emergence of behavioral disturbances. This article identifies treatment and management strategies for use of these agents.

Melinda S. Lantz, MD
Pui Yin Wong, MD

CHAPTER 38—DELIRIUM

KEY POINTS

- The new *Diagnostic and Statistical Manual of Mental Disorders, Fifth Edition (DSM-5)* criteria characterize delirium as a disorder of attention and awareness that develops acutely and tends to fluctuate.

- The first key step in delirium management is accurate diagnosis; several brief diagnostic assessments are available that operationalize the Confusion Assessment Method diagnostic algorithm after administration of a brief mental status examination that includes testing attention.

- All delirious patients require a thorough evaluation for reversible causes; all correctable contributing factors should be addressed.

- In addition to the established associations of delirium with death, functional decline, and nursing home placement, new evidence shows that patients with delirium are at increased risk of prolonged cognitive decline and dementia.

- Pharmacologic intervention should be reserved for key target symptoms that cannot be adequately managed with nonpharmacologic interventions; low-dose, high-potency antipsychotics are usually the treatment of choice.

- Proactive, multifactorial interventions have reduced the incidence, severity, and duration of delirium.

Delirium has been described in the medical literature for more than two thousand years. Despite this, it remains under-recognized and often inappropriately evaluated and managed. Clinicians call delirium by many different names; up to 30 synonyms exist in the peer-reviewed literature. *Acute confusional state* is the most common synonym, and the term still preferred today by some specialties, such as neurology. Other common synonyms include *acute mental status change*, *altered mental status*, and *toxic* or *metabolic encephalopathy*. The International Classification of Disease coding (ICD-10-CM) has one major code for delirium (R41.0), with multiple qualifiers and related codes under other entities.

INCIDENCE AND PROGNOSIS

Delirium is common and associated with substantial morbidity and mortality. Approximately one-third of patients ≥70 years old admitted to a general medical service experience delirium; one-half of these are delirious on admission to the hospital, while the other half develops delirium in the hospital. Among those admitted to intensive care units, the prevalence of delirium is much higher, and when rates for delirium are combined with those for stupor and coma, prevalence rates exceed 75%. Ten to fifteen percent of older adults presenting to the emergency department are delirious. In post-acute skilled-nursing facilities, approximately 15% of new admissions meet criteria for delirium. The prevalence of delirium at the end of life is reported to be as high as 85%, while the overall prevalence in the community is reported to be 1%–2%, largely among older patients recently discharged from the hospital.

Although delirium is traditionally viewed as a transient phenomenon, there is growing evidence that it may persist for weeks to months in a substantial portion of affected individuals (SOE=A). A systematic review found that persistence rates for delirium at hospital discharge and at 1, 3, and 6 months after discharge were 45%, 33%, 26%, and 21%, respectively. Risk factors for delirium persistence predominantly relate to predisposing factors, including advanced age, preexisting dementia, multiple comorbidities, and functional impairment, but also include severity of delirium and use of restraints. When delirium persists beyond 6 months, it is likely that the patient will have permanent cognitive decline, and the resulting condition should be called dementia/neurocognitive disorder or mild cognitive impairment (mild neurocognitive disorder), depending on its severity.

Evidence is mounting that delirium is strongly and independently associated with poor patient outcomes (SOE=A). A meta-analysis that included almost 3,000 patients followed for a mean of 22.7 months demonstrated that delirium was independently associated with an increased risk of death (OR 2.0; 95% CI, 1.5–2.5), institutionalization (OR 2.4; 95% CI, 1.8–3.3), and dementia (OR 12.5; 95% CI, 11.9–84.2). Further, rates of mortality, nursing-home placement, functional decline, and dementia are consistently higher in patients with persistent delirium than in patients whose delirium resolves more quickly.

DIAGNOSIS AND DIFFERENTIAL DIAGNOSIS

Under-recognition of delirium is a major problem, with only 12%–35% of all cases recognized in routine care. Several systematic reviews have recommended the Confusion Assessment Method (CAM) as the most useful bedside assessment tool for delirium (www.hospitalelderlifeprogram.org). Clinicians can establish

Table 38.1—Comparison of 4 Brief Instruments for Assessment of Delirium

Instrument	CAM-[a] based?	Process	Validation Study	Test Characteristics	Comments
CAM-ICU[b]	Yes	2 Steps: Administer RASS[c]— if markedly abnormal, stop, consider "delirious" Otherwise administer CAM-ICU[c]: Assess attention: HAVEAHAART and picture recognition task Assess disorganized thinking: follow commands, 4 yes/no questions Assess acute change, altered level of consciousness using the RASS	406 emergency department patients Mean age: 73.5 years Delirium: 12% Dementia: 6% Reference standard delirium diagnosis: Comprehensive 30-min assessment by psychiatrist using *DSM-IV* criteria Dementia diagnosis: medical record documentation	*Overall:* Sensitivity: 68%–72% Specificity: 99% *No dementia:* Sensitivity: 48% Specificity: 99% *Dementia:* Sensitivity: 94% Specificity: 83%	Designed originally for nonverbal patients in ICU. Applied to verbal patients in emergency department. Other studies report lower sensitivity.
B-CAM[d]	Yes	2 Steps: delirium triage screen: RASS plus "lunch" backwards If negative, stop. If positive, administer B-CAM: Similar to CAM-ICU except months of year backwards to July is substituted as attention task	Same study as above.	*Overall:* Sensitivity: 78%–82% Specificity: 96%–97% Results stratified by dementia not available	Modification of the CAM-ICU designed for verbal patients.
4AT[e]	No	Assess 4 items: Alertness: level of consciousness Orientation Attention Acute change/fluctuations	236 patients on acute geriatrics ward or a rehabilitation unit Mean age: 83.9 years Delirium: 12% Dementia: 31% Reference standard delirium diagnosis: Clinical assessment by geriatrician Dementia diagnosis: proxy interviews	*Overall:* Sensitivity: 90% Specificity: 84% *No dementia:* Sensitivity: 83% Specificity: 91% *Dementia:* Sensitivity: 94% Specificity: 65%	Brief instrument with a 0–12 score; scores ≥4 indicative of delirium
3D-CAM[f]	Yes	Assess 4 CAM diagnostic features: Acute change: 3 patient-reported symptoms Attention: days of week, months of year backward, digit span 3 and 4 backward Disorganized thinking: orientation to type of place, year, day of the week Observe level of consciousness Optional: 8 interviewer observations linked to CAM features, 1 proxy question	201 patients on an acute general medicine unit Mean age: 84.5 years Delirium: 21% Dementia: 28% Reference standard delirium diagnosis: patient assessment, proxy interview, medical record review. Diagnosis by expert panel using *DSM-IV* criteria Dementia diagnosis: patient, proxy interviews, medical record review	*Overall:* Sensitivity: 95% Specificity: 94% *No dementia:* Sensitivity: 93% Specificity: 96% *Dementia:* Sensitivity: 96% Specificity: 86%	Items selected using modern measurement methods including Item Response Theory. Assessment completed in median of 3 minutes.

NOTE: CAM = Confusion Assessment Method, RASS = Richmond Agitation and Sedation Scale

[a] Inouye SK, van Dyck CH, Alessi CA, et al. Clarifying confusion: the Confusion Assessment Method: a new method for detection of delirium. *Ann Intern Med*. 1990;113:941–948.

[b] Han JH, Wilson A, Graves AJ, et al. Validation of the Confusion Assessment Method for the Intensive Care Unit in older emergency department patients. *Acad Emerg Med*. 2014;21:180–187.

[c] Ely EW, Margolin R, Francis J, et al. Evaluation of delirium in critically ill patients: validation of the Confusion Assessment Method for the Intensive Care Unit (CAM-ICU). *Crit Care Med*. 2001;29:1370–1379.

[d] Han JH, Wilson A, Vasilevskis EE, et al. Diagnosing delirium in older emergency department patients: validity and reliability of the delirium triage screen and the brief confusion assessment method. *Ann Emerg Med*. 2013;62:457–465.

[e] Bellelli G, Morandi A, Davis D, et al. Validation of the 4AT, a new instrument for rapid delirium screening: a study in 234 hospitalised older people. *Age Ageing*. 2014;43:1–7.

[f] Marcantonio ER, Ngo L, O'Connor MA, et al. 3D-CAM: validation of a 3-minute diagnostic interview for CAM-defined delirium. *Ann Intern Med*. 2014;161:554–561.

the diagnosis of delirium by judging the presence or absence of the four key CAM features: acute change or fluctuating course, inattention, disorganized thinking, and 4) altered level of consciousness. Although the CAM can be completed by using observations from routine care, use of a formal mental status evaluation greatly improves detection and reliability of the assessment. Over the past 2 years, 3 brief assessment tools have been developed for assessment of delirium. These 3 assessment tools, along with the CAM-ICU, are described in Table 38.1. In the absence of a formal evaluation or when there is doubt, any older adult with acute change in mental status should be considered delirious, and evaluated and managed as described below.

To improve recognition of delirium, medical centers are starting to use standardized tools (see Table 38.1) to screen high-risk patients, such as those in the ICU or who have had major surgery or are very old. Such screening is particularly important for identifying cases of hypoactive delirium, which might otherwise go unnoticed by the care team. A brief but standardized screening assessment should be administered on a daily basis, or even more frequently. Frequent standardized assessment and documentation of mental status is also important to allow detection of acute changes and fluctuations, which are a key feature of delirium. There is no consensus on how to best implement widespread screening for delirium. It could be performed by physicians, nurses, or other hospital personnel; if performed by personnel other than the patient's physician or nurse, the results need to be promptly and reliably communicated to the primary care team to allow for timely intervention. Importantly, widespread screening needs to be coupled with education on best practices of delirium management (see below).

The differential diagnosis of delirium includes dementia, depression, and acute psychiatric syndromes. In many cases, it is not truly a "differential" diagnosis, because these syndromes can coexist and indeed are risk factors for one another. Instead, it is better thought of as a series of independent questions: Does this patient have delirium? Does he or she have dementia? Does he or she have depression? Does the patient have more than one disorder? The most common diagnostic issue is whether a newly presenting confused patient has dementia, delirium, or both. To make this determination, the clinician must ascertain the patient's baseline status. In the absence of prior knowledge or documentation of the patient's baseline cognitive function, information from family members, caregivers, or others who know the patient is essential. An acute change in mental status from baseline is not consistent with dementia and suggests delirium. In addition, a rapidly fluctuating course (over minutes to hours) and an abnormal level of consciousness are also highly suggestive of delirium. Depression can also be confused with hypoactive delirium. Finally, certain acute psychiatric syndromes, such as mania, can present similarly to hyperactive delirium. Hyperactive patients are best initially evaluated and managed as if they have delirium rather than attributing the presentation to psychiatric disease and potentially missing a serious underlying medical disorder.

THE SPECTRUM AND NEUROPATHOPHYSIOLOGY OF DELIRIUM

The classic presentation of delirium is thought to be the extremely agitated patient. However, agitated, hyperactive, or mixed delirium represents only 25% of cases, with the remaining having hypoactive ("quiet") delirium. Evidence suggests that hypoactive delirium is associated with an equal or poorer prognosis than delirium with hyperactive or normal psychomotor features (SOE=B). Potentially, one of the reasons for this poorer prognosis is that hypoactive delirium is less frequently recognized. As described above, special case-finding efforts are necessary to detect hypoactive delirium among high-risk older adults. If agitation is present, behavioral interventions may be necessary (see below), but such measures alone are not adequate treatment for delirium, and in some cases they can exacerbate or prolong delirium.

Although delirium is often said to be either present or absent, the number and severity of symptoms vary widely. To more completely describe delirium, several severity scales have been validated and published. The most recent scale, termed CAM-Severity (or CAM-S), is derived directly from the CAM and has both a long form that uses all 10 CAM delirium features (scored 0–19, 19 worst) and a short form that uses only the 4 CAM diagnostic features (scored 0–7, 7 worst). The CAM-S has excellent predictive validity (incremental beyond diagnosis) for several important clinical and health utilization outcomes. Patients who have some delirium features, but do not meet all diagnostic criteria, have subsyndromal delirium, which is renamed "attenuated delirium" in *DSM-5*. Regardless of its name, this entity has been associated with poor outcomes, although not as serious as full delirium. There is a gradient of worsening outcomes over the spectrum of delirium.

Research into the pathophysiology of delirium is accelerating rapidly but has not yet progressed to the point that it has an impact on clinical management. One of the best-documented mechanisms of delirium is cholinergic deficiency. This is seen classically in overdoses of anticholinergic medications such as

Table 38.2—Mnemonic for Reversible Causes of Delirium

Drugs	Any new additions, increased dosages, or interactions
	Consider OTC drugs and alcohol
	Consider especially high-risk drugs (Table 38.4)
Electrolyte disturbances	Especially dehydration, sodium imbalance
	Thyroid abnormalities
Lack of drugs	Withdrawals from chronically used sedatives, including alcohol and sleeping pills
	Poorly controlled pain (lack of analgesia)
Infection	Especially urinary and respiratory tract infections
Reduced sensory input	Poor vision, poor hearing (lack of glasses, hearing aids in the hospital)
Intracranial	Infection, hemorrhage, stroke, tumor
	Rare; consider only if new focal neurologic findings, suggestive history, or diagnostic evaluation otherwise negative
Urinary, fecal	Urinary retention: "cystocerebral syndrome"
	Fecal impaction
Myocardial, pulmonary	Myocardial infarction, arrhythmia, exacerbation of heart failure, exacerbation of COPD, hypoxia

atropine, which in severe cases can be reversed by administration of physostigmine. In addition, many medications not classified as anticholinergic (eg, antihistamines, certain opioids, and antidepressants) have substantial anticholinergic activity and can also precipitate delirium. Indices have been developed that enable clinicians to estimate the anticholinergic burden of a patient's medication regimen. Despite their potential ability to reverse cholinergic deficiency, the cholinesterase inhibitors donepezil, rivastigmine, and galantamine have not been effective for either the prevention or treatment of delirium (SOE=B).

A second potential mechanism of delirium is inflammation, which can be particularly important in postoperative patients and in those with cancer or infection. A growing body of literature has documented an association of delirium with increased levels of inflammatory markers, including C-reactive protein, interleukin-1β and 6, and tumor necrosis factor α. Inflammation can break down the blood-brain barrier, allowing toxic medications and cytokines greater access to the CNS. Once in the CNS, inflammation can cause direct toxicity to neurons, which may explain increased levels of neuronal injury markers such as S-100β in the serum of patients with delirium, and also the potential link between delirium and long-term cognitive dysfunction.

RISK FACTORS

In the absence of a clear neuropathophysiologic basis for delirium, the cornerstone of management of delirium focuses on the assessment and treatment of modifiable risk factors. Several consistent risk factors for delirium have been identified and classified into two groups: baseline factors that predispose patients to delirium, and acute factors that precipitate delirium. Predisposing factors include advanced age, preexisting dementia, preexisting functional impairment in activities of daily living, and high medical comorbidity. Male gender, sensory impairment (poor vision and hearing), depressive symptoms, laboratory abnormalities, and history of alcohol abuse have also been reported in some studies. Acute precipitating factors include medications (especially those that are sedating or highly anticholinergic), surgery, uncontrolled pain, low hematocrit level, bed rest, and use of certain indwelling devices and physical restraints. A useful model suggests that delirium develops when the sum of predisposing and precipitating factors crosses a certain threshold. In such a model, the greater the predisposing factors, the fewer precipitating factors are needed for delirium to develop. This would explain why older, frail adults develop delirium in the face of stressors that are much less severe than stressors that can cause delirium in younger, healthy adults. For a mnemonic for reversible risk factors for delirium, see Table 38.2.

DELIRIUM AND DEMENTIA

Although dementia is an established risk factor for delirium (SOE=A), evidence is increasing that the relationship may be bidirectional. As described above, a meta-analysis demonstrated that nondemented patients who develop delirium are at increased risk of incident dementia over the next 1–5 years (SOE=B). Most of these studies did not involve detailed testing of neuropsychologic performance before the onset of delirium, so it remains unclear whether delirium was the herald of previously unrecognized cognitive impairment (or other brain vulnerability), or whether the delirium itself set forth a CNS process that initiated or accelerated onset of dementia. Complementing these studies in nondemented patients is a growing body of literature demonstrating that patients with Alzheimer disease experience accelerated cognitive decline after an episode of delirium (SOE=B).

Although there is no doubt that delirium and Alzheimer disease are intertwined, several recent studies provide evidence that delirium may exert a negative long-term impact on cognitive function that is independent of Alzheimer disease. A recent study examined the 1-year cognitive trajectories of older cardiac surgery patients and found that delirium is associated with an acute decline in cognitive function and persistent deficits. Patients who did not develop delirium returned to their preoperative cognitive baseline by 1 month after surgery, whereas those with delirium had not returned to baseline 1 year after surgery. In a second recent study that measured cognitive function in survivors of an ICU stay 1 year later, 24% these patients were functioning at or below the level of patients with mild Alzheimer disease. This study was not restricted to older adults, and this level of cognitive dysfunction was seen in all age groups (as young as 18–45 years) and all levels of comorbidity. Finally, in an autopsy study in which the brains of patients with reported episodes of delirium during life with subsequent cognitive decline were examined, there was significant neuropathology that was independent of the typical findings of Alzheimer disease. Taken together, this evidence suggests that delirium is not just an unmasking of latent Alzheimer disease (SOE=B) and, therefore, efforts to prevent and treat delirium (see below) may have a significant public health impact by reducing the burden of cognitive impairment among older adults.

POSTOPERATIVE DELIRIUM

Delirium may be the most common complication after surgery in older adults. The incidence is 15% after elective noncardiac surgery and up to 50% after high-risk procedures such as hip fracture repair, aortic aneurysm repair, and coronary artery bypass grafting. In a prospectively validated clinical prediction rule for delirium after elective noncardiac surgery, 7 risk factors were identified preoperatively: advanced age, cognitive impairment, physical functional impairment, history of alcohol abuse, markedly abnormal serum chemistries, intrathoracic surgery, and aortic aneurysm surgery. Patients with none of these risk factors had a 2% risk of delirium, those with 1 or 2 risk factors had a 10% risk, and those with ≥3 risk factors had a 50% risk. More recently, a clinical prediction rule for delirium after cardiac surgery has been validated. Four risk factors were identified: cognitive impairment, history of stroke or transient ischemic attack, depressive symptoms, and low or high albumin.

In addition to baseline risk factors, intraoperative and postoperative management plays an important role in the development of delirium. Multiple studies demonstrate that the type or route of intraoperative anesthesia, whether general, spinal, epidural, or combined, has little impact on the risk of delirium (SOE=A). However, the total dose of anesthetic agents may play an important role (SOE=B) and efforts to reduce or titrate this dose to the lowest effective amount may reduce delirium. For instance, a randomized trial used Bispectral Index™ monitoring to titrate the dosage of intraoperative sedative medications among hip-fracture patients undergoing surgical repair using spinal anesthesia. Patients in the low-dose arm had a markedly reduced rate of postoperative delirium relative to the high-dose arm (19% versus 40%, $P<.01$).

Postoperative medication management also plays an important role in delirium. Postoperative use of benzodiazepines and certain opioids, especially meperidine, is strongly associated with development of delirium. Although pain medications can cause delirium, adequate pain management is also important, because high levels of postoperative pain have also been associated with delirium. Strategies to provide adequate analgesia with minimally effective doses of opioids should be used. These include the use of scheduled rather than as-needed dosing, patient-controlled analgesic pumps, regional analgesia, opioid-sparing analgesics, and nonpharmacologic approaches, such as ice packs. Low postoperative hematocrit level (<30%) has also been associated with postoperative delirium, although transfusions have not been shown to reduce delirium. The AGS recently published delirium management guidelines focused on surgical patients (see below).

Postoperative cognitive dysfunction (POCD) is a phenomenon that has received considerable attention, with a particular focus on long-term POCD after cardiac surgery. As opposed to delirium, POCD does not have *DSM-5* or ICD diagnostic criteria. POCD is usually defined by declining performance on serial testing with a neurocognitive battery, although there is no consensus as to how this measurement can be used. Interestingly, many studies of POCD have not included good measures of delirium, and many studies of postoperative delirium do not measure POCD. Results from studies that have both measures well integrated are just emerging. These suggest that delirium and POCD are associated but do not fully explain each other, ie, some patients with delirium do not go on to develop POCD, and some patients who develop POCD did not have delirium. Ongoing studies will further elucidate the complex relationship between these 2 entities.

EVALUATION AND MANAGEMENT

All patients with newly diagnosed delirium require a careful history, physical examination, and targeted laboratory testing. Most treatable causes of delirium lie outside the CNS, and these should be investigated first. Moreover, multiple contributing factors are often

Table 38.3—Management of Delirium

Step	Key Issues	Proposed Treatment
Identify and treat reversible contributors	Medications	Reduce or eliminate offending medications, or substitute less psychoactive medications.
	Infections	Treat common infections: urinary, respiratory, soft tissue.
	Fluid balance disorders	Assess and treat dehydration, heart failure, electrolyte disorders.
	Impaired CNS oxygenation	Treat severe anemia, hypoxia, hypotension.
	Severe pain	Assess and treat; use local measures and scheduled pain regimens that minimize opioids; avoid meperidine.
	Sensory deprivation	Use eyeglasses, hearing aids, portable amplifier.
	Elimination problems	Assess and treat urinary retention and fecal impaction.
Maintain behavioral control	Behavioral interventions	Teach hospital staff appropriate interaction with delirious patients; encourage family visitation.
	Pharmacologic interventions	Only if necessary, use low-dose high-potency antipsychotics (Table 38.5).
Anticipate and prevent or manage complications	Urinary incontinence	Implement scheduled toileting program.
	Immobility and falls	Avoid physical restraints; mobilize with assistance; use physical therapy.
	Pressure ulcers	Mobilize; reposition immobilized patient frequently and monitor pressure points.
	Sleep disturbance	Implement a nonpharmacologic sleep hygiene program, including a nighttime sleep protocol; avoid sedatives; minimize unnecessary awakenings (for vital signs, etc).
	Feeding disorders	Assist with feeding; use aspiration precautions; provide nutritional supplementation as necessary.
Restore function in delirious patients	Hospital environment	Reduce clutter and noise (especially at night); provide adequate lighting; have familiar objects brought from home.
	Cognitive reconditioning	Have staff reorient patient to time, place, person at least three times daily.
	Ability to perform ADLs	As delirium clears, match performance to ability.
	Family education, support, and participation	Provide education about delirium, its causes and reversibility, how to interact, and family's role in restoring function.
	Discharge	Because delirium can persist, provide for increased ADL support; follow mental status changes as "barometer" of recovery.

present, so the diagnostic evaluation should not be terminated because a single "cause" is identified. For key steps in the evaluation and management of delirium, see Table 38.3.

The history should focus on the time course of the changes in mental status and their association with other symptoms or events (eg, fever, shortness of breath, medication change). Because medications are the most common and treatable cause of delirium, a careful medication history, using the nursing administration sheets in the hospital or a "brown-bag" review in the outpatient setting, is imperative. In the outpatient setting, it is also important to review the patient's use of OTC drugs, herbal or other supplements, and alcohol. The physical examination should include vital signs and oxygen saturation, a careful general medical examination, and a neurologic and mental status examination focusing on tests of attention. The emphasis should be on identifying acute medical problems or exacerbations of chronic medical problems that might be contributing to delirium.

Laboratory tests and imaging studies should be selected based on the history and examination findings. Most patients require at least a CBC, electrolytes, and kidney function tests. Urinalysis, urine toxicology for drugs of abuse, blood alcohol level, tests for liver function, serum medication levels, arterial blood gases, as well as chest radiographs, an ECG, and appropriate cultures are helpful in selected situations. Cerebral imaging is often performed but is rarely helpful, except in cases of head trauma or new focal neurologic findings. In the absence of seizure activity or signs of meningitis, electroencephalograms and cerebrospinal fluid analysis rarely yield helpful results.

Delirious hospitalized patients are particularly vulnerable to complications and poor outcomes. Special care is needed and requires an interprofessional effort by clinicians, nurses, family members, and others. A multifactorial approach is the most successful, because many factors contribute to delirium; thus, multiple interventions, even if individually small, can yield marked clinical improvement (Table 38.3). If delirium is not diagnosed and managed properly, costly and life-threatening complications and long-term loss of function can result.

Modifying the risk factors that contribute to delirium is critically important. Some factors, such as age and prior cognitive impairment, cannot be modified. However, some predisposing factors, such as sensory impairment, can be modified through proper use of eyeglasses and hearing aids. Newly admitted older adults should be screened for cognitive loss, severity of illness, sensory deficits, and markers of dehydration with a goal

Table 38.4—Drugs to Reduce or Eliminate in Management of Delirium

Agent	Adverse Events	Possible Substitutes	Comments
Alcohol	CNS sedation and withdrawal	If history of heavy intake, careful monitoring and benzodiazepines for withdrawal symptoms	Alcohol history is imperative
Anticholinergics (oxybutynin, benztropine)	Anticholinergic toxicity	Lower dosage, behavioral measures	Rare at low dosages
Anticonvulsants (especially primidone, phenobarbital, phenytoin)	CNS sedation and withdrawal	Alternative agent or none	Toxic reactions can occur despite "therapeutic" drug concentrations
Antidepressants, especially tertiary amine tricyclic agents (amitriptyline, imipramine, doxepin)	Anticholinergic toxicity	Secondary amine tricyclics (nortriptyline, desipramine), SSRIs, or other agents	Secondary amines as good as tertiary for adjuvant treatment of chronic pain
Antihistamines (eg, diphenhydramine)	Anticholinergic toxicity	Nonpharmacologic protocol for sleep, pseudoephedrine for colds, nonsedating antihistamines for allergies	Must take OTC medication history
H_2-blocking agents	Possible anticholinergic toxicity	Lower dosage, antacids or proton-pump inhibitors	Most common with high-dosage intravenous infusions
Antiparkinsonian agents (levodopa-carbidopa, dopamine agonists, amantadine)	Dopaminergic toxicity	Lower dosage; adjusted dosing schedule	Usually with advanced disease and high dosages
Antipsychotics, especially low-potency anticholinergic agents and second-generation agents (clozapine)	Anticholinergic toxicity, CNS sedation	No agents or, if necessary, low-dosage high-potency agents	See note for Table 38.5 for warnings about second-generation antipsychotics
Barbiturates	CNS sedation, severe withdrawal syndrome	Gradual discontinuation or benzodiazepine substitution	In most cases, should no longer be prescribed; avoid inadvertent or abrupt discontinuation
Benzodiazepines	CNS sedation, potential for withdrawal	Nonpharmacologic sleep management, melatonin, ramelteon	Associated with delirium in medical and surgical patients
Chloral hydrate	CNS sedation	Nonpharmacologic sleep protocol, melatonin, ramelteon	No better for delirium than benzodiazepines
Nonbenzodiazepine hypnotics (eg, zolpidem)	CNS sedation and withdrawal	Nonpharmacologic sleep protocol, melatonin, ramelteon	Like other sedatives, can cause delirium
Opioid analgesics (especially meperidine)	Anticholinergic toxicity, CNS sedation, fecal impaction	Local and regional measures and nonpsychoactive pain medications (acetaminophen, NSAIDs) around the clock, reserve opioids for breakthrough and severe pain	Higher risk in patients with renal insufficiency; must consider risks versus benefit
Almost any medication if time course is appropriate			Consider risks and benefits of all medications in older adults

of addressing correctable risk factors proactively before the onset of delirium. Medications are the most common reversible causes of delirium. Anticholinergics, H_2-blockers, benzodiazepines, opioids, and antipsychotic medications should be replaced with medications that have no central effects. For example, H_2-blockers can be replaced by antacids or proton-pump inhibitors, and regular dosing of 650 mg of acetaminophen 3 or 4 times daily can reduce or eliminate the need for opioids in many patients (Table 38.4).

The delirious patient is susceptible to a wide range of iatrogenic complications, and careful surveillance is critical. Bowel and bladder function should be monitored closely, but urinary catheters should be avoided unless absolutely required for monitoring fluids or treating urinary retention. Bowel stimulants and fecal softeners can be used to prevent obstipation, particularly in those who are concomitantly using opioids. Complete bed rest should be avoided, because it can lead to increasing disability through disuse of muscles and development of pressure ulcers and atelectasis in the lungs. Physical exercise and ambulation prevent the deconditioning often associated with hospitalization. Malnutrition can be avoided through use of nutritional supplements and careful attention to intake of food and fluids. Some delirious patients may need assistance for eating.

Table 38.5—Pharmacologic Therapy of Agitated Delirium

Agent	Mechanism of Action	Dosage	Benefits	Adverse Events	Comments
Haloperidol[OL]	Antipsychotic	0.25–1 mg po, IM, or IV q4h prn for agitation	Relatively nonsedating; few hemodynamic effects	EPS, especially if >3 mg/d	Usually agent of choice[a]
Risperidone[OL]	Second-generation antipsychotic	0.25–1 mg po q4h prn for agitation	Similar to haloperidol	Might have slightly fewer EPS than haloperidol	Small trials[b]
Olanzapine[OL]	Second-generation antipsychotic	2.5–5 mg po, SL, or IM q12h, max dosage 20 mg q24h (cannot be given by IV infusion)	Fewer EPS than haloperidol	More sedating than haloperidol	Small trials[b]; oral formulations less effective for acute management
Quetiapine[OL]	Second-generation antipsychotic	25–50 mg po q12h	Fewer EPS than haloperidol; can be used in patients with Parkinsonism	More sedating than haloperidol; hypotension	Small trials[b]
Lorazepam[OL]	Benzodiazepine	0.25–1 mg po or IV q8h prn for agitation	Use in sedative and alcohol withdrawal; history of neuroleptic malignant syndrome	More paradoxical excitation, respiratory depression than haloperidol	Generally should not be used except for specific indications noted under "benefits"

NOTE: EPS = extrapyramidal symptoms
Use of all these drugs for delirium is an off-label indication. Because of the small number and size of trials investigating the use of these agents in the treatment of agitation in delirium, the SOE=B.

[a] In a randomized trial comparing haloperidol, chlorpromazine, and lorazepam in the treatment of agitated delirium in young patients with AIDS, all were found to be equally effective in treating symptoms of psychosis, but haloperidol had the fewest adverse events.

[b] Second-generation antipsychotics have been tested primarily in small equivalency trials with haloperidol and recently in small placebo-controlled trials in the ICU. The FDA requires a "black box" warning for all second-generation antipsychotics because of the increased risk of cerebrovascular events, stroke, and mortality in patients with dementia. First-generation antipsychotic agents also have an FDA "black box" warning regarding an increase in all-cause mortality among patients with dementia.

Managing Behavior in Delirium

Managing behavioral problems while ensuring both the comfort and safety of the patient can be challenging. The patient should be placed in a room near the nursing station for close observation. Nonpharmacologic behavioral measures provide orientation and a feeling of safety. Orienting items such as clocks, calendars, and even a window view should be made available. Patients should be encouraged to wear their eyeglasses and hearing aids. Physical restraints, which are often justified as a means to reduce the risk of patient self-injury, have actually been associated with increased injury (SOE=B). On the regular medical and surgical wards, use of restraints should be reduced, if not eliminated. In the ICU (where 1:1 or 1:2 nursing is available), restraints may be required to prevent the removal of important devices, such as endotracheal tubes, intra-arterial devices, and central intravenous catheters. Whenever restraints are used, the indicators for use should be frequently reassessed, and the restraints should be removed as soon as possible.

Medications used as chemical restraints extract a costly toll in accidents, adverse events, and loss of mobility and should also be avoided if possible. Pharmacologic intervention may be necessary for symptoms such as delusions or hallucinations that are frightening to the patient when verbal comfort and reassurance are not successful. Some delirious patients display behavior that is dangerous to themselves or others and cannot be calmed by a family member or aide. As for physical restraints, indications for pharmacologic intervention should be clearly identified, documented, and constantly reassessed. The lowest dose of the least toxic agent should be used for the shortest time possible. Daily renewal of orders for physical or chemical restraints is one way of ensuring they are stopped when no longer needed.

The literature on pharmacologic management of delirium is growing rapidly and is best understood keeping several important factors in mind: 1) Except in unusual cases (eg, alcohol withdrawal delirium), antipsychotics have a more favorable risk:benefit ratio than benzodiazepines or other sedatives. 2) All use of antipsychotics for delirium is off-label—there are no FDA-approved drugs for the indication of delirium. 3) Many drug treatment and prevention studies were conducted in mixed-age groups in the ICU; it is unclear whether the risk:benefit ratio for use of these drugs will be similar in older hospitalized patients on the general wards. 4) Many studies are not blinded, not placebo controlled, or corporate sponsored, raising concerns about validity. 5) The outcome of some studies is delirium severity; yet, existing delirium severity scales tend to weigh hyperactive symptoms too heavily, so that converting hyperactive delirium to hypoactive delirium (which has worse outcomes, as noted above) is measured as a reduction in severity.

A recent editorial summarized the case for the use (or non-use) of antipsychotics for prevention and treatment of delirium. A total of 7 high quality studies were identified, all published in the past 10 years, with 5/7 addressing prevention (administration of drugs before delirium onset) and 3/7 addressing treatment (1 study addressed both). Of the 5 studies that addressed prevention, 3 showed a reduced rate of delirium, and 2 did not. Of the 2 that did not, one showed reduced duration/severity. One study that showed reduced incidence showed increased duration and severity in the patients who developed delirium in the active treatment arm. Most of the studies showed no differences in other outcomes, such as ICU length of stay, total hospital length of stay, and mortality. Thus, the verdict on giving low-dose antipsychotics to high-risk patients to prevent delirium remains uncertain. In the absence of more definitive evidence, the prudent clinician would be skeptical about adopting this practice into routine care (SOE=C).

In terms of delirium treatment, the data is even more preliminary. Of the 3 high-quality studies noted above that addressed treatment, none demonstrated that antipsychotics reduce the duration of delirium, although some demonstrated a reduction in hyperactive symptoms. There was also no improvement in other outcomes such as mortality, ICU or hospital length of stay, or complications. The decision whether to use antipsychotics might come down to a trade-off between immediate reduction of bothersome symptoms of agitation, hallucinations, and delusions versus the potential risk of antipsychotic-induced complications, prolonged delirium, and long-term cognitive impairment. Until further data are available, this difficult trade-off should be made on a case-by-case basis (SOC=C).

If treatment with antipsychotics is warranted, the literature suggests that all of the drugs listed in the Table 38.5 are equally effective. The choice of agent is often made based on adverse effects. Drugs such as haloperidol and risperidone have the least sedation but greatest risk of extrapyramidal side effects, whereas quetiapine is most sedating and has the least extrapyramidal side effects. The availability of intravenous dosing may be important for patients in the ICU. Regardless of the drug selected, the initial dose should be as low as possible, because there is a wide variability in response. Another dose of the drug can always be administered, but once a dose is administered, it cannot be taken away. For the most part, dosing in delirium (as opposed to in dementia with behavioral disturbances) is on an as-needed basis, although patients with prolonged delirium with behavioral symptoms may need continual scheduled dosing. As noted above, these drugs should be stopped as soon as possible. In the rare circumstances that they are needed beyond hospital discharge, clear parameters for their discontinuation should be included in the discharge paperwork.

Family Counseling

It is important to stress to family members that delirium is usually not a permanent condition, but rather that it improves over time. Unfortunately, as described above, persistence of delirium is common. Thus, when counseling families, it is important to point out that many cognitive deficits associated with the delirium syndrome can continue, abating weeks and even months after the illness. Advanced age (≥85 years old), preexisting cognitive impairment, and severe illness (ICU stay) are risk factors for slow (or absent) recovery of cognitive function after delirium. Careful monitoring of mental status and providing adequate functional supports during this period are necessary to give the patient the maximal chance of returning to his or her baseline level.

Specialized intervention programs have been developed that aim to facilitate recovery after an episode of delirium. Studies of cognitive and physical rehabilitation are ongoing in the inpatient, postacute, outpatient settings. No definitive results are available, and these models must be evaluated and refined before widespread adoption.

Family members can play an important role in the hospital and postacute setting by providing appropriate orientation, support, and functional assistance. Hospitals are increasingly making provisions for family members to sleep overnight with relatives who are already delirious or at high risk of developing delirium. Although symptoms of delirium may persist, acute exacerbation of cognitive dysfunction is not expected during the convalescent period and therefore likely heralds a new medical problem. Families should be counseled to seek prompt medical attention if a patient's mental status acutely worsens.

Models of Care

A growing body of literature has focused on prevention and management of delirium. These studies can be best understood along a continuum, ranging from proactive interventions to prevent delirium or to reduce its severity and consequences, to reactive interventions designed to treat delirium after it has developed. The overall trend suggests that the more proactive, the more successful the intervention.

In a landmark 1999 study, a unit-based proactive multifactorial intervention termed HELP (the Hospital

Table 38.6—Key Recommendations of the AGS Guideline for Postoperative Delirium

Clinical Practice Guideline Summary

Eight *strong* recommendations: benefits clearly outweighed the risks, or the risks clearly outweighed the benefits.
- Multicomponent nonpharmacologic interventions delivered by an interprofessional team should be administered to at-risk older adults to prevent delirium.
- Ongoing educational programs regarding delirium should be provided for health care professionals.
- A medical evaluation should be performed to identify and manage underlying contributors to delirium.
- Pain management (preferably with nonopioid medications) should be optimized to prevent postoperative delirium.
- Medications with high risk of precipitating delirium should be avoided.
- Cholinesterase inhibitors should not be newly prescribed to prevent or treat postoperative delirium.
- Benzodiazepines should not be used as first-line treatment of agitation associated with delirium.
- Antipsychotics and benzodiazepines should be avoided for treatment of hypoactive delirium.

Three *weak* recommendations: current level of evidence or potential risks of the treatment did not support a strong recommendation.
- Multicomponent nonpharmacologic interventions implemented by an interprofessional team may be considered when an older adult is diagnosed with postoperative delirium to improve clinical outcomes.
- The injection of regional anesthetic at the time of surgery and postoperatively to improve pain control with the goal of preventing delirium may be considered.
- The use of antipsychotics (eg, haloperidol, risperidone, olanzapine, quetiapine, or ziprasidone) at the lowest effective dose for the shortest possible duration may be considered to treat delirious patients who are severely agitated or distressed or who are threatening substantial harm to self and/or others.

One "insufficient evidence" recommendation: current level of evidence or potential risks of the treatment did not support either a strong or weak recommendation.
- Use of processed electroencephalographic (EEG) monitors of anesthetic depth during intravenous sedation or general anesthesia may be used to prevent delirium.

Insufficient evidence to recommend either for or against the following:
- Prophylactic use of antipsychotic medications to prevent delirium
- Specialized hospital units for inpatient care of older adults with postoperative delirium

Reproduced with permission from American Geriatrics Society: Clinical Practice Guidelines for Postoperative Delirium, AGS Expert Panel on Postoperative Delirium.

Elder Life Program; [www.hospitalelderlifeprogram.org]) reduced the incidence of delirium among hospitalized patients ≥70 years old by 40% (matched OR=0.60; 95% CI, 0.39, 0.92; number needed to treat [NNT] = 19.6) (SOE=A). Six intervention components were used selectively on the basis of patient-specific risk factors determined at an admission assessment: cognitive impairment, sleep deprivation, immobility, visual impairment, hearing impairment, and dehydration. The HELP model was subsequently demonstrated to be cost-effective for hospitals in medium-risk patients, and for the health care system in all patients because of the large savings in postacute care. This model has now been disseminated widely, including in community hospitals and surgical patients.

A 2015 meta-analysis examined the effectiveness of multifactorial nonpharmacologic interventions for delirium, such as HELP. Of the 14 high-quality intervention studies identified, 11 studies demonstrated a significant reduction in delirium incidence (OR=0.47; 95% CI 0.38, 0.58), and 4 studies demonstrated a significant reduction in in-hospital falls (OR=0.38; 95% CI, 0.25,0.60) (SOE=A). There were also nonsignificant trends toward shorter hospital length of stay and reduced need for postacute nursing home placement.

Another approach with proven benefit for prevention of delirium is proactive geriatrics consultation. Two randomized trials demonstrated that this model of care can reduce the incidence of delirium in older patients undergoing hip fracture repair. In most cases, consultation began preoperatively and continued throughout the duration of hospitalization. Daily recommendations were based on a structured protocol that covers key elements in delirium prevention, such as limitation of psychoactive medications. The geriatrics consultation group achieved a 30%–40% reduction in the incidence of delirium (NNT=5.6) (SOE=A). Geriatrics-orthopedics services, in which hip fracture patients are comanaged by orthopedists and geriatricians, have been widely adopted.

Promoting better sleep in hospitals is an area of growing interest for prevention of delirium. The HELP model described above integrates a nonpharmacologic sleep protocol that involves trained volunteers offering patients warm milk, back rubs, and soothing music at bedtime; this is coupled with efforts to reduce noise and wake-ups in the middle of the night. This component of HELP substantially reduced the use of sedative-hypnotic medication, improved the duration and quality of sleep, and likely contributed to the overall reduction of delirium seen in this trial. There is a growing literature examining use of melatonin and its analogues for prevention of delirium. Thus far, the results are mixed, with two 2014 randomized trials showing contradictory results. In one, ramelteon (a melatonin analogue) was associated with a 91% risk reduction for delirium, whereas in the other, melatonin was not associated with any reduced risk of delirium. In sum, the literature suggests that promotion of good sleep hygiene and a reduction of sedative-hypnotics (both benzodiazepines and newer nonbenzodiazepine hypnotics) is beneficial for prevention of delirium (SOE=B), but it is unclear whether there is a role for alternative sleep-promoting agents (SOE=C). Finally, several studies have examined treatment of delirium using multifactorial strategies similar to those used for delirium prevention. For the most part, these have not yielded as dramatic benefits as the prevention models (SOE=B), although some have demonstrated improved recognition of delirium, reduction in delirium severity or duration, or faster cognitive recovery in the intervention group. New trials are underway to test treatment interventions.

QUALITY MEASURES AND CONSENSUS GUIDELINES

Recently, the American Geriatrics Society Section for Enhancing Geriatric Understanding and Expertise among Surgical and Medical Specialists (SEGUE) released new guidelines for prevention and management of postoperative delirium (Table 38.6). Although aimed specifically at the surgical setting, many of the recommendations in these guidelines are applicable to other patient populations. The level of evidence supporting various recommendations varies widely, from consistent randomized trials (SOE=A) to a reliance on best clinical practices (SOE=C).

CHOOSING WISELY® RECOMMENDATIONS

Delirium

- Avoid physical restraints to manage behavioral symptoms of hospitalized older adults with delirium.
- Do not use benzodiazepines or other sedative-hypnotics in older adults as first choice for insomnia, agitation, or delirium.

REFERENCES

- AGS Expert Panel on Postoperative Delirium. *Clinical Practice Guidelines for Postoperative Delirium in Older Adults*. New York: American Geriatrics Society; 2014.

    This paper presents clinical practice guidelines for prevention and treatment of postoperative delirium. A multidisciplinary panel performed a systematic literature review for all reported prevention and treatment strategies for postoperative delirium. Based on this evidence, interventions were graded as strong recommendations, weak recommendations, or insufficient evidence.

- Hshieh TT, Yue J, Oh E, et al. Effectiveness of multicomponent nonpharmacological delirium interventions: a meta-analysis. *JAMA Intern Med.* 2015;175(4):512–520.

    This paper presents the results of a meta-analysis examining the effectiveness of multifactorial nonpharmacologic interventions for delirium. Of 14 high-quality intervention studies identified, 11 studies demonstrated a significant reduction in delirium incidence (OR=0.47, 95% CI 0.38, 0.58), while 4 studies demonstrated a significant reduction in in-hospital falls (OR=0.38; 95% CI, 0.25, 0.60) (SOE=A). There were also nonsignificant trends toward shorter hospital length of stay and reduced need for postacute nursing home placement. This meta-analysis provides the strongest evidence to date of the effectiveness of nonpharmacologic approaches to prevent delirium and its associated poor outcomes.

- Inouye SK, Kosar CM, Tommet D, et al. CAM-S: development and validation of a new scoring system for delirium severity in 2 cohorts. *Ann Intern Med.* 2014;160(8):526–533.

    This study aimed to develop and validate a new delirium severity measure (CAM-S) based on the Confusion Assessment Method. Two cohorts of patients ≥70 years old were used, the first with 300 patients undergoing major surgery, and the second with 919 general medical patients. A 4-item short form and a 10-item long form were developed. The association of the maximum CAM-S score during hospitalization with hospital and post-hospital outcomes was evaluated. The CAM-S was associated with adjusted mean length of stay, which increased across levels of short-form severity from 6.5 days to 12.7 days (P for trend <.001), and across levels of long-form severity from 5.6 days to 11.9 days (P for trend <.001). CAM-S was also associated with adjusted relative risk of death or nursing-home residence at 90 days, which increased across levels of short-form severity from 1.0 (referent) to 2.5 (P for trend <.001) and across levels of long-form severity from 1.0 (referent) to 2.5 (P for trend <.001). The authors conclude that the CAM-S provides a new measure of delirium severity with strong psychometric properties and strong associations with important clinical outcomes.

- Inouye SK, Westendorp RG, Saczynski JS. Delirium in elderly people. *Lancet.* 2014;383(9920):911–922.

    This comprehensive systematic review summarizes the delirium literature in the areas of diagnosis, epidemiology, pathophysiology, and interventions. It concludes that delirium is an acute disorder of attention and cognition in adults ≥65 years old that is common, serious, costly, under-recognized, and often fatal. Diagnosis of delirium requires formal cognitive assessment and history of acute onset of symptoms. In terms of interventions, multicomponent nonpharmacologic risk factor approaches are the most effective strategies, and this article concludes there is no convincing evidence that pharmacologic prevention or treatment is effective. Delirium offers opportunities to elucidate brain pathophysiology, both as a marker of brain vulnerability and as a potential mechanism for permanent cognitive damage. Delirium provides a potent target for system-wide process improvements.

- Marcantonio ER, Ngo LH, O'Connor M, et al. 3D-CAM: derivation and validation of a 3-minute diagnostic interview for CAM-defined delirium. *Ann Intern Med.* 2014;161(8):554–561.

    This study aimed to derive the 3D-CAM, a new 3-minute diagnostic assessment for CAM-defined delirium, and to validate it against a clinical reference standard. The authors identified 20 items that best operationalized the 4 CAM diagnostic features to create the 3D-CAM. For prospective validation, 3D-CAM assessments were administered by trained research assistants, and the results were compared with a reference standard, which consisted of an extensive clinical delirium assessment with patient and family interviews and review of the medical record. The 201 participants in the validation study had a mean age of 84 years, and 28% had dementia. The reference standard assessment identified 21% with delirium. Median administration time for the 3D-CAM was 3 minutes (interquartile range, 2–5 minutes). Compared with the reference standard, 3D-CAM sensitivity was 95% (95% CI, 84%–99%), and specificity was 94% (CI, 90%–97%). The 3D-CAM performed well in patients with dementia (sensitivity 96%, specificity 86%) and without dementia (sensitivity 93%, specificity 96%). The authors conclude that the 3D-CAM operationalizes the CAM algorithm using a 3-minute structured assessment with high sensitivity and specificity relative to a reference standard and could be an important tool for improving widespread recognition of delirium among hospitalized older adults.

- Pandharipande PP, Girard TD, Jackson JC, et al. Long-term cognitive impairment after critical illness. *N Engl J Med.* 2013;369(14):1306–1316.

    This 1-year observational study enrolled 821 patients aged ≥18 years old admitted to ICUs with respiratory failure or shock. Baseline cognitive function was assessed by proxy report, and delirium was diagnosed using the Confusion Assessment Method for the ICU (CAM-ICU). Patients were assessed 3 and 12 months after discharge with the Repeatable Battery for the Assessment of Neuropsychological Status (R-BANS). The participants had only a 6% rate of cognitive impairment at baseline, but 74% developed delirium during the hospital stay. At 3 months, 26% had scores 2 standard deviations below the population means on the R-BANS, similar to scores for patients with mild Alzheimer disease. Deficits occurred in both older and younger patients and persisted, with 24% of all patients with assessments at 12 months having scores similar to those for patients with mild Alzheimer disease. A longer duration of delirium was independently associated with worse global cognition ($P=.04$) and worse executive function ($P=.007$) at 12 months. Use of sedative or analgesic medications was not consistently associated with cognitive impairment at 12 months. This study demonstrates that survivors of severe illness in medical and surgical ICUs are at high risk of long-term cognitive impairment, and that duration of delirium is the strongest risk factor for this impairment.

- Saczynski JS, Marcantonio ER, Quach L, et al. Cognitive trajectories after postoperative delirium. *N Engl J Med.* 2012;367(1):30–39.

    In this 1-year observational study of 225 patients ≥60 years old undergoing coronary artery bypass grafting or valve replacement surgery, cognitive trajectories of those who developed delirium after surgery were compared with that of those who did not. Patients were assessed with the Mini–Mental State Examination (MMSE) preoperatively; daily postoperatively; and at 1, 6, and 12 months after surgery. Delirium was diagnosed using the Confusion Assessment Method. The 103 patients (46%) who developed delirium had slightly lower preoperative MMSE scores (25.8 vs 26.9, $P<.001$) and a larger drop in cognitive function 2 days after surgery (7.7 vs 2.1 points, $P<.001$). Delirium was associated with an altered cognitive trajectory over 1 year after cardiac surgery. On average, patients who did not develop delirium returned to their preoperative baseline by 1 month after surgery, whereas on average those who developed delirium had not returned to their preoperative baseline 1 year after surgery. This is one of the first studies to link delirium with longer-term postoperative cognitive dysfunction.

Edward R. Marcantonio, MD, SM

CHAPTER 39—SLEEP ISSUES

KEY POINTS

- Comorbid psychiatric and/or medical conditions often contribute to the increased prevalence of insomnia in older adults.

- Compared with younger adults, older adults generally take longer to fall asleep at night and have more nighttime wakefulness and more daytime napping. An earlier bedtime and earlier wake time are also common.

- Older adults (especially older men) also have less N3, or slow-wave, sleep (which is the deeper stage of sleep) than younger adults.

- The appropriate treatment of sleep problems must be guided by knowledge of likely causes and potential contributing factors.

- Several trials, meta-analyses, and guidelines recommend behavioral interventions (eg, cognitive-behavioral therapy for insomnia) as first-line treatment for chronic insomnia in older adults.

Sleep problems are common among older adults, particularly those with other psychiatric and medical conditions. More than two-thirds of older adults with multiple comorbidities have sleep problems. The most common sleep complaints among community-dwelling older adults are difficulty falling asleep (around 40%), nighttime awakening (30%), early morning awakening (20%), and daytime sleepiness (20%). At least one-half of community-dwelling older adults use OTC and/or prescription sleeping medications.

EPIDEMIOLOGY

Epidemiologic studies in older adults have demonstrated an association between sleep complaints and risk factors for sleep disturbance (eg, chronic illness, multiple medical problems, mood disturbance, less physical activity, physical disability) but little association with older age, suggesting that these risk factors, rather than aging per se, account for much of the increase in sleep disturbance with age. However, certain primary sleep disorders do increase in prevalence with age, such as sleep-related breathing disorders (eg, sleep apnea), periodic limb movement disorder, restless legs syndrome, and circadian rhythm sleep disorders.

Insomnia is more common in women than in men at all ages (SOE=A). A meta-analysis of several epidemiologic studies from around the world found a risk ratio for insomnia in women compared with men that increased from young adulthood (risk ratio [RR]=1.28) to older age (RR=1.73). Self-reported sleeping difficulties are more common in older black Americans, particularly women and those with depression and chronic illness.

Late-life insomnia is often a chronic problem. In one British study, more than one-third of older adults with insomnia reported persistent severe symptoms at 4-year follow-up, and one-third of participants who reported use of prescription hypnotics were still using these agents 4 years later. Even among very old women (≥85 years old), there is evidence that more than 80% report sleeping difficulties, and many regularly use alcohol and/or OTC sleeping agents for sleep. Studies in the United States suggest that around 5% of older adults use sedative-hypnotics on a daily basis. Insomnia has been reported as a predictor of death and nursing-home placement (particularly in older men). In addition, in several epidemiologic studies, subjective sleep disturbance is associated with worse health-related quality of life in older adults (SOE=B). Recent evidence also suggests an association between worse sleep (measured subjectively and objectively) and subsequent cognitive decline in older adults, particularly older men.

CHANGES IN SLEEP WITH AGING

In general, older adults have decreased sleep efficiency (time spent asleep divided by total time spent in bed), stable or decreased total sleep time, and increased sleep latency (time to fall asleep) (Table 39.1). Older adults also often report an earlier bedtime and earlier morning awakening, more awakenings during the night, more wakefulness during the night, and more daytime napping. Notable age-related changes in sleep structure as measured by polysomnography include changes in both nonrapid eye movement (NREM, ie, stages N1, N2, and N3) and rapid eye movement (REM) sleep. Older adults have less N3, or slow-wave, sleep, which is the deeper stage of sleep, whereas the percentage of stage N1 and N2 sleep (the lighter stages of sleep) increases with age. The decline in slow-wave sleep begins in early adulthood and progresses throughout life, with a notable decline in middle age. Men have more decline in slow-wave sleep than women. Changes in REM sleep with age are less clear, but a decrease in REM sleep and an earlier onset of REM sleep in the night (ie, shorter REM latency) have been reported. Older adults also have a decrease in sleep spindles and K complexes on electroencephalography during sleep. In addition, older adults can have an advance in circadian rhythms of sleep and wake (ie, go to bed earlier, wake up earlier)

Table 39.1—Age-Related Changes in Sleep

Sleep Characteristic	Age-Related Change
Total sleep time	Decrease
Sleep latency (time to fall asleep)	Increase or no change
Sleep efficiency (time asleep over time in bed)	Decrease
Daytime napping	Increase
Stages N1 and N2	Increase
Slow-wave sleep (Stage N3)	Decrease
Percent rapid eye movement (REM)	Decrease
Wake after sleep onset	Increase

and a reduced amplitude in (ie, less robust) circadian rhythms.

There is some disagreement among experts as to whether the decreased sleep seen with aging is due to a decreased *ability* to sleep or a decreased *need* for sleep. After a period of sleep deprivation, older adults may actually show less daytime sleepiness, less evidence of decline in performance measures, and a quicker recovery of normal sleep structure than younger people. Older adults have more sleep disturbance with jet lag and shift work, which may reflect physiologic changes in circadian rhythms with age. In studies comparing good sleepers with poor sleepers, poor sleepers were found to take more medications, make more clinician visits, and have poorer self-ratings of health. In addition, as noted above, among older adults chronologic age per se does not seem to correlate with higher prevalence of poor sleep.

EVALUATION OF SLEEP

Symptoms of sleep disturbance in older adults can be identified with simple screening questions, such as asking whether the person is satisfied with their sleep, whether sleep or fatigue interferes with daytime activities, and whether a bed partner or others complain of unusual behavior during sleep, such as snoring, interrupted breathing, or leg movements. If the patient has a sleep complaint, having them keep a sleep log for 1–2 weeks can be helpful in obtaining a careful description of the sleep complaint. Each morning, the patient should record the time they went to bed the prior night, the estimated amount of sleep, the number of awakenings, the time of morning awakening, when they got out of bed for the day, and any symptoms that occurred during the night. Any medications or other agents taken for sleep and time spent napping during the day should also be recorded. The patient's sleep log should be supplemented by information from a bed partner (if available) or from others who may have observed unusual symptoms during the night. Examples of sleep logs and validated sleep questionnaires are available in the literature. The focused physical examination depends on evidence from the history. For example, reports of painful joints should be followed by a careful examination of the affected areas. Reports of nocturia that disrupts sleep should be followed by evaluation for cardiac, renal, or prostatic disease, or diabetes mellitus. Mental status testing should also be considered, with a focus on memory and mood problems, particularly depression. The findings of the history and physical examination should guide laboratory testing.

Polysomnography is indicated when a sleep-related breathing disorder (sleep apnea) or narcolepsy is suspected, or when there are symptoms of violent or injurious behaviors during sleep (SOE=A). Polysomnography may be indicated when other unusual behaviors occur during sleep or if periodic limb movement disorder is suspected (SOE=B). Portable sleep monitoring systems for use in the home have been developed and are used primarily when sleep apnea is suspected. Wrist activity monitors (ie, wrist actigraphy) estimate sleep versus wakefulness based on wrist movement. Wrist actigraphy can be used in identifying circadian rhythm disorders (SOE=A) and in nursing-home residents, in whom traditional sleep monitoring can be difficult to obtain (SOE=B).

COMMON SLEEP PROBLEMS

Insomnia

Insomnia disorder is defined by the *Diagnostic and Statistical Manual of Mental Disorders, Fifth Edition (DSM-5)* as a difficulty in initiating or maintaining sleep or waking up too early, which is associated with daytime impairment (such as fatigue, poor concentration, daytime sleepiness, or concerns about sleep). In addition to other features, diagnostic criteria also indicate that the sleep problems must occur at least 3 times per week and (to meet criteria for chronic insomnia) must have been present for at least 3 months. The prevalence of insomnia increases from about 10% in young adulthood to about 30% in those ≥65 years old. However, the prevalence of sleep complaints is even greater than the prevalence of insomnia disorder when strict diagnostic criteria are applied. Much of the increase in insomnia seen with older age seems to occur by middle age. In older adults in particular, insomnia generally coexists with other conditions, and older adults with insomnia are more likely to have medical and/or psychiatric illness than good sleepers. Other risk factors for insomnia include female gender, social isolation, low socioeconomic status, and use of multiple medications.

Some studies report that an associated psychiatric disorder is present in 30%–60% of patients presenting with insomnia. Depression is the most common and the most strongly associated comorbid psychiatric illness with insomnia, and most patients with depression also have sleep complaints. Common sleep complaints with depression include early morning awakening, increased sleep latency, and more nighttime wakefulness. Chronic insomnia is a risk factor for development of major depressive disorder in older (and younger) adults, and studies suggest that insomnia symptoms commonly precede the onset of depressive symptoms. In depressed older adults with sleep disturbance, treatment of depression can improve sleep complaints. Conversely, lack of attention to sleep complaints in older depressed adults can make depression less likely to respond to treatment. After depression, anxiety disorder is the psychiatric condition most commonly associated with insomnia symptoms, particularly difficulty falling asleep and early awakening. Caregiving is also associated with insomnia, and older caregivers report more sleep complaints than do noncaregivers of similar age. In one study, nearly 40% of older women who were family caregivers of adults with dementia reported taking a sleeping medication in the past month.

Many medical problems are associated with insomnia in older adults. Epidemiologic studies in older adults suggest a greater prevalence of insomnia in those with conditions such as hypertension, heart disease, arthritis, lung disease, gastroesophageal reflux, stroke, neurodegenerative disorders (eg, dementia, Parkinson disease), and other comorbid conditions. Common symptoms of medical illness that can contribute to sleep disturbance (particularly nighttime awakening) include pain, paresthesias, cough, nocturnal dyspnea, gastroesophageal reflux, and nighttime urination. In older adults with sleeping difficulties who describe pain at night, the painful condition should be assessed and managed. Nighttime urination is common in both older men and women and may be associated with insomnia and increased fatigue in the daytime.

Many medications can contribute to insomnia in older adults. Sleep can be impaired by diuretics or stimulating agents (eg, caffeine, sympathomimetics, bronchodilators, activating psychiatric medications) taken near bedtime. Some antidepressants, antiparkinson agents, antihypertensives (eg, propranolol), and cholinesterase inhibitors can induce nightmares and impair sleep. Required medications that are sedating (eg, sedating antidepressants) should be given at bedtime if possible. Chronic use of sedatives can cause light, fragmented sleep. For some sleeping medications, chronic use can lead to tolerance and the potential for increasing dosages. When chronic use of hypnotics is suddenly stopped, rebound insomnia can occur. Alcohol abuse is associated with lighter sleep of shorter duration. In addition, some older adults try to treat their sleeping difficulties with alcohol. Although nighttime alcohol causes an initial drowsiness, it can impair sleep later in the night. Finally, sedatives and alcohol can worsen sleep apnea; the use of these respiratory depressants should be avoided in older adults with untreated sleep apnea.

Sleep-Related Breathing Disorders

Sleep-related breathing disorders are characterized by disordered respiration during sleep. Limited evidence and even fewer guidelines are specific to older adults to guide the diagnosis and treatment of sleep-related breathing disorders, so management recommendations, in general, are based on findings from middle-aged or mixed aged populations. Central sleep apnea (CSA) syndromes are those in which respiratory effort is absent because of CNS or cardiac dysfunction. Obstructive sleep apnea (OSA) is characterized by an obstruction in the airway resulting in continued breathing effort but inadequate ventilation. In-laboratory polysomnography is the gold standard for diagnosis of these conditions (SOE=A). Portable devices that combine oximetry with additional measures (eg, heart rate, respiratory effort, nasal airflow) have shown some promise in diagnosing OSA in the home, but debate remains regarding the most appropriate use of these devices. These devices are less expensive, and monitoring can be performed more readily than in a sleep laboratory. The sensitivity of home testing may be lower than that of laboratory polysomnography (SOE=B). Therefore, in some cases negative home testing for sleep apnea may need to be followed by laboratory polysomnography to exclude sleep apnea.

In adults, CSA can be a primary disorder, secondary to neurodegenerative disease or stroke, or more commonly, the Cheynes-Stokes breathing pattern of heart failure. CSA is more common in older adults than in younger adults. Treatment of CSA associated with heart failure focuses on management of the heart failure. The role of positive-airway pressure (PAP) in treatment of patients with CSA and heart failure has been debated. However, evidence suggests that patients with CSA related to heart failure who are successfully treated with PAP to an apnea-hypopnea index (AHI) <15 have improved transplant-free survival (SOE=B). Therefore, recent guidelines recommend PAP therapy targeted to improve AHI in these patients. Nighttime oxygen supplementation can reduce the apnea and oxygen desaturation and has been recommended in CSA patients who are unable to tolerate PAP therapy (SOE=C). Adaptive servo-ventilation (ASV) is a form of ventilation that can normalize the breathing pattern in CSA patients; it has been suggested as an alternative to PAP (SOE=B), although it is much more costly than PAP therapy. In addition, it is worrisome that recent evidence found increased cardiovascular mortality among heart failure patients with a reduced left ventricular ejection fraction who were treated with ASV.

OSA is common among older adults, but reported prevalence varies considerably. Patients with OSA usually present with excessive daytime sleepiness and may be unaware of their frequent arousals at night. Patients can have morning headache, personality changes, poor memory, confusion, and irritability. A bed partner may report loud snoring, cessation of breathing, and choking sounds during sleep. OSA patients are generally obese, but there is less association between obesity and OSA in older age, and many older OSA patients have a normal BMI. Other reported predictors identified in community-dwelling older adults include falling asleep at inappropriate times, male gender, and napping. OSA should be considered in patients with treatment-resistant hypertension. The classic sleep apnea patient is an obese, sleepy snorer with hypertension. Large neck circumference has also been reported as a marker for sleep apnea in middle-aged adults but may not be a significant predictor of sleep apnea in older adults. Alcohol abuse and dependence is an important risk factor for sleep apnea, and sleep-disordered breathing is a significant contributor to sleep disturbance in men >40 years old with a history of alcoholism. Finally, there appears to be an association between sleep apnea and dementia. Of note, evidence suggests that OSA patients with mild-moderate dementia can tolerate PAP well, with acceptable adherence to treatment, improvement in OSA parameters, and some evidence of beneficial effects on cognition (SOE=B).

OSA is a treatable condition associated with cardiovascular disease, including hypertension, stroke, myocardial ischemia, arrhythmias, fatal and nonfatal cardiovascular events, and all-cause mortality (SOE=A). Recent evidence has further documented that PAP therapy (but not nocturnal supplemental oxygen therapy alone) reduces blood pressure in OSA patients with cardiovascular disease or multiple cardiovascular risk factors (SOE=A). OSA is also associated with motor vehicle accidents (SOE=A), and there is mixed evidence for a relationship with cognitive impairment (SOE=B). The importance of mild degrees of sleep-disordered breathing in older adults is unclear. In one study, no association was found between mild or moderate sleep-disordered breathing and subjective sleep-wake disturbance. The long-term consequences of asymptomatic OSA in older adults are also unclear.

Patients suspected of having OSA should be referred to a sleep laboratory for evaluation and, if the diagnosis is documented, treatment. As mentioned above, portable in-home monitoring devices are also available. Although controversial, recent evidence suggests that home sleep testing followed by use of auto-titrating PAP (autoPAP) treatment in patients diagnosed with OSA (ie, completely home-based diagnosis and treatment of OSA) may be noninferior to (the more costly) in-laboratory polysomnography testing for OSA and PAP titration. PAP therapy reduces sleepiness and improves quality of life in people with moderate and severe OSA (SOE=A). Older adults are likely to tolerate PAP as well as younger adults. Careful efforts to use devices (eg, variations in mask, humidification) that improve comfort may improve adherence with PAP. Early successful adherence (eg, within the first week of therapy) with PAP can predict long-term adherence with PAP treatment. Unfortunately, clinicians may not recommend PAP in older adults, perhaps because they assume that the treatment will not be tolerated or successful in this population.

Although most OSA patients are treated with continuous PAP (CPAP) therapy, other mechanical options are available as alternatives to CPAP. For example, bi-level PAP (biPAP) devices reduce expiratory pressure in an effort to increase comfort with PAP. Evidence suggests that biPAP does not improve efficacy or adherence in treatment of sleep apnea compared with CPAP (SOE=B), but these alternative devices can be appropriate in certain patients. Oral (ie, dental or mouth) appliances are also available, but PAP is more effective in improving OSA. Oral appliances are generally recommended only in patients with mild symptomatic OSA or in those unwilling or unable to tolerate PAP (SOE=B). Several upper airway surgical approaches have also been used, but evidence of effectiveness from large trials is limited. Other novel treatment options for OSA are under review, but the role of these therapies (particularly in older adults) remains unclear.

Periodic Limb Movements During Sleep and Restless Legs Syndrome

Periodic limb movements during sleep (PLMS) is a condition of repetitive, stereotypical leg movements that generally occur in non-REM sleep. PLMS increases in prevalence with age, but the significance of this is unclear, because many studies have found little relationship between PLMS and sleep disruption. In one study, evidence of PLMS was found in more than one-third of community-dwelling older adults. Some authors have suggested that the high prevalence of PLMS with age is associated with delayed motor and sensory latencies noted on nerve conduction testing. When PLMS is associated with clinical sleep disturbance or a complaint of daytime fatigue that is not better explained by another sleep disorder, this is termed periodic limb movement disorder (PLMD). Polysomnography is required to establish a diagnosis of PLMD.

Restless legs syndrome (RLS) is a condition of an uncontrollable urge to move one's legs at night, usually accompanied by an uncomfortable and unpleasant sensation of the legs that worsens with inactivity and improves with movement. The symptoms occur while the person is awake, and symptoms can also involve the arms. The diagnosis is based on the patient's description of the symptoms; polysomnography is not required to make the diagnosis. There may be a family history of the condition (particularly in patients with an earlier age onset of RLS) and, in some cases, an underlying medical disorder (eg, anemia, or renal or neurologic disease). RLS is 1.5 times more common in women than men, and evidence suggests that RLS prevalence increases with age. PLMS occurs in most (80%–90%) patients with RLS, but the presence of PLMS is not specific for RLS. RLS can also be seen in patients with dementia, in which the patient may not be able to adequately describe the symptoms. RLS should be considered in dementia patients who have signs such as rubbing or massaging of legs, increased motor activity (eg, pacing, wandering), and evidence of leg discomfort that occurs in the evening and/or with inactivity and improves with movement. Many medications can aggravate or induce RLS symptoms, such as antiemetics, antipsychotics, SSRIs, tricyclic antidepressants, and diphenhydramine. These and other medications should be addressed in patients with new or worsening RLS.

If pharmacologic treatment for RLS is indicated (because of severity of symptoms or significant effects on quality of life), dopaminergic agents are the initial agent of choice. An evening dose of a dopamine agonist (eg, pramipexole or ropinirole, about 1–2 hours before bedtime) is effective in treatment of RLS and PLMD (SOE=A). A nighttime dose of carbidopa-levodopa[OL] may also be effective (SOE=A) and can be used for patients who need medication infrequently (ie, for as-needed use). However, some patients describe a shift of their symptoms to daytime hours with successful treatment of symptoms at night; this problem (termed augmentation) appears more frequently with use of carbidopa-levodopa as treatment for RLS. RLS can be associated with iron deficiency, in which case RLS symptoms can improve with iron replacement therapy (SOE=B). Patients with RLS should be screened for iron deficiency. Of course, the cause of the iron deficiency should also be addressed. Gabapentin[OL] can also be effective (SOE=B), particularly in patients who cannot tolerate dopamine agonists. Benzodiazepines[OL] and opioids[OL] have also been used for RLS but likely carry greater risk of adverse effects in older adults. Recent guidelines suggest that there is insufficient evidence available to evaluate the use of pharmacologic therapy for patients with PLMD alone (ie, in the absence of coexisting RLS).

Circadian Rhythm Sleep Disorders

Disturbances in circadian rhythms of the sleep-wake cycle may be more common with advanced age. In particular, older adults are more likely to have an advanced sleep phase (ie, fall asleep early and awaken early) rather than a delayed sleep phase (ie, fall asleep late and awaken late), but a delayed sleep phase can be seen in older adults. Some individuals have extremely irregular sleep-wake cycles, including some patients with dementia and nursing-home residents. Some common changes in sleep pattern seen in older adults (such as increased daytime napping and disrupted nighttime sleep) can be due to alterations in circadian rhythms. Dementia is associated with sleep-wake cycle disturbance and frequent nighttime awakenings, nighttime wandering, and nighttime agitation.

A sleep log can help establish the presence of a circadian rhythm sleep disorder (SOE=B). Wrist actigraphy can also be useful for making a diagnosis (particularly in patients who are unable to complete a sleep log) and in monitoring treatment response in patients with a circadian rhythm sleep disorder (SOE=B), including older patients with dementia and nursing-home residents. Polysomnography is not routinely indicated in patients in whom a circadian rhythm sleep disorder is suspected, but referral to a sleep specialist may be indicated when symptoms do not respond to initial management, when the diagnosis is unclear, or when another sleep disorder is suspected (SOE=C). Treatment depends on the particular circadian rhythm sleep disorder. An advanced sleep phase may respond to appropriately timed (ie, evening) exposure to bright light (SOE=B). A delayed sleep phase may respond to appropriately timed morning bright light and/or evening melatonin (SOE=B).

REM Sleep Behavior Disorder

REM sleep behavior disorder (RBD) is characterized by excessive motor activities associated with dream enactment behavior during sleep and a pathologic absence of the muscle atonia that normally occurs during REM sleep. The presenting symptoms are usually vigorous sleep behaviors associated with vivid dreams, and patients may first present because of injuries (to themselves or their bed partner). The condition can be acute or chronic, and it is much more common in older men (in some series, >85% of cases are older men). There may be a family predisposition. Transient RBD has been associated with toxic metabolic abnormalities, primarily drug or alcohol withdrawal or intoxication. The chronic form of the disorder can be idiopathic but is increasingly recognized as associated with neurodegenerative disorders such as the synucleinopathies (eg, Parkinson disease, Lewy body dementia, multisystem atrophy) and other conditions. The RBD may predate (by many years) the development of the neurodegenerative disorder. Several psychiatric medications have been associated with RBD, including tricyclic antidepressants, monoamine oxidase inhibitors, fluoxetine, venlafaxine, cholinesterase inhibitors, and other agents. Polysomnography is indicated to establish the diagnosis. Removal of the offending agent is indicated for drug-induced RBD. Clonazepam[OL] is reported in the literature to be effective for treatment of RBD, with little evidence of tolerance to treatment effect over long periods of treatment, but older adults may be at increased risk of adverse events with this agent. Use of nighttime melatonin may be effective as an alternative treatment for RBD in older adults with coexisting neurodegenerative disorders (SOE=C). Environmental safety interventions are also indicated, such as removing dangerous objects from the bedroom, putting cushions on the floor around the bed, protecting windows, and in some cases, putting the mattress on the floor.

CHANGES IN SLEEP WITH DEMENTIA

Older adults with dementia have more sleep disruption and arousals, lower sleep efficiency, a higher percentage of stage N1 sleep, and more sleep fragmentation than nondemented older adults. Circadian rhythm sleep disorders are more common with dementia, resulting in excessive daytime sleeping and nighttime wakefulness. Cholinesterase inhibitors (often used in treatment of the symptoms of dementia) can exacerbate insomnia and cause vivid dreams; changing dose timing to morning hours can help alleviate this problem. Sedative-hypnotic agents have not been adequately tested in patients with dementia. As mentioned above, evidence suggests that those with coexisting OSA and mild to moderate dementia can tolerate PAP well, with improvement in OSA parameters and beneficial effects on cognition. Results of studies using melatonin for sleep disturbance in dementia have been mixed, but results of one large, randomized controlled trial in patients with Alzheimer disease suggested melatonin was not effective for sleep disturbance in these individuals (SOE=B). Bright light therapy has also been used in dementia patients, with some beneficial effects on sleep and circadian rhythms (SOE=B), but the most appropriate timing of the light exposure is unclear.

SLEEP DISTURBANCES IN THE HOSPITAL

Acute hospitalization can precipitate transient or short-term insomnia. This insomnia is likely multifactorial in origin and related to illness, medications, change from usual nighttime routines at home, and a sleep-disruptive hospital environment (eg, high noise levels at night). In one small uncontrolled study, nighttime melatonin levels increased in hospitalized older patients treated with daytime bright-light exposure. Another small study implemented "flexible medication times" that allowed inpatients to sleep longer in the morning, and their resulting in-hospital sleeping patterns were more similar to their at-home sleeping patterns. However, adherence with nonpharmacologic interventions can be difficult to achieve in the acute hospital. For example, one large clinical trial of nonpharmacologic interventions to prevent delirium in hospitalized older adults reported only a 10% adherence rate for the sleep protocol portion of the intervention. In a large study that tested the feasibility of a nonpharmacologic sleep protocol (consisting of a back rub, warm drink, and relaxation tapes) administered by nurses for hospitalized older adults, the use of sedative-hypnotic medications was successfully reduced; the sleep protocol had a stronger association with improved quality of sleep than the sedative-hypnotic medications.

Sleeping medications are commonly prescribed in hospitalized older adults. A large Belgian study of consecutively admitted patients at a university hospital found that 45% of patients took a sleeping medication while in the hospital, with greater use among patients ≥60 years old. In this sample, >15% of patients who were newly prescribed a sleeping pill while in the hospital reported that they planned to use the medication after discharge to home. In another study of hospitalized older adults in India, among those prescribed a benzodiazepine for sleep during their acute hospitalization, over half were not taking a sleeping pill before their admission. Unfortunately, clear guidelines are not available to guide the choice of a sleeping medication for hospitalized older adults. Benzodiazepine-receptor agonists are commonly used for insomnia in this setting, but prescribers should remember to try use of smaller dosages (than those used for younger adults) first, which are likely effective and safer in older adults. Sedating antihistamines (eg, diphenhydramine) should not be used as a sleep aid in hospitalized older adults because of possible complications related to anticholinergic adverse events (eg, delirium, urinary retention, constipation).

Sleep apnea is likely a common comorbidity in hospitalized adults, particularly among those with cardiac illness and stroke. In one study of older men on medicine wards in a Veterans Affairs hospital, survival among patients with heart failure and CSA was shorter than among heart failure patients without evidence of this disorder. Sleep apnea among stroke patients is associated with worse survival and less functional recovery. Sleep apnea patients should continue their use of PAP when hospitalized, particularly when sedating and narcotic medications are used and in the peri- and postoperative period.

SLEEP IN THE NURSING HOME

Nursing-home residents often have marked sleep disruption, frequent nighttime awakening, and excessive daytime sleeping. In one study, up to 70% of caregivers reported that nighttime difficulties played a significant role in their decision to institutionalize the older adult, often because the sleep of the caregiver was being disrupted. Once in the nursing home, many residents nap on and off throughout the day and wake up frequently during the night. One study found that 65% of residents reported problems with their sleep and that the use of hypnotic medications was common, but no association was found between the use of sedative-hypnotics and the presence, absence, or change in sleep complaints after 6 months of follow-up. In another study, the average duration of sleep episodes during the night in nursing-home residents was only 20 minutes. Nursing-home residents generally have little or no exposure to outdoor bright light, which likely exacerbates sleep-wake abnormalities. Other common conditions in nursing-home residents that can contribute to sleep disturbance include multiple physical illnesses, the use of psychoactive medications, debility and inactivity, large amounts of time spent in bed during the daytime, increased prevalence of sleep disorders, and environmental factors (eg, nighttime noise, light, disruptive nursing care).

Evidence suggests that sleep disturbance is also common among older adults in assisted-living facilities. In one prospective, observational cohort study, sleep disturbance was common in this population, and subjective and/or objective evidence of sleep disturbance was associated with more symptoms of depression, decline in functional status, and worse health-related quality of life over 6 months of follow-up.

MANAGEMENT OF INSOMNIA

Treatment of sleep problems in older adults must be guided by knowledge of likely causes and potential contributing factors. Sedative-hypnotics have a documented association with falls, hip fracture, and daytime carryover symptoms of sedation in older adults. However, there is also some evidence that untreated insomnia symptoms are associated with increased risk of falls in older adults. If the initial history and physical examination do not suggest a serious underlying cause of the sleep problem that should be addressed, a trial of improved sleep habits (eg, sleep hygiene techniques) is

Table 39.2—Measures to Improve Sleep Hygiene

- Maintain regular rising and bed time.
- Do not go to bed unless sleepy.
- Decrease or eliminate naps, unless necessary rest period.
- Exercise daily but not immediately before bedtime.
- Do not use bed for reading or watching television.
- Relax mentally before going to sleep; do not use bedtime as worry time.
- If hungry, have a light snack (except with symptoms of gastroesophageal reflux or medical contraindications), but avoid heavy meals at bedtime.
- Limit or eliminate alcohol, caffeine, and nicotine, especially before bedtime.
- Wind down before bedtime and maintain a routine period of preparation for bed (eg, washing up, going to the bathroom).
- Control the nighttime environment with comfortable temperature, quiet, and darkness.
- Try a familiar background noise (eg, a fan or other "white noise" machine).
- Wear comfortable bed clothing.
- If unable to fall asleep within 30 minutes, get out of bed and perform soothing activity such as listening to soft music or light reading (but avoid exposure to bright light).
- Get adequate exposure to sunlight or bright light during the day.

usually the best first approach and may improve mild symptoms of insomnia (Table 39.2), but more intensive behavioral treatment (as described below) is indicated for treatment of chronic insomnia. Providing simple sleep hygiene tips alone is generally not effective for chronic insomnia. If the person takes daytime naps, it is important to determine whether these are needed rest periods or due to inactivity, boredom, or sedating medications. Patients should be educated that daytime naps will decrease nighttime sleep.

Short-term hypnotic therapy may be appropriate in cases of transient, situational insomnia, particularly during bereavement, acute hospitalization, and other periods of temporary acute stress. Sedative-hypnotic medication treatment should not be withheld in situations when it is clearly indicated. People generally do not feel well if they do not sleep well. If a decision is reached to use a sedative-hypnotic in an older adult, the smallest dosage of the agent with the least risk of adverse events should be chosen. However, in older adults with chronic insomnia, sedative-hypnotic agents should be used cautiously because of the complications associated with their long-term use. The chronic use of benzodiazepines can lead to dependence or cognitive impairment. The newer, nonbenzodiazepine hypnotics have been tested in healthy older adults and seem to have less risk of daytime carryover and tolerance to

Table 39.3—Examples of Nonpharmacologic Interventions to Improve Sleep

Intervention	Goal	Brief Description
Stimulus control	To recondition maladaptive sleep-related behaviors	Patient is instructed to go to bed only when sleepy, not use the bed for eating or watching television, get out of bed if unable to fall asleep, return to bed only when sleepy, get up at the same time each morning, not take naps during the day.
Sleep restriction	To improve sleep efficiency (time asleep over time in bed) by limiting time in bed	Patient first keeps a sleep diary for 1–2 weeks to determine average total daily sleep time, then stays in bed only that amount of time plus 15 minutes, gets up at same time each morning, takes no naps in the daytime, gradually increases time allowed in bed as sleep efficiency improves.
Cognitive interventions	To change misunderstandings and false beliefs regarding sleep	Patient's dysfunctional beliefs and attitudes about sleep are identified (eg, "I'll sleep better if I spend more time in bed"); patient is helped to correct these maladaptive beliefs and attitudes, including education about changes in sleep that occur with aging
Relaxation techniques	To recognize and relieve tension and anxiety	In progressive muscle relaxation, patient is taught to tense and relax each muscle group; in electromyographic biofeedback, the patient is given feedback regarding muscle tension and learns techniques to relieve it; meditation or imagery techniques are taught to relieve racing thoughts or anxiety.
Cognitive-behavioral therapy	Combines features of several behavioral interventions	Typically combines stimulus control, sleep restriction, and cognitive interventions, with or without relaxation techniques. Often also includes sleep hygiene.
Bright light	To correct circadian rhythm causes of sleeping difficulty (ie, sleep-phase problems)	Patient is exposed to sunlight or a light box. For delayed sleep phase: early morning bright light; for advanced sleep phase: evening bright light; light intensity generally ≥2,000 lux. Appropriate time of day of the light exposure is important. Routine eye examination is recommended before treatment; do not use light boxes with ultraviolet exposure.

sedative effects. However, there has been little study of these (or other hypnotic) agents in older adults with significant medical comorbidity.

Behavioral and Nonpharmacologic Interventions

Extensive evidence has demonstrated that behavioral treatment of insomnia is effective in older adults, including those with insomnia comorbid with other conditions (SOE=A). It is important not to confuse these effective insomnia behavioral interventions with simple sleep hygiene, which is generally not effective when used alone for chronic insomnia. For a summary of such interventions, see Table 39.3. Several systematic reviews and meta-analyses of behavioral interventions for insomnia have been published; the strongest evidence currently supports cognitive-behavioral therapy for insomnia (which generally combines stimulus control, sleep restriction, and cognitive therapy) (SOE=A). These behavioral interventions produce reliable therapeutic benefits, including improved sleep efficiency, decreased nighttime wakefulness, and greater satisfaction with sleep; treatment is also helpful in reducing chronic hypnotic use. In at least 2 randomized trials of older adults with insomnia that compared cognitive-behavioral therapy with a prescription sedative-hypnotic agent, participants generally reported better improvement in their sleep patterns and more satisfaction with the cognitive-behavioral therapy (than with the sedative-hypnotic), and sleep improvements were better sustained over time with behavioral treatment. Recent evidence suggests that even brief behavioral treatments (eg, 2 in-person sessions plus 2 phone calls; 4 group sessions) are effective in older adults with chronic insomnia (SOE=A). Other recent research demonstrates that in older adults with osteoarthritis pain and insomnia, combined behavioral treatment for both pain and insomnia is effective in improving insomnia (SOE=B).

Several small studies have also tested the effectiveness of exposure to bright light (either natural sunlight or with commercially available light boxes) on the sleep of older adults with insomnia (SOE=B). Variable results have been reported for insomnia, with better results seen for circadian rhythm disorders. As mentioned above, appropriately timed morning bright light may be useful in delayed sleep phase, and evening exposure may be useful in older adults with an advanced sleep phase. Even short durations of bright light may be useful. One study reported beneficial effects in older adults using a visor, worn for only 30 minutes in the evening, that provided 2,000 lux to each eye.

There is less evidence to support other nonpharmacologic interventions for insomnia, but some patients may find these methods useful. For example, bathing before sleep may enhance the quality of sleep in older adults, perhaps related to changes in body temperature with bathing. Moderate-intensity exercise also improves sleep in healthy, sedentary adults ≥50 years old who reported moderate sleep complaints at baseline. However,

Table 39.4—Prescription Medications Commonly Used for Insomnia in Older Adults

Class, Medication	Starting Dose (mg)	Usual Dose (mg)	Estimate of Half-Life in Older Adults (hours)	Comments
Intermediate-acting benzodiazepine				
Temazepam	7.5	7.5–15	8.8	Psychomotor impairment, increased risk of falls. Caution suggested because of adverse cognitive and psychomotor effects in older adults. Guidelines recommend avoiding use in older adults.
Short-acting nonbenzodiazepines				
Eszopiclone	1	1–2	6	Increased risk of falls; may be associated with unpleasant taste, headache. Avoid administration with high-fat meal. Evidence for next day impairment of driving skills prompted lowering of recommended starting dose, especially in women.
Zaleplon (a pyrazolopyrimidine)	5	5–10	1	Increased risk of falls; occasional adverse effects include headache, dizziness, nausea, abdominal pain, and somnolence.
Zolpidem (an imidazopyridine)	2.5–5 (6.25 extended release)	5 (6.25 extended release)	3	Increased risk of falls. Available in extended release, as a dissolvable tablet, and as an oral spray. Complex sleep-related behaviors reported. Evidence for next day impairment of driving skills prompted FDA warning and the lowering of recommended starting dose, especially in women.
Melatonin receptor agonist				
Ramelteon	8	8	2.6	Dizziness, myalgia, headache, other adverse events reported; no significant rebound insomnia or withdrawal with discontinuation
Sedating antidepressants				
Doxepin	3	3–6	15.3 (doxepin); 31 (metabolite)	Somnolence/sedation, nausea, and upper respiratory tract infection reported; antagonizes central H_1 receptors (antihistamine); active metabolite; should not be taken within 3 hours of a meal
Mirtazapine[OL]	7.5	7.5–30	31–39	Increased appetite, weight gain, headache, dizziness, daytime carryover; long half-life may limit use in some older patients; lower doses tend to be more sedating than higher doses.
Trazodone[OL]	25–50	25–100	6 ± 2; may be prolonged	Orthostatic effects, increased risk of falls, risk of priapism in men; limited evidence for use in insomnia

strenuous exercise can interfere with sleep and should not be performed immediately before bedtime. Studies have also suggested beneficial effects on sleep with Tai Chi (SOE=B).

Nonpharmacologic interventions have been studied in institutional settings. In a study of institutionalized demented residents with sleep and behavior problems, morning exposure to bright light was associated with better nighttime sleep and less daytime agitation. In another study of ambient bright light therapy (2,500 lux delivered in the morning, evening, or all day) compared with standard lighting among older adults with dementia in a psychiatric hospital and a dementia-specific residential care facility, nighttime sleep increased significantly in participants exposed to morning and all-day light, with the increase most prominent in those with severe or very severe dementia. A study of residents with dementia and behavioral problems found that social interaction with nurses reduced behavioral problems and sleep-wake rhythm disorders in some residents. In a small trial, nighttime sleep increased and agitation decreased among nursing-home residents randomized to receive a daytime physical activity program plus nighttime intervention to decrease noise and light disruption. A trial that combined an enforced schedule of structured social and physical activity for 2 weeks in a small sample of assisted-living residents found that treated residents had enhanced slow-wave sleep and improved performance in memory-oriented tasks. Two large multicomponent nonpharmacologic interventions on sleep in nursing-home residents had mixed results, with greatest effects on decreasing daytime sleeping but little effect on nighttime sleep (SOE=B).

Pharmacotherapy

Pharmacotherapy is generally considered in individuals with transient sleep problems, such as problems associated with an acute stressor, or in individuals with chronic insomnia that has not responded to behavioral therapy. As mentioned above, if a decision is made to use a sedative-hypnotic in an older adult, the smallest dosage of an agent with the least risk of adverse events should be chosen and used for the shortest duration necessary. Short-acting sedative-hypnotic agents are recommended for patients with problems falling asleep, and intermediate-acting agents are recommended for patients with problems staying asleep (Table 39.4).

Benzodiazepines (eg, the intermediate-acting agents estazolam and temazepam) bind nonselectively to the gamma-aminobutyric-acid benzodiazepine (GABA-BZ) receptor subunits. As a class, these agents have potential adverse events, including confusion, rebound insomnia, tolerance (to treatment effects), and withdrawal symptoms on discontinuation. Older adults can be more sensitive to the sedating effects of benzodiazepines, with greater risk of confusion and falls (SOE=B). Long-acting benzodiazepines (eg, flurazepam, quazepam), in particular, should not be used in older adults. Short-acting agents appear to have less association with falls and hip fractures, presumably because of less daytime carryover, but at least one study demonstrated an association of short-acting agents with falls at night (SOE=B). However, agents with rapid elimination in general also result in the most pronounced rebound and withdrawal syndromes after discontinuation. Rebound insomnia after discontinuation of short-acting agents is dose dependent and can be reduced by tapering the dosage before discontinuing the drug.

The nonbenzodiazepine benzodiazepine-receptor agonists (NBRAs [eg, eszopiclone, zolpidem, zaleplon]) are structurally unrelated to benzodiazepines but bind to the GABA-BZ receptor with relative selectivity for sedative and amnestic properties. Evidence suggests that NBRAs are relatively well tolerated in healthy older adults (SOE=B), but evidence is limited in older adults with significant comorbidity. Zolpidem is a nonbenzodiazepine imidazopyridine. In older adults, studies suggest that zolpidem does not result in rebound insomnia, agitation, or anxiety when discontinued. Recent evidence of next morning impairment in driving ability (that the patient may not be aware of and that may increase risk of motor vehicle accidents) above a threshold blood level of zolpidem has prompted recommendations for use of lower doses of these agents, particularly in women, who clear zolpidem more slowly than men. Zaleplon is a nonbenzodiazepine hypnotic from the pyrazolopyrimidine class, which has also been studied for short-term use in older adults with insomnia. Because of their rapid onset of action, zolpidem and zaleplon should be taken only immediately before bedtime or after the individual has gone to bed and been unable to fall asleep. Eszopiclone is an s-isomer of the cyclopyrrolone zopiclone, and it has a longer duration of action than the other nonbenzodiazepines. Recent epidemiologic evidence suggests that nonbenzodiazepines may be associated with an increased age-adjusted risk of falling that is similar to that of the benzodiazepines. Given these and other findings, concerns remain regarding the risks of confusion, falls, and fracture with chronic use of NBRAs in older adults (particularly those who are frail), and caution is warranted even with these agents. The use of benzodiazepines and nonbenzodiazepine-receptor agonists should be limited to ≤6 months, because long-term use is associated with an increased risk of cognitive impairment and dementia.

A new class of hypnotic medications, orexin receptor antagonists, are reported to promote sleep at doses that do not disrupt cognition. Suvorexant is the first dual orexin receptor antagonist approved for treatment of insomnia in the United States; the potential role of this medication in treatment of older adults is not yet known.

The melatonin receptor agonist ramelteon does not act at GABA receptors; rather it is a selective MT1/MT2 receptor agonist. Ramelteon reduces sleep latency and increases total sleep time in older adults (SOE=B), without evidence of significant rebound or withdrawal effects with discontinuation.

The tricyclic antidepressant doxepin, which has been available for decades, is now available in a low-dose formulation (3–6 mg) approved for treatment of insomnia characterized by problems with sleep maintenance (SOE=B). At low dosages, doxepin selectively antagonizes H_1 receptors, which is believed to promote the onset and maintenance of sleep. Low dosages of other sedating antidepressants such as trazodone[OL] or mirtazapine[OL] at bedtime have been used as sleeping aids for many years, but there is limited evidence to support this practice (SOE=D). Sedating antidepressants have been suggested for use at low dosages as a nighttime aid for sleep in depressed patients receiving another antidepressant at therapeutic dosages during the daytime. Other indications include patients with a history of psychoactive substance use problems, lack of response to other sleeping medications, suspected untreated sleep apnea (in which further respiratory depression with certain other agents is a concern), and fibromyalgia (in which there is some evidence of antidepressant medication treatment effect). However, the adverse effects of sedating antidepressants may limit their usefulness.

Sedating antipsychotics[OL] are sometimes used for sleep complaints in patients with other serious psychiatric conditions that warrant treatment with an antipsychotic medication. Sedating antipsychotics should not be used in routine management of insomnia in older adults without serious psychiatric illness.

Chronic Hypnotic Use

In European studies, a relatively high prevalence of chronic sedative-hypnotic use in older adults (5%–8% in older men, up to 25% in older women) has been reported. There is strong epidemiologic evidence for increased morbidity and mortality with chronic use of prescription sleeping pills; however, much of this literature is older and predates the availability of newer, nonbenzodiazepine hypnotics, so the relationship between these hypnotics and morbidity/mortality is not clear. In addition, after tolerance to hypnotics develops, long-term use of these agents can actually make sleep quality worse. Data reported from a longitudinal study of older adults in Germany indicated a higher rate of sleep-related complaints in those who took sleeping medications than in those who did not.

Several studies have shown that the bulk of prescription sleeping medication use occurs among chronic users, and not those with transient sleeping difficulties. In a study in Spain, long-term use was 2–3 times more common in older adults than in middle-aged respondents. In studies in Canada and France, sleep-promoting medications were prescribed for ≥1 year in more than two-thirds of people who were taking these agents. Studies in the United States have also demonstrated more benzodiazepine use by older adults and by women, with chronic use being more common in older adults.

Methods to help older chronic hypnotic users reduce or eliminate their use of these agents have been reported (SOE=B). In general, tapering of the hypnotic in chronic users is necessary to prevent rebound insomnia and other adverse withdrawal effects. One reported strategy involved decreasing the hypnotic dose by one-half for 2 weeks, followed by full withdrawal (perhaps with the use of a substitute pill at night), which was effective in eliminating hypnotic use without adverse events on nighttime sleep, depressive symptoms, or daytime sleepiness. In another small controlled trial in which benzodiazepine use was tapered to complete withdrawal over as many as 6 weeks, more success was seen in those participants randomized to receive a nightly dose of 2 mg of controlled-release melatonin rather than placebo. At follow-up 6 months later, nearly 80% of those who successfully discontinued benzodiazepines continued to report good sleep quality. Cognitive-behavioral therapy, when combined with gradual tapering of the hypnotic dose, has also been demonstrated to be helpful in reducing or eliminating chronic benzodiazepine use (SOE=B).

Nonprescription Sleeping Agents

Nearly half of older adults report using nonprescription OTC sleeping agents; however, there is little evidence to support this practice. Commonly used nonprescription agents include sedating antihistamines, acetaminophen, alcohol, melatonin, and herbal products. Sedating antihistamines (eg, diphenhydramine) are common ingredients in OTC sleeping agents as well as in combination analgesic-sleeping agents that are marketed for nighttime use. Diphenhydramine has potent anticholinergic effects, and tolerance to its sedating effects develops after several weeks, so it is not recommended for older adults. Individuals with mild nighttime discomfort and mild insomnia may have adequate relief with a simple pain reliever (eg, acetaminophen) at bedtime. Although alcohol causes some initial drowsiness, it can interfere with sleep later in the night and can actually worsen sleeping difficulties. There is some evidence in older adults with insomnia that melatonin administration decreases sleep latency and wake time after sleep onset, and increases sleep efficiency (time asleep over time in bed), but results are mixed. However, there is evidence for effectiveness of melatonin in certain circadian rhythm sleep disorders. For example, blind people with abnormal circadian sleep-wake rhythms (eg, free-running rhythms not entrained to the external environment because of lack of light/dark perception) may correct with melatonin given at night (SOE=B). The melatonin dose in these studies has ranged from 0.5 to 10 mg, but lower doses may be most effective. Several weeks or months of treatment with nighttime melatonin may be required to correct the blind person's rhythm, and it is believed that melatonin treatment must be continued indefinitely, because the free-running rhythm will return if the melatonin is discontinued. Valerian is an herbal product with mild sedative action that has been marketed for insomnia. Its mechanism of action is uncertain, and it contains several potentially active compounds, with risk of adverse events. A systematic review found the existing evidence for efficacy of valerian to be inconclusive (SOE=C). Kava, another herbal product marketed for insomnia, has a significant risk of adverse events, including hepatotoxicity, and it is not recommended.

Choosing Wisely® Recommendations

Sleep Issues

- Do not use benzodiazepines or other sedative-hypnotics in older adults as first choice for insomnia, agitation, or delirium.

References

- Aurora RN, Chowdhuri S, Ramar K, et al. The treatment of central sleep apnea syndromes in adults: practice parameters with an evidence–based literature review and meta-analyses. *Sleep.* 2012;35(1):17–40.

  This paper provides evidence-based recommendations for management of central sleep apnea (CSA). Most of the evidence addresses CSA associated with congestive heart failure, in which optimizing therapy for heart failure is central to treating CSA. There is also evidence that continuous positive-airway presssure therapy targeted to achieve an apnea-hypopnea index <15 improves transplant-free survival in patients with CSA and heart failure. Other treatments are also described. Recommendations specific to treatment of CSA in older adults are not provided.

- Aurora RN, Kristo DA, Bista SR, et al. The treatment of restless legs syndrome and periodic limb movement disorder in adults—an update for 2012: practice parameters with an evidence-based systematic review and meta-analyses. *Sleep.* 2012;35(8):1039–1062.

  This paper provides evidence-based recommendations for treatment of restless legs syndrome (RLS). The dopamine agonists pramipexole and ropinirole are recommended for treatment of moderate to very severe RLS. Other treatment options are also described. There are no studies addressing the use of dopaminergic medications for treatment of periodic limb movement disorder alone (ie, without RLS), so this is not recommended. Recommendations specific to the treatment of RLS in older adults are not provided.

- Blackwell T, Yaffe K, Laffan A, et al. Associations of objectively and subjectively measured sleep quality with subsequent cognitive decline in older community-dwelling men: The MrOS Sleep Study. *Sleep.* 2014;37(4):655–663.

  This papers describes a population-based longitudinal study of cognitively intact community-dwelling older men (N=2, 822) who had subjective (ie, questionnaire) and objective (ie, actigraphy) measures of sleep during an ancillary visit of a larger study (Osteoporotic Fractures in Men [MrOS]). Two tests of cognitive function (Trails B and the Modified Mini-Mental State examination) were also performed. Among these men followed over 3.4 ± 0.5 years, objective measures of worse sleep (eg, reduced sleep efficiency, greater nighttime wakefulness) and poor self-reported sleep quality were associated with subsequent cognitive decline, particularly the Trails B (described as a measure of executive function).

- Buysse DJ, Germain A, Moul DE, et al. Efficacy of brief behavioral treatment for chronic insomnia in older adults. *Arch Intern Med.* 2011;171(10):887–895.

  This manuscript reports findings from a randomized controlled trial of a brief behavioral treatment for insomnia (consisting of individualized insomnia behavioral instructions delivered in 2 individual sessions and 2 telephone calls) compared with an information control condition (involving educational brochures on sleep and one follow up phone call). Both conditions were delivered by a mental health nurse practitioner. Participants (N=79) were older outpatients (mean age 71.7 years) with chronic insomnia. Compared with controls, participants in the intervention group had improvements in sleep based on self-reported measures and actigraphy, with improvements maintained at 6 months. This study suggests that this brief behavioral treatment improves insomnia in older adults.

- Diem SJ, Ewing SK, Stone KL, et al. Use of non-benzodiazepine sedative hypnotics and risk of falls in older men. *J Gerontol Geriatr Res.* 2014;3(3):158.

  This paper reports on analyses of data from community-dwelling older men (N=4,450) enrolled in the population-based prospective cohort study, Osteoporotic Fractures in Men (MrOS). The investigators analyzed data on use of nonbenzodiazepine sedative-hypnotics (eg, zolpidem, zaleplon, eszopiclone) and benzodiazepines (both determined by interview and verified by medication containers), and falls over 1-year follow-up (assessed by questionnaires performed 3 times per year). In these age-adjusted analyses, use of nonbenzodiazepine sedative-hypnotics was associated with an increased risk of falls similar to the risk of falls associated with use of benzodiazepines.

- Vitiello MV, McCurry SM, Shortreed SM, et al. Cognitive-behavioral treatment for comorbid insomnia and osteoarthritis pain in primary care: the lifestyles randomized controlled trial. *J Am Geriatr Soc.* 2013;61(6):947–956.

  This paper reports on the findings of a double-blind, cluster-randomized controlled trial in older adults (N=367, mean age = 73.1 years) with both osteoarthritis pain and insomnia with a 9-month follow-up period. Participants received either cognitive-behavioral therapy for pain and insomnia (CBT-PI), a cognitive-behavioral pain coping skills intervention (CBT-P), or an education only control (EOC) condition. Results demonstrated that CBT-PI reduced insomnia severity more than both the control (EOC) and the CBT-P conditions. Outcomes of pain severity and arthritis symptoms did not differ between groups. These findings suggest that cognitive-behavioral therapy for insomnia added to CBT-P improved insomnia in older adults with both pain and insomnia.

Cathy A. Alessi, MD, AGSF

CHAPTER 40—DEPRESSION AND OTHER MOOD DISORDERS

KEY POINTS

- Treatment of depression may require up to 12 weeks before remission is complete, but an initial response to medication should be seen within the first 4 weeks.

- In a substantial minority of cases, trials of more than one antidepressant or combination therapy with two antidepressants may be required before remission is achieved.

- Executive cognitive dysfunction is easily assessed and when present predicts poor response to medication as well as the need for adapted psychotherapy.

- Exercise reduces depressive symptoms and should be prescribed for all depressed older adults who are capable of increasing their level of physical activity.

- Bipolar depression in older adults may be more common than previously thought and should be treated with a mood stabilizer rather than an antidepressant.

EPIDEMIOLOGY

Depression is a leading cause of disability-adjusted life years lost across the life span and projected to be more so within a generation. Mood disorders are implicated in 10% of all hospitalizations. However, prevalence studies of community residents demonstrate surprisingly low rates of depressive disorders among those ≥65 years old. Only 1%–2% of women and <1% of men interviewed with standardized instruments met diagnostic criteria for major depressive disorder (SOE=A). Both current and lifetime prevalence rates for older adults are lower than those for middle-aged adults; furthermore, these relatively low rates persist after accounting for possible premature death and institutionalization, both of which can be associated with depression. Similarly, the incidence of first-episode major depressive disorder decreases after age 65. Data demonstrating that older adults are less likely to recognize depression and to endorse depressed mood offer one explanation for the lower prevalence and incidence of depressive syndromes among older community residents.

However, the prevalence of depressive symptoms that do not meet the threshold for a major depressive disorder as defined by the *Diagnostic and Statistical Manual of Mental Disorders, 5th Edition (DSM-5)* is substantial in older adults, with most studies reporting rates in the range of 15%. These subsyndromal states are not inconsequential. "Minor" or "subsyndromal" depression, defined variably as the presence of depressed mood with 2 or 3 additional symptoms of major depressive disorder has been associated with increased use of health services, excess disability, and poor health outcomes, including higher mortality. *DSM-5* uses a more descriptive, precise terminology to capture these depressive states and elevates them to the status of "other specified depressive disorder" in recognition of their associated morbidity.

The prevalence rates of both major and subsyndromal depression vary greatly by the setting in which older adults are seen and by methods used to identify cases. Increased rates of depression are found among older adults seen in health care facilities and inpatient settings. Major depressive disorder has been identified in 6%–10% of older adults in primary care clinics and in 12%–20% of nursing-home residents. More varied rates of 11%–45% have been reported among older adults requiring inpatient medical care. The reported prevalence rates of minor depression in outpatient medical settings have varied as well, with reported rates of 8% to >40%. Studies that count symptoms due to physical illness toward a diagnosis of depression can inflate prevalence rates among medical patients because of symptom overlap. In mental health settings, major depressive disorder is the most common diagnosis seen among older patients and accounts for >40% of outpatient caseloads and inpatient psychiatry admissions.

Studies show that risk factors for depression in older ethnic minority patients can differ from those in whites. For example, lack of spirituality was a risk factor for depression in black Americans but not in white Americans. In general, older adults of ethnic minorities exhibit less use of mental health services. Shorter length of residence in the United States as well as personal beliefs influence the use of mental health services among older immigrants and members of ethnic minority groups.

CLINICAL PRESENTATION AND DIAGNOSIS

The Geriatric Syndrome of Late-Life Depression

Although aging does not markedly affect the phenomenology of depression, older adults are more often preoccupied with somatic symptoms and less frequently report depressed mood and guilty preoccupations. Among those who do not acknowledge sustained sadness, a persistent loss of pleasure and interest in previously enjoyable activities (*anhedonia*) for at least 2 weeks is necessary for a diagnosis of major depressive disorder. The phrase "with seasonal pattern" may be added to recurrent major depressive disorder, but depression induced by the reduction in day length during winter is uncommon in older adults. Responses to a catastrophic loss such as bereavement, onset of crippling disability or illness, financial collapse, or natural disaster may include profound sadness, preoccupation with the event, impaired concentration, sleep disturbance, and loss of appetite—all consistent with the diagnosis of a depressive disorder. However, grief should be considered an appropriate and even adaptive response, rather than evidence of pathology. Nonetheless, when the response is out of proportion to personal expectations or cultural norms, or when there is a past history of depression, clinical judgment may dictate a diagnosis of major depression. When bereavement is associated with prolonged, nearly paralyzing preoccupation with the lost loved one, *DSM-5* places the condition under "other specified trauma- and stressor-related disorder" as a "persistent complex bereavement disorder."

The diagnosis of depression in physically ill older adults is confounded by the overlap among symptoms of major depressive disorder and somatic illness. Patients with advanced physical illness may be preoccupied with thoughts about death or worthlessness because of marked disability, yet not meet criteria for a major depressive episode. The *DSM-5* criteria require that the depressive symptoms are not a direct result of a general medical condition or medication used to treat it. The alternative diagnosis of mood disorder due to a general medical condition should be used for patients with depression that appears to result directly from a specific medical condition (eg, hypothyroidism, pancreatic cancer, end-stage renal disease). In either case, when symptoms are disabling, treatment should be offered.

Screening

Simply screening for the presence of depressed mood and anhedonia identifies most medically ill patients who also meet diagnostic criteria for major depressive disorder. These symptoms are less likely to be confounded by those of a medical illness. When the clinician fears an older adult is minimizing distress or associated disability, it is helpful to obtain further information from involved family members or caregivers. However, without a protocol for treatment initiation and response assessment or referral for mental health services, screening for depressive disorders in primary care or social service settings is ineffective. Informing the primary care clinician of the results of screening without linking to mental health consultation or referral too often leads to subtherapeutic dosages of an antidepressant, inadequate assessment of treatment response, and the patient's abandonment of therapy.

The nine items of the Patient Health Questionnaire (PHQ-9) cover the diagnostic criteria for major depressive disorder, and the initial two questions (the "PHQ-2") can be used for screening. In addition, serial administrations of the PHQ-9 can be used to reliably assess response to treatment. The parent instrument, the PRIME-MD, has also been validated using a telephone interview by a mental health specialist as the gold standard and adapted for computer-assisted telephone interviewing in population-based studies. Compared with in-person administration, telephone depression assessments do well in areas of item nonresponse, reliability, mean level of symptom severity, and proportion of respondents classified as depressed. The effect of sociodemographic characteristics is minimal to absent in both interview methods, and the instrument is available in Spanish. Telephone assessment may be viewed as less intrusive by the patient.

The PHQ-9 and PHQ-2 are available online in English and Spanish as public access (http://phqscreeners.com). Patients scoring a total of ≥3 on the depressed mood plus anhedonia questions on the PHQ-2 should be assessed with the remaining seven questions of the PHQ-9. Patients scoring 3 on the anhedonia questions alone should also be fully assessed. A complaint of depression need not be present for a diagnosis of major depressive disorder, provided the other symptoms significantly impair function and are not the direct result of somatic illness. For management based on PHQ-9 score, see Table 40.1.

At a score of ≥10, the PHQ-9 has good sensitivity and specificity for major depressive disorder among primary care patients versus a structured diagnostic interview conducted by a mental health professional. People scoring ≥15 and those with suicidal ideation may require psychiatric consultation. A change of 5 points is considered a minimal clinically important difference and evidence of response to treatment (Table 40.2). Remission is best defined as a total score of ≤5. When the score has changed by <5 points despite 4 weeks of treatment at recommended dosages, the medication should either be switched or combined with another antidepressant.

Another standardized instrument for evaluating depressive symptoms is the 15-item Geriatric Depression Scale (GDS) (www.stanford.edu/~yesavage/GDS.html; www.stanford.edu/~yesavage/GDS.english.short.score.html [accessed Jan 2016]). Although it offers the convenience of a "yes/no" response, and it is virtually free of somatic and sleep queries, it does not query suicidal or death ideation and is not useful for assessing treatment response. Those who acknowledge thinking they would be "better off dead" or "hurting yourself" should be asked about the presence of a firearm in the home. Firearms

Table 40.1—Indications to Start Antidepressant Therapy Based on Patient Health Questionnaire-9

PHQ-9 Score	Depression Severity	Clinician Response
1–4	None	None
5–9	Mild to moderate	If not currently treated, rescreen in 2 weeks. If currently treated, optimize antidepressant and rescreen in 2 weeks.
10–14	Major depressive disorder	Start antidepressant therapy.
≥15	Major depressive disorder	Start antidepressant therapy; obtain psychiatric consultation if suicidality or psychosis suspected.

For additional information, see http://phqscreeners.com.

Table 40.2—Prescriber Response Guidelines at 4 Weeks Based on the Patient Health Questionnaire-9 and the Sequenced Treatment Alternatives to Relieve Depression (STAR*D) Studies

PHQ-9 Score or Change	Outcome	Clinician Response
No decrease or increase	Nonresponse	Switch medication
Decrease of 2–4 points	Partial response	Add medication
Decrease of ≥5 points	Response	Maintain medication
Score <5	Remission	Maintain medication

For additional information, see http://phqscreeners.com.

are the leading means of suicide among older adults. The PHQ-9 and the GDS may be reliable when administered to people with mild to moderate dementia, but response to treatment with SSRI therapy in dementia with depression may be no better than with placebo (SOE=A).

Emerging evidence suggests that the diagnostic process for older patients should include an assessment of executive cognitive function. When present, executive dysfunction complicating depression predicts poor response to SSRI therapy and may be better addressed with psychotherapy (SOE=A).

Bipolar Disorder

Although the prevalence of bipolar disorder is low, the increasing numbers of older adults means both primary care clinicians and geriatricians will encounter more patients with a bipolar disorder, particularly bipolar depression. Bipolar disorders do not "burn out" in old age. Indeed, few patients with bipolar disorder recover full function despite symptom remission. Among those with bipolar disorder, mania is a more frequent cause of hospitalization than depression, but depression accounts for more disability. Late-onset mania is seen equally among men and women. Age has little impact on the symptom profile except for less sexual preoccupation among older adults. Impaired cognitive processing, executive dysfunction, and changes in subcortical brain structures are common, further reducing the chances of return to full function.

The *DSM-5* criteria for bipolar disorder type 1 (mania with or without depression) and type 2 (major depressive disorder without mania but with hypomania) are unchanged with age. The manic episode (prevalence 1 to 4 per 1,000) often presents with confusion, disorientation, distractibility, and irritability rather than with elevated, positive mood. The clinical interview can be characterized by irrelevant content delivered with an argumentative, emotionally intense yet fluent quality. Grossly unrealistic ideas concerning finances, travel, or plans for the future are common. Inflated self-esteem, grandiosity, and contentious claims of certainty in the face of evidence to the contrary are also seen. The unsuspecting examiner may be puzzled or irritated by the difficulty of the clinical interaction until the diagnosis of mania is considered.

The presence of psychosis, sleep disturbance, and aggressiveness may lead to the mistaken diagnosis of dementia or depressive disorder rather than mania. Because mania in late life is less frequent than depression or dementia, these patients are often treated with antipsychotics, antidepressants, or benzodiazepines, which provide partial relief. Late-onset mania is more often secondary to or closely associated with other medical disorders, most commonly stroke, dementia, or hyperthyroidism, and also with medications, including antidepressants, steroids, stimulants, and other agents with known CNS properties. A search for treatable components that contribute acutely to the person's disability should be pursued. Risk factors for cerebrovascular disease, including excessive use of alcohol or tobacco, suboptimal control of hypertension, hyperlipidemia, and other cardiovascular risk factors, should be explored. Careful inquiry of the family may reveal repeated hypomanic episodes that did not seriously impair the individual but in retrospect are clear indications of earlier disease. The difficulty of recognizing the diagnosis, care for contributing conditions, age-related vulnerability to adverse events of medication, and the frequency with which structural brain changes are associated all make treatment more difficult.

Occurring in approximately 0.5% of the U.S. population, bipolar disorder type II is characterized by recurrent major depressive episodes interspersed with periods of hypomania. Because interpersonal difficulties can be minimal, and some symptoms can temporarily increase performance with tasks, past episodes of hypomania may be unrecognized by the patient and family. Major depressive episodes also occur in bipolar disorder I, in which the occurrence of one or more manic episodes is the distinguishing diagnostic feature. There are also mixed states in which criteria for both mania and major depressive disorder are present. As a result, the term "bipolar depression" spans the spectrum of bipolar disorders.

Psychotic Depression

The recognition of psychotic depression has particular relevance for primary care clinicians. Patients with psychotic depression have sustained, fixed, false beliefs (delusions) in association with depressed mood. These delusions are often plausible and focused on physical or medical preoccupations, such as the belief that one's bowels are "blocked with cancer" or "I know there's something there and the doctors are just not telling me." Psychotic depression may be suspected when the irrational belief focuses on somatic symptoms or around fears of a serious physical condition when no medical evidence can be identified to support the belief. Patients with somatic delusions often visit multiple specialists and obtain repeated testing to identify problems that they "know" exist rather than for the purpose of seeking relief from persistent somatic "worries." Nearly 25% of older adults with somatic delusions are not diagnosed because of the lack of taking a thorough history, despite visits to other health care practitioners or specialists and multiple diagnostic tests and procedures. Recognition of the excess disability caused by somatic delusions will improve the rate of diagnosis and appropriate treatment of this type of depression.

TREATMENT

Overview

Although mood disorders are eminently treatable, effective treatment remains a goal not so easily attained. Only 50% of patients with major depressive disorder fully respond to initial antidepressant treatment (SOE=A). An additional one-third recover when the antidepressant is switched to another agent or is combined with a second antidepressant or psychotherapy. For those who do recover, 40%–60% experience recurrence depending on the severity of the initial episode and persistence of symptoms. Although a substantial number of patients with "subclinical," "subsyndromal," or "minor" depression experience a remission of symptoms without intervention, each category is associated with as much as a 5-fold risk of a subsequent major depressive episode. Poor self-assessed health, apathy, anxiety, executive dysfunction, and perceived lack of social support predict a less benign course. The onset of macular degeneration, stroke, and myocardial infarction are reliable indicators of depression risk, especially in the context of a prior history of mood disorder. Although the need to prevent mood disorders is substantial, success to date has been limited to reducing the progression of minor to major depressive disorder and to preventing recurrent episodes of major depressive disorder.

The current approach to mood disorders in late life includes a more aggressive acute phase of treatment to bring about remission of the current episode, continuation treatment for an additional six months after symptom remission to prevent relapse, and maintenance treatment to prevent recurrence. For patients with bipolar disorders or a history of depression complicated by psychosis, suicidality, or recurrent episodes, maintenance treatment should be provided for ≥3 years. However, the duration of maintenance therapy should be based on the frequency and severity of previous episodes and may need to be lifelong. Combined pharmacotherapy with psychotherapy is recommended for all patients with bipolar disorders and recurrent, severe psychotic or suicidal depression (SOE=B).

The First Weeks of Treatment

Substantial data indicate that 4 weeks is adequate to identify those patients who at 12 weeks will be nonresponders or partial responders (SOE=B). The sooner the response occurs, the sooner the remission is likely to be achieved. More severe depression at baseline is associated with slower response; higher self-esteem is associated with rapid response. At 4 weeks, one-third of medicated patients will be nonresponders, one-third will have responded fully, and one-third partially. As treatment duration extends, the response rate for both partial and nonresponders decelerates. The longer the patient remains symptomatic, the greater the indication that either the dosage or the medication should be changed. In addition, partial response predicts recurrence of a major episode of depression.

A visit or phone call sometime between the first and fourth week of treatment may have the added value of identifying those patients who ultimately will not respond as well as those who may never have started treatment. In the language of the patient response, partial response and remission are often referred to as "I'm better," "I'm still not myself," and "I'm well" (SOE=C). Assessing response to treatment need be no more burdensome than the decision to start treatment.

Table 40.3—Selected Antidepressants for Older Adults

Drug	Initial Dosage	Final Dosage	Comments/Precautions
SSRIs			
Citalopram	10 mg qam	20 mg qam	Risk of QT_c prolongation in doses >20 mg, nausea, tremor, hyponatremia, serotonin syndrome
Escitalopram	10 mg qam	10–20 mg qam	Nausea, tremor, serotonin syndrome; reduce dosage in renal insufficiency
Sertraline	25 mg qam	100–200 mg qam	Nausea, tremor, insomnia, serotonin syndrome
Selective Serotonergic and Noradrenergic Reuptake Inhibitors (SSRI/SNRI)			
Duloxetine	20–30 mg qam	60 mg qam	Drug interactions (CYP1A2, -2D6 substrate); chronic liver disease, alcoholism, increased serum transaminase; reduce dosage in renal insufficiency
Venlafaxine XR	37.5–75 mg qam	75–225 mg qam	Mild hypertensive; headache, nausea, vomiting; do not stop abruptly; reduce dosage in renal insufficiency
Vortioxetine	5 mg qam	10-20 mg qam	Nausea; no data available on doses >5 mg in older adults
Tricyclic Antidepressants (TCAs)			
Nortriptyline	10–25 mg qhs	25–100 mg qhs	Glaucoma, prostatic disease, diabetes; may be fatal in overdose; therapeutic window 50–150 ng/mL serum level
Others			
Bupropion	75 mg q12h 150 mg qam	150–300 mg 300 mg extended release qam	Agitation, insomnia, seizures
Mirtazapine	7.5 mg qhs	15–45 mg qhs	Dry mouth, weight gain, potential for neutropenia; reduce dosage in renal insufficiency

Pharmacotherapy of Single or Recurrent Episodes of Major Depression

Currently available antidepressants are thought to work through the enhancement of monoamine function by either blocking the reuptake or stimulating receptors of serotonin, dopamine, or norepinephrine. For a summary of antidepressants and adverse effects in older adults, see Table 40.3. Gastrointestinal distress is the most common transient adverse reaction to serotonergic agents. The syndrome of inappropriate antidiuretic hormone (SIADH) is a rare, life-threatening adverse reaction to serotonergic agents; it is generally treated with fluid restriction. The even rarer serotonin syndrome is difficult to diagnose and easily overlooked; it requires supportive care and treatment of associated symptoms (Table 40.4).

A series of reports from the Sequenced Treatment Alternatives to Relieve Depression (STAR*D) study team offer a genuine advance for older adults in primary care settings with a structured treatment protocol for use by clinicians. When remission was not achieved with use of the first SSRI in the STAR*D protocol (citalopram), augmentation with a non-SSRI (bupropion or buspirone) reliably achieved remission in one-third of patients. Stopping citalopram because of intolerability or lack of response and switching to bupropion, venlafaxine, or sertraline achieved remission in an additional one-fourth. For patients who could tolerate citalopram but did not achieve remission, augmentation with bupropion or buspirone was superior to switching to another agent. However, patients who did not tolerate citalopram did as well with sertraline as with bupropion or venlafaxine. There is also sufficient evidence form open-label trials

Table 40.4—Clinical Signs and Symptoms of Serotonin Syndrome

- Use of medication(s) with serotonergic activity
- Cognitive and behavioral changes: agitation, hyperactivity, worsening confusion, restlessness
- Diaphoresis
- Diarrhea and GI upset
- Fever usually >100.5° F (38° C)
- Hyperreflexia with or without myoclonus
- Incoordination, ataxia, or new onset of falls
- Ocular clonus
- Rhabdomyolysis
- Shivering
- Seizures
- Tremor

among older adults to recommend the antipsychotic aripiprazole for augmentation (SOE=B).

When psychosis complicates major depressive disorder, the evidence directing choice of pharmacotherapy for older adults is evolving. Electroconvulsive therapy (ECT) is effective for depression complicated by psychosis and is often considered the treatment of choice for patients with severe depression accompanied by suicidal thoughts and for those who do not respond to augmentation therapies (SOE=B). Yet, few patients or their family members will consider ECT without having exhausted other alternatives. In the multisite Study of Pharmacotherapy of Psychotic Depression (STOP-PD), remission was achieved in >60% of the geriatric patients who received a combination of sertraline and olanzapine over

12 weeks. Remission rates with combination therapy were substantially better than with sertraline alone. The average end-of-study daily doses were nearly 150 mg of sertraline and more than 12 mg of olanzapine. Therefore, although ECT remains an effective treatment option for late-life psychotic depression, intensive antipsychotic and antidepressant pharmacotherapy can be an effective initial strategy.

Pharmacotherapy of Mania

For a summary of treatment of bipolar disorders in older adults, see Table 40.5. Expert opinion, guidelines, and the Systematic Treatment Enhancement Program for Bipolar Disorder (STEP-BD) reports are in agreement that anticonvulsants, called mood stabilizers in this context, are preferable for both acute treatment and prevention of recurrence in late-life bipolar mania (SOE=A). The anticonvulsant divalproex is increasingly considered first choice for treatment and prevention of mania. A therapeutic blood level of 50-100 mcg/mL is considered both safe and efficacious. When the level is subtherapeutic and the patient response inadequate, the dose should be increased. When the level is at or above the upper limit and there is little or no response after 2 weeks, the drug trial should be declared a failure. Partial response accompanied by a blood level within the therapeutic range indicates the need to increase the dosage or add an antipsychotic. Divalproex inhibits hepatic enzymes that metabolize medications frequently used by older adults. Patients taking β-blockers, type 1C antiarrhythmics (eg, flecainide, propafenone), benzodiazepines, or anticoagulants should be monitored more closely until the divalproex dosage has been stabilized. Laboratory tests (including CBC with platelets, AST, ALT, and amylase) should be performed when treatment is started, when the dosage is increased, and at least every 6 months. Dosage reduction is indicated for tremor interfering with self-care, ataxia or unsteady gait, excess sedation, or heart rate <50 beats per minute. Divalproex should be held or discontinued if the following do not remit after dosage reduction or dosage withholding: platelet count <80,000/μL, or AST, ALT, or amylase ≥2-fold above upper limit of normal.

Response to divalproex requires at least a 3-week period, including titration to a therapeutic range. In the interim, individuals whose mania is exhausting or associated with overly aggressive behavior require an antipsychotic or benzodiazepine. A number of second-generation antipsychotics are approved by the FDA for treatment of mania (Table 40.5). Meta-analyses indicate that these second-generation antipsychotics appear to be equally effective (SOE=A) such that the choice of an individual agent is based on adverse-event profile.

However, the available data on the treatment of mania in these studies include few older adults.

Older adults who have had good results with lithium should not be switched to an alternative unless adverse events become disabling. Nonetheless, the use of lithium as initial treatment should be considered cautiously. Structural brain changes that may not be clinically apparent are associated with a higher risk of toxicity. Diabetes insipidus, hyperglycemia, thyroid abnormalities, severe tremor, confusion, heart failure, arrhythmia, and psoriasis are among the more frequent reasons for discontinuing lithium. Manifestations of lithium toxicity include GI complaints, ataxia, slurred speech, delirium, or coma. Toxicity in older adults can occur at plasma concentrations below the therapeutic threshold of 1 mEq/L. Mild tremor and nystagmus without functional consequences frequently accompany lithium treatment and should not be considered signs of toxicity. Dosage reduction is indicated for tremor interfering with self-care or resulting in ataxia or unsteady gait. The onset of diabetes insipidus can also be cause for discontinuing lithium.

Pharmacotherapy of Bipolar Depression

Similar to the case in the treatment of mania, there is a relative consensus that mood stabilizers are preferable to antidepressants for acute treatment and prevention of recurrence of late-life bipolar depression (SOE=B). Indeed, antidepressants should be used with caution in bipolar depression because of the risk of a manic reaction as well as other adverse events and lack of efficacy. However, the prescribing pathway for bipolar depression in late life is characterized more by off-label use of medications than by FDA-approved indications. Beyond the initial step of prescribing either lithium or lamotrigine, next steps are dictated by the patient's symptom profile. For episodes of depression in both bipolar types I and II in which the patient's history includes relatively less mania, the antidepressant bupropion is a reasonable addition. However, for instances characterized by mixed symptoms or more frequent episodes of mania, a second-generation antipsychotic or a second mood stabilizer is preferable. Purely on the basis of its adverse-event profile and the likelihood of drug interactions (Table 40.5), lamotrigine would appear to be preferable to lithium, divalproex, and carbamazepine for bipolar depression (SOE=D). Although lamotrigine may be given twice daily, its prolonged half-life, which requires slow titration, suggests once-a-day dosing may be adequate for older adults.

Titration should be conducted very carefully in patients who may also be taking hepatic cytochrome isoenzyme–inducing medications or valproic acid. In the absence of these, lamotrigine treatment can begin at 25 mg/d for 2 weeks, then 50 mg/d for 2 weeks,

Table 40.5—Medications Used to Stabilize Mood in Mania and Bipolar Depression

Drug	Initial Dosage (mg)	Final Dosage (mg)	Sedative Potential	Precautions	FDA-Approved Indications and Comments
Anticonvulsants					
Carbamazepine	100 q12h 100 qhs	500 q12h 800 hs	Moderate	Delayed onset of action, drug interactions, dizziness, unsteady gait, anemia; CBC and serum chemistries at baseline, then q6mo; enhances cytochrome P450 activity and decreases other drug concentrations	Acute manic and mixed bipolar I episodes; therapeutic concentration 4–12 mcg/mL
Divalproex sodium Extended-release Delayed-release	250 q12h 250 hs 250 hs	1,000 q12h 1,000 hs 500 hs	Moderate	Delayed onset of action, drug interactions, GI upset, tremor, weight gain, edema, thrombocytopenia, sedation; CBC and serum chemistries at baseline, then q6mo; inhibits hepatic enzymes and increases other drug concentrations; hepatotoxicity, pancreatitis; reduce dosage in renal insufficiency	Acute manic and mixed bipolar I episodes; better tolerated than carbamazepine; therapeutic concentration 50–100 mcg/mL
Lamotrigine	25 hs	100 q12h	Low	Headaches; prolonged half-life; appearance of rash calls for immediate cessation; clearance reduced by valproate	Bipolar I depression to prevent recurrence; does not alter cytochrome P450 activity
Antipsychotics					
Aripiprazole	5 qam	15 qam	Low	Prolonged half-life, may produce agitation at high dosages because of D_2 dopamine receptor agonist activity	Acute manic and mixed bipolar I episodes and for adjunctive treatment of major depressive disorder
Olanzapine	2.5 qhs	15 qhs	Moderate	Slightly anticholinergic as dosage increases, weight gain, metabolic syndrome, diabetes	Acute manic and mixed bipolar I episodes
Quetiapine	25 qhs	750 in divided doses	Moderate	Sedation, weight gain, metabolic syndrome, diabetes, arrhythmia	Acute manic and bipolar I and II depression; sedative; less extrapyramidal symptoms, tardive dyskinesia
Risperidone	0.25 qhs	6 in divided doses	Low	Extrapyramidal symptoms likely at doses >2 mg, weight gain, metabolic syndrome, diabetes	Acute manic and mixed bipolar I episodes
Lithium compounds					
Lithium carbonate Controlled-release	300 q24h 450 q24h	300 q8h 450 q12h	Low	Renal clearance is sole route of elimination; toxicity may appear below therapeutic range; mild tremor is a benign universal adverse event but not when excessive or combined with ataxia; polyuria, polydipsia may be signs of diabetes insipidus; nausea, vomiting are signs of toxicity; risk of hypothyroidism, renal impairment	Acute and maintenance therapy of mania in bipolar disorder; lowers risk of suicide; therapeutic level 0.6–1 mEq/L

then 100 mg/d for 1 week, then 200 mg/d for usual maintenance. As with most anticonvulsants, dosages should be reduced by approximately 50% for patients with moderate liver dysfunction and by approximately 75% for those with more severe dysfunction.

Electroconvulsive Therapy

ECT is highly effective for treatment of major depressive disorder and mania in older adults. ECT is the first-line treatment for patients at serious risk of suicide or life-threatening poor intake due to a major depressive disorder (SOE=B). Patients with delusional depression can demonstrate paranoia about their food or caregivers, precluding pharmacologic treatment because of unreliable oral intake. Also, delusional depression is less responsive to standard medication regimens. Therefore, ECT is generally the first-line treatment for these patients and is associated with response rates that approximate 80%.

The cognitive adverse events of ECT are the principal factor limiting its acceptance. Anterograde amnesia or the inability to learn new information can be pronounced initially, particularly during bilateral ECT, but improves rapidly after treatment is completed. Retrograde amnesia is more persistent, and the recall of events that immediately preceded ECT can be lost permanently. Although patients may complain that ECT has had a long-term effect on their memory, longitudinal studies have not demonstrated lasting cognitive effects; furthermore, improved memory, perhaps owing to recovery from depression, has been reported. There are few absolute medical contraindications other than the presence of increased intracranial pressure or unstable angina. Patients with coronary artery disease or cerebrovascular disease can be administered ECT safely by appropriate pharmacologic management of the autonomic responses that can occur during treatment. Nevertheless, a recent myocardial infarction or cerebrovascular event and unstable coronary artery disease increase the risk of complications. Right unilateral treatment produces fewer cognitive adverse events than bilateral treatment but is less effective unless doses markedly exceeding a patient's seizure threshold are used.

The selection of ECT over aggressive pharmacotherapy is generally made by weighing the risk of waiting for medication to work against the burden of hospital treatment, any medical conditions that can complicate general anesthesia, and fears of the patient and family. After a course of ECT, pharmacotherapy should be continued. Patients not responding to intensive antidepressant treatment before receiving ECT have lower acute response rates and are more likely to relapse subsequently, even when antidepressant treatment is continued with a new medication. Although maintenance ECT is sometimes used to prevent relapse, the burden that maintenance ECT places on patients and their families may limit its usefulness for long-term management of late-life major depressive disorder. However, some patients who respond uniquely well to ECT can tolerate maintenance ECT performed on an outpatient basis.

Repetitive Transcranial Magnetic Stimulation (rTMS)

rTMS is a newer treatment for depression in which an electrical coil is positioned over the left prefrontal cortex to generate a focal magnetic field. It is considered noninvasive and has also been studied in an array of psychiatric and neurologic conditions. Typically, treatments are delivered daily for 6 weeks or 30 treatments. Dropout rates and adverse reactions are comparable to those of placebo condition with sham rTMS. However, in a meta-analysis of 6 trials comparing ECT to rTMS, ECT showed greater remission rates. Response to rTMS in older adults is not as robust as in younger persons; only one large multisite trial did not show that younger age was a significant predictor of response (SOE=A). rTMS is not covered by either Medicare or Medicaid.

Psychosocial Interventions

Although evidence-based psychosocial interventions are not accessible to all depressed older adults, many components of the interventions have common sense appeal and can be incorporated into the practices of geriatricians and primary care clinicians. Studies demonstrating the efficacy of psychotherapy for major depressive disorder in older adults have included problem-solving therapy (SOE=B), cognitive-behavioral therapy, and interpersonal psychotherapy. Problem-solving therapy involves working with the patient to identify practical life difficulties that are causing distress and providing guidance to help the patient identify solutions. Therapy is generally conducted in 6 to 8 meetings spaced 1–2 weeks apart. Cognitive and interpersonal psychotherapy are also time-limited but less highly structured. Psychotherapy for minor depression has been promising, with efficacy demonstrated particularly in individuals who have suffered a loss; the goal is prevention of progression to major depressive disorder. Also, caregivers of older adults can develop depressive syndromes that benefit from psychotherapy. Psychosocial interventions can be effective without psychotropic medication. However, psychotherapy combined with an antidepressant has been associated with a longer period of remission after recovery from the acute episode (SOE=A).

Aerobic exercise is also prescribed as a treatment for mild to moderate depression in older adults who are capable of increasing their level of physical activity. It incorporates the concept of behavioral activation central to cognitive-behavioral psychotherapy. Exercise performed with a partner also adds to the perception of social support. Exercise in combination with antidepressants can yield faster, more lasting results than either alone (SOE=B). Encouraging physical activity should be part of the prescription for all depressed older adults.

Originally developed with younger and middle-aged patients, evidenced-based psychosocial interventions for bipolar depression are applicable to older adults. Intensive psychosocial interventions improve recovery of function and prevent hospitalization associated with recurrence (SOE=B). Improvements in relationships and life satisfaction associated with the interventions exceed those expected from improvements in mood alone. The interventions include family-focused treatment, interpersonal and social rhythms therapy, and cognitive-behavioral therapy as indicated based on individual needs.

For patients with available family, family-focused treatment emphasizes shared planning to prevent relapses, improved listening and communication, and problem-solving skills. In interpersonal and social rhythms therapy, interpersonal problems and difficulties maintaining a physiologically stabilizing schedule of sleep, waking, and activity are examined to minimize destabilizing social and interpersonal situations. In individual cognitive-behavioral therapy, patients and therapists discuss problem solving, cognitive restructuring, and behavioral activation exercises to reverse negative self-attributions and increase rewarding habits. Enthusiasm for these interventions must be tempered by the frequency with which cognitive impairment accompanies bipolar disorder. Nonetheless, the major components of these interventions have a common sense quality and can be applied in primary care.

Management of depression through a disease management model using behavioral health managers is being used more often. The behavioral health manager, usually a master's level social worker, psychologist, or nurse supervised by a psychiatrist, collaborates with the primary care clinician, patient, and family. Even when routine care is enhanced by improved access to psychiatric consultation, the collaborative disease management model proves superior. Most, if not all, of the patient screening, assessment, and follow-up are conducted over the phone by the behavioral health manager. Large-scale, multisite studies have shown greater rates of response and remission as well as lower levels of suicidality associated with the disease management model than enhanced routine care (SOE=A).

REFERENCES

- Alexopoulos GS, Raue PJ, Kiosses DN, et al. Problem solving therapy and supportive therapy in older adults with major depression and executive dysfunction: effect on disability. *Arch Gen Psychiatry*. 2011;68(1):33–41.

   In this study, >200 older adults with major depressive disorder and executive dysfunction were randomized to receive either 12 sessions of adapted problem-solving therapy or supportive psychotherapy. Both therapies reduced depression and disability in the first 6 weeks of intervention. The therapeutic advantage of problem solving over supportive therapy remained after 24 months. These results suggest an adapted psychotherapy for depression complicated by executive dysfunction offers emotional and functional advantages to a population likely not to benefit from pharmacotherapy.

- American Psychiatric Association. *Desk Reference to the Diagnostic Criteria from DSM-5*. Arlington, VA: American Psychiatric Association; 2013:93–114.

   Although the criteria for major depressive disorder were not changed for *DSM-5*, descriptions for other types of depression were altered to be more descriptive and precise. Dysthymia is now persistent depressive disorder characterized by depressed mood and two or more additional symptoms of major depression lasting ≥2 years. Major depressive episodes may occur within the duration of a persistent depressive disorder. The terms minor or subsyndromal depression were supplanted by 1) "recurrent brief depression," in which depressed mood and four additional symptoms lasting <2 weeks have occurred monthly for 12 consecutive months, 2) "short-duration depressive episode" lasting 4–13 days with depressed mood and four added symptoms, 3) "depressive episode with insufficient symptoms" lasting at least 2 weeks with depressed mood and at least one other symptom of a major depressive episode. These three forms of depression are meant to be exclusive of one another as well as major and persistent depression. Major depression may also be specified as "with anxious distress" if two additional symptoms such as tension, restlessness, foreboding, fear of losing control, and impaired concentration due to worry are present. When anxiety is marked, it may indicate a depressive episode of bipolar disorder in which a mood stabilizer is preferable to an antidepressant.

- Katona C, Hansen T, Kurre, C. A randomized, double-blind, placebo-controlled, duloxetine-referenced, fixed-dose study comparing the efficacy and safety of Lu AA21004 in elderly patients and major depressive disorder. *Int Clin Psychopharmacol*. 2012;27(4):215–224.

   In this double-blind, randomized, controlled study, 452 patients ≥65 years old from 7 countries were assigned to Lu AA21004 (vortioxetine 5 mg), duloxetine 60 mg, or placebo for 8 weeks, and efficacy, tolerability, and safety were evaluated. Inclusion criteria required a previous episode of major depression before age 60, Montgomery-Asberg Depression Rating Scale ≥26, and Mini–Mental Status Exam score ≥24. Both vortioxetine and duloxetine showed better efficacy than placebo at week 8. Both drugs also showed greater improvement in cognitive assessments (measures of processing speed, verbal learning, and memory) than placebo, but the effect was more pronounced with vortioxetine. The incidence of adverse effects with vortioxetine was comparable to that of placebo except for nausea. Duloxetine had higher adverse effects in general.

- Mulsant B, Blumberger D, Ismail Z, et al. A systematic approach to pharmacotherapy for geriatric major depression. *Clin Geriatr Med*. 2014;30(3):517–534.

   Differences between responses to antidepressants in routine care versus in experimental conditions are due to differences in the process of care rather than the medication. Response rates to placebo in randomized controlled trials with older adults exceed rates associated with medication in routine care. A systematic approach using more scheduled visits (4 to 6 in the first 6 weeks, and 6 to 12 over the next 8–12 weeks), with a predetermined duration (30–60 minutes), a treatment protocol with dose titration of a limited number of preselected antidepressants, treatment response monitored with validated scales, and psychoeducation are the components responsible for better outcomes. In addition, there is no evidence to support the choice of antidepressant based on the patient's symptom profile. Even when sleep disturbance is prominent, a more sedative antidepressant is not superior to a less sedating agent. The authors propose a stepwise approach with each step consisting of a 6-week trial of various medication(s), progressing to different agents as needed based on minimal or no response.

- Taylor WD. Clinical practice. Depression in the elderly. *N Engl J Med*. 2014;371(13):1228–1235.

   The author seeks to simplify the process of depression care with a stepped approach. SSRIs are considered first-line treatment not because of superior efficacy but because of tolerance and cost. Several drugs are discussed, including sertraline, escitalopram, duloxetine, venlafaxine, nortriptyline, and aripiprazole. Cognitive-behavioral therapy, interpersonal therapy, and problem-solving therapy may be considered first line treatment, but the evidence base for older adults is not representative of the population of older primary care patients; in addition, providers with the requisite skills may not be available.

Gary J. Kennedy, MD
Yara Bonet-Pagan, MD

CHAPTER 41—ANXIETY DISORDERS

KEY POINTS

- Late-life anxiety is often seen with other medical illnesses or depression.
- Comorbid medical problems that commonly lead to anxiety include cardiovascular and pulmonary disorders.
- SSRIs, including citalopram and sertraline, are often used as first-line treatment for anxiety in late life.
- Nonpharmacologic therapies, particularly cognitive-behavioral therapy and other types of psychotherapies, are beneficial in older adults.

The term "anxiety disorder" encompasses a spectrum of psychiatric illnesses that includes panic disorder, phobias, and generalized anxiety disorder. Older adults can suffer from the full spectrum of anxiety disorders, which are described in the *Diagnostic and Statistical Manual of Mental Disorders, 5th Edition (DSM-5)*. Older adults can experience a subjective feeling of anxiety that can meet a level of clinical concern that warrants treatment but does not necessarily fulfill the full diagnostic criteria for an anxiety disorder. Although such symptoms merit clinical attention, true anxiety disorders are the focus of this chapter. In addition, obsessive-compulsive disorders, including hoarding, as well as posttraumatic stress disorder will be discussed. These disorders are often associated with significant anxiety symptoms and were classified under the heading of "anxiety disorders" in previous editions of the *DSM*.

Because the published literature on anxiety disorders in older adults is limited, some of the characterizations and treatment strategies described are based on research conducted in younger populations. Such strategies have been modified to take into account the physiologic and psychologic differences between older and younger adults.

Numerous complexities are involved in a proper assessment of anxiety in older adults. Understanding the common issues faced in such an assessment will lead to a more accurate diagnosis and treatment plan. Examples of these complexities include differentiating anxiety disorders from symptoms related to medical conditions or medications, differentiating anxiety disorders from the appropriate ("normal") experience of anxiety associated with the stressors of late life, appropriately attributing the cause of anxiety to an adverse event of medication, and differentiating anxiety from depression. These common challenges are further complicated by the tendency of older adults to resist psychiatric evaluation because of stigma surrounding mental illness or frank denial of illness.

Assessment of anxiety in older adults generally begins with a clinical psychiatric interview to determine the course and nature of symptoms. The interview should include an evaluation of the patient's mental status, including appearance, stated mood, observed affect, and thought process. Consideration of the patient's social context and support systems is particularly relevant in the geriatric population. Assessment of any impairment in functioning related to the anxiety is an important part of the evaluation. A review of all medications, both prescription and OTC, should be done to exclude an alternative medical or pharmacologic explanation for what appears to be an anxiety disorder, or to identify an aggravating condition. Questioning should be done to explore substance use, because use of alcohol or other drugs can exacerbate anxiety symptoms, or may represent an attempt to self-medicate anxiety. Laboratory tests to check for common medical conditions such as renal, thyroid, or hematologic diseases are important. Urine toxicology should be considered in cases in which substance abuse or misuse is suspected.

Anxiety as a symptom related to a life stressor and clinical anxiety disorders are common problems. The ability to recognize and effectively treat anxiety in older adults is important, given the debilitating effects that an unhealthy level of anxiety can have in this vulnerable population.

CLASSES OF ANXIETY DISORDERS

The types of anxiety disorders as currently defined in *DSM-5* are discussed below.

Panic Disorder

Panic disorder is characterized by chronic, repeated, and unexpected panic attacks—spontaneous bouts of overwhelming and irrational fear, terror, or dread when there is no specific cause. During a panic attack, the person experiences a constellation of physical and cognitive symptoms that can include palpitations, sweating, trembling, shortness of breath, the feeling of choking, chest pain or discomfort, nausea or abdominal distress, dizziness or lightheadedness, feelings of derealization (ie, that oneself or others are unreal) or depersonalization (ie, feeling detached from oneself), paresthesias, chills or hot flashes, fear of losing control, "going crazy," or dying. A diagnosis of a true panic attack requires that at least 4 of the somatic symptoms listed above are experienced. Attacks are fairly brief, lasting typically 10–30 minutes. In between panic attacks, individuals with panic *disorder* worry excessively about when and where the next attack may occur and/or significantly change their behavior to avoid having an attack. A clinically significant degree of panic symptoms exists if the history reveals that recurrent and unpredictable panic attacks have occurred for at least 1 month and that time is being spent in worried anticipation of possible recurrence. Agoraphobia may be associated with panic disorder, but is now given a separate diagnosis. In the context of panic disorder, agoraphobia involves the persistent fear of situations that might trigger a panic attack, such as fear of having an attack in the mall or on pubic transportation, and therefore consistently remaining at home.

Individuals who experience one or more panic attacks may not necessarily warrant a diagnosis of panic disorder unless they are worrying about and changing their behavior because of fear of panic attacks. Panic attacks in late life often present with more limited symptoms, often related to one or two organ systems, such as shortness of breath, nausea, and diarrhea; the sensation of palpitations; or dizziness. These limited-symptom panic attacks may be accompanied by feelings of doom, dread, or fear of dying.

The literature suggests that the usual onset of panic disorder is between 15 and 40 years of age and that <1% will have a new-onset panic disorder after age 65, although a Canadian community health survey suggested that almost 25% of older adults with panic disorder in late life had onset after age 55. Panic disorder is considered fairly rare in older adults with a prevalence rate of 0.7% in adults >64 years old. Panic *attacks* in older adults are commonly associated with other psychiatric diagnoses, including major depressive disorder, as well as with medical illnesses, including COPD, hyperthyroidism, arrhythmias, irritable bowel syndrome, and pheochromocytoma.

Agoraphobia

In *DSM-5*, agoraphobia warrants its own diagnosis, separate and distinguishable from panic disorder. It is defined by marked anxiety about ≥2 of the following, including using public transportation, open spaces, enclosed spaces (shops, theaters), being in a crowd, and being outside unaccompanied. This fear is associated with being afraid of panic symptoms or severe embarrassment; the responses to the feared situations are consistent, persistent, and causes significant distress or impairment in social or occupational functioning. It may be associated with panic disorder. It usually begins in teens to mid 20s and is usually persistent. It is associated with significantly increased risk of depression. In older adults, it may be associated with a fear of falling.

Specific Phobia

A specific phobia is defined as a marked, persistent, excessive, unreasonable fear in the presence of or in anticipation of a particular distinct trigger, such as a specific person, animal, place, object, event, or situation. Examples of simple phobias include fear of snakes, mice, dogs, elevators, flying, or heights. Commonly, the person's anxiety level increases instantly when the feared trigger is encountered. Interestingly, he or she is able to identify this fear as unrealistic and unsupported, even though the cognitive and physiologic responses persist. Specific phobias often involve a great amount of anticipatory anxiety (ie, thoughts of the *possibility* of encountering the feared stimulus), and avoidance behaviors are likely to be reported. The consequence is that the person experiences a variety of personal difficulties as a result of the anxiety. These behaviors interfere with work and daily routines, and they decrease the person's opportunities to experience pleasurable situations (for fear that a trigger might be present). They can also contribute to secondary symptoms, such as frustration, hopelessness, and a sense of lack of control in one's life. The level of anxiety or fear usually varies as a function of both the degree of proximity to the phobic stimuli and the degree to which escape is limited. Specific phobias may be seen with panic disorder, with or without agoraphobia. Among older adults, especially in urban settings, fear of crime seems to be particularly prevalent, and it is important to explore whether this is a realistic fear or a phobia. Phobic disorders tend to be chronic and persist into old age. However, fear of falling is a specific phobia that is increasingly recognized to have an onset in later life. The prevalence of specific phobias in older adults is thought to be 3%–8%.

Social Anxiety Disorder

People with social anxiety disorder (social phobia) suffer from fears that they will behave in a manner that is inept or embarrassing while in a public place or setting. Commonly, the fear is that of trembling, blushing, or sweating profusely in social situations. Other common fears involve giving public speeches, going on dates, or simply socializing with others at a function or party. Similar to specific phobias, social anxiety disorder is often accompanied by a significant degree of anticipatory anxiety or avoidance, or both.

Although systematic studies of social anxiety disorder in older adults are lacking, epidemiologic data indicate that this disorder is chronic and persistent in old age (SOE=A). The 12-month prevalence in older adults is 2%–5%, and social anxiety disorder is more common in women, with some studies suggesting a 2:1 ratio of women to men. One Canadian study suggested that most social anxiety disorder begins in childhood, but onset after age 50 may occur in up to 10% of affected individuals. Common manifestations in old age include the inability to eat food in the presence of strangers, embarrassment concerning physical decline (tremor, vision, hearing) and, especially in men, being unable to urinate in public rest rooms. It is important to note that social anxiety disorder may be concurrent with medical conditions, depressive symptoms, and with alcohol misuse, and diagnosis may be obscured by changes in social environment or roles. Despite medical comorbidity, symptoms are out of proportion to actual disability.

Generalized Anxiety Disorder (GAD)

The distinctive symptoms of GAD include excessive anxiety and worry in addition to experiencing other symptoms, such as muscle tension, feeling easily fatigued, difficulty sleeping through the night, difficulty concentrating on a task, and feeling irritable or on edge. These symptoms need to have occurred for at least 6 months and must be accompanied by the sense that one cannot control the feelings of anxiety. In addition, these feelings of intense worry must concern intense worry over more than one activity. The worries are generally out of proportion to the stressors. Many older adults with GAD also have symptoms of depression. The clinician must try to distinguish between the two diagnoses. When these symptoms occur in the context of a major depressive disorder, it is the latter diagnosis that must be assigned, but it is not surprising that >25% of patients with major depressive disorder have symptoms that would qualify them for a diagnosis of GAD. Some studies suggest that GAD may be the most common anxiety disorder in older adults, with prevalence rates between 1.2% and 7.3%. That said, <1% of individuals >74 years old have new-onset GAD. Throughout the life span, the prevalence of GAD in women is twice that of men.

Obsessive-Compulsive Disorder (OCD)

OCD involves persistent thoughts (obsessions) and behaviors (compulsions) that are performed in an effort to decrease the anxiety experienced as a result of the obsessions. Obsessions are thoughts or ideas that come to a person's mind, often while completing a specific task or during a particular type of situation, that are generally experienced as intrusive. Compulsions are either clearly excessive or are not connected in any realistic way with the thought/obsession that they are designed to "neutralize." For example, a person may wash his or her hands repeatedly, for hours at a time, after shaking a stranger's hand; the unwanted thought is of possibly having been exposed to a disease. In this example, the act of washing is the compulsion. Other compulsive behaviors include turning lights on and off and checking locks on doors repeatedly. The obsessive-compulsive person may realize that this behavior is excessive but feels intense anxiety if he or she tries to control the compulsion. OCD is chronic and often disabling. Sufferers may spend many hours every day carrying out their compulsions. Depression and other symptoms of anxiety can also be comorbid illnesses in the older population.

In general, the prevalence of OCD is low, the 1-year prevalence being <1%. OCD first appearing in late life is unlikely. More commonly, new symptoms of obsessions may occur along with a depressive syndrome or early dementia. For example, obsessions about paying bills on time can occur in the context of difficulty in estimating time and planning.

Hoarding Disorder

Hoarding disorder is now recognized as a clinical disorder characterized in *DSM-5*. It is a late-life disorder that previously was thought to be related to OCD. However, hoarding was minimally responsive to OCD treatments. The key feature of hoarding disorder is the persistent difficulty discarding or parting with possessions regardless of actual value. These collected things may clutter and impede needed living space (eg, preventing the use of a kitchen, bathroom, or bedroom). In older adults, this syndrome is often referred to as senile squalor syndrome, or Diogenes syndrome, and is often characterized by extreme self-neglect. It often manifests itself with compulsive hoarding and the pathologic collection and storage of objects, often including items that have been collected from garbage cans and dumpsters and that the individual believes have value and meaning. The epidemiology is unclear; some surveys suggest a prevalence of approximately 5%. Unlike that of many psychiatric disorders, the prevalence is thought to be 3 times as common in adults aged 55–94 years old than in younger adults. The differential diagnosis of hoarding includes CNS disorders such as strokes or traumatic brain injury. In addition individuals with major depression who do not have the motivation to clean, those with physical limitations that impair them from cleaning, or those with frontotemporal dementia or Alzheimer disease would not merit a diagnosis of hoarding disorder.

Posttraumatic Stress Disorder (PTSD)

The distinctive feature of PTSD is that the person has experienced, either as a witness or a victim, a traumatic event to which he or she has reacted with fear and helplessness. Examples of such events include those that involve actual or threatened death or serious injury, other threats to personal integrity, witnessing an event that involves death or serious injury of another, or even hearing about death or serious injury of a family member or close associate. Commonly observed symptoms include the reexperiencing of the traumatic event, avoidance (both cognitively and behaviorally) of stimuli associated with the event, psychological numbing, and increased physiologic arousal. Reexperiencing can take the form of recurrent, intrusive recollections or images, thoughts, or even physical perceptions of the traumatic event. Such experiences are commonly termed flashbacks. Symptoms of hyperarousal include difficulty falling or staying asleep, hypervigilance, and exaggerated startle response. Nightmares, or recurrent distressing dreams of the traumatic event, are evidence of both hyperarousal and reexperiencing. Disorders often seen with PTSD include depression, panic disorder, and substance-use disorders. Symptoms must be present for at least 1 month and cause clinically significant distress or impairment in social, occupational, or other important areas of functioning. Individuals who experience these symptoms after a recent trauma (from 2 days to 1 month) are diagnosed with acute stress disorder. PTSD must be considered if distress persists for >1 month, and is considered chronic PTSD if the symptoms last for <3 months.

Although <50% of people exposed to a traumatic event go on to develop PTSD, those who experience symptoms of acute stress disorder are at higher risk than those who do not develop acute symptoms (SOE=B). In older adults, PTSD can have a delayed onset, eg, a new presentation of the disorder in a Holocaust survivor. It is postulated that lack of social supports in the context of new stressors in an older adult's life can contribute to such a presentation. PTSD symptoms have been suggested to be associated with increased cardiovascular events, as was seen in a prospective study from 2007.

The *DSM-5* now classifies PTSD in a new category of trauma-and stressor-related disorders.

COMORBIDITY

Depression with Marked Anxiety

Anxiety can be a prominent symptom of depression in many older adults. In fact, anxiety can be the presenting symptom that belies an underlying diagnosis of major depressive disorder. It is commonly believed that the expression of anxiety is more culturally acceptable in this cohort of older adults than the expression of depression. Patients presenting with a chief complaint of anxiety should routinely be evaluated for a major depressive disorder. Patients suffering from a combination of depressive and anxious symptoms can have clinically significant levels of distress despite the fact that they do not meet the full criteria for a diagnosis of either disorder.

Anxiety and Medical Disorders

Comorbid anxiety and medical disorders are commonly present. In many cases, medical illness can mimic an anxiety disorder in its presentation. Medical illness can also exacerbate a concurrent anxiety disorder, or vice versa. Finally, adverse effects of medications can produce or contribute to anxiety symptoms.

COPD is a common medical illness that can mimic an anxiety disorder. The common cold or influenza can aggravate a concurrent anxiety disorder. Other common medical illnesses that can cause or contribute to an anxiety disorder include cardiovascular or pulmonary conditions and hyperthyroidism. Medical illnesses that can be exacerbated by high levels of anxiety include angina pectoris or myocardial infarction.

Adverse effects of medications include those commonly encountered with thyroid hormone replacements, antipsychotics, caffeine, and theophylline, and can also be the primary cause of anxiety symptoms. Given the complicated clinical picture that results when anxiety and medical disorders coexist, a thorough assessment, including a clinical history, review of both prescribed and OTC medications and caffeinated beverages as well as herbal supplements (with an eye toward possible interactions), appropriate laboratory tests, and measurement of therapeutic medication concentrations when appropriate, is imperative before treatment begins. When medical illness and anxiety symptoms coexist, maximizing potential anxiolytic properties of a medical treatment should be considered. For instance, in the treatment of a patient with diabetic neuropathy and anxiety, it would be appropriate to consider maximizing the dosage of duloxetine to take full advantage of its anxiolytic effects.

PHARMACOLOGIC MANAGEMENT

Numerous drugs have been used over the years as anxiolytics: alcohol, barbiturates, antihistamines, benzodiazepines, antipsychotic medications, and β-blockers. Evidence to support the use of many of these agents is lacking. Although empirical studies of the use of medications in treating older adults were initially limited, the body of literature to support this practice is increasing, including several randomized controlled trials of the treatment of late-life anxiety disorders (most often GAD). For some disorders, the body of literature supporting the efficacy of these medications is gleaned from use in younger patients, modified by age considerations. For example, a study of time for treatment for an anxiety disorder suggested

Table 41.1—Treatment Strategies for Anxiety Disorders in Late Life

Disorder	First-Line Treatments	Second-Line Treatments or Adjunctive Therapies
Panic disorder, agoraphobia	SSRIs[a], SNRIs[a], CBT[a]	Benzodiazepines[b]
Social anxiety disorder	SSRIs[a] plus CBT[b]	Benzodiazepines[b]
Social anxiety disorder, specific type (eg, public speaking)	β-blockers[OL] plus CBT[b]	Buspirone[b]
Specific phobia (eg, rats, blood)	CBT[b] or PRN benzodiazepines[b]	SSRI[b]
Obsessive-compulsive disorder	SSRIs[a], SNRIs[b], CBT[b]	Clomipramine[b] (adverse effects in older adults)
Posttraumatic stress disorder	SSRIs[b], SNRIs[b]	CBT[b] Prazosin[b]
Generalized anxiety disorder	SSRIs[a], SNRIs[a], CBT[a] relaxation training	Benzodiazepines[b]
Anxiety and medical disorders	Identify and treat underlying cause; use SSRIs[a] or SNRIs[a] in primary anxiety disorder.	Benzodiazepines[b]
Depression with severe anxiety	SSRIs[a], SNRIs[a], CBT[a]	Buspirone[b], benzodiazepines[b]

NOTE: SNRIs=serotonin-norepinephrine reuptake inhibitors; CBT=cognitive-behavioral therapy
[a]SOE=A in studies of the geriatric population
[b]SOE=A in studies of the general adult population; insufficient studies in the geriatric population

that, in younger adults, if a patient responds, continuing on medication for a year decreases risk of relapse; this treatment recommendation should be considered with older adults as well. A brief description of the various classes of compounds currently favored as anxiolytics follows. For a summary of the treatment strategies for anxiety disorders in late life, see Table 41.1.

Antidepressants

Antidepressants have proved efficacious in treatment of panic disorder, OCD, GAD, and PTSD in younger patients. Studies have demonstrated that SSRIs, particularly citalopram, are safe and efficacious in specific treatment of late-life anxiety disorders. Given their relatively favorable adverse-event profile, the SSRIs should be considered the medications of choice for these disorders (SOE=A). Further, SSRIs should also be considered treatments of choice for depression with severe anxiety symptoms. Compounds such as venlafaxine and duloxetine (serotonin-norepinephrine reuptake inhibitors) should be considered as alternatives for those patients who do not respond to SSRIs or who experience adverse events.

Benzodiazepines

Over the past several decades, benzodiazepines have been the most commonly prescribed anxiolytics for both younger and older patients, but their use is now discouraged. When needed because symptoms are severe, benzodiazepines with shorter half-lives and without active metabolites, such as lorazepam and oxazepam, are preferable for treating older adults, because they are metabolized by direct conjugation, a process relatively unaffected by aging. However, the use of even short-acting benzodiazepines should be limited to <6 months because long-term use is fraught with complications, such as motor incoordination and falls, cognitive impairment, depression, and the potential for abuse and dependence.

Other Medications

Several studies have suggested that buspirone, an anxiolytic medication with some serotonin-agonist properties, is efficacious for treatment of GAD (SOE=A), although clinical experience is less positive. Buspirone appears to be a safer choice than benzodiazepines for patients taking several other medications or needing treatment for longer periods of time. One drawback of buspirone is the amount of time required to see a clinical response (approximately 4 weeks). At times, concomitant use of a short-acting benzodiazepine in the initial stage of treatment could be useful for some patients. Although antihistamines such as hydroxyzine[OL] and diphenhydramine[OL] are sometimes used to manage mild anxiety in younger patients, the anticholinergic properties of these agents can cause serious problems in older adults, in whom their use is not recommended. Second-generation antipsychotics, such as risperidone[OL], olanzapine[OL], and quetiapine[OL], are not recommended choices for treatment of a nonpsychotic older adult with an anxiety disorder.

PSYCHOLOGIC MANAGEMENT

Although pharmacotherapy is commonly the first-line treatment for late-life anxiety disorders, psychologic treatments are often efficacious, either alone or as adjuncts to medication (SOE=A). The psychotherapeutic remedies that have been most rigorously tested all fall under the rubric of cognitive-behavioral therapy. Techniques generally fall into 3 categories: 1) relaxation training used with music, visual imagery, aromatherapy, and instruction in relaxation techniques; 2) cognitive restructuring to help the patient identify triggers and stimuli that increase or sustain anxiety, gain more control over the effect of such stimuli, and develop a range of coping strategies and tools; and 3) exposure with response prevention (ie, the individual is exposed to the feared stimuli and prevented from performing a compulsive action), which is used with and particularly effective for OCD. Graded desensitization, which is used in panic and phobias, relies on exposure to gradually more anxiety-producing stimuli, with techniques to manage and tolerate the resultant anxiety.

Treatment of older adults typically includes a combination of these therapeutic approaches. Success depends on the appropriateness of the patient for psychotherapy (eg, patients with dementing disorders tend not to benefit from interventions that require remembering information and doing specific activities between sessions); the patient's support system, intellectual functioning, and level of motivation; the degree of coordination of care with medical professionals; and the nature of the disorder. Consultation with a mental health professional can assist in determining the appropriateness of a referral.

REFERENCES

- Andrescu C, Varon D. New research on anxiety disorders in the elderly and an update on evidence-based treatments. *Curr Psychiatry Rep.* 2015;17(7):53.

    This comprehensive review article provides an overview of the prevalence of a variety of anxiety disorders in late life and address often complex issues in identification and diagnosis. The increase in morbidity and mortality associated with anxiety in older adults is reviewed. Recent advances in treatment modalities, including medications in combination with CBT, relaxation, and home-based interventions, are discussed.

- Baldwin DS, Anderson IM, Nutt DJ, et al. Evidence-based pharmacological treatment of anxiety disorders, post-traumatic stress disorder and obsessive-compulsive disorder: A revision of the 2005 Guidelines from the British Association for Psychopharmacology. *J Psychopharmacol.* 2014;28(5):403–439.

    This is an evidenced-based review of treatment of anxiety disorders in patients across the life span. These consensus guidelines of medication algorithms are easily applied to primary care practices with serotonin-reuptake inhibitors useful as a first-line choice. Other agents, including serotonin-norepinephrine reuptake inhibitors, tricyclic antidepressants, and pregabalin, are also reviewed.

- Garrido MM, Kane RL, Kaas M, et al. Use of mental health care by community-dwelling older adults. *J Am Geriatr Soc.* 2011;59(1):50–56.

    In a sample of 1,681 community-dwelling older adults, only 6.5% of individuals made use of mental health services, whereas 66% of those with major depressive disorder and 73% of those with anxiety did not receive services. Use was associated with more household members, more years of formal education, and better self-care ability.

- Gould RL, Coulson MC, Howard RJ. Efficacy of cognitive behavioral therapy for anxiety disorders in older people: a meta-analysis and meta-regression of randomized controlled trials. *J Am Geriatr Soc.* 2012;60(2):218-229.

    This meta-analysis of 12 studies confirms the effectiveness of CBT for anxiety disorders in older adults but suggests that it is unclear if it is better than other active interventions for anxiety disorders in this population.

- Zhang X, Norton J, Carriere I, et al. Generalized anxiety in community dwelling elderly; prevalence and clinical characteristics. *J Affect Disord.* 2014;172C:24–29.

    This study of nearly 2,000 older adults revealed a lifetime prevalence of generalized anxiety disorder of 11%, with 25% reporting their first episode of anxiety after the age of 50. Comorbid major depressive disorder was noted among 14%, and 34% suffered from phobias. Despite the high prevalence of symptoms, only 34% received any type of treatment for these conditions.

Judith Neugroschl, MD

CHAPTER 42—SCHIZOPHRENIA SPECTRUM AND OTHER PSYCHOTIC DISORDERS

KEY POINTS

- Hallucinations are perceptions without stimuli that can occur in any sensory modality (ie, visual, auditory, tactile, olfactory, gustatory). In late life, multimodal hallucinations are common.

- Delusions are abnormal false beliefs that in late life are often paranoid or persecutory, such as a belief that one's safety is in jeopardy or that one's belongings are being stolen.

- Psychosis occurring for the first time in late life is often due to dementia or neurologic conditions such as Parkinson disease or stroke, as opposed to a primary psychotic disorder such as schizophrenia.

- Dementia with Lewy bodies is associated with characteristically vivid visual hallucinations, often including people or animals.

- When psychotic symptoms arise in the context of depression, the symptoms are often "mood congruent," such as delusions that one is penniless or that one is already dead.

Psychotic symptoms are defined as either *hallucinations*, ie, perceptions without stimuli, or *delusions*, ie, fixed, false, idiosyncratic ideas. Hallucinations are abnormal perceptions without stimulus that can be in any of the five sensory modalities (auditory, visual, tactile, olfactory, and gustatory). Delusions are false beliefs or ideas that are tightly held by the individual despite any evidence. Delusions can be suspicious (paranoid), grandiose, somatic, self-blaming, or hopeless. This chapter focuses on conditions in which psychotic symptoms are prominent and central to making the diagnosis. It only briefly discusses other disorders, such as dementia, delirium, and the mood disorders, in which psychotic symptoms can occur but the defining features are in the cognitive or mood realms.

Hallucinations and delusions occur in a variety of disorders. Evaluation of an older adult with hallucinations and delusions should begin with evaluation for underlying causes such as delirium, dementia, stroke, or Parkinson disease. An acute onset of cognitive change with inability to sustain attention and impaired level of awareness and/or arousal suggests delirium. Next, a primary mood disorder should be considered. Only after other causes are excluded should the diagnosis of a schizophrenia spectrum disorder be made. Delirium, most often superimposed on an underlying dementia, is the most common cause of new-onset psychosis in late life.

SCHIZOPHRENIA AND SCHIZOPHRENIA SPECTRUM SYNDROMES

Schizophrenia is defined as a chronic psychiatric disorder characterized by positive symptoms (eg, hallucinations, delusions, and disorganized speech, known as thought disorder) and negative symptoms (eg, social withdrawal and apathy). Mood disorder and cognitive disorder should be excluded before the diagnosis is made. In men, schizophrenia has a modal onset at age 18; onset after age 45 is uncommon. In women, modal age of onset is 28, and 20%–30% of cases begin after age 45. Approximately 85% of older adults with schizophrenia experienced onset of illness in early adult life. However, 10%–15% of cases of schizophrenia first come to clinical attention after patients are 45 years old. Schizophrenia with onset between the ages of 40 and 60 is called "late-onset schizophrenia," while patients with onset after age 60 are considered to have "very-late-onset schizophrenia-like psychosis."

In older adults, late-onset schizophrenia-like conditions are characterized by onset after age 40, prominent persecutory (paranoid) delusions, and multimodal hallucinations (SOE=C). For example, patients commonly complain that items are being stolen or report that they are being persecuted unjustly. Hallucinations often manifest in complaints, for example, that a neighbor is persistently banging on walls or the roof, that someone is pumping gas under the door, or that electrical sensations are being sent through the walls of the person's home and into his or her body. A schizophrenia-like psychosis can be diagnosed only when cognitive disorder, mood disorder, or other explanatory medical conditions such as delirium or focal brain pathology have been excluded.

The schizophrenia-like psychoses of late life differ from schizophrenia beginning in early life in two ways (SOE=C). First, thought disorder, a sign described as speech in which a series of thoughts are not connected to one another in a logical fashion, is much less common in older adults, comprising only 5% of cases. In early-onset schizophrenia, thought disorder is present in approximately 50% of cases.

Alcohol can induce a psychotic disorder marked by persistent auditory hallucinations in individuals who have a moderate or severe alcohol use disorder in the context of a clear sensorium (unlike delirium). When illogical speech occurs for the first time in late life, a delirium or dementia should be excluded. A second significant difference is the rarity of social deterioration and dilapidation among older adults with late-onset schizophrenia. Thus, personality and social functioning are often better preserved in late-onset cases. However, there is a dearth of long-term follow-up studies, so it is unknown whether social deterioration and personality changes occur after many years of symptoms.

Epidemiology and Clinical Characteristics

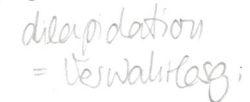

Late-onset schizophrenia is more common among women, whereas early-onset schizophrenia is equally common in women and men. The population-based incidence of late-onset schizophrenia is unknown, but the lifetime prevalence of schizophrenia is 1% among both men and women.

Late-onset schizophrenia-like psychoses affect predominantly women, with the female:male ratio ranging from 5:1 to 10:1. Many older adults with late-onset schizophrenia-like psychosis have been married at some time and have been able to hold responsible jobs and work efficiently, but premorbid isolation and "schizoid" (socially detached personality) traits are common. Studies report greater degrees of brain white matter hyperintensities on MRI scans in late-onset schizophrenia, a finding that suggests that brain vascular disease is a risk factor. However, this finding has not been adequately replicated, and other causes of white matter hyperintensities are plausible.

One condition that may be confused with late-onset schizophrenia is frontotemporal dementia, because it can involve features of socially inappropriate and odd behaviors as well as premorbidly odd or "schizoid" personality features.

Although many individuals with schizophrenia experience fewer hallucinations and delusions as they age, others remain significantly functionally impaired by psychotic symptoms. Moreover, older adults with schizophrenia have an increased risk of suicidal behavior than their peers without mental illness (SOE=C). Some individuals with schizophrenia experience remission of psychotic symptoms with aging, though this clinical remission may be temporary. Indeed, a recent longitudinal study of community-dwelling people with schizophrenia spectrum disorder found that remission status fluctuates over time. The study further found that remission status was affected by community support and integration, suggesting that social interventions help sustain clinical well-being in these older patients. In addition, individuals with early-onset schizophrenia have more cognitive deficits than patients with late-onset schizophrenia, although these cognitive changes remain relatively stable over time. Neither early-onset nor late-onset schizophrenia is considered a dementing illness, and rapid memory loss should prompt further evaluation for possible comorbid conditions, such as delirium or dementia. Recent studies indicate that older patients with schizophrenia have higher rates of dementia than persons without schizophrenia (SOE=B). They also have significantly higher rates of congestive heart failure, COPD, and hypothyroidism than individuals without schizophrenia, underscoring the importance of comprehensive health care for these older individuals (SOE=C).

Treatment and Management

Nonpharmacologic

Because suspiciousness and paranoid delusions are commonly the most prominent symptoms, the clinician's first task in treating late-onset psychosis is often to establish a trusting therapeutic relationship with the patient. On occasion, the suspicious ideas are conceivable (eg, the claim that the patient is being financially abused by a relative), but usually the delusions are bizarre and improbable. It is rarely effective to confront the patient with the unreality or implausibility of his or her ideas. The patient is more likely to respond positively if the clinician empathizes with the distress that the symptoms cause ("I can see how upset you are by all of this"). If patients ask whether the clinician "believes" them, a response such as, "I don't hear anything like that, but I appreciate the fact that you do" is both honest and empathetic. The symptoms are usually frightening and distressing to patients and can lead to unusual behaviors. For example, patients who develop concerns that their food is being poisoned may exhibit unusual eating habits or food avoidance. Furthermore, suspiciousness can isolate the patient from friends and family. Therefore, encouraging patients to maintain important relationships and seeking their permission to discuss the source of symptoms with close family members or friends can help patients maintain important, supportive relationships.

Pharmacologic

Clinical consensus and descriptive case series suggest that antipsychotic medications are as effective in late-onset schizophrenia as in early-onset cases (SOE=B). Most specialist clinicians recommend second-generation antipsychotic medications, because such agents are less likely to cause tardive dyskinesia (TD), an adverse event for which older age is a predisposing

Table 42.1—Dosing and Adverse Events of Commonly Used Antipsychotic Medications[a] for Psychotic Disorders

Medication	Starting Daily Dosage (mg)	Maximal Daily Dosage (mg)	Adverse Events		
			Extrapyramidal Signs[b]	Drowsiness	Weight Gain
Aripiprazole	2	15	++ (akathisia)	+	+
Asenapine	5	10	+	+++	++
Clozapine	12.5	100	+	+++	+++
Haloperidol	0.5	10	+++	++	+
Iloperidone	1	12	+	++	+
Lurasidone	40	80	+	++	+
Olanzapine	2.5	15	+	++	+++
Paliperidone	1.5	12	++	++	+
Perphenazine	4	32	++	++	++
Quetiapine	12.5	300	+	+++	++
Risperidone	0.25	4	++	+	++
Ziprasidone	20	120	+	++	+

NOTE: + = uncommon, ++ = somewhat common, +++ = common
[a] All listed medications have warning about hyperglycemia, cerebrovascular events, and increase in all-cause mortality in patients with dementia.
[b] Rigidity, parkinsonian tremor, dystonia, akathisia

factor. Dosages should be increased at semiweekly or weekly intervals as needed. While dosages are being titrated, patients should be monitored for emergence of extrapyramidal adverse events (eg, parkinsonian tremor, rigidity, dystonia) and other movement disorders. These should be treated by lowering the dosage and switching to an alternative antipsychotic if necessary. Polypharmacy should be avoided by reducing the dosage or switching the antipsychotic medication rather than by adding a medication for extrapyramidal symptoms. The more common adverse events with quetiapine are sedation and orthostatic hypotension; with risperidone, extrapyramidal symptoms; and with olanzapine, weight gain and sedation (Table 42.1).

No studies are available to guide the duration of treatment. Clinical experience suggests that patients who respond to antipsychotic medications should be continued on the minimal effective dosage for at least 6 months. Patients with early-onset schizophrenia and chronic stable symptoms may be able to tolerate a gradual reduction in dosage of antipsychotic medication. For all patients who relapse on treatment or who relapse when the dosage is lowered, maintenance treatment over a longer term (at least 1–2 years) is recommended (SOE=D). Patients should be monitored for emergence of TD, a syndrome characterized by repetitive involuntary movements of the oral and limb musculature. Rating scales for TD, such as the Abnormal Involuntary Movement Scale (AIMS [www.cqaimh.org/pdf/tool_aims.pdf]) or the Dyskinesia Identification System Condensed User Scale (DISCUS), are clinically useful and easy to administer in the office or institutional setting. If TD develops, the dosage of the antipsychotic medication should be lowered if possible. Depending on the duration of exposure, TD may worsen or appear when the antipsychotic is discontinued or the dosage is lowered, or when switching from one antipsychotic to another. At the time antipsychotic medications are started or as soon as symptoms improve enough so that the patient can understand the risk, the patient should be informed of the risk of TD and the possibility that it can be irreversible.

PSYCHOTIC SYMPTOMS

Psychotic symptoms can occur in a number of other disorders, in addition to schizophrenia.

Delirium and Delusional Disorder

Hallucinations, particularly visual hallucinations, can be a symptom of delirium, even when it is mild. The onset of delirium is usually acute, and there is generally an identifiable metabolic, pharmacologic, or infectious cause, or a combination of underlying causes. The hallmark feature of delirium is markedly impaired attention and impaired level of awareness. Typically, the mental status examination reveals multiple cognitive impairments and a diminished or waxing and waning level of consciousness with periods of lucidity and alertness alternating with periods of lethargy. Treatment of delirium involves treating the underlying medical condition(s) provoking the delirious state.

Some older patients present with long-standing chronic delusions without hallucinations. When these occur in patients with a normal mood and who do not have cognitive impairment, then a diagnosis of delusional disorder may be made. A recent study found that delusional disorder is more frequent among women but that men experience more severe symptoms. Most commonly, the delusions are persecutory or paranoid in nature, but delusions of jealousy or somatic delusions of bodily dysfunction also occur. Patients with somatic delusions may present to multiple health practitioners and request medical interventions. Management strategies include reassurance, amelioration of sensory deficits, and sometimes antipsychotic medication.

Mood Disorder

Psychotic symptoms, especially delusions, can be seen in major depressive disorder and in the manic phase of bipolar disorder. These delusions are described as "mood congruent." That is, in patients with depression, the delusional content usually reflects self-deprecation, self-blame, hopelessness, or the conviction of ill health. A patient may complain, for example, that he or she has no blood or that his or her intestines are not working; another patient may believe that he or she has caused a terrible wrong and deserves to be punished (a self-blaming delusion). Some patients become convinced that they are dying and nothing can be done to help them, although there is no physiologic evidence to support their concerns. Other common depressive delusions are the conviction that one has no insurance, no clothing, or no money when this is not true (delusion of poverty). Delusions congruent with mania are grandiose. Examples include the person's belief that he or she is infallible, can do impossible physical or intellectual activities, has skills and abilities that no other human being has, or is a special personage such as Jesus Christ. Treatment of psychotic symptoms in mood disorders includes antipsychotic medication as well as antidepressant or antimanic medications.

Dementia

Patients with dementia experience both hallucinations and delusions. These are usually less complex than the delusions seen in schizophrenia or mood disorder. Common delusions in dementia are the belief that one's belongings have been stolen or moved, or the conviction that one is being persecuted. Delusions that one's spouse is unfaithful (delusions of infidelity) are also common.

Management of psychosis in dementia is particularly challenging, because the use of antipsychotic medication warrants careful consideration of risks and adverse events. Nonpharmacologic interventions, such as redirection and reassurance, should be tried first. However, if the patient is physically aggressive or severely distressed by the psychotic symptoms, then a trial of low-dose antipsychotic medication is warranted (SOE=C). All antipsychotic agents carry an FDA warning regarding increased all-cause mortality in patients with dementia.

Second-generation antipsychotics have a class warning concerning the increased risk of developing hyperglycemia and diabetes in both younger and older patients with schizophrenia. The mechanism for these adverse events is unclear.

ISOLATED SUSPICIOUSNESS

Suspiciousness can be viewed as a personality trait, ie, an aspect of all human beings that varies among people in its degree of prominence. In one epidemiologic study, suspiciousness became more common in older Americans and affected 4% of those ≥65 years old. It is distinguished from psychotic disorders by the understandable nature of the ideas (eg, excessive worry about safety) and the absence of other psychotic or mood symptoms.

ISOLATED HALLUCINATIONS

Charles Bonnet Syndrome

Between 10% and 13% of patients with significant visual loss (bilateral acuity worse than 20/60) experience isolated visual hallucinations. These can take the form of shapes such as diamonds or rectangles but more commonly consist of complex silent hallucinations such as small children, multiple animals, or a vivid scene such as one would see in a movie. This condition, first described more than 200 years ago, goes by the eponym Charles Bonnet syndrome. The criteria for this syndrome are as follows:

- Silent visual hallucinations
- Partially or fully intact insight (the patient is aware that the perceptions cannot be real but still reports that they appear absolutely real and vivid)
- Visual loss
- Lack of evidence of brain disease or other psychiatric disorder

It has been suggested that this syndrome is a concomitant of the phantom limb syndrome caused by retinal lesions. However, visual hallucinations have also been reported in individuals with field defects caused by cortical lesions of the visual pathways.

The best treatment for Charles Bonnet syndrome is education, reassurance, and support. Patients should be informed that the hallucinations are a sign of eye disease, not mental illness. An occasional patient has partial insight or loses insight and becomes very distressed by this symptom. When this distress is significant or leads to dangerous behavior, a cautious trial of low-dosage second-generation antipsychotic medication is occasionally beneficial.

OTHER PSYCHOTIC DISORDERS

Psychotic Disorder Due to Another Medical Condition

It is appropriate to consider this diagnosis when a patient is experiencing hallucinations or delusions that are likely to be a direct result of another medical condition, rather than due to a psychiatric disorder such as schizophrenia or a mood disorder. Patients with Parkinson disease, stroke, and other brain disorders may experience delusions and hallucinations without prominent cognitive impairment or other evidence of psychiatric disorder (SOE=C). Delirium caused by a superimposed condition should be excluded. In patients with Parkinson disease, psychotic symptoms are common and may be secondary to a prescribed dopaminergic agent, although some patients experience visual hallucinations before any medications are started. Education and support should be offered to all patients with these symptoms. Judicious discontinuation or dosage reduction of nonessential antiparkinsonian medications often provides relief from psychotic symptoms. If patients experience significant emotional distress or if the symptoms lead to dangerous or upsetting behavior, cautious use of an antipsychotic medication is appropriate (SOE=B). Use of first-generation antipsychotic medications is usually avoided because of the potential for exacerbating parkinsonian symptoms (SOE=B). For patients with Parkinson disease and concomitant hallucinations or psychosis, quetiapine^{OL} 12.5–75 mg/d may be beneficial. Some patients require clozapine^{OL} 12.5–75 mg/d. However, patients taking clozapine should have a CBC with absolute neutrophil count done once a week for 6 months and then biweekly thereafter because of the risk of granulocytopenia. All patients taking clozapine must be enrolled in a national patient registry to ensure safe administration.

Dementia associated with Lewy bodies is increasingly recognized as an important cause of hallucinations in late life. The clinical scenario typically involves cognitive decline accompanied by motor features of parkinsonism. However, prominent visual hallucinations, which are often vivid and troubling, are a key part of the diagnosis.

Dementia associated with Lewy bodies presents a challenge similar to that of psychosis in Parkinson disease, because the medications in the class approved to treat psychosis (the antipsychotics) worsen the parkinsonian symptoms. At least two placebo-controlled clinical trials and multiple case studies report significant improvement through the use of cholinesterase inhibitors^{OL} (SOE=B). If an antipsychotic medication must be used, then the treatment strategies outlined above are appropriate if there is careful attention to the risk of extrapyramidal adverse events. Nonpharmacologic treatments include redirection, reassurance, and nonconfrontational explanation.

Substance/Medication-Induced Psychotic Disorder

Drugs of abuse, such as alcohol, cannabis, and cocaine, can cause persistent psychotic symptoms after the period of acute intoxication or withdrawal. Alcohol can induce a psychotic disorder marked by persistent auditory hallucinations in individuals who have a moderate or severe alcohol use disorder. Although substance use disorders are less frequent among older patients than in younger individuals, this is an area of growing concern. In addition, many classes of medications are associated with psychotic adverse events causing hallucinations or delusions. Older adults, especially those with CNS impairments, are particularly vulnerable. In a number of case reports, β-blockers such as metoprolol have been associated with persistent hallucinations and confusional states (SOE=C). In these cases, withdrawal of metoprolol resulted in rapid and complete resolution of psychosis. In addition, psychotic symptoms have been reported related to treatment with other medications such as dopaminergic agents, interferon, cyclosporine, and steroids. Antiarrhythmic agents, antiviral agents, opioids, antineoplastic agents, and other medications such as baclofen have also been associated with psychosis. In these instances, the appropriate therapeutic management is to reduce the dosage of or to discontinue the associated medication.

REFERENCES

- Cohen CI, Iqbal M. Longitudinal study of remission among older adults with schizophrenia spectrum disorder. *Am J Geriatr Psychiatry*. 2014:22(5):450–458.

    This report presents findings from the first long-term follow-up study of symptomatic remission of older patients with schizophrenia spectrum disorder in contemporary times. The study follows a baseline sample of 250 people over a mean follow-up period of 4.5 years. Previous cross-sectional studies had indicated that a significant percentage of patients with schizophrenia achieve symptomatic remission over time; the current study provides new information about the fluctuating course of remission status over time.

- Goldman JG, Holden S. Treatment of psychosis and dementia in Parkinson's disease. *Curr Treat Options Neurol*. 2014:16(3):281.

    This is an excellent review of the various types of psychotic symptom presentations seen in Parkinson disease and Parkinson dementia, as well a summary of evidence-based approaches to treatment.

- Hendrie HC, Tu W, Tabbey R, et al. Health outcomes and cost of care among older adults with schizophrenia: A 10-year study using medical records across the continuum of care. *Am J Geriatr Psychiatry*. 2014;22(5):427–436.

    This longitudinal, naturalistic observation data compares patients with schizophrenia with individuals without schizophrenia in a single health care system serving an economically disadvantaged population cohort.

- Iglewicz A, Meeks TW, Jeste DV. New wine in old bottle: late-life psychosis. *Psychiatr Clin North Am*. 2011:34(2):292–318.

    This excellent review summarizes the most common etiologies for late-life psychosis, including schizophrenia, delusional disorder, and dementia.

- Zilkens RR, Bruce DG, Duke J, et al. Severe psychiatric disorders in mid-life and risk of dementia in late-life (age 65–84 years): A population based case-control study. *Curr Alzheimer Res*. 2014:11(7):681–693.

    This large population case-control study in Western Australia looked at over 13,000 incident cases of dementia over a 10-year period compared with age- and sex-matched controls to examine the association of mid-life psychiatric factors with dementia.

Susan W. Lehmann, MD

CHAPTER 43—PERSONALITY AND SOMATIC SYMPTOM AND RELATED DISORDERS

Key Points

- Personality disorders persist into late life and pose complex challenges in patients across various medical and psychiatric settings.

- Personality disorders can be more difficult to detect in late life because of age-associated changes in symptoms, comorbid psychopathology, and lack of age-adjusted diagnostic instruments.

- The goal of treatment of personality disorders in late life is not to cure the disorder but to decrease the frequency and intensity of symptoms. To this end, both psychotherapeutic and psychopharmacologic strategies are needed.

- Somatic symptom and related disorders represent the presence of prominent physical symptoms or complaints that are associated with significant distress and impairment. The new diagnostic formulation de-emphasizes the previous focus on a lack of established underlying pathology.

- Treatment of somatic symptom and related disorders must attend to the affected individual's distress and belief in the veracity of his or her symptoms. Repeated reassuring clinical visits help to build a therapeutic relationship. Both psychotherapy and pharmacotherapy can be helpful for some individuals.

Personality Disorders

Personality refers to the unique characteristics and qualities that define an individual's ability to form relationships, cope with life stress, and approach the tasks of daily living. Personality disorders are defined in the *Diagnostic and Statistical Manual of Mental Disorders, 5th Edition* (*DSM-5*) by the presence of chronic and pervasive patterns of inflexible and maladaptive inner experiences and behaviors. These patterns lead to significant disruptions in several spheres of function, including cognitive perception and interpretation, affective expression, interpersonal functioning, and impulse control. Individuals with personality disorders are often distinguished by repeated episodes of disruptive or noxious behaviors and, as a result, they often receive pejorative labels, depending on their form. Descriptive terms often applied to those with personality disorders include "difficult," "dramatic," and "strange," to name just a few. The developmental roots of personality disorders are believed to lie in childhood and adolescence, but their features can present clinically at any age in adulthood. Personality disorders are influenced by both genetic and environmental factors.

The *DSM-5* describes 10 personality disorders, grouped into 3 broad clusters that are based on common phenomenology; however, they are no longer documented on a separate axis. For late-life features of all 10 personality disorders, see Table 43.1. Depressive and passive-aggressive personality disorders were 2 additional categories that were considered provisional in the previous edition of the *DSM* (*DSM-IV-TR*) but have not been included in *DSM-5* because of a lack of empirical support. Nonetheless, some clinicians continue to see older adults who present with the symptom constellations of these 2 personality disorders. Mixed diagnoses and those that do not fit into any existing category are labeled in *DSM-5* as "other specified personality disorder" and "unspecified personality disorder."

The *DSM-5* classification for personality disorders also includes the category of "personality change due to another medical condition" to represent emergent personality changes resulting from medical compromise. Such personality change has classically been described within the context of an "organic" personality disorder, but this term is no longer used in *DSM* nomenclature. Most often, personality changes with an "organic" source involve impairments in executive functioning, consisting of poor impulse control, poor planning, and greater vulnerability to irritability or agitation. Along these lines, Alzheimer disease and other dementias are often associated with personality changes, including apathy, egocentricity, and impulsivity. Frontal lobe injury can result in a disinhibited impulsive syndrome, or conversely, an apathetic, avolitional syndrome. Frontotemporal dementia has been associated with distinct personality changes, including impulsivity, disinhibition, apathy, and compulsive behaviors such as hoarding. Temporal lobe epilepsy can be associated with personality change, including emotional deepening, verbosity, hypergraphia, hypersexuality, and preoccupation with religious, moral, and cosmic issues. Other disorders found in older adults that are associated with personality disorders include brain tumors, multiple sclerosis, and encephalopathies.

Many older adults with personality disorders can easily become overwhelmed by age-associated losses and stresses, largely because they lack appropriate coping skills and the personal, social, or financial

Table 43.1—Features of Personality Disorders

Cluster/Disorder	General Features	Features Specific to Older Adults
Cluster A: Odd or Eccentric Behaviors		
Paranoid	Pervasive suspiciousness of the motives of others, which often leads to irritability and hostility	Increased risk of paranoid psychosis, agitation, and aggression
Schizoid	Disinterest in social relationships, coupled with isolative and sometimes odd behaviors	Poor, strained, or absent relationships with caregivers
Schizotypal	Characteristic appearance, behaviors, and beliefs that are strange, unusual, or inappropriate	Beliefs that can become delusional and lead to conflicts with others; relationships with caregivers can be strained or absent
Cluster B: Dramatic, Emotional, or Erratic Behaviors		
Antisocial	Poor regard for social norms and laws; lack of conscience and empathy for others; frequent reckless and criminal behaviors	Frequent remission of antisocial behaviors with less aggression and impulsivity
Borderline	Impaired control of emotional expression and impulses associated with unstable interpersonal relations, poor self-identity, and self-injurious behaviors	Persistent emotional lability and unstable relationships but less self-injurious and impulsive behaviors
Histrionic	Excessive emotionality and attention-seeking behaviors, sometimes appearing overly seductive or provocative	Behaviors that can become excessively disinhibited and disorganized, appearing hypomanic
Narcissistic	Pervasive sense of entitlement, grandiosity, and arrogance, coupled with lack of empathy	Can present as hostile, enraged, paranoid, or depressed
Cluster C: Anxious or Fearful Behaviors		
Avoidant	Excessive sensitivity to rejection and social scrutiny; social demeanor that can be timid and inhibited	Social contacts that can be extremely limited, providing for inadequate support
Dependent	Excessive dependence on others to help make decisions and provide support	Comorbid depression is common; clinical appearance often with demanding or clinging behaviors if dependency needs not met
Obsessive-compulsive	Pervasive preoccupation with orderliness and cleanliness; a perfectionistic, rigid, and controlling approach that can become more inflexible and indecisive under stress	Obsessive-compulsive traits can become exaggerated in efforts to maintain control over somatic and environmental changes

Descriptions of the clusters and of the disorders in each cluster are based on the *Diagnostic and Statistical Manual of Mental Disorders*. 5th ed. Washington, DC: American Psychiatric Association; 2013.

resources to buffer their losses. In particular, admission to a hospital or long-term care setting poses a unique stress on all individuals with personality disorders in late life. The loss of a familiar environment, personal items, privacy, and the control over one's schedule can lead to a sense of disorganization and displacement. Conflict in an institutional setting begins when patients with personality disorders try to cope with the stresses from their new environment by exaggerating their maladaptive behaviors. An obsessive-compulsive person may attempt to maintain a sense of control by demanding rigid adherence to schedules and rules of hygiene. Dependent individuals may feel helpless and panicked without enough attention to their needs, responding with clinging behaviors and excessive questions or requests for assistance. Paranoid, antisocial, and borderline patients may refuse to cooperate with treatment plans or institutional rules. Individuals with personality change, such as due to head trauma, often have great difficulty accommodating to age-related changes and may respond with characteristic labile or disinhibited moods and behaviors or, conversely, with an overall apathetic demeanor.

Epidemiology

Prevalence rates of late-life personality disorders in the community range from 5% to 13%, which is a slightly lower range than the 10%–20% prevalence estimates for individuals of all ages in the community. Prevalence rates in inpatient settings and with comorbid depression are much higher, ranging from 10% to >50%, depending on the method of diagnosis. The most common personality disorders in late life are dependent, obsessive-compulsive, paranoid, and unspecified. Although most research has demonstrated fewer diagnoses in older age groups, it is unclear whether this represents an actual difference in prevalence or merely reflects the fact that it is more difficult to make a diagnosis in late life. Some researchers have suggested that prevalence rates can be influenced by increased mortality among those with antisocial or borderline personality traits that are associated with higher rates of reckless, impulsive, and self-injurious behaviors. Other research exploring the neural substrates of emotion has demonstrated an attenuation of emotional reactivity in late life across a number of physiologic and behavioral parameters. These findings can partially explain the reduced prevalence of the more impulsive and emotionally reactive personality features, such as those associated with borderline personality disorder.

Diagnostic Challenges

Establishing a diagnosis of personality disorder in older adults can be especially challenging, because it requires a detailed, longitudinal psychiatric and psychosocial history. Older patients and their informants are not always able to provide sufficient history, especially when it may span ≥50 years. The history can be distorted by recall bias (the tendency to present more socially desirable traits) or memory impairment. Furthermore, schizotypal and paranoid individuals may be reluctant to engage in clinical interviews and share personal history, and antisocial and narcissistic individuals who lack insight into their problems may refuse to divulge relevant experiences. Records often do not provide sufficient information to determine prior personality dynamics. Remote diagnoses from previous decades cannot be easily correlated with current ones, because the diagnostic criteria for personality disorders have changed significantly in the past 50 years. As a result of all of these limitations, clinicians often are unable to make a diagnosis or end up making judgments based on insufficient information.

A further diagnostic challenge for clinicians is the need to isolate lifelong personality characteristics from a multitude of comorbid psychiatric and medical problems. Acute and chronic episodes of major depression, psychosis, and other major psychiatric disorders can considerably distort personality features. Even the current diagnostic nomenclature might serve to handicap late-life diagnosis because it is not age adjusted, and many criteria do not apply in late life. A final barrier to diagnosis can be present if the clinician erroneously considers all older patients to have disruptive personality features as a normal function of age. One future remedy for many of these challenges is to construct personality along several measurable dimensions, as opposed to retrospective categorization. *DSM-5* includes an alternative (but not yet adopted) dimensional model for personality disorders.

Differential Diagnosis

In clinical settings, it is important to remember that not every older patient with prominent or troubling personality features has a personality disorder. Those who demonstrate rigid and maladaptive personality traits but without the pervasiveness or severity as represented by *DSM-5* criteria are better described as suffering from certain personality traits or an adjustment disorder. An adjustment disorder might best characterize previously healthy and well-adjusted individuals who demonstrate acute changes in personality as a result of severe stresses. For example, physical pain and disability can lead to dependent or avoidant behaviors that resemble those seen in personality disorders but without the pervasive pattern and degree of maladaptiveness. Often, the symptoms of major psychiatric disorders and those of personality disorders overlap considerably, and without longitudinal history it can be difficult to distinguish between them. For example, the odd thinking and unusual perceptual experiences seen in psychotic disorders can resemble behaviors seen in schizotypal personality disorder. The emotional lability of bipolar states can mimic behaviors of borderline and histrionic diagnoses, and depressive symptoms from dysthymic and depressive disorders can be almost indistinguishable from depressive personality traits. Diagnosis of a personality disorder becomes more certain when seemingly acute behaviors emerge as enduring and pervasive personality traits. This process depends on the opportunity to observe a person over time and in multiple settings or situations.

Long-Term Course

Personality disorders can follow 1 of 4 possible courses: persist unchanged, evolve into a different form or major psychiatric disorder (eg, depression), improve, or remit. Few disorders have actually been studied over time, and rarely into late life. Several studies have suggested that personality disorders can enter a period of relative quiescence in middle age, with fewer and less intense symptoms and increased adaptation (SOE=C). However, this period may precede their reemergence in late life. Other researchers have proposed that personality disorders characterized by emotional and behavioral lability, including antisocial, borderline, histrionic, narcissistic, and dependent disorders, tend to improve over time, although patients remain vulnerable to depression. Personality disorders characterized by an overcontrol of affect and impulses, including paranoid, schizoid, schizotypal, and obsessive-compulsive personality disorders, are thought either to remain stable or to worsen in late life.

Only antisocial and borderline personality disorders have been looked at longitudinally, and both have shown symptom improvement and even remittance into middle and later life for a significant percentage of patients (SOE=B). At the same time, there can be persistent psychopathology that is not recognized within the context of existing antisocial or borderline diagnostic criteria. In other words, chronic personality dynamics can manifest in new behaviors. For example, those with antisocial personality disorders demonstrate less aggressiveness, violence, and criminal acts as they age but can still have antisocial tendencies expressed through substance abuse, disregard for safety, and noncompliance with institutional rules. Older borderline patients display less impulsivity, self-mutilation, and risk taking but more aging-related symptoms, such as the use of multiple medications and nonadherence with treatment.

Treatment

The treatment of personality disorders in late life is complicated and often has limited success. Given the chronic and pervasive nature of personality disorders, the overall goal of treatment in late life is not to cure the disorder but to decrease the frequency and intensity of disruptive behaviors. The first step should always be to clarify the diagnosis and then to identify recent stressors that may account for the current presentation. The resultant formulation can guide the selection of realistic target symptoms and therapeutic approaches, and allow a treatment team to anticipate future stressors. Treatment of personality disorders in late life uses the same basic approaches as with younger patients, but clinicians must incorporate a much broader understanding of the impact of age-related stressors and comorbid disorders. All forms of psychotherapy have been used to treat personality disorders in older adults, ranging from intensive and long-term insight-oriented approaches to equally intensive but more focused cognitive-behavioral models, such as dialectical behavior therapy. In late life, time and intensity of therapy may be more limited and, as a result, treatment must focus more on short-term approaches. Studies in adults generally find that comorbid personality disorders complicate the treatment of psychiatric illness, but that with consistent treatment, the prognosis is often favorable (SOE=B). The prognosis in late life is more guarded, especially for individuals with comorbid major depression. One study of older adults with major depressive disorder found that those with a concomitant personality disorder were less likely to benefit from psychotherapy.

In outpatient settings, control over a patient's environment is limited, and clinicians must therefore rely on one-to-one interventions (if the patient is willing to cooperate with treatment). With some patients, it may be necessary to convey a basic formulation of their behaviors, along with suggested approaches, to caregivers and affiliated health care professionals, such as primary care providers, social workers, and visiting nurses. This communication is important when patients are vulnerable to self-harm or likely to cause significant disruptions in other settings when they are not understood and approached in a therapeutic manner. For some therapeutic approaches that can be used with various personality disorders, see Table 43.2.

Long-term care settings allow more opportunities for intervention. A staff meeting or case conference often provides the best forum to discuss disruptive patients and to coordinate a consistent treatment plan. Disruptive behaviors can sometimes be traced to particular activities or staff interactions, which can be adapted as part of an overall treatment strategy. Sometimes, disengagement from patients reduces the intensity of disruptive interactions. In other situations, the continuity of staffing and of daily schedules is critical. In all situations, a treatment plan should be well documented and conveyed to the patient, as well as to all involved staff and caregivers. All plans must provide appropriate limits to ensure the safety of patients and staff. A written contract, signed by all parties, may be needed with nonadherent patients to eliminate ambiguity. Although it is important to involve family members in the treatment plan, clinicians must recognize that patients with personality disorders often have conflictual relationships with them. Attention should also be given to individual staff members who must work with difficult patients. These staff members need opportunities to discuss feelings of anxiety and frustration and to feel acknowledged and supported by administrative and other clinical staff.

Few studies have specifically evaluated pharmacologic strategies for personality disorders in late life, so extrapolation from guidelines used for younger people is needed. Psychotropic medications can be targeted at a particular personality disorder; specific symptoms or symptom clusters; or comorbid depression, anxiety, or psychosis. Again, the goal is not to cure the disorder but to reduce the frequency and intensity of targeted symptoms. Antidepressant medication can be helpful for the target symptoms of depression and anxiety found in most personality disorders (SOE=B). Mood stabilizers (eg, lithium carbonate[OL], carbamazepine[OL], divalproex sodium[OL], and lamotrigine[OL]) and antipsychotic medications can reduce mood lability and impulsivity in borderline patients, and they can be useful with similar symptoms in antisocial personality

Table 43.2—Therapeutic Strategies for Personality Disorders in Late Life*

Cluster A: Paranoid, Schizoid, Schizotypal Personality Disorders
- Always assess for and treat comorbid psychosis.
- Do not force social interactions but offer support and problem-solving assistance in a professional and consistent manner.
- Do not challenge paranoid ideation; instead, solicit and empathize with emotional responses to inner turmoil and fear of paranoid states.

Cluster B: Antisocial, Borderline, Histrionic, and Narcissistic Personality Disorders
- Assess for and treat underlying mood lability, depression, anxiety, and substance abuse.
- Adopt a consistent, structured, and predictable approach with strict boundaries to contain disruptive behaviors.
- Adopt a team approach with all involved clinicians to devise a common plan; avoid staff splits between "supporters" and "detractors" of the patient.
- Use behavioral contracts and authority figures when necessary to address recurrent disruptive behaviors.
- Do not personalize belligerent behaviors directed toward staff members; instead, provide opportunities for staff to discuss frustration and negative thoughts and emotions with professional colleagues.

Cluster C: Avoidant, Dependent, and Obsessive-Compulsive Personality Disorders
- Assess for and treat underlying anxiety, panic, and depression.
- Provide regularly scheduled clinical contacts rather than on an as-needed basis.
- When possible, provide case managers to solicit the needs of avoidant patients and to provide extra reassurance and attention to the needs of dependent and obsessive-compulsive patients.

*SOE=D

disorder (SOE=B). Antianxiety agents are commonly used for transient agitation seen in borderline, antisocial, narcissistic, and paranoid disorders, and they may reduce social anxiety and panic in avoidant and dependent patients (SOE=C). Antidepressants are used commonly to treat impulsive aggression as well as obsessive-compulsive personality symptoms, although efficacy has not been established for treatment of these symptoms (as it has been demonstrated for obsessive-compulsive disorder). Antipsychotic agents can treat the transient psychosis, agitation, and impulsivity seen in dramatic cluster and paranoid disorders, as well as the borderline psychosis and paranoia seen in cluster A disorders (SOE=B).

For personality disorders, psychotropic medications are best used as adjuncts to psychotherapy. In older adults, multiple medications should be avoided in general, and particularly when there is a history of nonadherence, confusion, or impulsivity. Attention must be given to potential interactions with multiple other medications used to treat medical disorders. It is important to obtain and document informed consent (or consent of family members or guardians) for the use of psychotropic medications when there is a history of dementia, recent delirium, paranoia, or conflictual doctor-patient relationships.

Finally, clinicians must recognize that in some cases it is best not to prescribe a psychotropic medication. Such cases include older adults with personality disorders and comorbid substance abuse, chronic nonadherence, or a history of or potential for abusive or self-injurious use of medications. Antisocial and borderline individuals often demonstrate such behaviors. Dependent patients often insist on medications as a means of fostering dependency on the clinician, and obsessive-compulsive patients can perpetuate a maladaptive relationship with the clinician through detailed and controlling discussions of medication management. In each example, medication management is corrupted by dysfunctional interpersonal behaviors that lie at the heart of personality disorders.

SOMATIC SYMPTOM AND RELATED DISORDERS

Somatic symptom and related disorders encompass a heterogeneous group of 5 diagnoses that have in common the presence of distressing physical symptoms, as well as abnormal thoughts, feelings, and behaviors in response to these physical symptoms. Previously, under *DSM IV-TR*, the somatic complaints occurred without objective organic causes; however, *DSM-5* does not require that the somatic symptoms be medically unexplained. Instead, somatic symptom disorder can also accompany a diagnosed medical disorder as long as the somatic symptoms are associated with significant emotional distress and impairment. The *DSM IV-TR* diagnoses of somatization disorder, undifferentiated somatoform disorder, hypochondriasis, and some presentations of pain disorder are now included under the *DSM-5* criteria as somatic symptom disorder. In somatic symptom disorder, the patient must have one or more distressing and/or disruptive somatic symptom(s) that is accompanied by at least one of the following: 1) concerns about the seriousness of the medical symptom that is out of proportion to what is typically experienced, 2) persistent high level of anxiety about the symptom, and/or 3) excessive time and energy focused on the somatic symptom. The clinician can also specify if the somatic symptom disorder occurs with predominant pain.

Illness anxiety disorder is a preoccupation with being susceptible to or having an illness. Patients with illness anxiety disorder tend to have milder somatic symptoms but higher anxiety levels than those with somatic symptom disorder. Symptoms must be persistent for ≥6 months, and patient behaviors can be described as care seeking or care avoidant. Conversion disorder is defined by one or more symptoms of altered voluntary motor and/or sensory function that causes significant social and occupational impairment and is not explained by a neurologic disease. Motor symptoms of conversion disorders may include weakness, paralysis, and abnormal movements (eg, tremor) and gait disorders. Sensory symptoms include changes in vision or hearing, or skin sensations. Psychological factors affecting medical conditions are psychological or behavioral factors that have an adverse effect on a diagnosed medical condition. For example, a patient may exacerbate symptoms of COPD because of anxiety, or a patient may manipulate insulin dosage in an attempt to lose weight. *DSM-5* also includes factitious disorders in this category, which are characterized by false symptoms associated with deception on the part of the patient. Patients with factitious disorder present as ill or injured without any obvious evidence of external reward or reinforcement. Distressing somatic symptoms that do not fit any of the above diagnoses are classified as other or unspecified somatic symptom and related disorders. Specific diagnostic criteria for these 5 conditions can be found in the *DSM-5*.

All of these disorders are especially relevant to geriatric care because affected older adults are seen in all health care settings, and they tend to overuse medical services. Somatic symptom disorders in late life have not been well studied, and existing research has usually focused on select diagnoses, such as hypochondriasis, in limited or biased samples. Research also has looked at somatic symptom reporting rather than at specific diagnoses. Prevalence rates in middle and late life have been found to be <1%, except for one study in which the prevalence rate for somatization disorder in women >55 years old seen in health care clinics was >36%. The presence of these disorders has not been found to be strongly associated with age, although there is weak evidence for a slight increase in hypochondriasis with age (SOE=C). However, increased somatic preoccupation and symptoms are associated with depression in late life, and older age of onset for depression may be most predictive. In addition to depression, increased somatic preoccupation is associated with the presence of neuroticism, a personality trait in which a person displays a tendency to experience more negative emotions. Somatic symptom disorders are found more commonly in women and in lower socioeconomic groups. Late onset may suggest associated neurologic illness.

A number of culture-bound psychiatric syndromes resemble somatic symptom disorders in that they involve somatic syndromes that lack an organic cause and often result from psychologic stress. They differ from somatoform disorders in that they are seen only in a specific culture and are often treated by folk medicine. Several examples included *dhat* (India) and *shenkui* (China), in which men suffer from fatigue, anorexia, and other vague somatic symptoms attributed by the patient to the loss of semen; *hwabyeong* (Korea), in which women suffer from insomnia, sighing, and a sensation of chest pressure in response to an emotional stress; and *susto* (Latin America), in which an individual presents with nervousness, insomnia, anorexia, and sometimes involuntary tics and diarrhea after a severely frightening experience.

Clinical Characteristics and Causes

Somatic symptom and related disorders, except for factitious disorder, do not represent intentional, conscious attempts by older adults to present factitious physical symptoms. Somatoform symptoms are experienced by the affected individual as real physical pain and discomfort, usually without insight into associated psychologic factors. Somatic symptom disorders do not represent delusional thinking as is seen in psychotic states, and they are different from psychosomatic disorders, which are characterized by actual disease states with presumed psychologic triggers. They also differ from malingering, with its intentional and fully conscious goal of avoiding a specific responsibility such as work. Rather, somatoform disorders represent a complex interaction between mind and brain in which an affected person is unknowingly expressing psychologic stress or conflict through the body. It is not surprising, then, that depression and anxiety are associated with increased somatic expressions. In late life, somatic symptom disorders, in particular illness anxiety disorder, can be a way for a person to express anxiety and attempt to cope with accumulating fears and losses. These may include fears of abandonment by family and caregivers, loss of beauty and strength, financial setbacks, loss of independence, loss of social role (eg, through retirement, loss of spouse, occupational disability), and loneliness. The psychologic distress and anxiety over such losses can be less threatening and more controllable when shifted to somatic complaints or symptoms. In turn, the resultant state of debility might be reinforced by increased social contacts and support.

The causes of somatic symptom disorders are usually multifactorial and are often rooted in early developmental experiences and personality traits. Psychodynamic approaches suggest that these disorders result from unconscious conflict in which intolerable impulses or affects are expressed through more tolerable somatic symptoms or complaints. One reason for this may be the presence of alexithymia, in which a person is unable to identify and express emotional states, so that the body becomes the available mode of expression.

Although psychodynamic explanations can apply across the life span, these conflicts often begin early in life, perhaps accounting for the relatively young age of onset for most somatic symptom disorders. In late life, psychologic conflict that results in significant depression and anxiety are, for the most part, the same conflicts that can lead to somatization. In addition, the presence of so many comorbid medical problems and the use of multiple medications can provide readily available somatic symptoms around which psychologic conflict can center. In long-term care, older adults are faced with many overwhelming losses, and their own bodies often serve as the last bastion of control. Somatic preoccupation thus serves as a means of coping with stress, even though it is maladaptive and can result in excessive and unnecessary disability.

Treatment

People with somatic symptom disorder do not usually present as such; by definition, they appear to have legitimate somatic complaints. It is only after repeated but fruitless evaluations, multiple and persistent complaints and requests, and sometimes angry and inappropriate reactions to treatment that clinicians begin to suspect a somatic symptom disorder. In some cases, the manner of presentation and symptom complex is more immediately suggestive of a particular somatic symptom disorder. In any event, it is important for the clinician to remember that from the perspective of the patient, the symptoms and complaints are quite real and disturbing. It is never wise to challenge the patient or to suggest that the symptoms are "all in your mind," even after diagnostic evaluation has made it obvious that psychologic factors are involved. The typical response to such advice is for the patient to seek additional opinions and medical tests, which in turn can perpetuate a cycle of somatization that never addresses the underlying issues.

Instead, the clinician should attempt to foster an ongoing, supportive, consistent, and professional relationship with the affected patient. Such a relationship serves to provide reassurance as well as to protect the patient from excessive and unnecessary medical visits and procedures. The clinician should focus on responding to individual complaints, perhaps with periodic but regularly scheduled appointments, and to set limits on evaluation and treatment in a firm but empathetic manner. This can be difficult to do when patients become demanding and attempt to consume excessive amounts of time, but the clinician must endeavor to remain professional, without personalizing the situation or feeling that he or she is failing the patient. Overall, the role of the clinician is to focus on reducing symptoms and rehabilitating the patient, and not attempting to force the patient to have insight into the potential psychologic nature of his or her symptoms. It would be hazardous to prematurely diagnose a somatic symptom disorder when there might actually be an underlying medical problem that has eluded diagnosis. For example, disorders such as multiple sclerosis, systemic lupus erythematosus, and acute intermittent porphyria commonly have complex presentations that elude initial diagnostic evaluation. Moreover, many somatic symptom disorders coexist with actual disease states; for example, many individuals with pseudoseizures also have an actual seizure disorder. At the same time, it is important for the clinician to set limits on what he or she can offer and to make appropriate referrals to specialists and mental health clinicians.

The mental health clinician should have an active role in addressing the somatic symptom disorder. Unfortunately, no particular treatment for any specific disorder has been found to have good efficacy, and most disorders tend to be lifelong. As a result, the goal of treatment is not to cure but to control symptoms. The clinician first forms a therapeutic alliance based on empathetic listening and acknowledgment of physical discomfort, without trivializing the somatic complaints. Sometimes an offer to review all available medical records can be a tangible way of conveying one's seriousness to the patient. Underlying anxiety and depression must be identified and treated with psychotherapy and, when necessary, antidepressant or antianxiety medications, or both. Cognitive-behavioral therapy focuses on identifying distorted thought patterns and triggers of anxiety, and then replacing them with more realistic and adaptive strategies. A mental health professional can assist in determining whether cognitive-behavioral therapy may be of benefit. In many cases, however, the supportive nature of regular visits to a primary care provider may be sufficient to meet the needs of individuals with somatic symptom disorders.

REFERENCES

- Black DW, Zanarini MC, Romine A, et al. Comparison of low and moderate dosages of extended-release quetiapine in borderline personality disorder: A randomized, double-blind, placebo-controlled trial. *Am J Psychiatry.* 2014;171(11):1174–1182.

    This is one of very few placebo-controlled trials of the use of quetiapine for primary borderline personality disorder that demonstrated reduced severity of borderline pathology as well as of verbal and physical aggression. Of note is that treatment with low-dose quetiapine (150 mg/d) was superior to placebo and to higher dosages (300 mg/d).

- Ingenhoven T, Lafay P, Rinne T, et al. Effectiveness of pharmacotherapy for severe personality disorders: meta-analyses of randomized controlled trials. *J Clin Psychiatry.* 2010;71(1):14–25.

    A meta-analysis of 21 placebo-controlled randomized trials of pharmacologic medications in borderline and schizotypal personality disorders between 1980 and 2007 found that antipsychotics benefitted cognitive-perceptual symptoms, mood stabilizers improved impulse dyscontrol, and antidepressants had mild effects on anxiety.

- Rabinowitz T, Hirdes JP, Desjardins I. Somatoform disorders. In: Agronin ME, Maletta GJ, eds. *Principles and Practice of Geriatric Psychiatry, 2nd Edition.* Philadelphia: Lippincott Williams & Wilkins; 2011:565–582.

    This review of somatoform disorders in late life includes illuminating data from the authors' own research to underscore many points. Keeping with the focus of the comprehensive textbook in which this chapter appears, clinical diagnosis and management are emphasized.

- Schuster JP, Hoertel N, Strat YL, et al. Personality disorders in older adults: findings from the national epidemiologic survey on alcohol and related conditions. *Am J Ger Psychiatry.* 2013;21(8):757–768.

    Taken from a large subsample of the massive National Epidemiologic Survey on Alcohol and Related Conditions, these data highlight the high degree of disability and multiple comorbidities of personality disorders in late life.

- Stevenson J, Datyner A, Boyce P, et al. The effect of age on prevalence, type and diagnosis of personality disorder in psychiatric inpatients. *Int J Geriatr Psychiatry.* 2011;26(9):981–987.

    This article identifies significant personality comorbidity across the life span, including inpatients up to 100 years old. Among older adults, 58.8% displayed a comorbid personality diagnosis, but clinician recognition of these comorbidities was <20%.

- Zweig RA, Agronin ME. Personality disorders. In: Agronin ME, Maletta GJ, eds. *Principles and Practice of Geriatric Psychiatry, 2nd Edition.* Philadelphia: Lippincott Williams & Wilkins; 2011:523–544.

    This comprehensive review of personality disorders in late life focuses on clinical diagnosis and management. Both psychotherapeutic and psychopharmacologic approaches are described in detail and supplemented with a practical table.

Marc E. Agronin, MD

CHAPTER 44—ADDICTIONS

KEY POINTS

- Alcohol and other substance abuse problems can remain undetected when screening questions are omitted during routine medical visits.

- Alcohol use can be an unrecognized cause of falls, cognitive decline, and medical problems (eg, anemia, increased results of liver function tests, hyponatremia, thrombocytopenia).

- It is important to consider a diagnosis of alcohol or benzodiazepine withdrawal in older adults who develop delirium with hospitalization or facility placement.

- Cognitive impairment from chronic alcoholism in older adults can improve with sustained abstinence.

- Inappropriate use of prescription drugs, including benzodiazepines and opioids, is often unrecognized.

- Smoking cessation efforts should persist throughout life.

The misuse of alcohol, psychoactive medications, illicit drugs, and nicotine has become a significant public health concern for the growing population of older adults. Substance use disorders among older adults is common, and older adults are particularly vulnerable to the cognitive and physical effects of these substances. Typically, substance use disorders are thought to develop only in those who use substances in large quantities and at regular intervals. Among older adults, however, negative health consequences have been demonstrated at consumption amounts previously thought of as light to moderate. A growing number of effective treatments for these problems lead not only to reduced substance use but also to improved general health. Both the risks and the emergence of new treatments underscore the need to identify problems and provide appropriate treatment for older adults suffering from the effects of substance misuse.

DEFINITIONS OF SUBSTANCE USE DISORDERS

Many older adults are not recognized as having problems related to their substance use, partly because the diagnostic criteria have been difficult to interpret and apply consistently to older adults. For instance, many older people drink at home by themselves; thus, they are less likely than younger drinkers to be arrested, get into arguments, or have difficulties in employment. Moreover, because many of the diseases potentially associated with substance use (eg, hypertension, stroke, and peptic ulcer disease) are common disorders in late life, the effects of substance use on older adults who have these other medical disorders can be overlooked. The literature indicates that older adults with alcohol use disorders are identified less often by clinicians and are less often referred for treatment than their younger counterparts.

Given the difficulties in applying this terminology to older adults, the *Diagnostic and Statistical Manual of Mental Disorders, 5th Edition (DSM-5)* represents a potential advance, because it no longer uses the terms substance "abuse" and "dependence." The diagnosis of a "substance use disorder" is now based on 11 criteria that encompass the following domains: impaired control, social impairment, risky use, and pharmacologic criteria. Severity is determined by the number of criteria met, from mild (2 or 3), moderate (4 or 5) to severe (≥6); legal problems are no longer a criteria.

Regardless of the diagnostic system, many experts advocate screening to identify those at risk of problem behaviors or who have at-risk or problem use. *At-risk use* is defined as any use of a substance at a quantity or frequency greater than a recommended level. The level of use is often determined empirically based on association with significant disability. For instance, the recommended upper limit of alcohol consumption for older adults has been established as no more than an average of 1 standard drink per day and no more than 2 episodes of binge drinking (≥4 drinks in a day) during a 3-month period. *Problem substance use* is defined as the consumption of any amount of an abusable substance that results in at least 1 problem related to this use. For example, the use of benzodiazepines by a patient who has a preexisting unsteady gait would be considered problem use.

On the other end of the spectrum, *abstinence* is defined as drinking no alcohol in the previous year. Approximately 60% of older adults are abstinent. If an older adult is abstinent, it can be useful to ascertain why alcohol is not used. Some individuals are abstinent because of a previous history of alcohol problems. For this reason, it is particularly important to obtain a history of both current and past use. Some older adults are abstinent because of recent illness; others have lifelong patterns of abstinence or low-risk use. Individuals who have a previous history of alcohol problems can require preventive monitoring to determine if any new stresses could exacerbate an old pattern. In addition, a previous history of at-risk drinking or alcohol dependence increases the risk of developing other mental health problems in late life, such as depressive disorders or cognitive problems, and can limit treatment response because of brain damage.

Low-risk or *moderate use* of alcohol is use that falls within the recommended guidelines for consumption and is not associated with problems. Older adults in this category not only consume amounts that fall within recommended drinking guidelines but also are able to reasonably limit their alcohol consumption (ie, they do not drink when driving a motor vehicle or boat, or when using contraindicated medications). However, a change in either physical health or prescription medications can increase even low-risk use to a problem level.

The most practical method for identifying individuals who could benefit from intervention is to determine the quantity and frequency of their substance use. This method has advantages over formal diagnostic interviews because of its brevity, easily interpretable results, and absence of stigmatizing language, such as "addiction," "alcoholism," or "alcoholic."

MAGNITUDE OF THE PROBLEM

Drug Use

Little is known about the epidemiology of substance use disorders other than alcoholism among older adults. The general belief is that older drug addicts are only younger addicts grown old and that few individuals initiate drug use in their later years. In the Epidemiologic Catchment Area study, lifetime prevalence rates of drug abuse and dependence were 0.12% for older men and 0.06% for older women, and lifetime history of illicit drug use was 2.88% for men and 0.66% for women. No active cases were reported in either gender. In contrast, a more recent study of an elder-specific drug program in a veteran population found that one-fourth had either a primary drug problem or concurrent drug and alcohol problems. This study may be a reflection of the growing number of older adults who used drugs during a time of expanded drug experimentation in the United States in the 1960s. Indeed, reports from the National Survey on Drug Use and Health suggest a rise in marijuana and cocaine use among individuals ≥50 years old, with the 1-year prevalence of marijuana use approaching 4% for the U.S. population aged 50–64 years, whereas use of illicit drugs has decreased in all younger age groups. Recent increases in hepatitis C among those ≥60 years old can reflect both a history of intravenous drug use, as well as increased risk of nosocomial infection with advanced age. Other studies to determine the prevalence and incidence of substance use disorders (in later life) involving nicotine, caffeine, and benzodiazepines are needed.

Medication Use

An increasing problem with the older age group is the misuse or inappropriate use of prescription and OTC medications, with 2.1% of adults aged 50 in the National Survey on Drug Use and Health reporting nonmedical use of prescription-type drugs, the most commonly used illicit class among those ≥65 years old. This problem includes the misuse of substances such as sedatives, hypnotics, narcotic and non-narcotic analgesics, diet aids, decongestants, and a wide variety of OTC medications. Community surveys have found that 60% of older adults are taking an analgesic, 22% are taking a CNS medication, and 11% are taking a benzodiazepine. Many medications used by older adults have the potential for inducing tolerance, withdrawal syndromes, and harmful medical consequences, such as cognitive changes, kidney disease, falls, and liver disease. A growing body of literature demonstrates a concerning increase in morbidity and mortality associated with misuse of prescription and nonprescription medications, even though this is not considered as a disorder in *DSM-5*.

Medication use by all older adults needs to be monitored carefully; prescribing potentially hazardous combinations of medications, medications with a high risk of adverse events, and ineffective or unnecessary medications should be avoided. A practical approach to monitoring psychoactive medications is to reevaluate the older patient's use every 3–6 months. Maintenance treatment should be continued only in those patients who have specific target symptoms and a documented response to the treatment. Patients who have no response or only a partial response should be reevaluated to consider the appropriate diagnosis and further care. In such cases, consultation with a geriatric mental health professional could be advantageous.

Alcohol Use

Community-based epidemiologic studies define the extent and nature of alcohol use in the older population by reporting percentages of abstainers, heavy drinkers, and daily drinkers. Abstention from alcohol ranges from 31% to 58%, and daily drinking ranges from 10% to 22% in samples of older adults. "Heavy" drinking, defined as a minimum of 12–21 drinks per week, is present in 3%–9% of the older population; alcohol abuse, as defined clinically, is present in approximately 2%–4%.

Longitudinally designed community studies give valuable insight regarding the natural course of drinking patterns in older age groups. Studies that examined longitudinal alcohol use indicate an incidence of heavy drinking of 0.2%–4% in older adults per year. Although older adults are likely to decrease the amount of alcohol consumed on a given day, the frequency or pattern of use changes very little over time.

Cultural and Demographic Factors

The prevalence of alcohol use and alcohol-related problems among older adults is much higher for men than for women. Among younger adults, however, the ratio of male to female drinkers has changed over the past several decades, with the result that more women present for treatment. These changes are likely to continue to be reflected in the next generation of older women. Similar patterns by gender are seen with illicit drug use, except that benzodiazepines are much more commonly used by older women than by older men.

Conclusions are less clear from the few studies addressing differences among various ethnic groups. Depending on the study, older black Americans and older Hispanic Americans consume amounts of alcohol similar to or lower than amounts consumed by older white Americans. The Epidemiologic Catchment Area data demonstrated significant differences in the 1-year diagnosis of alcohol abuse and dependence among black Americans (2.93% among men and 0.60% among women), white Americans (2.85% among men and 0.47% among women), and Hispanic Americans (6.57% among men and 0.36% among women). Increased leisure time and higher disposable income are more relevant risk factors for alcohol consumption among older adults than race or ethnicity.

Clinical Settings

Older adults constitute most admissions to acute care facilities and are frequent users of outpatient medical services, including primary care. The prevalence rates for alcohol problems among hospital populations are substantially higher than those among community dwellers. High prevalence rates for problems related to drinking are also becoming more common in retirement communities. Data from a survey of a Veterans Affairs nursing home demonstrated that 35% of patients interviewed had a lifetime diagnosis of alcohol abuse. A significant number of patients seen in outpatient clinics also have active alcohol use disorders. The high prevalence of alcohol-related problems in both hospital and outpatient populations underscores the need for thorough screening of older adults in medical settings.

The epidemiology of substance use suggests that the prevalence of misuse among older adults will likely increase as the baby boomers age. The growing numbers of patients in potential need of treatment will be paired with an ongoing shortage of providers trained in the treatment of older adults with mental health or substance use disorders. This growing public health problem is addressed in the recent Institute of Medicine report *The Mental Health and Substance Use Workforce for Older Adults: In Whose Hands?*

RISKS AND BENEFITS OF SUBSTANCE USE

Benefits of Alcohol Consumption

Moderate alcohol consumption among otherwise healthy older adults has been promoted as having significant beneficial effects, especially with regard to cardiovascular disease. Findings from the cardiovascular literature have led to a host of articles in the popular press espousing the benefits of alcohol use.

Alcohol in moderate amounts can promote relaxation and reduce social anxiety. And, somewhat surprisingly, a variety of observational and prospective, longitudinal cohort studies have found that infrequent or light alcohol consumption protects against incidence of cognitive impairment. However, the practice of recommending drinking to people who currently do not drink is not advocated. Many older adults do not drink because of past problems with drinking, family problems with drinking, the expense related to drinking, and the adverse effects of intoxication. There is no direct evidence to justify prescribing alcohol for individuals with heart disease or any other health condition.

Excess Physical Disability

Substance abuse has clear and profound effects on the health and well-being of older adults in all spheres of life. Older adults are particularly prone to the toxic effects of substances on many different organ systems because of both the physiologic changes associated with aging and the changes associated with other illnesses common in late life. The social and economic impact is also tremendous. Substance abuse has adverse effects on self-esteem, coping skills, and interpersonal relationships, which may be compounded by losses that are common in later stages of life.

Levels of alcohol consumption higher than 7 drinks per week, so-called at-risk drinking, have been associated with a number of health problems, including an increased risk of stroke caused by bleeding, impaired driving skills, and an increased rate of injuries such as falls and fractures (SOE=A). The risk of breast cancer in women who consume 3–9 drinks per week is approximately 50% higher than that of women who consume fewer than 3 drinks per week. Of particular importance to older adults are the potential harmful interactions between alcohol and both prescribed and OTC medications, especially psychoactive medications such as benzodiazepines and antidepressants. Alcohol also interferes with the metabolism of many medications, including warfarin.

Older adults who consume more than an average of 4 drinks per day or whose drinking has led to a diagnosis of alcohol dependence are at greatest risk of excess physical disability and physical illness related to drinking. The most common problems associated with alcohol dependence are alcoholic liver disease, COPD, peptic ulcer disease, and psoriasis. Moreover, unexplained multisystem disease should alert the clinician to probe more closely for alcohol use. With smoking, the risks are much clearer, including increased rates of pulmonary disease, especially cancer. Medications such as benzodiazepines are also associated with excess physical disability, increased rates of falls, and driving-related impairment. Research is beginning to demonstrate that the disability associated with these problems is also reversible with reduced substance use (SOE=B).

Mental Health Problems

Substance use can be a significant factor in the course and prognosis of nearly all mental health problems of late life. Use of alcohol, benzodiazepines, opioids, and cigarettes has been demonstrated to be related etiologically to mood disturbances, but these substances also complicate the treatment of concurrent mood disorders. Individuals with both alcoholism and depression have a more complicated clinical course of depression with an increased risk of suicide and more social dysfunction than nondepressed individuals with alcoholism. Overall, older adults with alcohol abuse or dependence are nearly 3 times more likely to have a lifetime diagnosis of another mental disorder. Alcoholism has been implicated in mood disorders, suicide, dementia, anxiety disorders, and sleep disturbances.

As might be expected, patients with alcohol-related dementia who become abstinent do not show a progression in cognitive impairment comparable to that of those with Alzheimer disease. The complex role of alcoholism in the development of Alzheimer disease is not fully understood, but alcoholism does lead independently to a syndrome of dementia. Interesting new hypotheses implicate glutamatergic toxicity, but overall, the mechanisms are not well understood. Clinical features supporting the diagnosis of alcohol-related dementia include end-organ damage (eg, liver disease), cognitive stabilization or improvement after abstinence, and evidence of cerebellar atrophy in brain imaging. Further research is needed to understand the potential benefits of long-term abstinence in alcohol-related dementia. Similarly, those with comorbid depression and alcohol use are likely to have better depression outcomes if they become abstinent. Moderate alcohol use has also been demonstrated to have negative effects on the treatment of late-life depression, further underscoring the need for reducing moderate use in the context of chronic health problems in older adults.

IDENTIFYING SUBSTANCE USE DISORDERS

Although clinical examination remains the most valuable tool for identifying substance use problems, screening instruments can help increase the sensitivity and efficiency of diagnosis. Several instruments have been developed for identifying alcohol use disorders, including self-administered questionnaires and laboratory studies. Self-administered questionnaires provide a rapid, sensitive, and inexpensive method of screening for alcohol problems. Two questionnaires have been developed with these principles in mind: the Michigan Alcoholism Screening Test (MAST)-Geriatric Version, and the AUDIT C (www.sbirttraining.com/sites/sbirt-training.com/files/MAST-G.pdf and www.integration.samhsa.gov/images/res/tool_auditc.pdf (accessed Jan 2016). Both of these instruments have high sensitivity and specificity for identifying alcohol misuse in middle-aged and older adults. The CAGE is a brief clinician-administered screening test that may be useful to identify problem drinking using a cutoff of 2 as a positive screen, although some suggest ≥1 should be considered positive if the prevalence is high in the population (www.uspreventiveservicestaskforce.org/Home/GetFileByID/838 (accessed Jan 2016).

Biologic markers of substance use can be useful in managing patients with known substance use disorders, but they have proved less valuable in detecting illness. These markers include γ-glutamyl transferase, which has a low sensitivity and a moderate specificity for diagnosing an alcohol use disorder; mean corpuscular volume, which has a low sensitivity but a high specificity; and carbohydrate-deficient transferrin, which has a low sensitivity and low specificity. These markers require further research but, clinically, any combination of macrocytic anemia, thrombocytopenia, and increased γ-glutamyl transferase should indicate the need for further screening. Urine drug screens are an effective method of screening for or identifying illicit drug use, as well as prescription drug use.

TREATMENT

Older adults with a substance use problem often need a variety of treatments. Therefore, it is important to have an array of services available for older adults that can be tailored to their individual needs and that have the flexibility to adapt to changing needs over time. The most important aspect of treating an older adult who is misusing a substance is to engage the individual in the intervention. Older adults engaged in treatment have been shown to have robust improvement, especially compared with younger cohorts. The spectrum of interventions for alcohol abuse in older adults range from prevention and education for those who are abstinent or low-risk drinkers, to minimal advice or brief structured interventions for at-risk or problem drinkers, to formalized alcoholism treatment for drinkers who meet criteria for abuse or dependence. The array of formal treatment options available includes psychotherapy, education, rehabilitative and residential care, and psychopharmacologic agents. An example of the necessity to tailor care is the contrast between the at-risk drinker or benzodiazepine user and the severely dependent patient. The at-risk user will not likely need the intensity of services required for the severely dependent patient. Indeed, requiring the at-risk drinker to accept a set of rigorous services can be more detrimental than helpful.

Dependency on medications such as benzodiazepines is managed by placing the patient on a 24-hour equivalent of the dosage of the drug on which the patient is dependent; tapering the dosage by 10% every three half-lives; and providing supportive counseling via groups, psychosocial support, and 12-step programs. Symptoms of withdrawal from narcotics can be controlled when necessary with oral clonidine[OL]. Assuring that the patient enters a long-term treatment program increases the likelihood of long-term success. For smoking cessation, it is important to prepare the patient for quitting by discussing management strategies before quitting, setting a quit date, and implementing a monitoring plan for maintaining success.

Detoxification and Stabilization

The assessment of any substance abuser starts with a thorough history, physical examination, and laboratory tests. The patient's potential to suffer acute withdrawal should also be assessed. Severe withdrawal such as that from alcohol use can be life threatening and warrants careful attention. Patients with severe symptoms of dependency or withdrawal potential and patients with significant medical or psychiatric comorbidity can require inpatient hospitalization for acute stabilization before implementing an outpatient management strategy. Detoxification is achieved by placing the patient on the minimal amount of drug that suppresses withdrawal symptoms and then decreasing the dosage by 10% every three half-lives. In general, longer-acting formulations of the drug being abused are preferred to shorter-acting formulations, but many clinicians find that prescribing the specific drug that a patient was abusing makes the process more acceptable to the patient and minimizes the time needed to determine the initial dose.

For patients who are hospitalized for an elective surgery or condition unrelated to the substance problem, remaining vigilant for any evidence of withdrawal is extremely important. Unrecognized alcohol withdrawal can result in serious morbidity and mortality in older adults. Early symptoms include tachycardia, diaphoresis, tremulousness, and hypertension. These symptoms can progress to overt delirium, psychosis, and seizures. Intravenous lorazepam[OL] is the most expedient intervention in this scenario, followed by oral lorazepam, in tapering dosages.

Outpatient Management

Traditionally, outpatient substance abuse treatment has been reserved for specialized clinics focused on substance abuse. However, it is becoming increasingly apparent that this model is inadequate in addressing the broader public health demand, and there is a need to involve a variety of clinicians and clinical settings to deliver substance abuse treatment. This is particularly important for older adults, who frequently seek medical services but rarely seek specialized addiction services. The traditional addiction clinic is focused on supportive group psychotherapy and encouragement to attend regular self-help group meetings such as Alcoholics Anonymous, Alcoholics Victorious, Rational Recovery, or Narcotics Anonymous. For older adults, peer-specific group activities are considered superior to mixed-age group activities. Outpatient rehabilitation, in addition to focusing on active addiction issues, usually needs to address issues of leisure time and social activity.

Clinicians should be wary of focusing on abstinence as the only positive outcome of treatment and should commend patients for making progress in decreasing use as well as stopping. This can be particularly relevant for misuse of medications such as benzodiazepines, because eliminating use may be more difficult. For benzodiazepines, the risk of adverse events such as falls is greater with higher dosages and with medications that have a longer half-life such as diazepam or clonazepam. Therefore, using medications with a half-life of 6–12 hours reduces the risks for that patient. If benzodiazepines seem to be indicated for an anxiety condition and treatment is started for the first time, shorter-acting agents that do not have active metabolites (eg, lorazepam) are preferred to long-acting preparations. However, for patients already receiving long-acting benzodiazepines (eg, diazepam at ≥50 mg/d), the risk of withdrawal complications is increased, and the dosage should be reduced very gradually. If the daily dose is greater than the equivalent of 100 mg of diazepam, then the patient should be hospitalized to start withdrawal. Ultimately, a transition to shorter-acting agents is ideal, but this should be done carefully and initially involve an equivalent dosage before any reductions are considered. The use of resources such as day programs and senior centers can be beneficial, especially for cognitively impaired patients. Social services, including financial support, are often needed to stabilize the patient in early recovery. Supervised living arrangements, such as halfway houses, group homes, nursing homes, and residing with relatives, should also be considered.

Brief Interventions

Low-intensity, brief interventions have been suggested as cost-effective and practical techniques that can be used as an initial approach in at-risk and problem drinkers in primary care settings. Studies of brief intervention have been conducted in a wide range of health care settings, from hospitals and primary health care locations to mental health clinics. Two trials of brief alcohol intervention with older adults have been reported. Both studies were randomized trials of brief intervention to reduce hazardous drinking by older adults, and both used advice protocols in primary care settings. These studies showed that older adults can be engaged in brief intervention protocols and that the protocols are acceptable in this population; drinking was substantially reduced among at-risk drinkers receiving the interventions than among a control group.

Pharmacotherapy

The use of medications to support abstinence may be of benefit, but it is not well studied. For strength of evidence, see Table 44.1. Small-scale studies have demonstrated that naltrexone for alcohol abuse is well tolerated and efficacious in older adults. Naltrexone is available in both oral and long-acting injectable forms. Studies of antidepressants, including the SSRIs, do not support widespread use of antidepressants as a treatment for alcohol misuse, although they can be effective in treating concurrent depression. Some of the general principles used in treating younger patients should be applied to older patients as well. For example, benzodiazepines are important in treatment of alcohol detoxification, but they have no clinical place in maintaining long-term abstinence because of their potential for abuse and for fostering further alcohol or benzodiazepine abuse. Disulfiram can benefit some well-motivated patients, but cardiac and hepatic disease limits its use by older adults who abuse alcohol. Acamprosate has not been studied in older adults. Methadone maintenance has proven efficacy in opioid dependence. Older adults can be started and maintained on methadone, following the same principles of use as in younger patients. Comorbid medical and psychiatric disorders must be identified and properly treated, and they may necessitate the need for referral to, or consultation with, a psychiatrist with expertise in these areas.

Buprenorphine, and buprenorphine with naloxone have been approved for outpatient treatment of opioid dependence. However, given the complexity of the treatment of opioid dependence, systematic training, practice, monitoring, regulation, and evaluation are necessary in a multidisciplinary treatment setting to optimize outcomes. Guidelines for developing treatment programs using buprenorphine are available on the website of the Substance Abuse and Mental Health Services Administration (http://buprenorphine.samhsa.gov/index.html [accessed Jan 2016]).

OTHER ADDICTIONS

Nicotine Dependence

Nicotine dependence is a chronic disease that typically requires multiple attempts to quit with repeated interventions over the life span. Smoking cessation at any age slows the decline in lung function, and aggressive cessation efforts are appropriate even in very old patients (>85 years). There is significant evidence to demonstrate that brief interventions performed at each office visit will promote smoking cessation (SOE=A). The basic elements of the approach are the "Five A's" from the Agency for Health Care Policy and Research:

- Ask patients about nicotine use at every office visit.
- Assess readiness to quit.
- Advise patients to quit.
- Assist patients in the quit attempt with aids such as a local cessation program and pharmacologic agents such as bupropion, nicotine replacement, or varenicline.
- Arrange both a quit date and a follow-up visit or contact to discuss the quit attempt.

Establishing abstinence from nicotine follows the same principles as that from other addicting substances. Initially, pharmacologic substitution with either nicotine gum or patch is followed by a gradual decrease in dosage. In several trials, antidepressant medications improved rates of continued abstinence, but only bupropion has been approved for this purpose by the FDA. Varenicline has not received specific attention in older adults but should be considered, because there is strong evidence for benefit in smoking cessation in younger adults (SOE=B). However, as of July 2009, the FDA requires a black box warning for varenicline because of neuropsychiatric symptoms, such as depression and suicidality. As with other abstinence regimens, psychotherapy plus pharmacotherapy is better than pharmacotherapy alone.

Gambling

Gambling in late life is less prevalent than in young adulthood. However, older adults who have engaged in

Table 44.1—Late-Life Addiction Treatment Research and Strength of Evidence

Indication	Treatment Strategy	SOE	Comments	Limits
Detoxification				
Alcohol	Substitution with benzodiazepine	A	Prevents sequela such as seizures, severe withdrawal symptoms; should be driven by specific plan and measurement of effects	Few specific studies in older adults, who may be at greater risk of idiosyncratic responses
	Gabapentin	C	Effective in several clinical trials	No studies specific to older adults
	Carbamazepine[OL] and other mood-stabilizing medications	D	Small-scale studies have shown promise, but these medications are somewhat more complicated to use.	Very limited evidence base for older adults
Benzodiazepines	Slow tapering	B	Effective in managing withdrawal	Limited evidence base for older adults; long-term outcomes not well correlated with success of detoxification
Opioids	Substitution/taper	B	Effective in managing withdrawal	Limited evidence base for older adults
Treatment Strategies				
Problem and at-risk drinking	Brief interventions	A	Randomized trials have showed efficacy in primary-care settings with less evidence in high-risk settings such as behavioral health, home care, and the emergency room.	Limited effect in those with alcohol dependence; limited dissemination
Alcohol dependence	Psychotherapy	C	Several naturalistic trials demonstrated increased adherence to treatment and generally better outcomes for older adults than for middle-aged adults. Individual therapy such as cognitive-behavioral therapy may be particularly effective.	Randomized trials designed to better understand age-dependent adherence and treatment outcomes are needed.
	Naltrexone	B	Well tolerated and showed some evidence of efficacy in post-hoc analyses.	
	Acamprosate	C	Inconsistent evidence base but approved for use	Very limited evidence base for older adults
	Disulfiram	C	Antabuse reaction can be particularly harmful for older adults with preexisting medical problems.	No age-specific studies or studies that have included significant numbers of older adults
	Topiramate	D	Not FDA approved but several positive clinical trials	Can cause cognitive effects and not studied in older adults
	Other agents	D	Antidepressants and mood-stabilizing agents are all used clinically but with an inconsistent evidence base.	No age-specific studies or studies that have included significant numbers of older adults
Nicotine dependence	Brief interventions	A	Less than for alcohol but consistent evidence for benefit	Limited evidence specifically for older adults
	Nicotine replacement	B	Strong evidence base for use	Limited evidence specifically for older adults
	Varenicline	B	Several evidence-based studies	Very limited evidence for older adults; case reports of depression and behavior disturbance
Opioid dependence	Methadone, buprenorphine	B	Strong evidence for decrease in use and improved function	Limited evidence base for older adults, many of whom have been on methadone for many years

problematic and compulsive gambling behaviors earlier in life often continue this pattern of destructive behavior. Gambling in late life, both recreational and problematic, is associated with a higher prevalence of mental and physical health problems (SOE=B). Many older adults report that gambling is a means of coping with loneliness and boredom, ie, a source of socialization. Regardless, clinicians should be mindful of asking about problematic gambling when taking a history. Such symptoms include preoccupation with gambling, restlessness or irritability when trying to quit, loss of control, need to bet more money with increasing frequency, "chasing" losses, and continuation of gambling despite negative social or occupational consequences. No medications have been helpful in reducing pathologic gambling behaviors. States that allow legalized gaming activities are required to post toll-free telephone numbers to access assistance with problematic gambling. Many 12-step programs are focused on problematic gambling. Older adults who engage in gambling activities should be screened for alcohol, smoking, and other substance use disorders. Referrals to community resources and 12-step programs may be useful.

REFERENCES

- American Psychiatric Association. Practice Guideline for the treatment of patients with substance use disorders, 2nd ed. *Am J Psychiatry.* 2007;164(4 Suppl):1–86.

    This comprehensive practice guideline includes sections devoted to the evaluation and treatment of substance use disorders in older adults. Detailed information is included on psychotherapy, marital and family therapy, and interdisciplinary approaches to treatment (although not specific to the needs of older adults). Medication management is reviewed at length. The American Psychiatric Association website (www.psych.org) provides ongoing updates to the practice guideline.

- Fiore MC, Jaen CR, Baker TB, et al. *Treating Tobacco Use and Dependence: 2008 Update.* Clinical Practice Guideline. Rockville, MD: U.S. Department of Health and Human Services. Public Health Service. May 2008.

    This comprehensive guideline addresses strategies and recommendations designed to assist clinicians in the assessment and treatment of tobacco use and dependence. Screening tools, brief interventions, pharmacotherapies, and more intensive interventions are reviewed. A section is devoted to the older smoker, and evidence-based strategies are provided.

- Institute of Medicine. *The Mental Health and Substance Use Workforce for Older Adults: In Whose Hands?* Washington, DC: National Academies Press, 2012 (www.iom.edu/Reports/2012/The-Mental-Health-and-Substance-Use-Workforce-for-Older-Adults.aspx).

    This comprehensive review of the epidemiology of late-life mental health and substance use disorders also discusses the type of treatment settings where patients receive care, anticipated demand for care and associated providers, and strategies to overcome the mismatch between care needs and workforce.

- Oslin DW. Evidence-based treatment of geriatric substance abuse. *Psychiatr Clin North Am.* 2005;28(4):897–911.

    This paper is a review of the evidence-based treatment literature for late-life addiction. It includes guidelines for the treatment of abuse of alcohol, prescription drugs, and heroin in older adults. Recommendations for screening are reviewed.

- Wu LT, Blazer DG. Substance use disorder and psychiatric comorbidity in mid and later life: a review. *Int J Epidemiol.* 2014;43(2):304–317.

    This update of the epidemiology of substance abuse among older adults reports that the prevalence is similar to depressive and anxiety disorders, making substance use disorders among the most common psychiatric disorders of older adults.

David W. Oslin, MD
Donovan Maust, MD, MS

CHAPTER 45—INTELLECTUAL AND DEVELOPMENTAL DISABILITIES

KEY POINTS

- Individuals with intellectual disability surviving into adulthood and old age are increasing in numbers.

- Maladaptive and challenging behaviors, as well as difficulties learning and retaining new skills of coping and adaptation, are significant problems for adults with intellectual disability and, consequently, for their caregivers.

- Receptive and expressive communication impairments and coexisting cognitive limitations can contribute to diagnostic and treatment difficulties for medical, psychiatric, and behavioral problems.

- Physiologic changes related to age as well as to disease states in individuals with intellectual disability can exacerbate or attenuate behaviors.

- Therapeutic interventions for maladaptive behaviors or psychiatric illnesses that coexist with intellectual disability can include medications and behavioral therapies.

- Individuals with intellectual disability often outlive their family caregivers, and caregiver succession planning is an important part of long-term management.

- The term developmental disability can describe a variety of medical conditions that are not defined by intellectual disability. However, these conditions can contribute to challenging behaviors and impact an individual's quality of life.

Intellectual disability, as used in the *Diagnostic and Statistical Manual of Mental Disorders, Fifth Edition (DSM-5)*, is defined as deficits in intellectual abilities that impact adaptive functioning in three areas: 1) conceptual skills, such as reading, writing, math, reasoning, and knowledge; 2) social and interpersonal skills, such as empathy, communication, and maintaining friendships; and 3) self-management skills, including personal care, recreation, and job skills. Cognitive processes such as attention and memory remain intact. Intellectual disability does not have a specific age requirement; however, the symptoms must occur during the developmental period and result in an inability to meet standards for personal independence. Diagnosis of an intellectual disability is based on the severity of the intellectual impairment and its impact on adaptive function and support needed. While the *DSM-5* no longer considers specific IQ scores in the grading of symptom severity, an IQ of approximately 70 or below based on formal testing is suggestive of an intellectual disability.

According to the *DSM-5*, the etiologies of intellectual disability are vast and include prenatal, perinatal, and postnatal causes. Examples of prenatal causes consist of genetic syndromes; brain malformations; and prenatal exposures to alcohol, drugs, or other toxins. Perinatal causes typically involve some type of trauma during labor and delivery, with resulting encephalopathy. Postnatal causes include factors such as hypoxic injury, traumatic brain injury, severe infections, and intoxications or poisoning (such as lead poisoning).

A demographic issue to remember is that not everyone with a developmental disability has intellectual disability. This chapter focuses on individuals with intellectual disability who may or may not have other comorbid conditions, such as cerebral palsy, epilepsy, and autism spectrum disorders.

PREVALENCE

The number of individuals with intellectual disability surviving into old age is increasing because of generally better health care overall, including earlier detection and treatment of some conditions. It is difficult to quantify the prevalence of older adults with intellectual disability because of methodologic considerations and heterogeneity of conditions; however, it is estimated that intellectual disability has a worldwide prevalence of approximately 1%. Prevalence rates vary by age and by severity of intellectual disability. Individuals with severe intellectual disability are estimated at 6 per 1,000. It is even more problematic to consider the issues from the perspectives of other cultures and standards in areas other than Europe and North America. More recently, there are studies from Australia, New Zealand, China, Taiwan, and Israel; however, there is very little information about prevalence, morbidity, and mortality of people with intellectual disability living in developing countries.

Life expectancy for individuals with intellectual disability has increased over time. In the 1930s, the average age at death for individuals with an intellectual disability was 19 years. In 1932, for children 10 years old, only 28% were expected to survive to age 60. By the 1990s, life expectancy had increased to 66 years. Although the life expectancy of individuals with intellectual disabilities has been increasing, particularly over the past 20 years, it continues to remain lower than that of the general population. In addition, those who are ≥50 years old are at increased risk of chronic, multiple comorbid medical conditions and are less likely to engage in health promotion activities.

Multimorbidity is associated with advanced age and severe intellectual disability. In a 2014 study in the Netherlands, 80% of individuals with intellectual disability who were ≥50 years old experienced two or more chronic medical conditions, and 47% had four or more chronic medical conditions.

Published estimates of the number of people of all ages with intellectual disability have ranged from 1% to 2% in the United States, with 2% used in some more recent reports. Regardless of the number, it is proposed to double for individuals ≥60 years old by 2030. In general, longevity decreases with severity of intellectual impairment, certain comorbid conditions (eg, seizure disorders, Down syndrome), and the general health of the population and socioeconomic status of the country or culture.

Intellectual Disability and Mental Illness

The literature on older adults with intellectual disability and mental illness (other than dementia) has been relatively sparse over the last few decades. This makes it even more problematic to determine accurate numbers for several reasons: definitions have changed (ie, through various editions of the *DSM* and various versions of the *International Classification of Diseases*), health care has improved, studies have been conducted in different countries or regions, standard methodologies are lacking, and the relative numbers of institutionalized versus community-based individuals have changed.

Over the last decades, several studies with diverse methodologies and equally uneven goals have been conducted, but there have been some common general conclusions, notably that the prevalence of psychiatric disorders among adults with intellectual disability is much greater than that of age-matched controls (SOE=B). Adults with intellectual disability have similar risk factors (biologic, psychologic, and social) for mental illnesses as their peers without disability but may have additional risks depending on the cause of their mental disability. Older adults who were raised in institutional settings or who have not benefitted from modern medical care are also at greater risk.

There are many reports of greater than expected rates of certain mental illnesses or behavioral disorders associated with specific physical illnesses or genetic disorders. For example, older adults with autistic spectrum disorders exhibit higher rates of compulsive behaviors requiring psychiatric treatment.

There is general agreement that among all groups of older adults with intellectual disability, behavioral problems are more common, or at least more commonly diagnosed, than are major psychiatric disorders, such as major depressive disorders and psychotic disorders. Some terms, such as "challenging behaviors," are used to describe various behavioral symptoms of autism and fragile X syndrome, whereas other behaviors may have a relationship to brain abnormalities or to impaired acquisition of typically learned social behaviors. Additionally, some behaviors are learned and, in some situations perhaps, discovered maladaptive or problem behaviors become symptomatic. Learned problematic behaviors are likely to occur from residing in an institutional setting for years.

There is nothing protective against a psychiatric disorder by virtue of having intellectual disability. The cloud of uncertainty is increased perhaps by lack of objective signs and an individual's ability to report their inner feelings. Some of life's stressors that are common for older adults may have a greater impact on those with intellectual disability. Loss of family or friends, income, residence, or vocational status may strain coping strategies as well as overwhelm caregivers or support systems, resulting in an overt decline in level of functioning or a worsening of symptoms.

Major psychiatric disorders are estimated to occur in about 10% of older adults with intellectual disability. Among the most common disorders is dementia. The presence of psychotic disorders increases with age as well. Some disorders are seen at a higher rate than in the general population, such as certain anxiety disorders. Mood disorders also continue into old age, and the management is complex if the individual's ability to participate in certain psychotherapies is limited. Some intellectual disabilities, such as Down syndrome, may increase the likelihood of some disorders such as obsessive-compulsive disorder, which may be three times more prevalent than in the general population. Again, the difference is in the presentation of symptoms in individuals with intellectual disability, and not in the possibility of psychiatric illness.

DIAGNOSTIC AND TREATMENT ISSUES

Clinicians face many diagnostic and treatment challenges when seeing patients with intellectual disability with or without comorbid issues of behavioral symptoms or mental illness. The best treatment requires an accurate, or at least the most likely, diagnosis, and that requires obtaining the best history. Unfortunately, all too often the patient's history and his or her subjective reporting are limited or unavailable. The availability of a family member or caregiver who knows the individual well is extremely valuable when making a diagnosis and developing an effective treatment plan.

Barriers to communication can exist for both clinician and patient. Under these circumstances, the clinician should try to be as effective as possible by recognizing the limitations of the patient. For the purposes of this discussion, these limitations are grouped into three broad categories: self-awareness, communication abilities, and diagnostic overshadowing.

For adult and older adult patients with intellectual disability, the clinician needs to estimate the degree to which the patient is aware of his or her problem, condition, or feelings. Barriers to that process of evaluation can come from the organic cause of intellectual disability or from the interviewer by asking questions that are too complex or by using vocabulary beyond the grasp of the patient.

The patient's receptive and expressive abilities need to be considered. These two abilities can be comparable in some individuals with intellectual disability or quite different in others with autism or fragile X syndrome. Differences in these abilities can be characteristic features for some conditions. The goal is to adapt the questions to fit the communication abilities of the patient. Collateral sources of information, such as family or caregivers who can provide histories, narratives, and other data, are critically important in both diagnostic and treatment considerations.

An enduring and important concept is that of diagnostic overshadowing, or the idea that the patient's symptoms and behavior are attributed to their intellectual disability, leaving comorbid conditions (including both medical and potentially other psychiatric conditions) undiagnosed and untreated. Such overshadowing is a barrier to critical thinking of the clinician and, therefore, clinicians should guard against it when presented with a difficult situation.

PSYCHIATRIC AND MENTAL DISORDERS IN AGING ADULTS WITH INTELLECTUAL DISABILITY

The prevalence of psychiatric disorders among adults with intellectual disability is about 5 times that of age-matched control groups. Depending on the exact population studied and the type of diagnoses included, rates range from 10% to 40%. It is, of course, more complicated, because human aging and pathologic processes are neither simple nor linear. In older adults with intellectual disability, the occurrence and severity of psychiatric disturbances can vary by age and comorbid conditions. For example, in a study of individuals with Down syndrome who subsequently developed Alzheimer disease, these individuals were far more likely to suffer from psychologic and behavioral symptoms with more rapid decline in functional status than those who did not develop dementia.

Some symptoms may improve as the patient ages or develops comorbid problems. In adults with Down syndrome, it is not uncommon to have complaints of significant obsessive and compulsive symptoms. This can be the primary focus of concern from young adulthood through the fifth or sixth decade of life or until symptoms of dementia become evident. As the dementia worsens, the anxieties of obsessions and compulsions can wane, and as memory function worsens, those symptoms are often lost or of little concern.

It is also true that some behaviors or conditions can worsen with age through various processes. Individuals with intellectual disability experience the same disorders of aging as others but possibly with reduced coping mechanisms. For example, they may be more affected by chronic pain conditions or by vision or hearing loss.

In lower-functioning individuals or in those with expressive communication disorders, a new behavioral concern can be a sentinel sign of a physical disorder. As a general rule, before determining that a new problem behavior should be the focus of a psychotropic medication or intervention, physical causes should be excluded. In particular, new-onset, self-injurious behavior can be an important clue to occult illness. Self-injurious behavior to the ears can be a sign of otitis externa or media. Self-injurious behavior to the eyes can be a clue to vision loss or changes. Delaying attention for a treatable vision condition, eg, presbyopia, can cause permanent loss through self-injury, such as a detached retina or corneal scarring.

Dementias

Individuals with intellectual disability have a higher prevalence of dementias overall than age-matched controls in the general population; this is especially true for dementia associated with Down syndrome (SOE=A). The challenge is to diagnose the condition correctly given the individual's baseline cognitive impairment and diminished reporting skills. All causes of dementia are possible, but some are more likely than others. The dementia of alcoholism is considered relatively rare given the lower rates of alcohol dependence (and other substance use disorders) in this particular population. Similarly, so-called "pugilistic dementia" is higher than might be expected in this population because of repeated self-injuring blows to the head from coup/contrecoup effects.

It has long been recognized that there is an association and a significantly increased risk of dementia and Down syndrome. Research has added imaging technology to the proof of common histologic pathology between Alzheimer disease and Down syndrome. Adults with Down syndrome are at increased risk of the early onset of Alzheimer disease, with nearly 100% already having developed the characteristic histologic neuropathology of plaques and tangles by age 40. However, it is not typical for individuals with Down syndrome to develop overt dementia at that young an age. Prevalence estimates vary by study, but it is common for at least 50% of adults with Down syndrome who are ≥60 years old to have clinical evidence of dementia (SOE=B).

Most individuals with Down syndrome and dementia die during the sixth decade. In a 2002 survey of nearly 18,000 individuals with Down syndrome compiled by the CDC for the years 1983–1997, the median age of death increased from 25 years of age in 1983 to 49 years of age in 1997. Based on data from death certificates, standardized mortality odds ratios (SMOR) of people with Down syndrome were more likely to show congenital heart defects (SMOR=29.1), dementia (SMOR=21.2), hypothyroidism (SMOR=20.3), or leukemia (SMOR=1.6) than those of people without Down syndrome. Apart from leukemia and testicular cancer, the risk of other malignant diseases was low in those with Down syndrome. Advancing age, presence of dementia, severity of intellectual disability, immobility, and institutional living were found to be significant predictors of mortality among individuals with Down syndrome.

The diagnosis of dementia among individuals with intellectual disability is made according to the same criteria as in the general population. The evaluation includes establishing presence of cognitive and adaptive deterioration; demonstration of deficits on examination (preferably with longitudinal follow-up showing progression of deficits); and exclusion of other possible causes of deterioration, such as medical or environmental factors, or other mental disorders, such as depression or delirium.

Interest has been growing in attempting to demonstrate the efficacy of medications such as cholinesterase inhibitors (donepezil, rivastigmine, galantamine) and the glutamate antagonist memantine in individuals with intellectual disability. The body of evidence is increasing for modest palliative efficacy in this population. One randomized trial showed minimal benefit with the use of donepezil[OL] for patients with Down syndrome who developed progressive dementia (SOE=C). Another study failed to demonstrate any benefit from use of memantine in a placebo-controlled randomized trial of patients with dementia secondary to Down syndrome (SOE=A). It may be that Alzheimer disease in Down syndrome is diagnosed relatively later in disease progression than in non–Down syndrome patients with Alzheimer disease, and potential benefits may be attenuated.

Adaptive Behavioral Difficulties

Adaptive behaviors are learned social and practical skills concerned with daily functions. Limitations in these skills have a negative impact on people's lives; however, these skill abilities are not fixed in place or easily assigned to a particular level of mental retardation. In general, the greater the severity of intellectual disability, the lower the level of adaptive abilities. However, these abilities can be improved over time with behavioral supports.

Adaptive behavior skills can be conceptual, such as in language, reading, and writing; social such as rules, self-esteem, and sense of responsibility; and practical such as job skills, eating, dressing, using the phone, or taking medications. As in any group, aging adults with intellectual disability can lose or become less adept with some adaptive behavior skills, significantly impacting quality of life.

Behavioral Disorders

Maladaptive behaviors are observable phenomena that are counterproductive or disruptive for the individual. Various other terms are sometimes used to describe these acts, including target behaviors (behaviors targeted for extinction) or challenging behaviors. As many as 50%–60% of adults with intellectual disability have a maladaptive behavior (such as withdrawal, self-injury, stereotypy) that is severe or that occurs frequently, and follow-up studies show that these behaviors can persist for years. The proportion decreases with age for various reasons, except in Down syndrome, in which the proportion is higher and the incidence of behavioral problems increases with the severity of intellectual disability. Aggression is seen with similar frequency in all age groups and has an extremely variable presentation.

Diagnosis and Treatment

The diagnosis of a mental disorder in an older adult with an intellectual disability is based on the same principles of history and examination that apply in the general population. However, as discussed above, the patient's presentation or reported symptoms can be different, and the perceptions of the clinician and the criteria used pose additional challenges.

Typically, it is difficult for patients to report their emotional or physical state because of impaired verbal skills or a limited awareness of their internal state. Often, mental disorders present as behavioral changes; therefore, the reports of family or other caregivers are extremely important. Their interpretation of an individual's behaviors or symptoms, as well as any physical or behavioral responses to therapeutic interventions, can be critically important.

It is important to not over-diagnose and therefore over-treat an individual's presentation. Because insight, judgment, and adaptive or coping skills are limited, individuals may be more likely to "act out," which may be incorrectly perceived as a serious symptom of illness when, in fact, it may just be frustration. Medication may not be called for in a situation in which supportive therapy and time could lead to resolution. Medication can be used, however, to create a window of opportunity to make behavioral supports or strategies more effective.

Changes in daily routines, staff, residential or vocational settings, or family health should be reported and considered as precipitating factors for all behavioral changes. The concepts of applied behavioral analysis are important tools to use in determining cause and effect of problem behaviors.

Maladaptive behaviors, such as aggression, can be common in individuals with intellectual disability and can be either a learned response or an impulsive response to a stressor. An appropriate treatment or response, as mentioned earlier, might be instructional or behavioral. Preferred behavior programs reward desirable behavior using positive reinforcement techniques.

Despite appropriate attempts to control physical aggression through behavioral methods, pharmacologic intervention may be necessary for the safety of the patient or those nearby. Very few medications are approved for the most common and challenging behaviors, and prescribing medications off-label is common. Medication management for symptoms of major mental illnesses in older adults with intellectual disability is not much different from that in the general population, keeping in mind the diagnostic caveats already mentioned.

A discussion of the various treatment options for such a diverse patient group is beyond the scope of this chapter. However, medication management is common in certain situations. Autism spectrum disorders probably represent the largest diagnostic group among aging individuals for whom medication management is common and difficult. Self-injurious behaviors are certainly the most common reason medications are considered; these behaviors include several potentially life-threatening behaviors that can damage to the brain, eyes, and ears, as well as have the potential for systemic infections.

There are a few good guidelines. When two medication options exist, a risk-benefit analysis should be done to identify the best choice, ie, the option that poses the least potential for harm with the greatest potential for benefit. Changing only one medication at a time decreases the number of variables. New medications should be started at a low dosage, and results monitored ("start low and go slow"). If possible, dosages of all medications should be tapered and, ultimately, pharmacotherapy discontinued. The use of antipsychotic medications should be avoided if possible, unless the presenting disorder includes distressing psychotic symptoms.

Medical Disorders

Adults with intellectual disability have more medical problems than age-matched individuals (approximately five medical conditions per person; those with more severe intellectual disability have more problems). Approximately two-thirds of those in a community setting have chronic conditions or major physical disability. It is estimated that 50% of these medical conditions go undetected. Prompt detection and treatment is associated with better survival. Visual or hearing impairments are more common in individuals with intellectual disability; they increase with age and affect approximately 25%.

Life expectancy decreases with increasing severity of intellectual disability and with other morbidity, such as inability to ambulate, lack of feeding skills, and incontinence. Life expectancy for adults with intellectual disability is about 65 years, with the most common causes of death being cardiovascular and respiratory disorders, cancer, and dementia (particularly in Down syndrome).

Social Conditions

At least 80% of adults with intellectual disability live at home and are cared for by aging family members; 20% live in residential programs. It is estimated that about 40% of eligible individuals may not be served by the formal service system. This situation often leads to a crisis when the parent is no longer able to provide adequate care or is unable to manage a behavioral problem. It is estimated that about half of intellectually disabled adults with a behavior problem eventually need a different living arrangement.

Typically, more than half of families have not made plans for the future care of adult relatives with intellectual disability. Patients in day programs or workshops do not typically have pensions or Social Security benefits to allow retirement. Not surprisingly, the degree of intellectual disability, physical health, and functional skills of the aging individual correlate with the degree of parental stress and burden, although maternal and family characteristics such as education and income are more correlated with overall life satisfaction and maternal well-being. A 2011 study demonstrated that as parents of individuals with intellectual disability aged, they had worse physical and mental health outcomes than parents of adult children without disabilities. Additionally, aging parents who continued to care for their adult child with intellectual disability at home were noted to be more socially isolated and have worse psychological functioning than parents who lived separately from their adult child. Care, support, and anticipatory guidance should be provided to the patient, family, and caregivers.

Table 45.1—Developmental Disabilities and Health Problems

System/Condition	Change with Developmental Disabilities	Management Strategies
Intellectual disability	Two-thirds of patients with developmental disabilities suffer from intellectual disability, many in the mild to moderate range.	Evaluation and referral to specialized services to maximize intellectual potential
Growth retardation	Usually found in patients with moderate to severe disabilities; it may present as short stature, inability to gain weight, lack of sexual development, or failure to thrive.	Medical evaluation for treatable causes
Sensory impairment	Nearly 90% of patients have impairments in hearing, vision, and speech. Strabismus is common, as is dysarthric speech.	Regular evaluation of hearing, vision, and speech; correction of deficits
Dental/oral conditions	Poor dentition and oral health are very common.	Oral hygiene and tooth brushing; regular dental visits
Thyroid	Thyroid problems can be a cause or a result of developmental disability.	Regular testing and treatment as indicated
Spinal deformities	Kyphosis, scoliosis, and lordosis are common among patients with muscle weakness and spasticity.	Monitoring of body habitus; physical therapy
Seizure disorders	Half of patients may suffer from some type of seizure disorder.	Diagnosis; anticonvulsant medications
Degenerative joint disease	Chronic muscle spasticity and mobility limitations often lead to osteoarthritis and joint disease. Strength and functional status may be prematurely impaired.	Physical therapy, occupational therapy, pain management
Osteopenia and osteoporosis	Lack of weight bearing leads to these chronic conditions in patients who are unable to ambulate.	Promotion of mobility (physical therapy); adequate calcium and vitamin D supplementation, screening and treatment of osteoporosis
Chronic pain syndromes	Muscle abnormalities and associated spinal deformities often result in chronic pain syndromes. Sensory abnormalities can result in the inability to describe the type, location, and source of the pain.	Regular monitoring of function and behavior to detect possible painful conditions; pain management
Functional decline	Aging patients with cerebral palsy and other similar conditions often develop fatigue, pain, weakness, and overuse syndromes that result in premature loss of function. This is referred to as *postimpairment syndrome* and often requires a reduction in work hours, increase in assistance or use of adaptive devices, and sometimes nursing-home placement.	Physical therapy, occupational therapy, pain management
Cardiac and pulmonary conditions	Patients with cerebral palsy and other similar physical disabilities typically require 3–5 times the energy level of unimpaired adults, predisposing patients to premature conditions of aging, such as hypertension, heart failure, and coronary artery disease.	Monitoring for hypertension, shortness of breath, angina; risk factor management; engaging in regular physical activity and healthy diet
GI conditions	Gastroesophageal reflux disease and constipation common; constipation can be chronic and severe.	Monitoring; medications, fiber-rich diet, exercise
Incontinence	Many patients are incontinent of bowel and bladder from childhood, but others develop these problems with age.	Screening for treatable causes; identifying functional impairments that can limit toileting
Depression and mood disorders	Patients with cerebral palsy are 4 times more likely to develop depression than age-compared other adults. The stress associated with multiple disabilities is a risk factor, as is the premature decline in functional status associated with the disorder.	Regular screening; counseling and/or medications for those diagnosed with mood disorder

Individuals with intellectual disability are now more likely to outlive their family caregivers, and caregiver succession planning becomes important for the clinician to address with the patient and the family before a crisis. A variety of alternatives for guardianship of person or property can provide for more flexible decision making, and save some time and money. Options include supported decision making; advance health care directives; appointment of a surrogate decision maker, power of attorney, and representative payee if income is primarily from the government; and establishment of trusts. Additionally, some organizations that coordinate care for individuals with intellectual disabilities provide medical and ethical review boards that can give guidance regarding treatment risks and benefits in the absence of a family decision maker. Guardianship of person, property, or both should be considered only if there is no less restrictive alternative and there is a significant need to safeguard the welfare of the disabled individual. State laws vary; however, information about adult public guardianship frequently can be obtained from state departments of aging and social services. Because guardianship is a legal proceeding in which a petitioner (often a family member or friend) asks the court to find that a person is unable to manage his or her affairs because of a disability, it is often advised to consult with an attorney.

DEVELOPMENTAL DISABILITIES AND COMORBIDITY

Some developmental disabilities may not cause an intellectual disability but nonetheless can contribute to other morbidities and challenging behaviors, resulting in reduced quality of life. Among these disabilities are cerebral palsy, seizure disorders, and a host of genetic disorders too numerous to mention. Some genetic disorders have significant variability in their impact on cognitive functioning; others once thought to affect only a single generation or gender are now thought to have broader implications, such as fragile X syndrome.

Seizure disorders can negatively impact an individual both directly (if the seizures are uncontrollable) or indirectly (through the medications needed for seizure control). Pre- and postictal states can be times of distinct vulnerability for some individuals. Chronic pain conditions associated with some developmental disabilities, such as the contractures of cerebral palsy, can be a source of medical and psychiatric morbidity. Medical conditions that require frequent hospitalizations or surgeries can carry a great behavioral cost to the individual.

In general, as the degree of cognitive impairment increases, the risk of morbidity due to physical causes increases. For the approximate prevalence and severity of some common conditions found in individuals with developmental disabilities with and without intellectual disability, see Table 45.1.

REFERENCES

- Coppus AM. People with intellectual disability: what do we know about adulthood and life expectancy? *Dev Disabil Res Rev*. 2013;18(1):6–16.

    This review article highlights that although the life expectancy of individuals with intellectual disabilities has increased over the past 20 years, it continues to remain lower than that of the general population. An evidence-based overview of multimorbidity and life expectancy of the 11 most common conditions associated with intellectual disability is summarized.

- Hemming K, Hutton JL, Pharoah PO. Long-term survival for a cohort of adults with cerebral palsy. *Dev Med Child Neurol*. 2006;48(2):90–95.

    This paper describes the increasing longevity of a group of children born with cerebral palsy. More than 90% of children with cerebral palsy live to at least 18 years old, and up to two-thirds have lived well into their 50s and 60s. This has created a significant need for health maintenance, wellness promotion, and care for the increasing needs of this population. As adults with cerebral palsy live longer, disorders such as osteoporosis, coronary artery disease, hyperlipidemia, and complications of spinal deformities, sensory loss, and spasticity are becoming increasingly problematic.

- Hermans H, Evenhuis HM. Multimorbidity in older adults with intellectual disabilities. *Res Dev Disabil*. 2014;35(4):776–783.

    This study describes how individuals with intellectual disability who are ≥50 years old are at increased risk of chronic mulitmorbidity (80% of the sample) and are less likely to engage in health promotion activities. Multimorbidity is associated with advanced age and severe intellectual disability.

- Livingston G, Strydom A. Improving Alzheimer's disease outcomes in Down's syndrome. *Lancet*. 2012;379(9815):498–500.

    This review and commentary highlights the increasing prevalence of adults who now live longer and develop Alzheimer disease (AD). More than half of adults with Down syndrome who reach the age of 60 years will develop AD. The need for more clinical trials using available agents is highlighted, as is the lack of efficacy of available agents, including cholinesterase inhibitors and memantine in the treatment of AD in this population.

- Moran JA, Rafii MS, Keller SM, American Academy of Developmental Medicine and Dentistry, et al. The National Task Group on Intellectual Disabilities and Dementia Practices consensus recommendations for the evaluation and management of dementia in adults with intellectual disabilities. *Mayo Clin Proc*. 2013;88(8):831–840.

    This national consensus statement of intellectual disability experts offers a step approach to the assessment and management of dementia among individuals with intellectual disabilities. It provides evidence-based recommendations regarding nonpharmacologic and pharmacologic management of dementia in this population.

- Seltzer MM, Floyd F, Song J, et al. Midlife and aging parents of adults with intellectual and developmental disabilities: impacts of lifelong parenting. *Am J Intellect Dev Disabil*. 2011;116(6):479–499.

    This longitudinal study focuses on the long-term outcomes of aging parents of individuals with intellectual disabilities. As parents aged, they had worse physical and mental health outcomes than parents of children without disabilities. Additionally, aging parents who continued to care for their adult child with intellectual disability at home were noted to be more socially isolated and have worse psychological functioning than parents who lived separately from their adult child.

Elizabeth Galik, PhD, CRNP
Andrew Warren, MB, BS, DPhil

CHAPTER 46—DERMATOLOGY

KEY POINTS

- Photoaging increases the fragility of the skin and decreases the elasticity/tensile strength of the skin.

- Older adults are at risk of xerosis and neurodermatitis, or lichen simplex chronicus.

- Venous insufficiency can cause stasis dermatitis and chronic leg ulcers. Treatment should begin by controlling venous hypertension with compression therapy.

- Ultraviolet (UV) light exposure and age are associated with increased incidence of skin cancers, including squamous cell carcinomas, basal cell carcinomas, and melanomas.

AGING AND PHOTOAGING

The incidence and prevalence of skin disease increase with aging and sun exposure. Dermatologic care of older adults requires an awareness of cutaneous changes of aging and the effects of cumulative UV radiation exposure, as well as knowledge of the common tumors, inflammatory diseases, and infections seen in this population. The skin of older individuals is characterized by several changes, including increased fragility, graying of hairs, and increased wrinkles, particularly at rest. Each of the skin layers changes with aging. In normal young skin, the epidermis interdigitates with the dermis. With time, the epidermis becomes flattened with reduced keratinocyte turnover and melanocyte numbers, contributing in part to the decreased rate of wound healing. In the dermis, the fibroblasts are elongated and collapsed. Types I and III collagen and microfibrils of elastin all decrease, leading to the appearance of laxity and atrophy. Changes in hair include graying, which is caused by changes in follicular melanocytes, and a decrease in scalp hair density secondary to a shortened length of anagen (the growth phase of the hair cycle) and an increased proportion of hairs in telogen (the resting phase). In aging skin, the number of immune antigen-presenting cells, such as Langerhans cells, decrease, which may have consequences for cutaneous immune surveillance.

Aging of skin is a result of both intrinsic and extrinsic factors. The largest contributor is the cumulative exposure to UV light. This leads to the clinical appearance of lentigines, guttate hypomelanosis, poikiloderma (areas of hyperpigmentation, hypopigmentation, and telangiectasia), laxity, yellow hue, and leathery appearance. *Photoaging* refers to the effects of UV exposure on skin. UV light appears to activate signaling pathways that lead to increased matrix metalloproteinase activity and decreased collagen production. In a vicious cycle, the fibroblasts become elongated and collapsed and respond by decreasing collagen production. UV light also causes DNA injury in part via oxidative damage, which likely also contributes to the aging phenotype. Cutaneous malignancies are also more common in photodamaged skin because of photocarcinogenesis and UV light–mediated immunosuppression.

Prevention of photodamage involves using broad-spectrum sunscreens (ie, sunscreens that protect against both UVA and UVB radiation), as well as avoiding direct sunlight and wearing protective clothing, including hats and sunglasses. Although various topical agents claim to decrease photodamage, only topical tretinoin has been shown to increase the thickness of the superficial skin layers, reduce pigmentary changes and roughness, and increase collagen synthesis (SOE=A). Topical and even oral antioxidants (particularly vitamins E and C) have been shown to have some photoprotective and chemoprotective capabilities. In addition, over 70 botanicals, including soy and green tea, are currently found in many cosmaceuticals, but pharmacokinetic, safety, and double-blinded efficacy studies are lacking.

Surgical options for treating photodamage include chemical peeling agents, dermabrasion, and laser resurfacing. All rely on the destruction of surface populations of keratinocytes, followed by repopulation with keratinocytes deep from within the sun-protected follicular structures. Controlled trials to evaluate the effectiveness of these expensive modalities are few and have been inconclusive. Lasers targeting the dermis (for wrinkles) and fat (for cellulite), radiofrequency systems, ultrasound technology, and photodynamic therapy are being studied as additional mechanisms to enhance the appearance of sagging skin.

Soft-tissue augmentation and facial volume restoration via injectable fillers composed of hyaluronic acid, calcium hydroxylapatite microspheres, or poly-l-lactic acid, can also reverse the degradation of extracellular matrix, in part by reversing the collapse of fibroblasts. One of the most popular cosmetic procedures is injection of a neurotoxin, botulinum toxin, that relaxes dynamic muscles and thereby reduces furrows and wrinkle lines. Complications of these treatments need to be discussed with patients and include the following: 1) bruising, swelling, injection site reactions, rarely granulomas, and reactivation of herpes with lip injections from filler injections, and 2) headaches or blepharoptosis, or both, with neurotoxins.

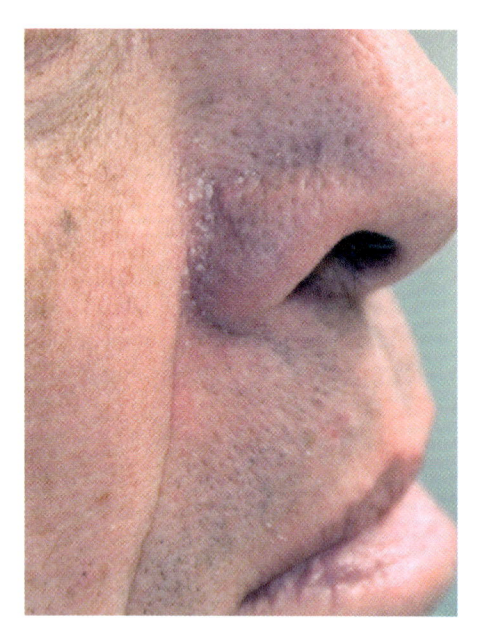

Figure 46.1—Seborrheic dermatitis. Erythema with greasy scaling noted along nasolabial folds.

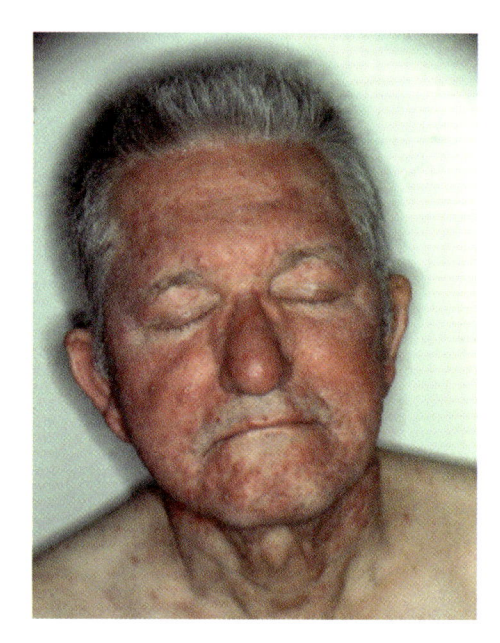

Figure 46.2—Rosacea. Diffuse erythema and erythematous papules and papulopustules are seen on the cheeks, forehead, and chin. The nose shows thickening of the skin and changes consistent with an early rhinophyma.

INFLAMMATORY AND AUTOIMMUNE SKIN CONDITIONS

Seborrheic Dermatitis

Seborrheic dermatitis (Figure 46.1) is a chronic inflammatory dermatosis characterized by symmetric pink patches with overlying greasy bran-like scaling distributed in the areas where sebaceous glands are found, namely on the scalp, the face, and sometimes the presternal chest and intertriginous areas. On the face, the lesions are found on the forehead, medial portions of the eyebrows, upper eyelids, nasolabial folds and lateral aspects of the nose, retroauricular areas, and occasionally the occiput and neck. At times, the lesions may be arcuate or petaloid, resembling flower petals. Occasionally, patients have features of both psoriasis and seborrheic dermatitis, particularly in the hairline and eyebrows, and this condition is therefore known as sebopsoriasis.

The pathogenesis of seborrheic dermatitis is unclear but may be related to the yeast colonies that normally colonize the skin, ie, *Malassezia furfur*. Seborrheic dermatitis is more prevalent in patients with Parkinson disease. Extensive and severe eruptions of seborrheic dermatitis often warrant an examination of HIV status. Rebound flares of seborrheic dermatitis can follow tapering of corticosteroid medications.

Although seborrheic dermatitis can be treated, it cannot be cured or eliminated. Treatment can be in the form of creams (face and body) or shampoos (scalp). Medications that target yeast, including selenium sulfide, ketoconazole, and various tar shampoos, are effective. In an acute flare, patients can be treated with mild topical corticosteroids such as hydrocortisone 1%; if treatment is unsuccessful, a trial of topical calcineurin inhibitors (eg cyclosporine, tacrolimus) can be tried. Aggressive topical or systemic therapy should be avoided because of risk of rebound.

Rosacea

Rosacea is a common condition in fair-skinned people. There are 4 subtypes with overlapping prevalence: erythematotelangiectatic rosacea has been reported in 96% of rosacea patients, papulopustular rosacea in 51%, phymatous rosacea in <5%, and ocular rosacea in 14%. In the erythematotelangiectatic subtype, there is persistent erythema of the central convex areas of the face (ie, nose, forehead, cheeks, and chin [Figure 46.2]), with telangiectasias and flushing. In the papulopustular subtype, there are follicular and nonfollicular papules and pustules in addition to the persistent erythema. In the phymatous subtype, there is sebaceous hyperplasia and thickening of the skin, in part due to recurrent flushing and edema; in some cases, this leads to rhinophyma ("bulbous" or "ruddy" nose). In ocular rosacea, irritation and burning of the eye can present as conjunctival injection, blepharitis, episcleritis, chalazion, or hordeolum. Other variants of rosacea include granulomatous rosacea, periorificial dermatitis, and pyoderma faciale.

Incidence of rosacea peaks in the third and fourth decades, but the disease is seen in young and older adults as well. The cause of acne rosacea is likely multifactorial, including contributions from vasodilatation, *Demodex* mites, and propionobacterium. In addition,

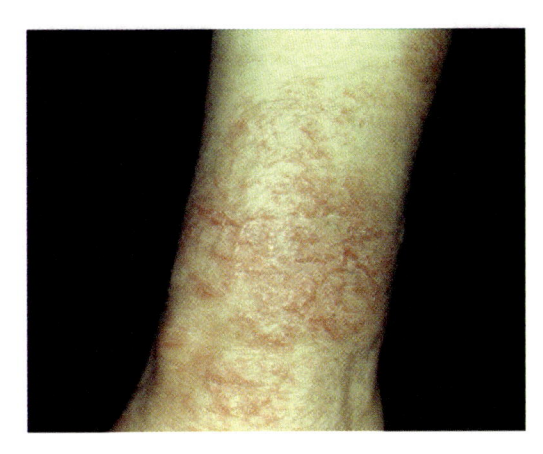

Figure 46.3—Eczema craquelé. Dry, erythematous, fissured, and cracked skin is seen on the lower legs of this patient.

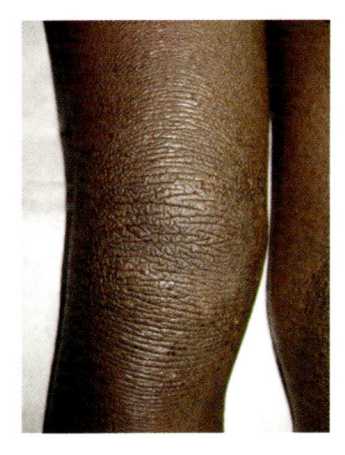

Figure 46.4—Lichen simplex chronicus. Chronic rubbing has caused the skin of this patient to become thickened and lichenified with an exaggeration of skin markings

thermal stimuli, sunlight exposure, and a number of medications can contribute to rosacea, including oral niacin and topical steroids. Often, seborrheic dermatitis and rosacea are seen together.

The treatment of rosacea depends on the subtype and severity. Topical antibiotics such as benzoyl peroxide, erythromycin[OL], and metronidazole can be used to treat papulopustular rosacea. Oral antibiotics such as tetracyclines (eg, doxycycline, minocycline) and macrolides are used to treat moderate to severe cases. Alternative therapies include topical azelaic acid, topical tretinoin, and oral isotretinoin[OL] for severe cases. For the persistent erythema, nasal decongestants such as oxymetazoline hydrochloride have shown some promise in small case series. For treatment of the telangiectasias, lasers, such as the potassium-titanyl-phosphate laser, intense pulsed light, and the pulsed dye laser, can be used. Rhinophyma can be treated with surgical reduction or electrosurgery.

Xerosis

Dryness of the skin, often a concern for older adults, is due to altered barrier function in the aging epidermis and a reduced ability to retain water. It is exacerbated by environmental factors such as decreased humidity; prolonged exposure to water, which can dilute out natural moisturizing factors; and use of harsh soaps, which can further damage the stratum corneum. During winter, when the heat is turned on, indoor humidity falls and dry skin conditions become more prevalent. Similarly, although summertime often is associated with an increase in ambient humidity outdoors, in many locations, indoor air conditioning can result in a drop in the humidity in home and office environments, causing dryness of the skin. Xerosis is often more pronounced on the legs. Depending on the severity of the dryness, xerosis can present as rough, itchy skin or as scales that give the skin a dry, cracked riverbed appearance known as *eczema craquelé* (Figure 46.3).

Treatment usually begins with avoiding the exacerbating factors mentioned above. Patients should be advised to take tepid showers and avoid using washcloths, sponges, or brushes to scrub the skin. Moisturizing agents, especially those containing lactic acid or α-hydroxy acids, can reduce roughness and scaliness. Moisturizing agents are often most helpful when applied immediately after a bath or shower. Home humidifiers may also be beneficial during seasons when home heating is being used. When irritation or inflammation is prominent, episodic use of mild topical corticosteroids for a short time provides relief.

Neurodermatitis

Neurodermatitis is a nonspecific term used to refer to chronic, pruritic conditions of unclear cause. Another commonly used term is *lichen simplex chronicus* (Figure 46.4). It is most common in adults >60 years old. The lesions show signs of chronic scratching, hyperpigmentation, and lichenification (increased skin markings), along with redness and scaling. Scratching these lesions is often satisfying and leads to a vicious cycle of skin changes and more pruritus. Treatment consists of potent topical corticosteroids (often under occlusion), emollients, and behavior modification. Other causes of pruritus such as irritant or allergic contact dermatitis, drug allergy, or xerosis must be excluded.

Intertrigo

Intertrigo (Figure 46.5) is any infectious or noninfectious inflammatory condition of 2 closely opposed skin surfaces (intertriginous area). It is more common in older adults because of the increased skin folds secondary to decreased dermal elasticity. Additional contributory factors include decreased mobility, moisture, friction, and poor hygiene. Factors that increase moisture (eg, obesity) or decrease immunity (eg, diabetes or systemic

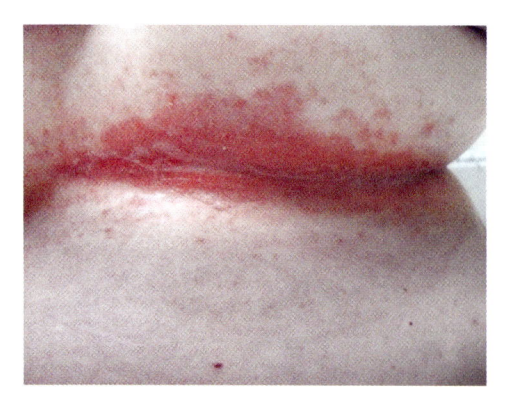

Figure 46.5—Intertrigo. Macerated skin under the breasts of an overweight woman.

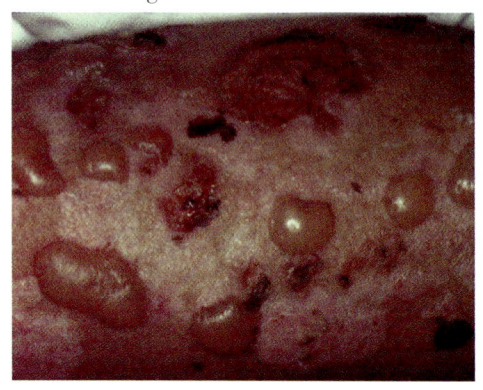

Figure 46.6—Bullous pemphigoid. Tense, fluid-filled, and hemorrhagic bullae on an erythematous base are seen on the trunk and extremities. Some of the bullae have ruptured and left a scab with crusting.

corticosteroids) predispose patients to develop intertrigo. Commonly involved areas, such as the inframammary area, abdominal folds, groin, and axillae, appear erythematous, macerated, moist, and mildly malodorous. Differential diagnosis includes seborrheic dermatitis and inverse psoriasis. Intertrigo often is associated with superficial infection with bacteria or *Candida*. Successful treatment involves decreasing moisture with topical drying agents, such as corn starch and antifungal powder (eg, miconazole or nystatin powder). Physical means of keeping the area dry include bed sheets/handkerchiefs to separate skin folds and frequent airing, or careful use of a hairdryer. If candidal intertrigo is suspected, treatment involves the topical polyene and azole antifungals, such as topical nystatin or ketoconazole. Occasionally, a very mild topical corticosteroid such as 1%–2% hydrocortisone is needed for a short period to reduce inflammation and irritation.

Bullous Pemphigoid

Bullous pemphigoid (Figure 46.6) is the most common autoimmune subepidermal blistering disease. It is a disease of older adults, with age of onset commonly >60 years. Clinically, the disease has diverse manifestations. Typically, bullous pemphigoid presents as an extremely pruritic eruption with widespread blister formation. The blisters are typically tense, often filled with clear fluid. The distribution is symmetrical and widespread, although the flexural areas and lower trunk may be favored. Mucous membranes are involved in up to one-third of patients. The blisters often resolve without scarring. Early or atypical lesions may be nonbullous with primarily urticarial lesions.

Bullous pemphigoid is a prototypical organ-specific autoimmune disease with a humoral and cellular immune response targeted against 2 antigens in the hemidesmosome. With the help of autoreactive T cells, pathogenic B cells produce antibodies that target these hemidesmosomal antigens. The antibodies trigger an inflammatory cascade of complement activation, the recruitment of neutrophils and eosinophils, and the elaboration of proteases. Bullous pemphigoid has been associated with medications, including diuretics, analgesics, antibiotics, and ACE inhibitors. Diagnosis is made by clinicopathologic correlation.

Although the disease may last for months to years, it is often self-limited. Treatment should be commensurate to the severity of disease. Limited, localized disease can be treated with potent topical corticosteroids, topical calcineurin inhibitors, and nicotinamide with tetracycline. Systemic corticosteroids are the mainstay of more extensive treatment. Steroid-sparing agents (eg, azathioprine[OL] and cyclophosphamide[OL]) are often used to avoid the adverse events of corticosteroids. Intravenous immunoglobulin and rituximab[OL], therapies that target the pathogenic antibodies and the pathogenic antibody-producing cells, have demonstrated efficacy but with some increased risk of adverse events (SOE=C).

Pruritus

Pruritus, a very common skin complaint, is associated with many cutaneous and systemic conditions. Severe pruritus can compromise quality of life. Pruritus can be idiopathic, related to a primary skin disease, or secondary to a systemic disease. In older adults, xerosis is the most common cause of chronic pruritus. However, evaluation must exclude other underlying pruritic dermatologic conditions, including infestations such as scabies; genetic or childhood diseases such as atopic dermatitis; and autoimmune blistering diseases, including bullous pemphigoid. Pruritus can be caused by medications (eg, dermal hypersensitivity reactions), related to chemical exposures (eg, irritant dermatitis or allergic contact dermatitis), or be a consequence of autosensitization to stasis dermatitis. Pruritus can be secondary to systemic diseases such as renal disease, cholestasis or chronic liver disease, thyroid disease, anemia, and occult malignancies. Finally, generalized pruritus can also be as-

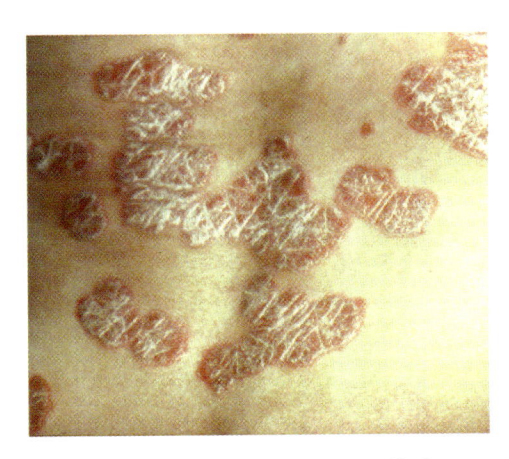

Figure 46.7—Psoriasis. Characteristic well-demarcated beefy red plaques with overlying silvery white scales are evident on the back of this patient.

sociated with generalized anxiety disorder, depression, and even psychosis, including delusions of parasitosis.

A thorough evaluation of pruritus in an older adult therefore includes a complete history and physical examination to exclude underlying and treatable skin disease. Distribution of the pruritus may help to determine the underlying cause. Involvement of flexural areas suggests atopic dermatitis or bullous pemphigoid, whereas primary involvement of the lower legs suggests an autosensitization to stasis dermatitis. Laboratory evaluation to exclude secondary causes includes a CBC and function tests of the liver, kidneys, and thyroid. It is also important to perform age-appropriate cancer screening, as warranted by the findings of above.

Treatment requires addressing the cause of the pruritus, if known, and relieving symptoms. If there is a primary dermatologic condition or a systemic disease, treatment should be tailored to the underlying disease. For example, prednisone may be warranted for bullous pemphigoid, and topical corticosteroids for atopic dermatitis. In addition, symptomatic relief often requires multiple modalities. Nonpharmacologic measures include open-wet dressings: in brief, a thin, white material such as a bed sheet can be moistened with lukewarm tap water and placed over the skin for 10–15 min; as the water evaporates, it can relieve pruritus. It is important to treat xerosis with frequent applications of emollients. Topical corticosteroids, such as 0.1% triamcinolone ointment, can also relieve xerosis and any underlying inflammation. Topical pramoxine, menthol in calamine preparations, and capsaicin[OL] cream can change the neurologic sensation of pruritus. These topical agents can also be used frequently with minimal adverse events in the short-term. Systemic therapy can include nonsedating oral antihistamines. Most trials investigating their use have used desloratadine in treatment of chronic idiopathic urticaria. It has significantly improved patient-reported pruritus, sleep disruption, and interference with daily activities with a low incidence of adverse events (SOE=A). Cetirizine, fexofenadine, and levocetirizine are also used for this purpose. In severe, refractory cases, including cases secondary to systemic disease, patients can be referred to a dermatologist for UVB phototherapy or oral thalidomide.

Psoriasis

Psoriasis (Figure 46.7) is a chronic inflammatory skin disease characterized by well-demarcated plaques with overlying silvery scale. Chronic plaque psoriasis is the most common variant, and it characteristically involves the scalp, the gluteal cleft, and extensor surfaces. Hands and feet can be involved, as well as the nails, which may portend psoriatic arthritis. The other psoriatic subtypes are as follows:

- Inverse pattern, in which lesions develop in skin folds, such as the neck, axillae, and genital area

- Guttate, in which small papules (approximately 1 cm or less) appear over the upper trunk and proximal extremities, usually after an infection

- Pustular, which is acute with generalized eruption of sterile pustules (2–3 mm) and fever

- Palmoplantar pustulosis, in which sterile pustules are confined to the palms and soles

- Erythrodermic psoriasis, in which the patient has generalized erythema

Psoriasis is common, affecting 2% of the population. The incidence is bimodal, first in the mid-20s and then at about 50–60 years of age. The cause is likely multifactorial. There is a strong genetic predisposition, with a multigene mode of inheritance, as well as a role for environmental factors. Triggers that initiate or exacerbate disease include physical trauma (known as Koebner phenomenon), infections (including streptococcal upper respiratory infections), stress, and medications (eg, oral corticosteroids, lithium, β-blockers, ACE inhibitors, NSAIDs). In psoriasis, the risk factors ultimately lead to activation and recruitment of autoreactive Th1 and Th17 T cells to the skin. Cytokines such as tumor necrosis factor-alpha (TNF-α) and IL-23 likely lead to activation of T cells, and IL-22 ultimately leads to increased keratinocyte proliferation.

Psoriatic arthritis, which is characterized by pain, swelling, and stiffness of affected joints, is also seen in 5%–35% of patients. Classically, psoriatic arthritis is an asymmetrical oligoarthritis of the small joints of the hands. Alternative patterns of presentation include inflammation restricted to the distal interphalangeal joints, symmetrical polyarthritis of the hands, and arthritis mutilans with telescoping of the involved digit.

Also, some patients suffer from back pain in the form of spondylitis or sacroiliitis.

Because of the wide clinical spectrum of disease, treatment should be tailored to the individual, with special attention paid to the risks and benefits for the older patient. Therapies directed at the skin are appropriate for patients with limited disease. These include topical treatments such as topical corticosteroids, vitamin D derivatives (eg, calcipotriene), topical retinoids (eg, tazarotene), salicylic acid, and tar compounds. Long-term use of topical steroids is limited by the risk of cutaneous atrophy. If topical therapy is unsuccessful or disease is extensive, phototherapy can be of benefit. UV light therapy, including narrow-band UVB therapy and psoralen with UVA light (PUVA), can be used alone or in conjunction with topical therapies. Patients receiving UV light therapy must be able to stand for the duration of the treatment. Risks include increased incidence of skin cancer.

For those with widespread and recalcitrant disease, systemic agents are available. Oral immunosuppressive agents, including cyclosporine and methotrexate, are effective but require careful monitoring for adverse events. Toxicities of cyclosporine include hypertension and renal dysfunction. Toxicities of methotrexate include bone marrow suppression, liver fibrosis, and interstitial lung pneumonitis. Oral retinoids such as acitretin can be used in conjunction with other therapies such as UV light.

Biologics can be effective in patients in whom traditional systemic therapies are either ineffective or contraindicated. Biologics include agents that block the cytokine TNF and T-cell surface molecules, including adhesion molecules and co-stimulatory molecules. The important adverse effects that have been most extensively related to TNF inhibitors include lymphoma, infections (especially tuberculosis reactivation and opportunistic fungal infections), congestive heart failure, demyelinating disease, a lupus-like syndrome, induction of auto-antibodies, and injection site reactions. In general, anti-TNF agents are contraindicated in those with a history of hepatitis C, multiple sclerosis, heart failure, and lymphoma. Antibodies targeting the common IL-12/IL-23 subunit (uztekinumab) have demonstrated remarkable efficacy and duration of response (up to 16 weeks from each treatment) in phase II and III studies. These antibodies are FDA approved, and many more new agents are under development.

Initiation of psoriasis involves both epithelial cells and immune cells; as a result of this interaction, psoriatic skin lesions and/or joint issues may develop, as well as an underlying systemic inflammatory disease with potential cardiovascular implications and risks. Therefore patients with psoriasis should be counseled about diet, exercise, and weight control.

Stasis Dermatitis

Stasis dermatitis can be an early sign of chronic venous insufficiency of the legs. Chronic venous hypertension, caused mostly by incompetency of the venous valves, is the initial trigger for stasis dermatitis. Venous hypertension slows down the flow of blood in the microvasculature, damages the permeability barrier of the small vessels, and allows for the passage of fluid and plasma proteins into the tissue, leading to edema and extravasation of erythrocytes. These processes lead to decreased oxygen diffusion and metabolic exchange and to activation and attraction of inflammatory cells and mediators to the site. Stasis dermatitis typically develops in the medial supramalleolar areas. It is often associated with intense pruritus. Initially, pitting edema to the ankle is noted, which is often worse later in the day. Over time, these events lead to progressive induration and adherence of the skin and subcutaneous tissues. Venous ulcers can develop spontaneously or secondary to trauma, arising most often in the supramalleolar areas.

The goal of therapy is to control the venous hypertension by regularly using compression bandages or stockings, elevating the legs at rest, and exercising the calf muscles to improve venous return. Topical treatment includes the judicious use of corticosteroids and emollients. Sensitization to ingredients in topical medications and emollients, including topical antibiotics, is common and frequently overlooked. Patch testing to exclude contact sensitization to these agents should be considered before use.

ULCERS

Venous and Arterial Ulcers

An ulcer is a wound with a loss of the epidermis. Ulcers of the lower leg are most often caused by vascular disease or neuropathy. Of leg ulcers caused by vascular disease, 72% are caused by venous disease, 22% have a mixed arterial and venous cause, and only 6% are caused by pure arterial disease. They have characteristic risk factors, morphologies, and distributions (Table 46.1).

Chronic leg ulcers are defined as open ulcers that fail to heal within a 6-week period. Treatment of the leg ulcers should be selected based on the cause of the ulceration. In addition to clinical criteria, ankle-brachial indices (ABI) can be used to determine the presence of underlying arterial disease; an ABI <0.8 is abnormal, and compression is contraindicated with an ABI <0.5.

For venous ulcers, venous hypertension can be reversed by either elastic compression, ie, compression stockings, or by inelastic compression, ie, Unna boot. Debridement of necrotic and fibrinous debris is important for reepithelialization and can be achieved by mechanical or chemical methods, eg, collagenase

Table 46.1—Characteristics of Venous, Arterial and Pressure Ulcers

Characteristic	Venous Disease	Arterial Disease	Pressure Ulcer
Signs and symptoms	Limb heaviness, aching leg edema that is associated with standing and is worse at end of day, brawny skin changes	Claudication (pain in leg with walking), ankle-brachial index <0.9, loss of hair, cool extremities	Partial- or full-skin thickness ulceration overlying points of pressure over bony prominences, commonly accompanied by pain
Risk factors	Advanced age, obesity, history of deep-vein thrombosis or phlebitis	Age >40 years old, cigarette smoking, diabetes mellitus, hyperlipidemia, hypertension, male gender, sedentary lifestyle	Bed-ridden or relatively immobilized patients; most often seen in older adults with poor nutrition
Location of ulcers	Along the course of the long saphenous vein, between the lower medial calf to just below the medial malleolus	Distal extremities, especially over bony prominences	Over bony prominences

treatment. Occlusive dressings can be used to help the wound heal; the type of dressing used depends on the ulcer type and amount of drainage. Surgical options include pinch grafts, split-thickness skin grafts, and allografts. Pentoxifylline^{OL} is a systemic agent with fibrinolytic and antithrombotic activities that has been reported to accelerate healing (SOE=C).

For arterial ulcers, the main goal is reestablishing the blood supply. Referral to vascular surgery is often warranted to consult for revascularization with arterioplasty or bypass surgery. To preclude worsening of disease and development of new ulcers, patients should be encouraged to reduce their risk factors for arterial disease, including smoking, hyperlipidemia, hypertension, and diabetes mellitus.

Pressure Ulcers

Tissue necrosis secondary to unrelieved pressure of soft tissue over a bony prominence for an extended period of time can result in a pressure (decubitus) ulcer. Areas most at risk when the patient is lying on their back include the heels, elbows, sacrum, coccyx, and scapular area. If the patient is chronically lying on his or her side, sites of potential pressure ulcers often include the lateral malleoli and greater trochanter. In addition to pressure, other elements involved in the cause of decubitus ulcers include shearing forces, friction, and increased moisture as due to perspiration or urine. Pressure ulcers can present as nonblanchable erythema of the intact skin to partial-thickness skin loss to full-thickness skin loss with necrosis that can extend to the muscle or bone. Treatment includes local wound care and alleviation of the persistent pressure by frequent position changes.

INFECTIONS AND INFESTATIONS

Herpes Zoster

Herpes zoster represents reactivation of the varicella zoster virus (VZV), the virus that is responsible for varicella, ie, chickenpox. Classically, it is a disease of older adults, with more than two-thirds of cases in patients >50 years old. The lifetime risk of reactivation of VZV is 20% in healthy adults and 50% in immunocompromised individuals. During primary infection, ie, varicella, VZV establishes a latent infection in sensory ganglia. Partly because of the decline in the cellular immune response associated with age or immunosuppressive conditions, the virus is reactivated and leads to painful ganglionitis. The infection spreads down the sensory nerve and is released around the sensory nerve endings in the skin, producing the characteristic lesions.

Usually, zoster begins with a prodrome of pain. In some people, the prodrome includes sensations of pruritus, tingling, tenderness, or hyperesthesia. The prodrome is followed by a painful eruption of grouped vesicles on an erythematous base, usually in a sensory distribution. In the localized form of zoster, the vesicles rarely cross midline (Figure 46.8). Rarely, prodromal pain is not followed by a cutaneous eruption, a condition called zoster sine herpete.

Herpes zoster infection has been associated with a number of complications, including post-herpetic neuralgia (PHN), scarring ophthalmic zoster, and Ramsay Hunt syndrome. The incidence and severity of PHN increase with increasing age and an immunocompromised state. In 7% of cases of herpes zoster, the ophthalmic branch of the trigeminal nerve is involved. Involvement of the nasociliary branch, which presents as vesicles in the pharynx and on the tip of the nose (known as Hutchinson sign), requires careful ophthalmic examination to monitor for complications, such as neurotrophic keratitis and ulceration, scleritis, uveitis, and ultimately blindness. In the Ramsay Hunt syndrome, the geniculate ganglion is involved. In addition to producing vesicles on the external ear or tympanic membrane, Ramsay Hunt is associated with facial palsy with or without tinnitus, vertigo, and deafness. Zoster is considered disseminated if it involves two noncontiguous dermatomes. In disseminated zoster,

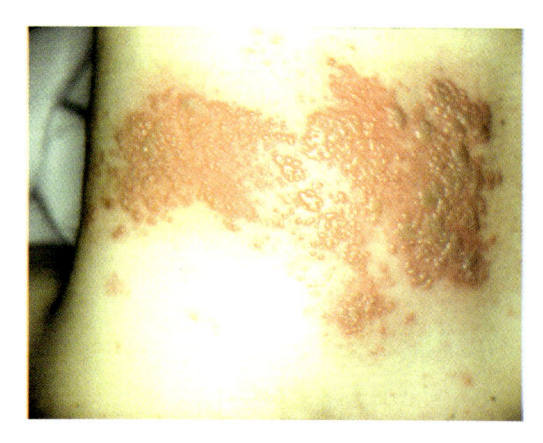

Figure 46.8—Herpes zoster. This patient has clusters of vesicles and pustules on an erythematous base involving a thoracic dermatome.

meningoencephalitis, hepatitis, and pneumonitis are also complications.

Although the symptoms of herpes zoster can be confused with a variety of conditions causing localized pain (ie, pleurisy, myocardial infarction, renal colic, cholecystitis, and acute glaucoma), the combination of the history and the characteristic physical examination (ie, the dermatomal distribution) facilitate the diagnosis. A Tzanck smear from the base of the vesicle can be performed to confirm the diagnosis. Detection of multinucleated giant cells suggests a herpes simplex or herpes zoster infection. Direct fluorescence antibody testing can be performed to confirm the presence of VZV. Polymerase chain reaction and viral cultures are the most sensitive means to confirm the diagnosis.

Early treatment with antiviral therapies, optimally within 72 hours of onset of rash, decreases disease duration and pain (SOE=A). FDA-approved therapies include acyclovir, famcyclovir, and valacyclovir; their use should be monitored in patients who have reduced renal function. A meta-analysis showed no benefit of adding oral corticosteroids to antiviral therapy for improving quality of life or reducing incidence of PHN. Intravenous antiviral therapy is reserved for immunocompromised individuals and for those who demonstrate signs of disseminated disease or complications. Most cases of acute herpes zoster are self-limited, but the probability of developing PHN increases with advanced age. PHN occurs in approximately 20% of zoster patients ≥70 years old and is difficult to treat. Acute herpetic neuralgia refers to pain preceding or accompanying the eruption of rash that persists up to 30 days from its onset. Subacute herpetic neuralgia refers to pain that persists beyond healing of the rash but that resolves within 4 months of onset. PHN refers to pain persisting beyond 4 months from the initial onset of the rash. Prevention of PHN can be attempted by vaccinating to decrease the incidence of acute zoster and PHN, by treating the acute zoster infection itself, or by treating acute zoster very early with preventive pain medications such as tricyclic antidepressants or anticonvulsants. Anticholinergic adverse events of tricyclics are common and may limit their use in older adults. In an animal study, early treatment with gabapentin reduced the incidence of delayed post-herpetic pain, but there are no clinical data in people for evaluating gabapentin in prevention of PHN.

Treatment of PHN can be challenging. Systematic reviews of randomized controlled trials of treatments of PHN with evaluation periods of >24-hour duration found no single best treatment. Tricyclic antidepressants[OL], opioids, topical capsaicin, gabapentin, topical lidocaine, pregabalin, and tramadol can alleviate the pain of PHN, but the long-term benefits of most therapies are not known and adverse events are common. Intrathecal methylprednisolone may relieve pain in patients refractory to the oral and topical measures discussed above.

Because of the high incidence and high morbidity associated with herpes zoster, prophylaxis by zoster vaccination is recommended for patients >60 years old. Even patients who have had zoster should be vaccinated to prevent future repeat episodes, according to the CDC. Vaccination is associated with a statistically significant decrease in zoster incidence and incidence of PHN (SOE=A). The vaccine is more effective in preventing zoster infection in patients 60–69 years old than in those ≥70 years old. However, it appears to prevent PHN to a greater extent in older research participants than in those 60–69 years old. In a large community-based study of participants ≥60 years old, herpes zoster vaccination was associated with a 55% reduced risk of herpes zoster in those who had received the vaccine compared with those who had not.

Candidiasis

Candidiasis has a wide spectrum of presentation. Cutaneous candidiasis is often seen in intertriginous areas; it can be superimposed on intertrigo caused by psoriasis or seborrheic dermatitis. *Candida* pustules can also develop on the backs of bedridden patients and on other areas prone to moisture and occlusion. In these areas, candidiasis is characterized by red patches, sometimes with erosions. Often, there are peripheral satellite pustules. Candidiasis can also affect the scrotum, the nails, the genital area, and corners of the lips, causing perleche. Oral thrush is an example of mucocutaneous candidiasis, seen most commonly in patients on corticosteroid inhalers, antibiotics, or immunosuppressive medications; or with concomitant systemic illnesses, such as diabetes mellitus. A potassium hydroxide preparation of skin scrapings of the involved site can confirm the diagnosis. The presence of spores and pseudohyphae is consistent with candidiasis.

Topical medications are generally effective and should be applied beyond the margins of the lesion. Most commonly used are topical polyenes such as nystatin, and topical azoles such as miconazole, clotrimazole, ketoconazole, and econazole. Other effective topical agents are terbinafine, butenafine, and ciclopirox. Topical therapies can be used twice a day until symptoms resolve and subsequently twice a week for prophylaxis as necessary. Pruritus, pain, and burning generally resolve with use of topical antifungal medications, although a low-dose topical corticosteroid can sometimes be used in conjunction. In patients with widespread candidiasis, oral therapy with an azole has a response rate of 80%–100%. Effective eradication of candidiasis generally also requires treating the underlying intertrigo by keeping the moist areas dry with drying agents and physical barriers to keep the skin folds separated (eg, bed sheets).

Scabies

Human scabies is a pruritic eruption caused by the mite *Sarcoptes scabiei* var *hominis*. The entire 30-day life cycle is confined to the human epidermis. After fertilization, adult female mites lay eggs, which mature over 10 days. For first-time infestations, sensitization can take 2–6 weeks; therefore, symptoms may not be seen until a month after infestation, making it difficult to make a diagnosis before disease spread. Scabies is spread primarily by person-to-person contact and is common in institutionalized older adults.

Scabies is characterized by intense pruritus, worse at night, and a symmetrically distributed cutaneous eruption. The eruption is most often characterized by small erythematous papules, sometimes accompanied by linear excoriations. The pathognomonic sign is a burrow characterized by a wavy, threadlike lesion about 1–10 mm long. The lesions are distributed over the interdigital webs, the flexural wrists, the umbilicus, the wrists, the ankles, and the feet. In men, lesions are also seen on the scrotum and penis. In women, the areolae, nipples, and genital areas are commonly affected. Immunocompromised patients can get crusted scabies, characterized by thousands of mites per gram of epidermis. Other manifestations include vesicles and indurated nodules. The lesions may be nonspecific, and the diagnosis should be considered in anyone with intense pruritus.

Diagnosis can be confirmed by microscopic examination of skin scrapings in mineral oil. This allows direct visualization of the adult mites, nymphs, eggs, or fecal matter (scybala). Occasionally, diagnosis can also be made by skin biopsy. Treatment includes topical creams such as 5% permethrin cream applied head to toe and left on for 8–14 hours, or systemic medications such as ivermectin (200 mcg/kg). Therapies are generally not effective against the eggs; therefore, a second treatment is needed 1–2 weeks later, after the eggs mature. Clothes, linens, and towels should be either washed in hot water and dried in high heat or left in a closed bag for 10 days to prevent reinfestation by fomites. In the absence of human contact, the mite cannot survive. Caregivers should also be treated because they are usually exposed, even though they may not have symptoms.

Louse Infestations

Lice can infest the body (pediculosis corporis), scalp (pediculosis capitis), or pubic hair (pediculosis pubis). With pediculosis corporis or capitis, lice are spread from person to person through physical contact or fomites. Pediculosis pubis is usually spread by sexual contact. In all cases, patients complain of pruritus of the involved areas, and there can be secondary infection. In pediculosis corporis, the lice feed on the body but live on clothing, where they lay eggs, often near the seams. In pediculosis capitis, the lice lay eggs on the proximal part of the hair shaft. The eggs (or nits) are visible as white specks cemented to the hair at an oblique angle. Patients with pediculosis pubis also have nits on the pubic hair and commonly have more organisms.

Treatment involves eradicating the lice and larvae, treating close contacts, and treating the secondary infection. Pyrethrin or its derivatives (permethrin) are ovicidal and can be used as a single 10-minute topical treatment. People who come into contact with the patient, including caregivers and those who share bedding, should be evaluated for lice and treated. Combs, brushes, hats, clothing, bedding, and towels must be washed with hot water.

BENIGN GROWTHS

Seborrheic Keratoses

Seborrheic keratoses (Figure 46.9) are benign growths that are extremely common in adults >40 years old. They are tan, gray, or black waxy or warty papules and plaques. They often have a stuck-on appearance with follicular prominence. They can be found anywhere on the body except on mucous membranes, palms, and soles. Occasionally, some lesions are darkly pigmented, and differentiation from a melanoma can be difficult without a biopsy. These growths can be removed for cosmetic purposes with cryosurgery or shave excision if necessary.

Cherry Angiomas

Cherry angiomas are the most common acquired cutaneous vascular proliferations. They usually appear

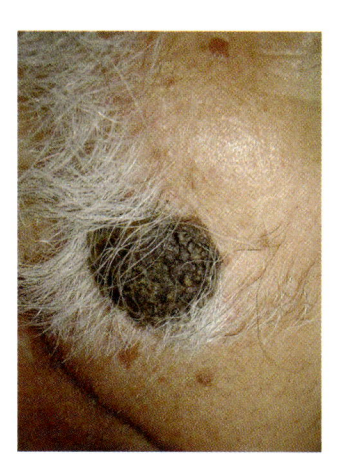

Figure 46.9—Seborrheic keratoses. These lesions present as waxy, warty, stuck-on papules in a variety of colors.

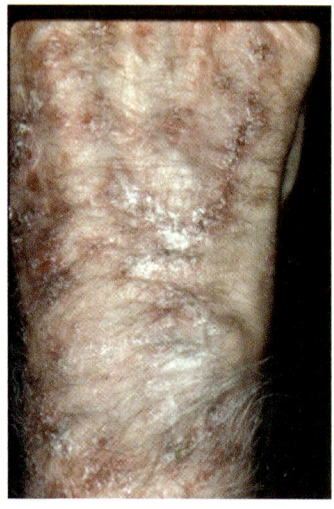

Figure 46.10—Actinic keratoses. These rough, scaly, red-brown macules on sun-exposed skin are premalignant.

in people in their 20s and increase in number over time. They are round to oval, bright red, dome-shaped or polypoid papules ranging in size from <1 mm to several millimeters. Cherry angiomas are benign, consisting of dilated, congested capillaries and postcapillary venules. However, they can bleed when traumatized. These lesions can be removed with excision, electrodessication, or laser ablation.

Actinic Keratoses

Actinic keratoses (Figure 46.10) are precancerous lesions caused by chronic UV radiation. They are seen in fair-skinned people and characterized by occasionally tender, rough, poorly circumscribed, erythematous papules with white or yellow scaling. They appear most often in areas with prolonged sun exposure, including the face, neck, ears, arms, and the dorsum of the hands. The scalp of alopecic men is commonly affected. Clinical variants include hypertrophic, pigmented, and lichenoid types. Some may have an overlying thick, hard, raised crust known as a *cutaneous horn*. Actinic keratosis or actinic damage of the lips is called *actinic cheilitis*.

Actinic keratoses are considered premalignant growths, precursors of squamous cell carcinoma. It is unclear how many progress to squamous cell carcinoma; reports vary from 0.24% to 20%. Actinic keratoses are treated to prevent progression to squamous cell carcinoma. They may respond to medical and surgical management. They can be easily treated in the office setting with cryotherapy (liquid nitrogen) or photodynamic therapy. Alternatively, they can respond to topical chemotherapeutic agents such as 5-fluorouracil, and immunomodulators such as imiquimod[OL]. When lesions are numerous, topical treatment with 5-fluorouracil or imiquimod is preferred over cryotherapy (SOE=B). These topical therapies are associated with a transient reaction characterized by bright erythema and discomfort.

SKIN CANCER

Basal Cell Carcinoma

Basal cell carcinoma (Figure 46.11) is the most common cancer in the United States. Although the tumors may be locally invasive, the risk of metastasis is low. There are many clinical subtypes, including nodular, superficial, and pigmented (which can be confused for melanoma). The three major clinical subtypes are the following:

- Nodular—the most common variant; appears as a waxy, translucent papule with overlying telangiectasias, often with central ulceration

- Morpheaform—has a scar-like appearance and can look atrophic

- Superficial—appears as an erythematous macule or papule with fine scale or superficial erosion often surrounded by telangiectasia

Risk factors for basal cell carcinoma include age, UV exposure, immunosuppression, genetic syndromes, and chemical exposures. Definitive treatment of basal cell carcinoma is surgical excision. Because of its higher cure rate, Mohs micrographic surgery is warranted for basal cell carcinomas that have indistinct borders, are >2 cm in diameter, are recurrent, or have high-risk histologic features (ie, morpheaform). An additional benefit of Mohs micrographic surgery is that it spares tissues and therefore can provide additional cosmetic benefits. Basal cell carcinomas that develop in poor surgical candidates can also be treated with ablative methods such as cryosurgery and radiation. Superficial basal cell carcinomas can be treated with less invasive techniques such as curettage with electrodessication and topical imiquimod therapy.

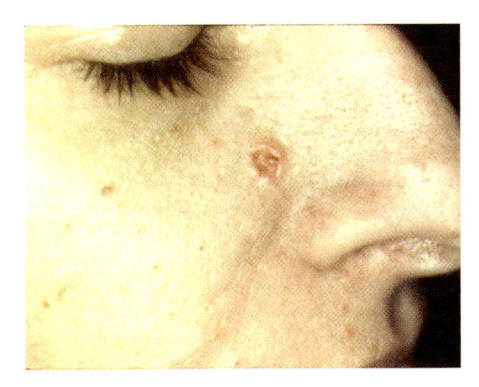

Figure 46.11—Basal cell carcinoma. This pearly, fleshy papule is ulcerated in the center and has a characteristic rolled border.

Squamous Cell Carcinoma

Squamous cell carcinoma is the second most common form of skin cancer. It generally presents as an occasionally tender, erythematous papule, plaque, or nodule with keratotic scale. The lesions can develop scaling and crusting. Squamous cell carcinomas are locally invasive and can cause subsequent tissue destruction. The risk of metastasis is low but higher than that of basal cell carcinomas; the risk increases with size of the tumor, high-risk histologic features (eg, poor differentiation, perineural invasion), depth of invasion, and location. Squamous cell carcinomas on the lip and ear can behave more aggressively. Squamous cell carcinomas also have a propensity to develop in longstanding, nonhealing wounds and in burn and radiation scars; these lesions are known as Marjolin ulcers and are associated with a higher risk of metastasis.

Like other nonmelanoma skin cancers, squamous cell carcinomas are associated with cumulative sun exposure and age. They tend to be found on sites chronically exposed to the sun, such as the face, the dorsum of hands, and arms. Additional risk factors include exposure to arsenic, ionizing radiation, and immunosuppression. Definitive treatment consists of surgical excision. In anatomically sensitive areas or with high-risk tumors, Mohs micrographic surgery is indicated. If surgery is contraindicated, palliative measures with lower cure rates (such as ionizing radiation) can be used.

Melanoma

Melanomas are malignant tumors of melanocytes. They have a higher risk of metastasis than basal cell carcinomas and squamous cell carcinomas. In addition to spreading locally, they are associated with distant metastases to the skin, brain, lung, liver, and small intestine. The tumors present usually as atypical pigmented lesions. There are 4 clinical types:

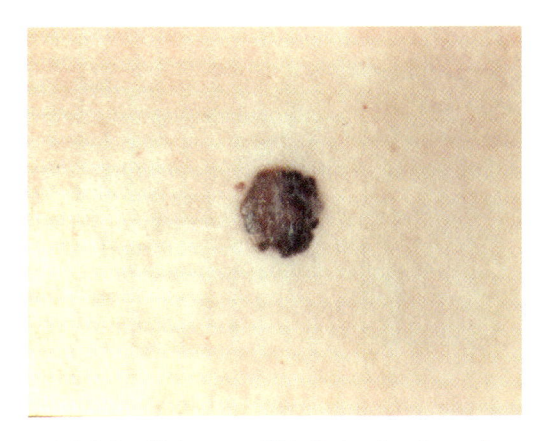

Figure 46.12—Melanoma. This lesion has irregular variegation in pigment (shades of brown and blue-black) as well as irregular borders, suggesting melanoma.

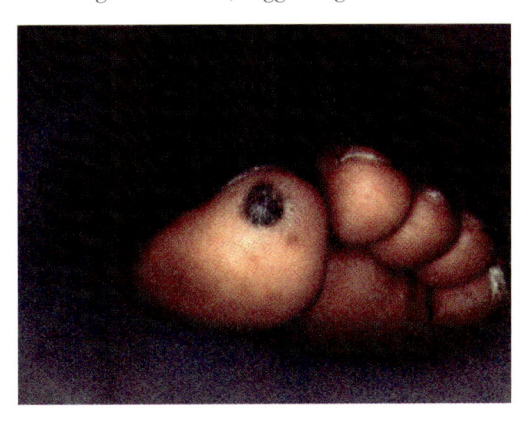

Figure 46.13—Acral lentiginous melanoma. This type of melanoma presents as a dark macular growth with irregular borders on volar surfaces of palms and soles (as in this case) and nails.

- Lentigo maligna—an irregularly shaped tan or brown macule that has been enlarging slowly; the type seen most commonly on atrophic, sun-damaged skin of older adults

- Superficial spreading—an irregularly shaped macule, papule, or plaque with great variation in color (Figure 46.12) and that can occur anywhere but most commonly on the trunk or proximal extremities

- Nodular—a papule or nodule, often brown, black or gray, that has been growing rapidly; can be red or amelanotic

- Acral lentiginous—a dark brown or black patch found on the palms, soles, or nail beds, with a pigmented streak of the cuticle known as Hutchison sign (Figure 46.13) found in all skin types; incidence is highest in adults ≥65 years old

The incidence of melanoma continues to increase. Mortality due to melanoma has also increased but at a lower rate, in part because of earlier detection.

Risk factors for melanoma include family history, fair skin type, red hair, history of dysplastic or numerous nevi, and sunlight exposure, particularly intermittent blistering sunburns in childhood.

Melanomas are usually asymptomatic. If detected early, they can be associated with a high rate of cure. Therefore, regular skin examinations and early recognition are important. A new pigmented skin lesion or a change in the color, size, surface, or borders of a preexisting mole should be biopsied. A useful mnemonic when examining skin for melanoma or atypical moles is ABCD: asymmetry, borders, color, diameter >6 mm.

Risk factors for metastases and mortality due to melanoma are depth of invasion, ulceration, and number of mitoses. Treatment is tailored to the perceived aggressiveness of the tumor. If caught early with a Breslow depth <1 mm, definitive treatment is surgical excision. If Breslow depth is ≥1 mm, standard treatment is wide excision, and sentinel node biopsy may be indicated. Adjuvant therapy such as interferon is sometimes used in cases with lymph node involvement. If there is evidence of distant metastases, treatment options include immunotherapy such as interleukin-2, pegylated interferon alpha-2b, and/or chemotherapy.

Until recently, 95% of patients with stage IV melanoma died within 5 years. In 2010–2011, two breakthroughs in treatment of metastatic melanoma engendered tremendous excitement. The first was FDA approval of ipilimumab, a monoclonal antibody that binds to cytotoxic T lymphocyte–associated antigen 4, which functions as a negative feedback mechanism within the immune system. Ipilimumab blocks this negative feedback and allows the T cells of the immune system to attack the melanoma cells. The second breakthrough was approval of vemurafenib, a drug that can inhibit mutated BRAF protein, which has been identified in >50% of melanomas. Melanoma cells with this mutation depend on activated signaling through the mitogen-activated kinase pathway. Vemurafenib is a potent inhibitor of melanoma cells with the BRAF V600E mutation and thus inhibits the kinase pathway, subsequently blocking proliferation of the melanoma cells. Recently, a new BRAF inhibitor (dabrafenib) in combination with a new MEK kinase inhibitor (trametinib) has shown enhanced clinical responses in patients with metastatic melanoma. Additionally, two drugs (pembrolizumab and nivolombab) that block the programmed cell death 1 (PD-1) receptor have been approved by the FDA for patients with advanced melanoma.

REFERENCES

- American Academy of Dermatology Work Group, Menter A, Korman NJ, Elmets CA, et al. Guidelines of care for the management of psoriasis and psoriatic arthritis: section 6. Guidelines of care for the treatment of psoriasis and psoriatic arthritis: case-based presentations and evidence-based conclusions. *J Am Acad Dermatol.* 2011;65(1):137–174.

    The authors presented evidence supporting the use of topical treatments, phototherapy, traditional systemic agents, and biological therapies for patients with psoriasis and psoriatic arthritis in 5 previous articles. In this sixth and final section, they present cases to illustrate how to practically use these guidelines in specific clinical scenarios. They describe the approach to treating patients with psoriasis across the entire spectrum of this disease from mild to moderate to severe.

- Beer KR. Combined treatment for skin rejuvenation and soft-tissue augmentation of the aging face. *J Drugs Dermatol.* 2011;10(2):125–132.

    Based on the author's experience and an extensive review of the literature, this paper discusses the use of combination therapies and techniques, as well as various products for skin rejuvenation of the aging face.

- Chang AL, Wong JW, Endo JO, et al. Geriatric dermatology part I and part II. *J Am Acad Dermatol.* 2013;68(4):521–542.

    The authors review age-related changes in the pharmacokinetics and pharmacodynamics of common medications used in dermatology. Renal function, liver toxicity, drug interactions due to polypharmacy, and ways to improve drug adherence are discussed. The cutaneous signs of mistreatment in older adults are also reviewed.

- Katalinic A, Waldmann A, Weinstock MA, et al. Does skin cancer screening save lives? An observational study comparing trends in melanoma mortality in regions with and without screening. *Cancer.* 2012;118(21):5395–5402.

    The authors performed skin cancer screening in a town in Germany for 1 year. They then compared trends in melanoma mortality in that town and in the adjacent regions where there was no access to skin cancer screening. In the town with screening, melanoma mortality declined by 47%–49%, whereas in the adjacent regions, the mortality rate was unchanged. These findings suggest that skin cancer screening can reduce melanoma mortality.

- Tseng HF, Smith N, Harpaz R, et al. Herpes zoster vaccine in older adults and the risk of subsequent herpes zoster disease. *JAMA.* 2011;305(2):160–166.

    In this Kaiser Permanente South California community-based study, 75,761 members ≥60 years old who received the herpes zoster vaccination were compared with 227,283 unvaccinated age-matched controls. Of 5,434 herpes zoster cases, there were 6.4 cases per 1,000 person-years among those patients who had been vaccinated versus 13.0 cases per 1,000 person-years among those who had not been vaccinated. The authors conclude vaccination was associated with a 55% reduction in the risk of developing herpes zoster.

- Yosipovitch G, Bernhard JD. Chronic pruritus. *N Engl J Med.* 2013;368(17):1625–1634.

    Chronic itching is commonly seen in older adults and reduces a patient's quality of life significantly. This review on chronic pruritus demonstrates the importance of careful evaluation for primary dermatologic (as xerosis, scabies, pemphigoid, etc) or systemic causes. Various topical and systemic therapies are also reviewed.

Jane M. Grant-Kels, MD

CHAPTER 47—DENTISTRY AND ORAL HEALTH

KEY POINTS

- Because teeth become less sensitive with age, it is not uncommon to observe profound yet asymptomatic untreated dental disease in older adults. This justifies the need for regular dental evaluations every 6–12 months and even more frequently if an individual's salivary flow is diminished as an adverse event of medication.

- Periodontitis caused by plaque formation within the gingival sulcus (that should be controlled with regular oral hygiene) can lead to loss of alveolar bone height, decreased support around the tooth, malposition, loosening, and eventual loss of the tooth. Prevention is possible with daily oral hygiene and regular examinations and cleanings. There is a growing body of evidence that bacteremia and circulating inflammatory factors due to periodontal infection are cofactors in multiple serious cardiovascular diseases.

- Dentures usually aid in speech and restore diminished facial contours, but improved ability to masticate is unpredictable and improved oral intake is a less likely outcome. Dental implants diminish patient's insecurity with their prosthetics but do not enhance eating ability or improve patients' dietary quality.

- Oral cancer screening can detect oral cancer early, potentially translating into improved outcomes and better survival rates.

- Antibiotic prophylactic coverage before invasive dental procedures to prevent infective bacterial endocarditis or infection of implanted prostheses (eg, prosthetic joints) is indicated only for specific high-risk situations. Patients at increased risk of these orally seeded infections should be counseled to maintain excellent oral hygiene to minimize incidence and severity of orally seeded bacteremia.

- Pulmonary pathogens responsible for institution-acquired pneumonia have been repeatedly documented as colonizing dental plaque on teeth and on pharyngeal mucosa. Daily oral hygiene in institutional health settings, such as hospitals (especially intensive care units) and nursing homes, is therefore an essential preventive measure that should be taught to direct care staff and its daily practice, whether by the patient or provided or assisted by staff, monitored as part of infection control.

- Osteonecrosis of the jaw has been reported in up to 5% of patients who have received extended intravenous treatment with bisphosphonates for management of bony metastases. This complication does not seem to affect those receiving bisphosphonates for osteoporosis to a greater extent than those not receiving bisphosphonates.

The oral cavity functions in initiating food intake, producing speech, and protecting the GI tract and upper airway. Dysfunction and disease in the mouth can therefore profoundly affect overall health and social functioning and can be particularly important for older adults who are frail or nutritionally at risk. Findings prevalent in older adults (eg, decay, missing teeth, periodontal disease, salivary hypofunction) do not represent normal aging, and individuals with such conditions should be urged, and assisted in their efforts, to obtain preventive and therapeutic care.

AGING OF THE TEETH

Most age-related changes in teeth are subtle (Table 47.1) but become significant in the presence of environmental factors or disease. For a combination of reasons, the teeth of older adults are typically less sensitive or wholly insensitive to temperature changes and, importantly, to the sensations that commonly herald dental disease in younger adults. It is not uncommon to observe profound yet asymptomatic untreated dental disease in older adults.

DENTAL DECAY

Dental *caries*, or decay, is a bacterially caused demineralization and cavitation that can attack teeth throughout life. *Recurrent caries* refers to decay at the interface between a dental restoration (such as a filling or crown) and the tooth. For the anatomy of the tooth, see Figure 47.1. Older adults have more restored teeth (and usually the restorations are older and more extensive) and thus are more likely to have recurrent caries. The teeth of older adults can have more caries of the root surfaces than are typically seen in younger adults because prior periodontal disease exposes the root surface, thereby predisposing it to demineralization and an increased risk of decay. Both recurrent and root caries are generally asymptomatic and can become advanced before discovery, often resulting in destruction of much or all of the tooth.

Untreated, advanced caries commonly results in necrosis of the remaining pulp, which usually leads to an acute or chronic dental abscess. These

Table 47.1—Clinical Significance of Selected Age-Related Changes in Oral Tissues

Tissue Affected	Nature of Change	Clinical Significance
Tooth dentin	Increased thickness	Diminished pulp space
	Diminished permeability resulting from sclerosis of dentinal tubules	Diminished sensitivity of dentin; diminished susceptibility to effects of bacterial metabolites; increased tooth brittleness
Dental pulp	Diminished volume	Diminished reparative capacity; diminished sensitivity and change in nature of sensitivity
	Shift in proportion of nervous, vascular, and connective tissues	Diminished reparative capacity; diminished sensitivity and change in nature of sensitivity
Salivary glands	Fatty replacement of acini	Possibly less physiologic reserve

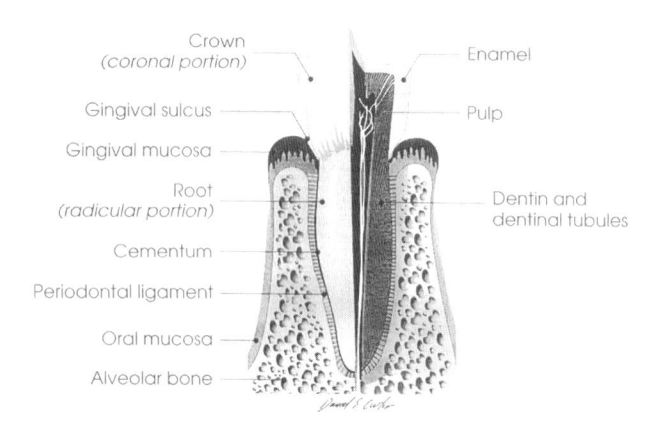

Figure 47.1—Dental and periodontal anatomy

infections may not present with pain, but they should not be ignored because severe metastatic infections of dental and oral origin have been reported in virtually every organ system. In particular, α-hemolytic (viridans) streptococci of the oral cavity have long been implicated in nearly one-third of the cases of bacterial endocarditis reported annually in the United States, and bacteria associated with dental abscesses (eg, *Staphylococcus aureus*) have been cultured from aspirates of infected hip arthroplasties.

The risk factors for dental caries are the same at any age, but many of the risk factors increase in prevalence with age. A primary risk factor is poor oral hygiene, which is common in older adults when visual acuity, manual dexterity, or arm flexibility is impaired, or when salivary flow is diminished. Another risk factor is frequent ingestion of sticky foods with a high content of sucrose, such as cake, candy, and cookies. Other risk factors include infrequent dental visits because of financial, access, or educational barriers; the presence of permanent or removable artificial teeth (more common with increasing age); and limited lifetime exposure to fluoride, widely used in the United States only in the past 50 years. White older Americans have a higher incidence of root caries than either black or Hispanic older Americans, but they are more likely to have received dental treatment for the lesions. Recurrent caries are also more common in white older Americans because of the greater likelihood that they have received prior dental treatment.

The prevention of caries involves daily oral hygiene with fluoride toothpaste, limitation of sugar intake, and regular dental examinations. The treatment of dental caries includes topical high-potency fluoride for remineralization, removal of demineralized tooth structure ("drilling"), and replacement of removed tooth structure with fillings or crowns. When caries involves the dental pulp, root canal treatment or tooth extraction becomes necessary.

DISEASES OF THE PERIODONTIUM

The investing tissues of the teeth, termed the *periodontium*, consist of the gingiva, the alveolar bone, and a collagenous sleeve (termed the *periodontal ligament*) located between the tooth root and the surrounding bone. Periodontal disease occurs when microorganic colonies (*plaque*) form on the teeth near the gingiva and between the gingiva and the root surface within the gingival sulcus. The most common form of periodontal disease is gingivitis, in which the inflammatory reaction to plaque is limited to the gingiva. Gingivitis develops more rapidly in older adults than in younger ones, but in both groups the changes—including gingival edema and light bleeding on brushing—rapidly resolve after plaque removal. If the inflammatory process extends to the periodontal ligament and alveolar bone, the process is termed *periodontitis*. In periodontitis, there is destruction of the hard and soft tissues of the periodontium due to immune-regulated osteolytic and proteolytic host defenses. In most adults, the process of periodontitis is marked by long periods of disease quiescence punctuated by bursts of localized destructive inflammation. The prevalence of active periodontitis is 20%–40% of dentate adults. By their 50s, more than 90% of Americans with teeth show ≥2 mm of lost alveolar bone height, the primary marker of prior periodontal disease activity. In advanced cases of periodontitis, the decreased support around a tooth leads to its malposition, loosening, and eventual loss.

Epidemiologic data and clinical observation support the concept that those who reach advanced age without significant periodontal bone loss will not likely experience a worsening of the disease in senescence. In contrast, other adults who have experienced a more rapid rate of bone loss commonly will have lost teeth in their 40s and 50s. In addition to age, risk factors for periodontitis include smoking and poor oral hygiene. Black and Hispanic Americans have a significantly higher prevalence of advanced periodontitis than white Americans. Preventing gingivitis and periodontitis is largely a matter of oral hygiene and regular dental examinations and cleanings. Managing periodontal disease involves debriding the roots below the gingiva, which may require surgical access. Adjunctive therapy with topical antibiotics such as chlorhexidine oral rinse (SOE=B) or systemic antibiotics such as minocycline (SOE=B) or metronidazole (SOE=C) can also be useful in periodontal therapy.

Periodontitis has long been reported to be worse in patients with poorly controlled diabetes mellitus. Investigations also support the contention that periodontitis, as a cause of chronic inflammation, impedes effective control of diabetes. Periodontal disease can be rapidly destructive in an individual whose immune system is impaired by disease or immunosuppressive therapy. Epidemiologic data also correlate osteoporosis and tooth loss due to periodontitis. Periodontal disease and the pathogens responsible for it have been linked epidemiologically and immunologically with coronary artery disease, peripheral vascular disease, cerebrovascular disease, and pneumonia. There is also epidemiologic association between gram-negative pneumonia, gram-negative periodontal pathogens, salivary hypofunction, and impaired swallowing (SOE=C). Numerous reports in the dental, infectious disease, and critical care literature demonstrate increasing prevalence of pulmonary pathogens from dental and oral plaque with increasing length of stay (SOE=B). Several studies have demonstrated significantly reduced incidence of institution-acquired pneumonia, reduced mortality, and reduced length of hospital stay in patients on ventilators (SOE=B) and those in nursing homes (SOE=C) when a program of daily oral hygiene is instituted.

The prevention and control of periodontal disease revolve around daily oral care, ie, tooth brushing and flossing to remove bacterial plaque on the teeth, particularly within the gingival sulcus. Properly used, electronic toothbrushes can facilitate oral hygiene for those with impaired manual dexterity and make plaque removal by caregivers easier and more effective as well. Regular dental evaluation, every 6–12 months, is important to ensure that the periodontium is healthy or to provide early intervention if it is not.

TOOTHLESSNESS

Advanced age was once considered synonymous with the need for false teeth, but that stereotype is fading. In the early 1960s, more than 70% of adult Americans ≥75 years old were edentulous. By the 1990s, fewer than 40% of this group were edentulous, most likely because of some level of preventive and restorative dental care in childhood or early adulthood.

Nevertheless, removal of one or more teeth in an older adult may be necessitated by various combinations of physiologic and behavioral factors. The leading cause is inability or unwillingness to access and pay for restorative dental treatment in the face of a symptomatic dental disease, usually stemming from dental caries. A second common cause is loosening of teeth as a consequence of periodontal disease, to the point that mastication becomes painful or ineffective. A third common cause is removal of otherwise healthy teeth that, because of the absence or loss of other teeth for the preceding or other reasons, would hinder the fabrication or function of a dental prosthesis to replace missing teeth.

Nearly 50% of Americans ≥85 years old have no natural teeth. There are unique problems associated with the edentulous state. Functionally, the teeth aid in mastication and enunciation. Aesthetically, the teeth support the lips and cheeks and keep the nose and chin a fixed distance apart. When a person has lost all teeth and there are no prosthetic replacements, the facial appearance is dramatically changed because of the lack of tissue support and the diminished vertical height of the lower half of the face. Chewing ability is severely compromised, yet the impact on nutritional intake is difficult to characterize. Several longitudinal studies have demonstrated correlation between loss of teeth and increased intake of carbohydrates and decreased intake of protein and selected micronutrients.

Removable dentures can aid in speech and restore diminished facial contours, but they are less predictably successful in restoring the ability to masticate. Edentulous people with dentures can generally eat a wider range of foods than edentulous people without dentures. Yet dentures restore, on average, only about 15% of the chewing ability of the natural dentition. The range of foods regularly eaten by denture wearers is significantly restricted compared with the dietary range of people with natural teeth. Denture wearers also have to chew more times before they swallow food, and they swallow their food in larger particles. Older adults and their clinicians who hope that dentures will restore oral intake in cases of malnutrition or unexplained weight loss are usually disappointed, whereas those who hope for a more socially acceptable appearance, clearer speech, and modest improvement in chewing comfort and range of dietary choices are more likely to be satisfied.

Dentures often are a considerable source of discomfort, dysfunction, and embarrassment for older adults. This is because the alveolar processes that originally held the natural teeth continually remodel and diminish in volume once the natural teeth are gone. For most individuals, dentures require frequent professional adjustment and periodic replacement. Alveolar ridge resorption is most severe in the oldest patients who have had the longest time without natural teeth; this effect is more pronounced in those with osteoporosis.

For health of the oral mucosa, dentures should be kept clean by being removed and cleaned after meals and soaked in a commercial disinfectant several times each week. Dentures should remain out of the mouth for several hours each day; most people choose to leave their dentures out during sleep. Fractured or broken dentures, as well as denture looseness or soreness, should be brought to a dentist's attention without delay. However, because neither dental services nor dentures are currently covered by Medicare and <10% of older Americans have private dental insurance, many older adults continue to use inadequate or even damaging dentures.

For the past 30 years, the dental profession has refined the placement and restoration of a variety of implanted devices that integrate with bone of the jaws and can more effectively anchor oral prostheses. Patients prefer dentures retained in this manner compared with mucosal-borne prostheses, but studies have not demonstrated enhanced chewing ability or significant improvements in dietary intake or quality. Rehabilitation with implants costs 3–20 times as much as traditional dentures and, therefore, is financially out of reach for many older adults.

SALIVARY FUNCTION IN AGING

Saliva is critical for protecting the tissues of the oral cavity and maintaining their function in speech, mastication, swallowing, and taste perception. Saliva buffers the intraoral pH, contains a wide spectrum of antimicrobial factors, remineralizes and lubricates the oral surfaces, and keeps the taste pores patent. In the absence of disease, the major salivary glands undergo regressive histologic changes with age. Yet data from the Baltimore Longitudinal Study on Aging and the Veterans Affairs Dental Longitudinal Study have demonstrated that with healthy aging, flow from the parotid glands under both resting and stimulated conditions remains essentially unchanged. In both studies, flow from the submandibular glands did not change with age. Data from other centers has shown a measurable but clinically minor decrease. It has been suggested that the major salivary glands demonstrate "organ reserve," in which the capacity of youthful glands exceeds ordinary demands, but that with age-related changes, functional reserves dwindle. By extreme old age, healthy glands function adequately under normal conditions but are more susceptible to factors that impede function, such as dehydration or drug-induced hypofunction.

Complaints of dry mouth are very common among older adults. The leading cause is an adverse event of medication. Commonly implicated are medications with anticholinergic effects, including antimuscarinic agents for urinary incontinence, tricyclic antidepressants, opioids, antihistamines, antihypertensives (including diuretics, ACE inhibitors, calcium channel blockers, and both α- and β-blockers), and antiarrhythmic agents. Separate studies have found that 72% of institutionalized older adults received at least one (and some as many as five) potentially xerostomic medications daily and that 55% of >4,000 rural community-dwelling older adults took at least one potentially xerostomic medication daily. Dry mouth can also be due to local disease, such as salivary gland tumors and blocked ducts, or to systemic disease. Sjögren syndrome affects approximately 3 million Americans, predominantly women, ≥50 years old. Cevimeline (30 mg q8h), a cholinergic agent, is approved for dry mouth in patients with Sjögren syndrome. Depression has been reported to diminish saliva flow, as have poorly controlled diabetes mellitus and hypothyroidism.

Dry mouth is also an adverse consequence of therapeutic irradiation of the head and neck. In the total dosage range administered for oral and oropharyngeal squamous cell carcinoma, salivary flow is commonly obliterated as a consequence of short-term direct effects on the glands and long-term fibrosis of their vascular supply. As a result, patients who have undergone radiation of the head can experience rapidly destructive dental caries and painful oral mucositis, which can affect nutritional status.

Treatment of older adults with dry mouth requires attention to both diagnosis and prevention. Diminished oral secretions increase the risk of serious oral disease. Medications that reduce salivary flow should be decreased, discontinued, or substituted for, if possible. Systemic causes, as well as a history of irradiation of the head and neck, should be excluded. Patients who have had irradiation should be considered for a 3-month course of oral pilocarpine (5–10 mg q8h), which may restore some salivary function. Saliva substitutes and oral lubricants, available without prescription and used as needed, can provide transient relief but replenish none of the protective properties of saliva. Patients should be counseled on the greatly increased risk of oral disease and educated on the need to limit dietary sugar, optimize daily oral hygiene practices, and have more frequent dental examinations.

COMMON ORAL LESIONS

Squamous cell carcinoma accounts for 96% of oral and oropharyngeal malignancies. Of the 28,000 new cases

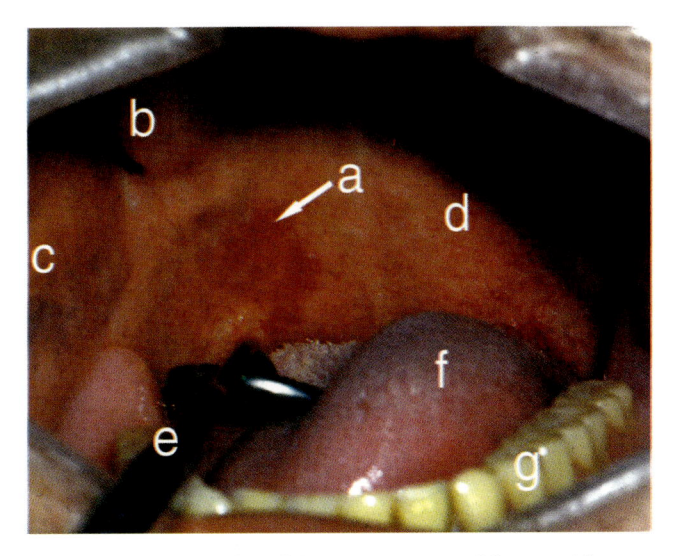

Figure 47.2—Erythroplakia in a 72-year-old man with a history of cigar smoking and alcohol abuse. Lesion confirmed by biopsy to be invasive squamous cell carcinoma, poorly differentiated.

Key: a = erythroplakia; b = right posterior maxillary alveolar ridge; c = inner aspect of right cheek; d = soft palate; e = tongue retractor; f = tongue dorsum; g = mandibular denture

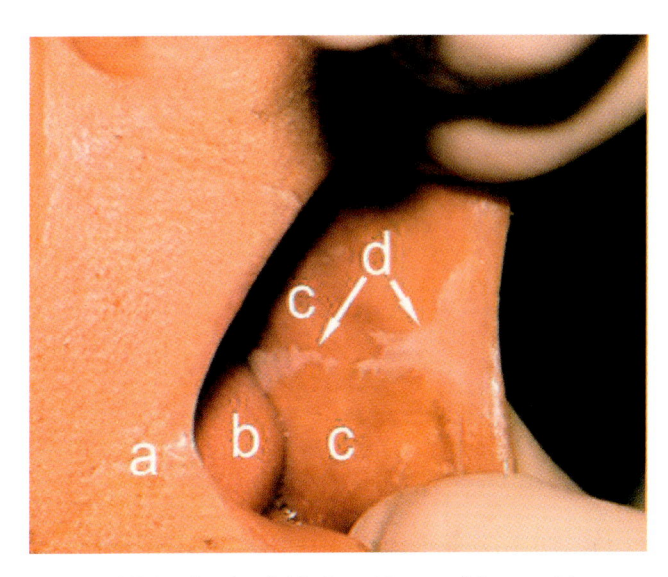

Figure 47.3—Leukoplakia in a 66-year-old man with a history of smoking. Lesion confirmed by biopsy to be carcinoma in situ.

Key: a = right lip commissure; b = tongue; c = inner aspect of left cheek; d = leukoplakia

of oral cancer reported in the United States annually, ≥95% occur in people ≥40 years old; age is the primary risk factor identified in epidemiologic analyses. The 5-year survival rate for white Americans is approximately 55% and for black Americans, 34%. Carcinoma of the lip, tongue, and floor of the mouth represents >65% of all oropharyngeal cases. Lip cancer affects men eight times more frequently than women; most other sites affect men at a ratio slightly below 2:1. Oral cancer is strongly linked with the use of tobacco, particularly cigarettes (SOE=A). Lip cancer is strongly correlated with pipe and cigar smoking (SOE=A). Alcohol is a potent cofactor that enhances the effects of tobacco. Other potential risk factors—dentures, poor oral care, oral viral disease (particularly human papilloma virus), oral lichen planus, and candidiasis—have been suggested, but none has shown the unambiguous associations of age, smoking, and alcohol use.

Oral malignancies appear clinically as painless red, white, or mixed red and white areas of the oral mucosa that may be ulcerated or indurated. Red and mixed lesions (termed *erythroplakia*) (Figure 47.2) display cellular atypia in as many as 93% of cases and should be biopsied immediately. White lesions (*leukoplakia*) (Figure 47.3) are malignant or premalignant <10% of the time and merit close monitoring; biopsy is indicated if a lesion does not resolve in 14 days or is increasing in size. Less invasive diagnostic tools can be used for determining whether a white or red lesion in the mouth merits biopsy, such as scraping (exfoliative cytology) and in situ staining. Early identification markedly improves outcome: 5-year survival without nodal involvement in white Americans is 80% and in black Americans is 69%, but survival rates decline with nodal involvement (41% and 30%, respectively) and with distant metastases (18% and 12%). A thorough oral cancer screening, which can be completed in <2 minutes, consists of a head and neck nodal assessment followed by inspection of the oral cavity using gauze to retract the tongue and tongue blades to enhance visualization of the cheeks, lips, and vestibules. Oral cancer screening is easy to learn, straightforward to perform, requires minimal instrumentation, and causes no discomfort to the patient; however, few older smokers receive oral evaluations as part of the routine physical examination.

The treatment of localized oral squamous cell carcinoma is generally surgical, although large but localized tumors can be managed with radioactive implants. More extensive disease necessitates surgery followed by beam irradiation. Concern over the deleterious adverse effects of irradiation (described in the preceding section) has led to the development of techniques that seek to limit destruction of healthy tissues surrounding a tumor. Radiation alone has been used to shrink inoperable tumors. Newer protocols combine surgery and chemotherapy with the goal of a cure.

Certainly not every oral lesion is malignant, but because most clinicians have not been trained to distinguish among different oral lesions or even normal oral anatomic structures, a brief overview is provided. Exostoses can form on either or both sides of the palatal suture at the crest of the roof of the mouth in about 20% of the population. Termed "torus" (plural "tori"), these also are commonly found on the medial aspects of the

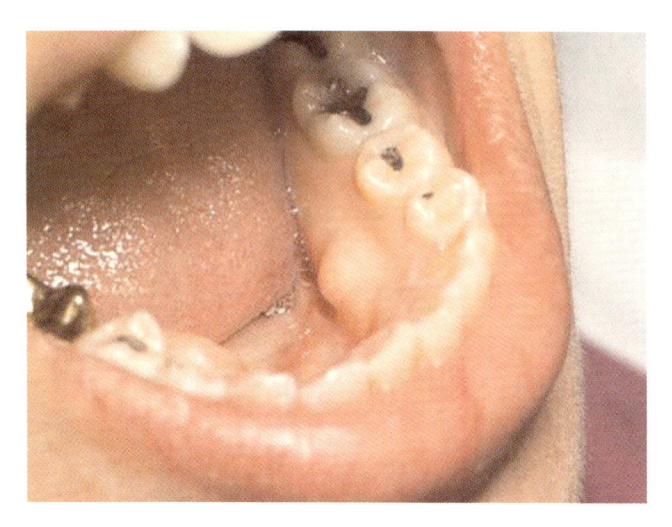

Figure 47.4—Mandibular torus

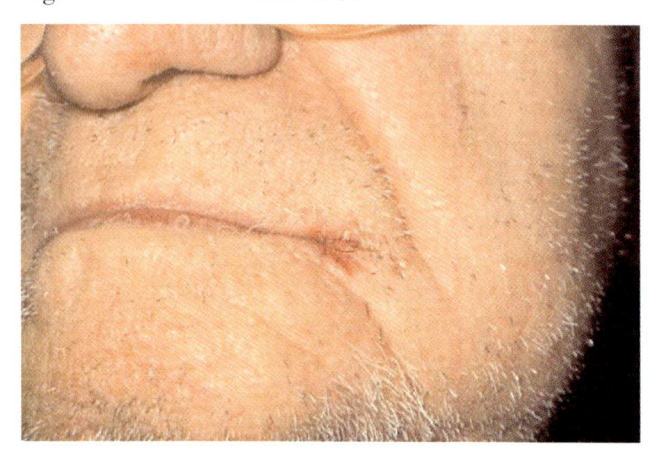

Figure 47.5—Angular cheilitis

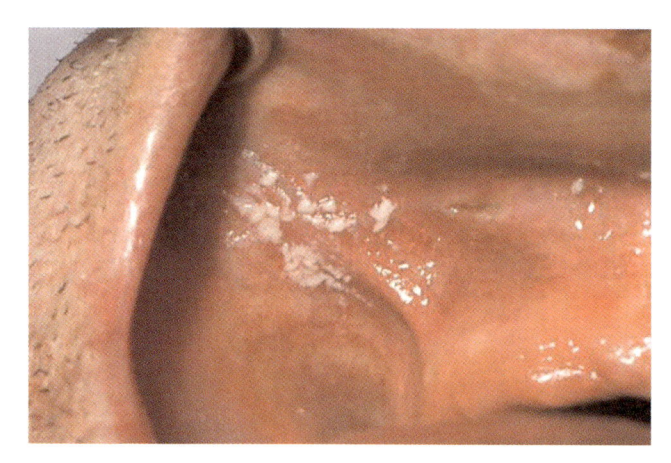

Figure 47.6—Thrush

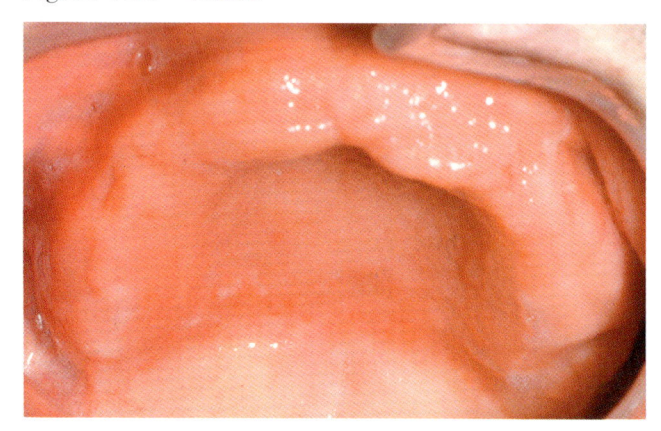

Figure 47.7—Denture stomatitis due to a maxillary complete (ie, replacing all the teeth of the upper jaw) denture

mandible as well (Figure 47.4). Tori can grow slowly throughout adulthood and sometimes reach dimensions that can predispose to trauma from food and impede swallowing.

The parotid ducts enter the mouth under small flaps of tissue termed Stenson's papillae, which are located lateral to the maxillary second molars. These can be distinguished from pathologic polypoid structures by applying gentle pressure to the preauricular area—saliva will be excreted only if the structure is Stenson's papilla.

The dorsum of the tongue in some individuals displays irregular patterns of hyperkeratotic and denuded reddened areas lacking lingual papillae. This presentation is variously termed geographic tongue (because the pattern looks map-like) and migratory glossitis (because the patterns change over time) and is no basis for concern.

Candidiasis presents as diffusely erythematous mucositis, cracking at the corners of the mouth (angular cheilitis [Figure 47.5]), curd-like white patches (thrush [Figure 47.6]), or erythema in denture-bearing areas (denture stomatitis [Figure 47.7]); it can be wholly asymptomatic or result in taste dysfunction, burning, itching, and pain. Older adults are particularly susceptible to candidiasis because of denture use, salivary hypofunction, the prevalence of diabetes mellitus, and the use of antibiotics for pulmonary and urologic diseases. Use of inhaled corticosteroids places oropharyngeal structures in the path of the spray, increasing their risk of localized candidal colonization. Management of candidiasis involves first excluding any immunopathologic cause for the disease, followed by administering topical or systemic antifungal agents and optimizing oral and denture hygiene.

Herpes simplex is a virus that resides preferentially in the trigeminal ganglion and periodically causes intraoral outbreaks. These outbreaks are limited to the hyperkeratotic areas of the palate (Figure 47.8), the gingiva, and the extraoral aspects of the lips. They begin as clusters of small, circular, red-rimmed yellowish blisters that burst and coalesce into irregular denuded lesions. They are highly contagious until healed. Herpes can be readily distinguished from another episodic, painful oral outbreak, aphthous ulcer (Figure 47.9), in

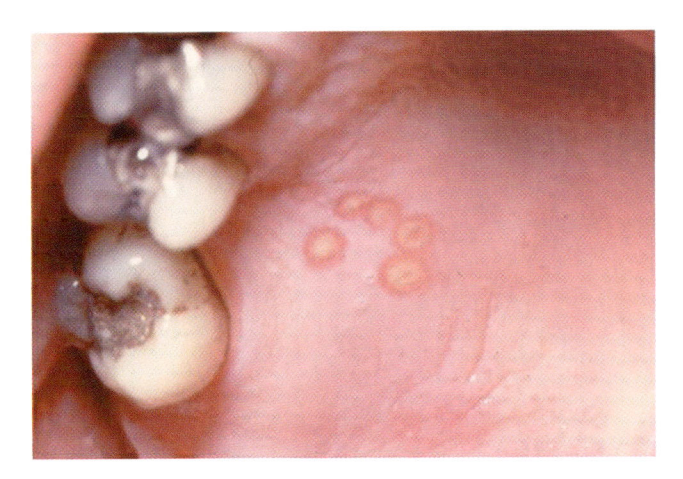

Figure 47.8—Early lesions of herpes simplex, right palate

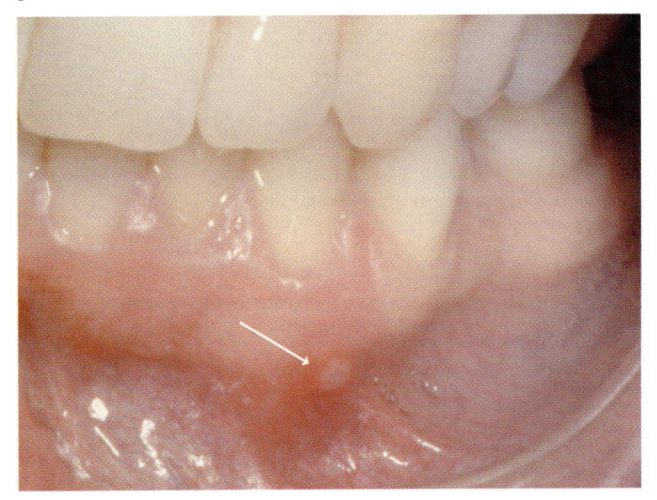

Figure 47.9—Aphthous ulcer

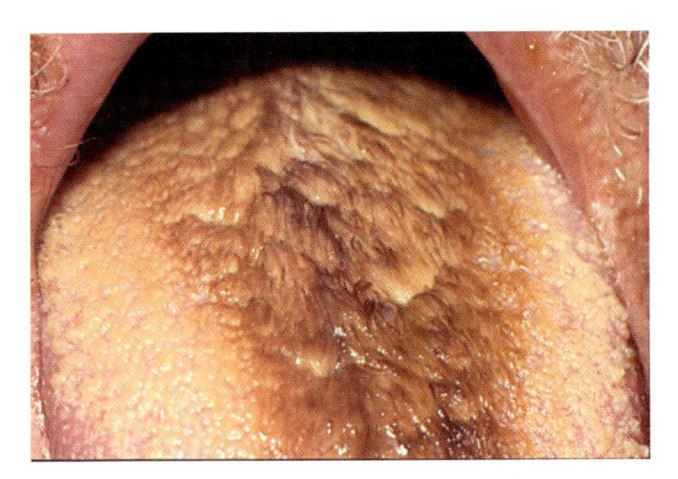

Figure 47.10—Black hairy tongue

that the latter tend to appear as isolated lesions and form only on the parakeratinized tissues of the mouth (ie, inner aspects of the cheeks and lips, floor of the mouth, and lateral border of the tongue). Aphthous ulcerations are not known to be contagious.

An idiopathic disruption of the desquamation of tongue filiform papillae (normally about 1 mm long), which seems to become more prevalent with advancing age, results in elongation of the papillae (to ≥3 mm) and the appearance of a "hairy tongue." This condition is prone to staining from a variety of foods (eg, tea, coffee), from tobacco use, and from medications (eg, bismuth). "Hairy tongue" can also serve as a substrate for bacterial and/or fungal growth. Any of these, all of which are exacerbated by salivary hypofunction, can confer on the tongue notable colorations (eg, "black hairy tongue" [Figure 47.10]), but none is associated with symptoms.

Burning mouth syndrome is a chronic orofacial pain disorder usually without other clinical signs. It typically affects women ≥50 years old, particularly in Asian Americans and Native Americans. The pain most commonly affects the lips, tongue, and palate. Multiple causes have been suggested, including xerostomia, denture use, candidiasis, nutritional deficiencies, and psychiatric disorders. Treatment is symptomatic and empirical.

CHEMOSENSORY PERCEPTION

Olfactory function declines with age. A decreased ability to identify odors and to rank their intensities affects both older men (to the greater extent) and women. Several medications have been implicated in olfactory dysfunction, as has Alzheimer disease, among other disorders common among older adults. Impaired olfaction in older adults has been anecdotally implicated as a risk factor for eating spoiled food or failing to notice gas leaks or domestic fires.

Taste perception changes with aging. The subjective perception of saltiness and sweetness blunts with advancing age. This change potentially has clinical significance, possibly playing a role in the tendency to oversalt foods or crave sweets.

Complaints of taste and smell dysfunction are common among older adults. Often the complaint derives from medication use, but other causes are possible (Table 47.2 and Table 47.3). Some medications may have no primary effect on taste but reduce saliva flow and lead to impaired taste perception. The sense of "taste" can actually be more accurately termed "flavor," ie, the full range of sensations that accompany eating, including temperature, texture, sound, and smell in addition to the perception of sweet, salt, sour, and bitter. Older adults are prone to impaired flavor perception because of changes in olfaction and oral stereognosis, salivary hypofunction, and the presence of dentures, which present physical and thermal barriers. Flavor enhancement strategies have had positive effects on both food preference and caloric intake among frail older adults.

Table 47.2—Medications That Interfere With Gustation (Taste) and Olfaction (Smell)

Gustation[a]		
Allopurinol	Diclofenac	Ofloxacin
Amiloride	Dicyclomine	Nifedipine
Amitriptyline	Diltiazem	Pentamidine
Ampicillin	Doxepin	Phenytoin
Baclofen	Enalapril	Propranolol
Buspirone	Fenoprofen	Ritonavir
Captopril	Hydrochlorothiazide	Saquinavir
Chlorpheniramine	Imipramine	Sulfamethoxazole
Desipramine	Nabumetone	Tetracyclines
Dexamethasone	Nelfinavir	Zidovudine

Olfaction[b]		
Amitriptyline	Dexamethasone	Morphine
Amphetamine	Enalapril	Pentamidine
Beclomethasone dipropionate	Flunisolide	Pirbuterol
	Flurbiprofen	
Codeine	Hydromorphone	

[a] Gustation: source lists >250 agents reported to disturb the sense of taste; agents listed are limited to those for which taste disturbance was determined objectively through threshold or intensity scaling or both, using one or more standardized solutions.

[b] Olfaction: source lists >40 agents reported to disturb the sense of smell; agents listed are limited to those for which olfactory disturbance was determined objectively through experiment or clinical trial.

SOURCE: Data from Schiffman SS, Zervakis J. Taste and smell perception in the elderly: effect of medications and disease. *Adv Food Nutr Res.* 2002;44:247–346.

COMMON MEDICAL CONSIDERATIONS IN DENTAL TREATMENT OF OLDER ADULTS

The mouth contains about 10^{11}–10^{13} microorganisms, and the rich vascular supply beneath the relatively delicate mucosal covering predisposes to episodes of orally seeded bacteremia. Approximately one-third of the reported cases of infective endocarditis are caused by organisms normally found only in the mouth. Case reports of prosthetic implants infected by organisms originating in infected oral tissues have for years compelled physicians and dentists to administer antibiotics prophylactically before invasive dental care for patients with such history. However, the recommendations from the American Heart Association in 2007 reflect that tooth brushing and eating in the presence of gingival inflammation are recognized to present, over time, as much as or a greater source of bacteremia than dental care, and that there is growing concern that widespread, short-term antibiotic treatment promotes the emergence of drug-resistant strains of microorganisms. Prophylactic coverage is now recommended only in specific high-risk situations. Although those recommendations are directed at preventing infective endocarditis, bacteremia-induced

Table 47.3—Nonpharmacologic Causes of Taste and Smell Dysfunction in Older Adults

Gustatory dysfunction
Oral causes:
  Burning mouth syndrome (chronic orofacial pain disorder without clinical signs)
  Candidiasis
  Laceration
  Malignancy
  Salivary hypofunction
  Therapeutic irradiation of head
  Thermal or chemical burn
Other causes:
  Alzheimer disease, other neurodegenerative disorders
  CNS tumor
  Endocrinopathies (eg, diabetes mellitus, Cushing syndrome, adrenocortical insufficiency, hypothyroidism)
  Head trauma
  Nutritional deficiencies (vitamin B_{12}, zinc)
  Psychiatric disorders
  Stroke

Olfactory dysfunction
Upper aerodigestive and respiratory causes:
  Dental infection
  Periodontal disease
  Poor oral hygiene, including poor denture hygiene
  Sinusitis
  Tobacco smoking or use of nasal snuff
  Tumor of airway or sinus
  Upper respiratory infection (bacterial or viral)
Other causes:
  Alzheimer disease, other neurodegenerative disorders
  CNS tumor
  Exposure to volatile or particulate toxins
  Head trauma
  Nutritional deficiencies (niacin, zinc)
  Psychiatric disorders
  Stroke

infections of prosthetic implants (such as joint arthroplasties, stents, vascular patches, and shunts) are less common than endocarditis, and the link between their occurrence and dental disease far more tenuous. As such, the case for antibiotic coverage in such situations is also less robust and should be the exception rather than the rule.

Correlation between length of stay in nursing homes, hospitals, and intensive care units, and colonization of dental and oral mucosal plaque with known pulmonary pathogens (SOE=B), is compelling justification for ensuring daily oral care is a required nursing task. Direct care staff should receive training, and the daily practice of such care carefully monitored as a component of infection control (SOE=B).

Because of the rich vascular supply of the head and neck, invasive dental treatment of a patient on anticoagulants presents particular risk of prolonged bleeding. Generally, if the INR is ≤3.5, the risk of uncontrolled oral hemorrhage is minimal and outweighed by the protective effects of anticoagulation (SOE=B).

The risk of precipitating a hypertensive episode or an ischemic cardiac event in a susceptible patient due to accidental intravascular injection of epinephrine as a part of dental care is quite remote and should not in general be of concern. The common forms of injectable local anesthetic solutions used by dentists do contain some vasoconstricting agent to prolong the anesthetic effect. The normal volume of an anesthetic carpule is 1.4 mL, and a typical epinephrine concentration is 1:100,000, representing 14 mcg per administration. Dental personnel are trained to aspirate (to ensure a blood vessel has not been entered) before injecting when administering local anesthetic as either a nerve block or for infiltration anesthesia. In general, the amount of endogenous epinephrine that might be secreted in response to pain induced by dental treatment (due to inadequate anesthesia) is likely far greater than would be introduced by dental personnel except in the unusual case of arterial infusion of a full carpule.

There are case reports in the medical and dental literature describing apparently spontaneous aseptic osteonecrosis of the mandible in patients who had been treated with bisphosphonates for management of bony metastases. Because the reports are relatively uncommon, formal epidemiologic determination of risk factors has been challenging. However, it does appear that bisphosphonates administered for osteoporosis are unlikely to result in osteonecrosis, that women are more likely affected than men, and that the mandible is more likely to be affected than the maxilla (SOE=C). Impending dental surgery in a patient who is likely to be treated with bisphosphonates for bony malignant disease should be completed before the chemotherapy. If dental surgery is undertaken in a patient with a history of high-dosage bisphosphonate therapy, the patient should be advised of the increased risk of osteonecrosis-related complications.

REFERENCES

- Legout L, Beltrand E, Migaud H, et al. Antibiotic prophylaxis to reduce the risk of joint implant contamination during dental surgery seems unnecessary. *Orthop Traumatol Surg Res*. 2012;98(8):910–914.

  As in endocarditis, antibiotic prophylaxis has been recommended to cover oro-dental surgery in immunosupressed patients with joint implants <2 years old, despite the lack of any formal proof of efficacy. This meta-analysis of the English and French literature explored the evidence on which this practice is based. Of 650 articles, 68 identified by a keyword search were analyzed regarding frequency and intensity of bacteremia of oro-dental origin, frequency of prosthetic joint infection secondary to dental surgery, and objective efficacy of antibiotic prophylaxis in dental surgery in patients with joint implants. Bacteremia of oro-dental origin is more frequently associated with everyday activities such as mastication than with tooth extraction. Epidemiologic studies of those with joint implant found that absence of antibiotic prophylaxis during oro-dental surgery did not increase the rate of prosthetic infection. The findings support existing guidelines that advise against antibiotic prophylaxis in oro-dental surgery in those with implants, regardless of implant age or comorbidity.

- Panwar A, Lindau R, Wieland A. Management for premalignant lesions of the oral cavity. A systematic review of salivary gland hypofunction and xerostomia induced by cancer therapies: management strategies and economic impact. *Expert Rev Anticancer Ther*. 2014;14(3):349–357.

  Premalignant lesions of the oral cavity present as visible abnormal areas of mucosa and may be a source of significant anxiety for the patient and the clinician. Suspicious lesions should be biopsied to evaluate for dysplasia. The risk of malignant transformation may relate to patient characteristics, environmental risk factors, and genetic alterations. Management of such lesions hinges on risk modification, surveillance, symptom management, and directed biopsies. Excision or ablation of dysplastic lesions is indicated. This article reviews the current evidence relating to management of premalignant lesions of the oral mucosa and makes recommendations for practitioners.

- Pichardo SE, van Merkesteyn JP. Bisphosphanate-related osteonecrosis of the jaws: spontaneous or dental origin? *Oral Surg Oral Med Oral Pathol Oral Radiol*. 2013;116(3):287–292.

  This retrospective review of 45 cases of bisphosphonate-related osteonecrosis of the jaws (BRONJ) sought to clarify whether onset of BRONJ predominantly occurs spontaneously or after dental treatment. The finding that 97.5% (n=44) of the cases studied had a clear temporal link to dental or oral surgical care is a sober reminder that, as uncommon as BRONJ is, when it occurs it invariably follows dental care.

- Wahl MJ. Dental surgery and antiplatelet agents: bleed or die. *Am J Med*. 2014;127(4):260–267.

  In patients taking antiplatelet medications who are undergoing dental surgery, physicians and dentists must weigh the bleeding risks in continuing antiplatelet medications versus the thrombotic risks of interrupting antiplatelet medications. Bleeding complications requiring more than local measures for hemostasis are rare after dental surgery in patients taking antiplatelet medications. Conversely, the risk of thrombotic complications after interruption of antiplatelet therapy for dental procedures is significant, although small. That is, there is a remote chance that continuing antiplatelet therapy will result in a (nonfatal) bleeding problem requiring more than local measures for hemostasis but a small but significant chance that interrupting antiplatelet therapy will result in a (possibly fatal) thromboembolic complication. The decision is simple: it is time to stop interrupting antiplatelet therapy for dental surgery.

Kenneth Shay, DDS, MS, AGSF

CHAPTER 48—PULMONOLOGY

KEY POINTS

- With age, forced vital capacity (FVC), forced expiratory volume in 1 second (FEV_1), and Pao_2 all decrease, while the alveolar-arterial gradient (A-a gradient) increases.

- Clinically significant dyspnea is often underreported and unrecognized in older adults.

- 5%–10% of people ≥65 years old meet the criteria for asthma.

- COPD is the third leading cause of death in older adults. Pharmacologic treatment of COPD chiefly consists of inhaled bronchodilators and steroids.

- Smoking cessation will slow the decline in lung function at any age.

AGE-RELATED PULMONARY CHANGES

Studies of age-specific changes in pulmonary function are limited because of potential confounding by common, important comorbidities experienced by older adults, including smoking-related diseases, occupational and industrial exposures, as well as other significant organ dysfunction such as heart failure, sarcopenia, or physical deconditioning. These study limitations notwithstanding, decrements in various aspects of pulmonary function have been demonstrated with aging.

Because of changes in connective tissue with age, the size of the airways is reduced and the alveolar sacs become shallower. Chest wall compliance is reduced as a consequence of kyphoscoliosis, calcification of the costal cartilage, and arthritic changes in the costovertebral joints. Sarcopenia results in intercostal muscle atrophy, and diaphragmatic strength is reduced by 25%. These processes result in a decline of FVC and FEV_1 of 25–30 mL/year in nonsmokers and approximately double that (60–70 mL/year) in smokers ≥65 years old. The normal A-a gradient increases with age and can be approximated by the following formula: (age/4) + 4 (in mmHg). The Pao_2 decreases with age and can be estimated by the equation: $Pao_2 = 110 - (0.4 \times age)$.

COMMON RESPIRATORY SYMPTOMS AND COMPLAINTS

There is a common misperception that older adults tend to overestimate or exaggerate respiratory symptoms; however, the opposite is more often true. Many older adults and their clinicians underestimate the importance of dyspnea, the cause of which may go undiagnosed until disease is advanced. This is partly because dyspnea is blamed on deconditioning and "normal" aging. Older adults often reduce their activity level to compensate for the often insidious decline in lung function and resultant disabling dyspnea. (Unfortunately, with increasing amounts of sedentary time, deconditioning may become a significant contributor to the problem.) Such changes in lifestyle often go unnoticed by family, the clinician, and even the patient. Pulmonary or cardiac disorders, or both, may underlie such modifications in lifestyle, and testing (eg, pulmonary function tests, chest radiography, or cardiac echocardiography) can reveal major abnormalities such as asthma, emphysema, pulmonary fibrosis, or pulmonary arterial hypertension. Another complicating feature of symptom recognition in older adults is that there is often more than one explanation for their problems. A patient may have overlapping symptoms of dyspnea, cough, and wheezing because of a combination of diseases such as asthma or emphysema, obstructive sleep apnea, heart failure, and gastroesophageal reflux.

Rhinosinusitis

Rhinitis complaints of older adults include a constant need to clear the throat, a sense of nasal obstruction, nasal crusting, facial pressure, and a decreased sense of taste and smell. Some changes in physiology and function of the nose accompany aging. As people age, the nose lengthens and the tip begins to droop secondary to weakening of the supporting cartilage. These physiologic changes can cause a restriction in nasal airflow. Resultant narrowing of the nasal passages can lead to complaints of nasal obstruction, which has been referred to as geriatric rhinitis.

There are no data to determine if either acute or chronic rhinosinusitis manifests any differently in older adults than in younger adults, so guidelines from the American Academy of Otolaryngology–Head and Neck Surgery do not advise different approaches to diagnosis or treatment based on age. Acute (<4 weeks in duration), subacute (4–12 weeks in duration), and chronic (>12 weeks in duration) rhinosinusitis are further subclassified as uncomplicated, when inflammation is restricted to the nasal cavity and sinuses, or complicated, when inflammation extends beyond these areas (eg, with soft-tissue or neurologic involvement). Older adults with sinusitis may report nasal discharge or crusting, sense of nasal obstruction, constant need to clear the throat, vague facial pressure, and decreased sense of smell and/or taste. Bacterial rhinosinusitis is associated with purulent nasal discharge and facial pain or pressure. Treatment may focus on pain relief with simple analgesics, as well as on relief of nasal obstruction by saline irrigation. Antibiotics are generally not prescribed for patients who have mild illness but are advised if symptoms persist for ≥7 days, or if the symptoms worsen at any time. Early treatment with antibiotics in patients with mild disease has been shown to be harmful (SOE=B). In patients with clear nasal discharge, the cause of the rhinosinusitis is likely viral, and treatment should be symptomatic only. Although topical α-adrenergic decongestants may be effective, their use should be restricted in older adults, particularly those with hypertension or voiding symptoms from prostate disease. Chronic rhinosinusitis may be treated with a variety of topical agents. A Cochrane review demonstrated that saline irrigation is more effective than placebo and offers a safe approach for many older adults. Topical nasal steroids are more effective than saline irrigation but may cause epistaxis and local irritation. Allergic causes of rhinosinusitis are best treated by avoidance of the inciting allergens if possible, although topical nasal steroids are often required. Anti-allergy medications may also have a role in treatment of allergic rhinosinusitis in older adults but should be used judiciously, because antihistamine formulations may also have undesired anticholinergic effects.

Dyspnea

Dyspnea becomes prominent in end-stage lung diseases such as COPD and idiopathic pulmonary fibrosis. Importantly, the level of dyspnea is the best predictor of quality of life, yet it does not correlate with either oxygenation or pulmonary function test results. A thorough history and physical examination can help tailor both testing and empirical treatment choices. For example, in an older adult presenting with dyspnea and associated nocturnal cough, common diseases such as asthma, emphysema, allergic rhinitis with postnasal drip, and gastroesophageal reflux disease should be considered first. Minimal testing (eg, pulmonary function tests only) followed by an empiric trial directed toward the most likely cause would be a reasonable approach. In the same patient, the presence of significant weight loss or constitutional symptoms (eg, fever, night sweats) could suggest other disease, such as malignancy or tuberculosis. At times, the particular language the patient chooses to describe the dyspnea can be revealing, such as "heavy" for cardiac dysfunction or deconditioning or "tight" for asthma. Common causes of dyspnea to consider in older adults include COPD, cardiac disease, asthma, interstitial lung disease, anemia, and deconditioning.

Chronic Cough

Fortunately, most patients can be reassured that chronic cough, although annoying, usually has a benign cause in individuals without a history of chronic lung disease or smoking. By far, the most common causes of chronic cough are postnasal drip, asthma, and gastroesophageal reflux. These three diagnoses account for >90% of the causes identified in most series, so a reasonable approach to the treatment of chronic cough is empiric treatment for these conditions (SOE=C). Not infrequently, a combination of these conditions may contribute to a single individual's cough, and treatment for multiple causes may be warranted when single therapies are ineffective. In older adults, the possibility of silent aspiration needs to be considered, especially in patients with frequent pneumonias, neurologic deficits, or residence in extended-care facilities. In these cases, videofluoroscopy (modified barium swallow) can evaluate oropharyngeal and esophageal aspiration. Fiberoptic endoscopic evaluation of swallowing can also be used to evaluate swallowing problems in the pharyngeal or laryngeal areas and can be performed at the bedside. Less common yet important differential diagnostic considerations of cough in older adults include medication effects (eg, ACE inhibitors), COPD and chronic bronchitis, heart failure, laryngeal dysfunction, *Bordetella pertussis* infection, chronic cough after viral upper respiratory tract infection or secondary bacterial infection, or respiratory tract anatomical abnormalities such as bronchiectasis or central airway tumors. A careful history and physical examination should help direct the diagnostic evaluation or empiric treatment of cough.

Wheezing

Although asthma is a common cause of wheezing in all age groups, it is not the principal cause in older adults, particularly if the wheezing is not associated with cough or dyspnea. Wheezing in older adults is more commonly caused by COPD or heart failure. ("Cardiac asthma" refers to wheezing arising from heart failure.) Other common causes of wheezing include postnasal drip and uncontrolled gastroesophageal reflux disease.

MAJOR PULMONARY DISEASES

Asthma

After childhood, the prevalence of asthma peaks again after the age of 65 years (late-onset asthma); 5%–10% of older adults meet criteria for airway obstruction and bronchial hyperreactivity, particularly in nonsmokers. Atopy and obesity are common in older adults with long-standing asthma. Asthma deaths in older adults account for >50% of asthma fatalities annually, and older adults with the disease have a 5-fold increased overall mortality compared with younger adults. This is likely due to reduced awareness of bronchial constriction on the part of the older adults (with attendant delays in seeking medical attention), as well as under-recognition and undertreatment on the part of clinicians. Asthma has a significant negative effect on quality of life in many older adults.

Population studies of asthma in older adults have shown that, unlike younger adults, who may need only symptomatic treatment, most older adults require continual treatment programs to control their disease (SOE=B). Overall, asthma management does not differ between older and younger people. Inhaled corticosteroids (or other controller drugs such as leukotriene-receptor antagonists) are the mainstay of therapy in both older and younger patients. The lowest effective dosage should be prescribed, and a spacer and counseling on rinsing of the oropharynx are important to avoid thrush. Oral corticosteroids are discussed in COPD, below. The bronchodilator response to inhaled β-agonists declines with age, but β-agonists are still the mainstay as-needed reliever medication for asthma treatment. The potential for adverse events of β-agonists—eg, hypokalemia or possible QT prolongation in cardiac patients on digoxin or other medications—warrants adequate controller drug use in older asthmatic patients to minimize their overreliance on the β-agonist. Use of long-acting β-agonists is helpful for long-term maintenance therapy and nocturnal symptoms. Anticholinergics can be considered in patients who cannot tolerate β-agonists. Biologic agents such as omalizumab can be used as an adjunct therapy for uncontrolled severe asthma despite maximal inhaler regimens in older asthma patients with increased serum immunoglobulin E (IgE) levels. In older adults, theophylline use is fraught with adverse events and drug interactions, and it should be considered as a third-line medication. Theophylline should be prescribed for use only once daily in the evening, for severe asthma or COPD, with a target serum level of 5–15 mg/L if tolerated.

In addition to pharmacologic treatment, asthma "action plans" should be developed and addressed in the event of worsening pulmonary symptoms. For an example of an asthma action plan, see Table 48.1. Patients should keep a copy of such a plan in a convenient location for easy reference.

Chronic Obstructive Pulmonary Disease

COPD is estimated to affect between 12.7–14.7 million adults in the United States, based on responses to the National Health Interview Survey and the Behavioral Risk Factor Surveillance System. COPD is the third most common cause of death after heart disease and cancer. The prevalence of COPD in adults ≥75 years old is at least 10%. Both the prevalence of COPD and its mortality are increasing, especially in older adults. Episodes of acute respiratory failure that require mechanical ventilation are associated with mortality rates ranging from 11% to 46%. The National Heart, Lung and Blood Institute estimated annual direct costs of COPD/asthma were $53.7 billion, with $20 billion required for prescription medications and $13 billion spent on inpatient hospitalizations. COPD is a leading cause of hospitalization in the United States; it accounts for 19.9% of the total hospitalizations for patients 65–75 years old and 18.2% for patients >75 years old. In one study, patients >65 years old who were admitted to an intensive care unit with COPD had a hospital mortality of 30% and a 1-year mortality of 59%.

Airflow limitation is a key feature of COPD, yet no single item or combination of items from the history and clinical examination can exclude it. For criteria often used to make the diagnosis of COPD, see Table 48.2. Because the FEV_1/FVC ratio decreases with age, using a fixed ratio to separate normal from obstructive creates a risk of over-diagnosis of COPD in older adults. Up to one-fifth of current smokers and one-seventh of individuals >50 years old who have never smoked can be misidentified as abnormal when a fixed cut-off is used. Other approaches to staging severity of COPD include using the lower limit of normal based on survey-derived survey estimates or distribution of Z-scores, similar to the strategies used in measuring bone mineral density or pediatric growth charts. The most recent recommendations for diagnosing COPD from the Global Initiative for Chronic Obstructive Lung Disease (GOLD) are to use a combined approach, including spirometric assessment of airflow obstruction (FEV_1), symptoms, and exacerbation history. Current guidelines recommend against screening asymptomatic older adults for COPD. In smokers, chronic cough is the most commonly reported symptom associated with COPD diagnosis. Wheezing noted on physical examination is the most potent predictor of airflow limitation; individuals with obstructive airflow limitation are 36 times more likely to have wheezing than those without this problem. Other findings associated with an increased likelihood of airflow limitation include a barrel-shaped chest, hyperresonance on percussion, and a forced expiratory time of >9 seconds measured during a clinical bedside examination.

Smoking cessation at any age slows the decline in lung function, and aggressive cessation efforts are appropriate even in the oldest patient. The "Five A's" method, from the Agency for Health Care Policy and Research, is a commonly used approach for addressing

Table 48.1—Example of an Asthma Action Plan

Green zone: Doing well

No cough, wheeze, chest tightness, or shortness of breath during day or night Can do usual activities *Peak flow:* ≥80% of my best peak flow	Take these long-term medications as prescribed: Medicine 1: how much, when to take it Medicine 2: how much, when to take it

Yellow zone: Getting worse

Cough, wheeze, chest tightness, or shortness of breath, *or* Waking at night due to asthma, *or* Can do some, but not all, usual activities *Peak flow:* 50%–79% of my best peak flow	Keep taking your Green zone medications and add quick-relief medication (a short-acting β_2-agonist). If your symptoms return to Green zone after 1 hour of above treatment, continue monitoring. If your symptoms do *not* return to Green zone after 1 hour of treatment, take another dose of the short-acting β_2-agonist and add oral steroid.

Red zone: Medical alert

Very short of breath, *or* Quick-relief medications have not helped, *or* Cannot do usual activities, *or* Symptoms are the same or get worse after 24 hours in the Yellow zone *Peak flow:* <50% of my best peak flow	Take a short-acting β_2-agonist and oral steroid. Then call your doctor *now*. Go to the hospital or call an ambulance if you are still in the Red zone after 15 minutes *and* you have not reached your doctor.

Table 48.2—GOLD[a] Guidelines for COPD

Key Factors for Considering a Diagnosis of COPD

Dyspnea	Progressive or worsens over time Worse with exercise Persistent (present daily) Described as "increased effort to breathe," "heaviness," "air hunger," "gasping"
Chronic cough	May be intermittent and nonproductive
Sputum production	Any pattern of chronic sputum production can indicate COPD
Risk factors	Tobacco smoke Occupational dusts and chemicals Smoke from home cooking and heating fuel Family history, genetic variant (α-1 antitrypsin deficiency)

Spirometric Classification of Airflow Obstruction in COPD (Post-Bronchodilator FEV_1)
FEV_1/FVC <70%[b] applies to each category

Mild	FEV_1 ≥80% predicted
Moderate	50% ≤ FEV_1 <80% predicted
Severe	30% ≤ FEV_1 <50% predicted
Very severe	FEV_1 <30% predicted or FEV_1 <50% predicted and chronic respiratory failure[c]

NOTE: FEV_1 = forced expiratory volume in 1 sec; FVC = forced vital capacity
[a] GOLD=Global Initiative for Chronic Obstructive Lung Disease
[b] Using the criteria FEV_1/FVC <70% may overdiagnose COPD in older, nonsmoking adults; some experts recommend using as the lower limit of normal the 5th percentile of the normal distribution of the FEV_1/FVC ratio for the reference (older) population. The Global Lung Initiative recommends using this 5th percentile value as the cutoff. Most recent GOLD recommendations for COPD diagnosis and severity assessment are to use a combination of spirometric classification, symptoms, and exacerbation history.
[c] Chronic respiratory failure entails the need for chronic invasive or noninvasive ventilator support.

smoking cessation with patients. The basic elements of the approach are:

- **A**sk patients about use of tobacco at every office visit.
- **A**ssess readiness to quit.
- **A**dvise patients to quit.
- **A**ssist patients in the quit attempt with aids such as a local cessation program and pharmacologic agents such as bupropion, nicotine replacement, or varenicline.
- **A**rrange both a quit date and a follow-up visit or contact to discuss the quit attempt.

The chief components of daily medication therapy in COPD consist of a β-agonist, ipratropium bromide or a long-acting anticholinergic medication (tiotropium, umeclidinium, aclidinium), or both in combination (Table 48.3 and Table 48.4). For more severe disease, the

Table 48.3—Inhaled Bronchodilators and Corticosteroids for COPD

Class	Medications	Duration (hours)	Dosage
Short-acting			
β_2-Agonists	Albuterol sulfate, levalbuterol, pirbuterol	4–6	2 puffs q6h
Anticholinergic	Ipratropium bromide	4–6	2 puffs q6h
Long-acting			
β_2-Agonists	Formoterol fumarate, salmeterol xinafoate	8–12	1 puff q12h
	Arformoterol	8–12	15 mcg nebulized q12h
	Indacaterol maleate	24	1 puff q24h
	Olodaterol	24	2 puffs q24h
Anticholinergic	Tiotropium bromide	>24	1 puff q24h
	Aclidinium	12	1 puff q12h
	Umeclidinium	24	1 puff q24h
Inhaled corticosteroid	Beclomethasone diproprionate	12	1 or 2 puffs q12h
	Fluticasone[OL]	12	1 or 2 puffs q12h[a]
	Budesonide[OL]	12	Nebulized, or 2 puffs q12h
	Mometasone furoate	24	1 or 2 puffs q24h

[OL] Off-label when used alone (not as a component of a combination product) for treatment of COPD.

[a] Also available in diskus form in 3 strengths, dosed 1 puff q12h.

use of the long-acting anticholinergic tiotropium with albuterol-only rescue inhalers or long-acting β-agonists such as salmeterol can achieve long-term control. Symptoms can be controlled in some patients with monotherapy, potentially improving long-term adherence by reducing the number of maintenance inhalers by one. Concern has been raised over risk of cardiovascular events associated with anticholinergic medications, although in a randomized controlled trial of 6,000 patients with COPD, tiotropium use was associated with decreased cardiovascular events compared with treatment with β-agonists, inhaled corticosteroids, and/or theophylline. Use of inhaled corticosteroids has been associated with some improvement in airway reactivity, frequency of exacerbations, and respiratory symptoms, but they have not been shown to impact the rate of decline in lung function (SOE=A). Combination therapy with inhaled corticosteroids and a long-acting β-agonist has been associated with better lung function and symptom control but not survival benefit. A landmark investigation documented that use of systemic corticosteroids (intravenous followed by oral) reduces the duration and recurrence of acute exacerbations of COPD for up to 6 months (SOE=A). Importantly, there is no benefit to a course of systemic steroids for >14 days for acute exacerbation of COPD.

A subset of patients with recalcitrant COPD experience frequent exacerbations or persistent symptoms despite the use of maximal inhaler therapy, and they may benefit from trial of additional treatments. Phosphodiesterase-4 inhibitors, such as roflumilast, have been shown to reduce exacerbations and improve quality of life when used as adjuvant therapy in patients with severe COPD. Prophylactic antibiotics may reduce exacerbation frequency but carry substantial risk of increasing bacterial drug resistance or secondary infections such as *Clostridium difficile* diarrhea. Theophylline may also be considered in patients with refractory COPD but should be used cautiously. Chronic systemic steroids are required for relatively few patients (5%–10%). The risks of peptic ulcer disease, hypertension, cataracts, diabetes mellitus, osteoporosis, psychosis, seizures, poor wound healing, infections, and aseptic necrosis of the hip must be carefully considered in these patients. Appropriate preventive measures should be taken in circumstances of prolonged use, such as monitoring for signs of osteopenia or osteoporosis; using the lowest possible dosage of corticosteroids; and using supplemental vitamin D, calcium, and perhaps a bisphosphonate for those at risk of osteoporosis.

Long-term oxygen therapy benefits patients who have a resting PaO_2 of ≤55 mmHg on ambient air (SOE=A). Use of oxygen for at least 15 hours per day improves survival, exercise tolerance, sleep, and cognitive function. Other possible beneficial interventions in older adults with COPD include pulmonary rehabilitation via exercise training, and respiratory therapy and education. Home-based, self-administered exercise and strength-building programs may also have a role in pulmonary rehabilitation of older adults with COPD. Palliative care consultation should be strongly considered for patients with refractory symptoms of dyspnea from COPD. Both major depressive disorder and anxiety are

Table 48.4—COPD Therapy[a]

Class	Treatment
Mild COPD	
$FEV_1 \geq 80\%$	Short-acting β_2-agonist or combination of short-acting β_2-agonist and anticholinergic, prn
	Smoking cessation
Moderate COPD	
$50\% \leq FEV_1 < 80\%$	Long-acting β_2-agonist or anticholinergic if needed for added benefit or if ≥2 exacerbations per year
	Smoking cessation
	Rehabilitation
Severe COPD	
$30\% \leq FEV_1 < 50\%$	Regular treatment with one or more bronchodilators[b], preferably long-acting β_2-agonist or anticholinergic
	Inhaled steroids[c] if significant symptomatic and PFT response or if ≥2 exacerbations per year
	Smoking cessation
	Rehabilitation
Very severe COPD	
$FEV_1 < 30\%$ *or*	Regular treatment with one or more bronchodilators[b], preferably long-acting β_2-agonist or anticholinergic
	(Consider adding a phosphodiesterase-4 inhibitor if chronic bronchitis or frequent exacerbations.)
$FEV_1 < 50\%$ plus chronic respiratory failure	Inhaled steroids[c] if significant symptomatic and PFT response or if repeated exacerbations
	Smoking cessation
	Treatment of complications
	Long-term oxygen therapy if respiratory failure
COPD exacerbation	
(acute increase in breathlessness, wheezing, cough, and sputum beyond normal day-to-day variation and leads to change in medication)	Increase dosage and/or frequency of β_2-agonists with or without anticholinergics.
	Use spacers or nebulizers for improved medication delivery.
	Add steroid (eg, oral prednisolone 30–40 mg/d for 5 days).
	Add antibiotics if increased sputum volume, increased purulence, and/or increased dyspnea or requiring mechanical ventilation (for specific agents, consider local bacterial resistance patterns and/or patient's prior sputum culture results).
	Supplemental oxygen (target saturation 88%–92%), monitor arterial blood gas
	CBC, chest radiograph, ECG
	Indications for noninvasive mechanical ventilation: severe dyspnea (respiratory accessory muscle use, paradoxical motion of abdomen, intercostal space retraction), respiratory rate ≥25 breaths/min, arterial pH ≤7.35, or pCO_2 45 mmHg
	Indications for invasive mechanical ventilation: unable to tolerate noninvasive (with or without hypoxemia), respiratory or cardiac arrest, loss of consciousness, gasping for air, massive aspiration, inability to clear respiratory secretions, severe hemodynamic instability, life-threatening ventricular arrhythmias

NOTE: PFT = pulmonary function test
[a] $FEV_1/FVC < 70\%$ for all levels of severity
[b] β_2-agonists, ipratropium, slow-release theophylline (caution in older adults with other conditions and taking other medications). Inhaled bronchodilators are preferred over oral because of efficacy and adverse effects. Avoid inhaled anticholinergics (ipratropium, tiotropium) in men with lower urinary tract obstructive symptoms.
[c] Consider osteoporosis prophylaxis.
SOURCE: Data from *Global Initiative for Chronic Obstructive Lung Disease (GOLD)*; 2014. www.goldcopd.org (accessed Jan 2016).

present in up to 40% of patients with COPD; these diagnoses should be screened for and treated appropriately. In older adults, anxiety is associated with diminished physical functioning and is a major predictor of emergency department visits and hospitalization. Pulmonary rehabilitation can improve respiratory function, as well as relieve depression and anxiety in patients with refractory COPD. By stimulating nasopharyngeal mechanoreceptors, a stream of air from an electric fan can help to relieve dyspnea in patients with refractory symptoms. When dyspnea persists despite these measures and maximal bronchodilator therapy, low-dose oral opiates can be used. Careful monitoring must accompany this treatment with attention to somnolence, neuropsychiatric adverse effects, and constipation.

Paramount to the care of older adults with asthma or COPD is adequate instruction in proper use of peak expiratory flow meters and inhalers. Neurologic, muscular, and arthritic diseases in older adults can lead to suboptimal timing and lack of coordination in proper use of inhaler devices. Only 60% of older adults have been reported to show adequate technique with a metered-dose inhaler; this number decreases to 36% when objective criteria are used. Although the use of spacers improves technique, 85% of older adults do not use the spacer when it is prescribed. Breath-activated dry-powder inhalers demand less coordination but require a certain minimal peak inspiratory flow for adequate drug delivery. The clinician should observe the patient actually using the inhaler; pharmacists may provide instruction in inhaler technique as well. Cost is another additional barrier to adherence in over one-quarter of patients with COPD, particularly when out-of-pocket costs exceed $20.

Patients with advanced-stage COPD and recalcitrant dyspnea may benefit from referral to palliative care. Characteristics of patients who may satisfy hospice prognostic criteria are dyspnea, hypoxemia despite supplemental oxygen, weight loss, poor functional status, and disease progression (manifested by repeated emergency department visits or hospitalizations).

Obstructive Sleep Apnea

Sleep-related breathing disorders are very common in older adults, and obstructive sleep apnea (OSA) is the most frequent. As in younger patients, OSA in older patients is more common in men. The estimated prevalence of OSA in older men ranges from 13% to 28% and in women from 4% to 20%. Age-related changes of respiratory anatomy and physiology, such as increased upper airway adipose tissue deposition and pharyngeal bony changes, may predispose older adults to sleep apnea. Body habitus as a risk factor for apnea is less important in older patients than in younger patients. In the Heart Health Study, although the overall prevalence of OSA did not differ by racial group, black women were significantly younger than white women at the time of diagnosis. Black patients with OSA are more obese and have higher rates of hypertension than white patients with OSA. Medications, alcohol consumption, and abnormal upper airway configuration are additional risk factors for OSA, with the latter issue particularly relevant in older adults. OSA has been associated with cerebrovascular accidents, myocardial infarctions, and a 3-fold increase in mortality (SOE=B). Untreated OSA is associated with significant cognitive impairment, including executive dysfunction, as well as depression in older patients. Most patients with OSA remain undiagnosed and therefore without treatment of this life-threatening, yet potentially treatable disease. Clinicians should consider the diagnosis in patients who have complaints of daytime somnolence, frequent daytime napping, or drowsiness while driving. A history of snoring or witnessed apneas or hypopneas by a bed partner should also prompt further evaluation. Treatment options include addressing upper-airway obstruction via weight loss, avoiding alcohol and sedatives, sleeping on one's side or upright, correcting metabolic disorders such as hypothyroidism, and using continuous positive-airway pressure (CPAP) via a nasal mask. To increase adherence to the use of CPAP, the treatment can be ordered with "nasal pillows" to increase comfort, and "ramping technique" to give a delayed rise in the applied pressure after the individual has fallen asleep. Diagnosis and treatment issues are generally the same for both young and old, and the major consideration for the primary clinician is to maintain a high index of suspicion for this disease.

Idiopathic Pulmonary Fibrosis

Among older adults, idiopathic pulmonary fibrosis (IPF) is the most common of the >100 causes of interstitial lung diseases. It has a mean age of onset of 55 years and is increasing in prevalence with the aging population. The disease shows a relentless progression, and its median survival is 3–5 years. Survival is even worse in patients with both IPF and pulmonary hypertension. Disease presentation is normally one of insidious dyspnea (often unrecognized because of a decrease in the activity level on the part of the patient) and nonproductive cough, with dry inspiratory rales on examination. Clubbing is often a prominent finding on physical examination in IPF (40%–70%), as opposed to emphysema, which rarely causes clubbing. (Discovery of clubbing in an emphysematous patient should prompt a search for another disease, such as occult lung cancer). Older adults often present with advanced disease because of the insidious onset of symptoms. IPF should be considered in older adults with a restrictive ventilatory defect or a reduced diffusing capacity on pulmonary function testing, or both. Chest radiographs often show reticular opacities in the mid and lower lung zones. High-resolution CT scans show characteristic areas of subpleural reticulation and honeycombing. Experienced pulmonologists and radiologists can often make the diagnosis based on clinical and radiographic findings.

In the past, oral corticosteroids (dosed at 0.5 mg/kg/d for 3–6 months) had been commonly used as initial therapy, but only 10%–20% of patients respond to these agents and adverse events are common. High-dose steroids are commonly used for acute exacerbations, although data supporting their use are lacking. Combination therapy with oral corticosteroids, azathioprine, and N-acetylcysteine had been used for several years. However, more recent trials showed that mortality, hospitalizations, and adverse events were higher in those treated with this combination. Although there is no medical cure for IPF, there have been some exciting discoveries for treatment. In randomized controlled trials, disease progression was significantly reduced in patients with mild-moderate disease treated with pirfenidone and nintedanib than with placebo; pirfenidone may reduce mortality. Although older age was not a specific focus, the mean age of patients enrolled in these trials was 66–68 years. GI adverse effects (nausea, diarrhea, increases in liver function tests) were the most common adverse drug-related events in trials of these drugs. In patients with IPF and pulmonary hypertension, a therapeutic trial of sildenafil may be reasonable in patients without contraindications. Treatment of GI reflux disease may also slow progression of disease.

Lung transplantation is the only treatment for end-stage IPF. However, risks associated with lung transplant need to be carefully considered, especially in patients ≥65 years old whose survival after transplant is lower than that of younger patients. With the advent of ongoing research trials and recent new treatment options for IPF, early referral to a subspecialist experienced in fibrotic lung diseases may be warranted. The primary care provider may initiate the evaluation by obtaining a history and searching for evidence of chemical exposure, smoking, asbestosis, connective tissue syndromes, chronic aspiration, or a family history of lung diseases. Chest CT and pulmonary function tests are helpful in guiding subsequent management decisions. Patients with advanced disease may benefit from a palliative care approach.

Venous Thromboembolic Disease

The incidence of venous thromboembolism (VTE), including deep venous thrombosis (DVT) and pulmonary embolism (PE), increases in older adults because of age-related risk factors, including changes in the hemostatic system that predispose to thrombosis; venous stasis related to illness, injuries (eg, hip fracture), and immobility (especially hospitalization and residence in long-term care); incompetence of the superficial and deep veins, including failure of the venous valves; and the high prevalence of systemic illnesses associated with thrombogenesis (eg, heart failure, cancer, neurologic diseases). Established risk factors for VTE include age >60 years, indwelling central venous catheters, surgery, trauma, chronic lung disease, dehydration, history of VTE, having a first-degree relative with VTE, increased fibrinogen level, activated protein-C resistance due to factor-V Leiden gene mutation, inflammatory bowel disease, obesity, rheumatoid arthritis, or treatment with various medications (aromatase inhibitors, hormone replacement therapy, megestrol acetate, selective estrogen-receptor modulators, or erythroid-stimulating agents with hemoglobin concentration >12 g/dL). The incidence of PE triples between the ages of 65 and 90 years and has a reported 10% recurrence rate within 1 year. Age >70 years has been independently associated with missed antemortem diagnosis of PE.

Symptoms and signs of VTE are similar in older and younger patients, but it is important to recognize that most patients with DVT or PE, or both, are asymptomatic; therefore, a high index of suspicion for these conditions must be maintained, particularly in hospitalized patients and in residents of transitional-care facilities and nursing homes. Physical examination findings of DVT include limb pain, tenderness, warmth, and edema. The clinical diagnosis of venous thrombosis is generally insufficiently accurate to exclude additional testing, because the signs and symptoms are nonspecific. The utility of most routine tests, including blood tests, arterial blood gases, chest radiographs, ECGs, and echocardiography for diagnosing VTE is quite low, and the presence of "normal" findings on each of these tests does not exclude a diagnosis of DVT or PE. The plasma d-dimer level, when performed using ELISA, has a high sensitivity for VTE but very low specificity in older adults; therefore, a normal d-dimer level in an older patient with low clinical suspicion for VTE essentially excludes the diagnosis. The upper limit of normal for d-dimer increases with age and can be estimated (in ng/mL) by multiplying age (in years) by 10. Increased D-dimer levels are common in older and hospitalized patients, particularly after surgery or in those who have been diagnosed with malignancy or renal insufficiency. Serum brain natriuretic peptide (BNP) and troponin are not sensitive or specific for pulmonary embolism but can inform risk stratification for patients with suspected PE.

Noninvasive tests for DVT include upper and lower extremity venous Doppler examinations, impedance plethysmography, and CT of the legs; rarely, contrast venography may be required to establish the diagnosis. When positive, noninvasive tests provide presumptive evidence for VTE, but negative tests do not exclude DVT or PE, especially in patients for whom the clinical suspicion is high. Similarly, ventilation/perfusion lung scanning and spiral CT of the chest are useful when the findings are unequivocally normal or abnormal. However, indeterminate ventilation/perfusion scans are common in older patients, and 2%–10% of patients with PE have false-negative spiral CT scans, depending on whether multidetector or single-detector scanners are used. Therefore, in patients in whom clinical suspicion of PE is high but noninvasive evaluations (which might include lower extremity ultrasound studies) are negative, pulmonary angiography should be performed as the definitive diagnostic procedure. Although clinicians are often reluctant to recommend pulmonary angiography, data from the PIOPED study indicate that this procedure is generally well-tolerated by older adults and that the risks of the procedure are lower than those of either empiric anticoagulation in patients without PE or not anticoagulating patients with PE. Magnetic resonance pulmonary angiography is reserved for patients who cannot undergo spiral ventilation/perfusion scans or CT scans for PE evaluation. However, the sensitivity and specificity of these scans are limited, especially for subsegmental emboli; thus, scan results should not be used to exclude PE if clinical suspicion is high.

Anticoagulants are central to VTE therapy, and their use is generally guided by the same principles for patients of any age. Because of reduced cardiopulmonary reserve in older patients, achieving satisfactory anticoagulation quickly may be particularly urgent to avoid major adverse hemodynamic or oxygenation defects. The trend toward increased use of low-molecular-weight heparin preparations for outpatients, while achieving anticoagulation with warfarin, is supported by large, well-designed randomized controlled trials (SOE=A). Weight-adjusted dosage of low-molecular-weight heparin can be safely used in older patients, except for those weighing <45 kg. Full-dose low-molecular-weight heparin adjusted for weight and renal function, subcutaneous fondaparinux adjusted for weight and renal function, and intravenous unfractionated heparin to maintain the activated partial thromboplastin time in the range of 50–70 seconds (1.5–2 times the control value) have been the mainstay of initial therapy (SOE=A for all). Because of risk of hemorrhage and mortality, unfractionated heparin is less favorable than low-molecular-weight heparin and fondaparinux. The oral factor Xa inhibitors apixaban, rivaroxaban, and edoxaban may also be used for initial therapy of VTE.

Long-term therapy for VTE may include warfarin, low-molecular-weight heparin, apixaban, rivaroxaban, edoxaban, or the direct thrombin inhibitor dabigatran. If warfarin is chosen, administration may begin on the same day as the initial (fast-acting) anticoagulant. The initial anticoagulant (eg, low-molecular-weight heparin) should be used for at least 5 days, which should include 1–3 days of overlap with warfarin while the INR is therapeutic. For patients with VTE and malignancy who do not have abnormalities in kidney function or contraindications to anticoagulation, clinical practice guidelines recommend low-molecular-weight heparin as both initial and chronic therapy for at least 6 months. Patients who are not candidates for anticoagulation should be considered for an inferior vena caval filter, recognizing that such devices reduce the risk of PE but may increase the risk of recurrent DVT and post-phlebitic syndrome.

Factor Xa inhibitors and direct thrombin inhibitors do not require routine blood work (eg, INR monitoring) and, unlike warfarin, do not require prolonged bridging therapy before becoming effective. Until recently, these agents did not have specific antidotes to treat significant and life-threatening bleeding events, leaving providers to consider expert opinion for the use of prothrombin complex concentrates for this purpose. However, idarucizumab, an antibody fragment, was recently shown to rapidly reverse the anticoagulant effects of dabigatran, with the effect evident within minutes and potentially lasting up to 24 hours.

Long-term anticoagulation (≥6 months) is preferred to shorter term (eg, 3 months) unless there are increased risks of bleeding. Patients with multiple ongoing risk factors for pulmonary thromboembolic disease may be considered for anticoagulation therapy for up to 2 years or longer. Recurrent pulmonary thromboembolism is usually treated with lifelong anticoagulation therapy (SOE=C). In addition to the above measures, regular exercise, such as walking, is recommended to reduce the risk of recurrent DVT, and elastic compression stockings are recommended for up to 2 years after an episode of DVT to reduce the risk of post-phlebitic syndrome.

VTE prophylaxis with subcutaneous unfractionated or low-molecular-weight heparin, fondaparinux, or intermittent pneumatic compression of the calves is indicated in all hospitalized older adults who are not fully ambulatory, as well as in transitional care and long-term care residents at increased risk of VTE.

REFERENCES

- Akgün KM, Crothers K, Pisani M. Epidemiology and management of common pulmonary diseases in older persons. *J Gerontol A Biol Sci Med Sci.* 2012;67(3):276–291.

    This review article discusses epidemiology, risk factors, treatment, and outcomes of 5 common pulmonary diseases (pneumonia, COPD, asthma, lung cancer, and idiopathic pulmonary fibrosis) in older adults.

- Albertson TE, Schivo M, Zeki AA, et al. The pharmacological approach to the elderly COPD patient. *Drugs Aging.* 2013;30(7):479–502.

    This article is a comprehensive review on the diagnosis and treatment of COPD in older patients and includes a discussion of symptom management and palliative care.

- Edwards BA, Wellman A, Sands SA, et al. Obstructive sleep apnea in older adults is a distinctly different physiological phenotype. *Sleep.* 2014;37(7):1227–1236.

    This article is one of the first to compare the unique pathophysiology of obstructive sleep apnea (OSA) in older adults versus younger patients with OSA, matched for gender and body mass index.

- Gooneratne NS, Vitiello MV. Sleep in older adults: normative changes, sleep disorders, and treatment options. *Clin Geriatr Med.* 2014;30(3):591–627.

    This comprehensive review of sleep disturbances that affect older adults includes insomnia and sleep apnea and outlines potential treatments, including cognitive behavioral therapy for insomnia.

- Greig MF, Rochow SB, Crilly MA, et al. Routine pharmacological venous thromboembolism prophylaxis in frail older hospitalized patients: where is the evidence? *Age Ageing.* 2013;42(4):428–434.

    This review includes epidemiology of deep venous thrombosis and pulmonary embolism in older hospitalized patients, reviews pros and cons of thromboprophylaxis in this population, and considers situations that may make routine thromboprophylaxis more risky in older patients.

- Lowery EM, Brubaker AL, Kuhlmann E, et al. The aging lung. *Clin Interv Aging.* 2013;8:1489–1496.

    This review article describes changes to the respiratory system that frequently develop with normal aging, the role of "inflamm-aging" and changes in lung immunity. The authors also focus on the impact and unique challenges of COPD diagnosis and treatment in aging individuals.

- Melani AS. Management of asthma in the elderly patient. *Clin Interv Aging*. 2013;8:913–922.

   This article reviews the treatment of asthma in older adults. It extensively reviews treatment options for asthma in older adults, including biologic agents and even bronchoscopic procedures for treating uncontrolled asthma.

- Yáñez A, Cho SH, Soriano JB, et al. Asthma in the elderly: what we know and what we have yet to know. *World Allergy Organ J*. 2014;7(1):8.

   This article reviews the epidemiology, diagnosis, and treatment of asthma in older adults and identifies key features to distinguish asthma from COPD. The immunologic mechanisms and the role of immunosenescence of asthma in older adults are reviewed extensively.

Kathleen M. Akgün, MD, MS
Margaret Pisani, MD, MPH

CHAPTER 49—CARDIOLOGY

KEY POINTS

- Increasing age is associated with extensive changes throughout the cardiovascular system that lead to a progressive decline in cardiovascular reserve capacity and to substantive alterations in the clinical presentation, response to therapy, and prognosis of cardiovascular disease in older adults.

- Older adults account for the majority of patients hospitalized with acute coronary syndromes (ACS), and approximately 80% of deaths attributable to ACS occur in patients ≥65 years old. Although the benefits of current treatments for ACS are generally similar in older and younger patients, older patients are at increased risk of major complications from therapeutic interventions.

- Atrial fibrillation (AF), the most common sustained dysrhythmia in clinical practice, increases in prevalence with age, and >50% of all patients with AF are ≥75 years old. Most older adults with AF respond to rate-control medications in conjunction with antithrombotic therapy, but some patients require antiarrhythmic drug therapy or other intervention to maintain sinus rhythm and alleviate symptoms.

- Calcific aortic stenosis (AS) is the most common valve disorder requiring intervention in older adults. Surgical aortic valve replacement (SAVR) is the primary treatment for AS in healthier older adults, while transcatheter aortic valve replacement (TAVR) is an effective alternative to SAVR in older adults at high risk of surgery due to comorbidity, frailty, or other factors.

- The prevalence of peripheral arterial disease (PAD) increases progressively with age, and the presence of PAD is often predictive of concomitant coronary artery and cerebrovascular disease. Management of patients with PAD should therefore include appropriate treatment of hypertension, dyslipidemia, diabetes, and tobacco abuse in accordance with existing practice guidelines.

EPIDEMIOLOGY

The prevalence of cardiovascular disease (CVD) increases progressively with age, exceeding 80% in both men and women >80 years old (Table 49.1). Similarly, the annual incidence of CVD increases from 1% in men 45–54 years old to 7.4% in men 85–94 years old, and from 0.4% in women 45–54 years old to 6.5% in women 85–94 years old. Because of the high prevalence of CVD in older age, adults ≥65 years old account for 71% of hospitalizations for CVD in the United States, including over 50% of percutaneous and surgical coronary revascularization procedures, 60% of defibrillator implantations, 71% of arterial endarterectomies, and 82% of permanent pacemaker insertions. In addition, women comprise an increasing proportion of cardiovascular hospitalizations and procedures with increasing age.

Over the past 50 years, lifestyle changes and medical advances have led to a progressive decline in age-adjusted mortality rates from CVD. Nevertheless, CVD remains the leading cause of death in the United States, accounting for approximately 31% of all deaths in 2011. Notably, cancer is the leading cause of death among adults up to age 75, and it is only after age 75 that CVD becomes the dominant cause of death. Thus, among 786,600 deaths in the United States from CVD in 2011, more than 80% occurred in adults ≥65 years old and 66% occurred in the 6% of the population ≥75 years old. Mortality rates from CVD are higher in men than in women at all ages, but women account for more than 50% of CVD deaths among adults ≥65 years old. CVD mortality rates are highest in black Americans, followed by non-Hispanic whites, Hispanic Americans, Native Americans, and Asians/Pacific Islanders. With the aging of the population, it may be anticipated that the absolute number of cardiovascular deaths in older adults will increase markedly over the next several decades.

EFFECTS OF AGING ON CARDIOVASCULAR FUNCTION

Normal aging is associated with diverse changes throughout the cardiovascular system (Table 49.2), and these changes are accentuated by common comorbid conditions, particularly hypertension, diabetes, obesity, and atherosclerosis.

Increased collagen deposition and cross-linking in concert with degenerative changes in elastin fibers contribute to increased stiffness of the large arteries with increasing age. These changes in turn lead to a gradual increase in systolic blood pressure

Table 49.1—Prevalence (percent of population) of Cardiovascular Disease in Americans by Age and Sex

Age Cohort	Men	Women
20–39 years old	11.9	10.0
40–59 years old	40.5	35.5
60–79 years old	69.1	67.9
≥80 years old	84.7	85.9

SOURCE: Data from NHANES 2009–2012.

Table 49.2—Principal Effects of Aging on the Cardiovascular System

Age Effect	Clinical Implication
↑ Arterial stiffness	↑ Afterload and systolic blood pressure
↓ Myocardial relaxation and compliance	↑ Risk of diastolic heart failure and atrial fibrillation
Impaired responsiveness to β-adrenergic stimulation	↓ Maximum heart rate and cardiac output; impaired thermoregulation
↓ Sinus node function and conduction velocity in the atrioventricular node and infranodal conduction system	↑ Risk of sick sinus syndrome, atrioventricular block, left anterior fascicular block, and bundle branch block
Impaired endothelium-dependent vasodilation	↑ Demand ischemia and risk of coronary artery disease and peripheral arterial disease
↓ Baroreceptor responsiveness	↑ Risk of orthostatic hypotension, falls, and syncope
↓ Exercise response (↓ maximal heart rate, maximal cardiac output, V_{O_2} max, coronary blood flow, peripheral vasodilation)	↓ Exercise capacity and ↑ cardiac complications (ischemia, heart failure, shock, arrhythmias, death) with illness

and increased impedance to left ventricular ejection (ie, increased afterload). Arterial pulse wave velocity, a marker of vascular stiffness, increases with age, and early reflection of the pulse wave from the periphery results in further impedance to left ventricular ejection in late systole.

Myocardial relaxation, an active, energy-requiring process, is attenuated with age because of impaired release of calcium from the contractile proteins at the end of systole coupled with delayed calcium reuptake by the sarcoplasmic reticulum. Increased interstitial collagen and adipose tissue result in increased myocardial stiffness, and this effect is potentiated by compensatory myocyte hypertrophy in response to increased afterload and myocyte apoptosis. The combination of impaired relaxation and decreased myocardial compliance results in decreased filling of the left ventricle during early and mid-diastole. These changes are accompanied by dilatation and hypertrophy of the left atrium with increased force of left atrial contraction to preserve left ventricular end-diastolic volume, a major determinant of stroke volume and cardiac output. These characteristic changes in left ventricular diastolic function and in the left atrium predispose older adults to the development of heart failure with preserved left ventricular ejection fraction (HFpEF) and atrial fibrillation.

Responsiveness to β-adrenergic stimulation declines with age. As a result, the maximal attainable sinus heart rate decreases with age in a roughly linear fashion, often approximated by the formula: maximal heart rate = 220 − age. Because cardiac output is the product of heart rate and stroke volume, it follows that maximal cardiac output decreases as age increases. In addition, peak ventricular contractility (mediated by $β_1$-adrenergic receptors) and peripheral vasodilation (mediated by $β_2$-adrenergic receptors) decline with age. The latter effect results in decreased blood flow to exercising muscles and also to the skin, leading to impaired thermoregulation.

Degenerative changes in and around the sinus node result in a progressive loss in function of sinus node pacemaker cells and partial or complete separation of the node from the surrounding atrial tissues. By age 75, more than 90% of sinus node pacemaker cells have lost the ability to initiate an electrical impulse. These changes lead to a gradual but progressive decline in sinus node function, often culminating in development of symptomatic "sick sinus syndrome," the leading indication for pacemaker implantation in older adults. Additional age-related changes in the conduction system include slowed conduction through the atrioventricular node and calcification of the cardiac skeleton, the latter resulting in increasing prevalence of infranodular conduction abnormalities such as left anterior fascicular block and bundle-branch block.

Endothelium-dependent vasodilation declines with age, primarily due to decreased nitric oxide synthase activity and the resulting decline in the availability of nitric oxide, the principal mediator of endogenous endothelial vasodilation. Because endothelium-dependent vasodilation is the primary mechanism for increasing coronary blood flow in response to increased myocardial oxygen demands, maximal coronary blood flow declines with age. As a result, older adults are subject to "demand ischemia" (ie, myocardial ischemia precipitated by a sudden increase in myocardial oxygen demand, eg, due to tachycardia or severe hypertension), even in the absence of coronary artery disease (CAD). In addition, because endothelial dysfunction contributes to the pathogenesis and progression of atherosclerosis, age-related endothelial dysfunction provides "fertile soil" for development of CAD and peripheral arterial disease. Of note, endothelium-independent vasodilation appears to be unaffected by age, so that the vascular response to exogenous nitrates, such as nitroglycerin, is similar in older and younger adults.

Aging is associated with myriad changes in peripheral responsiveness to neurohumoral stimulation. Among these, perhaps the most important from the cardiovascular perspective is diminished responsiveness of the carotid baroreceptors. As a result, older adults have decreased capacity to rapidly adjust heart rate, blood pressure, and cardiac output in response to abrupt changes in cerebral blood flow, as occurs, for example, during postural changes. Impaired baroreceptor responsiveness thus contributes to orthostatic hypotension and, consequently, to falls and syncope in older adults. Moreover, the age-related predisposition to orthostasis is aggravated by many medications commonly used to treat cardiovascular disorders, including diuretics, β-blockers, and vasodilators.

In healthy older adults, the changes described above have modest effects on cardiac hemodynamics and performance at rest; resting heart rate, ejection fraction, stroke volume, and cardiac output are well preserved even at very advanced age. However, the capacity of the cardiovascular system to respond to increased demands associated with exercise or illness decreases as age increases. As a result, peak aerobic capacity, as assessed by maximal oxygen consumption (Vo_2 max), declines inexorably with age. In the Baltimore Longitudinal Study on Aging, for example, maximal oxygen consumption in healthy men and women ≥80 years old without cardiovascular disease was roughly equivalent to that in middle-aged adults with New York Heart Association functional class II heart failure. Moreover, limited cardiovascular reserve renders older adults more vulnerable to cardiac complications, especially ischemia, heart failure, arrhythmias, shock, and death, in the context of cardiac or noncardiac stressors, such as uncontrolled hypertension, infections, surgical procedures, or anemia.

Age-related changes in other organ systems have important implications for diagnosis and treatment of cardiovascular disorders in older adults. These changes interact with the cardiovascular system to substantially alter the clinical features, response to therapy, and prognosis of older adults with prevalent cardiovascular diseases.

CARDIOVASCULAR RISK FACTORS

In general, the 4 major risk factors for cardiovascular disease—hypertension, diabetes mellitus, dyslipidemia, and smoking—exert significant influence on cardiovascular risk, even in older adults. In addition, because the incidence and prevalence of cardiovascular diseases are higher in older than in younger individuals, the absolute number of cases attributable to a given risk factor tends to increase with age. Moreover, because the prevalence of hypertension, diabetes mellitus, and dyslipidemia all increase with age, older adults are more likely to have multiple risk factors that act in concert with age-related cardiovascular changes to promote development and progression of heart and vascular disorders.

Hypertension

Pulse pressure (the difference between systolic and diastolic blood pressure) increases with age, and isolated systolic hypertension is the dominant form of hypertension in older adults, especially women. In the Framingham Heart Study and other epidemiologic studies, increased systolic blood pressure was identified as the strongest risk factor for incident cardiovascular disease in older adults, including those >80 years old (SOE=A). In some but not all studies, pulse pressure was equivalent or stronger than systolic blood pressure as a marker for cardiovascular risk. Although the prevalence of diastolic hypertension declines with age, its presence nevertheless confers increased cardiovascular risk independent of the systolic blood pressure, particularly in men.

Diabetes Mellitus

The prevalence of diabetes mellitus increases with age, at least up to age 80, and approximately half of all patients with diabetes in the United States are ≥65 years old. As in younger individuals, the impact of diabetes on cardiovascular risk is greater in older women than in older men. In the Framingham Heart Study, for example, the adjusted risk for incident coronary heart disease was 2.1 in older women with diabetes compared with 1.4 in older men with diabetes. Notably, the excess risk associated with diabetes was greater in both men and women >65 years old than in younger individuals.

Dyslipidemia

Population mean total serum cholesterol levels increase in men until approximately age 70 and then level off. In women, total cholesterol levels tend to rise rapidly after menopause and average 15–20 mg/dL higher than in men after age 60. Low-density lipoprotein (LDL) cholesterol levels track with total cholesterol levels in men and women, while high-density lipoprotein (HDL) cholesterol levels average about 10 mg/dL higher in women than in men throughout adult life. The strength of association between total cholesterol and LDL-cholesterol levels and incident CAD declines with age, especially after age 80, in part because of the confounding effects of comorbid conditions and nutritional factors. Nevertheless, low HDL-cholesterol levels (<40 mg/dL in men, <50 mg/dL in women) and high total cholesterol to HDL-cholesterol ratios (≥5.5 in men, ≥5 in women) remain independently associated with coronary events among adults at least up to age 85 years (SOE=A). In addition, clinical trials have demonstrated beneficial effects from lipid-lowering therapy with statins in moderate- and high-risk patients, ie, those with established coronary heart disease, diabetes, or multiple other risk factors (cerebrovascular or peripheral vascular disease, smoking, hypertension) up to 85 years of age (SOE=A). The value, however, of lipid-lowering therapy for primary prevention of cardiovascular disease in older adults, especially those >80–85 years old, remains uncertain.

Smoking

Unlike other risk factors, the prevalence of smoking declines with age, in part because of successful smoking cessation and in part because of premature deaths attributable to smoking. In 2013, approximately 10.6% of men and 7.5% of women ≥65 years old in the United States were active smokers, declining to <5% among individuals >85 years old. In most but not all studies, smoking remains a strong and independent risk factor for fatal and nonfatal cardiovascular disease events among older adults. Importantly, several large observational studies have shown that among older smokers, cessation is associated with substantial reductions in cardiovascular risk, relative to continued smoking, within 2–6 years.

Other Risk Factors

Obesity is associated with increased cardiovascular risk in young and middle-aged people, in part because of its association with hypertension, diabetes mellitus, and dyslipidemia. The importance of obesity as a cardiovascular risk factor among older adults, especially those >80 years old, is less clear. Indeed, among older adults with CAD, heart failure, or renal insufficiency, there is evidence that being overweight or mildly obese (ie, BMI 25–35 kg/m^2) exerts a favorable effect on prognosis, while being underweight (BMI <20 kg/m^2) confers the highest mortality risk (SOE=B). Although severe obesity (BMI ≥40 kg/m^2) is associated with worse outcomes in older adults with established cardiovascular disease, it is not clear that it portends an increased risk of incident cardiovascular disease at advanced age.

Low levels of physical activity are associated with increased risk of cardiovascular and all-cause mortality in people of all ages, and participating in a regular exercise program reduces risk across the age spectrum. Additional benefits of regular exercise include improved functional capacity and quality of life, improved control of other risk factors, and reduced depressive symptoms. Strength and balance training also reduce the risk of falls and fractures in older adults. Thus, in the absence of contraindications, older adults with or without CVD should be encouraged to participate in a regular exercise program that includes both aerobic and strengthening activities.

Increased levels of the inflammatory marker C-reactive protein (CRP) are associated with increased risk of incident CAD events and cardiovascular death in older adults, but the clinical utility of CRP in guiding management is undefined, and routine measurement of CRP is not currently recommended. Similarly, although increased levels of fibrinogen, d-dimer, and plasmin-antiplasmin complex have been associated with increased risk of myocardial infarction in older adults, measurement of these markers to identify patients at increased risk is not recommended.

The utility of assessing coronary artery calcium content by CT scanning is uncertain. Coronary artery calcium scores increase with age, while the correlation of calcium scores with the severity of clinically significant coronary artery stenoses declines with age. Nonetheless, calcium scores ≥100 (Agatston method) are associated with increased risk of incident coronary events in older adults, and higher scores predict greater risk. Despite this, routine use of CT scans to screen for CAD is not recommended, even in patients with multiple risk factors.

In the Cardiovascular Health Study, several subclinical markers of cardiovascular disease identified individuals at increased risk of subsequent cardiovascular events. These included increased carotid artery intima-media thickness assessed by carotid ultrasonography, increased left ventricular mass by echocardiography, borderline or decreased left ventricular ejection fraction, and decreased ankle-brachial index. As with CT scanning, the clinical use and cost-effectiveness of these measures require further study, but in patients with diabetes or multiple other risk factors, the presence of any of these markers may identify those likely to benefit from more aggressive management (SOE=C).

Pre-frailty and frailty are associated with increased risk for developing CVD, possibly because of the interplay of shared mechanisms, including chronic low-level inflammation and insulin resistance. The presence of frailty is also linked to increased morbidity, functional decline, and mortality in older adults with CVD. Whether interventions aimed at reducing frailty can diminish the risk of CVD and, conversely, whether prevention of CVD can reduce the risk of frailty, remain to be determined.

CORONARY ARTERY DISEASE

Epidemiology

In the United States, the incidence of nonfatal and fatal CAD has declined markedly over the past 5 decades. Nonetheless, autopsy studies indicate that up to 70% of adults ≥70 years old have significant CAD, defined as ≥50% obstruction of one or more coronary arteries. In men, the prevalence of clinically diagnosed CAD increases from 6.3% in those 40–59 years old, to 19.9% among those 60–79 years old, and 32.2% after age 80; among women, prevalence increases from 5.6% to 9.7%

and 18.8% across these age ranges. Notably, the annual incidence of nonfatal myocardial infarction (MI) or fatal coronary heart disease is higher in men than in women up to age 85, but after age 85 the reverse is true. The prevalence of angina pectoris increases with age and exceeds 10% in both men and women older than age 80. The incidence of angina pectoris peaks between the ages of 65 and 84 and decreases modestly thereafter. Of an estimated 700,000–800,000 fatal and nonfatal MIs occurring annually in the United States (excluding silent MIs), approximately two-thirds are in adults ≥65 years old, including more than 40% in those ≥75 years old. The proportion of MIs occurring in women increases progressively with age, exceeding 50% in those ≥75 years old. Mortality after acute MI increases exponentially with age, with up to 80% of MI deaths occurring in adults ≥65 years old, and approximately 60% occurring among those ≥75 years old.

ACUTE CORONARY SYNDROMES

The acute coronary syndromes (ACS) comprise unstable angina, non-ST-elevation MI (NSTEMI), and ST-elevation MI (STEMI). Unstable angina and NSTEMI are often considered together, because they are pathophysiologically similar and clinically difficult to distinguish at the time of presentation; the distinction depends on analysis of cardiac biomarker proteins (ie, troponin or creatine kinase).

Presentation

The proportion of patients with ACS who present with chest pain declines with age, especially after age 80, and shortness of breath is the most common initial symptom in patients >80–85 years old. Older ACS patients are more likely than younger patients to present with altered mental status, confusion, dizziness, or syncope, and the prevalence of these symptoms approaches 20% among patients ≥85 years old. The time from onset of symptoms to initial presentation at a medical facility also tends to be longer in older patients, in part due to the decreased prevalence of chest pain, although other factors likely contribute to delays.

The initial ECG is more likely to be nondiagnostic of ACS in older than in younger patients due to the higher prevalence of prior MI, conduction abnormalities (especially left bundle-branch block), left ventricular hypertrophy, and paced rhythm. In addition, the proportion of ACS associated with ST elevation declines with age, further reducing the diagnostic accuracy of the ECG. Importantly, the combination of presentation delays, altered symptomatology, and nondiagnostic ECGs often results in slowed initiation of treatment, thereby limiting the potential benefits of current therapies and contributing to higher complication rates and worse outcomes.

Therapy

All patients with suspected ACS, regardless of age, should immediately receive aspirin 160–325 mg (SOE=A). Oxygen should be administered to maintain an arterial oxygen saturation of at least 92% (SOE=B), but routine use of oxygen in patients with arterial oxygen saturations >92% is of unproven value and may be harmful (SOE=C). Patients with ongoing chest discomfort should receive intravenous nitroglycerin initially, followed by intravenous morphine if nitroglycerin is ineffective. Patients with ACS should also receive oral metoprolol or atenolol in the absence of contraindications (ie, heart rate <45–50 beats per minute, systolic blood pressure <100 mmHg, advanced heart block, moderate or severe heart failure, active bronchospasm). An ACE inhibitor should be administered to hemodynamically stable patients with adequate renal function (estimated creatinine clearance ≥30 mL/min), especially those with left ventricular (LV) systolic dysfunction, clinical heart failure, or both (SOE=A). An angiotensin-receptor blocker (ARB) may be substituted in patients with known intolerance to ACE inhibitors due to cough. Early administration of high-dose statin therapy (eg, atorvastatin 80 mg) has been associated with improved outcomes in some but not all studies, and some experts recommend its routine use; data in patients >75–80 years old are, however, very limited (SOE=C).

In addition to aspirin, current Class I recommendations for antithrombotic therapy in patients with ACS include a combination of a $P2Y_{12}$ inhibitor (clopidogrel 300 mg or 600 mg loading dose followed by 75 mg daily, or ticagrelor 180 mg loading dose followed by 90 mg twice daily) and a parental anticoagulant (enoxaparin, unfractionated heparin, bivalirudin, or fondaparinux). Enoxaparin and bivalirudin require dose reduction in patients with creatinine clearance <30 mL/min. Fondaparinux is not approved in the United States for treatment of ACS, and it is contraindicated in patients with creatinine clearance <30 mL/min and in those weighing <50 kg. Prasugrel and glycoprotein IIb/IIIa inhibitors are not recommended for routine use in ACS but may be appropriate in selected patients. Prasugrel has been associated with increased bleeding risk in patients ≥75 years old. In patients receiving clopidogrel, ticagrelor, or prasugrel who require coronary bypass surgery, these drugs should be discontinued for at least 5 days (clopidogrel, ticagrelor) or 7 days (prasugrel) before surgery, if feasible, to reduce the risk of perioperative bleeding.

Reperfusion therapy with percutaneous coronary intervention (PCI) or a fibrinolytic agent is indicated in patients presenting within 6–12 hours of onset of STEMI (or MI associated with new left bundle-branch block). PCI is the preferred reperfusion strategy; it has been associated with superior outcomes relative to fibrinolysis in patients up to 85 years old, provided the procedure can be performed within 90–120 minutes of the patient's arrival at the hospital. Fibrinolytic therapy reduces mortality in STEMI patients <75 years old, as well as in carefully selected patients ≥75 years old. The risk of intracranial hemorrhage after administration of a fibrinolytic agent increases with age, especially after age 75, and is higher with fibrin-selective agents, such as tissue plasminogen activator or reteplase, than with the nonselective agent streptokinase.

In the setting of non-ST-elevation ACS, early PCI has been associated with improved outcomes in high-risk patients, including older adults, especially those with ongoing ischemia, extensive ECG changes, decreased LV systolic function, or hemodynamic instability (hypotension, tachycardia, heart failure) (SOE=A). In hemodynamically stable older patients without active chest pain or major ECG abnormalities, an initial strategy of either optimal medical therapy or coronary angiography is appropriate. However, invasive management is not recommended in patients with extensive comorbidities in whom the benefits of revascularization are unlikely to outweigh the risks.

Routine use of antiarrhythmic agents, including lidocaine and amiodarone, is not recommended in patients with ACS. Similarly, intravenous magnesium and the combination of glucose-insulin-potassium are of unproven benefit. Dihydropyridine calcium channel blockers are contraindicated in patients with acute MI (SOE=A), and the use of diltiazem and verapamil should be limited to the treatment of supraventricular tachyarrhythmias (including atrial fibrillation and atrial flutter) in patients unresponsive to or intolerant of β-blockers. Digoxin is not indicated for patients with ACS, including those with heart failure, and it also has limited efficacy in treatment of atrial fibrillation.

After documented ACS, patients should be maintained on aspirin, a β-blocker, an ACE inhibitor (or ARB), and a statin in the absence of contraindications (SOE=A). Clopidogrel 75 mg, ticagrelor 90 mg twice daily, or prasugrel 10 mg (for patients <75 years old) is recommended for 12 months for all patients with ACS, whether or not PCI is performed. The duration of dual antiplatelet therapy (DAPT) may be shortened in patients at high risk of bleeding, especially those treated with bare metal stents. Conversely, selected patients may benefit from extended DAPT for up to 30–36 months. Patients with large anterior MIs associated with apical wall motion abnormalities should receive warfarin for 3–6 months to maintain an INR of 2–3 to reduce the risk of mural thrombus formation and embolization.

In addition, aggressive interventions should be undertaken to control all treatable cardiovascular risk factors, and appropriate recommendations about diet, exercise, and sexual activity should be conveyed before hospital discharge. Whenever feasible, patients should be referred to a structured cardiac rehabilitation program, because such programs have been associated with improved functional, emotional, behavioral, and clinical outcomes, including 25%–30% reduction in mortality, and the beneficial effects are at least as great in older as in younger patients (SOE=A).

Chronic Coronary Artery Disease

Presentation and Diagnosis

As is the case with ACS, older patients with chronic CAD are more likely than younger patients to present with exertional fatigue or shortness of breath rather than classical angina pectoris. Withdrawal from usual activities and other atypical manifestations of ischemia are also more common in older adults. In addition, older patients tend to present later in the course of disease, in part because more sedentary lifestyles result in delays in symptom onset or reduced symptom severity. Coronary angiographic studies and autopsy series indicate that older patients tend to have more severe and diffuse CAD, including more triple-vessel and left main CAD, as well as higher prevalence of prior MI and associated LV dysfunction.

The diagnosis of CAD is similar in older and younger adults, except that older adults have, on average, a higher pretest likelihood of having significant coronary obstructions. As a result, false-positive rates on stress tests tend to be lower in older adults, whereas false-negative rates tend to be higher. Diminished exercise capacity can also contribute to higher false-negative rates on exercise stress tests (but not pharmacologic stress tests) in older patients.

In most patients with stable symptoms thought likely to be due to coronary ischemia, a stress test is the initial diagnostic test of choice. When feasible, an exercise test is preferable to a pharmacologic test because it is more physiologic and provides additional information about exercise tolerance and the hemodynamic response to exercise not afforded by pharmacologic testing. In patients unable to exercise because of poor physical conditioning or comorbid illness (especially orthopedic or neurologic disorders), pharmacologic stress tests such as dobutamine echocardiography or adenosine (or regadenoson) thallium (or sestamibi) provide equivalent diagnostic sensitivity and specificity relative to exercise tests.

In patients with accelerating symptoms or a markedly abnormal stress test in whom coronary revascularization may be a suitable therapeutic option, coronary angiography provides definitive information about the precise location and severity of coronary stenoses. Although the risks of coronary angiography increase slightly with age, in experienced centers the procedure can be performed with very low risk of major complications (<2% combined risk of all major complications, including death), even in patients of very advanced age (ie, nonagenarians and older). The risk of serious bleeding is substantially lower when angiography is performed via the transradial rather than the transfemoral approach.

Medical Therapy

Control of risk factors is the foundation for reducing CAD progression in patients of all ages. Diabetes, hypertension, and lipid abnormalities should be treated in accordance with published guidelines. Individuals who smoke should be strongly encouraged to discontinue use of all tobacco products, and behavioral or pharmacologic support, or both, should be routinely offered to all patients who express an interest in smoking cessation. A diet low in saturated fat and cholesterol but high in fruits, vegetables, and whole-grain products should be prescribed, and patients should be encouraged to engage in at least 30 minutes of aerobic exercise, such as walking, at least 5 days per week. Modest weight reduction is advisable in patients who are markedly overweight (BMI ≥35 kg/m^2), but as noted above, the value of weight loss in older adults with lesser degrees of obesity has not been established.

All patients with chronic CAD should receive aspirin 75–162 mg/d (SOE=A). Lower dosages are associated with decreased incidence of GI intolerance and bleeding complications but possibly higher risk of aspirin resistance. In the small percentage of patients with true aspirin allergy or intolerance, clopidogrel 75 mg/d is a reasonable alternative. Although the combination of aspirin with either clopidogrel or warfarin is somewhat more effective than aspirin alone in reducing the risk of ACS in patients with CAD, the additional expense and higher risk of major hemorrhage makes combination therapy less desirable in the absence of specific indications (eg, clopidogrel after PCI or warfarin for atrial fibrillation).

Statin therapy is indicated for all patients with CAD, because statins have been shown to reduce mortality and major cardiac events regardless of the pretreatment LDL-cholesterol level (SOE=A). Current guidelines advocate use of a moderate to high dose statin (eg, atorvastatin 40–80 mg; rosuvastatin 20–40 mg) in older adults with established CAD, and no longer recommend treating to specific targets, such as LDL-cholesterol <100 mg/dL. Statins have been shown to improve clinical outcomes in trials involving CAD patients up to 85 years old, and observational studies support the use of statins for secondary prevention in these patients as well. Although altered hepatic metabolism and the use of multiple medications may place older patients at increased risk of statin-related adverse events, studies have not consistently shown an increased incidence of major statin toxicity in older adults. However, there is some evidence that statin-associated myalgias may be more common in older adults, perhaps because of reduced muscle mass. In addition, long-term statin use is associated with an increased risk of incident diabetes.

ACE inhibitors have been shown to reduce mortality and cardiovascular morbidity in patients up to 85 years old with CAD, peripheral arterial disease, or diabetes. Routine use of ACE inhibitors is recommended for most patients with established CAD in the absence of contraindications (SOE=A). ARBs are an acceptable alternative in patients unable to tolerate ACE inhibitors because of cough. Both classes of agents should be used cautiously, if at all, in patients with estimated creatinine clearance <30 mL/min (unless receiving dialysis). Renal function and serum potassium levels should be monitored when starting or titrating ACE inhibitors or ARBs.

Patients should be treated with a β-blocker for at least 3 years after an MI in the absence of contraindications or limiting adverse effects (SOE=A). In addition, β-blockers are indicated for all patients with an LV ejection fraction <40%, regardless of cause. β-blockers are also the most effective anti-ischemic agents and should be considered the medications of first choice for treatment of angina pectoris or other ischemic symptoms. The dosage of β-blocker should be titrated to maintain a resting heart rate of 50 to no more than 70 beats per minute. Up to 20%–30% of patients are unable to tolerate β-blockers because of adverse events, but there is no convincing evidence that older patients experience more adverse events than younger patients. Ivabradine, a novel agent for slowing heart rate, may be a useful adjunct to β-blockers in patients for whom a heart rate <70 beats per minute cannot be achieved with β-blockers alone. Studies of this drug have included a limited number of patients >75 years old.

Calcium channel blockers are effective anti-ischemic agents, either as first-line therapy in patients unable to take β-blockers, or in combination with either β-blockers or long-acting nitrates. Calcium channel blockers are relatively contraindicated in patients with heart failure or an LV ejection fraction <40%. Leg edema due to venodilation is a common adverse effect of dihydropyridine calcium channel blockers, whereas constipation is more common with the nondihydropyridines, especially verapamil; both problems appear to be more common in older patients.

Long-acting nitrate preparations, such as isosorbide mononitrate, are less effective anti-ischemic agents than β-blockers or calcium channel blockers, in part because of the high rate of tolerance that develops during long-term use and the need for a daily nitrate-free interval of at least several hours. These agents are therefore best used as adjunctive therapy in patients with persistent symptoms despite treatment with a β-blocker, calcium channel blocker, or both. Headache is the most common adverse effect associated with nitrates, but most cases resolve with continued use. Occasionally, patients develop hypotension, dizziness, falls, or syncope, most commonly on initiation of nitrate therapy.

Ranolazine, alone or in combination with conventional antianginal medications, reduces angina and improves exercise tolerance in patients with symptomatic CAD. In addition, the benefits of ranolazine are similar in older and younger patients. Ranolazine is generally well tolerated, although adverse events, including constipation and dizziness, tend to be more common in patients >70 years old than in younger patients. Ranolazine increases the QT interval slightly, but a significant proarrhythmic effect has not been reported.

Revascularization

Adults >65 years old currently account for over half of all PCIs and coronary bypass operations performed in the United States, and both of these procedures are now routinely performed in octogenarians. In patients with chronic CAD, the principal indications for coronary revascularization are to ameliorate symptoms that have not responded to maximally tolerated medical therapy and to improve quality of life. In patients <70 years old, clinical trials conducted more than 20 years ago demonstrated that coronary bypass surgery decreased mortality relative to medical therapy in patients with stenosis of the left main coronary artery, in patients with severe multivessel CAD and LV systolic dysfunction, and in other patient subgroups. The applicability of these findings to the current population of older patients is unclear, especially in light of the availability of more effective medical treatments. In addition, neither coronary bypass surgery nor PCI has been shown to reduce the risk of MI in patients with stable CAD. Conversely, complication rates, including mortality, increase with age after both PCI and coronary bypass surgery, especially among patients >80 years old. Nevertheless, despite the failure of revascularization procedures to reduce mortality or major coronary event rates in most patients with stable CAD, some trials have demonstrated improved symptoms and quality of life in older patients in whom aggressive medical therapy did not elicit an adequate response (SOE=A). Therefore, it is appropriate to offer revascularization on an individualized basis to older patients with persistent symptoms and impaired quality of life attributable to coronary ischemia.

Several trials have compared PCI and coronary bypass surgery in patients who are suitable candidates for either procedure. In general, long-term outcomes for the two approaches are similar. Short-term mortality, major complication rates (including cognitive dysfunction), hospital length of stay, and convalescence time are all increased with surgery relative to PCI, but the need for subsequent revascularization procedures and late mortality are higher after PCI. PCI is also somewhat less effective in relieving symptoms (SOE=A). In selected patients with diabetes and multivessel or left main disease, surgery appears to be associated with better outcomes than either PCI or medical therapy. Overall, in choosing between revascularization procedures, factors favoring PCI include severe CAD that is amenable to complete revascularization by PCI, increased risk of perioperative complications (eg, multiple comorbid conditions, renal insufficiency, frailty), and personal preference to avoid a major operation. Factors favoring bypass surgery include more severe CAD (especially if complete revascularization by PCI is unlikely), high-risk coronary anatomy (eg, left main disease or high-grade stenosis of the proximal left anterior descending artery not suitable for PCI), personal preference to minimize the need for subsequent revascularization procedures, and possibly diabetes. In all cases, the benefits and risks of all major therapeutic options—continued medical therapy, PCI, or bypass surgery—should be discussed in detail with the patient and family before deciding the best course of treatment.

An important consideration in assessing the risk of bypass surgery is the potential for postoperative cognitive impairment and functional decline. Up to 50% of older patients undergoing bypass surgery using extracorporeal circulation experience measurable cognitive impairment after surgery (SOE=B). Although most patients recover completely within 3–6 months, a small percentage demonstrate persistent cognitive dysfunction. Functional decline is also common after major cardiac surgery, and return to the preoperative functional status often takes several months; some patients experience irreversible functional loss. To minimize functional deficits, rehabilitation should be started in the hospital as soon as possible after surgery, and patients should be referred to a structured cardiac rehabilitation program after hospital discharge whenever possible.

VALVULAR HEART DISEASE

Valvular heart diseases include aortic stenosis (AS), aortic regurgitation (AR), mitral stenosis (MS), and mitral regurgitation (MR).

Epidemiology

The prevalence of AS increases with age, approaching 15% in octogenarians, and AS is the most common valvular abnormality requiring intervention in older adults. AS in patients >70 years old is usually due to fibrosis and calcification of a previously normal trileaflet aortic valve, rather than to a congenitally bicuspid valve or rheumatic disease, which are the most common causes in middle-aged adults.

AR may be acute or chronic, and the incidence of both increases with age. Although up to 30% of older adults have some degree of AR detectable by echocardiography, in most cases it is mild or moderate in severity, and only rarely is it severe enough to require surgical intervention. The most common causes of acute AR in older adults include infective endocarditis, dissection of the ascending aorta, malfunction of a previously implanted prosthetic valve (eg, dehiscence or thrombosis), and chest trauma. Chronic AR may be due to pathology of the valvular apparatus (eg, calcific or rheumatic valve disease, prior endocarditis, chronic malfunction of a valve prosthesis) or to dilatation of the aortic root resulting in poor coaptation of the valve leaflets (eg, from ascending aortic root aneurysm, sinus of Valsalva aneurysm, chronic ascending aortic dissection).

Rheumatic MS is uncommon in older adults in the United States, but occasionally patients in their 70s or 80s will present with symptoms attributable to previously undiagnosed rheumatic disease. Alternatively, the diagnosis may be established incidentally when a patient undergoes echocardiography for another reason (eg, new-onset atrial fibrillation). More commonly, MS in older adults is due to nonrheumatic calcification of the mitral valve annulus and subvalvular apparatus, leading to a narrowed orifice and decreased excursion of the valve leaflets.

MR of at least mild severity is present in up to one-third of older adults, but only a small proportion require surgical intervention. As with AR, MR may be acute or chronic. Causes of acute MR include papillary muscle dysfunction or rupture due to acute myocardial infarction, rupture of chordae tendinae related to myxomatous degeneration (ie, mitral valve prolapse), and destruction of the valvular apparatus due to infective endocarditis. Chronic MR may be due to myxomatous degeneration, annular dilatation associated with ischemic or nonischemic dilated cardiomyopathy, mitral annular calcification, rheumatic mitral valve disease, or prior endocarditis.

Diagnosis

The echocardiogram is the procedure of choice for diagnosing valvular disorders. For AS, it is essential for assessing disease severity, evaluating left ventricular function, and determining the presence of associated valvular lesions. Moderate AS is indicated by an aortic jet velocity (AJV) of 3–4 meters/second or an aortic valve area (AVA) of 1–1.5 cm^2; severe AS is indicated by an AJV >4 meters/second or AVA <1 cm^2. Occasionally, technical considerations or the presence of severe LV dysfunction preclude accurate echocardiographic assessment of AS severity; in these cases, right- and left-heart catheterization is definitive.

In patients with acute severe AR, echocardiography demonstrates a short duration AR jet with rapid deceleration, and premature closure of the mitral valve. In patients with severe chronic AR, the AR jet is typically more prominent and of longer duration, often persisting throughout diastole. The left ventricle is usually dilated and shows signs of diastolic volume overload. In advanced cases, there may be evidence of LV systolic dysfunction, as evidenced by a reduced ejection fraction.

Echocardiography is the definitive test for diagnosing MS, quantifying disease severity, and evaluating for the presence of other valvular lesions, especially MR. Severe MS is indicated by a mitral valve area <1 cm^2.

Echocardiography with Doppler assists in determining the cause and severity of either acute or chronic MR. Echocardiography also provides important information about left ventricular size and function, left atrial size, pulmonary artery pressure, and the presence and severity of other valvular lesions.

Clinical Features and Treatment

See Table 49.3.

TRANSCATHETER AORTIC VALVE REPLACEMENT (TAVR)

Until recently, surgical aortic valve replacement (SAVR) was the only effective treatment for severe AS, and numerous studies have demonstrated excellent outcomes after SAVR in appropriately selected older adults, including octogenarians. However, many older patients are either not suitable candidates for SAVR or decline to undergo the procedure due to high perioperative risk attributable to comorbidity or frailty. In the past few years, transcatheter aortic valve replacement (TAVR) with a bioprosthesis has been shown to be associated with improved outcomes relative to medical therapy in older adults who are not candidates for SAVR. TAVR is performed through an arteriotomy

Table 49.3—Cardiac Valvular Conditions

Condition	Symptoms	Findings	Treatment
Aortic stenosis (AS)	Angina, DOE, heart failure, light-headedness, presyncope/syncope	*Physical examination*: mid/late systolic ejection murmur radiating to carotids, S4 gallop, left ventricular heave *ECG*: LVH	*Medical*: no effective therapy *Percutaneous*: transcatheter aortic valve replacement in selected patients at intermediate to high surgical risk[a] *Surgical*: AVR[b] for severe AS with symptoms; bioprosthetic valves preferred in older patients[c]
Aortic regurgitation (AR)	Can be acute or chronic; asymptomatic or minimally symptomatic in mild/moderate AR; DOE, heart failure, angina in severe AR	*Physical examination*: ↑ pulse pressure, bounding/collapsing pulses, diastolic decrescendo murmur, systolic ejection murmur *ECG*: LVH (severe chronic AR), tachycardia (acute AR) *Chest radiograph*: cardiomegaly (severe chronic AR), pulmonary congestion (acute AR)	*Medical* (less severe cases): control of hypertension, preferably with a dihydropyridine calcium channel blocker, ACE inhibitor, or angiotensin receptor blocker (SOE=B); β-blocker in patients with symptoms or LV systolic dysfunction (SOE=B) *Surgical*: AVR[b] indicated for acute severe AR, symptomatic severe chronic AR, asymptomatic severe chronic AR with LVEF <50% or left ventricular end-systolic dimension ≥5 cm (all SOE=B)
Mitral stenosis (MS)	Gradually worsening DOE early, orthopnea and leg edema late, progressive decline in exercise capacity, fatigue	*Physical examination*: early diastolic opening snap, low-pitched ("rumbling") diastolic murmur at apex, pulmonary hypertension, right heart failure	*Medical*: diuretics for volume overload and β-blockers for decreased exercise tolerance associated with tachycardia *Percutaneous*: balloon valvuloplasty safe and effective, but most older adults are not good candidates because of extensive calcification and commissural fusion or concomitant mitral regurgitation *Surgical*: MVR[b] effective but with 5%–15% operative mortality in older patients
Mitral regurgitation (MR)	Can be acute or chronic; marked shortness of breath, orthopnea in acute severe MR; progressive DOE in chronic MR	*Physical examination*: pulmonary rales, tachycardia, narrow pulse pressure, S3, and short harsh systolic murmur in acute severe MR; holosystolic murmur radiating to axilla, S3, pulmonary hypertension, right heart failure in chronic severe MR	*Medical*: medical therapy as for heart failure with systolic dysfunction in patients with symptomatic chronic MR and LVEF <60% who are not candidates for intervention (SOE=B) *Percutaneous*: transcatheter mitral valve repair in selected patients (SOE=B) *Surgical*: mitral valve repair preferred over MVR[b] (SOE=B); bioprosthetic valves[c] preferred over mechanical valves in older patients; all effective with 5%–15% operative mortality in older patients. Operative mortality is lower for repair than replacement. Surgical intervention is indicated: ■ Urgently for acute severe MR with heart failure ■ Symptomatic patients with severe chronic MR and LVEF >30% (SOE=B) ■ Asymptomatic patients with severe chronic MR and LVEF 30%–60% and/or left ventricular end-systolic dimension ≥4 cm (SOE=B) ■ When mitral valve repair is deemed likely to be successful in asymptomatic patients with severe chronic MR and an LVEF ≥60% (SOE=B) ■ In patients with severe chronic MR and pulmonary artery systolic pressure >50 mmHg or new-onset atrial fibrillation with high likelihood of successful MV repair (SOE=B)

NOTE: DOE = dyspnea on exertion; LVH = left ventricular hypertrophy; LVEF = left ventricular ejection fraction; AVR = aortic valve replacement; MVR = mitral valve replacement

[a] Based on comorbidities and frailty.
[b] Older adults being considered for AVR and MVR should have coronary angiography first, because significant coronary artery disease is present in >50% of patients.
[c] After AVR with a bioprosthetic valve, antithrombotic therapy with aspirin 75–100 mg/d is recommended in the absence of risk factors for thromboembolism (SOE=B). After MVR with a bioprosthetic valve, anticoagulation to maintain INR of 2–3 is recommended for 3 months (SOE=C), followed by maintenance therapy with aspirin 75–100 mg/d in the absence of risk factors for thromboembolism (SOE=B).

or transapically and does not require either a median sternotomy or extracorporeal circulation. As a result, hospital length of stay tends to be shorter and functional recovery faster than with SAVR. Vascular complications and stroke are more common after TAVR; conversely, major bleeding and atrial fibrillation are more common after SAVR. One year outcomes, including survival and quality of life, are similar after either procedure, and benefits are maintained for at least 3–5 years.

INFECTIVE ENDOCARDITIS

Since the early part of the 20th century, infective endocarditis has undergone a transformation from a disease of young adults with rheumatic or congenital valve anomalies to one of older adults with degenerative valve disorders or prosthetic valves. Native-valve endocarditis is most commonly caused by *Streptococcus viridans* or *Staphylococcus aureus*. Enterococcal species and gram-negative bacilli, including gastrointestinal and genitourinary organisms, are also common causes of native valve endocarditis in older adults. Less frequently, infections are due to HACEK organisms (a group of gram-negative rods that primarily inhabit the oral cavity and include the genera *Haemophilus*, *Actinobacillus*, *Cardiobacterium*, *Eikenella*, and *Kingella*) or other atypical pathogens. Coagulase-negative staphylococci are a common cause of prosthetic-valve endocarditis, particularly in the first 60 days after valve replacement.

Endocarditis is often difficult to diagnose in older adults. Fever is less common than in younger patients, occurring in 55% versus 80%, respectively, as is leukocytosis, occurring in 25% versus 60%. Rates of positive blood cultures do not vary by age, but the sensitivity of transthoracic echocardiography is reduced to 45% in older patients (versus 75% in younger patients) because of the increased prevalence of calcific valve disease and prosthetic valves. Transesophageal echocardiography (TEE) improves the diagnostic yield for infective endocarditis, but the lack of positive findings on TEE does not exclude the diagnosis. TEE is of particular value in managing *S aureus* bacteremia. Thus, evidence for endocarditis on TEE supports prolonged antibiotic administration (4–6 weeks) versus short-course (2 weeks) therapy in the absence of endocarditis. TEE, however, is semi-invasive and costly.

Antibiotic treatment of infective endocarditis is directed at the identified pathogen or at the most likely causes if blood cultures are negative. Therapy is administered intravenously for 2–6 weeks. Surgical therapy should be considered in the presence of severe valvular dysfunction, recurrent emboli, marked heart failure, myocardial abscess formation, vegetations >1 cm in diameter, or fungal endocarditis. Surgery should also be considered when appropriate antibiotic treatment does not yield negative blood cultures. In the absence of major comorbidities, age does not appear to play a major role in mortality risk, with a 2-year survival of 75% for infective endocarditis in all age groups.

Recommendations for preventing endocarditis after dental procedures focus on providing prophylaxis only in the highest-risk patients (ie, those with a prosthetic valve, prior endocarditis, certain congenital heart diseases, or cardiac transplantation with valve disease). Recent guidelines have eliminated recommendations for prophylaxis for those undergoing gastrointestinal or genitourinary procedures.

CARDIAC ARRHYTHMIAS

Epidemiology

Age-related changes in the cardiac conduction system, coupled with the increasing prevalence of cardiovascular diseases at older age, lead to a progressive increase in the incidence and prevalence of conduction abnormalities and heart rhythm disturbances in older adults. In a cohort of 1,372 healthy adults ≥65 years old participating in the Baltimore Longitudinal Study on Aging (BLSA), >90% of men and women demonstrated supraventricular ectopic activity and >75% demonstrated ventricular ectopic activity on 24-hour ambulatory electrocardiographic recordings. In addition, almost 50% of men and women exhibited short runs of supraventricular tachycardia, and 13% of men and 4% of women had ≥3 consecutive ventricular premature depolarizations. In contrast, <0.5% of men and women in this cohort had runs of ≥5 beats of ventricular tachycardia. In a related study, approximately 4% of women >60 years old developed runs of ≥4 atrial premature beats during an exercise test, and the proportion of men with the same abnormality was found to increase with age, approaching 15% in those ≥80 years old.

In the absence of structural heart disease, the presence of supraventricular and ventricular arrhythmias had no effect on mortality or the incidence of cardiac events in BLSA participants, except that exercise-induced supraventricular tachycardia was associated with an increased risk of developing atrial fibrillation during follow-up. Conversely, in patients with prevalent cardiovascular disease, increased ventricular (but not supraventricular) ectopy was associated with an increased risk of cardiovascular mortality. In addition, although patients with preexisting atrial fibrillation were excluded from the BLSA ambulatory monitoring study, atrial fibrillation, whether paroxysmal or persistent, has been shown to be an independent predictor of increased mortality in both men and women (SOE=A).

Age-related degenerative changes in and around the sinoatrial and atrioventricular (AV) nodes lead to an increase in bradyarrhythmias with advancing age. Although resting heart rate is unaffected by age in healthy individuals, the incidence and prevalence of sinus node dysfunction ("sick sinus syndrome") and AV-nodal block increase progressively with age. As a result, >75% of permanent pacemakers are implanted in patients ≥65 years old, and approximately half are in patients ≥75 years old. The prevalence of infranodal conduction disorders, including left anterior fascicular block and left and right bundle-branch block, also increases with age.

Atrial Fibrillation

Atrial fibrillation (AF) is the most common sustained arrhythmia encountered in clinical practice. The incidence and prevalence of AF increase exponentially with age, such that the prevalence of AF in octogenarians is approximately 10%. Among older patients with valvular heart disease or HF, the prevalence of AF is even higher, approaching 30%. The prevalence of AF is higher in men than in women, and higher in whites than in other racial and ethnic groups. Currently, about half of patients with AF are ≥75 years old, and it is projected that by 2050 half will be ≥80 years old. AF confers relative risks of mortality of 1.10–1.15 in men and 1.20–1.25 in women.

The proportion of strokes attributable to AF also increases exponentially with age: AF accounts for about 1.5% of strokes in patients 50–59 years old but 23.5% of strokes in patients 80–89 years old. In addition, women with AF are at increased risk of stroke relative to men, especially after age 75, and the relative risk of stroke in women compared with that in men is approximately 1.8 in this age group.

Clinical Features

Symptoms related to AF are highly variable. Most commonly, patients experience palpitations, shortness of breath, or impaired exercise tolerance. However, some patients are entirely asymptomatic, whereas others present with acute pulmonary edema. Less commonly, stroke, transient ischemic attack, or an acute coronary syndrome may be the initial manifestation. Physical examination reveals an irregularly irregular rhythm with heart rates ranging from <60 beats per minute (eg, in patients with AV nodal dysfunction and in those taking a β-blocker) to >150 beats per minute. Increased systolic blood pressure is a common but nonspecific finding. Pulmonary crackles may be present in patients with acute HF, whereas a heart murmur may be heard in patients with valvular heart disease. Rarely, an enlarged or nodular thyroid may be detected, or signs of deep venous thrombosis may be evident, reflecting the association of hyperthyroidism and venous thromboembolism with this dysrhythmia.

Diagnosis and Evaluation

In patients with ongoing AF, the standard 12-lead ECG is diagnostic. Additional laboratory studies should include evaluation of serum electrolytes (especially potassium and magnesium) and an assessment of thyroid function. A transthoracic echocardiogram is indicated in all patients with new-onset AF to evaluate LV size and function, left atrial size, pulmonary artery pressure, and the cardiac valves. Further evaluation in selected cases might include a chest radiograph, serial cardiac biomarker proteins to exclude acute MI, a brain natriuretic peptide level, a d-dimer level, lower-extremity venous Dopplers, and an evaluation for pulmonary embolism.

Management

The objectives of therapy for AF include relieving symptoms and minimizing risk of thromboembolic events, particularly stroke. The principal strategies for relieving symptoms are control of heart rate and maintenance of normal sinus rhythm. Several clinical trials comparing "rate control" with "rhythm control" have consistently demonstrated that in patients who are asymptomatic or minimally symptomatic, therapy directed at controlling the heart rate with AV-nodal blocking agents such as a β-blocker, diltiazem, verapamil, or digoxin, alone or in combination, is associated with fewer hospitalizations and favorable trends in stroke and mortality rates relative to therapy directed at maintaining sinus rhythm using antiarrhythmic medications (SOE=A). Based on these findings, rate control in conjunction with systemic anticoagulation is the preferred treatment for AF patients with minimal or no symptoms. In general, β-blockers are the most effective agents for rate control, followed by diltiazem and verapamil. Digoxin is not recommended as first-line therapy but may be a useful adjunct in patients with persistently increased heart rates despite β-blockers or rate-lowering calcium channel blockers. In the Rate Control Efficacy (RACE-II) trial, lenient heart rate control (resting heart rate <110 beats per minute) was not inferior to strict heart rate control (resting heart rate <80 beats per minute) with respect to major clinical outcomes in patients with chronic AF (mean age 68 years). Based on these findings, guidelines have been modified to reflect the safety and efficacy of lenient rate control.

Patients who experience significant shortness of breath, fatigue, or exercise intolerance attributable to AF may be best managed with antiarrhythmic drug therapy aimed at maintaining sinus rhythm. Selection of an antiarrhythmic agent is challenging. Amiodarone is the most effective medication available, but it is associated with multiple adverse events (eg, thyroid dysfunction, neurologic disorders, pulmonary toxicity, ophthalmologic disturbances, liver function abnormalities), some potentially serious, as well as numerous drug interactions. Dronedarone, an amiodarone analogue, is less effective than amiodarone but has fewer adverse events. However, dronedarone is contraindicated in patients with advanced heart failure, and it may be associated with increased mortality, stroke, and hospitalizations for heart failure in older patients with chronic (permanent) AF. Sotalol is less effective than amiodarone and is contraindicated in patients with significant renal insufficiency. Flecainide and propafenone are contraindicated in patients with CAD or heart failure. Quinidine and procainamide have limited efficacy and are accompanied by relatively frequent adverse events, whereas disopyramide is generally contraindicated in older adults because of its anticholinergic effects. Dofetilide is moderately effective, but use of this drug is restricted in the United States, and it may be dispensed only by pharmacies and health care settings that are specially certified. Initiation of the drug requires hospitalization for a minimum of 2–3 days. Alternatives to antiarrhythmic drug therapy for maintenance of sinus rhythm include catheter ablation of the arrhythmogenic foci, usually through pulmonary vein isolation, and the surgical maze procedure. Pulmonary vein isolation has been associated with "cure" rates of >80% in younger patients with paroxysmal AF, but experience is limited with this procedure in older patients with persistent AF. Nonetheless, catheter ablation may be considered in older patients with refractory symptoms attributable to AF in whom antiarrhythmic drug treatment has not been successful and left atrial size is normal or only mildly increased. The maze procedure results in long-term maintenance of sinus rhythm in >90% of cases but requires open heart surgery; however, it is a reasonable option in older patients with AF undergoing open heart surgery for other indications if a surgeon with expertise in performing the procedure is available.

All older patients with paroxysmal or persistent AF require stroke prophylaxis, regardless of whether a rate-control or rhythm-control strategy is adopted. Prior to 2010, the two main options for stroke prophylaxis were warfarin titrated to maintain an INR of 2–3 and aspirin 75–325 mg/d, alone or in combination with clopidogrel. In patients with nonvalvular AF, numerous trials have shown that warfarin reduces the risk of stroke by 65%–70%, whereas aspirin reduces the risk by 20%–25% (SOE=A). In the past 5 years, 4 novel oral anticoagulants (NOACs) have been approved for use in the United States: dabigatran, rivaroxaban, apixaban, and edoxaban. The NOACs are all at least as effective as warfarin for stroke prevention in patients with nonvalvular AF, and are not inferior to warfarin with respect to major bleeding complications. In addition, dabigratan, rivaroxaban, and apixaban (but not edoxaban) have been associated with reduced risk of intracranial hemorrhage (ICH) relative to warfarin. The NOACs are administered in fixed dosages (with adjustment for renal function as described below) and do not require routine monitoring of INR or other coagulation parameters. The NOACs also have fewer interactions with other medications and foods than does warfarin. Disadvantages of the NOACs include inability to monitor level of anticoagulation and higher cost. Dabigatran and rivaroxaban are associated with higher risk of GI bleeding than warfarin, and dabigatran may also be associated with higher risk of MI. Recently, idarucizumab, an antibody fragment, was approved by the FDA as an antidote to dabigatran, and agents to reverse the anticoagulant effects of the other NOACs are under development.

Selection of a strategy for stroke prophylaxis is often challenging in older adults, who are at higher risk of both stroke and hemorrhagic complications than are younger patients. To aid in the decision-making process, it is helpful to stratify AF patients according to stroke risk, for which the $CHADS_2$ and CHA_2DS_2-VASc scores are widely used. $CHADS_2$ assigns 1 point for chronic heart failure, hypertension, age ≥75 years, and diabetes, and 2 points for prior stroke or transient ischemic attack. Annual stroke risk increases from about 2% in patients with a $CHADS_2$ score of 0 to about 18% in patients with a $CHADS_2$ score of 6. CHA_2DS_2-VASc is similar to $CHADS_2$ but assigns 2 points for age ≥75 years, 1 point for age 65–74 years, 1 point for vascular disease (coronary, peripheral, or aortic), and 1 point for female sex. CHA_2DS_2-VASc, has been shown to be more accurate than the $CHADS_2$ score in identifying patients at low risk of stroke. In general, patients with a CHA_2DS_2-VASc score of 0 are at very low risk of stroke, and the risks of systemic anticoagulation outweigh the benefits; therefore, either no antithrombotic treatment or aspirin only is appropriate in these patients. Similarly, patients with a CHA_2DS_2-VASc score of 1 are at relatively low risk of stroke, and current guidelines indicate that such patients can be managed with aspirin, warfarin, a NOAC, or no antithrombotic therapy. However, all women ≥65 years old and all men ≥75 years old have a CHA_2DS_2-VASc score of at least 2, and in most of these cases the beneficial effects of systemic anticoagulation outweigh the risks. In patients 65–74 years old who are not considered candidates for anticoagulation, the addition of clopidogrel to aspirin reduces the risk of stroke but increases the risk of bleeding. Importantly, among patients ≥75 years old, the value of aspirin, alone or in combination with clopidogrel, for reducing the risk of thromboembolic events is uncertain.

One of the most common reasons for not prescribing anticoagulation for older patients with AF is concern about the risk of falls and the potential for serious bleeding complications, particularly ICH. However, in most older patients with a CHA_2DS_2-VASc score ≥2, the risk of thromboembolic stroke exceeds the risk of fall-related intracranial bleeding, and it has been estimated that a patient would have to fall almost 300 times in 1 year for the risk of ICH to outweigh the benefit of stroke prevention. Therefore, in most cases the perception of high fall risk alone is insufficient justification for withholding anticoagulation.

The NOAC dabigatran is a direct thrombin inhibitor that is more effective than warfarin for reducing stroke risk and is also associated with a lower risk of intracranial hemorrhage. After oral administration, dabigatran has a predictable anticoagulant effect. As a result, it can be given at a fixed dose without laboratory monitoring. Drug-drug and drug-food interactions are substantially less frequent than with warfarin. Disadvantages of dabigatran include twice-daily dosing, relatively short duration of action (ie, missing doses may lead to subtherapeutic anticoagulation), inability to routinely monitor level of anticoagulation (the INR is unreliable and not recommended), requirement for dosage adjustment in patients with renal impairment (see below), and higher cost than warfarin. The most common adverse events with dabigatran are bleeding and dyspepsia, and older adults may be at increased risk of serious bleeding. The recommended dosage of dabigatran for patients with relatively preserved renal function (creatinine clearance ≥30 mL/min) is 150 mg q12h. For patients with creatinine clearances of 15–30 mL/min, the recommended dosage is 75 mg q12h. Dabigatran is not recommended for patients with more severe renal insufficiency.

Rivaroxaban, apixaban, and edoxaban are orally active reversible inhibitors of coagulation factor Xa. In a large randomized trial comparing rivaroxaban with warfarin in more than 14,000 patients with AF, of whom 77% were 65 years or older and 38% were 75 years or older, rivaroxaban was found to be not inferior to warfarin with respect to both prevention of thromboembolic events and bleeding complications. Results were similar in older and younger patients. Although bleeding risk was higher in older patients, the net benefit was similar across the age spectrum. The recommended dosage of rivaroxaban is 20 mg/d for patients with a creatinine clearance ≥50 mL/min and 15 mg/d for patients with a creatinine clearance of 15–50 mL/min; rivaroxaban is not recommended for patients with more severe renal impairment.

Apixaban was compared with warfarin in a randomized trial involving more than 18,000 patients with AF (median age 70 years, 31% ≥75 years old). Overall, apixaban was superior to warfarin with respect to thromboembolic events, major bleeding complications, and mortality. Results were consistent across age groups, and there was a clear advantage of apixaban both in patients 65–74 years old and in those ≥75 years old. The standard dose of apixaban is 5 mg twice daily; the dose should be reduced to 2.5 mg twice daily in patients with 2 or more of the following: age ≥80 years, weight ≤60 kg, and creatinine ≥1.5 mg/dL.

The most recent NOAC to gain FDA approval is edoxaban. In a randomized trial involving 21,105 patients with AF (median age 70 years, 40% ≥75 years), edoxaban was not inferior to warfarin with respect to prevention of stroke or systemic embolization, and it was superior to warfarin with respect to bleeding complications. Death from cardiovascular causes was also significantly lower in the edoxaban group. Results were similar in patients ≥75 years to those in younger patients. The dose of edoxaban is 60 mg/d for patients with creatinine clearance 50–95 mL/min and 30 mg/d for those with creatinine clearance 15–50 mL/min; edoxaban is contraindicated in patients with creatinine clearance <15 mL/min or >95 mL/min.

As with other antithrombotic agents, the main adverse events associated with rivaroxaban, apixaban, and edoxaban are bleeding complications. Other adverse events appear to be relatively infrequent, although additional experience is needed in a broader range of older patients with higher comorbidity burden than those enrolled in the clinical trials. These agents cost substantially more than generic warfarin. Despite their costs and complications, it seems likely that newer antithrombotic agents will play an increasingly important role in the management of older patients with AF over the next several years.

Other Supraventricular Arrhythmias

Atrial flutter most often occurs in older patients with concomitant AF, and for this reason management is similar to that for AF as discussed above. Occasionally, patients have incessant atrial flutter without evidence of AF. Patients with symptomatic persistent atrial flutter in whom response to medical therapy is not satisfactory should be considered for catheter ablation of the atrial flutter focus. This procedure is successful in alleviating atrial flutter in >70% of cases, although some patients subsequently develop atrial fibrillation.

Atrial tachycardia, AV-nodal reentrant tachycardia, accessory pathway–mediated supraventricular tachycardia, and multifocal atrial tachycardia are less common than AF and atrial flutter in older patients, especially after age 75. Management is similar for older and younger patients with these arrhythmias and generally involves treatment of the underlying condition and pharmacotherapy aimed at rate control or arrhythmia suppression. In selected patients with recurrent symptomatic episodes, antiarrhythmic medications or catheter ablation may be considered.

Ventricular Arrhythmias

In general, frequent ventricular premature beats, ventricular couplets, and short runs of nonsustained ventricular tachycardia require no specific therapy unless highly symptomatic, in which case β-blockers are the medications of first choice. Patients with longer episodes of ventricular tachycardia associated with dizziness or syncope should be referred to a cardiologist or electrophysiologist for consideration of antiarrhythmic drug therapy or an implantable cardiac defibrillator. In addition, patients with New York Heart Association class II–III heart failure, an LV ejection fraction of <35%, and a remaining life expectancy of at least 1 year may be considered for an implantable cardiac defibrillator, regardless of whether ventricular arrhythmias are clinically manifest.

Bradyarrhythmias

Increasing age is associated with a progressive increase in the incidence and prevalence of bradyarrhythmias. Patients with mild bradycardia (resting heart rate 50–60 beats per minute) are often asymptomatic; indeed, bradycardia may protect against the development of angina pectoris in patients with CAD. Patients with more marked bradycardia (resting heart rate 40–50 beats per minute) may experience fatigue, lightheadedness (especially on standing), or reduced exercise tolerance. Presyncope or syncope may occur in patients with profound bradycardia, manifested by a heart rate of <40 beats per minute or asystolic pauses of ≥3 seconds, whether due to sinus node dysfunction or heart block within the AV node or infranodal conduction system.

Diagnostic evaluation of patients with suspected symptomatic bradycardia should start with exclusion of significant electrolyte abnormalities, measurement of the thyrotropin level to exclude hypothyroidism, and a review of the patient's medications (including OTC medications and dietary supplements). The most commonly used medications associated with bradycardia in older adults are β-blockers (including eye drops), diltiazem, verapamil, clonidine, amiodarone and other antiarrhythmic agents, and cholinesterase inhibitors. In patients with orthostatic hypotension, presyncope, or syncope, blood pressure should be measured in the supine, sitting, and standing positions. Detection of significant orthostatic hypotension should prompt a search for potentially treatable causes, including adverse effects of medication(s), dehydration, or autonomic dysfunction (eg, due to diabetes, amyloidosis, parkinsonism, or other neurologic disorders). Patients with otherwise unexplained presyncope or syncope should undergo carotid sinus massage to evaluate for carotid hypersensitivity. An abnormal response to carotid massage is defined as unequivocal reproduction of the patient's symptoms (eg, syncope), asystole ≥3 seconds, or a decrease in systolic blood pressure ≥50 mmHg in the absence of symptoms or ≥30 mmHg in association with symptoms (eg, dizziness, presyncope).

In patients with intermittent symptoms, it is essential to establish a correlation between symptoms and bradyarrhythmias before considering pacemaker implantation. If symptoms occur daily or almost every day, an ambulatory monitor (for 24–48 hours) may be helpful for confirming or excluding bradycardia (or other heart rhythm disorder) as the proximate cause. In patients whose symptoms occur at least once a month (but not daily), a 30-day event monitor may provide a definitive diagnosis. In patients with rare (ie, less than monthly) but recurrent symptoms of a serious nature (eg, syncope with injury), an implantable loop recorder may be considered. These devices, which may be left in place for a year or longer, have increased diagnostic yield in patients with infrequent syncopal events. Head-up tilt testing may be useful in diagnosing vasovagal (neurocardiogenic) syncope in younger patients, but it is of limited use in older adults because of low specificity and a high prevalence of "false-positive" tests.

Invasive electrophysiologic (EP) testing is not usually indicated for the diagnosis of syncope or bradyarrhythmias. However, in patients with recurrent unexplained syncope and a nondiagnostic noninvasive evaluation, EP testing may be helpful, especially in patients with CAD or cardiomyopathy, or with evidence of infranodal conduction system disease (eg, right or left bundle-branch block). In such cases, EP testing may distinguish syncope due to bradycardia (eg, high-grade infranodal AV block) from that due to a tachyarrhythmia (eg, supraventricular tachycardia or sustained monomorphic ventricular tachycardia), thus facilitating appropriate therapy.

Management of bradycardia includes correction of any treatable causes (eg, hypothyroidism) and elimination of potentially offending medications, if possible. In patients with confirmed symptomatic bradycardia not amenable to conservative management, permanent pacemaker implantation is warranted. Class I indications for permanent pacing are listed in Table 49.4. In patients with sinus rhythm and preserved atrioventricular conduction (ie, normal PR interval and narrow QRS complex), atrial pacing is the preferred pacing mode. Patients with sinus rhythm but impaired atrioventricular conduction are often best served

Table 49.4—Class I Indications for Permanent Pacemaker Implantation for Bradyarrhythmias

- Sinus node dysfunction with documented symptomatic bradycardia, including frequent sinus pauses that produce symptoms (SOE=C)
- Symptomatic chronotropic incompetence (inability to increase heart rate commensurate with increased activity level) (SOE=C)
- Symptomatic sinus bradycardia or advanced AV block that results from required drug therapy for medical conditions (SOE=C)
- Third-degree or advanced second-degree AV block associated with symptomatic bradycardia or ventricular arrhythmias presumed to be due to AV block (SOE=C)
- Third-degree or advanced second-degree AV block in awake, symptom-free patients in sinus rhythm with periods of asystole ≥3 seconds or any escape rate <40 beats per minute, or with an escape rhythm that is below the AV node (SOE=C)
- Third-degree or advanced second-degree AV block in awake, symptom-free patients in atrial fibrillation with 1 or more periods of asystole ≥5 seconds (SOE=C)
- Second-degree AV block with associated symptomatic bradycardia (SOE=B)
- Third-degree AV block after catheter ablation of the AV junction (SOE=C)
- Second- or third-degree AV block during exercise in the absence of myocardial ischemia (SOE=C)
- Asymptomatic persistent third-degree AV block with average awake ventricular rates of 40 beats per minute or faster if cardiomegaly or left ventricular dysfunction is present or if the site of block is below the AV node (SOE=B)

by dual-chamber (ie, atrial and ventricular) pacing, whereas patients with bradycardia in the context of atrial fibrillation or atrial flutter should receive a single-chamber ventricular pacemaker. Dual-chamber pacemakers have been associated with reduced incidence of atrial fibrillation and heart failure relative to single-chamber ventricular pacemakers, but beneficial effects on mortality and stroke have not been demonstrated.

Tachy-Brady Syndrome

The tachy-brady syndrome is a common variant of "sick sinus syndrome," in which patients manifest both tachyarrhythmias (most commonly supraventricular tachycardia or atrial fibrillation) and bradyarrhythmias, either or both of which can result in symptoms. Treatment of the tachyarrhythmias with AV-nodal blocking agents or antiarrhythmic medications often exacerbates symptoms related to bradycardia, for which pacemaker implantation may be required.

PERIPHERAL ARTERIAL DISEASE

Peripheral arterial disease (PAD) encompasses disorders of the abdominal aorta, renal and mesenteric arteries, and the iliofemoral-popliteal arterial tree. The prevalence of PAD increases with age and is higher in men than in women. In one study, the prevalence of PAD increased from 5.6% in adults 38–59 years old, to 15.9% in adults 60–69 years old, and to 33.8% in adults 70–82 years old. In another study, the prevalence of symptomatic PAD in nursing-home residents with a mean age of 81 years was 32% in men and 26% in women. In addition to age, risk factors for PAD include hypertension, diabetes, smoking, and to a lesser extent in older adults, family history.

Abdominal aortic aneurysms (AAA) are usually asymptomatic in the early stages. As the aneurysm enlarges, patients may notice abdominal pulsations or experience back pain or abdominal discomfort. Symptoms of lower extremity PAD include claudication with exertion and skin changes related to chronically impaired circulation. In advanced cases, rest pain, ulcers, or dry gangrene may develop. Physical findings associated with PAD may include a pulsatile abdominal mass, bruits over the renal or femoral arteries (or both), diminished or absent peripheral pulses, and skin changes ranging from hair loss and hyperpigmentation to ulcers and gangrene.

Diagnosis

It is estimated that at least 50% of patients with PAD are either asymptomatic or attribute their symptoms to another disorder (eg, arthritis); this proportion is likely even higher in older adults because of a more sedentary lifestyle. Diagnosis of PAD therefore requires a high index of suspicion and a proactive approach. Current guidelines recommend a formal history and physical examination to screen for symptoms and signs of PAD in all adults 50–69 years old with risk factors for atherosclerosis, as well as in all individuals ≥70 years old with or without risk factors (SOE=C). Men ≥60 years old with a family history of AAA and men 65–75 years old who have ever been smokers should undergo an abdominal ultrasound to screen for the presence of AAA (SOE=B).

Individuals with symptoms or physical findings suggestive of PAD should undergo assessment of the ankle-brachial index (ABI), the ratio of the systolic blood pressure obtained at the ankle to the blood pressure obtained over the ipsilateral brachial artery. A normal ABI is 1.0–1.4, and an ABI <0.9 has been reported to be 95% sensitive and 99% specific for leg PAD. An ABI of 0.91–0.99 is considered borderline low, whereas an ABI >1.4 is usually associated with stiff, noncompressible arteries, which are commonly seen in older patients with atherosclerosis or long-standing hypertension. An ABI <0.40 is generally associated with critical PAD and severely impaired perfusion of the distal limb. In most cases, an exercise treadmill test is also recommended, preferably with pre- and postexercise ABIs, to assess the degree of functional impairment.

Patients with moderate or severe symptoms and an abnormal ABI should undergo additional evaluation if percutaneous or surgical revascularization is being contemplated. Imaging procedures that may be useful in selected cases include Doppler flow velocity measurements, ultrasonic duplex scanning, magnetic resonance angiography, and CT angiography. If revascularization is indicated based on symptoms and the results of noninvasive testing, contrast angiography is usually required before performing the revascularization procedure.

Treatment

PAD is considered a CAD risk-equivalent, indicating that patients with PAD have a ≥20% risk of experiencing a new coronary event within 10 years (SOE=A); in patients with comorbid diabetes or established CAD, the risk is even higher. Indeed, most deaths in patients with PAD are attributable to CAD or its complications (eg, heart failure, arrhythmias) rather than to PAD per se. The importance of PAD as a risk marker for CAD provides the rationale for the proactive approach to diagnosis described above, as well as for the aggressive treatment of prevalent cardiovascular risk factors. Thus, older patients with PAD should be treated with a moderate to high dose statin, and blood pressure should be treated in accordance with current guidelines. Smoking cessation should be strongly encouraged, and patients who indicate an interest in quitting should be offered counseling in combination with drug therapy.

In addition to risk factor management, patients with significant lower extremity PAD should engage in a regular exercise program, preferably under supervision (SOE=A). Exercise should include walking for at least 30–45 minutes at least 3 times a week for a minimum of 12 weeks (SOE=A). Data from multiple randomized trials and at least one large meta-analysis indicate that the beneficial effects of exercise on maximal walking capacity exceed those of available pharmacotherapies. In addition, the greatest improvements in walking ability occur in individuals who exercise to near maximal pain threshold for a period of at least 6 months.

Pharmacotherapy for PAD includes aspirin 75–325 mg/d to reduce the risk of MI, stroke, or vascular death (SOE=A). Clopidogrel 75 mg/d is a reasonable alternative to aspirin in selected patients (SOE=B). The combination of aspirin and clopidogrel may be considered in patients at high risk of vascular events and acceptably low risk of bleeding (SOE=B). In addition to antiplatelet therapy, routine treatment with an ACE inhibitor or ARB for the prevention of cardiovascular events is reasonable in patients with symptomatic PAD (SOE=B).

Currently, the only pharmacologic agent that has been shown to improve symptoms and walking distance in patients with claudication is the phosphodiesterase inhibitor (type III) cilostazol. At dosages of 100 mg q12h, cilostazol increases maximal walking distance by 40%–60%, and a therapeutic trial of this agent is recommended for patients with lifestyle-limiting claudication (SOE=A). Although cilostazol is generally well tolerated, it is not recommended in patients with heart failure. Pentoxifylline is another agent approved for use in patients with symptomatic PAD, but the clinical effectiveness of this drug appears marginal (SOE=C).

Revascularization is indicated for patients with severe symptoms attributable to PAD that have not responded to a trial of aggressive risk factor modification, exercise, and pharmacotherapy. Revascularization is also indicated for patients with critical-limb ischemia, defined as rest pain, ulceration, or gangrene; in this context, revascularization has been shown not only to improve symptoms but also to reduce the likelihood of subsequent amputation. The choice of revascularization procedure, ie, percutaneous transluminal angioplasty with or without stenting versus surgical revascularization, depends on lesion location and severity, likelihood of success, risk of major complications, and experience and technical expertise of the interventionalist and surgeon. Importantly, these two therapeutic approaches should be viewed as complementary rather than competing strategies, and the choice of procedure should be tailored to individual patient circumstances and preferences.

Indications for AAA repair include development of symptoms, rapid aneurysmal dilatation detected during serial assessments (≥1 cm in 1 year), and aneurysms ≥5.5 cm in diameter. Patients with asymptomatic AAAs 4–5.4 cm in diameter should undergo repeat evaluations at intervals of 6–12 months. The choice of open or endovascular surgical repair of AAAs is based on location of the lesion and patient comorbidities and prognosis. Open repair is favored for suprarenal AAAs and for patients with fewer comorbidities and a remaining life expectancy of >10 years, because this procedure has reduced rates of long-term leakage and rupture (SOE=B). Endovascular repair is suitable for patients with infrarenal AAAs and for those who have a higher surgical risk or shorter remaining life expectancy, because it is associated with lower perioperative complications and mortality (SOE=B).

Choosing Wisely® Recommendations

Cardiology/Coronary Artery Disease

- Do not order coronary artery calcium scoring for screening purposes in low-risk, asymptomatic individuals except those with a family history of premature CAD.

- Do not use coronary artery calcium scoring for patients with known CAD (including stents and bypass grafts).

- Do not routinely order coronary CT angiography for screening asymptomatic individuals.

- Do not perform stress cardiac imaging or advanced noninvasive imaging in the initial evaluation of patients without cardiac symptoms unless high-risk markers are present.

- Do not obtain screening exercise ECG testing in individuals who are asymptomatic and at low risk for coronary heart disease.

- Do not perform routine annual stress testing after coronary artery revascularization.

Cardiology/Valvular Heart Disease

- Do not perform echocardiography as routine follow-up for mild, asymptomatic native valve disease in adult patients with no change in signs or symptoms.

Cardiology/Peripheral Arterial Disease

- Refrain from percutaneous or surgical revascularization of peripheral artery stenosis in patients without claudication or critical limb ischemia.

REFERENCES

- Amsterdam EA, Wenger NK, Brindis RG, et al. 2014 AHA/ACC Guideline for the management of patients with non-ST-elevation acute coronary syndromes. *J Am Coll Cardiol*. 2014;64(24):e139–e228.

    The ACC/AHA guideline for the management of non-ST-elevation acute coronary syndromes includes a separate section devoted to the management of older adults and advocates a patient-centered approach that includes consideration of comorbidities, functional and cognitive status, life expectancy, and patient preferences.

- Fihn SD, Gardin JM, Abrams J, et al. 2012 ACCF/AHA/ACP/AATS/PCNA/SCAI/STS Guideline for the diagnosis and management of patients with stable ischemic heart disease. *Circulation*. 2012;126(25):e354–e471.

    The ACC/AHA guideline for the management of stable ischemic heart disease includes a section that focuses on management of older adults, acknowledging the importance of functional capacity, quality of life, goals of care, and end-of-life preferences in clinical decision-making.

- January CT, Wann LS, Alpert JS, et al. 2014 AHA/ACC/HRS guideline for the management of patients with atrial fibrillation. *J Am Coll Cardiol*. 2014;64(21):e1–76.

    The AHA/ACC guideline for the management of atrial fibrillation (AF) includes a section on AF in older adults, emphasizing that older patients are a heterogeneous population with high comorbidity burden and increased risk of stroke as well as adverse outcomes from medications and other interventions. The guideline also contains useful information on the new oral anticoagulants.

- Nishimura RA, Otto CM, Bonow RO, et al. 2014 AHA/ACC guideline for the management of patients with valvular heart disease. *J Am Coll Cardiol*. 2014;63(22):e57–185.

    The AHA/ACC guideline for the management of valvular heart disease points out that aortic stenosis is predominantly a disorder of older adults and that older adults have been well represented in clinical studies of this condition, including the recent transcatheter aortic valve replacement trials. Nonetheless, advanced age, comorbidity, and functional impairments are risk factors for adverse outcomes.

- O'Gara PT, Kushner FG, Ascheim DD, et al. 2013 ACCF/AHA guideline for the management of ST-elevation myocardial infarction. *J Am Coll Cardiol*. 2013;61(4):e78–140.

    Current ACC/AHA guideline for the management of patients with ST-elevation myocardial infarction acknowledges that older adults present challenges to diagnosis and management but generally recommends a similar approach to treatment across the age spectrum.

Michael W. Rich, MD, AGSF

CHAPTER 50—HEART FAILURE

KEY POINTS

- Heart failure (HF) is the leading cause of hospitalization in older adults and a major source of chronic disability.

- Compared with younger patients, older patients with HF are more likely to be women and more likely to have preserved left ventricular systolic function.

- ACE inhibitors, angiotensin-receptor blockers, β-blockers, aldosterone antagonists, and in selected patients hydralazine/nitrates reduce morbidity and mortality from HF with reduced ejection fraction (HFrEF). No pharmacotherapy for HF with preserved ejection fraction (HFpEF) has been definitively shown to reduce mortality.

- Optimal management of HF in older patients often requires a multidisciplinary approach.

EPIDEMIOLOGY

Heart failure (HF) currently affects approximately 5.1 million Americans, with >650,000 new cases diagnosed each year. HF costs in the United States exceed $30 billion annually, half of which is spent on hospitalizations, which number over 1 million annually and are associated with readmission within 1 month in up to 25% of cases. The incidence and prevalence of HF increase progressively with age, and HF is the leading cause of hospitalization and rehospitalization in older adults. The median age of patients hospitalized with HF is 75 years, and approximately two-thirds of deaths attributable to HF occur in patients ≥75 years old. In addition, HF is a major cause of chronic disability and impaired quality of life in older adults, and it is a common factor contributing to loss of independence and admission to long-term care facilities. Although the incidence of HF is somewhat higher in men, women comprise slightly over half of prevalent HF cases.

ETIOLOGY AND PATHOPHYSIOLOGY

The syndrome of HF in older adults is often multifactorial in origin. Hypertension is the most common antecedent cardiovascular condition in both men and women with HF, and it is the principal cause of HF in 60%–70% of women. In men, 30%–40% of HF is attributable to hypertension, and a similar proportion is attributable to coronary artery disease (CAD). Other common causes of HF in older adults include valvular heart disease and nonischemic dilated cardiomyopathy. Less common causes include hypertrophic cardiomyopathy, restrictive cardiomyopathy (eg, from amyloidosis), and pericardial disease. The rising prevalence of HF with increasing age reflects both age-related changes in cardiovascular structure and function that diminish cardiovascular reserve, and greater prevalence of those cardiovascular diseases (especially hypertension and CAD) that predispose to HF.

Distinguishing between HF patients with a left ventricular ejection fraction <40% (heart failure with reduced ejection fraction, or HFrEF) and those with a left ventricular ejection fracture >40%–50% (heart failure with preserved ejection fraction, or HFpEF) is clinically important. The terms HFrEF and HFpEF have supplanted the previous labels of "systolic" and "diastolic" heart failure. (One reason HFrEF is a more descriptive term than the old label "systolic HF" is that patients with this condition generally have impaired diastolic as well as systolic function.) HFpEF comprises approximately 50% of total HF prevalence and is associated with female sex, obesity, CAD, diabetes, dyslipidemia, atrial arrhythmias, and, most importantly, hypertension. Although nearly 90% of HF patients <65 years old have HFrEF, approximately 40% of men and two-thirds of women >65 years old with HF have HFpEF. The rising prevalence of HFpEF in older patients is due to age-related changes in left ventricular diastolic function and increased prevalence of hypertension, particularly for women.

CLINICAL FEATURES

As in younger patients, exertional shortness of breath, fatigue, orthopnea, and leg edema are the most common symptoms of HF in older adults. Exertional symptoms, however, may be less prominent in older patients because of a more sedentary lifestyle. Conversely, the prevalence of atypical symptoms increases with age, and older HF patients may present with decreased mental acuity, confusion, lethargy, irritability, anorexia, abdominal discomfort, or altered bowel function.

Classical physical findings of HF in younger patients include tachycardia, narrowed pulse pressure, increased jugular venous pressure, hepatojugular reflux, an S_3 gallop, moist pulmonary crackles, diminished breath sounds at the lung bases (due to pleural effusions), and pitting edema of the legs. Many or even all of these findings may be absent in older HF patients, especially those with HFpEF, in whom an S_3 gallop and signs of right-heart failure are not usually present. In addition, pulmonary crackles in older patients may be due to comorbid chronic lung disease or atelectasis, and peripheral edema may arise from hepatic or renal disease, venous insufficiency, hypoalbuminemia, or medications (especially calcium channel blockers).

Because the symptoms and signs of HF in older adults are often atypical and nonspecific, it is important for clinicians to maintain a high index of suspicion when an older patient presents with complaints that are vague, or the origins of which appear unrelated to the circulatory system.

DIAGNOSIS

The diagnosis of HF may be established on clinical grounds in patients presenting with a constellation of classical symptoms and signs. However, the diagnosis is often uncertain, and additional testing is required.

The standard chest radiograph remains a useful initial test for determining the presence of HF, with the appearance of cardiomegaly, pulmonary congestion, or pleural effusion suggesting the diagnosis. Competing diagnoses such as pneumonia can also be excluded. However, the chest radiograph may be difficult to interpret in older adults with chronic lung disease, kyphoscoliosis, or poor inspiratory effort. Moreover, the absence of pulmonary congestion on a chest radiograph does not exclude a diagnosis of HF.

The ECG may show evidence of left ventricular hypertrophy, acute ischemia or prior myocardial infarction, left atrial enlargement, or atrial fibrillation—all of which predispose to the development of HF—but the ECG is not usually helpful in establishing a diagnosis of either acute or chronic HF. Similarly, although it is appropriate to obtain a CBC, routine chemistry panel, thyroid studies, a urinalysis, and in selected cases, biomarkers of cardiac ischemia (ie, troponin, creatine kinase) in patients with suspected HF, in most cases these tests are insufficient to confirm or exclude the diagnosis.

B-type natriuretic peptide (BNP) and its precursor N-terminal pro-BNP (NT-proBNP) are generated by cardiac myocytes in response to myocardial stretch and are thus valuable laboratory tools for establishing the diagnosis of volume overload due to HF (either HFrEF or HFpEF) and for distinguishing shortness of breath due to HF from that attributable to noncardiac causes. Unfortunately, BNP and NT-proBNP levels increase with age (especially in women) and with decreasing renal function. As a result, the specificity of increased levels of these peptides for diagnosing HF decreases with age, and the clinical significance of an isolated increase of BNP or NT-proBNP in an older adult may be difficult to interpret. Despite these caveats, a BNP level <100 pg/mL in an older adult with suspected acute HF makes the diagnosis very unlikely (negative likelihood ratio approximately 0.1), whereas a BNP level ≥500 pg/mL is consistent with active HF (positive likelihood ratio approximately 6). Finally, BNP and NT-pro-BNP levels are lower in obesity and therefore may be less helpful in excluding the diagnosis of HF.

Once a diagnosis of HF has been established, it is important to determine the cause and to assess left ventricular function because these factors affect management. Echocardiography with Doppler is the preferred method for evaluating left ventricular function, because it provides concomitant detailed assessment of left and right ventricular size and wall thickness, systolic and diastolic function, atrial size, valvular function, intracardiac pressures, and the pericardium. MRI may be used in patients with inadequate echo images or to assess for infiltration or scarring of the myocardium. Radionuclide ventriculography is another alternative for quantitation of left ventricular ejection fraction (LVEF) in patients with inadequate echo images. In patients with suspected CAD who are suitable candidates for revascularization (including willingness to undergo further testing and interventions if clinically indicated), a stress test (echo or nuclear medicine) should be performed, followed by coronary angiography if the stress test indicates severe CAD, especially in a multivessel distribution.

MANAGEMENT

The goals of HF management are to decrease symptoms, improve quality of life, reduce acute exacerbations requiring hospitalization, and prolong survival. Hypertension, hyperlipidemia, and diabetes should be treated in accordance with current guidelines. Smoking cessation should be strongly encouraged and supported, and alcohol intake should be limited to no more than 2 drinks/day in men and 1 drink/day in women. NSAIDs should be avoided because they promote water and sodium retention, and they antagonize the effects of diuretics and renin-angiotensin system inhibitors. CAD should be treated with anti-ischemic medications and, if indicated, percutaneous or surgical revascularization. Similarly, valvular lesions should be managed in accordance with established practice guidelines. In patients with atrial fibrillation, the heart rate should be controlled, preferably with β-blockers. In selected cases, restoration and maintenance of sinus rhythm may be considered using either a pharmacologic or catheter-based approach, recognizing that rhythm control is not superior to rate control in patients with HF (SOE=B). Finally, patients should be screened for anemia and thyroid dysfunction, and appropriate therapy started if indicated.

Nonpharmacologic Therapy

HF patients have long been counseled to restrict dietary sodium intake to no more than 2 grams/day (SOE=C), but low-sodium diets have been linked to worse outcomes in several clinical trials and little data exist on optimal sodium intake. Sodium allowances should likely be individualized, taking into account volume status, serum sodium level, and severity of HF, particularly in older patients predisposed to hyponatremia. Fluid restriction is not usually necessary except in patients with advanced HF or hyponatremia, but patients should be advised to avoid excess fluid intake (ie, the oft-quoted dictum to drink 8–10 glasses of water every day does not apply to individuals with HF, renal insufficiency, or other fluid-retaining states). Exercise training or regular physical activity (eg, walking, stationary cycling, swimming, or water aerobics) has favorable effects on functional status in HF patients and is recommended by current HF guidelines (SOE=B). Exercise duration and intensity should be adjusted to the individual patient's level of conditioning, severity of HF, and comorbidities, but should be gradually increased over time, if possible, to achieve 30–60 minutes of aerobic exercise most days of the week. These activities should be complemented by stretching and strengthening exercises, as well as by gait and balance exercises if indicated. Cardiac rehabilitation for patients with stable symptoms and an LVEF ≤35% has been approved by CMS and most private insurance companies as an effective therapy for older HF patients.

Patients should be instructed to keep an ongoing record of their daily weight. Weights should be measured in the morning without clothes after going to the bathroom but before eating. A "dry weight" should be established (based on the home scale, not the office scale), and patients should be instructed to contact their clinicians if the weight varies by more than 2–3 pounds above or below the dry weight. Selected patients may be provided with detailed instructions for self-adjustment of diuretic dosages based on daily weights.

Older patients with moderate or advanced HF, multiple comorbidities, or a recent HF exacerbation requiring hospitalization may benefit from participation in a structured HF disease management program. Such programs offer enhanced education and follow-up, usually by an HF nurse specialist or interprofessional team, in some cases supplemented by telemonitoring devices. They have been shown to reduce hospitalizations and inpatient costs, as well as to improve quality of life in older HF patients (SOE=A) (see Recurrent Hospitalization section below for further discussion).

Pharmacotherapy of HFrEF

ACE inhibitors, angiotensin-receptor blockers (ARBs), aldosterone antagonists, and β-blockers have been shown to improve outcomes and reduce mortality in multiple large prospective trials involving a broad range of HF patients with decreased left ventricular systolic function (SOE=A), and these agents are now considered the cornerstone of therapy for HFrEF. Although older patients, especially those with multiple comorbid conditions, have been markedly under-represented in these trials, the available evidence indicates that the beneficial effects of these agents likely extend to older patients.

For a list of ACE inhibitors approved for the treatment of HF, along with recommended initial and maintenance dosages, see Table 50.1. In general, treatment of older HF patients should be started at the lowest dosage and gradually titrated to the maintenance dosage as tolerated. Contraindications to ACE inhibitors include known intolerance to these agents, hyperkalemia (serum potassium ≥5.5 mEq/L), hypotension (systolic blood pressure <80 mmHg), and severe renal insufficiency (estimated creatinine clearance <30 mL/min) in patients not currently undergoing dialysis. Common adverse events include cough in 5%–10% of patients during long-term treatment, mild worsening of renal function (often transient), hyperkalemia, hypotension, GI distress, and rarely angioedema. Renal function and potassium concentrations should be monitored at least weekly during initiation and titration of ACE inhibitor therapy.

ARBs are indicated as an alternative to ACE inhibitors in HF patients unable to tolerate the latter class of medications because of cough, allergic reactions, or GI disturbances. Contraindications and adverse events associated with these agents are otherwise similar to those of ACE inhibitors. In particular, the incidence of renal insufficiency, hyperkalemia, and hypotension is comparable with equivalent dosages of ACE inhibitors and ARBs. Combination therapy with an ACE inhibitor and an ARB increases the probability of adverse events without providing clear clinical benefit.

β-Blockers counteract the deleterious effects of chronic activation of the sympathetic nervous system in HF patients and have been shown to improve ventricular function and symptoms while reducing the risk of both sudden and non-sudden cardiac death (SOE=A). Unlike the case with ACE inhibitors and ARBs, the reduction in mortality of β-blockers is not thought to be a class effect and has only been demonstrated for carvedilol, metoprolol succinate, and bisoprolol. The treatment strategy of β-blockers is like that for ACE inhibitors and ARBs, starting at the lowest available dosage and gradually titrating to the maintenance dosage over several weeks (Table 50.1). The benefit of β-blockers is proportional to the degree of heart-rate reduction achieved, but there is no established "optimal" heart rate, and the potential benefit of dose escalation should be weighed against the risk of adverse effects. Contraindications to starting β-blocker therapy include severe decompensated HF, active bronchospastic lung disease, marked bradycardia (heart rate <45–50 beats per minute), relative hypotension (systolic blood pressure <90–100 mmHg), significant atrioventricular nodal block (PR interval ≥240 msec or higher degrees of block), and known intolerance to β-blockers. Occasionally, HF symptoms will worsen on initiation or titration of a β-blocker (and patients should be warned about this possibility), but in most cases this is a transient phenomenon and >80% of HF patients are able to tolerate long-term β-blocker therapy when judiciously initiated and titrated, even those whose treatment is started before discharge (during hospitalization for HF).

Diuretics are usually a necessary component of HF therapy, and they remain the most effective agents for relief of congestion and edema. Except for aldosterone antagonists (see below), diuretics have not been shown to reduce mortality. In general, the diuretic dosage should be adjusted to maintain euvolemia, manifested by the absence of pulmonary rales, an S_3 gallop, increased jugular venous pressure, hepatojugular reflux, and peripheral edema. In patients with equivocal findings, serial measurement of BNP may be useful for tracking volume status. Some patients with mild HF respond satisfactorily to a thiazide diuretic, but most require maintenance therapy with a loop diuretic, such as furosemide, bumetanide, or torsemide. Patients with advanced HF, concomitant renal insufficiency, or both, may be resistant to conventional dosages of loop diuretics; in these patients, the addition of metolazone at 2.5–10 mg/d is often effective, but careful monitoring of electrolytes is required. The principal adverse events associated with diuretic therapy are electrolyte disturbances, including hypokalemia, hyponatremia, and hypomagnesemia; close monitoring of these electrolytes, as well as renal function, is therefore warranted. Thiamine deficiency may occur during long-term treatment with loop diuretics and can contribute to apparent diuretic resistance. Although routine monitoring of thiamine levels is not recommended, supplemental thiamine in the form of a multivitamin is reasonable in older patients who require long-term therapy with a loop diuretic (SOE=D). Older patients as a group are also at increased risk of dehydration during diuretic treatment because of attenuation of the thirst response and diminished oral fluid intake, especially during periods of illness or increased ambient temperatures. Therefore, clinicians should remain vigilant for possible signs of dehydration, including excess weight loss during daily weight monitoring.

The aldosterone antagonist spironolactone has been shown to reduce mortality and hospitalizations in patients with New York Heart Association (NYHA) class III–IV HF (Table 50.2) and an LVEF <30% (SOE=A), with similar benefits in older and younger patients. Similarly, the selective aldosterone antagonist eplerenone has been associated with improved outcomes in patients with recent myocardial infarction complicated by HF or an LVEF <40%, as well as in patients with NYHA class II HF and an LVEF ≤35% (SOE=A). Based on these studies, spironolactone 12.5–25 mg/d or eplerenone 25–50 mg/d is recommended for patients with NYHA class II–IV HF and an LVEF ≤35%. Spironolactone and eplerenone are contraindicated in patients with serum creatinine ≥2.5 mg/dL or serum potassium ≥5 mEq/L. Older adults are at increased risk of worsening renal function and hyperkalemia during aldosterone antagonist therapy, and frequent monitoring of electrolytes and creatinine is necessary. Potassium supplementation can usually be discontinued in patients receiving an aldosterone antagonist, especially in combination with an ACE inhibitor or ARB. Up to 10% of patients develop painful gynecomastia during long-term treatment with spironolactone compared to <1% with eplerenone.

Before the advent of ACE inhibitors and β-blockers, the combination of hydralazine and isosorbide dinitrate was shown to reduce mortality relative to placebo in patients with HFrEF. Although a subsequent study

Table 50.1—Recommended Dosages of ACE Inhibitors, Angiotensin II Receptor Blockers, and β-Blockers in Patients with Heart Failure with Reduced Ejection Fraction (HFrEF)

Agent	Starting Dosage	Target Dosage
ACE Inhibitors		
Benazepril[a]	2.5 mg/d	40 mg/d
Captopril	6.25 mg q8h	50 mg q8h
Enalapril	2.5 mg/d	10–20 mg q12h
Fosinopril	5–10 mg/d	40 mg/d
Lisinopril	2.5–5 mg/d	20–40 mg/d
Moexipril[a]	3.75 mg/d	15 mg/d
Perindopril[a]	2 mg/d	8–16 mg/d
Quinapril	5 mg q12h	10–20 mg q12h
Ramipril	1.25–2.5 mg/d	10 mg/d
Trandolapril	1 mg/d	4 mg/d
Angiotensin II Receptor Blockers		
Candesartan	4 mg/d	32 mg/d
Eprosartan[a]	400 mg/d	400 mg q12h
Irbesartan[a]	75 mg/d	150–300 mg/d
Losartan[a]	25 mg/d	50–100 mg/d
Olmesartan[a]	20 mg/d	40 mg/d
Telmisartan[a]	20 mg/d	80 mg/d
Valsartan	20–40 mg q12h	160 mg q12h
β-Blockers		
Bisoprolol[b]	1.25 mg/d	10 mg/d
Carvedilol	3.125 mg q12h	25–50 mg q12h
Carvedilol ER	10 mg/d	80 mg/d
Metoprolol XL	12.5–25 mg/d	200 mg/d

[a] Not approved for HF by the FDA
[b] Not approved for HF by the FDA but has been shown to be effective in HF

Table 50.2—New York Heart Association Functional Class

Class	Symptoms
I	No symptoms and no limitation in ordinary physical activity Walking, climbing stairs, or doing household chores does not cause undue shortness of breath, palpitations, chest discomfort, or fatigue.
II	Slight limitation of physical activity Ordinary physical activity causes shortness of breath, palpitations, chest discomfort, or fatigue; able to walk >2 blocks and climb 2 flights of stairs.
III	Marked limitation of physical activity Less than ordinary physical activity (eg, walking <2 blocks) causes shortness of breath, palpitations, chest discomfort, or fatigue; no symptoms at rest.
IV	Severe activity limitation Unable to carry out any physical activity (eg, walking in the house, dressing, bathing, toileting) without shortness of breath, palpitations, chest discomfort, or fatigue; symptoms may be present at rest.

showed reduced mortality in patients treated with the ACE inhibitor enalapril compared to those treated with hydralazine and nitrates, retrospective analysis revealed that this difference was not evident in black participants. This observation led to a prospective trial conducted exclusively in self-described blacks who demonstrated additional survival benefit when hydralazine and nitrates were added to background therapy that included ACE inhibitors/ARBs and β-blockers. Based on these studies, the combination of hydralazine and nitrates is recommended for HF patients with contraindications to ACE inhibitors and ARBs (eg, severe renal insufficiency), and in blacks with advanced HF as an adjunct to ACE inhibitor and β-blocker therapy (SOE=A). The benefit of adding hydralazine and nitrates to ACE inhibitors and β-blockers in non-black patients has not been established. The starting dosage of hydralazine is 25–50 mg q8h, titrating to a maximal dosage of 100 mg q8h. The starting dosage of isosorbide dinitrate is 10 mg q8h, titrating to a maximal dosage of 30–40 mg q8h. Common adverse events associated with hydralazine include palpitations, nausea, and dizziness; rarely, a drug-induced lupus syndrome may occur during prolonged therapy at high dosage (≥300 mg/d). The most common adverse event from isosorbide dinitrate is headache, which usually resolves with continued use.

Digoxin improves symptoms and reduces HF hospitalizations in patients with HFrEF but does not decrease mortality. In fact, the drug may be less effective and even harmful in women with heart failure, and it has been associated with increased mortality in patients with atrial fibrillation. Digoxin nevertheless remains a reasonable therapeutic option in patients with persistent limiting symptoms or recurrent hospitalizations in whom the measures discussed above have not resulted in a satisfactory response. Retrospective analyses based on a large randomized trial suggest that the optimal digoxin concentration for improving clinical outcomes is 0.5–0.9 ng/mL, which is substantially lower than the "therapeutic range" previously reported by most clinical laboratories. Therefore, digoxin should be dosed to maintain the digoxin concentration <1 ng/mL, and a dosage of 0.125 mg/d is likely to be sufficient for most older patients with relatively preserved renal function, whereas a lower dosage (0.125 mg every other day) might be required in patients with renal insufficiency or low lean body mass. Adverse effects of digoxin include nausea, visual disturbances, and cardiac arrhythmias (bradyarrhythmias as well as supraventricular and ventricular tachyarrhythmias). However, with appropriate monitoring of the serum digoxin concentration, serious digoxin toxicity is infrequent, and there is no convincing evidence that older patients are at increased risk of life-threatening digitalis intoxication. Amiodarone, quinidine, and verapamil, as well as several other medications, are associated with up to a 2-fold increase in serum digoxin concentrations, and the dosage of digoxin should be reduced by 50% in patients receiving these medications.

Previous guidelines suggested consideration of antiplatelet or anticoagulant therapy for HF patients in normal sinus rhythm, even in the absence of compelling indications for treatment. However, although HFrEF patients are at increased risk of thromboembolic events, the only placebo-controlled trial of antithrombotic therapy in these patients showed no difference in a composite outcome that included stroke. Randomized trials comparing different antithrombotic strategies (aspirin, clopidogrel, warfarin) have also shown no benefit of one strategy over another. Moreover, among HF patients >60 years old, warfarin has been associated with increased bleeding without a corresponding reduction in thromboembolic events. Current guidelines therefore recommend against routine anticoagulation in HF patients in the absence of atrial fibrillation. For HF patients with comorbid atrial fibrillation, which includes nearly 30% of the geriatric HF population, long-term anticoagulation with warfarin or one of the newer oral anticoagulants is indicated in most cases.

In summary, optimal treatment of HFrEF usually requires a minimum of three medications and, in some cases, up to seven. Because HF in older patients almost never occurs as an isolated disease process, almost all patients are taking one or more additional medications for other coexisting illnesses. Thus, pharmacotherapy of the older HF patient is problematic from the perspective of adherence, high potential for drug interactions and adverse events, and cost. It is therefore essential that therapy be individualized,

Table 50.3—Pharmacotherapy Trials for Heart Failure with Preserved Ejection Fraction (HFpEF)

Trial[a, b]	Number of Patients	Age (years)	LVEF (%)	Treatment	Statistically Significant Outcomes Compared with Placebo
PEP-CHF	850	75 (72–79)	65 (56–66)	Perindopril	Heart failure hospitalization by 1 year HR 0.63 (0.41–0.97, P =.033)
CHARM-Preserved	3023	67 ± 11	54 ± 9	Candesartan	None
I-PRESERVE	4128	72 ± 7	60 ± 9	Irbesartan	None
SENIORS (EF >35% subgroup)	643	76 ± 5	49 ± 10	Nebivolol	None
TOPCAT	3445	69 (61–76)	56 (51–62)	Spironolactone	Heart failure hospitalization HR 0.83 (0.69–0.99, P=.04)
Aldo-DHF	422	67 ± 8	67 ± 8	Spironolactone	Reduced E/e' avg 1.5 (P<.001)
RELAX	216	69 (62–77)	60 (56–65)	Sildenafil	None
ESS-DHF	192	65 ± 10	61 ± 12	Sitaxsentan	Median 43-second relative increase in Naughton treadmill time (P=.03)
DIG Ancillary	988	67 ± 10	55 ± 8	Digoxin	None

NOTE: LVEF = left ventricular ejection fraction, E/e' avg = echocardiographic mitral inflow velocity/tissue Doppler velocity ratio, age and LVEF presented as mean ± SD or median (IQR), HR = hazard ratio (with 95% confidence interval)

[a] Trial acronyms: PEP-CHF (Perindopril in Elderly People with Chronic Heart Failure), CHARM-Preserved (Candesartan in Heart failure: Assessment of Reduction in Mortality and morbidity – Preserved LVEF), I-PRESERVE (Irbesartan in Heart Failure with Preserved Ejection Fraction Study), SENIORS (Study of the Effects of Nebivolol Intervention on Outcomes and Rehospitalisation in Seniors with Heart Failure), TOPCAT (Treatment of Preserved Cardiac Function Heart Failure with an Aldosterone Antagonist), Aldo-DHF (Aldosterone Receptor Blockade in Diastolic Heart Failure), RELAX (Phosphodiesterase-5 Inhibition to Improve Clinical Status and Exercise Capacity in Heart Failure with Preserved Ejection Fraction), ESS-DHF (Effectiveness of Sitaxsentan Sodium in Patients With Diastolic Heart Failure), DIG Ancillary (Digitalis Investigation Group Ancillary Trial)

[b] All-cause mortality was not significantly reduced in *any* trial.

taking into consideration the multiple and often competing factors that influence quality of life and other clinical outcomes in older adults with multiple chronic illnesses and limited life expectancy.

Pharmacotherapy of HFpEF

In contrast to HFrEF, relatively few clinical trials have been directed at treatment of HFpEF, and to date no trials have demonstrated a clear reduction in mortality with any pharmacologic intervention in patients with this condition (Table 50.3). Several antagonists of the renin-angiotensin system have shown a trend toward reduced hospitalizations, including the ARB candesartan (SOE=A) and the ACE inhibitor perindopril (SOE=B). In contrast, a large trial of the ARB irbesartan showed no effect on mortality, hospitalizations, or other cardiac outcomes in older adults with HFpEF (SOE=A). The TOPCAT trial showed that the aldosterone antagonist spironolactone did not reduce a composite outcome of cardiovascular death or hospitalization, but a small reduction in HF hospitalizations was noted (SOE=A). Conversely, a large retrospective registry study failed to demonstrate improved clinical outcomes, including hospitalizations, with the use of aldosterone antagonists among HFpEF patients ≥65 years old (SOE=B). Digoxin may reduce hospitalizations due to HF in patients with HFpEF, but this appears to be at the expense of increased hospitalizations for unstable angina (SOE=B). In a study of HF patients ≥70 years old, the β-blocker nebivolol was associated with an overall reduction in a composite outcome of all-cause death or hospitalization, but this difference was not statistically significant in a subgroup analysis of patients with LVEF ≥35% (SOE=B). The phosphodiesterase-5 inhibitor sildenafil had no effect on functional or clinical outcomes in the RELAX trial (SOE=B), whereas the endothelin A-type receptor antagonist sitaxsentan had a modest but significant effect on exercise performance in the ESS-DHF trial (SOE=C). Based on the available evidence, optimal therapy for HFpEF remains undefined. Current recommendations include aggressive treatment of hypertension and other risk factors, appropriate management of comorbid CAD, and maintenance of sinus rhythm or effective rate control in patients with atrial fibrillation (SOE=D). Diuretics should be used judiciously to maintain euvolemia while avoiding over-diuresis, because patients with HFpEF are often "volume-sensitive." The addition of an ACE inhibitor or ARB, and possibly a β-blocker (especially in patients with CAD), is appropriate to reduce the risk of hospitalization, recognizing that the impact of these agents on other clinically relevant outcomes is unproved.

Device Therapy, Mechanical Circulatory Support, and Heart Transplantation

The implantable cardioverter-defibrillator (ICD) has been shown to reduce mortality from sudden cardiac death in patients with HF (whether ischemic or nonischemic) and an LVEF of ≤35% (SOE=A). However, few older patients were enrolled in the ICD randomized trials, and a meta-analysis suggested that the benefit of ICDs in reducing mortality is lower in older than in younger patients, probably because of competing risks (SOE=A). In addition, major complications related to ICD implantation are 2-fold greater in patients ≥80 years old than in younger patients (SOE=B). Nonetheless 40%–45% of ICDs in the United States are implanted in patients ≥70 years old. Importantly, ICDs have not been shown to improve survival in patients with NYHA class I or IV HF, and there is no survival benefit within the first 12–18 months after implantation. Also, quality of life is impaired in patients who receive one or more ICD shocks, and up to 20% of shocks are inappropriate, ie, occurring in the absence of a life-threatening tachyarrhythmia.

Based on available evidence, prophylactic ICD placement is recommended in patients with NYHA class II or III HF, an LVEF ≤35%, and a remaining life expectancy with good functional status of at least 1 year. ICD implantation should be deferred for at least 40 days after acute myocardial infarction and for at least 90 days after a new diagnosis of dilated cardiomyopathy (in the latter case because left ventricular function often improves after initiation of β-blocker and ACE inhibitor therapy).

Given that HF patients >75–80 years old have limited remaining life expectancy, especially if they have multiple comorbid illnesses or frailty, and that ICDs may not reduce mortality in this age group, the selection of older patients for ICD therapy must be individualized, and a shared decision-making approach is recommended. Patients should be advised about the potential benefits and risks of ICD implantation, including the possibility of an adverse effect on quality of life. Although many older patients elect to forego ICD implantation after an informed discussion, those who desire an ICD should not be denied one solely on the basis of age, assuming that appropriate indications for the device are present. In these patients, it is appropriate to discuss circumstances under which the patient would want to have the device disabled, especially at end of life due to progressive HF or other terminal illness.

Cardiac resynchronization therapy (CRT) has been shown to improve symptoms, exercise tolerance, quality of life, and survival in selected patients with advanced systolic HF and persistent severe symptoms (NYHA class III or IV) despite conventional medical therapy (SOE=A). CRT involves placement of a biventricular pacemaker with one lead in the right ventricle and a second lead inserted retrograde into the coronary sinus to stimulate the left ventricle. CRT is indicated in patients with dyssynchronous left ventricular contraction, most commonly related to left bundle-branch block, which is present in up to 30% of patients with HFrEF. The basis for CRT, as the name implies, is to "resynchronize" left ventricular contraction, thereby increasing myocardial efficiency, stroke work, ejection fraction, and cardiac output. Although few older patients have been enrolled in the CRT trials, observational studies indicate that the benefits of CRT are age-independent (SOE=B). Therefore, because the main objective of CRT is to improve symptoms and quality of life, and because the risk of CRT is modest, it seems reasonable to offer CRT to older patients with severe left ventricular dysfunction, advanced HF symptoms, and evidence of left ventricular dyssynchrony (ie, left bundle-branch block with QRS duration ≥150 msec).

An advance in the management of HF patients who remain highly symptomatic despite optimal medical and device therapy is the development of implantable mechanical left ventricular assist devices (LVADs). LVADs reduce symptoms, increase exercise tolerance, and improve quality of life and survival in selected patients with HF and severe systolic dysfunction, including adults in their 70s and 80s. Although originally reserved for use as a "bridge" to heart transplantation, LVADs are now often implanted (ie, used as "destination therapy") to alleviate symptoms and improve quality of life in patients who are not transplant candidates. As a result, an increasing number of older adults are receiving LVADs, and this trend is likely to accelerate as the safety and efficacy of these devices continue to improve. Older patients are at increased risk of LVAD-related complications, particularly GI bleeding, and patients with advanced comorbidities or frailty may not be suitable candidates. Nonetheless, small studies of LVADs in highly selected septuagenarians and octogenarians have reported favorable effects on quality of life and survival, so age alone should not be considered an absolute contraindication to LVAD implantation.

RECURRENT HOSPITALIZATION

Recurrent hospitalization is common among patients hospitalized with HF. Approximately 20%–25% of such patients are readmitted within 30 days of discharge, and up to 50% are readmitted within 6 months. Prediction and prevention of early readmission has proven to be challenging, in part because less than half of patients readmitted within 30 days have HF as the primary reason for rehospitalization. Nonetheless, efforts to predict and prevent readmission have intensified following the October 2012 implementation of the Hospital Readmissions Reduction Program under the Affordable Care Act, which requires CMS to reduce payments to hospitals with excess readmissions.

Contributors to readmission may include biological factors (severity of heart failure, number and severity of comorbidities), patient behavioral factors (adherence to pharmacotherapy, adherence to diet and lifestyle), and health-care system factors (discharge practices, care transitions, outpatient care resources). Providers should consider the impact of therapeutic choices on comorbid conditions, with particular attention to renal function, anticoagulation, lung disease, and drug interactions. Patients who experience recurrent HF hospitalization should be questioned carefully and educated appropriately about adherence to the medication regimen, use of over-the-counter medications (especially NSAIDs and "dietary supplements"), dietary choices, and daily fluid intake. Patients should also be asked if they have been monitoring their weight and if there have been any recent changes. In patients who acknowledge nonadherence to the medication regimen or to sodium restriction, reasons for nonadherence should be explored. Reasons for medication nonadherence often include concerns about adverse events, cost, efficacy, and excessive number of pills. Nonadherence to sodium restriction may be rooted in lack of knowledge about the salt content of foods, inability to acquire low-sodium foods, frequent eating out, and altered sense of taste. If possible, strategies should be developed to overcome these barriers, and the importance of future adherence as a means to prevent subsequent admissions emphasized. An interprofessional team approach, including the physician, HF nurse specialist (if available), dietitian, social worker, pharmacist (preferably with expertise in geriatric drug prescribing), and home-health representative, is most likely to result in significant changes in health behavior, thereby fostering improved adherence, self-efficacy, and decreased risk of early readmission (SOE=A). When feasible, the patient's partner and family should be actively engaged in the evaluation and teaching process.

Health services research in the care of patients with HF is helping to clarify factors that reduce readmission risk. Practitioner-level factors associated with reduced readmissions include discharging patients on evidence-based therapies for chronic HF, such as ACE inhibitors and β-blockers (SOE=B). Hospital-level practices associated with fewer readmissions include partnering with community doctors and other hospitals to develop consistent strategies for reducing readmission, nursing supervision to coordinate medications, scheduling follow-up appointments before patient discharge, sending discharge information to the patient's primary care provider, and contacting patients about test results received after discharge (SOE=B). HF disease management programs, as described above, have a positive impact on near-term outcomes, but more intensive post-discharge and outpatient monitoring interventions, through structured telephone support and telemonitoring (with automated transfer of patient physiological data), do not clearly reduce mortality or rehospitalizations when added to optimal medical therapy and disease management programs (SOE=B). Implantable hemodynamic monitoring is a new technology that may play a role in following advanced HF patients to reduce readmissions (SOE=C), although to date only one device has gained FDA approval.

PROGNOSIS

The prognosis of older patients with HF is poor, with median survival rates of 2–3 years. However, the prognosis is also heterogeneous, with 25%–30% of patients dying within 1 year after initial diagnosis, 50% surviving 1–5 years, and 20%–25% surviving >5 years. Increasing age plays a critical role in prognosis; eg, in a study of Medicare beneficiaries hospitalized with HF in 2008, 1-year mortality rates in patients 65–74, 75–84, and ≥85 years old were 22.0%, 30.3%, and 42.7%, respectively. Women have somewhat better survival rates than men, as do patients with HFpEF versus those with HFrEF, but other outcomes, including hospitalization rates, functional status, and quality of life, do not differ significantly among these subgroups. Other factors that adversely affect prognosis include more severe symptoms (eg, higher NYHA functional class), lower systolic blood pressure, the presence of CAD (an important factor contributing to worse outcomes in men), diabetes (especially in women), peripheral arterial or cerebrovascular disease, cognitive impairment or dementia, renal insufficiency, anemia, and hyponatremia. Patients with higher BNP also have a worse prognosis, especially if the BNP remains substantially increased despite aggressive therapy.

END-OF-LIFE CARE

In light of the poor prognosis of older HF patients, it is appropriate to initiate discussions about end-of-life care early in the course of treatment and to readdress these issues as clinical circumstances evolve. Patients should be counseled to prepare an advance directive, which may include the appointment of a surrogate decision maker and the delineation of interventions desired or to be avoided in the event of clinical worsening and approaching death. Patients with ICDs should be asked to indicate under what conditions they would want the ICD turned off to avoid repetitive painful shocks at the end of life. For patients with particularly poor prognosis and remaining life expectancy of <6 months (eg, NYHA class IV symptoms despite appropriate medical therapy), clinicians should offer the option of a transition to palliative care and hospice as part of a candid discussion of prognosis and goals of care.

Choosing Wisely® Recommendations

Heart Failure/Device Therapy, Mechanical Circulatory Support, and Heart Transplantation

- Do not leave an ICD activated when it is inconsistent with the patient/family goals of care.

REFERENCES

- Afilalo J, Alexander KP, Mack MJ, et al. Frailty assessment in the cardiovascular care of older adults. *J Am Coll Cardiol.* 2014;63(8):747–762.

    This white paper from the American College of Cardiology provides an overview of the pathobiology, relationship to cardiovascular disease, and utility of frailty assessment in older patients, highlighting the incremental value of frailty assessment relative to simple age-based assessment for evaluating health status and risk in older patients with cardiovascular disease.

- Allen LA, Stevenson LW, Grady KL, et al. Decision making in advanced heart failure: A Scientific Statement from the American Heart Association. *Circulation.* 2012;125:1928–1952.

    This American Heart Association scientific statement provides the rationale, supporting evidence, and practical advice for the incorporation of shared decision making into the management of patients with advanced heart failure. Particular attention is given to palliative care and therapy-specific complications.

- Jurgens CY, Goodlin S, Dolansky M, et al; American Heart Association Council on Quality of Care and Outcomes Research; Heart Failure Society of America. Heart failure management in skilled nursing facilities: a scientific statement from the American Heart Association and the Heart Failure Society of America. *J Card Fail.* 2015;21(4):263–299.

    This scientific statement from the American Heart Association and Heart Failure Society of American provides a comprehensive review of the diagnosis and management of heart failure for residents of skilled-nursing facilities.

- Kirklin JK, Naftel DC, Pagani FD, et al. Sixth INTERMACS annual report: a 10,000-patient database. *J Heart Lung Transplant.* 2014;33(6):555–564.

    The most recent report of the Interagency Registry for Mechanically Assisted Circulatory Support (INTERMACS) provides data on complication rates and various outcomes, including quality of life, in left-ventricular assist device recipients stratified by age and comorbidities.

- Whellan DJ, Goodlin SJ, Dickinson MG, et al. End-of-life care in patients with heart failure. *J Card Fail.* 2014;20(2):121–134.

    This consensus document on end-of-life care in heart failure from the Quality of Care Committee of the Heart Failure Society of America discusses strategies to reduce symptoms, improve communication, and enhance delivery of patient-centered care, including palliative care and hospice, in heart failure patients approaching the end of life.

- Yancy CW, Jessup M, Bozkurt B, et al. 2013 ACCF/AHA Guideline for the Management of Heart Failure: A Report of the American College of Cardiology Foundation/American Heart Association Task Force on Practice Guidelines. *J Am Coll Cardiol.* 2013;62(16):e147–e239.

    The current American College of Cardiology/American Heart Association guideline for the diagnosis and treatment of heart failure includes sections addressing treatment of older patients, men and women, and ethnic minorities. The high prevalence of heart failure with preserved left ventricular ejection function in older adults is noted, as is the need for dosage adjustment of many heart failure medications in older patients with altered drug metabolism.

Justin M. Vader, MD
Michael W. Rich, MD, AGSF

CHAPTER 51—HYPERTENSION

KEY POINTS

- Age-related changes in blood pressure regulation lead to greater variability in blood pressure and postural changes. Multiple blood pressure readings, including home and postural measurements, are needed to accurately and safely diagnose and manage hypertension.

- Treating hypertension is beneficial, independent of age, and reduces stroke, heart failure, and cardiovascular and overall mortality.

- Choice of initial antihypertensive drug therapy should be individualized according to the patient's comorbidities.

- Caution is needed in treating frail older adults with antihypertensives. "Start low and go slow." Monitoring for falls, decrease in orthostatic blood pressure, and other adverse drug events is essential.

EPIDEMIOLOGY AND PHYSIOLOGY

Systolic blood pressure progressively increases with age, whereas diastolic blood pressure plateaus in the fifth to sixth decade. According to the National Health and Nutrition Examination Survey (NHANES) 2011–2012, 65% of noninstitutionalized adults ≥60 years old had hypertension. Over the last few decades, awareness and control rates of hypertension have improved significantly. The number of adults ≥60 years old who were aware of their hypertension was 86%, and the number of those receiving treatment was 82% in the same period. Close to 50% of older adults have their hypertension controlled.

The association between hypertension and cardiovascular, cerebrovascular, and renal diseases is well documented in older adults (SOE=A). Increased systolic blood pressure, especially in midlife, may also increase the risk of both age-related cognitive decline and cognitive disorders (SOE=B). Many observational studies have documented that the risk associated with hypertension does not decrease with age, although the association between hypertension and mortality is weaker in the very old. In 2003, the Seventh Report of the Joint National Committee on Prevention, Detection, Evaluation, and Treatment of High Blood Pressure (JNC-7) issued criteria defining hypertension (see Table 51.1). The 2014 Report from the Panel Members Appointed to JNC-8 did not address the definition of hypertension but recommended an age-based approach for managing hypertension, discussed below. Many factors contribute to poor rates of blood pressure control, including lack of awareness of having hypertension and misinformation on desired normal blood pressure goals; these issues appear to be particular barriers among older black and Hispanic women. Factors related to health care providers' practices and concepts about hypertension in older adults also contribute to the age-related disparities in control rates.

Vascular structural changes and neurohumoral alterations contribute to the progressive increase in blood pressure with aging. Large vessels become less distensible with age. This is related to structural changes in the media (elastin fracture, collagen deposition, and calcification), atherosclerosis, and endothelial dysfunction. These changes lead to increased peripheral vascular resistance and decreased vascular compliance, the physiologic hallmark of hypertension in older adults. Decreased sensitivity of the baroreflex, perhaps related to decreased arterial distensibility, contributes to an increase in blood pressure variability and sympathetic nervous system activity. The dynamic regulation of vascular tone is affected by impairments in vasodilator systems (eg, production of nitric oxide by vascular endothelial cells and vasodilation mediated by β-adrenergic receptors) and by heightened vasoconstriction mediated by α-adrenergic receptors. Changes in kidney function as well as in systems involved in sodium balance, such as the renin-angiotensin system, lead to an increase in salt sensitivity and the blood pressure response to dietary sodium. Approximately two-thirds of hypertensive older adults have salt-sensitive hypertension.

In addition to the increase in blood pressure level, blood pressure dysregulation in aging renders older adults at increased risk of orthostatic and postprandial hypotension. Maintaining normal blood pressure and cerebrovascular and coronary perfusion in the face of hypotensive stimuli related to postural challenge, meals, or medications requires the integrated coordination of multiple compensatory mechanisms both

Table 51.1—JNC-7 Classification of Blood Pressure Levels

Category	Systolic (mmHg)		Diastolic (mmHg)
Normal	<140	and	<90
Hypertension			
Stage 1	140–159	or	90–99
Stage 2	>160	or	>100

NOTE: Diagnoses should be based on the average of two or more readings taken at each of two or more visits after an initial screening.

centrally and peripherally. The age-associated decline in baroreflex sensitivity and changes in sympathetic nervous system function impair the dynamic regulation of blood pressure. Because of the blunted sensitivity of the baroreflex, a greater decrease in blood pressure occurs before heart rate increases and other compensatory mechanisms are activated. Other pathophysiologic changes that impair blood pressure regulation include arterial and cardiac stiffness and a decrease in early diastolic filling. Finally, changes in the circadian control of blood pressure predisposes older adults to higher relative night-time blood pressure and greater early morning blood pressure rise, both leading to increased risk of stroke and myocardial infarction.

CLINICAL EVALUATION

Accurate measurement of blood pressure is the most critical aspect of diagnosis of hypertension in older adults. Because variability in blood pressure increases with age, the diagnosis of hypertension requires at least 3 blood pressure readings taken on 2 separate visits. Ambulatory (home) 24-hour blood pressure monitoring is recommended for patients with extreme blood pressure variability or possible "white-coat" hypertension. Ambulatory blood pressure monitoring is also recommended for evaluation of resistant hypertension and when there is concern regarding hypotensive episodes, including postural hypotension. Additional clinically useful information derived from ambulatory blood pressure monitoring is the mean blood pressure over a 24-hour period and the diurnal blood pressure rhythm. A diminished nocturnal fall in blood pressure (<10% of waking values)—the non-dipping pattern—has been associated with higher cardiovascular risk. If 24-hour ambulatory blood pressure monitoring is not possible or not available, home-based blood pressure measurements using a calibrated blood pressure monitor may provide important information about the blood pressure in the non-clinical setting. Further, the use of home blood pressure monitoring facilitates partnerships between patients and their providers and family members. This provides an important aspect of the patient-centered medical home, in which both providers and patients are intimately involved in chronic disease management.

Indirect or cuff blood pressure measurements correlate very well with direct, intra-arterial measures in most older adults. In rare individuals, extreme rigidity of the peripheral arteries may prevent complete compression of the brachial artery when the cuff is inflated, resulting in a falsely high blood pressure measurement. This is referred to as *pseudohypertension* and should be considered in cases of what appears to be resistant hypertension or when there are marked adverse events—especially hypotension-related symptoms—when antihypertensive therapy is started. Clinicians should also be aware of an auscultatory gap, which can lead to underestimation of the true systolic blood pressure and can indicate arterial stiffness. This can be avoided by inflating the blood pressure cuff 40 mmHg higher than the pressure required to occlude the brachial pulse.

Once hypertension has been diagnosed, the remainder of the clinical evaluation focuses on excluding secondary forms of hypertension and risk stratification by identifying target-organ damage, other cardiovascular risk factors, and the presence of comorbid conditions. Although most hypertensive older patients have essential hypertension, secondary forms of hypertension should be suspected in the presence of malignant hypertension, a sudden increase in diastolic blood pressure, new worsening level of blood pressure control, or resistant hypertension (poorly controlled blood pressure on a regimen of 3 antihypertensive medications, including a diuretic). Renovascular disease is the most common secondary form of hypertension among older adults. Hyperaldosteronism, obstructive sleep apnea, and use of NSAIDs are other causes of secondary hypertension that can be reversed. Treatment decisions are based on both risk stratification and overall evaluation of the patient's remaining life expectancy and functional status. Higher risk strata are those with target-organ damage (eg, left ventricular hypertrophy) or comorbid illnesses such as diabetes mellitus and hyperlipidemia, renal disease, or congestive heart failure. In older adults, risk stratification should also include an overall evaluation of functional abilities, life expectancy, and personal health care wishes. Those who have a short remaining life expectancy or are extremely frail should be counseled and monitored closely for adverse events to medications. Final decisions regarding treatment or target blood pressure should be based on goals of care and patient/family preferences.

Hypertensive older adults should always be counseled about lifestyle modification because doing so may decrease the need for antihypertensive medications. Obtaining a lifestyle history, including smoking history, dietary intake of sodium and fat, alcohol intake, and level of usual physical activity is essential and should be a part of hypertension evaluation. Contrary to common belief, older adults are able and willing to change their lifestyle but require specific education and monitoring.

TREATMENT

Treatment of hypertension in healthy and robust older adults is safe and effective. Meta-analyses of more than 40 randomized clinical trials of antihypertensive therapy have provided compelling evidence that treatment is effective in reducing cardiovascular (eg, chronic heart failure) and cerebrovascular (eg, stroke) morbidity and mortality (SOE=A). In a meta-analysis of outcome trials in systolic hypertension among older adults, treatment was associated with significant reductions in overall mortality by 13%, cardiovascular events by 26%, and stroke by 30% (SOE=A). The treatment effect was largest in men, in those ≥70 years old, and in those who had greater pulse pressures.

In those ≥80 years old, the evidence is not as robust. Until the Hypertension in the Very Elderly Trial (HYVET) study was completed in 2007, few participants in randomized controlled trials of hypertension treatment were >80 years old and almost none were >85 years old. This randomized controlled trial of 3,845 participants >80 years old ended early when its data safety monitoring board identified a significant 21% reduction in total mortality (10.1% versus 12.2%, ARR 2.2%, NNT 45 over a median of 1.8 years) in the intervention (extended-release indapamide plus perindopril if needed to achieve a goal systolic blood pressure of 150 mmHg) relative to the placebo control group (RR 0.76; CI 95%, 0.62–0.93; P=.007). The treatment group also demonstrated improvements in fatal and nonfatal stroke (RR 0.59; CI 95%, 0.40–0.88; P=.009) and heart failure and reported fewer adverse events. It is important to note that the participants in this trial were generally healthy, community-living older adults; those with dementia, living in nursing homes, or an inability to walk were excluded. The study design also required participants to have a standing blood pressure >140 mmHg at entry into the trial. For these reasons, the HYVET study results cannot be generalized to apply to frail, very old individuals.

The JNC-8 recommends treating adults ≥60 years old to achieve a blood pressure below 150/90 mmHg (SOE=A). The below 150 mmHg target has been a source of controversy, and many other guidelines have recommended a target below 140 mmHg in those ≥60 years old. In JNC-8, the committee considered targeting lower systolic blood pressure (<140/90 mmHg) acceptable if treatment is not associated with adverse effects on health or quality of life (SOE=D). The Committee also recommended a target below 140/90 mmHg for those with diabetes mellitus using expert opinion evidence (SOE=D). An individual status-based approach to managing hypertension in older adults is recommended in which both age and health status (rather than age alone) are considered when initiating or continuing antihypertensive therapy and in defining the blood pressure target of therapy.

Treatment should focus on systolic blood pressure because among older hypertensive adults, it is a stronger predictor of adverse outcomes than diastolic blood pressure. Some studies have shown increased mortality with blood pressure reduction below a certain threshold—especially diastolic blood pressure (<60 mmHg)—creating a J-shaped curve in relation to mortality (SOE=B). The significance of these concerns remains controversial. The relationship between lower diastolic blood pressure and increased cardiovascular morbidity when diastolic blood pressure is below 60–70 mmHg was observed in the Systolic Hypertension in the Elderly Trial and in the INVEST trial. The latter included only hypertensive patients with coronary artery disease. In a meta-analysis of individual's data from hypertension trials, a J curve was noted in both treated and untreated patients. It is possible, as concluded by the authors of this meta-analysis, that this J-curve is explained by poor health. Yet it seems reasonable to attempt to avoid excessive reductions in diastolic blood pressure (eg, diastolic levels <60–65 mmHg), especially in individuals with coronary heart disease.

Further complicating the issue of blood pressure targets for treatment are the preliminary results of the Systolic Blood Pressure Intervention Trial (SPRINT). In this trial, 9,361 participants >50 years old, 2,636 of whom were ≥75 years old, were randomized to treatment systolic blood pressure target groups of <140 mmHg and <120 mmHg. In September 2015, SPRINT was stopped early because of an observed 25% relative risk reduction (0.54% per year absolute risk reduction) of cardiovascular events and death in the latter group. The incidence of hypotension, syncope, electrolyte abnormalities, and acute kidney failure was significantly higher in the intensive treatment group, while there was no difference observed in the rate of injurious falls. The findings were consistent across age strata. Patients with diabetes or prior stroke were not enrolled in the trial, and residents of assisted-living facilities and nursing homes were also excluded.

Concerns about falls and use of antihypertensive therapy have been generated from observational studies (SOE=C). Yet, as found in SPRINT, clinical trials have not demonstrated an increased risk of falls. The differences between populations studied may explain this discrepancy, with clinical trial enrollees being healthier than those included in analyses of Medicare or other datasets. Hence, caution should be exercised when treating older adults with anti-hypertensive medication who report falling or who are at increased risk of falls.

Lifestyle Modification

Nonpharmacologic therapy is an important adjunct to drug treatment in all patients because of synergistic effects with antihypertensive drugs and the benefits realized through reduction in other cardiovascular risk factors. Lifestyle modifications that target the typical characteristics of the older hypertensive adult—overweight, sedentary, and salt-sensitive—are likely to be

Table 51.2—General Treatment Recommendations for Hypertension

- Begin with a nonpharmacologic approach.
- Base drug selection or combination therapies on individual patient characteristics.
- Use a low-dose thiazide-type diuretic, long-acting calcium channel blocker, ACE inhibitor, or angiotensin-receptor blocker as the first choice for initial pharmacologic therapy.
- When starting drug therapy, begin at half the usual dosage, increase dosage slowly, and continue nonpharmacologic therapies.
- Treatment goals should be gauged by systolic blood pressure and based on the patient's comorbidity profile.
- Avoid excessive reduction in diastolic blood pressure (<60–65 mmHg).

effective. The randomized Trial of Nonpharmacologic Interventions in Elderly study, which evaluated the effects of dietary sodium restriction and weight loss in older adults, demonstrated that relatively modest reductions in dietary sodium intake (1.8 g/d) and in body weight (4 kg) are accompanied by a 30% decrease in the need to reinitiate pharmacologic treatment. A meta-analysis of randomized trials assessing the effects of dietary sodium restriction demonstrated a significant reduction in systolic (a mean decrease of 3.7 mmHg for each decrease of 2.4 g/d of sodium) but not in diastolic blood pressure (SOE=A). This differential reduction in systolic pressure is particularly well suited for the older hypertensive patient. Stress-reduction techniques and increasing potassium intake in the form of fruits and vegetables also lower blood pressure. Increasing physical activity is particularly critical, because the benefit of exercise may surpass lowering blood pressure to affect other domains such as balance and cognitive function (SOE=C).

Pharmacologic Treatment

The general approach to pharmacologic management of older hypertensive adults is similar to that presented in the JNC-8. General principles regarding drug selection are reviewed here and summarized in Table 51.2. Initial drug choice is influenced by the presence or absence of comorbid conditions (eg, diabetes mellitus, coronary artery disease or history of myocardial infarction, heart failure, prostatism), cost, and compliance. A once-a-day regimen with long-acting medications is more likely to be successful. Medications should be started at the lowest dosage and cautiously increased during follow-up visits (every 4–6 weeks). If the response is inadequate or there is evidence of adverse events, a drug from a different class can be substituted. However, before adding new drugs, the following should be considered: polypharmacy, nonadherence, and drug interactions.

Thiazide-type diuretics, calcium channel blockers, angiotensin-receptor blockers (ARBs), and angiotensin-converting enzyme (ACE) inhibitors are all effective as initial treatment in non-black older adults (SOE=A). In black older adults, thiazide-type diuretics or calcium channel blockers may be preferred (SOE=B). Centrally acting agents (eg, clonidine, methyldopa) and α-blockers are not recommended as first-choice (SOE=A). β-Blockers in noncardiac patients are also not recommended as first-choice agents. Many older patients will not reach their systolic blood pressure goal on a single medication, and additional medications may be necessary.

Diuretics

Therapy with low-dose thiazide-type diuretics (eg, chlorthalidone ≤25 mg/d, or the equivalent) has demonstrated significant benefits in mortality, stroke, and coronary events in randomized clinical trials in older hypertensive adults (SOE=A). The adverse-event profile includes hypokalemia, hyperuricemia, hypomagnesemia, hyponatremia, and possible glucose intolerance. Adverse events are more likely to occur with higher dosages, so lower dosages are recommended. Adequate potassium replacement during diuretic-based treatment decreases the risk of arrhythmias and glucose intolerance. Thiazide diuretics are also well suited for use in combination therapies because of synergistic effects with other classes of antihypertensive medications. Loop diuretics may be used for hypertension but are usually reserved for those with heart failure or chronic kidney disease. Their adverse-event profile includes increasing glucose concentration, headaches, ototoxicity, and electrolyte disturbances. Aldosterone antagonists (spironolactone, eplerenone) are also useful in hypertension and may be used in those prone to hypokalemia.

ACE Inhibitors

ACE inhibitors block the production of angiotensin II and are effective in lowering blood pressure in hypertensive older adults. They lower peripheral vascular resistance through their humoral and structural effects on the vasculature without causing reflex tachycardia as seen with direct vasodilators. They are also effective in slowing the progression of hypertension nephrosclerosis and are particularly advantageous in those with concomitant diabetes or heart failure (SOE=A). Their use in African Americans has been questioned, but data from the African American Study of Kidney Disease and Hypertension (AASK) trial showed a significant beneficial effect in African Americans (SOE=A). Their adverse-event profile includes cough, hyperkalemia, angioedema, renal insufficiency (especially in those with renal artery stenosis), and in rare instances neutropenia and agranulocytosis. Black Americans are at greater risk of cough and angioedema than white Americans.

Angiotensin-Receptor Blockers

ARBs block the effect of angiotensin II on the type 1 angiotensin receptor. ARB therapy may be considered as first line or as an alternative to an ACE inhibitor, especially in those with diabetes, heart failure, or microalbuminuria. ARBs are excellent choices for those who cannot tolerate ACE inhibitors (SOE=A).

Renin Inhibitors

Renin inhibitors (eg, aliskiren) are approved for hypertension treatment. They are as effective as ACE inhibitors or ARBs in their blood pressure lowering effects, with the advantage of no dose-related increases in adverse events in older adults (SOE=B). However, no long-term outcome data are available for older adults, and renin inhibitors are significantly more expensive than other antihypertensives. They are associated with diarrhea, and there are no data on safety in those with a glomerular filtration rate <30 mL/min/1.73 m^2.

Calcium-Channel Antagonists

Therapy with long-acting dihydropyridine calcium-channel antagonists (CCAs) (nifedipine-like) is effective in reducing stroke risk in hypertensive older patients (SOE=A). CCAs in combination with ACE inhibitors have been shown to be superior to the diuretic–ACE inhibitor combination in patients with multiple vascular risk factors. Because of age-related changes in the pharmacokinetics of CCAs, lower dosages should be used. Adverse events are related to vasodilator mechanisms and include ankle edema, headaches, and postural hypotension. CCAs are also associated with constipation. Non-dihydropyridine CCAs can suppress left ventricular function and may precipitate heart block in older adults with conduction defects. Unless there is a strong indication for their use (eg, symptomatic supraventricular tachycardia, rate-controlled atrial fibrillation), they should be avoided as first choice for hypertension management. Short-acting CCAs should not be used to treat hypertension.

β-Receptor Antagonists

Several meta-analyses have questioned the efficacy of β-blockers in treating uncomplicated hypertension. Compared with placebo, β-blockers, especially atenolol, provide no reduction in all-cause mortality and myocardial infarction in older adults, and only modest reduction in stroke, which is smaller than the risk reduction seen with other antihypertensives (SOE=A).

Based on available evidence, β-blockers are not preferred as first-line agents, unless there is a strong indication, such as heart failure, prior myocardial infarction, acute coronary syndrome, stable angina, prevention of perioperative cardiac complications, or hypertrophic obstructive cardiomyopathy. Because of their effectiveness in management of symptomatic coronary artery disease, in secondary prevention after myocardial infarction, and in management of heart failure, β-receptor antagonists should be considered for older adults whose hypertension is complicated by these comorbid conditions (SOE=A).

α-Receptor Antagonists

α-Receptor antagonists are not appropriate for first-line therapy of hypertension. The treatment arm that included participants randomized to therapy with the α-receptor antagonist doxazosin in the ALLHAT study was stopped early because of a higher rate of cardiovascular complications, including a 2-fold greater likelihood of being hospitalized for heart failure. α-Receptor antagonist therapy might be considered as part of a multidrug regimen, especially in those with prostatism, because these drugs have been shown to be efficacious in improving obstructive urinary symptoms.

Other Classes

Direct vasodilators (hydralazine and minoxidil) are considered last-line therapy because of their toxic adverse-event profile, which includes tachycardia, arrhythmia, and fluid retention. Centrally acting agents (eg, clonidine) are also poorly tolerated in older adults and can be associated with sedation, bradycardia, and reflex hypertension, as well as tachycardia if abruptly stopped. Alpha-beta blockers have an antihypertensive effect, but their tolerability is an issue in older adults. Labetalol is useful in hypertensive urgencies and carvedilol in heart failure with reduced ejection fraction. Both may be associated with weakness and significant orthostatic hypotension.

Follow-Up Visits

Attempts to reduce blood pressure to target levels too rapidly are unnecessary and likely deleterious. For most patients, an interval of 4–6 weeks between visits is appropriate to determine the need for dosage adjustment. However, it may take up to 10–12 weeks for full pharmacodynamic effect after starting a medication or increasing a dosage. At all follow-up visits, it is imperative to determine both supine and standing blood pressure measurements. It is good practice to adjust antihypertensive drug dosages to achieve the target (seated) blood pressure only after determining whether postural hypotension is present.

Blood pressure monitoring outside the clinic setting may be essential, especially in those who cannot tolerate even small doses of antihypertensives. Home blood pressure monitoring may also aid in promoting adherence to therapy (SOE=B). If available, an interprofessional geriatric team is well suited to provide a well-rounded approach to hypertension management (eg, nurses to provide feedback on degree of blood pressure control, dietitians to review dietary information and adherence, pharmacists to promote adherence to the medical regimen, and social workers to review the financial burden associated with medical therapy). Models of care such as the patient-centered medical home or community-based medical care may offer additional advantage in hypertension management (SOE=C).

When a patient's blood pressure has not been successfully reduced to the target level, cautiously increasing the dosage, adding another medication (particularly a thiazide diuretic if the patient is not already taking one), or switching to another class of medication should be considered. Patients should also be counseled to continue their lifestyle modifications. Achieving the target blood pressure goal may take many months. When this goal is not attained despite adherence to a 3-drug regimen, an evaluation for refractory or resistant hypertension (especially renovascular disease, hyperaldosteronism, and sleep apnea) should be considered. After more than a year of appropriate stable blood pressure control, step-down treatment may be considered; dosages may be decreased cautiously, with close blood pressure monitoring. Patients who have successfully modified their lifestyle (eg, weight loss) are most likely to be able to reduce their dosage or eliminate antihypertensive medications.

SPECIAL CONSIDERATIONS

Hypertensive Emergencies and Urgencies

Increased blood pressure per se in the absence of signs or symptoms of target-organ damage does not constitute a hypertensive emergency. Rapidly and too aggressively decreasing blood pressure in a patient with incidentally discovered increased blood pressure is potentially harmful and can cause complications, such as coronary or cerebral hypoperfusion syndromes (SOE=B).

Examples of true hypertensive emergencies in older adults include hypertensive encephalopathy, acute heart failure with pulmonary edema, dissecting aortic aneurysm, and unstable angina. These patients present with symptoms and signs of vascular compromise of affected organs. Management of these emergencies requires an acute hospital setting, with parenteral administration of a short-acting antihypertensive agent and continual blood pressure monitoring to immediately reduce blood pressure, although not initially to a normal target level.

Blood pressure should not be lowered emergently more than 25% within the first 2 hours, with a goal of achieving 160/100 mmHg gradually over the first 6 hours of therapy (SOE=D).

Hypertension in the Long-Term Care Setting and Frail Older Adults

Approximately one-third to two-thirds of residents in long-term care facilities have hypertension. Special considerations are warranted in the care of residents with respect to making the correct diagnosis and defining the goals of therapy and its effects on quality of life. Blood pressure measurements in long-term care settings may not be accurate because of measurement errors and the temporal variability in blood pressure, particularly in relation to meals. Blood pressure appears to be highest in the morning before breakfast. Postprandial hypotension is common among long-term care residents, affecting about one-third of this population. It has been associated with otherwise unexplained syncope and found to be a significant independent risk factor for falls, syncope, stroke, and overall mortality.

Several factors should be considered in management of hypertension in this setting. First, the advanced average age and comorbidity of residents in long-term care facilities raises controversy surrounding the question of whether the benefits of antihypertensive therapy extend to this population. If the beneficial effects of treatment are less evident, the potential adverse events and risks of therapy should be weighed more heavily in defining the goals of therapy. Even an intervention as seemingly innocuous as a sodium-restricted diet needs to be evaluated in the context of the high prevalence of protein-energy malnutrition among nursing-home residents. Second, the average resident in long-term care takes 9 or 10 medications, and most have 3 or more comorbid conditions. The addition of an antihypertensive medication increases the possibility of an adverse event in this frail, at-risk group. A study of 1,130 frail individuals ≥80 years old (the Predictive Values of Blood Pressure and Arterial Stiffness in Institutionalized Very Aged Population [PARTAGE] multicenter, longitudinal study) found a significant increase in mortality in those receiving more than 2 antihypertensive medications and a systolic blood pressure below 130 mmHg. Hence, avoiding aggressive blood pressure control (eg, avoiding systolic blood pressure <130 mmHg) is likely to be the safer approach in this population. Third, several studies have identified the use of antihypertensive medications, particularly vasodilators, as a risk factor for falls in this high-risk population, experiencing an average of 2 falls each year (SOE=B). It is therefore important to assess both postural and postprandial blood pressure in this population. Further, the evidence for a mortality or morbidity benefit in frail older adults is lacking. In observational studies, older adults who could not walk more than 6 meters (20 feet) in <8 seconds demonstrated no association between blood pressure and mortality. In particular, in those with severe physical frailty, higher blood pressure may be linked with lower mortality (SOE=B). Therefore, it is critical to assess functional levels and expected survival in frail patients before starting or continuing antihypertensive therapy.

Renal Artery Stenosis

Atherosclerotic renal artery stenosis (defined as ≥50% narrowing) is present in 7% of older adults and in 25% of those with a serum creatinine >2 mg/dL. In older adults, renal artery stenosis is a common contributor to resistant hypertension and may lead to cardiac destabilization syndromes such as heart failure exacerbation, cardiac ischemia, and "flash" pulmonary edema. Detection can be performed by Doppler ultrasonography and CT or MR angiography. Medical therapy includes lifestyle change and blood pressure medications. Percutaneous renal artery revascularization and stenting is an additional treatment option, but the clinical benefit for stenting is limited. Both the Cardiovascular Outcomes in Renal Atherosclerotic Lesions (CORAL; mean age=69.1 years) and Angioplasty and Stenting for Renal Artery Lesions (ASTRAL; mean age=70 years) studies failed to demonstrate a benefit for stenting on either cardiovascular or renal outcomes (SOE=B). Better patient selection using dynamic or physiologic effects of the renal artery stenosis (eg, flow reserve or a translational pressure gradient >20 mmHg) may improve clinical response (SOE=C). Clinically, selecting those with resistant hypertension (use of 3 medications including a diuretic), ischemic renal disease with bilateral stenosis, or cardiac destabilization syndromes (flash pulmonary edema or ischemic cardiac events) should be evaluated for potential stenting (SOE=C). Stenting is limited by the development of intra-stent restenosis; hence, the risk of secondary interventions should be weighed against the modest clinical benefit observed in clinical trials.

Choosing Wisely® Recommendations

Hypertension

- Do not screen for renal artery stenosis in patients without resistant hypertension and with normal renal function, even if known atherosclerosis is present.

REFERENCES

- Aronow WS, Fleg JL, Pepine CJ, et al. ACCF/AHA 2011 Expert Consensus Document on Hypertension in the elderly: a report of the American College of Cardiology Foundation Task Force on Clinical Expert Consensus documents developed in collaboration with the American Academy of Neurology, American Geriatrics Society, American Society for Preventive Cardiology, American Society of Hypertension, American Society of Nephrology, Association of Black Cardiologists, and European Society of Hypertension. *J Am Coll Cardiol*. 2011;57(20):2037–2114.

    This comprehensive consensus statement provides both a review of the current evidence and clinical expert opinion about hypertension and aging. It suggests that lowering blood pressure is generally safe and leads to improved overall outcomes in older adults. The evidence is robust for those <80 years old but weaker in those ≥80 years old. According to the Hypertension in the Very Elderly Trial (HYVET), lowering blood pressure below 150/80 mmHg in those ≥80 years old is associated with improved cardiovascular morbidity and mortality. The summary also provides a review of antihypertensive medications and summarizes the evidence behind their recommendations.

- Beckett NS, Peters R, Fletcher AE, et al. Treatment of hypertension in patients 80 years of age or older. *N Engl J Med*. 2008;358(18):1887–1898.

    This landmark study, the Hypertension in the Very Elderly Trial (HYVET), was designed to address the risks and benefits of antihypertensive therapy in patients ≥80 years old, predominantly in Eastern Europe and China. A total of 3,845 participants were randomized to active therapy (extended-release indapamide plus an ACE inhibitor, perindopril, if needed) or placebo and followed for primary outcomes of fatal or nonfatal stroke. At 2 years, there was a 15/6 mmHg difference in blood pressure between the two groups; target blood pressure (150/80 mmHg) was met in 20% of the placebo group and in 48% of the active treatment group. Most (75%) patients were receiving both study drugs. In addition to the 21% reduction in overall mortality, the active treatment group also demonstrated a 30% decrease in fatal and nonfatal stroke and a 64% decrease in heart failure. The estimated NNT to prevent one stroke in 2 years is 94 patients. Based on the study's entry criteria, its participants were healthier than the general very old population and, consequently, its findings may not generalize broadly to this population.

- James PA, Oparil S, Carter BL, et al. 2014 Evidence-based guideline for the management of high blood pressure in adults: report from the panel members appointed to the Eighth Joint National Committee (JNC 8). *JAMA*. 2014;311(5):507–520.

    The report from panel members appointed to the Eighth Joint National Committee (JNC) provides treatment guidelines applicable to older hypertensive adults. In contrast to prior JNC recommendations, a target blood pressure below 150/90 mm Hg is recommended in those ≥60 years old. More than one antihypertensive medication is often needed to achieve the target blood pressure. An individualized approach to therapy based on the patient's risk factors and comorbidities is emphasized. Also new to the report is the removal of β-blockers as first-line therapy; they are not recommended for blood pressure lowering unless the patient has heart disease (coronary artery disease, congestive heart failure).

- Lipsitz LA. A 91-year-old woman with difficult-to-control hypertension: a clinical review. *JAMA*. 2013;310(12):1274–1280.

    A case-based presentation of the age/health status approach to hypertension management in those ≥80 years old is described.

This paper provides an example case, an overview of the literature, and a summary recommendation about managing the very old with hypertension.

- Ritchie LD, Campbell NC, Murchie P. New NICE guidelines for hypertension. *BMJ*. 2011;343:d5644.

    The National Institute for Health and Clinical Excellence (NICE) in the United Kingdom released an update on the management of hypertension. According to this update, blood pressure targets were relaxed for those ≥80 years old to less than 150/90 mmHg. The guidelines acknowledge that achieving a target blood pressure of 140/90 mmHg is challenging and should strike a balance between lowering blood pressure and development of symptoms and issues with adherence. Another major change is related to first-line treatment, in which calcium channel blockers and ACE inhibitors are now considered equally effective as thiazide diuretics. Finally, the NICE guidelines advocate the use of ambulatory blood pressure monitoring to identify "white-coat" hypertension because of its cost effectiveness. This may be particularly useful in older adults in whom polypharmacy and risk of drug adverse events may be higher than in younger hypertensive adults. JNC-8 is expected to have similar but not identical recommendations.

- Wright JT Jr, Fine LJ, Lackland DT, et al. Evidence supporting a systolic blood pressure goal of less than 150 mm Hg in patients aged 60 years or older: the minority view. *Ann Intern Med*. 2014;160(7):499–503.

    In this article, a subgroup form the JNC-8 panel provided a counterargument for increasing the target blood pressure from less than 140 mmHg to less than 150 mmHg in those ≥60 years old: "We, the panel minority, believed that evidence was insufficient to increase the SBP goal from its current level of less than 140 mmHg because of concern that increasing the goal may cause harm by increasing the risk for CVD and partially undoing the remarkable progress in reducing cardiovascular mortality in Americans older than 60 years. Because of the overall evidence, including the RCT data reviewed by the panel, and the decrease in CVD mortality, we concluded that the evidence for increasing a blood pressure target in high-risk populations should be at least as strong as the evidence required to decrease the recommended blood pressure target."

Ihab Hajjar, MD, MS, FACP, AGSF

CHAPTER 52—GASTROENTEROLOGY

KEY POINTS

- Although physiological changes of aging can affect GI function, most GI symptoms and signs are due to pathologic conditions and should be evaluated accordingly.

- Medications used to treat many illnesses that affect older adults can cause GI symptoms and disorders.

- Geriatric patients often present with atypical symptoms of GI disorders and with more severe disease, creating diagnosis challenges and urgency.

- Older patients can tolerate many treatments for GI diseases as well as younger patients but may be more susceptible to medication adverse events.

The structure and function of the GI tract are affected both by physiological changes of aging and by the effects of accumulating disorders involving many organ systems. In association with advancing age, changes in connective tissue can limit the elasticity of the gut and changes in the nerves and muscles can impair motility. Disturbances of epithelial, muscle, or neural function may all result from age-related enteric neurodegeneration and loss of excitatory enteric neurons. Accumulating chronic conditions are often associated with increased use of medications by older adults, many of which have direct effects on intestinal mucosa and motility. Some disease states, such as atherosclerosis and diabetes mellitus, can adversely influence GI function and lead to symptoms and complications. GI problems can quickly compromise the older adult's ability to maintain adequate nutrition, leading to fatigue and weight loss.

DISORDERS OF THE ESOPHAGUS

Dysphagia

Dysphagia refers to the subjective sensation of difficulty swallowing and may be due to any disruption in the swallowing process. The prevalence of dysphagia in patients ≥ 65 years old has been reported to be 15%–40% in the outpatient setting and up to 60% in older adults living in nursing homes. Physiological or anatomical abnormalities along any portion of the esophagus, including the upper and lower sphincters, may lead to the sensation of difficulty swallowing. Dysphagia is typically classified as oropharyngeal or esophageal. Although there are physiological changes associated with aging that may lead to dysphagia, this is considered an alarm symptom that must prompt evaluation and should never be attributed to normal aging without an appropriate evaluation.

Oropharyngeal dysphagia (often referred to as transfer dysphagia) is characterized by the inability to initiate a swallow or transfer food from the mouth to the esophagus. In addition to the sensation of dysphagia, typical symptoms include coughing, choking, nasopharyngeal regurgitation, aspiration (with or without subsequent pneumonia) and retained food in the mouth after an attempted swallow. In patients with advanced dementia, oropharyngeal dysphagia may result from apraxia and be misinterpreted as a refusal to swallow. Multiple changes in the physiology of the aging gut as well as specific disorders may lead to oropharyngeal dysphagia. Physiological studies have shown reduced tongue strength, reduced pharyngeal wall contraction, decreased salivary flow, and impaired gag reflexes in healthy older adults, all of which likely contribute to dysphagia. Poor dentition may lead to inadequate mastication of food bolus and contribute as well. Neurologic disorders (such as stroke, Parkinson disease, Alzheimer dementia, myasthenia gravis) and malignancies of the oropharynx are common causes of oropharyngeal dysphagia. Structural abnormalities such as a Zenker diverticulum or prominent cervical osteophytes are also common in this age group.

In contrast, esophageal dysphagia typically presents as the sensation of food getting stuck in the esophagus (or chest) several seconds after initiating a swallow. Age-related physiologic changes such as decreased salivary flow and loss of neurons in the myenteric and submucosal plexus lead to altered motility and contribute to the high rates of dysphagia among older adults. Further, medications can exacerbate these changes, often through anticholinergic effects. The etiology of esophageal dysphagia is usually subclassified into motility disorders, structural disorders, and infectious diseases. Dysphagia for both solids and liquids from the onset usually implies a motility disorder of the esophagus. Common primary motility disorders include achalasia, nonspecific peristaltic disorders (ineffective esophageal motility), and hypertensive or spastic disorders (nutcracker esophagus, distal esophageal spasm). The most well-described motility disorder, achalasia, occurs most commonly in patients under the age of 60 years. However, due to its chronic benign nature, the prevalence rises with age. Less is known about the epidemiology of the nonspecific motility disorders, which may be the presenting problem in systemic disorders such as scleroderma. In contrast, dysphagia for solids that progresses later to involve liquids suggests mechanical obstruction. In

Table 52.1—Evaluation of Dysphagia

Type of Dysphagia	Test/Procedure	Comments
Oropharyngeal	Videofluoroscopy	Assesses swallowing mechanics, detects aspiration, evaluates effects of various barium consistencies
	Nasopharyngolaryngoscopy	Evaluates oropharynx, larynx, and perilaryngeal regions for masses, pooled secretions, or retained food
	Fiberoptic endoscopic swallowing evaluation	Assesses for masses, pooled secretions, retained food, and sensory functioning of swallowing structures
Esophageal	Barium esophagram	Assesses structural abnormalities and changes suggestive of underlying motility disorders
Both types	Upper endoscopy	Identifies structural abnormalities, allows for biopsy and histologic examination, and can perform therapeutic procedures such as dilatation

the older age group, multiple causes of mechanical obstruction are seen. Malignancy must be excluded in all patients. The most common cancers tend to be adenocarcinomas occurring in the distal esophagus often in the background of Barrett changes. Benign strictures may be due acid to reflux, prior radiation, or pill-induced esophageal injury. Extrinsic compression may be due to variant vasculature, a large aortic aneurysm, an enlarged left atrium, or extra-esophageal malignancies such as lymphoma. Dysphagia accompanied by odynophagia (painful swallowing) is suspicious for an infectious etiology, such as a viral or fungal infection. Candidal infections are the most common and often seen in the setting of systemic immunosuppression or with use of steroids administered via inhaler. Common viruses are the herpes simplex virus, which can be seen in immunocompetent older adults, and cytomegalovirus, which is typically found only in immunosuppressed patients.

The evaluation of dysphagia is typically multimodal. See Table 52.1 for testing options.

Treatment of dysphagia depends on the underlying cause. A medication review should be done, particularly focusing on anticholinergic drugs that may worsen dysphagia. Treatment of oropharyngeal dysphagia may require swallowing rehabilitation or dietary modifications such as thickening liquids, or careful hand feeding with a spoon, cup, or straw. In cases in which dementia is the cause of dysphagia, the placement of a percutaneous gastrostomy with tube feeding has not demonstrated improvement in survival, function, or symptoms, and tube feeding is recognized as a risk factor for aspiration (SOE=B). Multiple treatment options exist for achalasia. Injection of the lower esophageal sphincter with botulinum toxin may provide months of symptomatic relief in patients who are not surgical candidates. In most patients, however, definitive treatment with surgical or endoscopic myotomy is indicated (SOE=A). Calcium channel blockers or phosphodiesterase inhibitors (such as sildenafil[OL]) may provide relief in various spastic motility disorders (SOE=B). Treatment of malignancy is primarily surgical, often with adjunct chemotherapy and/or radiation. However, in nonadvanced cancers or in patients who are not surgical candidates, endoscopic treatments may be available for curative or palliative intent. Strictures are treated with endoscopic dilation, with a very high success rate, although they often require ongoing medical treatment of the underlying cause as well (eg, reflux). Infectious causes require targeted antiviral or antifungal therapy.

Gastroesophageal Reflux Disease

Gastroesophageal reflux disease (GERD) is defined as symptoms or complications resulting from the reflux of gastric contents into the esophagus or beyond to the oropharynx, nasopharynx, larynx, or lung. GERD is the most commonly seen upper GI condition in primary care. Among adults ≥65 years old, symptoms of heartburn or acid regurgitation occur at least weekly in 20% of the population and at least monthly in 59%. Prolonged pH studies show that esophageal acid exposure frequency and duration increases with age, and endoscopic data suggest that esophagitis is more severe in older adults. However, likely because of decreased pain perception in this age group, the severity of symptoms often does not correlate with the severity of disease.

Multiple potential factors aggravate GERD in older adults, including frequent inappropriate transient lower esophageal sphincter relaxations, medications known to decrease lower esophageal sphincter tone, higher prevalence of hiatal hernia, impaired esophageal peristalsis, and decreased salivary volume and bicarbonate concentration.

Heartburn is the characteristic symptom of GERD, described as a "burning" sensation in the chest, often rising from the epigastrium. Symptoms often occur or are worse after a meal, and patients may note certain food triggers (eg, spicy foods, citrus or acidic foods, fats, caffeine, or alcohol) that reliably bring on the symptoms. Older patients may present with atypical or extraesophageal manifestations of GERD, sometimes without accompanying heartburn. These so called atypical or extraesophageal symptoms include dyspepsia, epigastric pain, nausea, bloating, belching, asthma, chronic cough, and laryngitis or voice changes. Many older adults with longstanding disease marked by atypical symptoms delay in seeking care and first present with alarming symptoms such as dysphagia, odynophagia, or vomiting.

Diagnosis of GERD, especially in the older population, may be difficult. Guidelines allow for a presumptive diagnosis of GERD in the setting of typical symptoms and recommend initial treatment with an empiric trial of acid-suppression therapy. In the general population, empiric treatment with a proton-pump inhibitor (PPI), as a test for GERD, has a sensitivity of 68%–83% (SOE=A). Current guidelines do not differentiate diagnosis in older adults from any other age group. Older adults may benefit from earlier endoscopic evaluation, because they may have vague or mild symptoms despite the presence of severe esophagitis and even complications of GERD. Patients with alarm signs or symptoms, or those with longstanding reflux, should undergo endoscopy to exclude severe esophagitis, strictures, Barrett esophagus, dysplasia, and malignancy. Patients who do not respond to a trial of PPI and/or do not have endoscopic findings to explain their symptoms warrant further testing. Evaluation with 24-hour pH-impedance testing can confirm or exclude acid and nonacid reflux. Prolonged pH monitoring for 48–96 hours using a wireless pH capsule can identify acid reflux in patients who do not have daily symptoms. Esophageal manometry is used to document the presence of effective esophageal peristalsis in patients in whom antireflux surgery is being considered and to exclude an underlying esophageal motility disorder, such as achalasia, as the cause of the symptoms.

The primary goals of treatment are to reduce symptoms and prevent complications. Although evidence for the effectiveness of lifestyle and dietary modifications is limited, these nonpharmacologic interventions are still considered first-line therapy. Obesity has been associated with increased risk of GERD, and weight loss has been shown to decrease reflux symptoms; thus, for obese patients with GERD, weight loss is recommended. Elevating the head of the bed and avoiding meals within 2–3 hours before bedtime should be recommended for patients with nocturnal symptoms. Medications that reduce lower esophageal sphincter tone or acidify gastric contents should be avoided when possible. These include anticholinergics, benzodiazepines, opiates, nitrates, and calcium channel antagonists. Elimination of food triggers such as chocolate, caffeine, spicy foods, citrus foods, or carbonated beverages is recommended only in patients who can identify an exacerbation in symptoms with specific foods. Antacids, alginic acid, or OTC histamine$_2$-receptor antagonists (H$_2$RAs) may be helpful in relieving mild, transient reflux symptoms (SOE=B). The duration of action of each of these is limited, as is their ability to achieve healing of erosive esophagitis.

Antisecretory therapy in the form of PPIs is the treatment of choice for patients with moderate to severe GERD or GERD with any complication (SOE=A). PPIs achieve healing of erosive esophagitis in >80% of patients, compared with 50%–60% with H$_2$RAs, regardless of age. Available PPIs include omeprazole, esomeprazole, lansoprazole, dexlansoprazole, pantoprazole, and rabeprazole. Omeprazole, esomeprazole, and lansoprazole are currently available as OTC formulations. There are no clinically important differences in symptom relief with any of the above PPIs given once daily. As recommended in current guidelines, an 8-week course of once-daily PPI should be administered in most patients. PPIs should be taken 30–60 minutes before a meal for maximal pH control. If acute medical therapy alleviates symptoms, a trial off medication can be considered after symptoms have resolved. Maintenance PPI therapy should be administered for GERD patients who continue to have symptoms after PPI is discontinued, and in patients with complications including erosive esophagitis and Barrett esophagus. Recurrence of symptoms is common after therapy is stopped, and lifelong therapy may be needed. Intermittent therapy with an H$_2$RA or PPI may be successful in some patients with mild to moderate symptoms, while maintenance daily PPI therapy is needed in those with severe symptoms. A dosage increase or change in PPI can be attempted in patients who only partially respond to a PPI. Patients who do not respond to PPIs should be referred for evaluation with endoscopy, pH monitoring, and/or manometry.

Antisecretory therapy, specifically with PPIs, is associated with potential risks. Case reports have shown association between long-term PPI use and lowered vitamin B$_{12}$ levels in older adults. A relationship between antisecretory therapy and infections, specifically pneumonia and enteric infections (particularly *Clostridium difficile*), has been raised because of the loss of the gastric acid barrier; however, the data are mixed. Concerns have also been raised regarding blunted calcium absorption in the setting of acid suppression and long-term effects of PPIs on bone mineral density. However, the data regarding this association have been conflicting, and current guidelines state that even patients with known osteoporosis can stay on PPIs and that concern for hip fractures and osteoporosis should not affect the decision to use PPIs in the average patient. Regardless, it is reasonable to adjust the regimen in patients with known osteoporosis risk factors. For PPI users who require calcium supplementation, a soluble form such as calcium citrate is preferred. Concerns have been raised about the interaction between PPIs (which inhibit the hepatic cytochromic P450 system) and the anti-platelet medication clopidogrel. This concern was borne out of pharmacokinetic platelet aggregation studies as well as observational data which suggested an increased risk of cardiovascular events in patients taking PPIs. However, a large number of subsequent studies, including several randomized controlled trials and meta-analyses showed no increased risk of cardiovascular or cerebrovascular or mortality events and revealed a lower rate of gastrointestinal bleeding in PPI users. Thus it is not recommended to routinely stop or avoid PPI use in patients on clopidogrel.

Surgical treatment of GERD is generally reserved for selected patients with large hiatal hernias or in whom the diagnosis is confirmed and for whom lifestyle changes and antisecretory therapy alone do not resolve symptoms. Studies on antireflux surgery in older adults show high success rates with mortality and morbidity similar to those of younger patients.

Drug-Induced Esophageal Injury

Several medications are known to cause direct injury to the esophageal mucosa. Older adults are at increased risk of pill-induced injury because of several factors, including polypharmacy, impaired esophageal peristalsis, and decreased salivary flow. Increased age alone has been shown to be a risk factor for pill retention. These factors increase contact time between the caustic (typically acidic) contents of the medications and the mucosa, allowing for a chemical injury. The site of injury is commonly at the level of the aortic arch, of an enlarged left atrium, or of the esophagogastric junction, areas with a potentially decreased lumen circumference.

Antibiotics have been commonly implicated in pill esophagitis. Tetracyclines, particularly doxycycline, are the most common antibiotics that induce esophagitis. All NSAIDs, including aspirin, can damage the esophageal mucosa. Other common offenders include potassium chloride, ferrous sulfate, quinidine, and bisphosphonates. Bisphosphonates appear to be of particular concern, because they have been reported to induce severe esophagitis, often with an affected surface area much larger than that of the offending tablet. Gelatin capsules are of particular concern.

The diagnosis of pill esophagitis is often clinical. The typical presenting symptom is odynophagia. Patients often recall having ingested a medication known to cause injury, often with little or no water or immediately preceding bedtime. Upper endoscopy is the most sensitive diagnostic tool and may reveal a discrete ulcer of variable size with normal surrounding mucosa. Endoscopy is needed if the diagnosis is not clear from the clinical history or in cases of severe symptoms.

Affected mucosa typically heals within a few days to a week without intervention. Symptoms seem to resolve as quickly. Patients should avoid the offending medication, if possible, until symptoms resolve. Otherwise, specific treatment is not typically required. Acid suppression (with PPIs or H$_2$RAs), topical anesthetics (such as lidocaine), and sucralfate suspension or slurries (to provide a protective coating) are often given, but their use is off-label and little evidence exists to show efficacy. In severe disease, patients may be unable to tolerate any oral intake and should be admitted for parenteral hydration. Underlying dysmotility should be evaluated and treated if suspected to prevent recurrence as should strictures, which may be the cause of or result of pill-induced injury.

Patients should be instructed to drink plenty of water (at least 8 ounces) with each pill and to sit or stand upright for at least 30 minutes after pill ingestion. This will allow gravity to facilitate esophageal emptying. For patients with known esophageal disorders, alternative medications or liquid forms should be considered.

DISORDERS OF THE STOMACH

Dyspepsia

Dyspepsia implies chronic or recurrent pain or discomfort in the upper abdomen, more specifically bothersome postprandial fullness, epigastric pain, or epigastric burning. These symptoms are common (with up to 40% of the general population affected during their lifetime), and the differential diagnosis for these symptoms is broad, which often makes diagnosis difficult. The most common diseases associated with dyspepsia are peptic ulcer disease, gastroesophageal reflux, biliary colic, or medication-induced discomfort. Some would consider gastritis due to *Helicobacter pylori* as a potential cause for symptoms but this is debated. Esophageal, gastric, or duodenal malignancies have all been seen in patients presenting with dyspepsia. Patients in whom structural disease is excluded meet the criteria for functional dyspepsia.

Although an empiric trial with antisecretory therapies is often used, prompt endoscopy should be considered in older adults because of the increased rate of organic disease (including malignancy) in this age group. Endoscopy for evaluation of dyspepsia in older adults has been shown to obtain diagnostic information in >90% of patients and is associated with a significant reduction in PPI use and an improvement in quality-of-life measures (SOE=B). Endoscopy has been shown to be safe in older adults who are otherwise healthy. The risk of endoscopy in elderly patients with cardiac, pulmonary or other systemic disease depends on disease severity. The decision to perform endoscopy should be made on a case-by-case basis.

H pylori testing should be performed in all patients with dyspepsia, with a 13C-urea breath test or fecal antigen test along with biopsies at the time of endoscopy. Treatment for *H pylori* in patients with ulcers will result in healing and elimination of symptoms in a large majority of patients. Large or nonhealing ulcers should be biopsied to exclude malignancy. Data are conflicting on whether treating *H pylori* in patients with nonulcer or functional dyspepsia reduces symptoms. Many in practice treat these patients in hope that eradication will reduce or eliminate symptoms. Those who are negative for *H pylori* should be given a 2-month empirical trial of a PPI (SOE=B).

Patients with a normal upper endoscopy should be considered for further testing (including abdominal imaging and a gastric emptying study). Imaging should include an abdominal sonogram to rule out hepatobiliary disease, which can mimic dyspepsia. Further imaging with a CT scan can be considered, but is recommended in patients with weight loss, severe pain or other alarm features. A gastric emptying study can be performed in any patient with dyspepsia and a normal endoscopy, but may be most useful in patients who describe early satiety or vomiting. Ultimately, patients with no identified organic disease are classified as having functional dyspepsia. These patients can also be given a trial of PPI, although the rate of symptom improvement is low. Tricyclic antidepressants[OL] have been shown to be efficacious in the general population but are not recommended for use in older adults.

NSAID-Induced Gastric Complications

All NSAIDs, including aspirin, are capable of causing considerable injury to the gastric and duodenal mucosa. Age is an independent risk factor for NSAID-induced complications, and older adults experience considerable morbidity and mortality due to this class of medications.

The common gastroduodenal adverse effects of NSAIDs are dyspepsia (associated with gastritis and duodenitis) and peptic ulcer disease (PUD), with associated pain, bleeding, and perforation. The pathogenesis of NSAID-induced injury appears to be due to the systemic effect of the medications, although local effects do play a role. Many NSAIDs are carboxylic acids and exert local injury on contact with gastric and duodenal mucosa. However, most NSAID toxicity appears to occur through the cyclooxygenase pathway. Cyclooxygenase-1 (COX-1) is a constitutive enzyme used by healthy gastric and duodenal mucosa in production of mucosal-protective prostaglandins. Prostaglandins protect the upper GI mucosa by decreasing acid production, increasing local mucin and bicarbonate secretion, and enhancing local blood flow and oxygen supply. NSAIDs induce injury by inhibiting COX-1 and disrupting these protective mechanisms.

In addition to age ≥65 years, risk factors for NSAID-induced disease include high-dose NSAID use, a prior history of PUD, and concurrent use of two NSAIDs (typically, low-dose aspirin in addition to another NSAID). Patients also taking anticoagulants, glucocorticoids, antiplatelet medications (such as clopidogrel), or SSRIs (which have weak antiplatelet activity) appear to have an increased risk of bleeding with NSAIDs. The presence of *H pylori* infection appears to have a synergistic effect on the risk of ulcer disease and bleeding in the setting of NSAID use. Several preventive strategies are available to minimize risk of GI complications in patients who must use NSAIDs. Enteric-coated NSAID formulations appear to reduce endoscopic evidence of injury but do not protect against GI bleeding, and their use is not enough to provide adequate protection in patients at risk. Switching to NSAIDs that selectively inhibit COX-2 (such as celecoxib) is associated with a 40% reduction in bleeding risk but at a potentially higher risk of cardiovascular events. Concurrent use of PPIs while on NSAIDs has been shown to be a safe and effective strategy in reducing complications, with some case series showing no gastric ulcers in patients using PPIs while on NSAIDs. Similarly, the prostaglandin E analogue misoprostol has been shown to reduce serious GI complications by >50% (SOE=A). The AGS Beers Criteria recommend the use of PPIs or misoprostol in older adults requiring chronic NSAID therapy.

Peptic Ulcer Disease

Peptic ulcers are GI mucosal defects created in part by acid injury. Although ulcers can be seen throughout the GI tract, the term peptic ulcer usually refers to ulcers in the stomach and duodenum. Ulcers in the esophagus may be acid related but are not typically called peptic. Rates of PUD have been falling over the past several decades. Nonetheless, PUD is still a common disorder, and the incidence and complications of PUD both increase with age. In the United States, *H pylori* infection is responsible for about 80% of duodenal ulcers and 60% of gastric ulcers. The vast majority of ulcers in *H pylori*–negative patients are due to NSAIDs. Ulcers may be asymptomatic and found on upper endoscopy performed for other indications. In symptomatic PUD, common presentations are dyspepsia, bleeding, anemia, and acute abdominal pain.

Peptic ulcers are diagnosed via endoscopy, which has a sensitivity of >90% and also allows for treatment of bleeding lesions (and lesions at high risk of bleeding). Equally important, endoscopy allows for biopsies to differentiate benign ulcers from gastric cancers as well as to exclude an underlying *H pylori* infection. Clinicians should have a low threshold for repeat endoscopy in older patients with gastric ulcers to confirm ulcer healing and to exclude malignancy, because initial biopsies for gastric cancer can have a sensitivity as low as 70%.

Once a diagnosis of PUD is made, PPI therapy should be instituted. All PPIs are effective in inducing ulcer healing with rates of 80%–100% at 8 weeks (SOE=A). All patients with peptic ulcers who are infected with *H pylori* should undergo therapy to eradicate the infection. In such patients, PPI therapy can be stopped after *H pylori* treatment if ulcers were small and the patient is otherwise at low risk of bleeding. *H pylori* eradication should be confirmed with a post-treatment urea breath test or fecal antigen test. Patients with NSAID-induced PUD should remain on antisecretory therapy indefinitely if they are to remain on NSAIDs. PPI treatment once a day is sufficient in these patients.

Biliary Disease

Gall stones primarily form in the gallbladder and are often asymptomatic. However, when they obstruct the cystic duct, common bile duct or ampulla, symptoms and complications can occur.

Gall stone disease encompasses a variety of disorders, including biliary colic, cholecystitis, cholangitis, and gall stone pancreatitis. Biliary colic is typically due to a stone transiently obstructing the cystic duct (during a gallbladder contraction) and results in severe, epigastric or right upper quadrant pain that lasts for ~30–60 minutes. Cholecystitis and cholangitis are due to stones obstructing the cystic duct and common bile duct, respectively, and are associated with inflammation and/or infection of the biliary tree. In addition to pain, these may cause a full spectrum of infectious symptoms, including fever, delirium, and shock. Older adults may present atypically, without pain or fever, and with only advanced symptoms such as delirium or hypotension.

The evaluation of biliary disease includes appropriate blood tests (including liver function tests, amylase, and lipase) as well as imaging. The initial imaging of choice in all patients is an abdominal ultrasound, which can have a sensitivity of >80% and a specificity of nearly 100% for gall stone disease. Abdominal CT can better visualize the pancreas and can identify common bile duct stones often missed by ultrasound. Magnetic resonance cholangiography is a highly-sensitive imaging modality for the biliary system and may be used when suspicion of ductal stones is high, but the above imaging studies are nondiagnostic. Advanced imaging, with endoscopic ultrasound or endoscopic retrograde cholangiopancreatography, is limited to cases with a very high suspicion of gall stone disease and negative imaging or for those patients requiring endoscopic therapy.

Gallstones can be found in 35% of women and 20% of men by 70 years of age because of an age-related increase in the lithogenicity of bile. Although many older adults with cholelithiasis are asymptomatic, biliary disease is the predominant indication for urgent abdominal operations in this population; in adults >80 years old, hepatobiliary disease accounts for 20% of all abdominal surgeries. In general, asymptomatic patients with gall stones can be observed. Patients with symptomatic cholelithiasis should undergo laparoscopic cholecystectomy if they are surgical candidates because of the high rate of complications such as cholecystitis, cholangitis, and pancreatitis. In the rare older patient who is unable to undergo surgery, treatment with ursodeoxycholic acid or lithotripsy, or both, may be attempted, although efficacy rates are low. In patients with common bile duct obstruction due to gall stones, endoscopic sphincterotomy and bile ductal drainage is adequate in preventing recurrent cholangitis, and the gallbladder may be left in situ. In older adults presenting with biliary pain who have had a cholecystectomy, a retained common bile duct stone should be suspected and evaluated by endoscopic retrograde cholangiopancreatography, magnetic resonance cholangiography, or endoscopic ultrasonography.

The possibility of cancer should be considered in any older adult with biliary symptoms. For patients with malignant jaundice, treatments are mostly palliative, with either surgery or percutaneous or endoscopic stenting. Such drainage improves quality of life, decreases pruritus, and improves nutritional state, but does not improve survival.

Pancreatitis

Acute pancreatitis is any acute inflammatory process affecting the pancreas. It is a common cause of presentation to the emergency department for abdominal pain and can range in severity from mild to life threatening. The epidemiology of pancreatitis is complex due to the multiple underlying etiologies. However, the incidence does appear to increase with age.

The three most common causes of pancreatitis are alcohol abuse, gallstones, and medications. Alcohol, the most common cause of pancreatitis in the young, appears to cause only a minority of acute pancreatitis in patients over the age of 65. Gallstones are a common cause of pancreatitis in all age groups, but become increasingly prevalent with age (as noted in the biliary disease section above). Finally, a significant portion of elderly patients are classified as having an "idiopathic" cause, although the vast majority of these are likely to be medication induced. Medications associated with pancreatitis include diuretics such as furosemide, statins, certain antibiotics, and many cardiac medications.

Patients with pancreatitis typically present with epigastric abdominal pain radiating to the back and worsening with food intake. As in many diseases, geriatric patients may present with delirium. The diagnosis requires any 2 of the 3 following criteria: classic pain, increase in the serum amylase or lipase to ≥3 times than the upper limit of normal, or classic findings of acute pancreatitis on imaging (CT, MRI or ultrasound). Once the diagnosis is made, the evaluation of acute pancreatitis is typically straightforward. Routine history-taking is needed to assess the patient's alcohol exposure and medication use. Hepatic enzymes levels should be obtained, with an increase in the transaminases or bilirubin suggesting gallstones as the cause of the pancreatitis. A sonogram of the gallbladder should be obtained to identify gallstones.

The bedrock of treatment for acute pancreatitis is volume resuscitation with intravenous fluids. Fluid replacement should be aggressive as patients are often severely volume depleted (typically, rates of 5 to 10 mL/kg/hour are given). Fluid status should be checked regularly, with blood tests and lung exams to ensure adequate replacement without inducing fluid overload. Pain control with opiates is important as uncontrolled pain can trigger further hemodynamic instability. Nutrition has been an area of debate. Although bowel rest is critical in the initial stages of pancreatitis, recent data have shown that early refeeding (24-48 hours in most cases) is beneficial. Management of severe pancreatitis, such as necrotizing pancreatitis, pancreatitis with evidence of other end-organ compromise, pancreatitis that does not appear to be improving in the first 24 hours or any other concerning features, should be managed by a specialist. In these cases, consultation with the gastroenterologist early in the admission is critical.

DISORDERS OF THE COLON

Constipation

Chronic constipation affects about 30% of adults ≥65 years old, more commonly women. The rate can be even higher in hospitalized or nursing home patients (with up to 50% of patients affected). Constipation has been defined as a fecal frequency of <3 times per week. However, some individuals may complain of lumpy or hard feces, straining at defecation, or a sense of incomplete defecation despite a daily bowel movement.

Common primary causes of constipation include functional constipation (in which no specific etiology is identified), slow-transit constipation (or colonic inertia), and pelvic floor dyssynergia. Metabolic causes include hypothyroidism, hypercalcemia, and diabetes. Structural lesions, such as strictures, malignancy, and rectal prolapse are relatively uncommon, but important to exclude. Many medications have been implicated in constipation. Calcium supplements (and antacids containing calcium or aluminum), iron supplements, anticholinergics, opiates, and smooth muscle relaxants (such as calcium channel blockers) are commonly used medications with known constipating effects. In many older adults, lack of mobility, poor diet with limited fiber intake, and inadequate fluid intake play a major role in constipation.

Evaluation of constipation relies foremost on the history and physical examination. Patients should be asked about fecal frequency and consistency, straining, and if they use any maneuvers to assist with defecation. Alarm signs or symptoms, such as bleeding, weight loss, or a recent change in fecal caliber should be elicited. A complete review of medications, including nonprescription medications, should be performed. Further evaluation can be pursued, if needed, based on this initial basic assessment. For many older adults, adjusting medications and/or a trial of fiber or laxatives may be sufficient to treat the constipation. If this empiric trial is not successful, more invasive testing is required. A basic metabolic evaluation, including measurements of thyroid-stimulating hormone and calcium should be considered. Patients with alarm signs or symptoms, patients with abrupt onset of symptoms, or those are have never had colorectal cancer screening should undergo colonoscopy. In patients who do not respond to dietary changes, fiber supplementation or a trial of stool softeners or laxatives as outlined below, anorectal manometry and a rectal balloon expulsion test should be performed to exclude dyssynergia or pelvic floor dysfunction and a colonic transit study (Sitz marker study) could be considered to assess colonic motility. The reported prevalence of pelvic floor dysfunction is as high as 50% in elderly patients with constipation. There are conflicting data on the prevalence of slow colonic motility in this age group, although it is considered a common problem.

Management of constipation depends on the results of the above evaluation and is often multimodal. In all patients, medications should be reviewed and adjusted as needed to eliminate those that may induce constipation. An increase in fluid intake, dietary fiber intake, and physical activity should be recommended, often with a fiber supplement as well (typically psyllium husk). Patients who respond poorly or who do not tolerate fiber may require laxatives. Osmotic laxatives, such as polyethylene glycol, are safe and effective used on a daily basis. Use of stimulant laxatives such as bisacodyl and senna 2 or 3 times a week is generally safe, although they can be associated with cramping and have been associated with electrolyte abnormalities with long-term use. Stool softeners, such as docusate sodium, have minimal to no effect and should generally be avoided (SOE=B). Saline laxatives (such as magnesium

Table 52.2—Management of Chronic Constipation

Step	
Step 1	Reduce or stop constipating medications if possible, consider metabolic causes of constipation (hypothyroidism, hypercalcemia), consider structural evaluation to exclude obstructive lesions.
Step 2	Increase fluid intake to ≥1,500 mL/day, increase physical activity if possible, increase dietary fiber to 6–25 g/day.
Step 3	Add a bulking agent, eg, psyllium.
Step 4	Add an osmotic agent, eg, sorbitol 70% solution or polyethylene glycol.
Step 5	Add a stimulant laxative, eg, bisacodyl or senna, 2 or 3 times per week.
Step 6	Add a colonic secretagogue, eg, lubiprostone or linaclotide.
Step 7	For refractory cases not responding to the above steps, consider: 1) referral for anorectal manometry, balloon expulsion test, and/or defecography with pelvic physical therapy and/or surgical evaluation as indicated based on findings; 2) addition of an enema (water or saline, 2 times weekly as needed, follow electrolytes carefully); and/or 3) surgical evaluation for subtotal colectomy.

hydroxide) have not been well-studied in the geriatric population, are associated with a risk of hypermagnesemia, and should be avoided if possible.

Patients with slow-transit constipation should be treated similarly. If first-line laxatives fail, newer pharmacologic agents, typically colonic secretagogues such as lubiprostone or linaclotide, should be considered (SOE=A). Although they appear to be safe and effective in the general population, these agents have not yet been studied extensively in older adults and should be used with caution. Patients with slow-transit constipation with severe, longstanding symptoms who do not respond to these therapies may ultimately require surgery (typically a subtotal colectomy). However, this is considered a treatment of last resort.

Patients with defecatory disorders identified by anorectal manometry and a balloon expulsion test should be referred for pelvic floor retraining and biofeedback. This can be done in addition to the therapies used in normal-transit and slow-transit constipation.

Tables 52.2 and 52.3 provide a stepwise approach for treatment of chronic constipation. Depending on the response to each step, the underlying colonic motility or any identified anorectal disorders, these treatments can be combined or attempted in concert with one another.

Fecal impaction is common in older adults with constipation of any etiology. This should be treated first by manual disimpaction to fragment large fecal boluses and then followed by several warm-water enemas to help evacuate the rectum. After local disimpaction, a polyethylene glycol preparation should be used to cleanse the entire colon. Long-term management involves treating the underlying cause of constipation and typically adding a daily polyethylene glycol laxative to the patient's medication regimen. Weekly cleansing enemas can be considered in those with recurrent fecal impaction.

Fecal Incontinence

Fecal incontinence is a disturbing disability, affecting quality of life and often leading to social isolation. Multiple definitions of fecal incontinence exist, but in general it is defined as the involuntary passage or the inability to control passage of fecal material through the anus. This problem can be subcategorized as major incontinence (involuntary excretion of feces) or minor incontinence (seepage of liquid feces, staining of undergarments, or inadvertent escape of flatus). Fecal incontinence affects 2%–7% of adults, mostly older adults in poor general health, and is a common cause of nursing-home placement. Women are disproportionately affected. Patients are reluctant to discuss this disorder with clinicians because of embarrassment and social stigma, resulting in substantial delays in treatment.

Fecal continence depends on many factors, such as physical and mental function, fecal consistency, colonic transit, rectal compliance, internal and external anal sphincter function, and anorectal sensation and reflexes. Normal defecation is a complex sequential process that starts with the entry of feces into the rectum, leading to reflex relaxation of the internal anal sphincter. If defecation is desired, the anorectal angle is voluntarily straightened, and abdominal pressure is increased by straining. This results in descent of the pelvic floor, contraction of the rectum, and inhibition of the external anal sphincter, which causes evacuation of the rectal contents. Fecal incontinence may thus occur with a disruption of any of the above processes and it is often a multifactorial issue.

The history and physical examination often provide clues to the cause of fecal incontinence. A description of the incontinence should be obtained. The history should determine if the incontinence is of a large volume of stool, small volume, or simple staining of the underwear and if it occurs chronically or only with increased intra-abdominal pressure (such as with laughing or coughing). Additional important historical details to obtain include coexisting diarrhea, an obstetric history, and concomitant conditions such as diabetes, neurologic disorders, and spinal cord injury. The examination should note sphincter tone, appropriate perineal descent, any rectal prolapse, and perineal sensation. A flexible sigmoidoscopy may be considered to exclude inflammation or tumor. The next step is anorectal manometry, which measures resting anal sphincter tone, squeeze pressure, the rectoanal inhibitory reflex, rectal sensation, and

Table 52.3—Medications for Chronic Constipation

Medication	Onset of Action	Starting Dosage	Site and Mechanism of Action
Bulk laxatives			
Methylcellulose (eg, Citrucel)	12–24 h (up to 72 h)	1 heaping tablespoon with 8 oz water q8–24h	Small and large intestine; holds water in feces; mechanical distention
Psyllium (eg, Metamucil)	12–24 h (up to 72 h)	1 or 2 capsules, packets, or teaspoons with 8 oz water or juice q8–24h	Small and large intestine; holds water in feces; mechanical distention
Polycarbophil (eg, FiberCon)	12–24 h (up to 72 h)	1,250 mg q6–24h	Small and large intestine; holds water in feces; mechanical distention
Osmotic laxatives			
Polyethylene glycol (eg, Miralax)	24–96 h	17 g powder q24h (~1 tablespoon) dissolved in 8 oz water	GI tract; osmotic effect
Lactulose	24–48 h	15–30 mL q12–24h	Colon; osmotic effect
Sorbitol 70%	24–48 h	15–30 mL q12–24h; max 150 mL/d	Colon; delivers osmotically active molecules to colon
Colonic secretagogue			
Lubiprostone (Amitiza)	48–96 h	24 mcg q12h with food	Enhances chloride-ion intestinal fluid secretion; does not affect serum sodium or potassium concentrations; for idiopathic chronic constipation
Linaclotide (Linzess)	48–96 h	145 mcg or 290 mcg daily (30 minutes before breakfast)	Enhances chloride-ion intestinal fluid secretion by increasing intracellular cGMP
Stimulant laxatives			
Bisacodyl tablet (eg, Dulcolax)	6–10 h	5–15 mg × 1	Colon; increases peristalsis
Bisacodyl suppository (eg, Dulcolax)	15–60 min	10 mg × 1	Colon; increases peristalsis
Senna (eg, Senokot)	6–10 h	2 tablets or 1 teaspoon qhs	Colon; direct action on intestine; stimulates myenteric plexus; alters water and electrolyte secretion

rectal compliance. This test requires complete cooperation by the patient and will not be appropriate for many patients, particularly those with moderate or advanced dementia. The results often identify pelvic floor disorders that may be treated with physical therapy aimed at the specific abnormalities identified. Pelvic floor physical therapy also depends on intensive cooperation and involvement by the patient and would not be performed in uncooperative or demented patients. Abnormalities of the anal sphincters, the rectal wall, and the puborectalis muscle identified on anorectal manometry can be further evaluated by use of endorectal ultrasound. Typically, a defect in the internal anal sphincter is associated with low resting sphincter pressure, whereas defects in the external sphincter are associated with lower anal squeeze pressure.

Medical therapy is aimed at treating the underlying cause when possible, improving fecal consistency, and reducing fecal frequency. Fecal bulking agents (eg, methylcellulose) and antidiarrheal medications (including loperamide and diphenoxylate/atropine) can be effective first-line agents. Diphenoxylate/atropine should be used with caution in older adults because of its anticholinergic effects. Biofeedback therapy, which includes anal sphincter strengthening and rectal sensory conditioning, is painless, safe, and often effective in patients who have no structural defect. Patients in whom conservative measures fail, or who have anal sphincter defects, may benefit from injectable sphincter bulking agents or surgery. Bulking agents are injected submucosally at the site of sphincter weakness and may be best reserved for those with mild incontinence (eg, seepage) (SOE=B). Surgery allows for repair of the sphincter or construction of a neosphincter and can be effective in appropriate candidates.

Chronic Diarrhea

Chronic diarrhea is defined as a decrease in fecal consistency lasting for >4 weeks. Diarrhea is associated with decreased quality of life and significant morbidity and sometimes mortality in older adults. There are many potential causes of chronic diarrhea and evaluation can be challenging. The presenting history is essential in narrowing the differential diagnosis and helping to target the evaluation.

Common causes of chronic diarrhea are irritable bowel syndrome, lactose or other food intolerance, inflammatory bowel disease (typically Crohn disease), malabsorption syndromes (such as celiac disease, small-intestinal bacterial overgrowth, and chronic pancreatitis), and chronic infections (such as recurrent *C difficile*, amebiasis, giardiasis, *Cryptosporidium*, Whipple disease, and *Cyclospora*). Microscopic colitis (lymphocytic and collagenous colitis) is common in this age group and should be strongly considered in those with endoscopically normal colons. Many medications, including OTC medications, herbs, and supplements are associated with development of diarrhea. Common medications include SSRIs, PPIs, and certain oral hypoglycemic and chemotherapeutic agents. OTC medications or supplements include vitamin C or magnesium-containing antacids. Clinicians should be aware that diet drinks, foods, or even chewable medications containing sorbitol or other artificial sweeteners can cause chronic diarrhea.

A thorough medical history is essential to define fecal consistency, volume, and frequency, and the presence of urgency or fecal soiling. Fecal incontinence is frequently confused with diarrhea in older adults. Malodorous feces and weight loss may suggest fat malabsorption, whereas visible blood suggests inflammatory bowel disease. If the diarrhea occurs during fasting or at night, a secretory etiology (eg, neuroendocrine tumor) needs to be considered. Large-volume watery diarrhea is more likely to be due to a small-intestinal disorder or microscopic colitis, whereas small-volume frequent diarrhea with tenesmus reflects distal colonic inflammation. All medications must be reviewed and patients asked specifically about nonprescription medications and "sugar-free" or diet food products.

Depending on the initial history and physical examination, the diagnostic approach to chronic diarrhea is complex and multifaceted, involving fecal analyses, exclusion of infectious causes, structural evaluation by colonoscopy with appropriate biopsies, small-bowel capsule endoscopy and/or radiography, and abdominal CT imaging. Guidelines for diagnosis and management of diarrhea have been published (www.gastro.org/guidelines) [accessed Jan 2016]). Treatment of chronic diarrhea depends on the underlying diagnosis and may require referral to a specialist.

Diverticular Disease

The prevalence of diverticular disease is age dependent, seen in 30% by age 60 and increasing to 65% by age 85. Although most patients remain asymptomatic, 20% develop diverticulitis, and 10% may develop diverticular bleeding. Therefore, the mere presence of diverticulosis does not require specific therapy. A diet high in fiber appears to be associated with a reduced risk of developing diverticular disease and may reduce the risk of subsequent complications.

Uncomplicated diverticulosis is often an incidental finding on screening sigmoidoscopy, colonoscopy, or cross-sectional imaging, such as a CT scan. Some patients may complain of nonspecific abdominal cramping, bloating, flatulence, and irregular bowel habits. Diverticular bleeding is usually painless and self-limited, and it rarely coexists with acute diverticulitis. Diverticulitis usually presents with left lower quadrant pain, although nausea, vomiting, constipation, diarrhea, and dysuria or frequency may occur, particularly in women. The physical examination usually reveals left lower quadrant tenderness, a tender mass, and abdominal distention. Generalized tenderness suggests perforation and peritonitis. Low-grade fever and leukocytosis are common, but their absence in older adults does not exclude the diagnosis. Urinalysis may reveal sterile pyuria induced by adjacent colonic inflammation; the presence of mixed colonic flora on urine culture suggests a colovesical fistula. Other potential complications include perforation, obstruction, and abscess formation.

CT scanning is the optimal imaging choice in suspected acute diverticulitis. CT features of acute diverticulitis include increased density of soft tissue within pericolic fat and colonic diverticula, thickening of the bowel wall, soft-tissue masses (phlegmon), and pericolic fluid collections (abscess formation). CT can also identify peritonitis, obstruction, and fistula to the bladder, vagina, and abdominal wall. However, in approximately 10% of patients, diverticulitis cannot be distinguished from colon cancer, because both may show focal thickening of the bowel wall. In such cases, on resolution of the acute inflammation, a colonoscopy is indicated. In older adults, CT-guided percutaneous drainage of localized abscesses may obviate emergent surgery and eventually permit single-stage elective surgical resection.

Most (85%) patients with simple diverticulitis respond to medical therapy. Patients with complicated diverticulitis usually require surgery. Indications for emergency surgery are free perforation with peritonitis, obstruction, clinical deterioration or lack of improvement with conservative management, and an abscess that cannot be drained percutaneously. Indications for elective surgical intervention are recurrent or intractable symptoms, persistent mass, obstruction, and fistula or abscess formation.

Mild diverticulitis with left lower quadrant pain, low-grade fever, and minimal physical findings is often treated on an outpatient basis, with clear liquids and oral antibiotics, such as ciprofloxacin 500 mg q12h or metronidazole 500 mg q8h, or both. Hospitalization is needed only if no improvement is seen. Once the episode resolves, solid food is reintroduced and the colon is evaluated, preferably by colonoscopy. For patients with moderate to severe symptoms, treatment with bowel rest, fluids, and intravenous antibiotics is initiated, with the aim to avoid urgent surgery. Antibiotics should be active against gram-negative rods and anaerobes. If there is no improvement, either the diagnosis is incorrect or an abscess, peritonitis, fistula, or obstruction is present. Older immunosuppressed patients with multiple underlying medical conditions may present with minimal symptoms or signs, even in cases of frank peritonitis, and the diagnosis is commonly delayed. In such cases, early surgical intervention should be considered. Diffuse peritonitis requires fluid resuscitation, broad-spectrum antibiotics, and emergency laparotomy. Colonic resection removes the septic focus, corrects the obstruction or fistula formation, and restores bowel continuity. In most elective cases, resection and primary anastomosis are possible if the disease is well localized or has significantly resolved.

After successful medical therapy of the first episode of diverticulitis, one-third of patients will remain asymptomatic, another third will have episodic abdominal cramps (painful diverticulosis), and the remaining will proceed to a second attack of diverticulitis. Therefore, elective surgery is not necessary for all patients with diverticulitis who respond to medical therapy. If surgery is performed, progression of diverticulitis in the remaining colon occurs in only 15%, and the need for further surgery is reduced to <10%.

Irritable Bowel Syndrome

Irritable bowel syndrome (IBS) is a functional GI disorder with remissions and exacerbations, characterized by abdominal pain, bloating, and either constipation or diarrhea, or both. Although the pathogenesis is incompletely understood, IBS appears to result at least partly from altered bowel motility, visceral hypersensitivity, and enhanced perception by the brain of many visceral stimuli. A common mediator for all these abnormalities is serotonin, and serotonin-receptor agonists and antagonists are used in management of IBS. Although psychosocial factors are commonly involved in IBS, they are not known to have a causative role.

Because the clinical symptoms characteristic of IBS are not specific, it is important to be mindful of features that are not consistent with IBS. These include weight loss, first onset of symptoms after age 50, nocturnal diarrhea, family history of cancer or inflammatory bowel disease, rectal bleeding or obstruction, and laboratory abnormalities (eg, anemia, leukocytosis, abnormal chemistries, positive fecal cultures, or the presence of parasites in the feces). In older patients, the diagnosis should be made only after other conditions (ie, ischemia, diverticulosis, colon cancer, or inflammatory bowel disease) have been carefully excluded. An appropriate evaluation of an older adult with symptoms consistent with IBS should include a colonoscopy and often an upper endoscopy. A CT scan of the abdomen should be considered. Small-bowel imaging, either with CT enterography, MRI enterography, or video capsule endoscopy should be performed in patients with symptoms, signs, or laboratory values suggestive of possible small-bowel disease. These include patients with weight loss, iron-deficiency anemia, or diarrhea that is unexplained by endoscopy and colonoscopy.

If the history, physical examination, and laboratory or imaging studies are negative, the diagnosis of IBS can then be made and subcategorized as IBS with constipation (IBS-C), IBS with diarrhea (IBS-D), or IBS with alternating constipation and diarrhea (IBS-M or IBS mixed).

Treatment depends on IBS subtype. Reassurance is necessary in all subtypes to clarify that, although it may impact quality of life, IBS is not life threatening and repetitive testing is unnecessary and may be harmful. Dietary changes may be useful in all subtypes of IBS, with many patients responding well to increased fiber intake. In patients with diarrhea, a 3- to 6-week trial of a lactose-free diet may identify patients with concomitant lactose intolerance (calcium supplementation should be considered in patients on a long-term lactose-free diet). Some specific diets have been studied for IBS. A gluten-free diet has been shown to be helpful in some randomized trials, although no specific data are available in older adults. A diet low in fermentable oligo-, di- and monosaccharides and polyols (FODMAP diet) has been shown to be effective in reducing IBS symptoms in a few high-quality trials, but again no data exist specifically in the geriatric population. These diets should be instituted with the aid of a nutritionist, because they can be very restrictive and difficult to maintain and pose a risk of nutritional deficiencies. Probiotics (specifically, bifidobacterium-containing formulations) have been used in treatment of all subtypes of IBS with anecdotal efficacy, but available data do not support routine use. Antibiotics have been used, with randomized trials showing significant improvement in global symptoms of IBS with a short course of the nonabsorbable antibiotic rifaximin (SOE=A). However, the long-term efficacy of rifaximin is unknown. Antispasmodic agents, typically short-acting intestinal smooth-muscle relaxants, should be used with caution to treat the pain of IBS, because they act via anticholinergic properties and may have systemic adverse effects. Tricyclic antidepressants have been shown to be efficacious in treatment of global symptoms of IBS in younger populations, but these drugs should be avoided in older adults if possible. Less consistent data are available for nontricyclic antidepressants such as SSRIs.

IBS-C can be treated similarly to chronic constipation. Of the constipation medications, specific consideration should be given to linaclotide, because in the general population it appears to have an analgesic effect independent of its effect on constipation (SOE=A). However, its use in older adults has not been systematically evaluated. IBS-D may respond to fiber-bulking agents such psyllium, because they help normalize fecal consistency. Loperamide, an antidiarrheal opiate agonist, has been shown to be effective in randomized controlled trials. Bile acid sequestrants, such as cholestyramine or colestipol, can be effective as well. They should not be taken with other medications, because they can bind and block absorption of those drugs. Finally, a serotonin antagonist, alosetron, available on a compassionate use basis from the FDA, is highly effective but should be used with extreme caution, because it may precipitate intestinal ischemia.

Occult Gastrointestinal Bleeding

Older adults commonly have a positive fecal occult blood test (FOBT) or are diagnosed with unexplained iron-deficiency anemia, or both. Although colorectal cancer is a leading concern, other causes (of which there are many) include esophagitis, peptic ulcers, esophageal and gastric malignancies, intestinal or colonic angiodysplasia, benign colon polyps, inflammatory bowel disease, or hemorrhoids. A positive FOBT should not be attributed to esophageal varices or colonic diverticula, because it is rare for such lesions to bleed in an occult fashion. The presence of a positive FOBT warrants evaluation and should not be attributed to aspirin or other antiplatelet or anticoagulant use.

Detection of fecal occult blood using a standard guaiac-based test has a low sensitivity and a high rate of false-positive results, leading to more invasive and expensive tests. Newer fecal immunochemical tests are more specific (they respond only to human globin and not to animal source of heme), but they miss upper GI sources of blood loss (as the globin is digested in transit) and can be expensive. Despite these limitations, an annual FOBT is currently recommended as one method of screening for colon cancer and has been associated with up to a 33% reduction in mortality from colon cancer. Because of the high prevalence of colorectal cancer and/or adenomatous polyps in older adults with a positive FOBT, a colonoscopy should be performed and, if negative, consideration given to an upper endoscopy. If symptoms of upper GI disease are present, there is a high likelihood for a positive endoscopy. However, in older adults at risk of colon cancer, the presence of an upper GI lesion should not preclude evaluation of the colon. Patients with normal upper and lower endoscopy should be considered for evaluation for a small-bowel source using video capsule endoscopy, followed if necessary by balloon enteroscopy. The most common cause of bleeding from the small bowel is angiodysplasia, followed by tumors or ulcers that are commonly caused by NSAIDs. Unrecognized gluten-sensitive enteropathy can result in iron-deficiency anemia, because iron is absorbed in the proximal small bowel, and multiple biopsies should always be taken from the duodenum to confirm this diagnosis histologically.

In one prospective study in which patients with iron-deficiency anemia were evaluated with colonoscopy and endoscopy, followed by radiographic examination of the small intestine if these tests were negative, a source of bleeding was identified in 62% of cases. A lesion was seen on colonoscopy in 25%, on upper endoscopy in 36%, and on both in 1% of patients. Peptic ulcer disease was the primary abnormality in the upper GI tract, but cancer was detected on colonoscopy in 11% of patients.

Colonic Angiodysplasia

The terms *angiodysplasia*, *arteriovenous malformation*, and *vascular ectasia* are often used interchangeably. These aberrant vessels are dilated, thin-walled vascular structures in the mucosa and submucosa that are lined by endothelium or by smooth muscle. Although they are mostly tortuous veins, arteriovenous communications or enlarged arteries may be present, leading to brisk bleeding. The pathogenesis of angiodysplasias is not well understood. They are commonly seen in association with certain systemic disorders, including end-stage renal disease and aortic stenosis and appear to increase with age. When angiodysplasias occur in the setting of a known syndrome, such as Osler-Weber-Rendu syndrome or scleroderma CREST variant, they are typically referred to as telangiectasias.

Angiodysplasias are seen most often in the cecum and ascending colon, where they may cause bleeding, particularly in patients ≥60 years old. However, angiodysplasias are seen throughout the GI tract and may be multiple or coexist in several different regions of the GI tract. They may be asymptomatic or cause occult or clinically overt GI bleeding.

Angiodysplasias are usually diagnosed during endoscopy or colonoscopy, appearing as 5- to 10-mm cherry-red, ectatic blood vessels radiating from a central vascular core. Angiodysplasias can also be diagnosed by angiography. If they are serendipitously detected during routine endoscopy or colonoscopy, angiodysplasias do not require treatment. However, an actively bleeding angiodysplasia should be treated. Whether angiodysplasias were the cause of bleeding in patients who have stopped bleeding and, in particular, in patients who are found to have both angiodysplasias and diverticula is a more difficult problem. In such cases, bleeding from angiodysplasias is almost always from the cecum or ascending colon.

Many endoscopic ablation techniques have been used in treatment of angiodysplasias. Although acute bleeding can be successfully controlled with these approaches, rebleeding is common either from the same site or from coexisting angiodysplasias elsewhere in the bowel. Angiography may localize the site of active bleeding and allows embolization or infusion of vasopressin. Surgical resection is definitive for lesions that have been clearly identified as the source of bleeding. However, recurrent bleeding may occur from other proximal or distal lesions in >30% of cases. Hormonal therapy with estrogen (with or without progesterone) has also been used in women, but its benefit should be weighed against the potential risks of thromboembolic disease, estrogen-dependent tumors, and uterine bleeding. Other medical therapies include angiogenesis inhibitors (such as thalidomide) and octreotide, each with limited, but supportive, evidence. Iron supplementation should be given to all patients with chronic bleeding from angiodysplasias and may be the only treatment needed in patients with limited, occult bleeding (SOE=B).

Colonic Ischemia

Ischemic colitis is the most common form of intestinal ischemia and typically affects patients >65 years old. Colonic ischemia usually occurs in the setting of an acute but temporary reduction in blood flow to the colon. In the vast majority of cases, the effect is transient and symptoms resolve without long-term sequela. However, up to 15% of patients can present with life-threatening ischemia or colonic gangrene, which is associated with high mortality.

Any low-flow state can cause ischemic colitis, including dehydration, infection, or medication-induced hypotension. Risk factors for colonic ischemia include known cardiovascular disease, prior vascular surgery, hemodialysis, and thrombophilia. Ischemia usually affects "water-shed" segments of the colon, such as the splenic flexure and the rectosigmoid junction, where collateral blood flow is limited.

The presentation of ischemic colitis depends on the severity of hypoperfusion. In the typical, nonocclusive presentation, patients will complain of acute, crampy abdominal pain followed by hematochezia. Diagnosis is often made radiographically, with CT showing segmental thickening of the affected watershed region in the appropriate clinical setting. Colonoscopy, if performed, reveals segmental edema, hemorrhages, gray-black pseudomembrane formation, and focal ulcers, mostly in the region of the splenic flexure and typically sparing the rectum.

Treatment is mostly supportive with intravenous fluids and treatment of the underlying cause of the low-flow state. In the minority of cases when life-threatening ischemia occurs (suggested by peritoneal signs, fever, marked leukocytosis, increased lactate and/or a lack of response to fluid resuscitation), emergent surgery and broad-spectrum antibiotics are required. However, in these cases, morbidity and mortality can be as high as 75% even with rapid surgical intervention.

Acute Colonic Pseudo-Obstruction

Acute colonic pseudo-obstruction (Ogilvie syndrome) is manifested by acute massive dilation of the colon without evidence of mechanical obstruction. In older adults, it is often related to neurologic disease such as Parkinson or cerebrovascular disease, trauma, recent orthopedic surgery, or use of narcotics. Infections, particularly *C difficile*, and colonic ischemia can cause colonic dilation and need to be excluded. Ogilvie syndrome presents clinically with abdominal distention, often with accompanying pain. Patients may have a lack of fecal output or a paradoxical "postobstructive" diarrhea. The diagnosis is made with an abdominal radiograph and confirmed with a CT scan to exclude an underlying obstruction. Treatment is initially supportive and aimed at addressing underlying precipitating factors such as poor mobility, narcotic use, or metabolic disturbances that may exacerbate gut dysmotility (such as hypokalemia or hypomagnesaemia). Patients who do not respond to conservative measures in the first 24 hours, who have abdominal pain, or who have significant (>10 cm) dilation of the colon should receive further care. Treatment with neostigmine, an acetylcholinesterase inhibitor, can produce rapid and sustained colonic decompression but must be performed in a monitored setting because of the risk of bradycardia and hypotension. In extreme cases (or when neostigmine is contraindicated), colonoscopy can provide temporary decompression. Placement of a colonic tube at the time of colonoscopy can provide longer-term decompression. Surgical decompression is rarely used and reserved for only severe cases unresponsive to all other measures.

CHOOSING WISELY® RECOMMENDATIONS

Gastroenterology

- For pharmacologic management of GERD, use lowest dosage needed to achieve symptom control.

- For diagnosis of IBS, exclude ischemia, diverticulosis, colon cancer, and inflammatory bowel disease by physical examination and testing (colonoscopy, CT scan, or small-bowel series). Do not repeat CT unless major changes in clinical findings.

REFERENCES

- Caglia P, Costa S, Tracia A, et al. Can laparoscopic cholecystectomy be safely performed in the elderly? *Ann Ital Chir.* 2012;83(1):21–24.

    In clinical practice, there is always concern when considering surgery in an older patient, even when it would be clearly indicated in a young patient. This retrospective study examined the safety of laparoscopic cholecystectomy in patients >70 years old with symptomatic gallstones and found a low morbidity and mortality rate.

- Cardoso RN, Benjo AM, DiNicolantonio JJ, et al. Incidence of cardiovascular events and gastrointestinal bleeding in patients receiving clopidogrel with and without proton pump inhibitors: an updated meta-analysis. *Open Heart.* 2015 Jun 30;2(1):e000248.

    This updated meta-analysis of the interaction between proton pump inhibitors (PPIs) and clopidogrel confirms the cardio- and cerebrovascular safety of PPI use in patients on clopidogrel and shows a decreased rate of GI bleeding in patients who take both medications than in those on antiplatelet therapy alone.

- Khan A, Carmona R, Traube M. Dysphagia in the elderly. *Clin Geriatr Med.* 2014;30(1):43–53.

    An up-to-date overview of the etiologies and evaluation of dysphagia in older patients, this review describes the types, causes, and pathophysiology of dysphagia focusing on the presentation of older patients. Appropriate evaluation, including when to obtain GI consultation (and the tests performed by the gastroenterologist) are reviewed. A brief overview of treatment strategies in common disorders is discussed.

- Lanza FL, Chan FK, Quigley EM. Guidelines for prevention of NSAID-related ulcer complications. *Am J Gastroenterol.* 2009;104(3):728–738.

    This set of guidelines reviews risk factors for NSAID-induced GI toxicity (for which age >65 years old is an independent risk factor) and proposes an algorithm for choosing selective or nonselective NSAIDs and an appropriate preventive strategy.

- Pardis DS. Microscopic colitis. *Clin Geriatr Med.* 2014;30(1):55–65.

    This review of microscopic colitis, with a focus on the older population, details the two types of microscopic colitis (collagenous and lymphocytic), with their histopathologic differences, clinical presentation, diagnosis, and treatment.

- Soumekh A, Schnoll-Sussman FH, Katz PO. Reflux and acid peptic disease in the elderly. *Clin Geriatr Med.* 2014;30(1):29–41.

    This review of reflux in the geriatric population focuses on key differences in the assessment and management of reflux in this group compared with the average population. Recommendations from the most recent guidelines on the management of GERD are discussed.

Amir E. Soumekh, MD
Philip O. Katz, MD

CHAPTER 53—NEPHROLOGY

KEY POINTS

- As people age, their kidneys become less able to maintain homeostasis in response to physiologic stress.

- Serum creatinine is a poor marker of kidney function. Kidney function is best approximated by the estimated glomerular filtration rate (eGFR).

- Causes of acute kidney injury are divided into prerenal azotemia, urinary tract obstruction, and intrinsic kidney disease, which may be glomerular, tubulointerstitial, or vascular in origin.

- Chronic kidney disease (CKD) is very common in older adults and is classified into stages based on eGFR. Preventing progression of CKD is important at any age.

- Referral to a nephrologist is recommended when eGFR decreases to <30 mL/min (Stage 4 CKD) for help in management of CKD-related complications and discussions regarding dialysis and transplantation.

KIDNEY ASSESSMENT

Measures of Kidney Function

Serum creatinine has been traditionally monitored to assess kidney function, but creatinine alone can be misleading. Muscle mass, the source of serum creatinine, declines with age, especially in frail older adults. Because the decline in muscle mass occurs in parallel with the decline in kidney function, many older adults maintain a relatively stable serum creatinine even as their kidney function, or glomerular filtration rate (GFR), falls significantly. Therefore, kidney function can be profoundly impaired, despite a "normal" serum creatinine concentration. For example, an 80-year-old woman with a serum creatinine of 1.5 mg/dL has an eGFR of ~33 mL/min, a level at which many renally cleared medications must be dose adjusted to prevent toxicity. Cross-sectional studies have shown a progressive decline in GFR after the age of 40 in both men and women, averaging a decline of ~8 mL/min per decade.

There is an ongoing search for novel molecules that might prove useful in assessing kidney function. The best studied is cystatin C, a small protein that comes from all nucleated cells. Similar to creatinine, it is cleared by the kidneys such that the serum level increases as kidney function decreases. Because it comes from all nucleated cells, cystatin C is less affected by aging and changes in muscle mass.

Because direct measurement of GFR is not practical in the clinical setting, formulas for estimating GFR have been developed. Estimation formulas account for the patient's age and thus the decline in muscle mass with aging. Examples include the Cockcroft-Gault, Modified Diet in Renal Disease (MDRD), and CKD-Epi equations. The Cockcroft-Gault formula is mathematically straightforward but may not be as accurate in patients with advanced CKD. The MDRD equation was developed using measured GFR as the gold standard, but it is not accurate when GFR is >60 mL/min. The more recent CKD-Epi equation is a variation of the MDRD that is accurate across the spectrum of GFR values. There are now 2 variations of the CKD-Epi formula that use cystatin C. One of these uses cystatin C alone and is not better than the CKD-Epi creatinine equation. The version that takes into account both creatinine and cystatin C has been shown to be more accurate and may be best used to confirm the GFR in patients with moderate CKD to clarify prognosis. The National Kidney Foundation has an online calculator that provides an estimate of GFR by the MDRD and the various CKD-Epi equations (www.kidney.org/professionals/KDOQI/gfr_calculator).

As suggested by the National Kidney Foundation, many clinical laboratories now provide an estimated GFR (eGFR), usually based on the CKD-Epi formula, along with measurements of serum creatinine. This reported eGFR is valid only when the serum creatinine is stable. It may also be unreliable in patients who have more or less muscle mass than average patients their age. Examples include very obese patients, those with cachexia, and amputees. In these situations, another way to estimate the GFR is by measuring creatinine clearance based on a 24-hour urine collection. However, under most circumstances, a 24-hour urine collection is not recommended because of frequent errors in collection and misleading results. Having a close approximation of a patient's GFR is essential for medication dosing, as well as for avoiding nephrotoxins that pose increased risk to patients with already tenuous renal function.

Measures of Urinary Protein Excretion

Proteinuria is an important sign of kidney damage, as well as a risk factor for vascular events and progression of CKD. There are several methods of measuring urinary protein excretion. The standard urine dipstick is a simple screening test but is insensitive for low levels of proteinuria, which may be seen in early kidney disease. Importantly, dipsticks only react with negatively

Table 53.1—Physiologic Changes in Kidney and Related Endocrine Function with Aging

Function	Mechanisms	Clinical Significance
↓ GFR	Advanced glycation end products Comorbidities Medication use	Chronic kidney disease ↑ risk of acute kidney injury
↓ diluting capacity	↑ ADH secretion Comorbidities (CHF, liver, renal disease) Medications (thiazide diuretics)	↑ risk of hyponatremia
↓ concentrating ability	↓ sensitivity of kidney to ADH ↓ tonicity of the renal medulla ↓ ADH at night in nocturnal polyuria syndrome	↑ risk of hypernatremia Poor compensation for volume depletion Nocturia
↓ sodium conservation	↓ sodium reabsorption ↓ plasma renin activity ↓ production of aldosterone ↑ atrial natriuretic hormone	Volume depletion Osmotic diuresis Nocturia
↓ sodium excretion	↓ suppression of plasma renin activity with sodium loading	Salt sensitive hypertension Edema
↓ ammonium production and generation of bicarbonate	↓ plasma renin activity ↓ production of aldosterone ↓ GFR	Metabolic acidosis

Note: ADH=antidiuretic hormone

charged proteins, principally albumin, and fail to detect positively charged proteins such as light chains, which may indicate multiple myeloma. The urine microalbumin/creatinine ratio has been recommended as the best screening test for low levels of albuminuria in high-risk individuals. Microalbuminuria is defined as 30–300 mg/g creatinine, and frank albuminuria is >300 mg/g creatinine. Urine albumin/creatinine ratio provides an estimate of 24-hour albumin excretion. A 24-hour urine collection is generally not recommended to quantify proteinuria because of inaccuracy due to frequent errors in technique.

METABOLIC AND VOLUME DISORDERS

Older adults are vulnerable to metabolic and volume derangements for a number of reasons. Age-related anatomic, hemodynamic, and hormonal changes affect crucial functions that maintain homeostasis of fluids, electrolytes, volume, and acid-base balance. Under normal conditions, the aging kidney is usually able to maintain homeostasis; however, under stress, the adaptive response to maintain homeostasis is impaired. See Table 53.1 for examples of kidney-related physiologic changes with aging.

Disorders of Water Balance: Hyponatremia and Hypernatremia

Changes in Antidiuretic Hormone (ADH) with Aging
Serum sodium concentration is abnormal in >25% of older adults presenting acutely to the hospital. Increasing age is a strong independent risk factor for both hyponatremia and hypernatremia. Water balance is regulated through the effects of ADH, or vasopressin, which is released from the posterior pituitary in response to increased blood tonicity and hypernatremia. ADH binds receptors in the kidneys, leading to reabsorption of water through water channels and, thus, concentrated urine. ADH is normally suppressed in hyponatremia, leading to a dilute urine and excretion of excess water. Severe volume depletion, through the action of the baroreceptors in the aortic arch and carotid bodies, is a nonosmotic stimulus for ADH release and causes retention of water at the expense of maintaining a normal serum sodium concentration. In older adults, alterations in the ADH system have clinical implications, as discussed below. In addition, decreased ADH secretion at night can lead to nocturia with significant urine volumes, termed the nocturnal polyuria syndrome.

Hyponatremia
Hyponatremia has been reported to occur in 11.3% of hospitalized geriatric patients and in up to 22.5% of older adults in long-term care facilities. Older adults tend to have normal to increased basal ADH secretion, with increased ADH response to osmoreceptor stimulus, which results in impaired urinary diluting capacity and, thus, diminished ability to excrete a free water load. This can lead to hyponatremia if water intake is excessive. Many medications and common comorbidities in older adults also contribute to increased incidence of hyponatremia.

Early recognition and treatment of hyponatremia are critical to avert serious complications and neurologic sequelae, so it is essential to be aware of its varied symptoms and signs. Hyponatremia causes an osmotic shift of water from the extracellular to the intracellular space, which can lead to brain edema and symptoms of apathy, disorientation, lethargy, muscle cramps, anorexia, nausea, agitation, headache, seizures, and coma. Even when mild and apparently asymptomatic, hyponatremia is associated with deficits in gait and attention, falls, and increased fracture risk in older adults (SOE=A). Overt symptoms are more likely to develop when the sodium concentration acutely falls below 125 mEq/L. The only manifestations of chronic hyponatremia may be lethargy, confusion, and malaise.

The first step in determining an underlying cause is obtaining the serum osmolality. If the serum is hypertonic due to an osmotically active substance such as glucose, the hyponatremia does not cause osmotic shifts or symptoms. If the hypertonicity is due to osmotically inactive molecules, such as urea or alcohols, symptoms do occur. In pseudohyponatremia, the serum osmolality is normal, but an excess amount of the plasma volume is taken up by increased lipids or proteins, for example in multiple myeloma. The plasma sodium appears low, but the serum sodium is normal and there are no symptoms. Most hyponatremia is hypotonic, with low serum osmolality. After considering serum osmolality, the next step in diagnosis is determining the patient's volume status.

Hyponatremia with Volume Depletion

Older adults are prone to volume depletion due to a number of factors, including comorbid conditions, medications (particularly diuretics), and hormonal changes including decreased aldosterone secretion and exaggerated atrial natriuretic hormone release. Significant volume depletion leads to release of ADH in response to signals from baroreceptors in the aortic arch and carotid bodies. ADH stimulates the kidneys to concentrate the urine, and if a patient takes in free water, the serum sodium drops. The patient appears volume depleted, showing typical signs such as tachycardia, orthostatic hypotension, and lack of edema. In this situation, the patient is sodium avid, as evidenced by urine sodium concentration <10 mEq/L. Once intravascular volume is repleted with isotonic fluid, ADH is suppressed and the kidneys excrete the excess water, leading to correction of hyponatremia.

Hyponatremia with Volume Overload

Common conditions include heart failure and hypoalbuminemic states such as cirrhosis and the nephrotic syndrome. In these conditions, a decrease in effective arterial volume stimulates the renin-angiotensin-aldosterone system (RAAS), thus promoting salt retention and edema. The urine sodium concentration is typically <10 mEq/L. A decreased effective circulating volume causes the baroreceptors to stimulate ADH release, again leading to concentrated urine and water retention. Patients are edematous and usually quite thirsty. The serum sodium drops with excessive intake of free water. Treatment includes fluid restriction and loop diuretics.

Hyponatremia with Normal Extracellular Fluid Volume

There are a number of causes of euvolemic hyponatremia, including kidney disease, thiazide diuretics, hypothyroidism, adrenal insufficiency, the syndrome of inappropriate antidiuretic hormone (SIADH), and a reset osmostat.

Thiazide diuretics are an important cause of euvolemic hyponatremia in older adults and have been implicated in ~30% of cases. Thiazides lead to decreased sodium reabsorption in the distal convoluted tubule, the diluting segment of the nephron, and thus impair the kidney's ability to maximally dilute the urine and excrete a water load. The effect is reversible when the thiazide is discontinued.

SIADH is a common cause of hyponatremia in older adults. Most cases are mild and relatively asymptomatic but, as stated above, may increase the risk of falls, gait impairment, and difficulty sustaining attention in older adults. In this condition, ADH is released despite euvolemia and hyponatremia. Because the patient is euvolemic, there is no stimulus for sodium retention, and urine sodium concentration reflects sodium intake. Urine sodium is usually >40 mEq/L on a typical American diet but can be low if the patient consumes a very low sodium diet. Another clue is a urine uric acid <4 mg/dL. Pulmonary and brain pathology, including infections and malignancy, may cause SIADH. Medication-related causes include SSRIs, sulfonylureas, carbamazepine, oxcarbazepine, and tricyclic antidepressants. In addition, several agents potentiate the action of ADH, including nicotine, morphine, cyclophosphamide, and vincristine. SIADH is managed by discontinuation of offending medications, fluid restriction, and loop diuretics. Occasionally, demeclocycline or lithium is used to decrease ADH response. Drugs that block the ADH receptor, such as tolvaptan, are approved for treatment of both euvolemic and hypervolemic hyponatremia but are extremely expensive and thus not commonly prescribed. Additionally, the adverse effects of tolvaptan on older adults are not well known, because the mean age range of participants was 60–65 years old in clinical trials that demonstrated its efficacy and effectiveness.

Reset osmostat refers to a type of SIADH in which the set point for ADH release is lower than the usual serum sodium value of 140 mEq/L. In this situation, serum sodium is maintained at a lower than normal value. For example, if the set point is 132 mEq/L, ADH is released in response to serum sodium >132 mEq/L, resulting in concentrated urine and water retention until the serum sodium returns to the set point. In patients with this condition, ADH is suppressed when the sodium drops below the set-point, and for this reason, these patients are able to excrete a water load in <4 hours. A very dilute urine, or a low ADH level after water loading, suggests the diagnosis. Because the resultant hyponatremia is stable and chronic, it does not cause symptoms.

Treatment of Severe or Symptomatic Hyponatremia

Urgent or emergent treatment is indicated when hyponatremia is severe (serum sodium <120 mEq/L) or symptomatic and warrants admission to the hospital for management. Because hyponatremia is usually caused by an inability of the kidneys to excrete a water load, free water restriction is important in managing all forms of hyponatremia. In patients with hypovolemia, isotonic saline is sufficient to correct the hyponatremia, because euvolemia restores osmotic regulation of ADH. In patients with SIADH, administration of isotonic saline can worsen hyponatremia as the salt is excreted and water is retained. Such patients, as well as any patient with symptomatic hyponatremia, warrant treatment with intravenous hypertonic saline. In patients treated with either isotonic or hypertonic saline, volume status and sodium levels should be reassessed frequently. Volume overload and pulmonary edema must be avoided. Additionally, overly rapid correction of chronic hyponatremia can result in osmotic demyelination and a devastating locked-in syndrome called central pontine myelinolysis. The goal is to raise serum sodium concentration by ~0.3–0.4 mEq/hr, though in severe symptomatic hyponatremia, a small bolus of 3% saline given over minutes to raise the sodium a few mEq/L acutely is safe and can alleviate symptoms.

The amount that a liter of given IV fluid would raise the serum sodium can be calculated using the following Adrogue-Madias formula:

$$\text{Change in serum sodium} = \frac{(\text{infusate sodium} - \text{serum sodium})}{(\text{total body water} + 1)}$$

The infusate sodium depends on which fluid is administered: isotonic 0.9% saline has a sodium concentration of 154 mEq/L, whereas hypertonic 3% saline has a sodium concentration of 513 mEq/L. In calculating total body water, it is important to keep in mind that in older adults the percentage of body weight that is water is less than that in younger adults. In men, total body water decreases from 0.6 to 0.5 × body weight in kg, while in women the figure decreases from 0.5 to 0.4–0.45 × body weight.

An example is useful to illustrate the point. Consider an 80-kg older man with a serum sodium concentration of 117 mEq/L who is having seizures. Hypertonic saline is indicated. How much would a liter of hypertonic saline raise the serum sodium concentration? The formula yields (513 − 117) / (40 + 1), or 9.7 mEq/L. The rate of infusion can be calculated to achieve the desired rate of rise in serum sodium concentration.

The formula provides only a starting point for management of severe hyponatremia because patients are not closed systems, taking in fluid and losing variable amounts of salt and water in the urine. For this reason, serum sodium concentrations should be monitored with serial blood tests to guide adjustments to therapy.

Hypernatremia

Serum sodium concentration can increase from either a net loss of water or a gain of sodium from ingestion. Despite increased ADH secretion, older adults have diminished sensitivity to ADH, which contributes to decreased ability to concentrate the urine. Adequate free water intake is necessary to maintain normal sodium concentration, but older adults often have an impaired thirst mechanism that can result in inadequate fluid intake despite dehydration. Patients with a diminished level of consciousness or immobility with decreased ability to obtain access to free water are at greatest risk of dehydration and hypernatremia. Comorbidities such as infections, fever, dementia, and neurologic disorders increase risk of hypernatremia. In addition, medications that can cloud the sensorium, osmotic diuretic agents, tube feedings containing high protein and glucose, and bowel cathartics increase risk of hypernatremia in older adults and should be used carefully.

Hypernatremia can lead to severe neurologic sequelae, including obtundation, stupor, coma, and death. Mortality can be as high as 70%. Free water deficits should be corrected by encouraging oral fluid intake, or if the patient is unable to take adequate fluid by mouth, administration of intravenous or enteral free water. Free water deficit should be replaced over 72 hours and can be calculated as follows:

$$\text{Free water deficit (L)} = ([\text{serum sodium}/140] - 1) \times \text{total body water}$$

The response to free water should be monitored and ongoing water losses should be added to the replacement as necessary to improve the water deficit over time.

Disorders of Sodium Balance: Hypovolemia and Hypervolemia

Hypovolemia differs from dehydration in that it implies a sodium deficit in addition to water. Older adults are at increased risk of volume depletion due to decreased activity of the RAAS, as well as increased atrial natriuretic hormone. Acute illness such as gastroenteritis can be a precipitating cause. Diuretics and cathartics can also contribute, as can a very low sodium diet. Symptoms include dizziness and fatigue. Signs include low blood pressure, tachycardia, orthostatic hypotension, and decreased skin turgor. Laboratory clues include hyponatremia, hypokalemia, metabolic alkalosis, and increased BUN/creatinine ratio. Treatment is aimed at replacing both salt and water, because giving water alone will precipitate hyponatremia.

Hypervolemia is a common problem and may be related to underlying conditions such as congestive heart failure, pulmonary hypertension, venous insufficiency, and hypoalbuminemic states such as malnutrition, cirrhosis, and the nephrotic syndrome. Excessive sodium intake invariably contributes to edema. A number of commonly prescribed medications can lead to salt and water retention, especially NSAIDs, thiazolidinediones (pioglitazone), and vasodilators such as calcium channel blockers, hydralazine, and minoxidil. Treatment consists of treating underlying conditions, discontinuation of offending medications if possible, and judicious use of diuretics. Loop diuretics are effective, whereas thiazide diuretics alone are often insufficient, particularly in the setting of diminished GFR. In diuretic-resistant cases, combinations of diuretics may be necessary, but combined use of loop and thiazide diuretics can lead to profound hypokalemia and hypomagnesemia. Loop diuretics can also be used in combination with potassium-sparing diuretics such as spironolactone or eplerenone to mitigate electrolyte derangements.

Disorders of Potassium Balance

Most potassium in the body is intracellular. Derangements in serum potassium concentrations may be caused by shifts of potassium in and out of cells, as well as by excessive potassium intake or potassium losses. Kidneys regulate potassium concentrations in the collecting tubule where aldosterone acts to reabsorb sodium, thereby creating an electrochemical gradient drawing potassium and hydrogen into the urine.

Hypokalemia in older adults occurs for a number of reasons. Because of decreased ability to conserve sodium, older adults are at increased risk of volume depletion, leading to stimulation of the RAAS, which causes sodium retention and potassium loss. GI losses from vomiting, diarrhea, and fistula drainage similarly cause hypokalemia through volume depletion and secondary activation of the RAAS. Medications such as loop and thiazide diuretics, and cathartics lead to potassium loss. Inadequate intake of potassium can also contribute to the development of hypokalemia. Treatment consists of correcting volume depletion, discontinuing offending medications if possible, and increasing potassium intake. When potassium loss has occurred over time, the total body potassium deficit can be quite significant.

Several factors contribute to the increased risk of hyperkalemia in older adults, including an age-related decline in aldosterone levels, leading to decreased potassium excretion in the collecting duct. This is often seen in patients with diabetes and in those with CKD associated with metabolic acidosis, known as type IV renal tubular acidosis (RTA), or hyporenemic hypoaldosteronism. For a number of commonly prescribed medications that contribute to hyperkalemia, see Table 53.2.

Hyperkalemia may be spurious due to hemolysis of the specimen, so abnormal values should be repeated. Pseudohyperkalemia refers to hyperkalemia that develops in the serum separator tube in the setting of markedly increased WBC or platelet counts as seen in some hematologic malignancies. In this situation, the potassium level should be checked in a sample from a heparinized tube to avoid the spurious hyperkalemia.

The urgency of treatment of hyperkalemia in older adults varies with the cause, duration, and presence of signs indicating cardiac toxicity (peaked T waves, widened QRS interval, arrhythmias). In cases of severe hyperkalemia, hospital admission is warranted. Calcium is given intravenously to stabilize the myocardium while medications, including intravenous insulin and glucose, sodium bicarbonate, and nebulized albuterol,

Table 53.2—Common Medications that Cause Hyperkalemia

Medication	Mechanism
ACE inhibitors and ARBs	Decrease aldosterone production
Aldosterone antagonists	Decrease sodium reabsorption and potassium excretion
Amiloride, triamterene	Decrease sodium reabsorption and potassium excretion
β-blockers	Decrease renin release, decrease β receptor–mediated shift of potassium into cells
Heparin	Interferes with aldosterone production
Trimethoprim, pentamidine	Triamterene-like effect
NSAIDs	Decrease percent GFR

Note: ACE=angiotensin-converting enzyme, ARB = angiotensin II receptor blockers, GFR=glomerular filtration rate are given to shift potassium into cells. Medications that remove potassium include diuretics and sodium polystyrene (Kayexalate). Dialysis may be necessary in severe cases, especially when kidney function is poor.

In less severe and chronic cases, offending medications should be decreased or stopped, at least temporarily. Additional treatment includes a low potassium diet, and diuretics may also be used to increase renal potassium excretion. In cases of type IV RTA, sodium bicarbonate administration lowers serum potassium. Fludrocortisone, a synthetic mineralocorticoid, causes sodium retention and potassium loss but can exacerbate edema and hypertension. Sodium polystyrene should not be used on a chronic basis because of the risk of bowel toxicity.

Disorders of Acid-Base Balance

Older adults are at increased risk of both metabolic acidosis and metabolic alkalosis. Metabolic acidosis may occur as a result of decreased aldosterone production, particularly in the setting of an increased acid load as seen in a high-protein diet, or bicarbonate loss through the GI tract. As described above, medications that inhibit the RAAS or sodium reabsorption in the distal tubule lead to metabolic acidosis and hyperkalemia. The presentation is similar to a type IV RTA, which is often seen with CKD and diabetes. Type IV RTA, a relatively common syndrome, can be recognized by the presence of hypokalemia and a non-anion gap metabolic acidosis. A type II proximal RTA is sometimes seen in older adults as a result of myeloma or amyloid, and is often associated with Fanconi syndrome, in which diffuse proximal tubular dysfunction leads to glucosuria, amino aciduria, and loss of other ions such as calcium, phosphorus, and magnesium. Severe metabolic acidosis may lead to shortness of breath as the respiratory system attempts to blow off CO_2. Chronic acidosis also contributes to bone loss, because the acid is buffered in the bones, leading to hypercalciuria and increased risk of kidney stones. Studies suggest that chronic acidosis can also lead to progression of CKD. Acidosis is usually treated with administration of exogenous base, either as sodium bicarbonate tablets or powder, or citrate salts.

Metabolic alkalosis often occurs as a result of volume depletion and diuretic use, both common in older adults. Volume depletion leads to increased RAAS activity. As the kidney reabsorbs sodium, potassium and hydrogen are secreted into the urine. Vomiting and nasogastric tube suction of gastric contents lead to loss of hydrogen and can also precipitate metabolic alkalosis. Severe metabolic alkalosis may decrease respiratory drive, which can precipitate respiratory acidosis and may impair the ability to remove intubated patients from mechanical ventilation. Treatment includes cessation of diuretics and administration of saline to volume-depleted patients. In the case of volume-overloaded patients, a limited course of treatment with the carbonic anhydrase inhibitor acetazolamide can cause renal bicarbonate loss.

SECONDARY HYPERTENSION AND RENAL ARTERY DISEASE

The prevalence of hypertension increases with advancing age, affecting about two-thirds of patients >65 years old. Older adults are at increased risk of hypertension for a number of reasons, including increased arterial stiffness and impaired sodium handling leading to salt sensitivity. Most hypertension is idiopathic, or essential, but occasionally secondary causes are discovered, such as renal artery disease, mineralocorticoid hypertension (Conn syndrome), hypercortisolism (Cushing syndrome), or pheochromocytoma. CKD is a more common cause of secondary hypertension. Secondary causes should be suspected in patients with new onset, very severe, or accelerated hypertension.

There has been a great deal of controversy over blood pressure targets for hypertensive patients. The most recent guideline issued by the Eighth Joint National Committee, published 2014, significantly relaxed blood pressure targets to 150/90 mmHg for nondiabetic patients aged ≥60 years old. For diabetic patients and those <60 years old, the target is 140/90 mmHg. The guideline does not recommend reducing medications for patients >59 years old already on medications and stable with a blood pressure <140/90 mmHg.

Renal Artery Disease

Atherosclerotic renovascular disease is primarily an illness of older adults, because most risk factors increase with age and include smoking, hypertension, hyperlipidemia, diabetes mellitus, and dissecting aortic aneurysms. Renovascular disease is closely associated with other vascular disease and is present in 24% of those undergoing coronary angiography (SOE=A). Mortality is typically related to cardiovascular events rather than to renal impairment. Stenosis of the renal artery needs to be >70%–80% of the luminal area to decrease renal blood flow. The decreased blood flow causes activation of the RAAS and systemic hypertension in an attempt to restore renal perfusion.

Renal artery stenosis should be suspected in patients with other documented vascular disease, and in the setting of new-onset hypertension; acceleration of previously controlled hypertension; resistant hypertension, defined as inability to control blood pressure despite maximal doses of 3 blood pressure medications; or progressive azotemia after starting an ACE inhibitor or an angiotensin-receptor blocker (ARB). Diagnostic test options include CT or MR angiography, nuclear renal scanning after administration of an ACE inhibitor, or renal angiography, the gold standard. The decision to image rests on whether a diagnosis would change management.

Medical management includes blood pressure control, and given that RAAS activation is a central cause of hypertension in this setting, treatment regimens should include an ACE inhibitor or ARB. With severe bilateral stenosis, RAAS blockade can cause progressive acute kidney injury (AKI). Although 2%–6% of patients treated with an ACE inhibitor or an ARB have an increased serum creatinine concentration as an expected complication of therapy, modest increases in creatinine should not deter prescribing these medications, which reduce morbidity and mortality in patients with hypertension and vascular disease (SOE=A for ACE inhibitors, SOE=B for ARBs).

Renal artery angioplasty, with or without stenting, has been advocated as a means to reduce blood pressure and blood pressure medication burden, as well as to stem progression of ischemic kidney disease. Renal angiography carries significant risk, including contrast-induced nephropathy and atheroembolic disease. Renal function declines abruptly in ~25% of patients after revascularization. Numerous case series of angioplasty with stenting show complication rates of 0–8% for embolization, 0–3% for dialysis, 0–4% for death, and 11%–26% for restenosis over an average of 10 months. In most patients, pill burden from antihypertensive agents is only minimally decreased. The CORAL trial, a landmark study, showed no benefit for renal artery stenting in addition to medical management in terms of major cardiovascular or renal outcomes. Thus, renal angiography and stenting is not indicated except in extreme cases of uncontrollable hypertension or progressive kidney failure from severe stenosis.

HEMATURIA AND NEPHROLITHIASIS

Hematuria may be microscopic, seen only by urinalysis, or gross, which is visible to the naked eye as pink, red, or brown urine. Urinary blood can come from anywhere along the urogenital tract, from the kidneys, to the collecting system, to the external genitalia. Hematuria from glomerular disease is often associated with proteinuria, and is distinguishable on urinalysis by dysmorphic red cells (acanthocytes) and red cell casts. Blood from elsewhere in the urinary tract may be due to infection, stones, arteriovenous malformations, or neoplasms. The likelihood of an associated malignancy increases with age. In one cohort of patients in their 60s, gross hematuria was associated with malignancy in 28.9% of men and 21.1% of women, whereas malignancy was diagnosed in 7.9% of men, and 4.5% of women with microscopic hematuria.

The evaluation for hematuria includes a urine culture and microscopic evaluation of the urine. Imaging depends on the clinical setting. A plain abdominal radiograph (kidney, ureture, bladder) may be sufficient to detect kidney stones, although a CT scan without contrast or an ultrasound is often done and is more sensitive. A CT scan with contrast is helpful to exclude an enhancing kidney or other mass, but it should be done in conjunction with a CT without contrast to also exclude stones. Urology consultation and cystoscopy is often recommended to further exclude a bladder or other collecting system malignancy.

ACUTE KIDNEY INJURY

Acute kidney injury (AKI) is defined as an acute increase in creatinine, and also by oliguria criteria, or <5 mL/kg/hr urine output over at least 6 hours. The incidence of severe AKI has increased in recent years, by one estimate 10% per year between 2000 and 2009. AKI occurs with increased frequency in the geriatric population, and even minor increased in creatinine have been associated with increased risk of prolonged hospitalization and death. In the setting of severe AKI, dialysis is sometimes indicated to support patients while treatment of underlying conditions is under way, awaiting recovery of renal function. Recovery is variable and depends on the specific cause of the injury. Mortality for older adults who develop dialysis-requiring AKI has been estimated at 31%–80%. The decision whether to undertake dialysis should be individualized and is discussed in detail below.

The differential diagnosis of AKI is typically categorized into prerenal, intrinsic renal, and postrenal causes. Intrinsic renal disease is divided into tubulointerstitial, glomerular, and vascular disease. The most common cause of AKI in older adults is acute tubular necrosis, followed by prerenal azotemia.

Prerenal Azotemia

Prerenal azotemia is among the most common causes of AKI in older adults. It is due to decreased renal blood flow from intravascular volume depletion or heart failure, and is often exacerbated by intrarenal hemodynamic changes caused by medications such as ACE inhibitors, ARBs, and NSAIDs. The diagnosis is suspected based on history and physical examination. Additionally, laboratory results such as a BUN:creatinine ratio >20 and fractional excretion of sodium (FE_{Na}) <1% suggest the diagnosis. It should be noted that a low FE_{Na} can be seen in other conditions, such as acute glomerulonephritis, contrast nephropathy, interstitial nephritis, and urinary tract obstruction. Therefore, a low FE_{Na} is not necessarily diagnostic of prerenal azotemia.

Older adults are at increased risk of prerenal azotemia for a number of reasons. Physiologic changes described earlier (Table 53.1) can contribute to volume depletion. Acute illness leading to poor oral intake, GI fluid loss, and comorbidities such as congestive heart failure and renal artery disease are additional risk factors. Many older patients take diuretics that can lead to volume depletion, as well as ACE inhibitors, ARBs, and NSAIDs, which decrease glomerular filtration pressure and impair renal autoregulation that normally maintains GFR when renal blood flow is decreased. Finally, older adults may have reduced access to fluids because of cognitive, physical, and/or environmental factors.

Treatment involves discontinuing or reducing offending medications and restoring intravascular volume. Prerenal azotemia caused by hypoalbuminemic states such as cirrhosis and nephrotic syndrome may require a colloid infusion to improve intravascular volume. If the AKI is purely prerenal, kidney function should improve rapidly with volume resuscitation.

Cardiorenal Syndrome

Cardiorenal syndrome refers to acute and chronic kidney injury that occurs in systolic or diastolic heart failure, and carries a poor prognosis. It is caused by some combination of diminished forward flow from decreased cardiac output leading to prerenal azotemia, and increased central venous pressure leading to renal congestion and decreased glomerular filtration pressure. Treatment is aimed at optimizing cardiac function, typically with diuretics and afterload-reducing agents. Inotropic support is occasionally used to aid with diuresis. As above, medications that impair renal autoregulation should be discontinued or the dosage reduced.

Obstructive Uropathy

Urinary tract obstruction is a common and often reversible cause of AKI in older adults. Obstruction can occur either at the level of the bladder outlet or the ureters. Because one kidney is usually sufficient to maintain GFR, unilateral ureteral obstruction does not tend to cause severe AKI, unless there is a solitary functioning kidney to begin with. The diagnosis is made by a high index of suspicion and an abdominal and pelvic ultrasound or CT scan.

Bladder outlet obstruction is more frequent in men but can occur in both genders. In men, bladder outlet obstruction from benign prostatic hyperplasia is the most common cause of obstructive uropathy. Symptoms include urinary hesitancy, a sensation of incomplete emptying of the bladder, and nocturia. Complete obstruction is obvious, but even partial obstruction can lead to back pressure through the collecting system and decreased kidney function. Treatment options include α-adrenergic blocking agents such as tamsulosin, 5-α reductase inhibitors such as finasteride, cessation of anticholinergic medications, and transurethral resection of the prostate. Functional bladder outlet obstruction can occur in both genders and is caused by anticholinergic medications such as narcotic analgesics, antihistamines, and antidepressants. Other causes of bladder outlet obstruction with a higher prevalence in older adults include bladder carcinoma and urethral stricture.

Ureteral obstruction is often caused by stones, strictures, or retroperitoneal malignancies, such as lymphoma, bladder carcinoma, or rectal tumors. Once the diagnosis of ureteral obstruction is made, additional imaging may be required to establish a cause, and urology consultation for further management is warranted. Treatment options include ureteral stenting and percutaneous nephrostomy placement.

INTRINSIC RENAL DISEASE

Tubulointerstitial Disease

Acute Tubular Necrosis (ATN)

Ischemia is the most common cause of ATN in older adults. Prerenal azotemia and ATN occur on a continuum depending on the severity and duration of hypoperfusion, and evolution of prerenal azotemia to frank ATN is more common in older patients with AKI (23%) than in younger ones (15%). Renal hypoperfusion to the degree required to cause severe ATN usually occurs in the setting of marked systemic hypotension and shock, although even less severe hypotension can cause ATN in those accustomed to very high blood pressure and in those with renal artery disease. Additionally, a number of medications and toxins have been associated with ATN, including aminoglycoside antibiotics, vancomycin, amphotericin B, and radiocontrast agents.

ATN is diagnosed based on urine sediment findings that include renal tubular epithelial cells and granular "muddy brown" casts. In the setting of oliguria, calculating FE_{Na}, or fractional excretion of urea nitrogen if the patient has recently been exposed to diuretics, can help distinguish prerenal azotemia from ATN. In prerenal azotemia, the kidneys are sodium avid, and FE_{Na} is <1%. In ATN, the kidneys are not able to retain sodium, and FE_{Na} is >2%. Diuretics impair sodium retention by the kidneys, so a high FE_{Na} in a patient on diuretics is not helpful in distinguishing between prerenal azotemia and ATN. However, a low FE_{Na} despite diuretics points to sodium avidity and argues against ATN. Fractional excretion of urea has been used in place of FE_{Na} in the setting of diuretic use; <25 is consistent with prerenal azotemia, and >35 suggests ATN.

Treatment of patients with ATN is generally supportive. Interventions should include optimization of hemodynamics to ensure renal perfusion and avoidance of nephrotoxins. Medication dosing should be adjusted to the level of renal function to prevent toxicity and further renal injury. Diuretic use in ATN does not improve or harm prospects for renal recovery and may be helpful to manage volume overload unless aggressive diuresis contributes to recurrent hypotension. ATN is often reversible over days to weeks, and dialysis may be required to support patients with severe ATN.

Acute Interstitial Nephritis

Acute interstitial nephritis is increasingly common in older adults. It manifests as AKI and is most commonly an allergic response to medication, although there are other causes such as viral infections. A diagnostic clue is sterile pyuria, with WBC casts on urinalysis. The CBC with differential may show eosinophilia, and eosinophils may be evident in the urine by special stain. Any medication can cause interstitial nephritis, but antibiotics are most commonly implicated, particularly β-lactam antibiotics and fluoroquinolones. Therapy consists of discontinuing the offending agent. Recent retrospective data suggest that a course of corticosteroids may speed recovery and lead to a more complete resolution of kidney injury. A kidney biopsy is usually indicated to confirm the diagnosis before initiating high-dose steroids because of their toxicity.

Multiple Myeloma

Multiple myeloma is a plasma cell dyscrasia with increasing prevalence in advancing age and is associated with a number of renal manifestations, including AKI. The malignant plasma cells generate monoclonal proteins that can form casts that obstruct renal tubules, a condition called myeloma kidney. The abnormal proteins can also deposit in the renal parenchyma, termed light-chain or heavy-chain deposition disease, or form fibrils that deposit as amyloid. These conditions are associated with heavy proteinuria, sometimes in the nephrotic range. Severe hypercalcemia can also result from development of lytic bone lesions, which can lead to renal vasoconstriction, volume depletion, and prerenal azotemia.

The diagnosis is suspected in the setting of acute or chronic kidney disease, a low serum anion gap, hypercalcemia, an increased protein gap (plasma total protein more than twice plasma albumin), anemia, and bone pain. Laboratory testing includes serum and urine electrophoresis, immunofixation studies, serum free light chains, β-2 microglobulin, and serum immunoglobulins.

A skeletal survey may show characteristic lytic bone lesions. Diagnosis is confirmed with a bone marrow biopsy. Treatment consists of chemotherapy agents, such as melphalan and prednisone, and may result in improvement of the associated kidney problems.

Vascular Disease

Atheroembolic disease occurs when cholesterol microemboli lodge in the small vessels of the kidneys and cause progressive damage. A major risk factor is angiography such as cardiac catheterization. The use of warfarin for anticoagulation is a risk factor for spontaneous atheroembolic disease. After angiography, kidney dysfunction can be delayed and is often slowly progressive. It can be confused with contrast-induced ATN but is less likely to improve over time. Patients may exhibit skin manifestations of *atheroembolism*, or livedo reticularis. Eosinophilia may be present, and serum complements can be transiently decreased.

Thrombotic microangiopathy causes AKI, because platelet microthrombi occlude small renal arterioles. The diagnosis is suspected in the setting of hemolytic anemia and progressive thrombocytopenia. Classic examples include thrombotic thrombocytopenic purpura (TTP) and hemolytic uremic syndrome (HUS), but a similar presentation can occur in the setting of malignant hypertension, catastrophic antiphospholipid antibody syndrome, and scleroderma renal crisis. Several medications have been associated with TTP, including mitomycin C, gemcitabine, cisplatin, clopidogrel, cyclosporine, and quinine. "Typical" TTP-HUS is associated with decreased levels of the von Willebrand factor cleaving protease ADAMTS-13. "Atypical" TTP-HUS associated with normal ADAMTS-13 levels is more common in older patients and is associated with malignancy. Treatment for thrombotic microangiopathy includes plasma exchange.

Occlusion of a large renal artery can occur in the setting of renal artery stenosis, or as a result of embolic phenomena related to atrial fibrillation or paradoxical venous thromboembolism through a patent foramen ovale. Acute renal artery occlusion causes renal infarction with pain, hematuria, and loss of GFR. If the infarction is unilateral and the other kidney is still functioning, the decrease in GFR is often not dramatic, and kidney function tends to improve as the functioning kidney hyperfilters to compensate for lost renal parenchyma. Increased lactate dehydrogenase is a diagnostic clue. It is confirmed with imaging studies such as an ultrasound with Dopplers, CT with contrast, or a nuclear renal perfusion scan. Treatment includes anticoagulation in the setting of ongoing risk of embolic phenomena, and consideration of angiography with stenting.

Glomerular Disease

Glomerulonephritis can cause both AKI and CKD. Glomerulonephritis is divided into rapidly progressive glomerulonephritis (RPGN), acute nephritic syndrome, nephrotic syndrome, asymptomatic hematuria and/or proteinuria, and chronic glomerular disease. Of these, RPGN and acute nephritic syndrome are causes of AKI. Kidney biopsy in the geriatric population is generally as safe as in younger patients and is often critical in guiding appropriate management of glomerular disease.

RPGN is the most common form of acute glomerulonephritis in older adults, accounting for 40%–50% of biopsies in some series. Clinically, the decline in renal function begins insidiously and progresses rapidly over days to weeks, leading to end-stage renal disease (ESRD) if untreated. Histologic examination reveals glomerular cellular crescents and necrosis, commonly affecting more than half of the glomeruli. There are 3 patterns seen on immunostaining of biopsy tissue. The most common pattern, seen in up to 75% of cases, is "pauci-immune" glomerulephritis, with negative immunostaining. This is usually caused by antineutrophil cytoplasmic antibody (ANCA)-associated vasculitis, either granulomatosis with polyangiitis (formerly called Wegener's), or microscopic polyangiitis. The second pattern consists of linear staining for IgG along the basement membranes, which is characteristic of anti-glomerular basement membrane, or Goodpasture's, disease. The third pattern reveals immune complexes in the capillary walls and mesangia, which are seen in several conditions including lupus nephritis, IgA nephropathy, and infection-associated glomerulonephritis. Therapy for RPGN includes intravenous steroids followed by oral steroids and additional immunosuppression (eg, cyclophosphamide, rituximab). Plasmapheresis is often used in severe acute cases. Once remission is achieved, treatment is usually maintained with a prolonged course of azathioprine or mycophenolate.

Acute nephritic syndrome classically presents with decreasing kidney function, hematuria with dysmorphic red cells and red cell casts on urine microscopy, variable proteinuria, hypertension, and fluid retention. Symptoms of systemic disease, such as staphylococcal or streptococcal infection, or vasculitis may be prominent. The diagnosis may be delayed in older adults because of incorrectly attributing symptoms to common conditions such as urinary tract infection, heart failure, or venous stasis disease.

A proliferative acute glomerulonephritis can occur in the setting of various infections, such as streptococcal infection of the throat and skin but also with staphylococcal infections. Postinfectious glomerulonephritis is generally self-limited. Treatment is supportive, and the prognosis is generally favorable, although the risk of acute complications such as a fatal exacerbation of heart failure is increased.

IgA nephropathy (Berger disease) is another common cause of proliferative glomerulonephritis in the geriatric population. It presents as acute or chronic nephritic syndrome with variable proteinuria. Chronic interstitial scarring on biopsy, and proteinuria >500 mg/day are risks for progression to ESRD. IgA nephropathy may be primary or secondary due to cirrhosis, celiac disease, or HIV infection. Other infectious causes of IgA nephropathy include cytomegalovirus, *Haemophilus parainfluenzae*, *Staphylococcus aureus*, disseminated tuberculosis, and toxoplasmosis. Treatment generally consists of controlling the underlying conditions, blood pressure control using ACE inhibitors if possible, and management of CKD.

NEPHROTIC SYNDROME

Nephrotic syndrome consists of urinary excretion of >3.5 g of protein per day, with associated hypoalbuminemia, hyperlipidemia, and edema. Hematuria is variably present but not to the degree seen in acute nephritic syndrome. Very heavy proteinuria is associated with a hypercoagulable state and increased risk of deep-vein thrombosis, pulmonary embolism, and renal vein thrombosis. Hypertension and progressive kidney disease are also seen in about one-third of cases in older adults. Nephrotic syndrome can result from primary glomerular disease or secondary to systemic disease such as infection, malignancy, exposure to allergens or medications, diabetes, or hypertension. In most cases of nephrotic syndrome, a renal biopsy is indicated for early diagnosis and appropriate therapy. Therapy for nephrotic syndrome includes blood pressure control, use of RAAS blockers, sodium restriction, and statins for hyperlipidemia. Anticoagulation is considered when plasma albumin is <2.8 g/dL.

Membranous Nephropathy

Membranous nephropathy is the most common histopathology in the geriatric population, found in 20%–40% of biopsies performed for nephrotic syndrome. Although most patients have idiopathic disease, the 2 most common causes of secondary membranous nephropathy are NSAID use and malignancy. Primary membranous nephropathy has been associated with an antibody to the phospholipase A2 receptor-1 in 70%–80% of cases, although an assay for the autoantibody is not routinely available yet. Approximately 7%–20% of patients with membranous nephropathy have been associated with solid organ tumors, particularly of the lung, colon, rectum, breast, and kidney, which are sometimes discovered after nephrotic syndrome develops. Therefore, malignancy should be considered in older adults with membranous nephropathy.

The prognosis for older adults with membranous nephropathy is quite variable and correlates with the severity of the proteinuria and the degree of hypoalbuminemia. About a third of cases resolve without therapy, and a third have continued proteinuria without declining kidney function. The other third have a progressive decline in kidney function. For these high-risk patients, first-line therapy options include a calcineurin inhibitor, either cyclosporine or tacrolimus, with or without low-dose steroids, or cyclic corticosteroids and cytotoxic agents. The latter regimen is associated with increased risk of leukopenia and infection in older patients. There is a risk of relapse with either regimen. Second-line agents include rituximab or ACTH gel.

Focal Segmental Glomerulosclerosis

Focal segmental glomerulosclerosis (FSGS) in older adults presents as insidious onset of nephrotic syndrome, usually with abnormal GFR, and associated hypertension. Primary FSGS is idiopathic, whereas secondary causes include infections such as hepatitis B, parvovirus, or HIV, malignancies including lymphoma, and medications such as pamidronate. Secondary FSGS also occurs with morbid obesity and many forms of advanced CKD as remaining nephrons are injured as they hyperfilter to maintain GFR. Basic treatment principles include correcting reversible causes, controlling blood pressure, using ACE inhibitors or ARBs to minimize proteinuria, and moderately restricting dietary protein. In primary disease, a prolonged course of steroid therapy may be helpful but is often not well tolerated due to adverse effects and long-term risks such as osteoporosis and pathologic fractures. Calcineurin inhibitor therapy with lower dose steroids is another option if GFR is not markedly impaired.

Minimal Change Disease

Minimal change disease (MCD) can be idiopathic or associated with hypersensitivity reactions, hematologic malignancies, or drugs, particularly NSAIDs. In older adults, MCD usually presents with abrupt onset of full-blown nephrotic syndrome and normal blood pressure. Compared with that in younger patients, the risk of AKI is increased; it occurs in 30% of older patients and is usually reversible. Treatment typically consists of a prolonged course of high-dose steroids. Up to 80% of older patients respond to initial steroid therapy, but relapse rates are as high as 33%. In steroid-dependent cases, and when steroids are not tolerated, other agents such as calcineurin inhibitors or cyclophosphamide may be tried. Steroid resistance suggests that the true diagnosis may be FSGS rather than MCD.

Amyloidosis and Other Protein Deposition Diseases

Systemic amyloidosis is common in older adults with nephrotic syndrome. A renal biopsy or abdominal fat pad biopsy should be stained with Congo red or thioflavine T to evaluate for amyloidosis. Renal tissue should also be examined by electron microscopy for myeloid fibrils. Paraproteinemia can be found in up to 68% of patients with primary amyloidosis. Therefore, both serum and urine immunoelectrophoresis should be performed in all older adults with nephrotic syndrome. If findings are abnormal, bone marrow biopsy should be done to exclude multiple myeloma. Treatment with an appropriate chemotherapy regimen can delay progression to ESRD.

CHRONIC KIDNEY DISEASE

Kidney function as measured by GFR declines on average 8 mL/min per decade after age 40. Renal glomerular and tubulointerstitial fibrosis increases with age, leading to nephron dropout and CKD. CKD has many causes in older adults, including diabetes, hypertension, glomerulonephritis, obstructive uropathy, and chronic interstitial nephritis often due to medications such as NSAIDs. CKD in older adults frequently manifests with a decompensation of preexisting medical illness such as heart failure, diabetes mellitus, hypertension, or dementia.

Data from the National Health and Nutrition Examination Survey (NHANES) 2007–2012 suggest that 33% of patients >60 years old have CKD and 23% have an eGFR <60 mL/min. The incidence varies among ethnic and racial groups. Diabetes and hypertension, both important causes of CKD, are more common in black, Hispanic, and some Native American populations. Black Americans with diabetes or hypertension are more than twice as likely to develop kidney failure than other ethnic or racial groups, and the odds increase for individuals with a first-degree relative on dialysis for any reason.

Chronic Kidney Disease Classification

In 2002, the National Kidney Foundation (NKF) through the Kidney Disease Quality Initiative (KDOQI) established a classification system for CKD and issued related clinical practice guidelines (Table 53.3). CKD is defined as either kidney damage or decreased kidney function, with eGFR <60 mL/min for ≥3 months. The NKF KDOQI staging system is based on estimated GFR. Most older adults have a GFR <60 mL/min, and there is ongoing debate whether this represents disease or is related to normal aging. Revisions to the KDOQI classification used in the Kidney Disease: Improving Global Outcomes (KDIGO) CKD Work Group 2012 Guidelines have divided Stage 3 CKD into 3A and 3B, again based on GFR, and

Table 53.3—Stages of Chronic Kidney Disease

Stage	Description	GFR (mL/min/1.73 m²)
1	Kidney damage with normal or ↑ GFR	≥90
2	Kidney damage with mildly ↓ GFR	60–89
3A	Mildly to moderately ↓ GFR	45–59
3B	Moderately to severely ↓ GFR	30–44
4	Severely ↓ GFR	15–29
5	Kidney failure (end-stage renal disease)	<15

Note: GFR = glomerular filtration rate; chronic kidney disease is defined as either kidney damage or decreased kidney function, with eGFR <60 mL/min for ≥3 months.

SOURCE: National Kidney Foundation. NKF KDOQI Guidelines, 2002, and the KDIGO Guidelines, 2012.

have added a term for the degree of proteinuria. Of note, older patients with Stage 3A CKD (eGFR 45–60 mL/min) and no albuminuria are unlikely to suffer complications of CKD or to progress to ESRD.

Management

In older adults, treatment approaches should be based on preserving remaining renal function and limiting complications. Basic treatment principles include correcting reversible causes, controlling blood pressure, using RAAS blockers to decrease proteinuria, controlling diabetes, and moderately restricting dietary protein. Detailed clinical guidelines are available on the NKF website at www.kidney.org.

Declines in GFR are accompanied by a broad range of complications, including hypertension, anemia, malnutrition, metabolic bone disease, neuropathy, depression, impaired functional status, and increased cardiovascular morbidity and mortality. Early recognition of impaired kidney function allows for the screening and management of these complications, improving outcomes. NKF guidelines recommend referral to a nephrologist when a patient reaches Stage 4 CKD for management of complications such as acidosis, phosphorus retention, and anemia. A nephrologist can also guide discussions regarding dialysis preparation and options for transplantation.

Risk of Cardiovascular Events

Patients with CKD of all stages are at increased risk of cardiovascular events, including myocardial infarction, stroke, and death. They are far more likely to die of cardiovascular disease than to require dialysis. Reduction of morbidity and mortality in CKD therefore requires aggressive management of cardiovascular disease risk factors. This includes blood pressure control, lipid-lowering therapy, smoking cessation, and attention to diet and exercise.

Medication Use in Chronic Kidney Disease

Prescribing medications for older patients with CKD is complicated by diminished renal clearance compounded by age-associated changes in pharmacokinetics and pharmacodynamics. Many medications or their metabolites are renally excreted, and extreme care must be taken to dose these medications appropriately to avoid renal and systemic toxicity. Dose adjustments may vary based on GFR, and some may be contraindicated at low GFRs. A good practice is to verify renal dosing of any new medication being prescribed.

Additionally, certain medications, particularly NSAIDs, are potentially nephrotoxic and should be avoided or used with extreme care in patients with CKD. NSAIDs can predispose to prerenal azotemia and ATN, cause acute and chronic interstitial nephritis, and exacerbate hypertension and fluid overload. Other examples of nephrotoxic agents include radiocontrast agents, gadolinium, aminoglycosides, and amphotericin B.

Anemia

Anemia screening should start when patients reach Stage 3B CKD. Anemia in this setting is typically normochromic, normocytic, and primarily caused by decreased production of erythropoietin by the kidneys. It is important to exclude other causes before treatment is initiated. In older adults, this would entail checking vitamin B_{12}, folate, thyrotropin, and iron studies, including ferritin and transferrin saturation. In cases of iron deficiency, a bowel evaluation should be considered.

Erythropoiesis-stimulating agents (ESAs), such as recombinant erythropoietin, are often used to treat CKD-associated anemia. The main goal of this therapy is to prevent the need for blood transfusions, which carry the risk of allosensitization of potential kidney transplant recipients, and transfusion-related infections. In 2006, two large randomized control trials (CREATE and CHOIR) demonstrated that attempts to normalize hemoglobin with erythropoietin increased vascular events, particularly stroke. Taken altogether, the evidence demonstrates inconsistent quality-of-life benefit, and potential harm in terms of mortality, cardiovascular, or renal outcomes with higher hemoglobin goals. In light of this evidence, the 2012 KDIGO anemia guidelines recommend individualized consideration of ESA initiation in CKD nondialysis-dependent patients when the hemoglobin concentration is <10 g/dL. The guidelines also recommend against maintaining hemoglobin levels >11.5 g/dL through ESA use. Of note, the FDA labels advise against ESA use to achieve and maintain hemoglobin levels >11 g/dL. The NKF-KDOQI expert group, in its commentary on the KDIGO guidelines, cite a lack of strong evidence to support the upper treatment limit of 11.5 g/dL.

For ESAs to be effective, patients must have adequate iron stores to support accelerated erythropoiesis. Approximately 50% of patients who reach ESRD are iron deficient. Iron should be replaced before starting ESA therapy for anemia, with goal ferritin >100 ng/mL and transferrin saturation >20%. Most patients can tolerate oral iron, although it often causes constipation. In very advanced kidney disease, intestinal iron absorption is impaired. In this situation, or with symptomatic anemia, iron sucrose can be given intravenously, which is better tolerated than older iron preparations.

Calcium, Phosphorus, and Renal Bone Disease

Abnormalities of calcium, phosphorus, and parathyroid hormone (PTH) are common in patients with a GFR <60 mL/min/1.73 m^2 and begin early in CKD. These abnormalities have been blamed for the increased risk of vascular calcification and cardiovascular morbidity and mortality in patients with CKD. Screening for metabolic derangements begins in Stage 3 CKD. Serum phosphorus concentrations often remain normal as PTH increases to stimulate the kidneys to excrete excess phosphorus. Dietary phosphorus intake should be restricted if the PTH is increased, even if serum phosphorus remains normal. Phosphorus binders should also be considered when the PTH is increased. Phosphorus concentrations should be maintained between 2.7 and 4.6 mg/dL in patients with Stage 3 or 4 CKD. In Stage 5 CKD, phosphorus goal is considered ≤5.5 mg/dL.

The management of CKD-related mineral bone disorder is complex. Markedly increased PTH is associated with high bone turnover disease, which increases fracture risk. Increased PTH can be suppressed with vitamin D preparations, specifically active vitamin D metabolites, such as 1,25-dihydroxyvitamin D (calcitriol). However, administration of vitamin D can cause hypercalcemia. If this develops, the calcimimetic cinicalcet can be used to suppress PTH and lower serum calcium as well as phosphorus. Overaggressive suppression of PTH leads to low bone turnover disease, also known as adynamic bone disease, which causes dense, brittle bones, and thus increased fracture risk.

In the older population, CKD-related mineral bone disorder is associated with increased fracture risk 4 times that of age-matched controls. Older adults with CKD often also have osteoporosis, which presents diagnostic and management challenges. In patients with advanced CKD, dual-energy x-ray absorptiometry (DEXA) scanning is not a reliable indicator of fracture risk. Bisphosphonates are the recommended treatment of choice for osteoporosis in the early stages of renal impairment, although data on their use in CKD populations is sparse. Small studies have shown measurable increases in bone mineral density and reductions in fractures in patients on dialysis (SOE=C). Bisphosphonates are also efficacious in the transplant population. Bisphosphonates are contraindicated in adynamic bone disease, because they inhibit osteoclastic bone resorption. Calcitonin is probably safe in patients with adynamic bone disease, but no efficacy data are available (SOE=D). No safety or efficacy data are available on the use of estrogens and their derivatives in CKD.

Depression

Depression is common in any population suffering from chronic disease but has been underrecognized in the CKD population, especially those on dialysis. In one study, 13% of dialysis patients were diagnosed with depression, whereas 43% tested positive on a randomly administered depression screening test, suggesting that the true rate of depression is 3 times that of the recognized rate. Therefore, screening for depression in patients with CKD and in those on dialysis is warranted. Depression can be difficult to diagnose in the dialysis population, because the vegetative symptoms can be similar to those of uremia or insufficient dialysis. Functional and cognitive decline are particularly common presenting symptoms in older adults with kidney disease.

Most depression screening instruments have been validated in the kidney failure population. Very low doses of SSRIs can safely be used for treatment. Shorter-acting sertraline and citalopram are considered relatively safe in this population; long-acting medications such as fluoxetine and paroxetine should be avoided.

Nutrition

Dietary requirements for patients with CKD are complex. Intake of protein, phosphorus, and potassium all need to be controlled while maintaining adequate energy intake. Once a patient reaches Stage 4 CKD, an experienced renal dietitian should be involved in the patient's nutritional management. The recommended protein intake for patients with Stage 4 CKD is 0.8 g/kg/day. Limiting protein intake delays the incidence of ESRD and also helps with control of phosphorus and reduces metabolic acidosis. Dietary recommendations limit phosphorus intake to 800–1,000 mg/day, although the benefits of severe dietary restrictions in frail or institutionalized older adults have not been proved. Overaggressive dietary restriction has the potential to cause malnutrition and its complications.

Adequate nutrition and dietary therapy in older adults with advanced CKD is complicated by many common age-related factors. Lack of transportation, lower income, and loss of social/family support can compromise access to therapeutic food choices. Loss of teeth, impaired sensory function, and medications that reduce appetite or cause nausea can also impede adequate nutritional intake. Comorbid conditions such as depression, cognitive deficits, mobility impairment, or loss of function from stroke, arthritis, or Parkinson disease pose obstacles to appropriate food preparation. Referral to a dietician can be helpful in these circumstances.

END-STAGE RENAL DISEASE (ESRD)

Epidemiology

ESRD is to a large extent a disease of the older population, and more than 38% of ESRD patients are ≥65 years old. Although the incidence rates of ESRD in older adults have plateaued in recent years, the number of affected individuals continues to increase as the population ages. In recent years, there has been a trend to offer dialysis to older and sicker patients. A disproportionate amount of Medicare resources pay for the care of dialysis patients, who experience increased hospitalization rates and many complications of their disease.

Renal Replacement Therapy

The mean age at the start of renal replacement therapy is 62.3 years for men and 63.4 years for women. The KDOQI guidelines suggest that patients who progress to Stage 4 CKD should be referred to a nephrologist for assistance in managing related complications and discussions regarding preparations for ESRD. Historically, there was an emphasis to start patients on dialysis in early Stage 5 CKD, but this has not shown a benefit in morbidity or mortality. Dialysis is initiated when clear indications arise, usually with an eGFR <10 mL/min. An alternative is nonaggressive renal care, ie, a palliative approach that may include hospice.

The decision to pursue dialysis is highly individualized and should always include a cogent discussion regarding the patient's goals of care and potential benefits and harms. ESRD results in a number of complications, including metabolic abnormalities, difficulty with blood pressure and fluid management, and eventually symptomatic uremia with anorexia, nausea, sleep disturbance, myoclonic jerks, serositis, altered mental status, and death. Dialysis ameliorates these symptoms, prolongs life in patients with ESRD, and has the potential to improve both quality of life and functional status. However, a number of recent studies have shown diminished benefit of dialysis in older adults, especially those with poor functional status. A study of 3,702 nursing-home residents on dialysis showed a 1-year mortality rate of 58%, and only 13% maintained functional status after 1 year of dialysis compared with 3 months before initiation of hemodialysis. In patients who live independently, a large percentage experience functional decline and become more dependent during the first year of dialysis. Geriatric syndromes, such as frailty and falls, become more prevalent. In a study of patients with ESRD who chose dialysis despite physician recommendations for nonaggressive renal care, average survival was 8.3 vs. 6.3 months. Patients who chose dialysis in this situation often had increased hospitalizations and interaction with the health care system at the end of life.

Both hemodialysis and peritoneal dialysis have disadvantages to consider. Hemodialysis-related difficulties include a substantial time commitment, the need to travel to a dialysis facility, discomfort related to muscle cramps, fatigue after treatment, and dangerous variations in blood pressure that lead to subacute cognitive decline and cardiac damage. Peritoneal dialysis–related difficulties include the need to store supplies at home, daily dialysis often requiring assistance from caregivers, increased protein loss, and risk of infection.

Kidney Transplantation

More than 80,000 patients are currently on the kidney transplant wait list, and the list grows every year. Older patients, including those in their seventies, are increasingly considered for transplantation. As in younger patients, mortality rates in older patients with transplants are considerably less than in those on dialysis. Remaining life expectancy doubles for a dialysis patient once moved from the wait list to transplantation. Suitable older patients and their families should be encouraged to explore the option of transplantation before the need for dialysis arises.

Older patients undergo the same transplantation evaluation process as younger patients. However, older patients are more likely than younger patients to have vascular contraindications to transplantation, as well as other contraindications such as cancer and dementia. Less than 5% of dialysis patients >70 years old are active on a renal transplant list. Older renal transplant recipients demonstrate lower acute rejection rates, lower incidence of chronic rejection, and higher risk of infection and sepsis than younger recipients, and they have greater survival probability than patients remaining on dialysis even when corrected for levels of comorbidity (SOE=A).

In December 2014, the United Network for Organ Sharing kidney allocation system for deceased donor kidneys was changed. The new system relies on life expectancy scores for candidates and on quality scores for available kidneys. Age figures prominently in the calculation of life expectancy scores, and older patients no longer have access to kidneys that are expected to function the longest, leaving these organs for younger, healthier recipients. The wait time for a deceased donor kidney can be 4–5 years or longer, depending on the region of the country where a patient is listed. Living donor kidney transplantation remains an excellent option, because there is no waiting time once the donor and recipient are cleared for surgery.

Nonaggressive Renal Care and Hospice

Patients with advanced CKD who opt for nonaggressive renal care have several options for symptomatic treatment. Medications such as diuretics can help manage fluid overload and hyperkalemia. A low-protein diet can limit production of uremic toxins and stem-related symptoms. Administration of iron and erythropoietin can limit symptomatic anemia. Unnecessary medications such as statins and some blood pressure medications should be stopped. Death may occur as a result of cardiac arrhythmia related to hyperkalemia, or as a result of other metabolic complications. As uremia progresses, patients usually stop eating, become sleepy and confused, and then comatose.

Once a chronic dialysis patient stops dialysis, death usually occurs within 7–14 days. Most people who choose to withdraw from dialysis are >65 years old. The decision to stop can be precipitated by a catastrophic insult such as a major stroke or myocardial infarction, but in almost half of cases, failure to thrive is the driving reason. About 20% of the dialysis cohort withdraws from dialysis in any given year. Of the patients who choose to withdraw from dialysis, less than half use hospice. Patients receiving hospice care are far more likely to die at home; in a 2006 study, only 22.9% of patients receiving hospice care who withdrew from dialysis died in the hospital versus 69% of nonhospice patients. Geriatricians have an important opportunity to guide nephrologists, as well as patients and their families, when nonaggressive renal care and/or hospice may be the best option.

CHOOSING WISELY® RECOMMENDATIONS

Nephrology

- Do not use antimicrobials to treat bacteriuria in older adults unless specific urinary tract symptoms are present.
- Avoid NSAIDs in individuals with hypertension or heart failure or chronic kidney disease of all causes, including diabetes mellitus.
- Do not initiate erythropoiesis-stimulating agents to patients with chronic kidney disease with Hb ≥10 g/dL without signs or symptoms.
- Do not perform routine cancer screening for dialysis patients with limited life expectancies without signs or symptoms.

REFERENCES

- American Society of Nephrology Geriatric Nephrology Curriculum, 2009. Available (free) at www.asn-online.org/education/distancelearning/curricula/geriatrics (accessed Jan 2016).

  This online text consisting of 38 chapters addresses various aspects of caring for older adults with kidney disease, including age-related changes to the kidney, drug dosing, fluid balance disorders, and renal replacement therapy.

- Anderson S, Eldadah B, Halter JB, et al. Acute kidney injury in older adults. *J Am Soc Nephrol*. 2011;22(1):28–38.

  This review summarizes the current literature and knowledge gaps in the impact, causes, diagnosis, and management of acute kidney injury in older adults.

- Cooper CJ, Murphy TP, Cutlip DE, et al. for the CORAL Investigators. Stenting and medical therapy for atherosclerotic renal-artery stenosis. *N Engl J Med*. 2014;370(1):13–22.

  This clinical trial randomly assigned 947 participants with mean age 69 years, atherosclerotic renal artery stenosis, and either systolic hypertension while taking ≥2 antihypertensive medications or chronic kidney disease, to medical therapy plus renal artery stenting vs medical therapy alone. Participants were followed over a median period of 43 months for adverse cardiovascular and renal events. There was no difference between groups in the primary composite end point (death from cardiovascular or renal causes, myocardial infarction, stroke, hospitalization for congestive heart failure, progressive renal insufficiency, or the need for renal replacement therapy), the individual components of the primary end point, or all-cause mortality.

- Kidney Disease: Improving Global Outcomes (KDIGO) CKD Work Group. KDIGO 2012 clinical practice guideline for the evaluation and management of chronic kidney disease. *Kidney Int Suppl*. 2013;3:1–150.

  This clinical practice guideline provides comprehensive recommendations and the evidence base for the diagnosis and management of chronic kidney disease and related complications.

- Kliger AS, Foley RN, Goldfarb DS, et al. KDOQI US commentary on the 2012 KDIGO clinical practice guideline for anemia in CKD. *Am J Kidney Dis*. 2013;62(5):849–859.

  This National Kidney Foundation-Kidney Disease Outcomes Quality Initiative group of experts reviews the evidence for select KDIGO anemia guidelines and provides commentaries and qualifications.

- Thorsteinsdottir B, Swetz KM, Albright RC. The ethics of chronic dialysis for the older patient: time to reevaluate the norms. *Clin J Am Soc Nephrol*. 2015;10(11):2094–2099.

  This article considers the decision of initiating dialysis in older adults through an ethics lens and provides a recommended approach to starting and discontinuing hemodialysis in this population.

- Uhlig K, Boyd C. Guidelines for the older adult with CKD. *Am J Kidney Dis*. 2011;58(2):162–165.

  This article discusses the shortcomings of clinical guidelines and makes recommendations regarding the application of chronic kidney disease guidelines to older adults.

Joshua I. Bernstein, MD
Josette A. Rivera, MD

CHAPTER 54—GYNECOLOGY

KEY POINTS

- Many older women do not spontaneously discuss gynecologic problems with their health care providers, yet many of these problems are treatable.

- Symptomatic urogenital atrophy is common in postmenopausal women and is readily reversed with administration of local estrogen.

- Half of all cases of invasive cancer of the vulva are in women >70 years old.

- Pessaries can improve comfort and bladder function in some older women with pelvic organ prolapse.

- Any abnormal genital bleeding in a postmenopausal woman should be evaluated.

Most older women do not seek regular gynecologic care, perhaps in part because they are reticent about discussing personal gynecologic problems. Consequently, important and treatable disorders often go undiagnosed until they become severely disabling. For example, although urinary incontinence affects 16 million adults in the United States, the average time between onset and reporting to a physician is 8.5 years; gynecologic problems such as genital prolapse and atrophic vaginitis often exacerbate urinary incontinence. Full gynecologic examination should be a routine part of a complete history and physical examination for all older women who are amenable to screening.

HISTORY AND PHYSICAL EXAMINATION

The American College of Obstetrics and Gynecology recommendations for primary care of women ≥65 years old include inquiring not only about routine gynecologic issues but also about involuntary loss of urine or feces, sexual behavior patterns and potential exposure to sexually transmitted diseases, and use of alternative medical treatments.

Nongynecologic medical problems that can have significant gynecologic effects should be noted in the history. For example, breast cancer therapy typically leads to severe urogenital atrophy. Obesity can result in hyperestrogenic states and possible endometrial hyperplasia due to peripheral conversion of androgens to estrogen. Osteoporotic lordosis causes increased intra-abdominal pressure and resultant predisposition to genital prolapse. Previous obstetrical events can cause neuromuscular damage to the pelvic floor and eventual development of urinary incontinence and genital prolapse. A variety of systemic illnesses and dermatoses may contribute to vulvovaginal disorders.

If a woman is on systemic hormone replacement therapy (HRT), the regimen should be reviewed annually to ensure adherence, need for continued therapy, and absence of adverse events. If the uterus is present, estrogen must be combined with a progestin to prevent development of endometrial intraepithelial neoplasia (formerly referred to as endometrial hyperplasia). The route of administration of estrogen therapy may be reassessed because of observed differences of oral and non-oral therapy on the vascular and other systems. The history should also include inquiry about abdominal distention, early satiety, new onset pelvic pain, and abnormal vaginal discharge or bleeding (signs of gynecologic malignancies). The pelvic examination also presents an opportunity to discuss sexual function with the patient. Although a relative paucity of available, sexually capable men may limit an older woman's sexual activities, many older women are interested in maintaining sexual relationships. Issues related to sexual activity such as atrophy-related dyspareunia, postcoital bleeding, and sexually transmitted diseases should be addressed. Many women require reassurance that enjoyable sexual activity is possible and normal at their age. Also, women who maintain regular sexual activity are less likely to have significant vaginal atrophy.

Most ambulatory older women can assume the lithotomy position for a pelvic examination. Skeletal lordosis and other spine disease may require varying degrees of head elevation while the patient is supine. The dorsal position, in stirrups for a pelvic examination, requires flexion and external rotation of the hips. For patients with osteoarthritis who find the lithotomy position uncomfortable or impossible to assume, an alternative position should be used. The left lateral decubitus position is one alternative. The patient lies on her left side, with knees flexed. The upper hip (right) is flexed to a greater degree and the right leg is elevated, exposing the perineum. An adequate speculum and bimanual examination can usually be done in this position. A bedbound patient can be examined by positioning an inverted bedpan under the sacrum to elevate the pelvis. Some very immobile women can be examined in the supine position by carefully inserting the small Pederson speculum upside down. Because the vaginal introitus can be small and stenotic, smaller speculums may be needed. Loss of vaginal depth may not allow full insertion of the speculum, and digital palpation before inserting the speculum is a useful maneuver. Water-based lubricants facilitate the examination and can be used even if a Pap smear will be performed.

Pelvic examination of older women should include the following:

- Examination of the vulva for excoriations, changes in surface texture, abnormal pigmentation, erythema, or raised lesions
- Examination for signs of urogenital atrophy (including urethral caruncle and vulvovaginal mucosa that is thin, dry, and pale) as well as loss of vaginal rugations and reduced vaginal caliber and depth
- Valsalva maneuver performed by the patient to evaluate for pelvic organ prolapse and urinary incontinence
- Careful palpation for pelvic masses or ovarian enlargement on bimanual examination
- A Pap smear if indicated

Bimanual examinations and perineal inspection performed annually can detect vulvar, vaginal, or ovarian pathology. A rectal examination can also be performed at the same time to identify masses, detect occult bleeding, and evaluate the anal sphincter.

Ovaries become smaller with aging, and any palpable adnexal tissue should prompt consideration of malignancy. Although uterine fibroids are common, any increase in uterus size should be investigated. An ovarian or uterine mass should be evaluated by transabdominal or, anatomy permitting, transvaginal pelvic ultrasound to elucidate details such as size and location, sonolucency, and vascular flow. Additional investigation with the use of MRI as well as serum tumor markers can be useful. In some cases, a benign nature cannot be established with confidence, and further surgical evaluation ultimately depends on clinical judgment.

TREATMENT OF MENOPAUSAL SYMPTOMS

Estrogen is labeled by the FDA for treatment of menopausal vasomotor symptoms and urogenital atrophy and for prevention of osteoporosis, but HRT has historically been used for other reasons as well.

Menopause on average occurs at age 51 in the United States. With a life expectancy of approximately 80 years, the average American woman is postmenopausal for one-third of her life. In light of the risks and benefits of HRT found in the Women's Health Initiative (WHI) Trial, many women and their clinicians choose to treat or prevent the sequelae of estrogen deficiency in menopause. The clinician should be aware of more recently published reassuring data, including WHI stratification studies and other post-WHI literature. Individualization of therapy is essential. Strategies for risk reduction include consideration of the following:

- route of administration of estrogen
- dosage
- duration of use
- selection of the progestational agent (when the uterus is intact)

Along with mood changes and sleep disorders, vasomotor symptoms or hot flushes are among the most common symptom of the climacteric, occurring in up to 80% of perimenopausal women. On average, vasomotor symptoms have been cited to persist for 5–10 years or longer, and the duration is inversely proportional to age of onset of menopause. In a small minority of women, symptoms may be lifelong. Although the pathophysiology of the vasomotor response remains incompletely understood, vasomotor symptoms are usually relieved within the first few weeks of HRT (SOE=A). Low-dose therapy can be started, and estrogen dosages titrated until symptoms improve. When estrogen is contraindicated or not acceptable, alternatives shown to have some efficacy include SSRIs[OL] and SNRIs[OL], GABA-analogues such as gabapentin[OL] and pregabalin[OL], and various progestins. Clonidine[OL], methyldopa[OL], vitamin E, or herbal remedies such as yams and black cohosh have also been tried with inconsistent evidence to support their use (SOE=C). Recently, the FDA has warned the compounding pharmaceutical industry against making claims that "bio-identical compounded" hormone preparations are more effective and/or safer than traditional FDA-approved hormone products because of lack of head-to-head comparison trials.

UROGENITAL ATROPHY

The lower genital tract is exquisitely sensitive to estrogen. Urogenital atrophy occurs in all postmenopausal women. Proliferation and maturation of the vaginal epithelium depends on adequate estrogen stimulation. With reduced estrogen production, genital blood flow decreases, leading to further decline in delivery of estrogen to those tissues. This reduction in microvascularity leads to vaginal dryness, mucosal pallor, decreased rugation, mucosal thinning, inflammation with discharge, and ultimately decreased vaginal caliber and depth. With progressive atrophy, the vaginal Pap smear–maturation index shows atrophic changes with a decrease in mucosal superficial cells and an increase in intermediate and basal cells. Vaginal pH can be measured using pH paper; a reading >5.0–5.5 usually denotes significant atrophy. Many women experience dyspareunia, burning, and even vaginal bleeding in some cases. Urethral mucosal atrophy leads to urinary urgency, frequency, nocturia, and predisposition to recurrent UTIs.

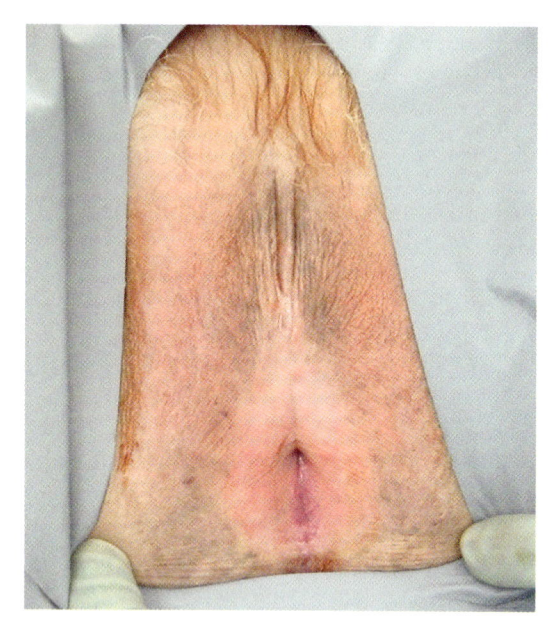

Figure 54.1—Severe labial fusion due to advanced atrophy and lichen sclerosis

See Figure 54.1 to illustrate severe labial fusion due to advanced atrophy and lichen sclerosis.

These changes are readily reversed by administration of topical estrogen (SOE=A). The intravaginal use of low-dose estrogen cream or tablets, as infrequently as 2 nights per week, allows topical estrogen therapy with minimal (if any) absorption into the circulation, endometrial proliferation, or other systemic effects. The available prescription estrogen creams appear to be therapeutically equivalent. Patients complaining of irritation and burning from these creams may better tolerate compounded estradiol or estriol in a hypoallergenic medium. The estrogen ring can be used for 3 months per ring. Estrogen cream is also an excellent lubricant for use during pessary insertion. In women concerned about systemic absorption of locally administered estrogen, serum estradiol levels can be monitored at baseline and 6–8 weeks after initiation of therapy; dosage can be reduced if any significant rise in levels is noted. In February 2013, the FDA approved the use of a SERM, ospemifene, for treatment of dyspareunia related to atrophic changes.

VULVOVAGINAL INFECTION AND INFLAMMATION

Postmenopausal women are susceptible to a broad range of vulvovaginal infections. Candidal infection, common in diabetic and obese patients who are plagued with moisture and irritation, can be treated with oral, intravaginal, and topical antifungal agents. Increasing resistance of *Candida* spp to commonly used azole therapy, including miconazole, terconazole, and oral fluconazole, has been reported. This is especially problematic in non-*albicans* species, including *C glabrata*, *C tropicalis*, *C parapsilosis*, and several even more rare species. When prescribing vaginal therapy, women should be questioned about their ability to insert a vaginal applicator before beginning therapy. For women with severe stenosis, a syringe (10 mL) can be filled with antifungal cream and attached to a urethral catheter (14 Fr.) for intravaginal administration. Topical corticosteroids can be used to hasten relief of symptoms of vulvar irritation but should be avoided as sole agents in vulvovaginal infections. Combination therapy with estrogen plus an antifungal cream may be necessary, because older women commonly have more chronic, untreated candidal infections that spread from the vulva to the inguinal areas.

Other vaginal infections such as *Trichomonas* and *Gardnerella* vaginosis that are common in women of reproductive age are less common in older women, likely because of the higher vaginal pH. Bacterial vaginosis is rarely seen in postmenopausal women. A wet preparation revealing sheets of inflammatory cells without bacterial forms can represent advanced atrophy rather than an infectious cause. In women with inflammatory atrophy, the vagina will look inflamed with the presence of petechiae and serous exudate, rather than thin, pale, and dry as is typical in advanced atrophy. Local estrogen cream may thus need to be considered as well. Clinicians should not be hesitant to inquire about sexual practices when a woman presents with recurrent vaginal infections, vesicular lesions, or other changes suggestive of a sexually transmitted disease.

DISORDERS OF THE VULVA

With aging, the skin of the vulva loses elasticity, and the underlying fat and connective tissues undergo degeneration, with loss of collagen and thinning of the epithelial layer. Consequently, postmenopausal women not on estrogen are predisposed to a variety of dermatologic disorders. The assessment of vulvar complaints must include direct examination. Any pigmented lesion should be carefully evaluated by a gynecologist or dermatologist knowledgeable in gynecologic skin lesions. Most will prove to be benign lentigo or postinflammatory hyperpigmentation. The vulva, however, representing only 1% of the total skin surface, will contain 2% of all melanomas. Biopsy should always be considered in uncertain cases.

Vulvar skin irritation can result from a variety of agents and causes burning, itching, and edema. Hygienic products used for urinary and fecal incontinence can lead to chemical irritant dermatitis. Treatment of incontinence and protection of the delicate mucosa and skin with fastidious hygiene and topical emollients is important. Vulvar burning or pain is rarely due to estrogen deficiency, and this complaint should be investigated rather than treated with ever-increasing dosages of estrogen.

Vulvodynia, a chronic vulvar pain syndrome, is seen in both pre- and postmenopausal women. The International Society for the Study of Vulvovaginal Diseases (ISSVD) categorizes vulvodynia as either generalized or localized. The condition is further divided into provoked (sexual, nonsexual), unprovoked, or mixed. Treatment of vulvodynia can be challenging and should be approached in a comprehensive manner that may include tricyclic antidepressants, GABA-analogues, certain muscle relaxants, SSRI and SNRI agents, local anesthetic agents (all off label), and others. Other treatment modalities may include pelvic floor rehabilitation therapy, administered by a therapist specifically trained in pelvic disorders. Additionally, sexual counselors, mental health care providers and pain management specialists are incorporated into the patients' treatment plan, because a team approach yields better outcomes. A thorough evaluation should be performed to exclude disorders presenting with a similar clinical picture such as pudendal neuralgia, contact irritant mucositis, vulvar vestibulitis, and other neuropathic disorders.

Vulvar excoriation can result from scratching of an inflamed vulva, often with lichen simplex chronicus. Local corticosteroids such as hydrocortisone 1% ointment applied daily, and sitz baths, combined with fastidious genital hygiene, can help alleviate vulvar irritation. Any chronically irritated area should be biopsied to exclude a malignancy.

Nonneoplastic Vulvar Lesions

Lichen sclerosus causes over one-third of all vulvar dermatoses and can extend beyond the vulva to the perirectal areas. Squamous cell carcinoma of the vulva can arise in 4%–5% of patients with untreated lichen sclerosus. There is epithelial thinning with edema and fibrosis of the dermis. It can progress to shrinkage and resorption of the labia, severe clitoral phimosis with reduction in introital caliber. Lesions are typically shiny, white or pink, and parchment-like; they can be asymptomatic but usually cause itching, vaginal soreness, and dyspareunia. Diagnosis is confirmed on biopsy of the involved vulvar areas. Recommended treatment involves application of an ultra-potent topical corticosteroid such as clobetasol propionate 0.05%. Patients should be counseled on the proper use of these ointments, ie, initially twice a day and gradually less frequently. Once improvements are noted, reducing the strength of the steroid or the frequency of application should be advised. Periodic visits to assess compliance, exclude new lesions, and monitor for skin thinning are important. Further measures include wearing cotton underwear and avoiding irritant soaps. Topical emollient agents can also be helpful.

Lichen simplex chronicus, known for very intense pruritus, including nocturnal itching (sometimes described as the end of the itch-scratch cycle), has been previously described by many other terms, including neurodermatitis and squamous hyperplasia. Lichen simplex chronicus is a localized type of atopic dermatitis that can arise from either extrinsic or intrinsic insults. This condition can present as hyperplastic, corrugated, and elevated areas found only on keratinized skin. Biopsy may precede treatment, although many specialists recognize and treat the disorder without tissue sample. Topical mid-potency corticosteroids such as triamcinolone 0.1% twice daily for a few weeks (or longer with thick lesions) typically resolve the lesions; intermittent therapy may be necessary to sustain the therapeutic effect. It is essential not only to remove all irritants or allergens but also to control itching with the cautious use of antihistamines to allow for healing of the involved skin. Cloth gloves are still often recommended to reduce skin trauma from inadvertent scratching during sleep.

Other problematic vulvar lesions include lichen planus, which presents as bright red, moist lesions of the vulva or vagina that can also be erosive, and often result in significant discomfort and scarring. Ultra-potency corticosteroids applied topically and hydrocortisone applied intravaginally are recommended. Bacterial infection is quite common with vaginal lichen planus and should be cultured and treated appropriately. Compromised coital ability due to infection a well as severe stenosis of the vagina is often addressed through surgery or vaginal dilation. Although lichen planus and certain cases of lichen sclerosus may sometimes be difficult to distinguish clinically, the hallmark distinction is that lichen sclerosus does not involve the vagina and extragenital lesions are rare, whereas lichen planus frequently involves the vagina and extragenital sites such as the oral cavity.

Vulvar Neoplasia

The classification system used by the ISVVD revised the nomenclature of vulvar intraepithelial neoplastia (VIN) in 2004. The older terms VIN 1, 2, or 3 have been replaced by VIN "plain" type versus VIN differentiated (d-VIN). Plain-type VIN is related to human papilloma virus, occurs in younger women, and tends to be multifocal. It also tends to be indolent and infrequently becomes invasive. It includes warty, baseloid, and mixed types. In contrast, d-VIN does not appear to be related to human papilloma virus, most commonly presents as a unifocal lesion, and is often seen within a background of lichen sclerosus.

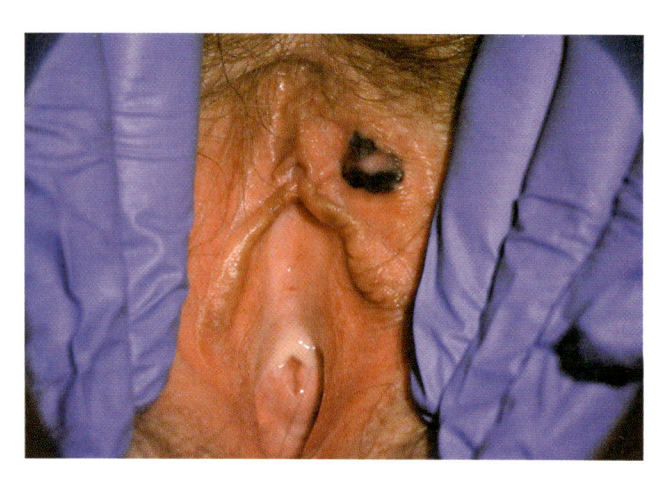

Figure 54.2—Vulvar melanoma, typical appearance of this unusual pigmented lesion

Because benign, premalignant, or malignant vulvar lesions may have similar clinical appearances, all suspicious, unusual, or symptomatic vulvar lesions should be biopsied. The prognosis of d-VIN is less predictable, but it does tend to be more aggressive in progression to invasive squamous cell carcinoma. The gold standard for treatment of unifocal d-VIN is surgical incision with margins of 0.5–1 cm. Surveillance for recurrence is recommended. Referral to a gynecologic oncologist should be considered if malignancy is suspected.

Invasive cancer of the vulva is an age-related malignancy; half of all cases occur after age 70. The vast majority are squamous cell carcinomas. Malignant melanoma, sarcoma, basal cell carcinoma, and adenocarcinoma account for <20% of cases. See Figure 54.2 for a typical appearance of vulvar melanoma. Treatment involves surgery (radical vulvectomy), occasionally accompanied by radiation.

DISORDERS OF PELVIC FLOOR SUPPORT

Genetic predisposition, gravity, the upright posture, childbearing, and other activities that increase intra-abdominal pressure cause progressive weakening of the connective tissue and muscular supports of the genital organs and can lead to genital prolapse. Constipation, chronic coughing, and heavy lifting commonly increase intra-abdominal pressure. Common symptoms of prolapse include pelvic pressure, lower back pain, urinary or fecal incontinence, difficulty with rectal emptying, or a palpable mass. Traditional classification of vaginal prolapse includes differentiated protrusion of the posterior vaginal wall (enterocele or rectocele), descent of the anterior vaginal wall (cystocele), and prolapse of the vaginal apex. These conditions are demonstrated by having the patient bear down or cough

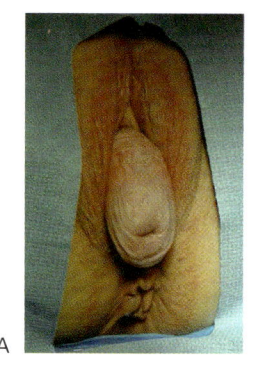

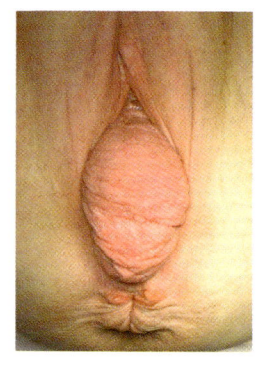

Figure 54.3 A and B—Complete uterine and vaginal vault prolapse representing complete eversion of vaginal canal

while in the dorsal lithotomy position, but the full extent of prolapse is often better appreciated with a standing Valsalva maneuver. Vaginal prolapse represents a pelvic organ hernia to, or through, the vaginal introitus. See Figure 54.3a and Figure 54.3b to illustrate complete uterine and vaginal vault prolapse.

The International Continence Society and the American Urogynecologic Association adopted a rather complex prolapse classification system (Pelvic Organ Prolapse Quantification [POPQ]) that is based on measurement of the distance between vaginal anatomic sites and the hymenal ring, as well as on vaginal length and perineal dimensions. The purpose of this classification, which is used by specialty societies, is to more objectively and reproducibly describe the degree of prolapse.

Progression of mild prolapse can be slowed with adequate estrogenization and Kegel exercises to strengthen the pelvic floor musculature (SOE=C). Genital prolapse does not always lead to bladder dysfunction and should not be assumed to be the cause of incontinence. Correcting advanced prolapse can cause or exacerbate urinary incontinence by "unkinking" the urethra or bladder neck. However, large cystoceles or rectoceles can produce urinary retention, and reduction of the cystocele can restore normal bladder function.

Pessaries

Pessaries are commonly used in an effort to delay or avoid surgery. Their use in older women may be indicated to provide comfort and restore bladder function when comorbid illness makes surgery undesirable (SOE=C). Such women may elect long-term pessary use under medical supervision. Available pessaries are made from rubber, plastic, or silicone. A variety of shapes and sizes are available: donuts, rings, cubes, inflatable balls, and foldable models.

The choice of pessary is influenced by the degree of prolapse, presence of incontinence, type of accompanying tissue relaxation, and ease of care.

Patients with prolapse and no incontinence require only space-occupying types (ie, donut). Those with stress incontinence benefit from a foldable lever-type, which restores bladder neck support. Ring pessaries are easier to insert and remove and may be preferred by older women, especially those who used a contraceptive diaphragm in their youth. For those with advanced degrees of apical or anterior wall prolapse, a more rigid pessary (ie, gelhorn) may be needed. Although more difficult to insert and remove, this pessary type is very popular because of its high degree of efficacy. Self-care can be more challenging. Cube pessaries should be used with caution because they can adhere to the vaginal walls (because of the suction effect) and result in infection and, when removed, mucosal ulcerations.

Pessary selection is a learned art, but even in experienced hands often proceeds by trial and error and may require multiple office visits; the optimal pessary fits snugly but comfortably and allows voiding and defecating without difficulty. Having patients use the commode, and also walk up and down stairs before leaving the clinic may help the clinician determine if a pessary is appropriate and may save a return visit. After pessary selection and insertion, clinical follow-up within a few days is essential to ascertain satisfactory usage. After initial fitting and recheck, pessaries should be removed, cleaned, and the vaginal walls inspected.

Pessary care requirements often influence the selection of a device and the amount of follow-up required. If an older woman's mobility or manual dexterity permits, she should remove the pessary 2 nights per week, wash it with soap and water, and reinsert it with a water-soluble lubricant after arising in the morning; she should use 1 g vaginal estrogen cream the 2 nights the pessary is out. Women who cannot perform this level of self-care should be assisted at periodic office visits (ie, every 6–12 weeks) or by a visiting nurse. All women with pessaries should be instructed to report any unusual odor, discharge, bleeding, or discomfort, and any changes in bladder or bowel function, and all should have a pelvic examination once or twice a year. If discomfort is present or the device becomes uncomfortable, a different size or type should be tried. Pessaries do not work as well with marked vaginal outlet relaxation. If a pessary is left in place for long periods without monitoring, fistulation can develop, or fibrous tissue can form around the pessary, and removal under anesthesia may be necessary.

Surgery for Prolapse

Surgical treatment of vaginal prolapse can be classified as either reconstructive or obliterative. Reconstructive procedures are designed to restore normal anatomy, whereas obliterative procedures result in total or partial closure of the vaginal canal. Vaginal reconstructive procedures include sacrospinous ligament fixation (for apical prolapse), anterior repairs (for a cystocele), and posterior repairs (for a rectocele). These can safely be done under regional anesthesia, which minimizes anesthetic risks. Abdominal reconstructive procedures include sacrocolpopexy (for apical prolapse) and paravaginal repairs (for a cystocele), which typically require general anesthesia. Urinary and fecal incontinence procedures can also be performed at the time of the prolapse surgery.

Obliterative procedures are restricted to older women who are not, and will not be, sexually active. In a LeFort colpocleisis, the anterior and posterior vaginal walls are sutured together, obliterating the vaginal canal. Two slender "canals" are left along the vaginal sidewalls to allow for recognition of infection or uterine bleeding. The simplicity and safety are very attractive, because the procedure can be done under regional or local anesthesia in the outpatient setting. Incontinence procedures can be done at the same time. In most cases, preexisting urinary retention or voiding dysfunction resolves once the prolapse is corrected. A recent large case series demonstrated the effectiveness and low morbidity of the LeFort procedure.

The use of mesh materials (as in hernia surgery) implanted using surgical kits became popular during the 1990s as minimally invasive procedures for prolapse. Recognition of mesh-related complications, including exposure through the vaginal walls and painful contraction, has recently led to markedly reduced use of vaginal mesh products.

Limiting physical activities (anything that would increase intra-abdominal pressure) for 6–12 weeks after surgery, performing pelvic floor exercises, and using vaginal estrogen cream are key to optimizing the success rate of surgical therapy. Many pelvic reconstructive surgeons insist that tobacco-using patients stop smoking, and chronic sneezing or coughing patients start therapy for those disorders before surgery. The impact on quality of life after prolapse surgery can be quite remarkable, because a large, exteriorized prolapse can markedly limit a woman's ability to participate in physical and social activities. Depending on the vaginal segment prolapsed and its degree of prolapse, success rates after surgical repair can vary from >90% (vaginal apex and posterior wall) to 60%–80% (anterior wall) (SOE=A).

Age, in itself, is not a contraindication to surgery for genital prolapse. When a proven protocol for perioperative care, including preoperative medical clearance, regional anesthesia, infection prophylaxis, and deep-vein thrombosis prophylaxis, is followed, vaginal surgery offers a safe alternative to pessary use for older women with symptomatic genital prolapse.

Table 54.1—Causes of Postmenopausal Vaginal Bleeding

Cervical	Carcinoma
	Cervicitis
	Polyp
Endocrinologic	Exogenous hormones
	Perimenopausal ovarian function
Ovarian	Functioning ovarian tumor
Uterine	Endometrial atrophy
	Hyperplasia
	Neoplasia
	Polyp
	Submucosal leiomyoma
Vaginal	Atrophy
	Inflammation
	Tumor
	Ulceration
Vulvar	Carcinoma
	Laceration or ulceration
	Urethral caruncle
Other	Coagulation disorder
	Rectal lesion
	Urinary tract infection

POSTMENOPAUSAL VAGINAL BLEEDING

Postmenopausal bleeding (defined as bleeding after 1 year of amenorrhea) occurs in a significant number of older women. The challenge is not only to exclude gynecologic malignancies but also to alleviate the symptoms and eliminate the cause of benign conditions. Causes of bleeding can be grouped according to anatomic areas and endocrine dysfunction (Table 54.1). Not all complaints of postmenopausal bleeding are related to the reproductive organs. Occasionally rectal or urinary tract bleeding may be misinterpreted by the patient or her caregiver as genital bleeding; therefore, if genital blood cannot be identified, the clinician should evaluate those sites. For confirmed postmenopausal genital bleeding, proper evaluation involves a complete pelvic examination (looking for any vulvar, vaginal, cervical, or uterine source) and directed diagnostic studies. The endometrium can be evaluated for presence of endometrial hyperplasia and cancer by measuring the endometrial thickness with ultrasound imaging and by performing an endometrial biopsy. Although neither technique has a 100% sensitivity or specificity, an endometrial thickness of <3 mm on transvaginal ultrasonography strongly suggests a benign etiology. However, if there is any uncertainty, a biopsy is indicated. In patients unable to tolerate an endometrial biopsy, an outpatient hysteroscopy and/or curettage should be considered. Diffuse thickening is usually more amenable to office endometrial biopsy, whereas focal lesions are better evaluated and biopsied hysteroscopically. New techniques to ablate the endometrial lining by heat, cold, or radiotherapy, can be helpful in women who have persistent bleeding that is poorly tolerated or is resulting in anemia and has been proved to be nonmalignant. Endometrial fibroids or benign polyps can be excised hysteroscopically. However, those modalities are infrequently used in postmenopausal women.

If endometrial cancer is diagnosed, the patient should be referred to a gynecologic oncologist for management. This will most likely require total hysterectomy with bilateral salpingo-oopherectomy and pelvic lymph node sampling. Until recently, this required an open laparotomy, but recent data on the use of less invasive laparoscopy or robotic surgery for older patients has demonstrated decreased postoperative morbidity, including reduced blood loss, lower rate of ileus, and shorter hospital stay. As with any other malignancy, management depends on tissue histology, degree and depth of invasion, and overall stage.

Leiomyosarcoma, cancer of the uterine myometrium and a relatively rare cancer, has received much attention recently because of the recognized possible dissemination of cancerous cells with use of a tissue morcellator for extraction of the uterus during laparoscopic surgery. Thus, when minimally invasive laparoscopic hysterectomy surgery is performed, removal of the surgical specimen should be performed vaginally or through a small abdominal incision to prevent dissemination.

The most common cause of postmenopausal uterine bleeding is an atrophic endometrium. As suggested above, cervical lesions, including infections, polyps, and malignancies, must be excluded. Of major importance, abrasions and lacerations that may be due to sexual assault or abuse must be carefully excluded, irrespective of the history provided by patient or caregivers. If abuse is suspected, reporting to local authorities is mandatory.

Exogenous hormone replacement is also a common cause of benign postmenopausal bleeding. Women using combined estrogen-progesterone replacement therapy (assuming adequate dosing of progesterone) actually have a lower risk of uterine cancer than women not using HRT. However, any unscheduled or otherwise suspicious bleeding should be evaluated. Women on cyclic hormone therapy who bleed at predicted and anticipated progestin-withdrawal times generally do not require evaluation, unless the characteristics of the withdrawal bleeding substantially change. Some specialists recommend biopsy if any bleeding, even in the presence of a normal ultrasound, persists longer than 6 months.

REFERENCES

- Committee on Gynecologic Practice; American College of Obstetricians and Gynecologists. Committee opinion #509: Management of vulvar intraepithelial neoplasia. *Obstet Gynecol*. 2011;118(5):1192–1194.

    This article summarizes the conclusions and recommendations of the Committee on Gynecologic Practice of the American College of Obstetricians and Gynecologists and the American Society for Colposcopy and Cervical Pathology on the management of vulvar intraepithelial neoplasia (VIN). This includes the classification, prevention, diagnosis, and treatment of VIN. The article specifically advocates for treatment of all cases of VIN.

- Committee on Gynecologic Practice; American College of Obstetricians and Gynecologists. Society of Gynecologic Oncology. Committee opinion #631. Endometrial intraepithelial neoplasia. *Obstet Gynecol*. 2015;125(5):1272–1278.

    Endometrial hyperplasia can be a precursor to endometrial cancer. Assessment of abnormal bleeding in peri- and postmenopausal women is key to identification of histologic evidence of precancerous tissue. This committee opinion delineates recommended approaches to this common condition.

- Kuncharapu I, Majeroni BA, Johnson DW. Pelvic organ prolapse. *Am Fam Physician*. 2010;81(9):1111–1117.

    This article reviews pelvic organ prolapse, a condition most commonly seen in older women. The epidemiology, etiology, clinical presentation, treatment, and follow-up of pelvic organ prolapse are detailed, including a discussion of pessary selection and fitting.

- Murphy R. Lichen sclerosus. *Dermatol Clin*. 2010;28(4):707–715.

    Lichen sclerosus is a chronic inflammatory dermatosis that occurs frequently in postmenopausal women. This review article summarizes the pathogenesis, clinical features, histology, disease complications, treatment investigations/failures, and follow-up/prognosis of this complex and chronic skin disease.

- Stewart KM. Clinical care of vulvar pruritus, with emphasis on one common cause, lichen simplex chronicus. *Dermatol Clin*. 2010;28(4):669–680.

    Vulvar pruritus is a common and distressing condition that can be caused by a wide variety of conditions, including candidiasis, contact dermatitis, lichen simplex chronicus, and lichen sclerosus. This review article first explores the patient history, physical examination, and differential diagnosis of vulvar pruritus. It subsequently focuses on lichen simplex chronicus, particularly emphasizing symptom relief and control.

- Zebede S, Smith AL, Plowright L, et al. Obliterative LeFort colpocleisis in a large group of elderly women. *Obstet Gynecol* 2013;121:1–7.

    LeForte colpocleisis represents a frequently forgotten option for older women with advanced degrees of pelvic organ prolapse. This paper represents the largest series published to date, demonstrating the safety and efficacy of this technique.

Jay R. Trabin, MD, FACOG
G. Willy Davila, MD

CHAPTER 55—PROSTATE DISEASE AND CANCER

KEY POINTS

- A number of treatment options exist for benign prostatic hyperplasia (BPH), including watchful waiting, medications, minimally invasive procedures, and more extensive operations. The choice is influenced by the extent of symptoms, the presence of complications from outflow obstruction, and patient preferences.

- The use of 5α-reductase inhibitors for BPH is indicated especially when the prostate gland is large.

- Men should be well informed about the risks and benefits of prostate-specific antigen (PSA) screening before making a decision whether or not to be screened for prostate cancer.

- Several treatment options exist for men with localized prostate cancer, including watchful waiting, resection of the gland and seminal vesicles, and radiation therapy. How the patient balances the potential benefits and burdens of the various options will influence the choice of therapy.

- For patients with chronic prostatitis, efforts should be made to identify the causative organism, and even with a prolonged course of appropriate antibiotics, a cure can be expected in fewer than half the patients.

With advancing age, the prevalence of prostate diseases increases dramatically. The three most common conditions are BPH, prostate cancer, and prostatitis. Self-reported prostate disease affects about 3 million American men. BPH develops in over half of men ≥65 years old and affects the overwhelming majority of men >85 years old. Prostate cancer is the second leading cause of cancer death in men, and many men have asymptomatic or low-grade tumors that cause few or no health problems. The prevalence of prostatitis is similar to that of ischemic heart disease or diabetes mellitus.

BENIGN PROSTATIC HYPERPLASIA

Epidemiology

BPH is a noncancerous enlargement of the epithelial and fibromuscular components of the prostate gland. The epithelial component normally makes up 20%–30% of prostate volume and contributes to the seminal fluid. The fibromuscular component comprises 70%–80% of the prostate and is responsible for expressing prostatic fluid during ejaculation. Age and long-term androgen stimulation induce development of BPH. Microscopic appearance of BPH can be seen as early as age 30, is present in 50% of men by age 60, and is present in 90% of men by age 85. In half of these cases, microscopic BPH develops into palpable macroscopic BPH. Of those with macroscopic BPH, only half develop clinically significant disease that is brought to medical attention. BPH is one of the most common conditions in aging men; in the United States annually it accounts for more than 1.7 million office visits and 250,000 surgical procedures.

Prostatism, or Lower Urinary Tract Symptoms

The symptoms of BPH are nonspecific; other diseases can result in identical symptoms. The pathophysiology of BPH symptoms is not completely understood, but presumably it involves the periurethral zone of the prostate gland, which results in obstructed urine flow and compensatory responses of the bladder, such as hypertrophy and decreased capacity. The urethral obstruction has both mechanical (obstructing mass) and dynamic (smooth muscle contractions) components. The resulting lower urinary tract symptoms are divided into irritative (eg, frequency, urgency, nocturia) and obstructive (eg, hesitancy, intermittency, weak stream, incomplete emptying) manifestations. These 7 lower urinary tract symptoms compose a quantitative symptom index for assessing severity and monitoring treatment response, which was developed by the American Urological Association and adopted by the World Health Organization, known as the International Prostate Symptom Score. Although tracking symptom severity is useful in the longitudinal management of patients, symptom severity has not been found to correlate with prostate size, urine flow rates, or postvoid residual volume. BPH primarily affects quality of life, although complications such as recurrent urinary tract infection, bladder stones, urinary retention, chronic renal insufficiency, and hematuria can develop.

Diagnosis

Differential diagnosis of lower urinary tract symptoms includes endocrine disorders (especially diabetes mellitus), neurologic disorders, urinary tract infections, sexually transmitted diseases, kidney or bladder stones, overactive bladder, and medications (especially medications with anticholinergic and diuretic effects). Overactive bladder and BPH are both very common and may coexist. If the lower urinary tract symptoms are primarily storage issues (frequency, urgency, nocturia), then overactive bladder may be considered the primary diagnosis. When voiding symptoms, such as poor flow or hesitancy are present, then the focus is placed on BPH. Digital rectal examination (DRE) can be unremarkable or reveal an

Table 55.1—Management Options for Benign Prostatic Hyperplasia

Category	Interventions	Rationale	Comments
Lifestyle modification	Reduce nighttime fluids to manage nocturia; eliminate bladder irritants (eg, caffeine, alcohol, nicotine)	Factors outside the urinary tract contribute to urinary symptoms	Often sufficient management for mild symptoms; complements management for moderate to severe symptoms
Pharmacologic management	α-Adrenergic antagonists Selective $α_1$: prazosin[OL] Long-acting selective $α_1$: terazosin, doxazosin Slow-release, long-acting selective $α_1$: tamsulosin, silodosin, alfuzosin	Relaxation of smooth muscle in hyperplastic prostate tissue, prostate capsule, and bladder neck decreases resistance to urinary flow	Adverse events: dizziness, mild asthenia, headaches, postural hypotension (reduced with careful dosage titration, not present with slow release selective $α_1$ agents), abnormal ejaculation, rhinitis
	5α-Reductase inhibitors: finasteride, dutasteride	Reduced tissue levels of dihydrotestosterone result in prostate gland size reduction	Most effective for men with larger prostates (>40 g); results may not be evident for up to 6 months
	Phosphodiesterase-5 inhibitor: tadalafil	PDE-5 activity in bladder neck, prostatic urethra, and prostate musculature contributes to urinary symptoms	Effective for men with or without erectile dysfunction; only drug that can treat both conditions
Surgery	Transurethral resection of the prostate; transurethral incision of the prostate; open prostatectomy; transurethral vaporization of the prostate; stent placement	Removal or expansion of periurethral prostate tissue reduces obstruction to urinary flow	Indicated for recurrent urinary tract infection induced by benign prostatic hypertrophy, recurrent or persistent gross hematuria, bladder stones, renal insufficiency

enlarged, smooth, rubbery, symmetrical gland. Urinalysis is routinely performed to evaluate for urinary tract infection, hematuria, and glycosuria. This minimal testing is usually sufficient for a provisional diagnosis and empiric therapy. Additional subsequent tests include postvoid residual urine volume (often done by office or bedside bladder scan), urine flow rates, and pressure flow studies. These tests can be considered when the diagnosis is uncertain or an invasive treatment is being planned.

Treatment Approaches

BPH therapy depends on the patient and is driven by the impact of symptoms on the patient's quality of life (Table 55.1). All patients should be educated regarding lifestyle modification by adjusting fluid intake (eg, avoiding caffeine) and avoiding medications (especially anticholinergics) that aggravate symptoms. Men with mild to moderate symptoms may be satisfied with lifestyle modification only. Both medical and surgical treatments are also available, with medication the usual first approach. Indications for surgical treatment include patient preference, dissatisfaction with medication, and refractory urinary retention, as well as renal dysfunction, bladder stones, recurrent urinary tract infections, or hematuria if these are clearly due to prostatic obstruction.

Medical Treatment

The two main pharmacologic approaches are α-adrenergic antagonist and 5α-reductase inhibitor therapy (SOE=A).

α-Adrenergic antagonists, or α-blockers, are directed at the dynamic component of urethral obstruction. Smooth muscle of the prostate and bladder neck has a resting tone mediated by α-adrenergic innervation. α-Blockers relax the smooth muscle in the hyperplastic prostate tissue, prostate capsule, and bladder neck, thus decreasing resistance to urinary flow. Of the two major α-adrenergic receptors, $α_1$ receptors predominate in the prostate. α-Blockade development for BPH therapy has progressed from selective $α_1$ agents (eg, prazosin) to long-acting selective $α_1$ agents (terazosin, doxazosin) and then to slow-release, long-acting selective $α_1$ agents (tamsulosin, alfuzosin, silodosin). The most common adverse events of $α_1$ agents are dizziness, mild asthenia (fatigue or weakness), and headaches. Postural hypotension occurs infrequently and can be minimized by careful dosage titration of terazosin and doxazosin; slow-release agents do not require dose titration. Ejaculatory dysfunction is common with these agents, but alfuzosin does not have this effect. For patients undergoing cataract surgery, intraoperative floppy iris syndrome (IFIS), characterized by sudden intraoperative iris prolapse and pupil constriction, is a potential risk of all α-blockers, with the greatest frequency and severity of IFIS among those using tamsulosin (SOE=B).

The enzyme 5α-reductase is required to convert testosterone to the more active dihydrotestosterone. Finasteride and dutasteride are inhibitors of 5α-reductase and reduce tissue levels of dihydrotestosterone, thus reducing prostate gland size. Improvements in symptom scores and urine flow rates may not be evident for up to 6 months. The 5α-reductase inhibitors are most effective in men with larger prostates (>40 g, about the size of a plum) (SOE=A). Because

5α-reductase inhibitors reduce serum PSA levels by an average of 50%, after 6 months of therapy men receiving prostate cancer surveillance will need a new baseline serum PSA determination.

When used together over years, the α-adrenergic antagonists combined with 5α-reductase inhibitors have been shown to be safe and to reduce clinical progression of BPH better than either agent alone (SOE=A). In particular, a lower risk of urinary retention, urinary incontinence, renal insufficiency, and recurrent bladder infections is associated with combination therapy. Trials of BPH therapy with the herbal preparation *Serenoa repens*, or saw palmetto, show conflicting results. Limited data from smaller studies suggested that it improves urinary symptoms and flow measures in men with BPH. However, a recent Cochrane review found that compared with placebo, *S repens* monotherapy does not improve urinary symptoms or maximal urinary flow rate even at double and triple the usual dosage.

Anticholinergic agents have a role in managing lower urinary tract storage symptoms in men with BPH. Used alone, or in combination with α-blockers, anticholinergic medications do not seem to significantly increase postvoid residual urine volumes or provoke acute urinary retention (SOE=A).

Many men experience both BPH and erectile dysfunction, and BPH medications can negatively impact erectile function. Shared pathogenetic mechanisms have been proposed for BPH/lower urinary tract symptoms and erectile dysfunction. Tadalafil is now FDA approved for both BPH and erectile dysfunction. Research continues to explore the role of phosphodiesterase-5 (PDE-5) inhibitors alone, or in combination with conventional BPH treatments, in relieving lower urinary tract symptoms in men with BPH, with or without erectile dysfunction. Caution is advised when using PDE-5 inhibitors and α-blockers because of possible additive effects of hypotension.

Surgical Treatment

Surgical management includes transurethral resection of the prostate (TURP), transurethral incision of the prostate (TUIP), open prostatectomy, transurethral vaporization of the prostate, and device insertion such as stent placement. Surgical approaches offer the best chance for symptom improvement but also have the highest rates of complications. The benefits of various surgical treatments are generally considered equivalent, but complication rates differ. TURP is the standard of care to which other BPH treatments are compared, and it has an 80% likelihood of successful outcome in properly selected patients (SOE=A). Usually performed under spinal anesthesia, TURP involves passage of an endoscope through the urethra to surgically remove the inner portion of the prostate. Long-term complications can include retrograde ejaculation, urethral stricture, bladder neck contracture, incontinence, and impotence. TUIP is an endoscopic procedure via the urethra to make one or two cuts in the prostate and prostate capsule, relieving urethral constriction. Limited to use in small prostate glands (<30 g), TUIP offers lower rates of retrograde ejaculation, bleeding, and contractures. Open prostatectomy involves removal of the inner portion of the prostate through a retropubic or suprapubic incision. It is best used for patients with larger prostates or with complicating conditions such as bladder stones or urethral strictures. Open prostatectomy is associated with incisional morbidity, longer hospitalization, and greater risk of impotence. Transurethral vaporization of the prostate uses a high-energy electrode inserted via the urethra to vaporize the prostate. This approach has little bleeding but creates more prolonged irritative voiding. Prostatic stents are used to maintain expansion of the prostatic urethra and have both temporary and permanent uses.

Management of Acute Urinary Retention

Acute urinary retention (AUR), considered a urologic emergency, is characterized by a sudden and painful inability to pass urine. Up to a third of men undergoing TURP present with AUR. AUR may be the result of natural progression of BPH, or it may be precipitated by surgical procedures, infection, or medications. Immediate management of AUR consists of bladder decompression, usually with a urethral catheter. Subsequently, conservative management is common with a trial of catheter removal after 1–3 days. Starting therapy with $α_1$ blockers before catheter removal improves the chances of success (SOE=B). The catheter should be removed as soon as possible, because this is the most effective means of reducing the incidence of catheter-associated urinary tract infections.

PROSTATE CANCER

Incidence and Epidemiology

Prostate cancer is the most common noncutaneous cancer and the second leading cause of cancer deaths among men in the United States. Since 2010, it has been estimated that over 200,000 men would be diagnosed with and over 30,000 men would die annually from prostate cancer. Incidence increases with age; prostate cancer is rare in men <40 years old. A prevalence study, reported in 2008, of 340 healthy men scheduled for organ donation found the prevalence of prostate cancer was 0.5% in men <50 years old, 23.4% in men 50–59 years old, 35% in men 60–69 years old, and 45.5% in men >70 years old. Earlier autopsy studies that included debilitated men had found prevalence rates as high as 80% in men >80 years old. The incidence of disease varies according to race, with black Americans having the highest risk in the world. Among black men, prostate cancer occurs at an earlier age, has a higher mortality rate, and tends to be at a more advanced stage at diagnosis. Family history is a contributing factor. Men with one first-degree relative affected have more than a 2-fold increased risk (SOE=B). Androgens are necessary for prostate cancer pathogenesis; the disease does not occur in men castrated before puberty. History of sexually transmitted infection can be associated with an increased risk of prostate cancer (SOE=B). The association between prostate cancer and omega-3 fatty acid intake, alcohol intake, or vasectomy is inconclusive.

Symptoms

Cancer usually arises in the peripheral zone of the prostate. Most men, especially those with early-stage, potentially curable disease, are asymptomatic. Prostate cancer spreads by 3 routes: direct extension, the lymphatics, and the bloodstream. Direct invasion of the urethra and bladder can lead to irritative voiding symptoms, urinary incontinence, and hematuria. Extension of disease to adjacent nerves can cause impotence and pelvic pain. Nodal metastasis can cause extrinsic ureteral obstruction. Leg edema can develop from lymphatic obstruction. Hematogenous metastasis to bone can cause severe local pain, normochromic normocytic anemia, pathologic fractures, and spinal cord compression. Less commonly, hematogenous metastasis involves viscera, namely the lung, liver, and adrenal glands.

Screening Controversy

The benefit of early detection and the best approach to treatment of prostate cancer are controversial. There is a large reservoir of prostate cancer that does not need to be diagnosed because most men with prostate cancer die with the disease, not from it. However, the well-recognized burden of progressive prostate cancer is a potential impetus for early detection and management.

Results of two prospective, randomized controlled trials of prostate cancer screening report somewhat conflicting findings. The Prostate, Lung, Colorectal, and Ovarian Cancer Screening Trial found no significant difference in prostate cancer mortality between screened and unscreened groups after 7–10 years of follow-up. The European Randomized Study of Screening for Prostate Cancer, which was actually a collection of smaller trials in different European countries, found a 20% decrease in prostate cancer mortality in the screened subgroup aged 50–64 years old over a mean of 9 years of follow-up; the absolute risk difference associated with screening was 0.071%, meaning that 1,410 men would need to be screened and 48 additional cases of prostate cancer would be treated for every prostate cancer death prevented. Both trials documented significantly increased prostate cancer incidence associated with screening. Men who were >74 years old at baseline were not enrolled in either trial. The two trials had significant methodologic differences, particularly for inclusion criteria, enrollment size, frequency and mode of screening, definition of a positive PSA level, and follow-up.

Screening for prostate cancer remains a somewhat controversial topic with different recommendations and guidelines from various task forces and specialty societies. In 2012, the U.S. Preventive Services Task Force issued updated recommendations giving routine screening for prostate cancer a "D" rating, meaning that "there is moderate or high certainty that the service has no benefit or that the harms outweigh the benefits." The U.S. Preventive Services Task Force noted that "The reduction in prostate cancer mortality 10 to 14 years after PSA-based screening is, at most, very small, even for men in the optimal age range of 55 to 69 years." Major guidelines from oncology, urology, and primary care recommend some level of shared decision making for PSA screening for prostate cancer. The American Cancer Society guideline recommends that men discuss screening with their clinicians to make an informed decision, starting at age 50, or younger if risk factors are present. The American Urological Association guideline recommends shared decision making for screening in men aged 55–69 years old, with the screening decision based on patient values and preferences. The American College of Physicians guideline recommends that clinicians inform men 50–69 years old about limited potential benefits and substantial harms of screening for prostate cancer, and recommends against PSA screening in men who do not express a clear preference for screening.

Screening and Diagnostic Tests

DRE allows palpation of the posterior surfaces of the lateral lobes of the prostate, where cancer most often begins. Cancer characteristically is hard, nodular, and irregular. Although DRE is less sensitive than PSA in detecting prostate cancer, it can sometimes detect cancers in men who have a normal PSA level. However, its use as a single screening test is greatly limited, because parts of the prostate gland cannot be palpated. About half of the cancers thought to be limited to the prostate on the basis of DRE are found during surgery to have already spread. DRE has many false-positive results; only about one-third of men with positive DRE tests have prostate cancer on biopsy. Local extension of prostate cancer into the seminal vesicles can often be detected by DRE, which may be valuable in staging of disease. Thus, despite its limitations, DRE has a role in prostate

Table 55.2—Staging Systems for Prostate Cancer

TNM Stage	Jewett-Whitmore Stage	Description
T_1	A1, A2	Tumor is an incidental finding.
T_{1c}		Tumor is identified by needle biopsy as a follow-up to screening that detected increased PSA.
T_2	B1, B2	Tumor is palpable, confined to prostate.
T_3	C1, C2	Tumor extends beyond the prostate capsule, may involve seminal vesicles.
T_4	C2	Tumor invades adjacent structures (eg, bladder neck, rectum, pelvic wall).
N	D1	Lymph node metastasis present.
M	D2	Distant metastasis present.

NOTE: TNM = tumor, regional node, metastasis

SOURCE: For further details, see AUA Prostate Cancer Clinical Guidelines Panel. *Report on the Management of Clinically Localized Prostate Cancer*. Baltimore, MD: American Urological Association; 1995.

cancer staging and in screening asymptomatic patients who choose to be screened.

The serum PSA test is not specific for prostate cancer. PSA increases in benign conditions of the prostate, namely, hypertrophy and prostatitis, and in transient response to conditions such as ejaculation and prostatic massage. The sensitivity of the PSA test is also imperfect. Decreased PSA values have been associated with acute hospitalization and use of medications such as 5α-reductase inhibitors and saw palmetto. PSA levels are normal in 30%–40% of men with cancer confined to the prostate (ie, false-negative tests). The reported positive predictive value of PSA in screening studies is 28%–35%; about one-third of men with increased PSA levels have prostate cancer demonstrated by fine-needle biopsy.

Several approaches to improve the accuracy of PSA testing have been developed. PSA density is derived from the PSA concentration divided by the volume of the prostate gland (measured by ultrasound). Prostate cancer results in higher PSA levels per unit volume than BPH and should therefore yield a higher PSA density. The PSA rate of change or velocity is more specific for prostate cancer than a single PSA measurement. Using a PSA velocity value of ≥0.75 ng/mL/year achieves 90% specificity, whereas using a single PSA level >4 ng/mL achieves 60% specificity. This high specificity for PSA velocity is realized even in serum PSA levels in the normal range (<4 ng/mL). Another approach involves age-adjusted PSA reference ranges, because PSA values increase with age. Finally, the ratio of free to complexed PSA can be measured, recognizing that PSA bound to α_1-antichymotrypsin accounts for a larger proportion of total PSA with prostate cancer than with BPH.

Abnormal DRE or PSA tests lead to transrectal ultrasound-guided biopsy of the prostate for pathologic diagnosis. Cancer can appear as a hypoechoic density, but ultrasonography is not specific enough to be used as a screening tool. Any suspicious areas (by DRE or ultrasound) are biopsied. In addition to, or in the absence of suspicious areas, spring-loaded core needle biopsies are routinely taken from the base, middle, and apex of each lobe (6 samples total, termed sextant biopsy). Sextant biopsy can be enhanced by extended biopsy schemes that sample more gland areas, particularly the lateral aspects. In a systematic review, prostate biopsy schemes that consist of 12 cores (standard sextant biopsy plus laterally directed cores) achieved a reasonable balance between cancer detection rates and adverse events.

Grading

The Gleason grading system is the most commonly used system based on the histologic appearance of prostate cancer. The Gleason grade ranges from 1, or well differentiated, to 5, or poorly differentiated. The Gleason score is the sum of the two most common Gleason grades observed. The Gleason score ranges from 2 to 10. Gleason scores are sometimes grouped as 2–4, well differentiated; 5–7, moderately differentiated; and 8–10, poorly differentiated. Well-differentiated tumors have a favorable prognosis; poorly differentiated tumors, an unfavorable prognosis (SOE=A). Most clinically detected tumors are moderately differentiated.

Staging

Staging of prostate cancer is necessary for planning disease management. Two classification systems are used: the tumor, regional node, metastasis (TNM) system and the Jewett-Whitmore (ABCD) system (Table 55.2). Usually detected by transurethral resection of the prostate, incidentally discovered cancers are staged according to the amount of tissue involved (T_1 or A). Stage T_{1c} reflects the growing number of tumors detected because of an increased PSA level. Tumors detectable by DRE and confined to the prostate (T_2 or B) are subdivided on the basis of the amount of tumor that is palpable. Staging is also based on the degree of extension and invasion of surrounding structures in tumors that extend beyond the prostatic capsule (T_3 to T_4 or C) and on presence of metastasis (M_1 or D).

The initial staging evaluation includes PSA level, DRE findings, transrectal ultrasonography results, and Gleason score. Routine bone scans should not be performed on low-risk patients with newly diagnosed prostate cancer who have a PSA ≤10 ng/mL and a Gleason score ≤6 (SOE=C). For patients electing active treatment, surgical assessment of lymph node involvement (pelvic lymphadenectomy) is performed by itself or in conjunction with prostate surgery or implantation of radioactive seeds. CT scans are often used for active treatment planning.

In the past, CT scans, MRI scans, pedal lymphangiography, and pelvic lymph node dissection were routinely used in various combinations to evaluate the extent of prostate cancer. In the initial staging evaluation of patients with prostate cancer, these tests should be eliminated, because they have been associated with unacceptably high false-negative and false-positive results. A subset of patients appears to benefit from CT scans combined with fine-needle aspiration. Patients who have a PSA >25 ng/mL, a Gleason score >6, and a palpable abnormality on DRE are recommended to undergo a CT scan with fine-needle aspiration if a lymph node >6 mm is present (SOE=D). Many of these patients will be diagnosed with nodal metastasis and are thus spared the need for bilateral pelvic lymph-node dissection and its associated morbidity.

Management of Localized Disease

Localized cancer lends itself to cure, but the prevalence of men dying with prostate cancer (often asymptomatic) but not from the disease questions the necessity of treatment. There remains a lack of evidence that treatment prolongs life when treatment is compared with watchful waiting. Thus, 3 approaches to localized prostate cancer are routinely advocated: watchful waiting, radical prostatectomy, and radiation therapy (Table 55.3).

Watchful waiting (also called *expectant* or *conservative management; surveillance*) is the approach offered most commonly to men with <10 years of remaining life expectancy, who have significant medical comorbidities, or whose tumor is small and well to moderately differentiated. Conservative management studies have shown that 10-year disease-specific survival is 89%–96% for men with Gleason score 2–5 tumors, 70%–82% for men with Gleason score 6 tumors, 30%–58% for men with Gleason score 7 tumors, and 13%–40% for men with Gleason score 8–10 tumors. Because most men with prostate cancer are asymptomatic, watchful waiting attempts to spare men the burden of unnecessary treatment. However, waiting for symptoms in men with prostate cancer before starting treatment means sacrificing the opportunity for cure. Patients are offered palliation if and when symptoms develop. Active surveillance combines the concept of expectant management with the option for deferred curative intent treatment. The optimal selection criteria and surveillance strategy for active surveillance have not been defined. Active surveillance selection criteria include cases detected by PSA screening with Gleason scores <7 and small volume involvement (<3 of 6 biopsy cores, <50% malignant involvement within each core). The National Comprehensive Cancer Network guidelines for active surveillance suggest serum PSA measurement as often as every 3 months, DRE as often as every 6 months, and repeat prostate biopsy as often as every 12 months (SOE=C).

Radical prostatectomy involves surgical removal of the entire prostate gland and the seminal vesicles. It can be performed through a perineal (incision near the rectum) or retropubic (lower abdominal incision) approach. The perineal approach allows an easier vesicourethral anastomosis and less bleeding, whereas the retropubic approach allows access to the pelvic lymph nodes and spares the neurovascular supply to the corpora cavernosa (with improved potency). The major complications of radical prostatectomy are urinary incontinence and erectile dysfunction. Surgery is thought to have the highest incidence of sexual dysfunction after treatment. In a population-based study of 1,291 men undergoing radical prostatectomy for clinically localized prostate cancer, 59.9% reported erections not firm enough for sexual intercourse and 8.4% were incontinent 18 months later (SOE=C). After radical prostatectomy, men are more likely to experience stress incontinence, with symptoms ranging from occasional leakage to no urinary control. Bladder neck contractures also occur, resulting in obstructive voiding symptoms and urinary retention. The relationship between these symptoms and sense of bother is not direct; for example, those with the most leakage may have little bother, whereas those with minimal leakage may report substantial bother.

Data regarding the benefits of radical prostatectomy are still lacking. Two randomized controlled trials have compared radical prostatectomy with watchful waiting. In one study of 695 men with 10-year follow up, prostatectomy and watchful waiting both reduced death from prostate cancer (10% and 15%, respectively) and distant metastases (15.2% and 25.4%, respectively). In the second study of 142 men, no statistically significant differences in survival were found; however, the study lacked sufficient power to detect moderate treatment differences. Both studies were conducted before prostate cancer detection with PSA testing was available. Two surgical improvements currently under investigation to reduce morbidity include the laparoscopic approach and robotic assistance. The laparoscopic approach has

Table 55.3—Management Approaches for Prostate Cancer

Management	Description	Comments	Selected Potential Adverse Effects
Localized			
Watchful waiting	Prostate cancer is not treated until symptoms develop.	Offered to men with <10 years of remaining life expectancy; significant medical comorbidities; small, well-differentiated tumors; or unwillingness to bear treatment burdens. Awaiting symptoms sacrifices opportunity for cure.	Anxiety
Active surveillance	Prostate cancer treatment is delayed until evidence of disease progression.	Offered to men with cancer detected by PSA screening, Gleason score <7, small volume involvement	Anxiety, discomfort of serial PSA, DRE, and prostate biopsies
Radical prostatectomy	Surgical removal of entire prostate gland and seminal vesicles	Offered to men who have no surgical contraindications. Adverse effects realized immediately.	Erectile dysfunction, urinary incontinence
External beam radiation therapy	Standard regimen delivers 6,000–7,000 rads of pelvic radiation over 5- to 8-week period.	Radiation reaches tissues outside the prostate, including pelvic lymph nodes. Adverse effects occur initially from radiation-induced inflammation, then develop over time as scar tissue develops.	*Acute:* proctitis, urethritis *Chronic:* erectile dysfunction, urinary incontinence, bowel dysfunction
Brachytherapy	Radioactive seeds (eg, iridium, palladium) are implanted into the prostate gland using CT scan guidance.	Improvements in prostate imaging allow uniform distribution of seed, overcoming past limitations. Adverse effects occur initially from radiation-induced inflammation, then develop over time as scar tissue develops.	*Acute:* prostatitis, urinary retention, hematuria *Chronic:* erectile dysfunction, urinary incontinence, bowel dysfunction
Locally Advanced			
Radiation therapy	See external beam radiation (above).	Offered to men with prostate cancer extending beyond capsule or into seminal vesicles. Asymptomatic cancer period may be prolonged.	See external beam radiation (above).
Androgen deprivation	Hormone therapy can be combined with radiation therapy.	Neoadjuvant androgen deprivation provides additional benefit toward increased survival and freedom from metastases; because of adverse effects, controversy exists regarding early versus delayed use of androgen deprivation.	Erectile dysfunction, loss of libido, loss of stamina, increased fatigue, hot flashes, diminished muscle mass, premature osteoporosis
Advanced/Metastatic			
Complete androgen ablation	Combined approach of reducing androgens to castration levels and inhibiting binding of androgen to its receptor	Includes orchiectomy or LHRH agonists with antiandrogens	Erectile dysfunction, loss of libido, loss of stamina, increased fatigue, hot flashes, diminished muscle mass, premature osteoporosis
Orchiectomy	Surgical castration	Oldest, safest, least expensive approach; rejected by half of American men	Erectile dysfunction, loss of libido, loss of stamina, increased fatigue, hot flashes, diminished muscle mass, premature osteoporosis
LHRH agonists	Chemical castration	Alternative to surgical castration, equally effective; causes initial increase in serum testosterone levels	Erectile dysfunction, loss of libido, hot flashes, gynecomastia, insomnia, GI upset, dizziness
Antiandrogens	Inhibit binding of androgen to its receptor	Used at initiation of LHRH-agonist therapy to block effect of increased testosterone levels; used after castration to block effect of residual small amount of androgen being produced by adrenal glands	Erectile dysfunction, loss of libido, gynecomastia, insomnia, GI upset, dizziness
Other	Symptom-specific approaches used as indicated	For example, focal radiation therapy can be provided to the site of a bony metastasis to reduce both pain and risk of fracture.	Intervention specific

NOTE: LHRH = luteinizing hormone-releasing hormone

raised concerns of poorer results related to positive surgical margins, return of continence, and preservation of potency. Robotic approaches have not shown advantage in hospital length of stay, postoperative pain, or blood replacement (SOE=C). Long-term outcomes are not yet known for either the laparoscopic or robotic approach. Thus, radical prostatectomy can be offered to men with locally confined disease, with >10 years of remaining life expectancy, and without contraindications to undergoing surgery (SOE=B).

Radiation therapy is provided through external beam radiation or through implantation of radioactive sources (known as *brachytherapy*). The standard regimen of external beam radiation delivers a total of about 6,000–7,000 rads over 5–8 weeks. Hypofractionated schemes use higher doses per fraction that achieve biologically similar doses over 4–5 weeks. Pelvic lymph nodes can be radiated as well. Proctitis and urethritis are common acute adverse events. Chronic complications include erectile dysfunction, urinary incontinence, and chronic proctitis. The incidence of urinary stress incontinence after radiation therapy is significantly less than with surgery but that of irritative voiding dysfunction is greater. Bowel dysfunction, uncommon after surgery, affects more than half of patients after radiation. Bowel symptoms include diarrhea, rectal urgency, and fecal soiling. Most patients classify these bowel symptoms as minor with little to no effect on quality of life. Conformal radiation therapy is a mode of high-precision external-beam radiation that uses high-resolution CT scan data and advanced computer technology to conform the radiation dose to the 3-dimensional configuration of the tumor. This newer technology shows promise in reducing complications and adverse events. Local control and cancer survival rates appear to be comparable to those of radical prostatectomy, at least for the first 5–8 years (SOE=C). Comparisons between treatments are difficult, because men undergoing radiation treatment tend to be older, less medically fit, and usually have not been pathologically staged.

Brachytherapy involves retropubic or perineal implantation of radioactive seeds, usually iridium or palladium. Improvements in 3-dimensional imaging of the prostate through CT scan or ultrasound guidance have allowed more uniform distribution of seeds throughout the prostate and overcome many of the past limitations of brachytherapy. Potency is better preserved with seed implants. Urinary symptoms include frequency, dysuria, and urge incontinence. Bowel symptoms include rectal urgency and rectal bleeding. The morbidity of seed implants appears to improve over time after the initial seed placement and associated prostate inflammation and swelling. In retrospective series, it appears that brachytherapy is comparable to radical prostatectomy and external beam radiation for low-risk disease.

However, brachytherapy outcomes appear less favorable for men with tumors that have a higher Gleason score or with higher pretreatment PSA levels (SOE=C).

Management of Locally Advanced Prostate Cancer

Locally advanced prostate cancer extends beyond the capsule or invades the seminal vesicle, without evidence of distant or nodal metastasis. Radiation therapy is the recommended treatment, and neoadjuvant androgen deprivation provides additional benefit toward increased survival and freedom from metastases (SOE=B). However, controversy exists as to when androgen deprivation should be started. Patients may have a prolonged asymptomatic cancer period, but significant negative quality-of-life changes from long-term androgen deprivation occur, including loss of stamina, increased fatigue, hot flashes, diminished muscle mass, and premature osteoporosis. Although radiation therapy with neoadjuvant androgen deprivation is a standard approach for locally advanced disease, some advocate that patients should be given the choice of early versus delayed androgen deprivation.

Management of Advanced Disease

Advanced disease is treated with androgen ablation and symptom-specific approaches, such as focal radiation therapy to painful bone metastasis. Androgen ablation aims to eliminate prostate cancer growth stimulation and includes orchiectomy or luteinizing hormone-releasing hormone (LHRH) agonists with antiandrogens. Orchiectomy and LHRH agonists are equally effective at reducing androgens to castration levels. Orchiectomy is the oldest, safest, least expensive approach but is rejected by nearly half of American men. LHRH agonists such as leuprolide and goserelin result in castration levels about 1 month after an initial increase in serum testosterone levels. Antiandrogens (eg, flutamide) are often given before starting LHRH agonists to blunt the effects of the initial testosterone increase. Antiandrogens inhibit the binding of androgen to its receptor. After castration, a small amount of adrenal androgen exists and may allow continued stimulation of prostate cancer growth. Antiandrogens can be combined with chemical or surgical castration, a practice called *complete androgen ablation*. Survival rates for antiandrogens alone are inferior to those for chemical or surgical castration alone; complete androgen ablation offers slight improvement in survival over that offered by castration only (SOE=B).

Radiation therapy is useful for relieving the pain of isolated bone metastasis and reducing the risk of fracture of bones with significant destruction. Diffuse bone metastases require alternative approaches. Bone-seeking radiopharmaceuticals such as strontium or radium can be beneficial for pain control (SOE=B). Androgen deprivation decreases bone pain in two-thirds of symptomatic patients (SOE=B). Bisphosphonates also decrease bone pain (SOE=B).

PROSTATITIS

Etiology

Prostatitis is an inflammatory condition of the prostate that can result from acute bacterial, chronic bacterial, or nonbacterial causes. The most common sources of acute or chronic infection are ascending urethral infection or reflux of infected urine into the prostatic ducts, or both. Direct extension or lymphatic spread from the rectum or hematogenous spread also occurs. Acute prostatitis is an infectious process that is more common in younger men than in older men. Pathogens in men ≤35 years old often include *Neisseria gonorrhea* and *Chlamydia trachomatis*. In older men, acute prostatitis is associated with indwelling urethral catheter use, and coliforms are the suspected bacterial cause. In >80% of patients with prostatitis, no infectious agent is identified.

Diagnosis

Acute bacterial prostatitis is characterized by fever, chills, dysuria, and a tense or boggy, extremely tender prostate. Because bacteremia can result from manipulation of the inflamed gland, minimal rectal examination is indicated. Gram stain and culture of the urine can identify the causative agent.

Chronic bacterial prostatitis presents classically as recurrent bacteriuria caused by the same organism, although most patients do not have this presentation. Patients have varying degrees of obstructive or irritative voiding symptoms and perineal pain. The prostate often feels normal. First-void or midstream urine is compared with expressed prostatic secretion or urine collected after prostatic massage. The expressed sample should reveal leukocytosis and the causative agent. Sterile expressant with leukocytosis suggests nonbacterial prostatitis.

Treatment

Acute bacterial prostatitis is treated with antibiotics and can require hospitalization. The severe inflammation allows antibiotics to penetrate the prostate, and prompt response to empiric therapy is expected. CT or MRI should be considered to evaluate for an abscess if recovery is delayed. Antibiotic selection should be based initially on results of a urine Gram stain, with subsequent consideration of sensitivity profiles. Fluoroquinolones are highly effective in most cases.

Antibiotics are less effective for chronic bacterial prostatitis because of their poor penetration of the prostate. Prolonged therapy (6–16 weeks) offers a cure rate of 30%–40%. Continuous low-dose antibiotic suppression therapy can be offered to those with frequent symptomatic relapse. Total prostatectomy offers cure but at a high risk-to-benefit ratio. Transurethral resection of the prostate is safer but cures only one-third of patients.

Nonbacterial prostatitis is treated symptomatically. A small percentage of cases can involve occult infections, and empiric antibiotic therapy is often used. Efforts to reduce pain and discomfort include anti-inflammatory agents, sitz baths, fluid adjustments (avoid caffeine), anticholinergic agents, and α-adrenergic antagonists.

CHOOSING WISELY® RECOMMENDATIONS

Prostate Disease

- Do not perform PET, CT, and radionuclide bone scan in the staging of early prostate cancer at low risk of metastasis.
- A routine bone scan is unnecessary in men with low-risk prostate cancer.
- Do not order creatinine or upper-tract imaging for patients with benign prostatic hyperplasia.
- Do not treat an increased PSA with antibiotics for patients not experiencing other symptoms.

REFERENCES

- Anothaisintawee T, Attia J, Nickel JC, et al. Management of chronic prostatitis/chronic pelvic pain syndrome: A systematic review and network meta-analysis. *JAMA*. 2011;305:78–86.

    This article provides a systematic review of randomized controlled trials comparing drug treatments in chronic prostatitis/chronic pelvic pain syndrome. α-Blockers, antibiotics, and combined therapy achieve the greatest improvement in symptoms scores compared with placebo. Anti-inflammatory agents have lesser benefit.

- MacDonald R, Tracklind JW, Wilt TJ. *Serenoa repens* monotherapy for benign prostatic hyperplasia (BPH): an updated Cochrane systematic review. *BJU Int*. 2012;109(12):1756–1761.

    This article provides a review of the evidence for the effectiveness and harms of *Serenoa repens* (saw palmetto) monotherapy for treatment of lower urinary tract symptoms (LUTS) in men with BPH. Compared with placebo, *Serenoa repens* therapy does not improve LUTS, even at double and triple the usual dose. The adverse events from *Serenoa repens* therapy are generally mild and comparable to those from placebo.

- Moyer VA. Screening for Prostate Cancer: U.S. Preventive Services Task Force Recommendation Statement. *Ann Intern Med*. 2012;157(2):120–134.

    This article provides a review of the evidence that lead to the 2012 updated USPSTF recommendation against routine prostate cancer screening in men of all ages. The new level "D" rating means "there is moderate or high certainty that the service has no benefit or that the harms outweigh the benefits." This article also provides a response to public comments on the draft version of this recommendation that was posted on the USPSTF website from October 11 to December 13, 2011.

- Paolone DR. Benign prostatic hyperplasia. *Clin Geriatr Med*. 2010;26(2):223–229.

    This article provides a review of the epidemiology, evaluation, and both medical and surgical therapeutic approaches for benign prostatic hyperplasia.

- Qaseem A, Barry MJ, Denberg TD et al; Clinical Guidelines Committee of the American College of Physicians. Screening for prostate cancer: a guidance statement from the Clinical Guidelines Committee of the American College of Physicians. *Ann Intern Med*. 2013;158(10):761–769.

    This article provides a critical review of 4 available guidelines from the American College of Preventive Medicine, American Cancer Society, American Urological Association, and U.S. Preventive Services Task Force to help guide clinicians in making decisions about screening for prostate cancer.

- Thompson IM, Goodman PJ, Tangen CM, et al. Long-term survival of participants in the Prostate Cancer Prevention Trial. *N Engl J Med*. 2013;369(7):603–610.

    This article provides data from an extended period of follow-up of men randomized to treatment with finasteride or placebo. Finasteride reduced the risk of prostate cancer by about one-third; however, high-grade cancer was more common in the finasteride group. After 18 years of follow-up, there was no significant between-group difference in the rates of overall survival or survival after the diagnosis of prostate cancer.

Lisa J. Granville, MD, AGSF, FACP

CHAPTER 56—SEXUALITY

KEY POINTS

- Normal age-associated changes lead to decreased sexual interest and ability; however, complete sexual dysfunction is not a part of healthy aging.

- Physiologic changes in sexual response occur in both men and women. It is important to distinguish between normal age-associated changes and pathologic conditions that can be related to medications or medical disorders.

- Sexual activity in older adults typically must be planned. Success requires privacy, longer foreplay, help with vaginal lubrication, and understanding of the impact of aging and disease on sexual function.

- Many older women have sexual dysfunction but do not report it to their primary care providers unless asked.

- Multiple effective options are available to treat male and female sexual dysfunction.

- Sexuality is an important part of quality of life for many older adults; treatment of sexual dysfunction can lead to improvements in quality of life.

- Prevention of sexually transmitted infection is still important despite older age.

MALE SEXUALITY

Age-Associated Changes

As men age, their sexuality changes. The frequency of sexual intercourse and the prevalence of engaging in any sexual activity decrease. Young men report having intercourse 3 to 4 times per week, whereas only 7% of men 60–69 years old and 2% of those ≥70 years old report the same frequency. Among men 60–70 years old, 50%–80% engage in any sexual activity, a prevalence rate that declines to 15%–25% among men ≥80 years old (SOE=A). However, sexual interest often persists despite decreased activity. The man's level of sexual activity, interest, and enjoyment in his younger years often determines his sexual behavior with aging. Factors contributing to a man's decreased sexual activity include poor health, social issues (eg, living in adult child's home), partner availability, decreased libido, and erectile dysfunction (ED. Although men 75–85 years old continue to prefer vaginal intercourse, approximately 50% report difficulty with erectile function.

Aging is associated with changes not only in sexual behavior but also in the stages of sexual response. During the excitement phase, there is a delay in erection, decreased tensing of the scrotal sac, and loss of testicular elevation. The duration of the plateau stage is prolonged, and preejaculatory secretion is decreased. Orgasm is diminished in duration and intensity, with decreased quantity and force of seminal emission. During the resolution phase, detumescence and testicular descent are rapid. The refractory period between erections is also longer. However, erectile failure is not a part of healthy aging but rather is frequently caused by age-associated disease or its treatment (eg, radical prostatectomy for prostate cancer) (SOE=B).

Erectile Physiology and Dysfunction

Penile rigidity results from a complex interaction between the brain, spinal cord, testosterone, neurotransmitters, arterial inflow, and venous outflow. In brief, testosterone, mental health, and an attractive partner typically stimulate sexual interest (libido). Fantasy, visual, tactile, or other erotic stimuli (eg, erotic scents or sounds) trigger neural impulses from the brain or spinal cord to the penis. Neural impulses cause release or synthesis of various neurotransmitters (eg, nitric oxide, cGMP), which induce arterial vasodilation and increased penile arterial inflow. Increasing arterial inflow results in penile tumescence, which impedes venous outflow. As the intrapenile (ie, intracavernosal) pressure equilibrates to mean arterial pressure, the penis becomes rigid. Thus, there are many steps along the path that can be broken and result in ED.

ED, the inability to achieve or maintain an erection adequate for vaginal intercourse, is the most common sexual problem of older men. The prevalence of ED increases with age; by 70 years of age, 67% of men have ED. This high prevalence is important; in a study comparing affected and unaffected men, men with sexual dysfunction reported impaired quality of life. For a summary of the causes of sexual dysfunction in men, see Table 56.1.

The most common cause (30%–50%) of ED in older men is vascular disease (SOE=A). Risk of vascular ED increases with traditional vascular risk factors, eg, diabetes mellitus, hypertension, hyperlipidemia, and smoking. In fact, ED is a predictor of future major atherosclerotic vascular events (ie, myocardial infarction and stroke).

Obstruction from atherosclerotic arterial occlusive disease likely impedes the intracavernosal blood flow and pressure needed to achieve a rigid erection. In addition, atherosclerotic disease can cause ischemia of trabecular smooth muscle and result in fibrotic changes

Table 56.1—Causes of Sexual Dysfunction in Older Men

Causes (in order of prevalence)	Characteristics
Vascular disease	■ Gradual onset Vascular risk factors: diabetes mellitus, hypertension, hyperlipidemia, tobacco use
Neurologic disease, eg, radiation therapy, spinal cord injury, autonomic dysfunction, surgical procedures	■ Gradual onset for progressive conditions; sudden onset for injury or surgery Neurologic risk factors: diabetes mellitus; history of pelvic injury, surgery, or irradiation; spinal injury or surgery; Parkinson disease; multiple sclerosis; alcoholism Loss of bulbocavernosus reflex
Medications, eg, anticholinergics, antihypertensives, cimetidine, antidepressants	■ Sudden onset Lack of sleep-associated erections or lack of erections with masturbation Temporal association with a new medication
Psychogenic, eg, relationship conflicts, performance anxiety, childhood sexual abuse, fear of sexually transmitted diseases, "widower's syndrome"	■ Sudden onset Sleep-associated erections or erections with masturbation are preserved
Hypogonadism	■ Gradual onset Decreased libido more than erectile dysfunction Small testes, gynecomastia Low serum testosterone concentration
Endocrine, eg, hypothyroidism, hyperthyroidism, hyperprolactinemia	■ Rare, <5% of cases of erectile dysfunction

leading to failure of venous closure mechanisms, ie, inability to impede venous outflow necessary for equilibration to mean arterial pressure causing penile rigidity. Venous leakage leading to vascular ED can also result from Peyronie disease, arteriovenous fistula, or trauma-induced communication between the glans and the corpora. In anxious men who have excessive adrenergic-constrictor tone and in men with injured parasympathetic dilator nerves, ED can result from insufficient relaxation of trabecular smooth muscle.

The second most common cause of ED in older men is neurologic disease (17%–37%). Disorders that affect the parasympathetic sacral spinal cord or the peripheral efferent autonomic fibers to the penis impair penile smooth muscle relaxation and prevent the vasodilation necessary for erection. In patients with prostate cancer, all forms of (curative) treatment frequently cause neurogenic erectile failure (brachytherapy or external radiation, 50%; radical prostatectomy with nerve sparing, 45%–80%) and pain on orgasm (SOE=B). Common health problems such as diabetes mellitus, stroke, and Parkinson disease can cause autonomic dysfunction that results in erectile failure. Finally, surgical procedures such as cystectomy and proctocolectomy commonly disrupt the autonomic nerve supply to the penis, resulting in postoperative ED.

Numerous commonly used medications have been associated with ED for which the mechanism, for the most part, is unknown. In approximately 5% of men with ED, the ED is drug-induced. Medications with anticholinergic effects, such as antidepressants, antipsychotics, and antihistamines, can cause ED by blocking parasympathetic-mediated penile artery vasodilatation and trabecular smooth muscle relaxation. Almost all antihypertensive agents have been associated with ED; of these, clonidine and thiazide diuretics have higher incidence rates, whereas ACE inhibitors and angiotensin-receptor blockers have lower incidence rates (SOE=B). One mechanism by which antihypertensives can cause ED is lowering blood pressure below the threshold needed to maintain sufficient blood flow for penile erection, especially in those men who already have penile arterial disease. OTC medications such as cimetidine and ranitidine can also cause ED. Cimetidine, an H_2-receptor antagonist, acts as an antiandrogen and increases prolactin secretion; thus, it has been associated with loss of libido and erectile failure. Ranitidine can also increase prolactin secretion, although less commonly than does cimetidine.

The prevalence of psychogenic ED correlates inversely with age. In approximately 9% of men ≥65 years old with ED, the ED is psychogenic. Psychogenic ED can develop via increased sympathetic stimuli to the sacral cord, inhibiting the parasympathetic dilator nerves and thus inhibiting erection. Common causes of psychogenic ED include relationship conflicts, performance anxiety, childhood sexual abuse, and fear of sexually transmitted diseases. Older men may have "widower's syndrome," in which the man involved in a new relationship feels guilt as a defense against subconscious unfaithfulness to his deceased spouse.

Hyperthyroidism, hypothyroidism, and hyperprolactinemia have been associated with ED. However, <5% of ED is caused by endocrine abnormalities. Thus, endocrine evaluation of men with ED but intact libido is of limited value (SOE=B).

The role of androgens in erection is becoming clearer. Hypogonadism is moderately common in older men. Hypogonadal men show smaller and slower developing erections in response to fantasy, which is improved with androgen replacement. However, even men with castrate levels of testosterone can attain erections in response to direct penile stimulation. It may be that erection from direct penile stimulation is less androgen dependent, whereas erection from fantasy is more androgen dependent. Nevertheless, testosterone is necessary for intracavernosal nitric oxide synthesis. Thus, testosterone plays a large role in libido and a smaller role in erectile function. For example, hypogonadal men do respond better to phosphodiesterase inhibitors after testosterone replacement therapy. However, men with ED and normal testosterone serum concentrations do not benefit from testosterone supplementation. Rather, giving eugonadal men testosterone supplementation may increase libido and vascular risk without improving erectile function.

Evaluation of Erectile Dysfunction

The initial step is to obtain a sexual, medical, and psychosocial history. Sexual history should clarify whether the problem consists of inadequate erections, decreased libido, or orgasmic failure. The onset and duration of ED, the presence or absence of sleep-associated erections, and the associated decline in libido are clues to the likely cause.

Sudden onset (in the absence of pelvic surgery) suggests psychogenic or drug-induced ED. A psychogenic cause is likely if there is a sudden onset but retention of sleep-associated erections or if erections with masturbation or a different partner are intact (SOE=A). If sudden-onset erectile failure is accompanied by lack of sleep-associated erections and lack of erection with masturbation, temporal association with new medication should be investigated. A gradual onset of ED associated with loss of libido suggests hypogonadism. Gradual onset associated with intact libido (most common presentation) suggests vascular, neurogenic, or other organic causes.

Medical history is directed at discerning those factors likely to be contributing to ED. Vascular risk factors include diabetes mellitus, hypertension, coronary artery disease, peripheral arterial disease, hyperlipidemia, and smoking. Neurogenic risk factors include diabetes mellitus; history of pelvic injury, surgery, or radiation; spinal injury or surgery; Parkinson disease; multiple sclerosis; or alcoholism. An extensive medication review, including OTC medications, is essential. Finally, the psychosocial history should assess the patient's relationship with the sexual partner, the partner's health and attitude toward sex, economic or social stresses, living situation, alcohol use, and affective disorders.

On physical examination, attention should be paid to signs of vascular or neurologic diseases. Peripheral pulses should be palpated. Signs of autonomic neuropathy (eg, orthostatic hypotension and absent heart rate response to standing) and loss of the bulbocavernosus reflex suggest neurologic dysfunction. The genital examination includes palpating the penis for Peyronie plaques and assessing for testicular atrophy. A femoral bruit and diminished (or absent) pedal pulses suggests arterial insufficiency. An absent bulbocavernosus reflex suggests penile neuropathy. A loss of secondary sexual characteristics, small testes, and gynecomastia suggest hypogonadism or hyperprolactinemia.

Appropriate laboratory evaluations are those that target relevant comorbid conditions such as diabetes mellitus and vascular disease or that evaluate neurologic disorders if suggested by the physical examination. The measurement of serum testosterone should be considered in the setting of other symptoms of androgen deficiency. As in women, men at risk of sexually transmitted infections (STIs) should be offered counselling and testing for HIV and other STIs. In 2009, the American College of Physicians recommended universal HIV screening up to age 75; in 2013, the United States Preventive Services Task Force (USPSTF) recommended universal screening up to age 65 and screening adults >65 years only if at increased risk of infection.

An at-home therapeutic trial of a phosphodiesterase inhibitor (sildenafil or vardenafil) is considered first-line evaluation and treatment. The initial dose should be low (sildenafil 25–50 mg or vardenafil 5–10 mg) in men suspected of having neurogenic ED. A poor response suggests vasculogenic ED. Further therapeutic trial with sildenafil at 100 mg or vardenafil at 20 mg may prove to be effective. An at-home therapeutic trial using tadalafil (5–10 mg) can be considered, but its long half-life complicates matters if an adverse event occurs with the first dose.

More extensive diagnostic tools are available but not commonly used. Nocturnal penile tumescence testing is of little value, except to confirm a psychogenic cause. The penile-brachial pressure index can be helpful in assessing arteriogenic ED. This index measures the loss of systolic pressure between the arm and the penis. When measured before and after exercise, it can be used to assess for a pelvic steal syndrome, which is the loss of erection associated with initiation of active pelvic thrusting, presumably due to the transfer of blood flow from the penis to the pelvic musculature. More invasive and expensive tests such as Doppler ultrasound to assess penile arterial function, dynamic infusion cavernosometry to assess venous leakage syndrome, and

Table 56.2—Treatment Options for Erectile Dysfunction

Treatment	Route/ Administration	Onset	Duration of Action	Dosage	Selected Adverse Events
Sildenafil	Oral	60 min	4 h	25–100 mg	Headache, flushing, rhinitis, dyspepsia, transient color blindness; contraindicated with nitrate use and α-blockers
Vardenafil	Oral	45 min	4 h	5–20 mg	Headache, flushing, rhinitis, dyspepsia; contraindicated with nitrate use and α-blockers
Tadalafil	Oral	45–60 min	24–36 h	5–20 mg	Headache, dyspepsia, flushing, rhinitis; contraindicated with nitrate use and α-blockers
Avanafil	Oral	30 min		100 mg	Headache, flushing, prolonged erection; contraindicated with nitrate use and α-blockers
Vacuum device	External	<5 min	30 min	—	Petechiae, bruising, painful ejaculation
Papaverine[OL]	Intracavernosal	10 min	30–60 min	15–60 mg	Prolonged erection, fibrosis, ecchymosis
Alprostadil	Intracavernosal	10 min	40–60 min	5–20 mcg	Prolonged erection, pain, fibrosis
Phentolamine[OL]	Intracavernosal	10 min	30–60 min	0.5–1 mg	Prolonged erection, fibrosis, headache, facial flushing
Medicated urethral system for erection (MUSE)	Intraurethral	10–15 min	60–80 min	250–1,000 mcg	Penile pain or burning, hypotension
Penile prosthesis	Surgical		replacement in 5–10 years	—	Infection, erosion, mechanical failure
Sex therapy	Counseling	weeks	years	weekly	Anxiety

NOTE: Above treatments, excluding sex therapy, are effective for neurogenic causes and may be helpful for arteriogenic and venogenic etiologies. Vacuum device and sex therapy are effective for psychogenic causes.

penile arteriography are generally reserved for research or penile vascular surgery candidates.

Treatment of Erectile Dysfunction

Multiple effective therapeutic options are available for the treatment of ED. Treatment should be individualized and based on cause, personal preference, partner issues, cost, and practicality (Table 56.2).

Oral therapy for ED with sildenafil, vardenafil, tadalafil, or avanafil has revolutionized treatment of male sexual dysfunction. Sildenafil is a type-5 phosphodiesterase inhibitor that potentiates the penile response to sexual stimulation. It improves the rigidity and duration of erection. It is taken 1 hour before sexual activity and has no effect until sexual stimulation occurs. Because absorption is attenuated when sildenafil is ingested with a fatty meal, patients need to be educated about this issue. Vardenafil is a more potent and specific phosphodiesterase inhibitor. A lower effective dose and better adverse-event profile (no effect on color vision) make vardenafil a reasonable option. Tadalafil is a longer-acting phosphodiesterase inhibitor with an adverse-event profile similar to that of vardenafil but with the added potential problem of muscle pain. Avanafil is a more recently approved phosphodiesterase inhibitor; it is taken 30 minutes before sexual activity. All four of these agents are contraindicated for concomitant use with nitrate medications, because the combination can produce profound and fatal hypotension. In addition, combined use of α-blockers with phosphodiesterase inhibitors should be done with caution, starting with the lowest dose of either. Choosing among these phosphodiesterase inhibitors should likely be based on price and patient preference. All phosphodiesterase inhibitors result in sufficient penile rigidity for an approximately 50% success rate at vaginal intercourse. Because of the longer duration of action of tadalafil, men tend to select it when given the choice (SOE=B).

Vacuum tumescence devices are another option. The apparatus consists of a plastic cylinder with an open end into which the penis is inserted. A vacuum device attached to the cylinder creates negative pressure within the cylinder, and blood flows into the penis to produce penile rigidity. A penile constriction ring placed at the base of the penis then traps the blood in the corpora cavernosa to maintain an erection for about 30 minutes. The vacuum device is effective for psychogenic, neurogenic, and venogenic ED, but it requires manual dexterity. Local pain, swelling, bruising, coolness of penile tip, and painful ejaculation are potential adverse events. It is important to remove the constriction ring after 30 minutes. This device is not recommended for men on anticoagulant therapy or with a history of bleeding disorders.

Intracavernosal injection of vasoactive drugs such as papaverine, phentolamine, and alprostadil are effective in producing erections adequate for sexual activity (SOE=A) but are used much less frequently since oral therapy has become available. Alprostadil, which is the only agent approved by the FDA for intracavernosal injection, produces erections that last 40–60 minutes. Phentolamine[OL] is mainly used in combination therapy with papaverine[OL] or alprostadil, or both. Potential adverse events are bruising, ecchymoses or hematoma, local pain, fibrosis from repeated injections, and priapism. Alprostadil appears to cause less scarring and priapism than papaverine. If an erection lasts >4 hours, detumescence is necessary by aspiration of blood from the corpora cavernosa or injection of phenylephrine because of the potential for intracavernosal hypoxia and fibrosis of trabecular smooth muscle, which can prevent future erections. In general, intracavernosal therapy should probably be reserved for patients in whom oral therapy with a phosphodiesterase inhibitor is not effective. Alprostadil can also be administered intraurethrally using a medicated urethral system for erection (MUSE). This system contains a small pellet of alprostadil that is placed within the urethra and is rapidly absorbed through the urethral mucosa to produce an erection within 10–15 minutes. Possible adverse events are penile pain, urethral burning, and a throbbing sensation in the perineum. The sexual partner may also experience burning or irritation if the intraurethral alprostadil is expelled during sexual activity.

Testosterone supplementation increases libido and can improve ED in men with true hypogonadism (SOE=B). However, as mentioned above, it has little value in eugonadal men with ED. Testosterone is available as an intramuscular injection (testosterone enanthate or cypionate), buccal patch, transdermal patch, and gel. Possible adverse events associated with testosterone include polycythemia, prostate enlargement, gynecomastia, and fluid retention. It is important to perform a digital rectal examination to assess the prostate and obtain a baseline prostate-specific antigen level before beginning therapy. If prostate-specific antigen or hematocrit increases with testosterone therapy, it usually does so within 6 months. Therefore, these levels should be checked every 3 months during the first year of therapy, then every 12 months thereafter.

Surgical implantation of a penile prosthesis is another therapeutic option. Mechanical failure, infection, device erosion, and fibrosis are possible complications. However, since the availability of alprostadil and, more recently, phosphodiesterase inhibitors, surgical implantation of a penile prosthesis is rarely done (ie, used in men with severe arterial occlusive disease). Nevertheless, long-term patient satisfaction with penile prosthesis is actually higher than with oral therapy (SOE=B). Penile revascularization surgery has limited success.

Men with psychogenic ED should be referred to a mental health or other professional specializing in treatment of sexual disorders for further evaluation and treatment.

FEMALE SEXUALITY

Age-Associated Changes

Many factors play an important role in the sexual response of older women, including changes that occur with menopause, cultural expectations, relationship problems, previous sexual experiences, chronic illnesses, and depression. American women live about 29 years after menopause and outlive their spouses an average of 8 years. Although the frequency of intercourse decreases with aging, sexuality remains important for older women. Among 513 women 75–85 years old in the National Social Life, Health and Aging Project (NSHAP), 37.2% were married, 1.2% were living with a partner other than their spouse, and 16.7% reported sexual activity with their spouse or other partner in the previous year. Of those who were sexually active with their spouse or other partner, 54.1% reported sexual activity at least 2 or 3 times per month. Among those women who had a spouse or other partner but had been sexually inactive in the previous 3 months, 64.8% attributed the inactivity to the partner's physical health problems or limitations and 24.8% to their own health problems.

The female sexual response cycle changes with aging. During the excitement phase, the clitoris may require longer direct stimulation, and genital engorgement is decreased. Vaginal lubrication is reduced, although with increased foreplay and gentle stimulation, lubrication is usually adequate for intercourse. During the plateau phase, there is less expansion and vasocongestion of the vagina. During orgasm, fewer and weaker contractions occur, although older women can still achieve multiple orgasms. Occasionally during orgasm, older women experience spastic and painful contractions of the uterine musculature. During the resolution phase, vasocongestion is lost more rapidly. Most of these changes are thought to be due to a decline in serum estrogen concentration after menopause, but a vasculogenic component can contribute to postmenopausal sexual dysfunction.

Female Sexual Dysfunction

For the most part, menopause is accompanied by decreased sexual function, with decreased sexual interest, responsiveness, and coital frequency. In addition, there is an increase in urogenital symptoms, often not discussed with the clinician. For example, in the NSHAP, among women 75–85 years old who were sexually active, the most common sexual problem was lack of interest (49.3%), followed by difficulty with lubrication (43.6%), inability to climax (38.2%), lack of pleasure during sex (24.9%), and dyspareunia (11.8%).

Dyspareunia, defined as pain with intercourse, can be due to organic or psychologic factors, or a combination. For example, a woman can experience an episode of dyspareunia because of postmenopausal vaginal atrophy. With each subsequent sexual encounter, she anticipates pain, causing inadequate arousal with decreased lubrication. Because of this cycle, she continues to experience dyspareunia, even after the vaginal atrophy has been treated. The most common organic cause of dyspareunia is vaginal atrophy (also referred to as vulvovaginal atrophy or atrophic vaginitis) due to estrogen deficiency. It affects up to 45% of postmenopausal women. Because of lack of estrogen, the vaginal epithelium becomes thinner and pH rises from a premenopausal value of 3.5–4.5 to a postmenopausal range of 5.0–7.5, which increases the risk of bacterial colonization and urinary tract infections. Other causes of dyspareunia include inadequate lubrication, localized vaginal infections, cystitis, Bartholin cyst, retroverted uterus, marked uterine prolapse, endometriosis, pelvic tumors, excessive penile thrusting, or vaginismus (involuntary muscle spasms).

Systemic or local estrogen therapy can improve symptoms of vaginal atrophy, but it has little effect on libido or sexual satisfaction (SOE=B). Libido is thought to depend on testosterone (even in women), rather than on estrogen. The ovaries and adrenals are the main sources of androgens in women. The effects of female androgen deficiency were originally identified in women treated for advanced breast cancer with oophorectomy and adrenalectomy. When deprived of androgens, these women reported loss of libido. Hypoactive sexual desire disorder (HSDD) is defined as decreased libido that causes personal distress and is not due to a psychiatric or medical illness or a substance (such as medication). HSDD is thought to be due to low testosterone. Because there are no normative data on plasma total and free testosterone in women and no well-defined clinical syndrome of androgen deficiency, the Endocrine Society has not recommended making a diagnosis of androgen deficiency in women. In August 2015, the FDA approved flibanserin to treat acquired, generalized hypoactive sexual desire disorder in premenopausal women. This is the first FDA-approved medication for sexual desire disorders. Use of alcohol is contraindicated when using flibanserin because of increased and more severe serious adverse effects of hypotension and syncope. No postmenopausal women were enrolled in the studies submitted for FDA approval.

Older women commonly have multiple medical conditions, some of which affect sexuality. However, scientific studies on the effect of chronic diseases and medications on the sexuality of older women are limited. Women with diabetes mellitus are less likely to be sexually active, and report decreased libido and lubrication and longer time to reach orgasm. Rheumatic diseases affect sexuality via functional disability. After mastectomy for breast cancer, 20%–40% of women experience sexual dysfunction, possibly because of disruption of body image, marital and family problems, spousal reaction, adjuvant therapy, or the psychologic impact of a breast cancer diagnosis. Several drugs can adversely affect sexual function, including antidepressants (with higher rates for SSRIs and lower rates for bupropion), antihypertensives, antipsychotics, antiestrogens, antiandrogens, anticholinergic drugs, narcotics, alcohol, and illicit/recreational drugs. Psychosocial factors also have an important role in sexual dysfunction. Women commonly marry men older than themselves and live longer than men. Consequently, heterosexual older women are likely to spend the last years of their lives alone. Even when a partner is available, he might have erectile dysfunction (ED). Finally, lack of privacy can be a problem when an older couple lives with their children or in a nursing home.

Evaluation and Treatment

Taking a sexual health history is the most important step of the evaluation. Careful and sensitive questioning can detect problems that a woman might not otherwise volunteer. In a survey of postmenopausal women, 43% experienced menopause-related vaginal discomfort; of these, 40% reported it affected their sex life but 66% did not discuss the condition with their clinician because of embarrassment and 33% expressed preference for the clinician to initiate the discussion. About half of the women did not know that topical treatments are available for vaginal discomfort. Clinicians should ask about dyspareunia, lack of vaginal lubrication, quality of the relationship and sexual communication with the partner, and previous negative experiences, such as rape, child abuse, or domestic violence. Medications should be carefully reviewed. A woman with dyspareunia should undergo a pelvic examination to exclude organic causes. Older women who have risk factors for sexually transmitted infections (STIs) should be offered counselling and testing for HIV and other STIs. It is important to note that older

Table 56.3—Treatment Options for Sexual Dysfunction in Older Women

Symptom	Possible Cause	Therapy
Decreased desire	Low testosterone from natural or surgical menopause	Testosterone[OL] is not recommended by the Endocrine Society
	Chronic illness	Treatment of underlying illness
	Depression	Antidepressant medication
	Relationship problems	Marital therapy
	Medications	Review of drug regimen
Decreased lubrication	Vaginal dryness or atrophy from postmenopausal status	Longer foreplay, regular intercourse, moisturizers/lubricants, low-dose topical estrogens
	Antiestrogens and anticholinergic medications	Review of medications, including OTC drugs
Delayed or absent orgasm	Neurologic disorders, diabetes	Treatment of underlying illness
	Psychologic problems	Cognitive-behavioral therapy, masturbation, Kegel exercises
Pain with intercourse	Organic cause	Treatment of underlying physical condition
	Vaginal dryness, atrophy	Longer foreplay, regular intercourse, moisturizers/lubricants, low-dose topical estrogens, oral estrogen-receptor modulator (ospemifene)
	Vaginismus (involuntary vaginal contractions)	Psychotherapy, cognitive-behavioral therapy

adults have increased potential to acquire STIs. Longer, more active living combined with increased rates of divorce increases the number of new sexual partners. Postmenopausal atrophic changes in the vaginal mucosa may lead to microabrasions during intercourse. Older adults may find negotiating safer sex unfamiliar and challenging, lack knowledge about HIV/AIDS risk factors, and are less likely to use condoms.

Decreased lubrication, vaginal discomfort, itching, and dyspareunia due to vaginal atrophy respond well to topical estrogen therapy (SOE=A). In the United States, there are three topical estrogen formulations that are considered "low-dose," because they cause minimal systemic absorption without significant proliferation of the endometrial lining. A low-dose conjugated estrogen cream regimen is 0.5 g once daily 21 days on/7 days off (cyclic regimen) or 0.5 g twice weekly (continuous regimen). The plastic applicator is calibrated in 0.5-g increments with a minimum of 0.5 g and a maximum of 2 g. It can be difficult for an older woman to self-administer the 0.5-g dose accurately, but doses >0.5 g are not considered "low-dose" and may have systemic effects. The low-dose vaginal estradiol ring releases estradiol at 7.5 mcg/d; the ring is replaced by the patient or physician every 90 days. Although the ring is left in the upper third of the vagina for 3 months, it does not interfere with intercourse. The estradiol vaginal tablet (10 mcg) is placed in the vagina daily for 2 weeks, then 1 tablet twice a week. The estradiol ring and tablet are better tolerated than topical estrogen creams because of ease of use and comfort. In the 2013 Position Statement on the management of vulvovaginal atrophy, the North American Menopause Society recommends discussing with the patient's oncologist before starting a woman with breast cancer on topical estrogen because of lack of safety data beyond 1 year. The 2015 American Geriatrics Society Beers Criteria notes that vaginal estrogens for the treatment of vaginal dryness are safe and effective; women with a history of breast cancer who do not respond to nonhormonal therapies are advised to discuss the risk and benefits of low-dose vaginal estrogen (dosages of estradiol <25 mcg twice weekly) with their health care provider. For mild symptoms of vaginal atrophy or if the patient is not a candidate for or does not want to use topical estrogen, nonhormonal vaginal moisturizers (eg, Replens) with the addition of lubricants during intercourse can provide some symptom relief but are not effective in reversing the atrophic changes. An alternative for women with atrophic vaginitis who do not like to use topical agents is the oral selective estrogen-receptor modulator (SERM) ospemifene. It was approved by the FDA in 2013 for moderate to severe dyspareunia due to vaginal atrophy. In a 12-week randomized trial, ospemifene administered orally at 60 mg/d improved symptoms of dyspareunia and improved vaginal epithelium and pH. It caused a slight increase in endometrial thickness from baseline, but biopsies did not show endometrial hyperplasia or carcinoma. Although ospemifene is effective, long-term safety data are lacking. Systemic adverse effects include hot flashes and increased risk of thromboembolism.

Importantly, local stimulation through regular intercourse helps maintain a healthy vaginal mucosa. Longer foreplay allows more time for vaginal lubrication in older women, just as older men often need longer and more direct stimulation to achieve an adequate erection.

Decreased libido without identifiable cause may respond to testosterone, but no androgen preparation is approved by the FDA for hypoactive sexual desire disorder in women. In several placebo-controlled, randomized trials, low-dose testosterone patch[OL] delivering 300 mcg/d dosed twice weekly or daily improved sexual desire in women with natural or surgical menopause and on systemic estrogens (SOE=A). Androgenic adverse events such as acne and hirsutism were uncommon, and concentrations of high-density lipoprotein cholesterol did not decrease as in studies with oral methyltestosterone. More recent studies demonstrated that the testosterone patch is also effective in women with natural or surgically induced menopause who have decreased libido and are not taking estrogens. Although the testosterone patch seems effective (SOE=A), there are only limited data on its long-term safety in women. One study showed the testosterone patch was safe and effective after 4 years of use in women taking oral estrogens.

Finally, older women should receive education about male sexual aging in addition to female sexual aging. Otherwise, an older woman might mistakenly attribute her partner's diminished erection and need for more genital stimulation to her own inability to arouse her partner. Other psychologic issues, including depression, history of sexual abuse, and relationship problems, should be addressed and treated with antidepressants, psychotherapy, and marital therapy, as necessary (SOE=C). A sex therapist can be identified on the website of the American Association of Sex Educators, Counselors, and Therapists (www.aasect.org). For a summary of treatments for female sexual dysfunction, see Table 56.3.

REFERENCES

- Avanafil (Stendra) – another PDE5 inhibitor for erectile dysfunction. *Med Lett Drugs Ther*. 2014;56(1442):37–38.

    This issue of the Medical Letter evaluated the new PDE5 inhibitor (ie, avanafil), comparing it to the other already available PDE5 inhibitors. All PDE5 inhibitors have a similar onset of action, but tadalafil has a much longer duration of action. All have an efficacy rate of 60%–70%, and cost varies from $21–$38 per dose; vardenafil is least expensive and tadalafil is most expensive. All PDE5 inhibitors should be avoided in patients taking nitrates and used with caution in patients taking α-blockers. All except sildenafil should be avoided in patients with severe hepatic or renal impairment.

- Lindhal SH. Reviewing the options for local estrogen treatment of vaginal atrophy. *Int J Womens Health*. 2014;6:307–331.

    Vaginal atrophy affects up to 45% of postmenopausal women and causes vaginal dryness, burning, and dyspareunia with possible bleeding during intercourse or touching. This is a literature review on topical estrogens for vaginal atrophy. Low-dose conjugated estrogen cream, low-dose estradiol vaginal ring, and estradiol vaginal tablets are effective, well tolerated, and safe in studies that lasted up to 1 year. No randomized trials have been done on low-dose vaginal estradiol cream, which therefore cannot be recommended. According to the 2013 recommendations of the North American Menopause Society, a progestogen is not needed when using low-dose vaginal estrogens.

- Maciel M, Lagana L. Older women's sexual desire problems: biopsychosocial factors impacting them and barriers to their clinical assessment. *Biomed Res Int*. 2014:2014:107217.

    Sexual activity has positive effects on older adults' physical health; therefore, health care providers should not hesitate to raise the topic of sexual health. Several medical and psychological factors have a negative effect on older women's sexual desire, including hormonal changes with menopause that may cause changes in the genitourinary system, decreased body image and self-worth in part due to social contexts and norms, quality of intimate relationships, erectile dysfunction in the sexual partner or lack of a partner, and religiosity and cultural aspects. Furthermore, health care providers are less likely to ask about sexual problems in older women than in older men because there is no "magic pill" for female sexual dysfunction. They also may have inadequate training and/or an ageist attitude toward older women's sexuality.

- Portaman D, Palacios S, Nappi RE, et al. Ospemifene, a non-estrogen selective receptor modulator for the treatment of vaginal dryness associated with postmenopausal vulvar and vaginal atrophy: a randomized, placebo-controlled, phase III trial. *Maturitas*. 2014:78(2):91–98.

    Ospemifene is a selective estrogen-receptor modulator (SERM) that was approved by the FDA in 2013 for moderate to severe dyspareunia due to vaginal atrophy. In this 12-week trial, 314 postmenopausal women with vulvovaginal atrophy and moderate to severe vaginal dryness were randomized to oral ospemifene at 60 mg/d or placebo. In the treatment group, 34% of the patients were considered "responders" with improvement of vaginal dryness and vaginal epithelium compared with 7% in the placebo group ($P<.001$). In the treatment group, 7.5% of women reported hot flushes, and there was one serious adverse event—deep vein thrombosis—probably related to the treatment. Ospemifene caused a slight increase in endometrial thickness from baseline, but biopsies did not show endometrial hyperplasia or carcinoma.

- Work Group for the HIV and Aging Consensus Project. Summary report from the Human Immunodeficiency Virus and Aging Consensus Project: Treatment strategies for clinicians managing older individuals with the human immunodeficiency virus. *J Am Geriatr Soc*. 2012;60(5):974–979.

    It is estimated that by 2015, 50% of the HIV population in America will be ≥50 years old. In 2010, a special meeting convened at the White House on HIV and Aging. This collaboration between the American Geriatrics Society and the American Academy of HIV Medicine focused on developing clinical treatment strategies. In recognition of the rapidly evolving developments in this field, an online site was created on which information is frequently updated (www.AAHIVM.org/hivandagingforum).

Angela Gentili, MD
Thomas Mulligan, MD, AGSF

CHAPTER 57—MUSCULOSKELETAL PAIN

KEY POINTS

- The most common cause of pain in older adults is related to musculoskeletal issues. Osteoarthritis accounts for most cases of knee pain.

- Back problems are the third most common reason for clinician visits by older adults.

- Lumbar spinal stenosis pain is characterized by back pain radiating into the buttocks or legs that is worse on standing and walking, particularly downhill, and is relieved with sitting.

- About 25% of women will experience a vertebral compression fracture in their lifetime.

GENERAL PRINCIPLES FOR DIAGNOSIS

Pain is a major issue for many older adults, and the most common cause is a musculoskeletal problem. Systemic analgesics have significant adverse effects in older adults and are often ineffective in position-associated musculoskeletal pain. A musculoskeletal problem is treated most effectively if the specific cause can be identified. The search for this cause can be both challenging and rewarding. This search requires knowledge of the referral patterns of pain for musculoskeletal conditions and expertise in performing a joint and manual muscle examination. The "gold standard" for determining the cause of this pain is the physical examination, complemented by a good history, and not an imaging or laboratory study such as MRI or rheumatoid factor. The history should elucidate the patient's story of the musculoskeletal complaint and its characteristics. What symptoms accompany the pain? What brings on the pain? Is the pain exacerbated when going from lying to sitting, ascending or descending stairs, standing, or walking? Is the pain worse in the morning, midday, or nighttime? Does the pain radiate? Does the pain cause the patient to cease the activity associated with the pain?

The pattern of the pain is also important. Pain that is gradual at onset and progressively worsens raises concern for a systemic condition such as a tumor or infection. Pain that is relatively abrupt at onset and related to position is more typical of mechanical pain. Some mechanical pain, such as rotator cuff tendonitis, is worse at night, interrupting sleep. Many musculoskeletal conditions produce pain at sites quite distant from the structure involved. The referral patterns of musculoskeletal conditions have been mapped out by numerous investigators. Neck conditions produce pain throughout the trapezius and retroscapular region. Shoulder and neck disease can cause pain throughout the arm. Lumbar spine disease can produce discomfort in the back and legs, whereas pain in the buttock, thigh, groin, and knee may originate from the hip.

When an older adult presents with pain in more than one joint, a systemic process may be considered; however, older adults often have multiple mechanical problems in different sites of the body. For example, many older adults may have osteoarthritis of the knees and hips along with tendonitis of the rotator cuff structures. Others might have inflammatory arthritis with involvement of the knees and shoulders. The physical examination is the most effective way of distinguishing a systemic process from multiple mechanical problems.

Careful observation of the patient's mobility is the first objective step in the search for the cause of the pain. Does the patient have a limp, spending less time on one leg than the other when walking? Does he or she have difficulty picking up a leg when going from a sitting to a supine position? Is the pain reproduced by ascending or descending stairs?

The next step is to perform a thorough physical examination, focusing on an assessment of joints and muscle groups. A manual muscle examination can identify patterns of weakness associated with musculoskeletal problems. The joint examination should focus on malalignment and swelling of joints, whether the swelling is soft tissue or bony enlargement, decreased range of motion, and patterns of joint involvement consistent with specific conditions. For example, generalized osteoarthritis affects the distal interphalangeal joints, proximal interphalangeal joints, the first carpal-metacarpal joint, hips, knees, and tarsal-metatarsal joints of the foot. This condition does not involve the metacarpal-phalangeal joints, wrists, shoulders, or ankles.

Diagnostic imaging and laboratory tests should be ordered only after a list of potential diagnoses has been formulated from the history and physical examination. Ordering these tests before establishing the differential diagnosis is costly, may expose the patient to risks of radiation and contrast material, and can mislead the clinician, often directing the process down the wrong path. These tests are very often abnormal in asymptomatic patients. In one study, 50% of asymptomatic individuals >60 years old had abnormal MRIs of the lumbar spine. The incidence of abnormalities on cervical spine radiographs and MRIs in older adults without neck pain is also very high.

EVALUATION AND MANAGEMENT OF REGIONAL MUSCULOSKELETAL COMPLAINTS

Neck Pain

Determining the cause of neck pain in older adults can be challenging. Four general conditions can produce pain in the neck and upper body region: systemic disease, cervical myelopathy, cervical radiculopathy, and mechanical neck disease.

A number of systemic conditions, particularly polymyalgia rheumatica, rheumatoid arthritis, and other inflammatory conditions, can cause this pain. These conditions usually produce systemic symptoms and signs, other joint complaints, and prolonged morning stiffness. Inflammation in the small joints of the hands and wrists can be a key to the diagnosis. These patients typically have symmetric loss of range in motion of the cervical spine. Laboratory tests of inflammation, such as the C-reactive protein and erythrocyte sedimentation rate, are often increased.

The myelopathy produced by cervical stenosis does not always cause neck pain. Rather, it is often characterized by a spastic gait disturbance and weakness in the lower extremities with upper motor neuron signs, including hyperreflexia, increased muscle tone, and positive Babinski signs. This condition can also produce lower motor neuron findings in the upper extremities. Thus, physical examination findings of lower motor neuron disease in the upper extremities and upper motor neuron disease in the lower extremities suggest cervical stenosis. Bladder symptoms include urgency, frequency, or retention. This condition should be identified as early as possible, because it is a potentially reversible cause of leg weakness and spasticity. The clinical course is quite variable. Of note, the same neurologic pattern is seen in amyotrophic lateral sclerosis.

Cervical radiculopathy is characterized by pain in the neck and arm, sensory loss, loss of motor function, and reflex changes in the affected nerve-root distribution. It is usually due to encroachment of the neuroforamina of the cervical spine. The C7 nerve root is most frequently affected. Pain that is reproduced by rotating the head or bending it toward the symptomatic side suggests this diagnosis. Most patients improve with symptomatic treatment, and only a relatively small number require surgery.

Most older adults with neck pain have nonspecific mechanical disease of the cervical spine. Cervical disc displacement appears to be a frequent cause of these complaints. Cervical disc disease can be referred into several regions. C2-C3 disease is felt in the occiput; C3-C4 and C4-C5 problems are referred into the posterior and lateral aspects of the neck; C5-C6 lesions are referred into the trapezius and upper cervical regions; C6-C7 disease is felt in the retroscapular region, often as far down as the mid to lower thoracic region. Cervical spine disease produces not only pain in those regions but also local muscle spasm and tenderness. This referred tenderness is often mistaken for the "trigger points" of fibromyalgia. Physical examination often shows asymmetric loss of range of motion of the cervical spine and weakness of the muscles innervated by cervical nerve roots, such as elbow extension and finger abduction in patients with C7, C8, and T1 disease.

There are little hard data on the effectiveness of one therapy versus another in the management of nonspecific neck pain. The Bone and Joint Decade 2000–2010 Task Force on Neck Pain suggested that manual therapy and exercise are more effective than alternative strategies. Although several studies have shown that spinal manipulation and exercise programs are helpful, virtually all these studies were done on patients ≤65 years old. Surgery is rarely if ever indicated for pain and should be considered only if there are significant, persistent, and worsening neurologic signs. Patients with significant neurologic findings associated with cervical spinal stenosis should be evaluated for possible surgery.

Shoulder Pain

The shoulder is a complex structure. The shoulder girdle is composed of 3 bones (the clavicle, scapula, and proximal humerus) and 3 joints (the glenohumeral, sternoclavicular, and acromioclavicular). Periarticular structures that often cause shoulder pain include the 3 rotator cuff tendons that insert on the greater tuberosity of the humerus (the supraspinatus, infraspinatus, and teres minor tendons), the subacromial bursa, and the biceps tendon. Joint problems can affect the acromioclavicular joint and the glenohumeral joint.

The first step in examination of the shoulder is to assess the passive range of motion of the glenohumeral joint, as well as check for a "painful arc." The examiner places one hand on the superior spine of the scapula and passively abducts the arm. The point at which the scapula starts to rise is the point of glenohumeral abduction. This is normally approximately 90 degrees. External or lateral rotation is checked by rotating the arm in that direction until tightness is felt. External rotation is usually approximately 90 degrees and internal rotation, approximately 80 degrees. At the same time that the examiner is abducting the arm, he or she should check for the presence of a "painful arc." This sign is present if the patient has discomfort when the arm is passively abducted from 45 degrees to 120 degrees. This finding indicates disease of 3 of the rotator cuff tendons (supraspinatus, infraspinatus, teres minor) or the subacromial bursa.

Common causes of shoulder pain include acromioclavicular disease, adhesive capsulitis, biceps tendonopathy and tendon rupture, and rotator cuff tendonopathies and tears.

Acromioclavicular Disease

The acromioclavicular joint is often affected by trauma as well as osteoarthritis. Patients complain of anterior shoulder pain, which is usually referred directly to the acromioclavicular joint.

Adhesive Capsulitis (Frozen Shoulder)

Adhesive capsulitis is characterized by loss of passive range of motion of the glenohumeral joint. Patients with shoulder injuries, tendonitis, or other conditions often lose mobility in this structure. Radiographs are normal. The natural history of this condition is good, although it may take up to a year to restore the range of motion of the shoulder.

Biceps Tendonopathy and Tendon Rupture

Tendonitis of the biceps muscle produces pain over the anterior aspect of the shoulder that is aggravated by lifting and pulling. This condition is diagnosed if pain is reproduced by resisting elbow flexion, shoulder flexion (bringing the arm forward with the elbow straight), or wrist supination with the patient's elbow by his or her side. The biceps muscle has a long and short head, and the long head often ruptures. This rupture produces an indention of the proximal biceps and a palpable mass of the distal biceps (positive "Popeye" sign). The strength loss with this rupture is relatively insignificant and does not require surgical repair.

Rotator Cuff Tendonopathies and Tears

These conditions are characterized by shoulder pain that is aggravated by pulling, lifting, or holding the arm above the shoulder level, as well as by lying on the affected side. This condition should be considered if the patient has a "painful arc." Tendonitis is suggested if the pain can be reproduced by resisting the active range of motion of the affected tendon (abduction for supraspinatus and external rotation for infraspinatus and teres minor). The pain from this condition is usually felt in the deltoid area and often down as far as the elbow. The supraspinatus is the most common tendon involved, and it can be evaluated with the "empty can" sign. The patient places a straight arm in 90 degrees of abduction and 30 degrees of forward flexion and then internally rotates the arm until the thumb is pointing down. The patient resists the clinician's attempts to push down the arm.

Pain without weakness is consistent with tendonopathy, whereas weakness is consistent with a tendon tear.

Rotator cuff tendonitis is typically treated with NSAIDs, physical therapy, and/or local subacromial corticosteroid injections. In one study, there was no difference at 1 year between patients treated with corticosteroid injections versus physical therapy. These patients, however, were all <65 years old. Because of the complications of NSAIDs in older adults, corticosteroid injections are often used for tendonitis. Although such injections may be helpful in reducing pain early on, mobilizing exercises alone are a reasonable approach to this condition.

Patients with persistent rotator cuff tendon symptoms may have tears of the tendon. Rotator cuff tears are common in older adults and may be insidious in onset. They cause recurring shoulder pain as well as loss of function. These conditions are diagnosed if active range of motion is less than passive range of motion of the glenohumeral joint, there is a positive "drop arm" sign (patient is unable to hold the arm in the abducted position against gravity), or the patient has significant weakness when performing the "empty can" sign. MRI is a definitive method of diagnosing these tears. Surgery should be considered if patients have substantial functional loss from a tendon tear or persistent pain that has not responded to conservative therapy.

Elbow Pain

Pain in the elbow region can result from a cervical radiculopathy or be referred from subacromial bursitis or rotator cuff tendonitis. Elbow pain can also be caused by arthritis of the elbow, olecranon bursitis, "tennis elbow" or lateral epicondylitis, and "golfer's elbow" or medial epicondylitis.

The synovial structure of the elbow must be evaluated to diagnose arthritis of this joint. The examiner should follow the lateral aspect of the humerus down the forearm with his or her thumb until finding the lateral epicondyle. There should be an indentation below that epicondyle and then a second bony structure below that indentation. If that structure rotates when the patient's wrist is rotated, it is the radial head. The examiner should run his or her thumb between the radial head and the olecranon. This space is where the synovial outpouching of the true elbow joint is felt. Swelling or induration of this region indicates an elbow joint process. Elbow disease usually limits flexion and extension of the elbow.

Olecranon bursitis causes swelling over the tip of the olecranon. This condition can be caused by trauma, gout, pseudogout, or infection. Asymptomatic swelling of that bursa can also occur. Infection of the bursa usually results from contiguous spread of infection from the skin, whereas infection of the elbow joint itself usually comes from an endovascular source. The best method of determining the cause of either bursitis or arthritis is to aspirate the bursa or joint and to examine the fluid for white cells, infection, or crystals.

"Tennis elbow", or lateral epicondylitis, is due to irritation of the wrist extensor tendons close to their insertion on the lateral epicondyle of the humerus. Tenderness may be found over the lateral aspect of the elbow. This diagnosis is made if the patient's elbow pain is reproduced by resisting extension of the patient's wrist.

"Golfer's elbow" occurs over the medial epicondyle. This condition is diagnosed if the patient's elbow pain is reproduced by resisting flexion of the wrist and is often accompanied by tenderness over the medial epicondyle.

Infection of the olecranon bursa can be treated with oral antibiotics and drainage of the bursa (outpatient). Steroid injections are not effective for lateral epicondylitis. Although there are little controlled data on their efficacy, physical therapy and counter-force braces placed 6–10 cm distal to the elbow joint are often suggested for this condition. Arthritis of the elbow joint should be treated in a manner appropriate for the underlying condition. Local corticosteroid injections are often helpful for patients with gout or pseudogout of this joint.

Hand and Wrist Pain

A variety of rheumatic and neurologic conditions can cause hand and wrist pain. As noted above, generalized osteoarthritis does not typically involve the metacarpal phalangeal joints and wrists. Osteoarthritis is treated with analgesics or anti-inflammatory drugs.

Synovial thickening of these joints indicates an inflammatory arthritis. Symmetric decreased range of motion of the wrists, in the absence of significant trauma, also suggests inflammatory joint disease. Monoarticular arthritis of the wrist is frequently caused by gout or calcium pyrophosphate deposition disease (pseudogout). In older adults, gout frequently affects the distal and proximal interphalangeal joints that are already involved in generalized osteoarthritis. Crystal-induced arthritis of the wrist (gout or pseudogout) can be effectively treated with a local steroid injection into the wrist.

De Quervain tenosynovitis produces pain along the radial aspect of the wrist, increased when grasping objects. This condition is caused by stenosing inflammation of the tendon sheath located over the radial styloid, which contains the abductor pollicis longus and extensor pollicis brevis tendons. Pain is produced when a clinched fist is deviated quickly in an ulnar direction. De Quervain tenosynovitis responds well to a corticosteroid injection into the tendon sheath.

Carpal tunnel syndrome is a common cause of hand pain. Patients complain of numbness and pain over the palm of the hands. Classically, the thumb and medial two fingers as well as the medial half of the ring finger are involved, but most patients cannot make this distinction. The pain is often increased in the morning; patients often drop objects because of this pain, which may radiate up the arm. The Tinel test for carpal tunnel syndrome involves tapping the medial aspect of the wrist with a reflex hammer. The test is positive if the hand has pain or paresthesias in the fingers innervated by the median nerve. In the Phalen maneuver, the patient hyperflexes his or her wrist by placing the backs of the hands against each other with the elbows in a flexed position. Pain or paresthesias in the fingers with 1 minute of wrist flexion is a positive test. The usual approach to treatment of carpal tunnel syndrome is splinting of the wrist. If splinting is ineffective, a corticosteroid injection into the carpal tunnel space can be tried. If this therapy is ineffective, surgery is the next option.

Ulnar neuropathies are common in peripheral neuropathies and can also be caused by trauma at the elbow area. Patients develop numbness and tingling on the lateral aspect of the hand. The diagnosis is confirmed if the patient has weakness of finger abduction but not elbow extension.

A "trigger finger" causes difficulty opening up a flexed finger. The syndrome is due to a combination of a flexor tendon nodule and thickening or fibrosis of the sheath in which this tendon travels. This combination results in a "mouse trapping" effect, in which the tendon is caught in a flexed position.

Dupuytren contraction of the palm of the hand produces painless deformities. These contractions cause thickening and fibrosis of the palmar fascia sheath, often with "puckering" of the skin over the flexor tendon. Flexion contractures of the fingers may result.

Thigh Pain

Thigh pain can be caused by such conditions as hip or back disease, trochanteric bursitis, a hernia, referred pain from abdominal viscera, femoral neuropathy, bone conditions, and vascular insufficiency.

Hip disease is a common cause of thigh pain as well as pain in the groin, buttock, and knee. The pain often comes on with walking and is relieved with sitting and lying. Patients may complain of significant pain on the first few steps after getting up from a sitting position. If the pain is significant, the patient usually limps, spending less time bearing weight on the affected side. If the disease is severe, it produces a short stride, because the hip is the "hinge" joint that controls the length of the stride. If the patient develops a flexion contracture of the hip, he or she will bend forward while walking.

The physical examination is the best method to diagnose hip disease. If the range of motion of the hip is normal, it is unlikely that this the hip joint is the cause of the pain. The patient should be placed in a supine position. The examiner places one hand on the pelvis and gently abducts the hip. Abduction of the hip is reached when the pelvis starts to tilt. This is normally approximately 40 degrees. The examiner should also be able to flex the hip beyond 110 degrees. With the hip flexed, the foot should be moved toward the midline (external rotation). Normal external rotation should be 50–60 degrees. Internal rotation is when the heel is moved away from the midline and is normally 15–20 degrees.

The most common cause of hip disease in older adults is osteoarthritis. Plain radiographs of the hip may not display significant changes in patients with early osteoarthritis, and cartilage can be seen only on an MRI. If the patient has significant signs and symptoms of hip arthritis with an unimpressive radiograph, then an MRI may be indicated.

Medical therapies for osteoarthritis of the hip are limited. In one study, physical therapy did not result in better improvement in pain or function than sham treatment. Although NSAIDs are effective in the treatment of osteoarthritis, their adverse effects limit their use in older adults. Corticosteroid injections, given under fluoroscopic guidance, can be an effective treatment of pain in hip osteoarthritis, with benefits lasting up to 3 months. Although medical therapies have a limited role in this condition, surgical approaches can be very effective. The success rate of a hip arthroplasty for osteoarthritis of the hip is high.

Lumbar spine disease commonly causes thigh pain, which often occurs with standing and walking. Pain can be felt on the lateral aspect of the hip and into the thigh region. The physical examination is key to this diagnosis, because the straight leg raise test is often positive. Many patients with lumbar spine disease will have subtle weakness of the great toe extensor, hip abductor, and hip extensor, because the L4-L5 and L5-S1 regions are the most common ones involved in lumbar spine disease.

Trochanteric bursitis pain is felt in the lateral thigh and may radiate down the lateral aspect to the knee. It is usually worse when rolling over on that side at night or after prolonged sitting, and it may be reproduced by resisting abduction of the hip. The most characteristic physical feature is local tenderness. This tenderness is usually felt approximately 1.5 inches below the superior portion of the trochanter.

The femoral nerve can produce pain in the thigh area, particularly in patients with diabetes, retroperitoneal hemorrhages, or metastatic cancer. Patients have pain over the anterior aspect of the thigh, not affected by movement. These patients may have altered sensation over the anterior aspect of the thigh and a decreased quadriceps reflex. This condition causes focal weakness of the hip flexor and knee extensor muscles, because both of these muscle groups are innervated by the femoral nerve.

Pain in the groin and upper thigh area may be due to an inguinal or femoral hernia. Discomfort is increased when intra-abdominal pressure is increased, which can occur with straining, prolonged standing, or heavy lifting. Although incarceration and strangulation of these hernias are rare, this complication requires urgent attention and surgery. The diagnosis of an inguinal or femoral hernia is best made on physical examination with the finding of a groin bulge or a discrete groin impulse that increases with cough or a Valsalva maneuver.

A number of visceral problems in the abdomen can produce leg pain. A psoas abscess can produce hip and leg pain. This pain is increased when the psoas muscle is stretched or extended, which occurs with extension of the hip. Psoas abscess pain is typically diminished with hip flexion.

Although peripheral arterial disease typically causes calf pain, it can cause thigh and buttock pain. Two studies have demonstrated that approximately 40% of patients with claudication have pain in the proximal aspect of the leg. Claudication produces pain and discomfort in the legs when walking but not when standing or sitting. The pain worsens if the patient walks up a hill quickly and should disappear within 10 minutes after standing still.

Patients with bone disease of the pelvis or femur can also develop pain in the thigh. A number of cancers, such as breast, prostate, lung and kidney, can produce metastatic lesions in these bones.

Knee Pain

Knee pain greatly limits the function of many older adults and can also be referred from the hip and back. The most common cause of this pain is osteoarthritis. In some cases, however, patients may have radiographic findings of osteoarthritis of the knees, but their pain may be caused by other conditions such as gout, pseudogout, or anserine bursitis.

Several structures around the knee can cause knee pain. The prepatellar bursa is located directly on top of the patella. The infrapatellar bursa is just inferior to the patella. The anserine bursa is on the medial aspect of the knee approximately 2 finger breadths below the joint line. The patient can often localize the site of the pain over the anterior, medial, or posterior aspect of the knee. Anterior pain can be due to prepatellar or infrapatellar bursitis or to irritation of the patellofemoral compartment of the knee. Patellofemoral pain can be reproduced by placing fingers firmly on the superior aspect of the patella and then asking the patient, lying supine, to press his or her knee into the bed. This maneuver contracts the quadriceps muscle, and the patella is a sesamoid bone within this muscle. When the quadriceps muscle contracts, the patella moves in a superior fashion. Pressure on the patella will reproduce pain from the patellofemoral component of the knee. Patellofemoral pain often radiates down to the anterior aspect of the lower leg and is usually worse on prolonged knee flexion (eg, sitting in a theater or airplane) or when the patient is descending stairs.

Pain on the medial aspect of the knee can be caused by conditions such as osteoarthritis of the medial compartment of the knee, medial meniscal disease, irritation at the attachment of the medial meniscus to the medial collateral ligament, or from irritation of the anserine bursa. Patients with a varus or "bow-legged" appearance have significant medial joint space narrowing due to osteoarthritis. Meniscal disease can be diagnosed by reproducing the patient's pain with a combination of extension and rotation of the knee. Patients with irritation at the attachment of the medial meniscus to the medial collateral ligament often have night pain in the medial aspect of the knee. There is usually tenderness along the medial joint line, and patients frequently put a pillow between their knees at night.

The first step in management of osteoarthritis of the knee should be quadriceps-strengthening exercises and weight reduction. NSAIDs can be effective, but their use is limited by their adverse effects in older adults. Interarticular injections of corticosteroids are effective but on average last only 4 weeks, although response is more prolonged in some patients. Although the use of hyaluronic acid injections is somewhat controversial, their adverse effects are limited and they may offer a more prolonged response than corticosteroid injections. They can be considered in patients for whom surgical intervention is not an option. These injections have fewer adverse effects than daily use of NSAIDs.

Many patients with osteoarthritis have evidence of meniscal disease. Caution is warranted when considering surgical interventions for meniscal abnormalities. A study has demonstrated that arthroscopic partial meniscectomy was no more effective than physical therapy for meniscal tears in patients with knee osteoarthritis.

Anatomists, noting that the combined insertion of the medial hamstring muscles (gracilis, semitendinosis and semimembranosus) on the tibia resembled a "goose's foot," named this region "pes anserine." The anserine bursa is located directly over that combined insertion, approximately 2 finger breadths below the medial joint line on the medial aspect of the tibia. Marked local tenderness at the region can indicate a bursitis. This condition often responds to a local injection of a corticosteroid and lidocaine.

Pain is often felt in the popliteal region if there is significant swelling or inflammation of synovial tissue. Sometimes this swelling can produce an outpouching in the popliteal area known as a popliteal or Baker cyst. This diagnosis is made by palpating a cystic mass in the popliteal space. These cysts sometimes rupture, causing swelling and pain in the calf, producing a "pseudothrombophlebitis" syndrome.

It is important to determine if the patient has a knee effusion, signifying that the problem is likely intra-articular. If there is pain and a joint effusion, the most important step is to aspirate the joint fluid and have it analyzed, looking for WBCs, crystals, and infection. The WBC count in the synovial fluid is very important. Patients with a mechanical disease such as osteoarthritis and meniscal irritation will have a bland fluid with a WBC count of <2,000 cells/mL. Any condition that produces inflammation of the joint, such as rheumatoid arthritis, gout, pseudogout, or infection, will produce a synovial fluid WBC count of ≥2,000 cells/mL.

Back Pain

Back problems are the third most common reason for clinician visits by older adults. The evaluation of back pain in older adults requires a careful history, because systemic conditions have a history quite distinct from that of mechanical pain (see Table 57.1). Several of the specific mechanical causes of back pain have characteristic historical features. Although systemic causes of pain are uncommon, they are more prevalent in older adults than in younger ones. There are also a number of specific causes for pain in older adults, including lumbar spinal stenosis, osteoporotic vertebral compression fractures, and osteoporotic sacral factures, that are rarely seen in younger individuals. The acuity and positional relationship of the pain provide useful diagnostic historical clues (see Table 57.2).

Low back pain is rarely associated with inflammatory arthritis. Although ankylosing spondylitis, psoriatic arthritis, and Reiter syndrome can produce back pain, this involvement is not seen with rheumatoid arthritis, systemic lupus, polymyalgia rheumatica, or other inflammatory conditions. Systemic conditions such as tumors and infections of the spine generally have an insidious onset of pain that becomes more and more persistent and severe over time. This pain is usually nonpositional, can occur at night, and may be associated with systemic symptoms or signs. The likelihood of cancer as a cause of back pain increases in adults >50 years old, those with a previous history of cancer, and those with pain that persists for longer than 1 month.

Fever, discrete local vertebral tenderness, pain in the upper lumbar or thoracic area, and nonpositional pain may indicate vertebral infection. Approximately

Table 57.1—Conditions Causing Back Pain in Older Adults

Condition	History	Examination	Laboratory Tests, Imaging
Tumor	Persistent, progressive pain at rest; systemic symptoms	No focal abnormalities	Anemia, increased ESR, abnormal bone scan or MRI
Infection	Persistent pain, fever; at-risk patient (eg, indwelling catheter)	Tender spine	Increased ESR, WBC count; positive bone scan or MRI
Unstable lumbar spine	Recurring episodes of pain on change of position	Pain going from flexed to extended position	MRI or CT showing one disc space narrowed and sclerotic spondylolisthesis
Lumbar spinal stenosis	Pain on standing and walking relieved by sitting and lying	Immobile spine; L4, L5, S1 weakness	MRI or CT scan showing stenosis
Sciatica	Pain in posterior aspect of leg; may be incomplete	Often positive straight leg raise; L4, L5, S1 weakness	Variable diagnostic imaging findings
Vertebral compression fracture	Sudden onset of severe pain; resolves in 4–6 weeks	Pain on any movement of spine; no neurologic deficits	Vertebral end-plate collapse; compression fracture seen on plain film
Osteoporotic sacral fracture	Sudden lower back, buttock, or hip pain	Sacral tenderness	H-shaped uptake on bone scan

NOTE: ESR = erythrocyte sedimentation rate

Table 57.2—Assessment of Lower Back Pain in Older Adults

Symptoms	Conditions
Acute pain	Vertebral compression fracture Disc displacement Osteoporotic sacral fracture Visceral origin (eg, aortic aneurysm)

Positional pain
  Increased with standing and walking and relieved with sitting
  Brought on by bending, lifting, or unguarded movements
	
	Lumbar spinal stenosis
	Unstable lumbar spine

Persistent pain (gradually increasing, nonpositional)	Tumor Infection

10% of older adults with endocarditis have back pain. Infection should be evaluated as a source of back pain in patients at risk of endovascular infections, such as those on hemodialysis, with chronic indwelling intravenous access catheters, or with a history of intravenous drug abuse.

A number of visceral problems, such as abdominal aortic aneurysm, bladder distention secondary to urinary retention, uterine fibroids, pancreatic cancer, or other intra-abdominal infections or tumors, can present with back pain. Referred pain from these conditions should be suggested by the historical pattern of the pain, the absence of positional changes, and a normal examination of the lumbosacral spine. Patients with a known cancer with likelihood of spread to the bones should be urgently evaluated if they develop back pain.

On physical examination of older adults with back pain, the back, hips, legs, and gait should be evaluated. Examination of the hips, described above, is important, because many patients with back, buttock, and leg pain have hip disease. Gait evaluation should note if the patient bends forward as he or she walks, has a short stride, or spends less time on one leg than the other (limp).

The patient should next be examined in the upright position. The back should be moved through all 4 planes of movement of the lumbar spine: side flexion to the right, side flexion to the left, forward flexion, and extension. The pain of lumbar spinal stenosis is often produced by spinal extension. Asymmetric limitation of the range of motion of the lumbar spine, or reproduction of the pain with these maneuvers, may indicate mechanical disease of the lumbar spine (see Table 57.3).

Straight leg raise tests can be helpful if positive. However, the most helpful physical finding in patients with possible back disease is subtle weakness of the L4-L5 and L5-S1 muscles. L4-L5 weakness is demonstrated by weakness of the great toe extensor and hip abductor. The ankle dorsiflexor is also innervated by L4-L5, but this muscle is quite strong and subtle weakness may be difficult to elicit. L5-S1 weakness is demonstrated by involvement of the hip extensors. This is easily tested by attempting to pull up the leg at the ankle when the patient is trying to hold the leg on the bed. Normally,

Table 57.3—Physical Examination of Older Adults with Lower Back Pain

Sign	Condition
Paravertebral muscle spasm	Mechanical disc disease*
Asymmetric range of motion of the lumbar spine	Mechanical disc disease Unstable lumbar spine
Spinal tenderness	Vertebral compression fracture Infection
Weakness of L4-L5 and L5-S1 muscles	Mechanical disc disease Lumbar spinal stenosis
Normal examination of lumbar spine	Osteoporotic sacral fracture Hip disease Tumor Referred visceral pain

*Not caused by tumor, infection, spinal stenosis, or fracture

Table 57.4—Innervation of Lower Extremities

Function	Muscle	Peripheral Nerve	Nerve Root
Great toe dorsiflexion	Extensor hallucis longus	Deep peroneal	L5
Ankle dorsiflexion	Tibialis anterior	Deep peroneal	L4, L5
Ankle eversion	Peroneus longus, brevis	Superficial peroneal	L5, S1
Ankle plantar flexion	Gastrocnemius, soleus	Tibial	S1, S2
Knee extension	Quadriceps	Femoral	L3, L4
Hip flexion	Iliopsoas	Femoral	L2, L3
Hip adduction	Adductor magnus, brevis, longus	Obturator	L3, L4
Hip abduction	Gluteus medius	Superior gluteal	L4, L5
Hip extension	Gluteus maximus	Inferior gluteal	L5, S1

the patient can successfully resist this maneuver (see Table 57.4).

In the setting of acute back pain, the *Choosing Wisely* recommendation to wait 6 weeks before performing diagnostic imaging tests is appropriate to limit the use of CT scans, MRIs, and plain radiographs in younger patients, but older adults commonly have red flags that warrant imaging without delay. A plain radiograph of the lumbar spine can detect a vertebral compression fracture and should be obtained in older women, and in older men with risk factors for osteoporosis, if the discovery of a compression fracture will change management. Other red flags that would prompt early imaging include acute neurologic deficit, bowel or bladder dysfunction, fever, and history of cancer.

Specific Conditions Causing Back Pain in Older Adults

Lumbar Spinal Stenosis

Lumbar spinal stenosis is a common cause of back pain in people in their late 80s and 90s. The clinician must ensure, however, that the patient has the clinical picture of this syndrome, because lumbar spinal stenosis is frequently seen on spine imaging in patients without these features.

The stenosis results from a narrowing of either the central or lateral aspect of the lumbar spinal canal. Osteophytes of the facet joints often impinge on nerve roots of the lower lumbar region when they travel in the lateral recess of the canal. This space can also be compromised by lumbar disc displacement into the canal.

The characteristic symptom of lumbar spinal stenosis is pain in the back radiating into the buttocks or legs that is worse on standing and walking, particularly downhill, and is relieved with sitting. A similar clinical syndrome can be seen in patients with osteoarthritis of the hips. The anatomy of the lumbar spine explains the symptoms: flexion of the lumbar spine results in an increase in spinal cord volume and a decrease in nerve root bulk, whereas extension of the lumbar spine results in a decrease in spinal canal volume and an increase in nerve root bulk. Therefore, positions that flex the spine, such as sitting, bending forward, walking up hill, or lying in a flexed position, all relieve symptoms. Positions that extend the spine, such as prolonged standing, walking, and walking downhill, exacerbate the symptoms.

Patients with lumbar spinal stenosis may develop sciatic pain with standing and walking. Pain in the calf when walking can mimic the claudication of arterial insufficiency and is referred to as pseudoclaudication. Patients with arterial insufficiency usually get relief of claudication when they stop walking and stand still. Patients with lumbar spinal stenosis usually do not get relief unless they sit down. Patients who can flex their spine when walking with a shopping cart or walker often can walk much further without pain. Patients with this condition usually have progressive and consistent symptoms. There is often subtle weakness of the muscles innervated by the L4, L5, and S1 nerve roots.

Given the pathophysiology of this condition, with bony encroachment into the lumbar canal, it is not surprising that conservative therapy has limited use. There is no clear evidence that physical therapy, exercise regimens, or medications alter the natural history of this condition. A study of epidural steroid injections for spinal stenosis demonstrated minimal or no short-term benefit compared with epidural injections of lidocaine alone. A randomized multicenter study did demonstrate that surgical treatment was more effective than conservative therapy. For patients who are not candidates for spinal surgery, the use of a rolling walker with an attached seat can be very helpful. This device can substantially improve quality of life and mobility of patients with this condition.

Sciatica

In addition to the pseudoclaudication syndrome, older adults can also develop a typical sciatica syndrome similar to that seen in younger individuals. Acute sciatica usually occurs spontaneously, with no obvious causal event. This pain can be felt in any position and is usually not relieved with sitting. The neuropathic component of this pain often causes a good deal of night discomfort. The clinical course in younger people is quite variable. In a review of patients in placebo groups, 50% were significantly improved in 10 days, whereas 80% had remission of symptoms within 8 weeks in another study. No studies have specifically evaluated sciatica in older adults.

Osteoporotic Vertebral Compression Fractures

About 25% of women will experience a vertebral compression fracture in their lifetime. This condition is unique in that only one-third of patients with these fractures have symptoms, but these symptoms can be quite severe. The onset of pain is typically abrupt with pain felt deep in the site of the fracture. The pain is usually worse on standing and walking and relieved with lying down. Although the pain may radiate to the flank or legs, neurologic sequelae are unusual. The diagnosis is usually made on a plain radiograph of the lumbar or thoracic spine.

The natural history of this pain in most individuals is good. In one study, analgesic use decreased by 16% at day 5 and by 33% at day 14. In another study, patients in the control group had a significant reduction in pain by 3 months. Patients usually have restricted activity for approximately 1 month after a fracture. Patients with these fractures are more likely to have further fractures, become more disabled, and have a higher mortality rate than those without fractures. It is hard to determine whether these fractures are markers of or actually causative of frailty.

There has been a good deal of controversy about the role of vertebroplasty and kyphoplasty in management of these patients. There is general consensus that conservative management with analgesics is successful in roughly two-thirds of patients with these fractures. Most authors indicate that the use of vertebroplasty and kyphoplasty should be reserved for patients who do not respond to conservative management. However, there is no clear evidence that these procedures are better than sham procedures for patients with chronic pain secondary to vertebral compression fractures. A number of studies have shown that calcitonin has analgesic effect in management of these fractures. The most important intervention for patients with vertebral compression fractures is treatment for osteoporosis. Hip fractures have significantly more adverse effects than vertebral compression fractures.

Osteoporotic Sacral Fractures

Osteoporotic sacral fractures in older women can cause spontaneous buttock, pelvic, and low back pain. Sacral tenderness on physical examination is usually present. The incidence of associated additional osteoporotic fractures is high. Plain radiographs are usually negative. Technetium bone scans demonstrate a characteristic H-shaped uptake over the sacrum. A CT scan shows displacement of the interior border of the sacrum. The pain usually resolves over 4-8 weeks.

Nonspecific Low Back Pain

Many older adults have nonspecific low back pain that is mechanical in origin. Although much has been learned about specific conditions that affect the back in older adults, such as lumbar spinal stenosis and vertebral compression fractures, very little is known about nonspecific mechanical low back pain, other than that these conditions are quite common and relatively short-lived. In the Framingham study, 22% of patients ≥68 years old had back pain on most days. A 10-year study of 550 community-dwelling adults ≥70 years old documented 1,528 episodes of low back pain severe enough to restrict activity. Of these episodes, 80% lasted less than 1 month and only 6.4% lasted longer than 3 months.

As in younger individuals, the best way to determine the probable cause of the pain in older adults is the history and physical examination. Diagnostic images demonstrate many abnormalities in asymptomatic patients. It is thus difficult to ascribe the pain to one of these abnormalities.

Mechanical pain usually has a relatively sudden onset and is exacerbated by positions that stress the lumbar spine such as going from supine to sitting, getting in and out of bed, bending, lifting, or putting on socks and shoes. If there is weakness of the L4-5 and L5-S1 innervated muscles, the pain is likely due to a displacement of disc material. Herniation of the nucleus pulposus is unlikely in older adults, because the water content of this structure decreases dramatically with age. It is no longer gel-like and, therefore, much less apt to herniate.

> **CHOOSING WISELY® RECOMMENDATIONS**
>
> *Musculoskeletal Pain*
>
> - Avoid NSAIDs in individuals with hypertension, heart failure, or chronic kidney disease of all causes, including diabetes mellitus.
> - Do not perform imaging for lower back pain within the first 6 weeks unless red flags are present (severe or progressive neurologic deficits or when serious underlying conditions are present).

REFERENCES

- Bennell KL, Egerton T, Martin, J, et al. Effect of physical therapy on pain and function in patients with hip osteoarthritis. *JAMA*. 2014;311:1987–1997.

    In this controlled trial of physical therapy versus sham therapy for patients with hip osteoarthritis, physical therapy did not result in greater improvement in pain or function than the sham treatment (inactive ultrasound and inert gel).

- Bronfort G, Evans R, Anderson AV, et al. Spinal manipulation, medication, or home exercise with advice for acute and subacute neck pain. *Ann Intern Med*. 2012;156:1–10.

    In this controlled trial of spinal manipulation therapy, medication, and home exercise with advice for patients with acute and subacute neck pain, spinal manipulation had a significant advantage over medication. No important differences in pain were found between spinal manipulation therapy and home exercise with advice. Both exercise and manipulation were superior to medications.

- Friedly JL, Comstock BA, Turner JA, et al. A randomized trial of epidural glucocorticoid injections for spinal stenosis. *N Engl J Med*. 2014;371:11–21.

    Patients with lumbar spinal stenosis, leg pain, and disability were randomized to receive epidural injections of glucocorticoids plus lidocaine or lidocaine alone. At 6 weeks follow-up, there was no significant difference in disability score or the intensity of leg pain in the two groups.

- Graven-Nielsen T. Arendt-Nielsen L. Assessment of mechanisms in localized and widespread musculoskeletal pain. *Nat Rev Rheumatol*. 2010:6:599–606.

    This article reviews the manifestations, assessment methods, and mechanisms underlying localized and widespread musculoskeletal pain. It includes a number of studies done over the years on referred pain and pain perception. This is a good review of the topic of referred pain.

- Katz JN, Brophy RH, Chaisson CC, et al. Surgery versus physical therapy for a meniscal tear and osteoarthritis. *N Engl J Med*. 2013;368:1675–1684.

    This study evaluated the outcomes in patients with knee osteoarthritis and a meniscal tear. Patients were randomized to surgery and a physical therapy regimen. After 6 months, there were no significant differences between the study groups in functional improvement. However, 30% of the patients assigned to physical therapy alone underwent surgery within 6 months.

- Makris UE, Fraenkel L. Han L, et al. Epidemiology of restricting back pain in community-living older persons. *J Am Geriatr Soc*. 2011;56:610–614.

    In this prospective cohort study, 550 community-living men and women ≥70 years old were followed for 10 years; 77% of men and 81% of women had at least one episode of back pain that restricted activity. The median duration was 1 month, and only 6% of back pain episodes lasted for ≥3 consecutive months. This study demonstrates that most back pain in older individuals has a good natural history and lasts <1 month.

Leo M. Cooney, Jr., MD

CHAPTER 58—RHEUMATOLOGY

KEY POINTS

- Osteoarthritis is the most common cause of chronic pain among older adults and leads to considerable morbidity and disability.

- History and physical examination remain the most important tools in diagnosing and distinguishing among the rheumatologic diseases, although laboratory tests and imaging studies can be helpful to confirm clinical suspicion.

- When developing treatment plans for older adults with rheumatologic disease, it is important to keep in mind each patient's comorbid medical conditions, functional status, and the potential for drug-drug and drug-disease interactions.

- Interventions ideally use a multimodal approach, including pharmacologic and nonpharmacologic treatments as well as rehabilitation modalities

OSTEOARTHRITIS

Osteoarthritis (OA) is the most common source of joint pain, and chronic pain, among older adults. Recent estimates suggest OA affects approximately 27 million people in the United States alone. Depending on the source of data and which joint is involved, OA is present in 50%–90% of older adults. OA is the principal cause of knee, hip, and back pain in older adults, and it is expected to increase in both incidence and prevalence as the population ages. Yet, caution needs to be exercised to avoid the reflexive conclusion that all joint pain in the geriatric age group is necessarily the result of underlying OA. Differential diagnosis of OA includes inflammatory and crystal arthritides, as well as septic arthritis and bone pain due to malignancy.

Cartilage degeneration is the hallmark of OA, with fibrillation and ulceration that begins superficially and eventually extends into deeper layers. However, evidence indicates that OA is not a purely degenerative disease restricted to the cartilage; subchondral bone abnormalities and focal synovial inflammation have also been seen in pathologic specimens. These pathologic characteristics are thought to arise as a result of repetitive cycles of degradation and repair responses that eventually become inadequate to maintain joint health. Inflammatory cytokines, matrix-degrading metalloproteinase enzymes, and chondrocyte apoptosis are likely contributors to this process.

OA commonly affects the hands, knees, hips, and cervical and lumbar spine, but it can develop in any joint that has suffered injury or other disease. On examination, bony enlargement and crepitus suggest OA. In the fingers, bony enlargement occurs in the distal interphalangeal joint (Heberden nodes) and in the proximal interphalangeal joints (Bouchard nodes). Osteophytes are the radiographic counterpart of this enlargement, and asymmetric joint space narrowing is common (Figure 58.1). Joint tenderness and warmth may appear, but true synovitis suggests an alternative or concomitant diagnosis. Advanced imaging studies are generally not indicated in patients with OA, although MRI can be helpful in certain circumstances. MRI should not be used as an initial diagnostic tool in the evaluation of chronic joint pain. Rather, MRI is typically reserved for patients who are experiencing progressing neurologic deficits or are considering surgical intervention.

The objectives of OA management are to alleviate painful symptoms, prevent disease progression, maximize function, and minimize disease-related complications. Obesity is a modifiable risk factor for OA, and weight reduction can help reduce pain and improve function in patients with OA of the knee, hip, or spine. Use of thermal agents is recommended for relief of pain and stiffness related to hand, knee, and hip OA, although patients should be cautioned regarding the risk of burning the skin if heating agents are used. Assessment of the older adult with OA should include evaluation of the patient's ability to perform daily activities. Many assistive devices can be recommended, including jar or bottle openers, walking aids, braces, and insoles, depending on the activity that is most difficult for the patient. In knee OA, braces can alleviate patellofemoral symptoms by improving patellar tracking and can provide a greater sense of joint stability by improving joint proprioception. Specific orthoses designed to reduce medial knee pain by unloading the medial compartment of the knee include a valgus unloader brace and a lateral wedge insole. A well-designed running shoe can also lessen pain and damage by decreasing the impact transmitted during ambulation. Finally, a properly fitted and used cane can provide stability as well as unloading the symptomatic knee or hip.

Physical activity is a critical component in the treatment of OA-related pain. Regular physical activity is associated with decreased pain, improvement in functional status, and decreased disability. The CDC and Arthritis Foundation recommend a minimum of 150 minutes (2.5 hours) of moderate intensity aerobic exercise along with two days of muscle strengthening exercise per week to improve pain and functioning in patients with OA, although these guidelines do not apply specifically to older adults. For patients with significant

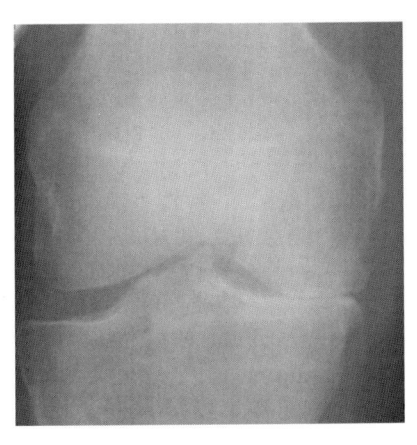

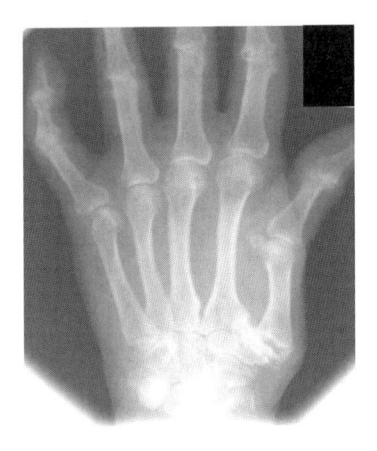

Figure 58.1—*Left:* Radiographic osteoarthritis of the knee with medial compartment osteophytes, joint space narrowing, and sclerosis. *Right:* Radiographic osteoarthritis of the hand with osteophytes, asymmetric joint space narrowing, and sclerosis of varying degrees of the thumb base (carpometacarpal joint) and proximal interphalangeal joints

pain and disability, achieving this level of activity may initially be difficult. Some studies suggest that simply adopting a more active lifestyle can improve pain and functional status; for example, one study found walking >6,000 steps per day to be protective against developing functional limitation related to OA. Additionally, regular physical activity has the additional benefit of promoting weight loss, which can further improve pain control. A multimodal interdisciplinary approach, including referral to physical and occupational therapy, is key in management of chronic pain related to OA. Physical and occupational therapists can help older adults maintain and often improve their functional status by implementing individualized therapy programs, assessing ability to perform activities of daily living (ADLs), providing recommendations about assistive devices to improve functioning, and training patients and caregivers in fall prevention.

The American Geriatrics Society (AGS) 2009 guidelines on the management of persistent pain (www.americangeriatrics.org/files/documents/2009_Guideline.pdf) is an appropriate resource to consult when managing OA-related pain. Traditionally, first-line therapy has been "around the clock" dosing of acetaminophen, with a maximum daily dose of 4 g in 24 hours; however, more recent evidence suggests that this therapy is not as effective as previously thought. Topical therapies (eg, analgesic balms, capsaicin, topical NSAIDs) can be helpful in hand or knee OA (SOE=C). NSAIDs should be used with caution in older adults because of known GI and renal adverse effects. NSAIDs can be used for an acute flare of OA, but use should be limited to the lowest dose and shortest duration possible. A proton-pump inhibitor should be added for GI protection if NSAIDs are used for longer duration. Tramadol can be tried for pain refractory to optimal acetaminophen or NSAID dosing. Low-dose narcotic medications may be considered in those who do not respond to acetaminophen, NSAIDs, or tramadol. Use of opioid medications for OA should be limited to those whose quality of life is significantly impacted by pain, and risks and benefits of use must always be considered. Studies evaluating glucosamine and chondroitin sulfate for pain have conflicting results, with more recent higher quality studies showing no superiority over placebo for patients with knee OA (SOE=A). Glucocorticoid injections are a reasonable treatment option for knee OA, and studies suggest they provide short-term relief that is superior to placebo. However, data supporting long-term relief from steroid injections are limited. Hyaluronic acid and hyaluronan polymers given in a series of weekly injections in the knee are approved for intra-articular viscosupplementation therapy; however, they are not shown to be more effective than placebo. For hip OA, glucocorticoid steroid injections have been shown to provide only temporary relief as compared with placebo. Prior studies have suggested that use of intra-articular steroids for hip OA could increase risk of postoperative infection after hip arthroplasty; however, evidence of this association is limited.

Surgical interventions, most commonly joint replacement, can be considered for patients with advanced OA who are 1) refractory to conservative management, 2) have identified clear impairments in function and reduced quality of life as a result of the OA, 3) are deemed appropriate surgical candidates, or 4) are aware of and motivated to participate in postsurgical rehabilitation. Arthroscopic debridement for knee OA is usually reserved for patients who report mechanical symptoms (eg, locking, "giveway" weakness), but effectiveness has not been proved (SOE=C), and initial treatment with physical therapy has shown similar outcomes when compared with surgical intervention. Total joint arthroplasty can be considered in patients with more extensive, disabling disease of the knee or hip. Although surgery remains the definitive intervention, it should be performed when the patient is likely to be able to withstand both the surgery and the ensuing rehabilitation.

RHEUMATOID ARTHRITIS

Although less prevalent than osteoarthritis, rheumatoid arthritis (RA) is an important disease in older adults. Up to 40% of patients with RA are >60 years old; some of these individuals have aged with the disease, whereas 20%–55% develop RA later in life. As with OA, the incidence and prevalence of RA in older adults is expected to increase as the population ages. Compared with the general population, patients with RA have an increased incidence of cardiovascular disease and an increased risk of premature death.

Most older adults with late-onset RA present similarly to young adults, with acute seropositive inflammatory polyarthritis that involves the small joints of the hands and feet. Those who develop RA in later life have marked early morning stiffness and prominent upper extremity pain, especially involving the shoulders, wrists, metacarpophalangeal and proximal interphalangeal joints. There are two additional seronegative presentations that are unique to older adults. The "RS3PE" syndrome consists of remitting seronegative symmetrical synovitis with pitting edema, and accounts for approximately 10% of late-onset inflammatory arthritis cases. Additionally, there is an acute onset, seronegative, inflammatory arthritis of the shoulder and hips similar to polymyalgia rheumatica (PMR), which accounts for approximately 25% of late-onset RA cases and can be difficult to distinguish from PMR. In fact, descriptive studies suggest that late-onset RA should be considered in the differential diagnosis of PMR and vice versa. Other diseases that mimic RA include calcium pyrophosphate dihydrate deposition disease (CPPD) and polyarthritis related to malignancy.

As with young adults, the diagnosis of RA relies on history, physical examination, radiologic, and laboratory criteria. When compared with younger adults, older adults more frequently present with constitutional symptoms such as malaise, fever, fatigue, and weight loss, in addition to the characteristic synovitis of RA. Older adults with RA are also more likely to have a higher initial erythrocyte sedimentation rate (ESR). Evaluation of possible RA in older adults should include checking autoantibodies, including rheumatoid factor (RF) and anti-cyclic citrullinated peptide/protein antibodies (anti-CCP or ACPA). However, prevalence of autoantibodies increases with age, so caution should be exercised in interpreting individual laboratory abnormalities, particularly a positive RF. A positive anti-CCP antibody has improved specificity to RF alone. Radiographic evaluation can be helpful to demonstrate erosions or deformities that appear in more aggressive and long-standing disease.

Assessment of disease activity in RA includes symptoms (including reports of impairment or disability), physical examination, laboratory data, and imaging. This should be done on the initial visit and routinely thereafter to assess response to treatment. Symptoms to assess include pain intensity and location, duration of morning stiffness, severity of fatigue, and functional status. Physical examination includes a systematic examination of the number of tender and swollen joints, as well as evaluation for extra-articular manifestations, including rheumatoid nodules and other cutaneous manifestations, interstitial lung disease, pleuropericardial disease, vasculitis, ocular disease, and neuropathy. Routine laboratory monitoring includes acute phase reactants, such as ESR and C-reactive protein (CRP), which can serve as markers of disease activity, as well as CBCs, metabolic panels, and liver function tests to evaluate for potential toxicity if the patient is on disease-modifying antirheumatic drugs (DMARDs). Radiographs may be obtained periodically to assess for progression of disease.

Descriptive studies suggest that patients with seropositive RA, even if of late onset, should be managed aggressively, including use of DMARDs (SOE=B). Similar to management of RA in younger adults, treatment of RA in older adults should be started as soon as the diagnosis is made, with the goal of achieving remission or the lowest level of disease activity possible. Initial approach to treatment should include initiation of one or more oral DMARDs, depending on disease severity and comorbidities. In general, patients should be optimized on triple therapy with oral DMARDs before moving on to biologic treatments. Methotrexate is well tolerated, but older adults may require a lower dose; it should be given with daily folic acid supplementation. Cases of lymphoproliferative disease have been reported with long-term methotrexate treatment. Hydroxychloroquine is well tolerated, but patients must be monitored for retinal toxicity, which is problematic if macular degeneration is present at baseline. Safety and efficacy of sulfasalazine in older adults appears to be similar to that in younger adults, although dosing should be adjusted for renal function. Leflunomide has been demonstrated to prevent radiographic progression in younger adults, but experience is minimal in older adults (SOE=B). It has a relatively fast onset of action (about 4 weeks) compared with other DMARDs; however, its half-life is longer. Older agents, such as penicillamine, gold, and cyclophosphamide, are less well tolerated by older adults and are rarely used.

Many biologic agents for RA are now available, but experience with these agents in older adults is limited, so their use is generally reserved for those in whom conventional triple therapy with oral DMARDs has not been effective. These agents, given via subcutaneous injection or infusion, work by inhibiting tumor necrosis factor α (etanercept, infliximab, adalimumab, golimumab, and certolizumab), antagonizing the interleukin-1 receptor (anakinra), serving as a fusion protein co-stimulation modulator via inhibition of CD28 (abatacept), inhibiting janus kinase (JAK inhibitor [tofacitinib]), or binding the CD20 antigen on B-lymphocytes (rituximab). Infliximab, adalimumab, and rituximab all increase the risk of granulomatous infections with organisms such as *Mycobacterium tuberculosis*, atypical mycobacteria, yeast, *Listeria,* and *Nocardia*. Infliximab can also cause postinfusion fever, chills, headache, chest pain, and dyspnea. All of the biologic agents have been associated with bacterial respiratory tract infections. B lymphocyte–depleting therapies, such as rituximab, have been associated with reactivation of hepatitis B, especially when used in combination with prednisone. Patients taking these medications should be screened before initiating therapy, as there are now excellent medications for suppressing reactivation (eg, entecavir or lamivudine).

Low-dose prednisone (10–20 mg/d) may be used as the primary treatment for seronegative PMR-like disease and the "RS3PE" syndrome. However, in contrast to classic PMR, late-onset RA may not respond promptly to low-dose prednisone. Further, prednisone alone is often not sufficient in managing seropositive RA but may be useful as an adjunctive agent. In general, chronic use of prednisone should be avoided, because its use is associated with increased risk of infectious complications, fluid retention, and osteoporosis.

GOUT

Gout is a crystal-induced arthropathy that is more common in older adults than in younger adults. The global burden of gout is increasing, particularly in high-income countries; this has been attributed both to the aging of the population as well as rising rates of obesity. Hyperuricemia and gout are associated with cardiovascular disease and metabolic syndrome. Women generally do not develop gout until menopause, at which time the rate in women approaches that in men. Polypharmacy, including diuretic use, and higher incidence of renal and hepatic impairment also predispose older adults to accumulation of uric acid and development of gout.

Gout can cause both severe pain and disability. The clinical characteristics of gout can differ appreciably in older adults. Gout can present as a subacute smoldering oligoarthritis affecting larger joints like knee, wrist, shoulder, and ankle, rather than as an acute, monoarticular, and incapacitating attack, as in classic podagra affecting the first metatarsophalangeal joint. Tophaceous deposits in the distal and proximal interphalangeal joints can be mistaken for, or coexist with, osteoarthritis. Similarly, tophi at the extensor surfaces can be confused with rheumatoid nodules. Acute attacks can be precipitated by trauma, acute nonarticular illness requiring hospitalization, and abrupt changes in uric acid concentration (as can be seen with dehydration and particularly after surgery or admission for congestive heart failure with aggressive diuresis). An acute gout flare is characterized by abrupt onset of intense inflammation and pain, typically reaching maximum intensity within 12–24 hours, with resolution of symptoms within 7–10 days, even without treatment.

Gout is a microscopic diagnosis, requiring demonstration of monosodium urate crystals from synovial fluid or an aspirate of a tophus. Sodium urate crystals are needle-shaped, strongly negatively birefringent and can be demonstrated in synovial fluid obtained during an acute flare or in the intercritical phase. Radiographs may show juxta-articular erosions of the involved joints. An overhanging edge (ie, Martel sign) can be seen and is helpful in distinguishing gout from RA erosions. With rare exception, asymptomatic hyperuricemia precedes the development of gouty arthritis. Increased serum uric acid, along with a clinical history of episodic mono- or oligoarthritis (often podagra) is highly suggestive of gouty arthritis. However, hyperuricemia is not uniformly present at the time of an acute gout attack, and the presence of hyperuricemia alone neither confirms a diagnosis of gout nor necessitates starting urate-lowering medication.

Patients with gout should be counseled regarding lifestyle modifications that can help prevent recurrent episodes of gout. These interventions include weight loss, avoidance of purine-rich foods such as shellfish, mollusks, organ meats, and full-fat dairy products, and avoidance of alcohol, particularly beer, which is especially purine rich. The importance of these lifestyle modifications should be reinforced at each follow-up visit, because these changes can be difficult to implement and sustain but can be invaluable in prevention of future attacks. Topical therapy with ice is an important and effective adjunctive therapy for an acute gout attack. In patients with recurrent attacks, discontinuation of medications that increase uric acid accumulation should be considered; however, this is not always feasible in older adults with multiple comorbidities. Diuretics, niacin, and low-dose aspirin are among the medications that may predispose a patient to developing a gout attack.

Treatment of gout in older adults must be individualized, taking into account the potential for drug-drug and drug-disease interactions. An acute gout attack may be managed with a short-acting NSAID in those who can tolerate it, keeping in mind the potential for serious cardiovascular, GI, and renal adverse effects in older adults. Intra-articular glucocorticoids (assuming septic joint has been excluded) are preferred for attacks involving one joint such as the knee, ankle, or wrist. Alternatively, short-term oral glucocorticoids tapered over 5–10 days are preferred in managing a polyarticular gouty flare. Glucocorticoids may be preferable to NSAIDs in the treatment of gout in older adults with multiple comorbidities, because the typical complications of steroid use are generally not seen with short-term treatment. Colchicine can also be used to treat an acute gouty attack, although its use is often limited by presence of renal impairment. Previously, colchicine was dosed every 1–2 hours until resolution of symptoms or onset of adverse effects; however, this aggressive regimen has proved to be both excessive and poorly tolerated in older adults. Current evidence suggests that doses as low as 0.6 mg q8–24 hours can be effective in treating an acute attack.

Medications such as allopurinol, febuxostat, or probenecid are uric acid–lowering therapies used for longer term management. Chronic use of uric acid–lowering agents should be considered in patients with more than 2 attacks in a year, evidence of tophi, or erosive disease. Historically, these medications are not initiated during an acute gout attack; however, there is limited evidence showing that doing so would worsen the acute attack (so long as abortive therapy is also prescribed). Probenecid works as a uricosuric agent but is ineffective if creatinine clearance is <30–40 mL/min. Allopurinol and febuxostat lower serum uric acid via inhibition of xanthine oxidase and are beneficial in management of chronic gout; the dosage should be adjusted in patients with renal or hepatic impairment. Because uric acid–lowering therapy is initiated with the goal of lowering serum uric acid levels to 5–6 mg/dL, it is important to educate the patient that this drop in serum uric acid may precipitate a flare. Therefore, it is reasonable to use a prophylactic agent such as colchicine at dosages as low at 0.6 mg/d, renal function permitting, or low-dose prednisone for several months as the uric acid lowering therapy is titrated up. If the patient develops an acute gout attack while on a uric acid–lowering agent, it is important to continue taking the medication daily while adding an abortive treatment. While patients are on uric acid–lowering therapies, serum uric acid as well as renal and liver function should be monitored. During dosage titration, these values should be checked every 1–2 months, but frequency of testing may be reduced once on a consistent dose if uric acid is at goal and other values remain stable.

CALCIUM PYROPHOSPHATE DIHYDRATE DEPOSITION DISEASE

Calcium pyrophosphate dihydrate deposition disease (CPPD), like gout, is a crystal-induced arthropathy that is more common in older adults. CPPD, also known as "pseudogout," causes synovitis that can mimic RA, inflammatory osteoarthritis, gout, or septic arthritis. CPPD is associated with disorders of calcium metabolism (eg, hypomagnesemia, hypophosphatemia, and hyperparathyroidism), hypothyroidism, and hemochromatosis. CPPD of the wrist can mimic RA but can be distinguished by prominent synovitis and chondrocalcinosis of the wrist and/or metacarpophalangeal joints; it is rheumatoid factor and anti-CCP antibody negative. CPPD can also mimic inflammatory osteoarthritis but with rapid joint destruction of the wrist, patellofemoral knee compartment, and hip joint.

CPPD can result in an acute, intermittently inflammatory arthritis of the knee, hip, wrist, and metacarpophalangeal joints, with elbow, shoulder, and ankle involvement less common. CPPD can mimic an acute gout attack with sudden onset of pain and swelling that coincide with or immediately follow an acute illness or traumatic event such as surgery. When fever is present, distinguishing CPPD from septic arthritis is imperative, and diagnostic arthrocentesis is indicated.

Arthrocentesis with crystal analysis is diagnostic and useful to distinguish CPPD from gout and infection. CPPD crystals are weakly positively birefringent rhomboids or squares. CPPD is commonly suspected by the radiographic finding of chondrocalcinosis on plain films (Figure 58.2), which appears as a stippled or linear calcification of the articular cartilage of the knee, wrist, hip, shoulder, and symphysis pubis.

Intra-articular steroid injection can result in significant relief of painful symptoms with CPPD and may be the preferred management option if one joint is involved. Short-acting NSAIDs and oral steroidal agents are also useful in management of CPPD in patients who can tolerate them (SOE=C). Evidence for use of colchicine in CPPD is limited, and its use is largely based on anecdotal evidence and extrapolation from gout treatment. Oral colchicine may be used to treat acute flares of CPPD and is typically dosed 0.6 mg q8–24 hours, similar to acute gout treatment. Colchicine can also be useful to prevent future acute episodes of CPPD, typically at doses of 0.6 mg q12–24 hours.

POLYMYALGIA RHEUMATICA

Polymyalgia rheumatica (PMR) is an inflammatory rheumatic disease unique to older adults. PMR occurs almost exclusively in patients aged ≥50 years old,

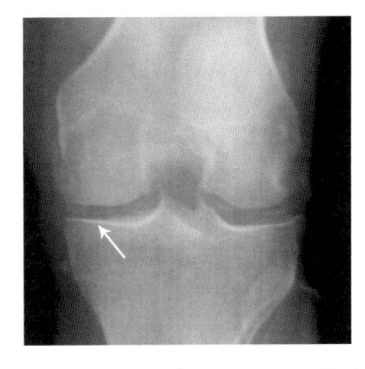

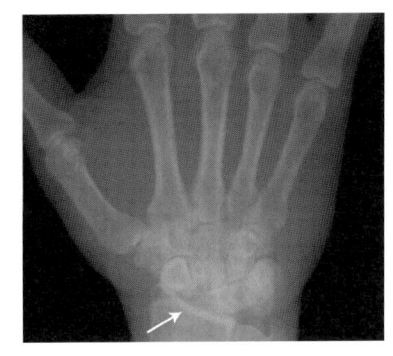

Figure 58.2—*Left:* Chondrocalcinosis of the meniscus. *Right:* Chondrocalcinosis of the triangular fibrocartilage of the wrist distal to the ulna

with most affected patients aged >70 years old. PMR is a relatively common condition, second in incidence only to RA among all of the inflammatory autoimmune rheumatic disorders. Approximately 53 new cases develop per 100,000 persons per year, with an estimated prevalence of 600 cases per 100,000 and higher prevalence with increasing age. Approximately 10%–20% of patients with PMR also have giant cell arteritis (GCA), whereas up to 50%–60% of patients with GCA will have symptoms of PMR. As such, diagnosis of one condition should prompt evaluation for the other.

PMR is characterized by persistent pain or stiffness of bilateral upper arms, shoulders, hips, or thighs that is accompanied by significant morning stiffness and constitutional symptoms of fatigue, low-grade fever, anorexia, and weight loss. In 2012, the European League Against Rheumatism (EULAR) and the American College of Rheumatology (ACR) released guidelines for the classification of PMR. Although these criteria were developed as a research tool, rather than specific diagnostic criteria, this classification system can be helpful in assessing patients with suspected PMR. Criteria require age ≥50 years old, bilateral shoulder pain or aching not explained by another etiology, and increased ESR and/or CRP. If all 3 required criteria are present, the diagnosis of PMR is then suggested based on a scoring system that includes morning stiffness that lasts >45 minutes, negative RF and/or anti-CCP antibodies, pain or limited range of motion of the hips, or absence of other joint involvement. Addition of ultrasound findings of unilateral or bilateral subdeltoid bursitis, biceps tenosynovitis, glenohumeral synovitis, hip synovitis, or trochanteric bursitis increases specificity of the criteria.

Differential diagnosis of PMR is broad, including RA (particularly the RS3PE and polymyalgia rheumatic variations), dermatomyositis, polymyositis, fibromyalgia, drug-induced myalgia or myositis, multiple myeloma, osteoarthritis, depression, vasculitis, hypothyroidism, and endocarditis. Initial evaluation in older adults with suspected PMR should focus on history, physical examination, and laboratory findings to exclude alternative diagnoses. Patients frequently lack physical evidence of an inflammatory arthritis of the small hand joints, distinguishing PMR from RA, and they also have normal muscle bulk and strength, unlike in the inflammatory myopathies. Laboratory evaluation in PMR is typically characterized by increased ESR and/or CRP, along with negative RF, anti-CCP, and ANA, and normal levels of muscle enzymes. However, it is important to keep in mind the increasing prevalence of positive RF and ANA with age, independent of the presence of autoimmune disorders. Plain radiographs of involved joints should not reveal abnormalities, and the arthritis of PMR is not characterized by erosions. As noted in the EULAR/ACR criteria, ultrasound can be helpful in differentiating PMR from other noninflammatory conditions, although it is less helpful in distinguishing PMR from RA. Recent studies of PMR have confirmed the presence of synovitis identical to that seen in RA, with synovial thickening, effusions, and lymphocytic synovial infiltration.

Corticosteroids are the cornerstone of treatment of PMR. Doses required for treatment of PMR are much lower than those used in treatment of GCA. Symptoms should typically respond dramatically and quickly, within 7 days or less, to doses of prednisone of ~10–20 mg/d. Concomitant GCA or an alternative diagnosis of RA should be considered in patients whose response to therapy is incomplete or not sustained. The duration of treatment required varies considerably, from 3 months to several years. Dosage reduction of steroids should be gradual, with periodic monitoring for symptom recurrence and laboratory studies (CRP, ESR) suggesting recurrence. For a starting dose of 20 mg daily, it is recommended to taper by 2.5 mg per week until a dose of 10 mg is reached. Taper should then be slowed further, decreasing by 1 mg every month. However, dose reduction should be individualized, based on signs and symptoms of inflammation. Typically, addition of an adjunctive agent such as methotrexate is not necessary initially, because PMR characteristically responds well to steroids alone. However, in patients at high risk of complications from prolonged glucocorticoid use, or who are unable to taper the dose effectively, methotrexate can be considered as a steroid-sparing agent. Osteoporosis prophylaxis with a bisphosphonate is recommended for patients on prednisone dosages of ≥7.5 mg/d for ≥3 months.

GIANT CELL ARTERITIS

Giant cell arteritis (GCA) is a granulomatous vasculitis that involves large and medium-sized arteries. Like PMR, GCA is a disease unique to older adults, occurring almost exclusively in patients ≥50 years old, and increasing in incidence with age. As noted previously, the overlap between GCA and PMR is notable; therefore, patients with PMR with any symptoms above the neck should have a temporal artery biopsy to evaluate for GCA.

The most well-known presentation of GCA is that of cranial arteritis that may result in visual loss; however, GCA may also present initially with extracranial arteritis, systemic inflammatory symptoms, PMR, or any combination of these manifestations. Head and neck manifestations of GCA include headache, scalp tenderness, jaw or tongue claudication, diplopia, and prominent tender, erythematous, or nodular temporal arteries, which are typically pulseless. Constitutional symptoms, including fatigue, malaise, weight loss, and fever, are common and may be the only manifestations of GCA. Optic nerve pallor or swelling portends ischemia with impending blindness that warrants immediate glucocorticoid therapy. GCA can also present as sudden blindness with no prior systemic illness. GCA may present with claudication in the arms, respiratory symptoms, transient ischemic attack, stroke, peripheral neuropathies, syncope, ischemic necrosis of tongue or scalp, or rarely myocardial infarction. Aortic aneurysm, predominantly thoracic, is a late manifestation of GCA even when previously appropriately treated. The incidence of aneurysm in GCA is about 10%, with discovery of thoracic and abdominal aneurysm occurring at a median of 5.8 and 2.5 years, respectively, after GCA diagnosis.

Laboratory evaluation of patients with suspected GCA is characterized by increased ESR and/or CRP. Patients may have other laboratory manifestations of systemic inflammatory disease, including anemia of chronic inflammation, thrombocytosis, leukocytosis, hypoalbuminemia, and increased alkaline phosphatase. Serologic tests are generally not helpful in establishing the diagnosis of GCA, although a proportion of patients are anti-phospholipid or anti-ferritin antibody positive.

Although presumptive diagnosis of GCA is made based on history, physical examination, and laboratory findings, temporal artery biopsy is the gold standard for diagnosis. In fact, biopsy is the only test able to definitively diagnose GCA. A specimen several centimeters in length should be obtained from the symptomatic side and immediately processed by frozen-section staining of multiple cross- and longitudinal sections. Because of the focal and segmental nature of GCA, inflammation may be missed with initial biopsy; a section of the contralateral side can be obtained if the initial specimens are negative. Histologic examination shows vasculitis with mononuclear cell infiltrates and giant cells. Evidence of vasculitis without giant cells suggests other diagnoses (eg, polyarteritis nodosa) that may require cytotoxic therapy. Ultrasound, angiography, MRI with gadolinium, and positron emission tomography have been investigated as diagnostic modalities for demonstrating vascular inflammation; however, none has replaced biopsy as the gold standard diagnostic test.

Preferably with a positive biopsy confirming GCA, but often with a convincing history and symptoms (and negative biopsy), patients suspected of having GCA should start treatment with prednisone to reduce the risk of sudden blindness. If necessary, prednisone may be started before biopsy; fortunately for diagnostic purposes, pathologic evidence of GCA persists for up to 2 weeks after prednisone therapy has been started. Prednisone is given at a dosage of 40–60 mg/d and should be maintained for at least 1 month before considering dosage reduction. Initial treatment with intravenous glucocorticoids may be considered in patients presenting with transient or permanent vision loss, diplopia, transient ischemic attack, or stroke. Treatment typically continues for approximately 1–3 years. Long-term glucocorticoid therapy warrants prophylaxis for osteoporosis. Published studies of methotrexate as a steroid-sparing agent have not consistently demonstrated a benefit. In addition, concomitant administration of low-dose aspirin has been shown to decrease the risk of vision loss and cranial ischemic complications. Relapses are fairly common in patients with GCA, affecting 25%–65% of patients. Monitoring for return of symptoms of PMR or temporal arteritis, increase of inflammatory markers, and radiographic screening for aortic aneurysms should continue after immunosuppressive therapy is discontinued.

SYSTEMIC LUPUS ERYTHEMATOSUS

Systemic lupus erythematosus (SLE) is an autoimmune multisystem disease that most commonly affects women of child-bearing age, yet up to 20% of cases are seen in older adults. When onset is after 50 years of age, the condition is referred to as "late-onset lupus." Late-onset lupus shows less of a female predominance than traditional SLE.

In contrast to SLE in younger patients, late-onset lupus is characterized by a more insidious onset, less major organ involvement, and lower disease activity, making definitive diagnosis challenging. Late-onset lupus may present initially with vague symptoms, including fatigue, fever, weight loss, arthralgia, and myalgia, invoking a broad differential diagnosis. Late-onset lupus should be considered in the differential diagnosis of rash (need not be malar in distribution), nonerosive arthritis, serositis (pleuritis, pericarditis), cytopenias (leukopenia, hemolytic anemia, or thrombocytopenia), neuropsychiatric symptoms (cognitive, seizures), sicca symptoms (in the absence of medication-induced dry mouth), and Raynaud phenomenon. Renal involvement (eg, urinary casts, proteinuria) is less common in older lupus patients than in younger lupus patients. Additional physical findings can include periungual or palmar erythema, asymptomatic oral or nasal ulcers, and livedo reticularis; when present, these should raise suspicion of anticardiolipin antibody syndrome (venous or arterial thromboembolic phenomena).

The more characteristic features of SLE, such as malar rash, photosensitivity, arthritis, and nephritis, are less common at presentation of late-onset lupus, and older patients typically fulfill fewer ACR criteria for the classification of SLE than younger patients. In contrast, pulmonary involvement and serositis seem to be more common in late-onset lupus. These differences in the presentation of late-onset lupus can contribute to a significant delay in diagnosis.

Diagnosis of SLE, particularly in older adults, requires a detailed history, thorough physical examination, and laboratory investigation. Evaluation can be guided by the 1997 ACR criteria for the classification of SLE, which requires presence of any combination of 4 of 11 laboratory, examination, and historical criteria. History and physical examination should evaluate for rash, oral or nasal ulcers, nonerosive arthritis, evidence of serositis, cognitive or neurologic disorders, history of sicca symptoms that are not medication induced, and history of Raynaud phenomenon. Initial laboratory investigation should include a CBC to evaluate for cytopenias, metabolic panel, and urinalysis. Patients should undergo serologic testing for ANA, anti-double-stranded DNA, and anti-Smith antibodies. In late-onset lupus, patients are less likely to have positive anti-ribonucleoprotein or anti-Smith antibodies, but they are more frequently positive for rheumatoid factor (RF), ANA, anti-Ro/Sjögren syndrome (SS) A, and anti-La/SSB. Anti-double-stranded DNA and hypocomplementemia, both useful in monitoring disease activity in younger patients, are less frequently found in older patients.

Given the frequency of polypharmacy in older adults, it is especially important to distinguish late-onset lupus from drug-induced lupus erythematosus, although this is often clinically difficult. Both have a positive ANA test, although drug-induced lupus erythematosus is associated with a speckled pattern with antihistone antibodies.

Renal biopsy should be pursued to evaluate patients with proteinuria or who have active urine sediment to determine the underlying histopathology before starting treatment. Patients with evidence of thromboembolic disease should undergo serologic evaluation for antiphospholipid syndrome, which requires measurement of lupus anticoagulant, IgG and IgM anticardiolipin antibody levels, and IgG or IgM anti-β2 glycoprotein antibodies on 2 separate occasions at least 12 weeks apart.

Treatment of SLE, especially in older adults, should be based on the individual's specific disease manifestations, with careful surveillance for adverse effects of treatment. Treatment recommendations are based entirely on extrapolation from younger adults; no studies of these therapies have been conducted in older adults with lupus (SOE=D). If not contraindicated, short-acting NSAIDs can be used to treat arthritis and serositis in older adults who can tolerate them. It is important to use a gastroprotective proton-pump inhibitor if NSAID use is prolonged. Hydroxychloroquine is effective in managing skin and joint manifestations (200–400 mg/d). However, before hydroxychloroquine is initiated, older adults should be evaluated for age-associated macular degeneration, because this is a contraindication to its use. Patients should also be monitored annually for visual field deficits possibly related to drug-induced retinopathy while receiving hydroxychloroquine. Low-dose corticosteroid use may be considered in patients with symptoms refractory to hydroxychloroquine, although long-term use of steroids in older adults is associated with significant adverse effects that may outweigh potential benefits. Depending on the organ system involved and disease manifestation, methotrexate[OL], azathioprine[OL], mycophenolate mofetil[OL], or cyclosporine[OL] can be of benefit as corticosteroid-sparing agents, although safety of these drugs has not been studied specifically in older adults. Patients who have evidence for antiphospholipid syndrome should receive preventive anticoagulant as well as immunosuppressive therapy. High-dose steroids and cyclophosphamide are reserved for severe neuropsychiatric and renal manifestations of SLE.

SJÖGREN SYNDROME

Sjögren syndrome is a systemic, multiorgan chronic disease characterized by lymphocytic infiltration of exocrine glands. Sjögren syndrome may develop alone or in conjunction with other rheumatologic diseases, including RA, lupus erythematosus, scleroderma, or inflammatory myopathy, in which case it is classified as secondary Sjögren syndrome. The presence of palpable purpura and C4 hypocomplementemia are recognized as potential predictors for development of lymphoma.

The most well-known manifestations of Sjögren syndrome are symptoms of keratoconjunctivitis sicca, including ocular and oral dryness (xerophthalmia and xerostomia, respectively), which result from destruction of lacrimal and salivary glands. These symptoms are relatively common in older adults, and initial evaluation should focus on excluding drug-induced sicca symptoms, particularly due to anticholinergic adverse effects, as well as age-related exocrine gland fibrosis or fatty infiltration, or other underlying connective tissue syndromes. It is important to remember that Sjögren syndrome is not limited to the lacrimal and salivary glands; it may present with dysphagia, weight loss, vaginal dryness, or sexual dysfunction. Sjögren syndrome may also cause extraglandular disease, including renal, bladder, liver, biliary, thyroid, nervous system, and skin manifestations. As such, Sjögren syndrome should be considered in patients with interstitial lung disease, malabsorption, CNS disease that mimics multiple sclerosis, unexplained renal, liver, or thyroid disease, or rash.

Evaluation of a patient with possible Sjögren syndrome includes an ophthalmologic examination with a Schirmer test and slit-lamp examination to assess for corneal damage and confirm the presence of keratoconjunctivitis. Laboratory evaluation should include ANA, anti-Ro/SSA, anti-La/SSB, and RF (usually positive). Biopsy of a salivary gland may show focal lymphocytic sialadenitis, whereas either sialometry or salivary gland scintigraphy can be used to assess salivary gland function. Biopsy of a skin rash can verify the presence of cutaneous vasculitis.

Sugar-free candies and artificial saliva can alleviate symptoms of xerostomia. Patients should be counseled on the importance of maintaining good dental health to prevent caries (they are at higher risk with xerostomia), gum disease, and dental erosions. Pilocarpine and cevimeline can be used to treat xerostomia; however, their use in older adults is limited by cholinergic adverse effects. Symptomatic treatment of xerophthalmia consists of lubricating ointments and artificial tears. Punctal plugs can be tried to retain tears. Ophthalmic cyclosporine or tacrolimus can be used to treat inflammatory eye disease. Treatment of an underlying inflammatory disease (eg, RA, systemic lupus erythematosus, myositis, or scleroderma) will usually improve symptoms as well.

POLYMYOSITIS AND DERMATOMYOSITIS

Inflammatory muscle diseases, including polymyositis and dermatomyositis, form a heterogeneous and uncommon group of skeletal muscle diseases. Incidence of these diseases peaks in adults in their 50s, but they can occur at any age, and studies suggest that up to 20% of cases occur in adults ≥65 years old. Inclusion body myositis is another type of idiopathic inflammatory myopathy that can be seen in older adults. In contrast to polymyositis and dermatomyositis, inclusion body myositis may be more insidious in onset, affects men more frequently than women, and causes both proximal and distal muscle weakness. Response to steroids or other immunosuppressive therapy is generally poor in inclusion body myositis, with disease progression despite treatment.

Muscle weakness is the central feature of polymyositis and dermatomyositis, and it is most prominent in the proximal muscle groups. Patients report difficulty with tasks such as standing from a chair, ascending stairs, or lifting a light package above the head. Muscle tenderness is usually not a manifestation and should raise suspicion of other conditions. Arthritis, when present, is inflammatory and occasionally erosive, suggesting overlap with RA. Esophageal dysmotility can cause dysphagia, hoarseness, and aspiration. Arrhythmia, symptoms of congestive heart disease, dyspnea on exertion, or persistent cough can also be present and suggest cardiac muscle involvement or coexistent interstitial lung disease. Pulmonary involvement, including interstitial lung disease and diaphragmatic insufficiency, is a poor prognostic sign associated with increased morbidity and mortality. Raynaud phenomenon or Sjögren syndrome can also be present. Dermatomyositis is characterized by a facial rash that can involve the eyelids (heliotrope) or the nose and malar areas, or be more generalized. Rash can also be apparent over the neck and upper torso in sun-exposed areas. Gottron papules (skin thickening over the metacarpophalangeal and interphalangeal joints) can also be seen.

Differential diagnosis of myositis includes endocrine, metabolic, musculoskeletal, and medication-related disorders, including thyroid disorders, diabetes, vitamin D deficiency, electrolyte abnormalities, PMR, and medication adverse effects from steroids or statins. Statins are perhaps the most widely used medication with risk of toxic myopathy, with increased risk in older adults; statins have been associated with myalgia in 5%–10% of patients, myositis in 1%, and rhabdomyolysis in 0.1%, and up to 25% may develop exercise-related muscle cramping or pain. In patients with suspected myositis, initial evaluation should focus on excluding other more common causes of muscle weakness before pursuing invasive testing with muscle biopsy. Serum levels of muscle enzymes (creatine kinase, aldolase, and sometime transaminases) are usually increased in myositis; normal levels suggest an alternative diagnosis. Electromyographic testing is used to exclude neuropathy and to identify the presence of an irritable myopathy. MRI using fat-suppression sequences helps to confirm myositis and can help to select which muscle to biopsy. Muscle biopsy remains the gold standard to confirm the diagnosis and also to distinguish among the subtypes of myositis. A diagnosis of polymyositis warrants an evaluation for cardiac and pulmonary disease. A diagnosis of dermatomyositis, and less so with polymyositis, warrants heightened suspicion for an underlying malignancy. Dermatomyositis and polymyositis have been associated with increased incidence of underlying colon, lung, breast, prostate, ovarian, and uterine cancers. However, extensive evaluation for occult malignancy is costly and is not without risks. It is recommended that patients with dermatomyositis and polymyositis simply undergo age-appropriate cancer screening, although physicians should keep in mind this increased incidence of malignancy when evaluating any new or abnormal signs or symptoms.

Response to therapy in older adults with polymyositis and dermatomyositis is lower than that in younger adults. Glucocorticoids are the initial therapy for polymyositis and dermatomyositis. Oral prednisone at 1 mg/kg/d is a typical starting dosage; for severe disease, an initial dose of methylprednisolone 1,000 mg IV is often used over 3 consecutive days. Prednisone can be tapered after an initial phase of improved muscle strength and normalized muscle enzyme concentrations. However, prolonged glucocorticoid use at high dosages can result in a myopathy with resultant proximal muscle weakness. Therefore, tapering the total dose by 10%–20% per month should be attempted. Methotrexate[OL], given orally or parenterally, in a weekly pulse regimen can be combined with corticosteroids and can also have a steroid-sparing effect in long-term therapy. Weekly oral methotrexate[OL] or mycophenolate mofetil[OL] may be effective in managing refractory skin manifestations of dermatomyositis. Because of hepatic and pulmonary toxicity of methotrexate, azathioprine[OL] may be a favorable alternative in patients with interstitial lung disease or underlying liver disease. Intravenous immunoglobulin can be an effective therapy in refractory dermatomyositis and is generally considered relatively safe, although older adults are at increased risk of renal failure and thrombotic events.

Supervised exercise over 6-week and 6-month study periods has proved beneficial in polymyositis (SOE=B), improving function without aggravating underlying disease.

FIBROMYALGIA

Fibromyalgia is a pain syndrome that incorporates both physical and psychological components. Because of its heterogeneous presentation, fibromyalgia can be challenging to diagnose and manage, particularly in older adults. Generalized body pain is the hallmark of fibromyalgia, which can be associated with various other complaints, including mood disturbance, fatigue, cognitive disorders, and a variety of somatic symptoms, including but not limited to irritable bowel syndrome, fatigue, muscle pain, headache, and sleep disturbance.

Fibromyalgia is a clinical diagnosis, which was redefined by the 2010 ACR criteria. Diagnosis is made on the basis of Widespread Pain Index and Symptom Severity scores, with symptoms present for at least 3 months and no other explanation for symptoms. Diagnosis of fibromyalgia no longer includes tender point examination, which was previously included in 1990 diagnostic criteria. Thorough history and physical examination are central to the diagnosis of fibromyalgia. Aside from generalized soft-tissue sensitivity, physical examination in patients with fibromyalgia should be normal for age. Importantly, patients with fibromyalgia will not have evidence of inflammation or synovitis on physical examination. Likewise, laboratory abnormalities such as an increased ESR or CRP should prompt investigation for an alternative diagnosis.

It is especially important in older adults to ensure that the diagnosis of fibromyalgia is accurate and that symptoms cannot be attributed to another condition. Diagnosis of fibromyalgia is complex in older adults, because widespread pain is more common in this population, and older adults may have multiple comorbid conditions with overlapping symptoms. Chronic pain from a variety of sources, including osteoarthritis, neuropathy, and degenerative spinal disease, may coincide with fibromyalgia, making differentiation of the source of chronic pain challenging. Differential diagnosis in fibromyalgia includes musculoskeletal, endocrine, psychiatric, and medication-related disorders, including RA, PMR, myositis, osteoarthritis, hypothyroidism, vitamin D deficiency, depression, and medication adverse effects (eg, from statins, bisphosphonates, and proton-pump inhibitors).

Pathophysiology of fibromyalgia remains unclear, but current theories suggest central pain sensitization as a result of dysregulation of pain processing. Although up to one-third of patients may have a clear inciting event, most patients with fibromyalgia have no identifiable cause.

Treatment of fibromyalgia, particularly in older adults, should be focused on nonpharmacologic therapies. Studies have shown that physical activity, patient education, and cognitive behavioral therapy can improve symptoms. When encouraging physical activity in patients with chronic pain syndromes, it can be helpful to distinguish between "hurt" and "harm." Although increasing activity may temporarily cause increased physical pain, it can be reassuring to emphasize that pain is not necessarily harmful, and that in the long-term, physical activity is an essential component of managing this condition. Increasing physical activity slowly and in small increments that are easily sustainable in daily life is critical. It is important to use a multimodal approach to treat fibromyalgia; chronic pain, sleep disturbances, and depression and anxiety must each be addressed individually to optimize efficacy of treatment.

Few pharmacologic treatments have proved effective in treatment of fibromyalgia. There are 3 FDA approved medications for fibromyalgia: pregabalin, duloxetine, and milnacipran. Other medications, including acetaminophen, anticonvulsants, antidepressants, and weak opioids such as tramadol, have been used in treatment of fibromyalgia, although studies have not specifically evaluated their use in older adults. Most medications used in treatment of fibromyalgia provide only modest benefits despite carrying considerable risk of adverse effects, including sedation, cognitive deficits, insomnia, balance impairment, and falls. Pharmacologic therapy should be individualized based on specific symptoms, and medication regimens should be frequently reassessed to evaluate for effectiveness and adverse effects. Perhaps the most crucial aspect of treatment of fibromyalgia is formation of a therapeutic alliance between physician and patient. By setting realistic expectations, expressing commitment to finding solutions, and, most importantly, being available to provide support and reassurance, physicians can ultimately help improve treatment outcomes for their patients with chronic pain syndromes.

Choosing Wisely® Recommendations

Rheumatology

- Use biologic DMARDs only after failure of nonbiologic DMARDs.

References

- Ferrell B, Aregoff CE, Epplin J, et al. Pharmacological management of persistent pain in older persons. *J Am Geriatr Soc.* 2009;57(8):1331–1346.

    This publication provides an update to the 2002 American Geriatrics Society clinical practice guidelines for the management of persistent pain in older adults, which incorporates new evidence and novel pharmacologic agents. The guideline reviews currently available, evidence-based therapies for chronic pain, with recommendations provided by expert consensus with specific focus on treating older adults.

- Hochberg MC, Altman RD, April KT, et al. American College of Rheumatology 2012 recommendations for the use of nonpharmacologic and pharmacologic therapies in osteoarthritis of the hand, hip, and knee. *Arthritis Care Res.* 2012;64(4):465–474.

    This is an update of the 2000 ACR recommendations for hip and knee OA, with additional new recommendations specifically regarding hand OA in older adults. These recommendations, made via consensus judgment of clinical experts, were generated through systematic evidence-based literature review of common pharmacologic and nonpharmacologic treatment modalities.

- Khanna D, Fitzgerald JD, Khanna PP, et al. 2012 American College of Rheumatology guidelines for management of gout. Part 1: systemic nonpharmacologic and pharmacologic therapeutic approaches to hyperuricemia. *Arthritis Care Res.* 2012;64(10):1431–1446.

- Khanna D, Khanna PP, Fitzgerald JD, et al. 2012 American College of Rheumatology guidelines for management of gout. Part 2: therapy and anti-inflammatory prophylaxis of acute gouty arthritis. *Arthritis Care Res.* 2012;64(10):1447–1461.

    The American College of Rheumatology provides clinical guidance for the management of gout. Recommendations were generated via expert consensus judgment based on systematic, evidence-based literature review. The recommendations focus on approaches to managing both acute gouty arthritis and chronic (tophaceous) gout, including uric acid–lowering therapies.

- Makris UE, Abrams RC, Gurland B, et al. Management of persistent pain in the older patient: a clinical review. *JAMA.* 2014;312(8):825–836.

    This review article provides a stepwise approach to management of persistent pain in the older adult patient, with a focus on both pharmacologic and nonpharmacologic treatment modalities. The article also highlights common barriers to managing pain in older adults, common comorbidities that complicate management, and a suggested approach to improve treatment outcomes.

- Nakasato Y, Yung RL, eds. *Geriatric Rheumatology: A Comprehensive Approach.* New York: Springer; 2011.

    This textbook specifically addresses the presentation and management of rheumatologic conditions in older adults. A broad range of rheumatologic disorders are covered, including rheumatoid arthritis, systemic lupus erythematosus, crystal arthropathies, myopathies, Sjögren syndrome, polymyalgia rheumatic, giant cell arteritis, and others.

- National Institute for Health and Care Excellence (NICE). *Osteoarthritis: Care and Management in Adults.* Clinical Guideline 177; 2014. www.nice.org.uk/guidance/cg177 (accessed Jan 2016).

    The NICE clinical guideline provides evidence-based recommendations for the management of osteoarthritis using both pharmacologic and nonpharmacologic approaches. This guideline also provides a particularly holistic approach to management, specific focus on older adults, as well as an overview for consideration of surgical intervention in the management of osteoarthritis.

- Overman RA, Toliver JC, Yeh JY, et al. United States adults meeting 2010 American College of Rheumatology criteria for treatment and prevention of glucocorticoid-induced osteoporosis. *Arthritis Care Res.* 2014;66(11):1644–1652.

    This guideline provides recommendations for the treatment and prevention of osteoporosis in patients on chronic glucocorticoid therapy. Recommendations are provided based on age and risk of fracture as calculated by the FRAX risk score.

Una E. Makris, MD, MCS
Janna Hardland, MD

CHAPTER 59—PODIATRY

KEY POINTS

- Foot and ankle problems are common in older adults. Early diagnosis and effective treatment are critical to maintaining function and quality of life.

- Long-term effects of common structural foot deformities, including collapsing pes plano valgus, cavus foot, and equinus deformity, cause significant disability in older adults.

- Skin disorders of the foot are common in older adults. Complete assessment of the skin of the foot is necessary to identify skin conditions and potential malignancies.

- Systemic diseases can have long-term effects on the foot and ankle.

- Structural changes not improved with shoe changes and/or OTC inserts may require referral to an orthopedic surgeon or podiatrist.

- Surgical intervention for treatment of foot deformities can alleviate pain and improve function in older adults who are appropriate surgical candidates. Most surgical interventions in older adults can be performed under local anesthesia.

Foot problems can have a significant effect on the functional capacity of older adults and negatively impact their quality of life. Left untreated, these problems can lead to inactivity, morbidity, and even death.

Foot problems vary in severity from dry xerotic skin on the plantar surface of the foot to an infected, limb-threatening diabetic foot ulcer in a patient with peripheral arterial disease. In general, most foot problems are musculoskeletal and/or dermatologic in nature, although vascular, neurologic, and systemic diseases can also affect the foot. Complicating the situation is the fact that many older adults are not in the habit of inspecting their feet, or may lack the flexibility and mobility to do so effectively. Unless they are experiencing pain or discomfort, they may not notice or may ignore pathologic changes that are developing.

Therefore, clinicians treating older adults should be conscious of the potential for foot problems and make an effort to determine whether any of these conditions, or predisposing factors exist. Once identified, specific problems should be treated or the patient referred to the appropriate specialist, depending on the preliminary presentation or diagnosis.

Not all older adults are similarly affected by foot problems. The prevalence of foot problems in older adults varies by level of disability and site of care. Studies of a variety of health care settings (including nursing homes, inpatient facilities, and outpatient settings) and examination of age- and morbidity-specific populations have confirmed that the prevalence of foot pathology increases with age. Approximately one-third of the geriatric population has some foot pathology, with a higher incidence in those residing in a medical facility such as a nursing home or hospital.

The most common problems identified by these studies are nail disorders, corns/calluses, hammertoes, plantar fasciitis, hallux valgus, and flat feet. Studies of the geriatric population demonstrate that foot complaints can inhibit daily activities such as getting out of a chair, walking, and climbing stairs. The resulting decrease in mobility can exacerbate other age-related conditions and lead to loss of muscle, a decrease in cardiovascular function, and weight gain. Foot complaints are also associated with increased risk of falling in the aging population.

THE ROLE OF THE PRIMARY CARE CLINICIAN IN FOOT CARE

Because older adults may not always be vigilant when it comes to the health of their lower extremities, primary care physicians should regularly assess their geriatric patients' feet. Practitioners should pay close attention to foot conditions and the complications of systemic diseases (such as arthritic changes, neurologic disorders, diabetes mellitus, peripheral arterial disease, and mental health issues) that can manifest as foot symptoms and signs. Primary care clinicians should recognize common foot problems and refer patients for podiatric care and management in a timely and appropriate manner. The health, quality of life, and functional capacity of older adults can be significantly improved by early detection and comprehensive management of foot problems (SOE=D).

COMMON DEFORMITIES OF THE FOOT

Most foot deformities derive from the longstanding effects of a pathologic foot. A pathologic foot is one that abnormally distributes weight during walking and other movement, creating stress on the musculoskeletal structure of the foot and often resulting in pain. Over an extended period, this physical stress on the foot may result in arthritis, tissue atrophy, and subluxation of foot joints.

This disability is created by two pathologic foot types (Figure 59.1): collapsing pes plano valgus (low arch morphology) and cavus foot (high arch morphology).

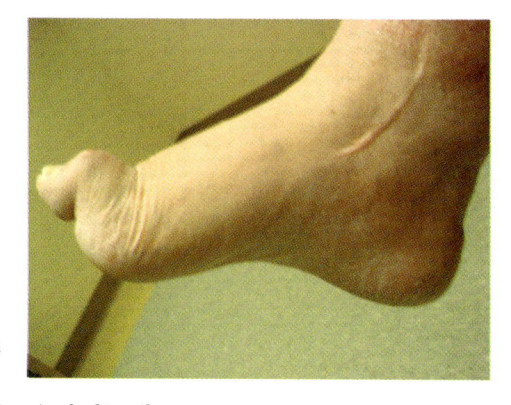

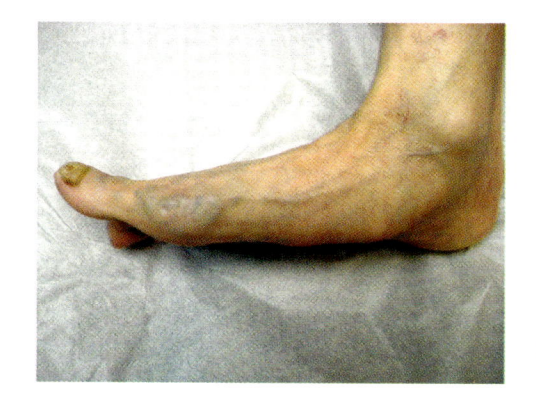

Figure 59.1—Arch disorders

A. A higher than normal arch (cavus deformity) can lead to pes cavus, which is commonly associated with neurologic change. In older adults, excessive pressure is usually placed on the metatarsal heads. With atrophy of the plantar fat pad and displacement, pressure is increased, which can predispose to pain and ulceration.

B. A flat arch (pes planus) can lead to collapsing pes plano valgus, ie, a flattening of the medial longitudinal arch (flat feet) along with pronation, demonstrated by a lateral deviation of the Achilles tendon and an outward and rotational deformity of the foot.

Equinus, the effect of a tight heel cord or Achilles tendon, is a deforming force that can be identified in both pes planus and pes cavus foot types.

Collapsing pes plano valgus is generally seen in a foot type with an unstable medial longitudinal arch, which leads to a "flat foot." The instability can occur in the talonavicular joint, the navicular cuneiform joint, and/or the first metatarsal cuneiform joint. This instability causes the forefoot to abduct on the rearfoot, and the rearfoot to go into valgus attitude in respect to the ankle joint. When the patient is standing, the longitudinal arch collapses on the weight-bearing surface, resulting in the subluxation of joints and leading to arthrosis.

Early in life, this deformity is usually quite flexible and can be treated with functional orthoses to help support the arch. However, later in life, the foot becomes more rigid and is better treated with an accommodative orthosis that absorbs the abnormally high pressure on the pes planus foot type. The condition can be congenital or acquired, but the extent of the deformity depends on activity level, body type, types of shoe worn, etc. Patients with this type of foot often have a number of other associated deformities, including posterior tibial tendon dysfunction, hallux valgus (bunion deformity), lesser metatarsal phalangeal joint dislocations (chronic dislocation of the toe joints), hammertoes, and neuromas.

The cavus foot type is generally rigid and a very poor shock absorber. It also can be congenital. If acquired later in life, it usually has a neurologic origin. Cavus foot often has a component of metatarsus adductus (inward orientation of the metatarsal bones). Older adults with this foot type generally experience loss of the fat pad in both the heel and the submetatarsal head region or ball of the foot. Associated deformities include cocked hallux (hammertoe of the great toe), sagittal dislocation of the metatarsal phalangeal joints, metatarsalgia, mid-foot dorsal exostoses (bone spurs), and rigid hammertoe deformities.

An equinus deformity is commonly seen in a pes planus or cavus foot, but it can also be seen in a foot with a normal appearance. It prevents weightbearing on the ball or heel of the foot, so a patient with an equinus deformity bears most of his or her weight on the toes when walking (just as a horse bears most of its weight on the front of its hoof). Equinus may involve a tightness of either the gastrosoleal complex or the gastrocnemius muscle complex, and this tightness can cause various conditions, including Achilles tendinitis, plantar fasciitis, metatarsalgia, and hammertoe deformities.

Common Associated Deformities

Specific associated deformities can develop due to the pathomechanics of the general deformities. See Table 59.1.

For other disorders of the foot, see Table 59.2.

Chronic Dislocated Metatarsal Phalangeal Joint

The end-stage of a hammertoe deformity is a chronically dislocated joint, a condition that is not uncommon in older adults and is caused by long-term biomechanical pathology in the forefoot. This is also seen sometimes at an earlier age in patients with rheumatoid arthritis. The toe generally dislocates on top of the metatarsal head, which places pressure on the ball of the foot. When this occurs on the second toe, it is usually associated with a hallux valgus deformity and can result in a cross-over deformity (Figure 59.2).

Metatarsal phalangeal joint dislocations are a source of chronic pain and can cause plantar ulcerations, especially in those who suffer from neuropathy. Patients developing metatarsal phalangeal joint dislocations

Table 59.1—Common Disorders of the Forefoot, Midfoot, and Rear Foot

Location/Disorder	Definition or Description
Forefoot	
Bunion	Prominent and dorsal medial eminence of the first metatarsal; associated with hallux valgus, ie, deviation of the tip of the great toe, or main axis of the toe, toward the outer or lateral side of the foot
Digiti quinti varus	Valgus displacement or splaying of the fifth metatarsal, with a resulting varus or inward deviation of the fifth toe
Dislocation of lesser metatarsal phalangeal joint	Toe joint is out of its socket.
Hallux abducto valgus	An alternative clinical diagnosis for hallux valgus, or bunion. There is a varus splaying of the first metatarsal with a valgus and rotational deformity of the phalanges of the great toe.
Hallux limitus and rigidus	A degenerative joint change involving the first metatarsal phalangeal joint, resulting from dorsal spurs, with a marked limitation or absence of any range of motion. The difference between hallux limitus and rigidus is based on the radiographic interpretation and difference in function.
Hammertoe	Muscle tendon imbalance causing contraction of the proximal or distal interphalangeal joint, or both
Tailor's bunion	Prominence of the dorsal lateral aspect of the fifth metatarsal head
Valgus position	Frontal plane position in which pressure is inwardly directed in the foot
Varus position	Frontal plane position in which pressure is outwardly directed in the foot
Midfoot	
Metatarsalgia	Pain in the forefoot near the heads of the metatarsals
Morton neuroma/syndrome	A congenital shortening of the first metatarsal shaft, which creates an abnormal metatarsal arc. Excessive weight is placed on the second metatarsal head during gait and stance. The dynamics and pathomechanics of the foot are modified and can lead to hallux valgus, abducto valgus, or rotational deformity of the hallux.
Tibialis posterior dysfunction	Chronic rupture or weakening of the tibialis posterior tendon secondary to long-term pes planus
Rear foot	
Calcaneal spur/heel spur	A calcification of the attachment of the plantar fascia, usually at the medial plantar tuberosity of the calcaneus. The spur projects anteriorly and is the consequence of chronic repetitive trauma or stress resulting from biomechanical and pathomechanical change. When ligamentous calcification occurs, inflammation and associated pain at the attachment result. This may be referred to as heel pain syndrome and may be related to plantar fasciitis.
Equinus	Tight Achilles tendon
Haglund deformity	A hyperostosis of the posterior and superior portion of the calcaneus, enlarging the calcaneus, which can in turn place pressure on the attachment of the Achilles tendon. The presence of the deformity also can produce a pressure area for the heel counter of the shoe. It is easily demonstrated on a lateral radiograph of the foot and can be associated with tendinitis or bursitis.
Plantar fasciitis	Inflammation and pain involving repetitive microtrauma to the plantar fascia, particularly at its posterior calcaneal attachment; associated with biomechanical and pathomechanical changes in the function of the foot. It is related to calcaneal spurs, ligamentous calcification, and tissue atrophy.
Tarsal tunnel syndrome	An entrapment neuropathy of the posterior tibial nerve

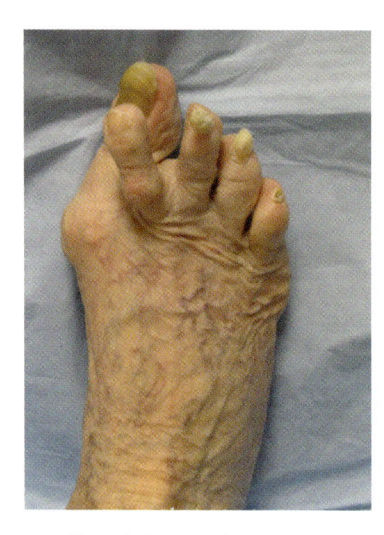

Figure 59.2—Hallux abducto valgus with crossover toe deformity

usually require shoes with increased toe box height to reduce dorsal pressure. When shoes can no longer control symptoms and skin breakdown, surgical reconstruction of the joint(s) may be necessary (SOE=A).

Hallux Limitus

Hallux limitus is an arthritic condition involving the first metatarsal phalangeal joint. Normal motion of the first metatarsal phalangeal joint generally ranges from 35 to 75 degrees. Hallux limitus occurs when there are clinical findings of arthritis, including crepitus and a decrease in the normal range of motion. Hallux rigidus is present when there is very little motion and the joint is essentially functioning as if it were fused.

The cause of hallux limitus is thought to be sagittal plane instability in the first toe (the first metatarsal has increased dorsiflexion and plantar flexion), resulting in hypermobility. This causes elevation of the first toe and impingement of the joint and, over time, results in an arthritic joint. Traditional treatment consists of orthoses that prevent motion at the first metatarsal phalangeal joint and thereby relieve pain. In a study of >700 patients, more than half were successfully treated with conservative orthotic therapy, indicating that this is a viable approach as an initial treatment (SOE=B).

An alternative approach in patients who still have some motion at the joint is to construct an orthosis with a first ray cut-out. This plantarflexes the first metatarsal and places the joint in a mechanically better position as the patient shifts his or her weight from the heel to the ball of the foot when walking. Surgical treatment of hallux limitus can range from removal of bone spurs (cheilectomy) and joint implants to osteotomies and arthrodesis of the joint. Surgery can successfully reduce symptoms and increase function (SOE=B).

Hallux Valgus

One-third of people >65 years old have a hallux valgus deformity, or bunion. The hallux valgus deformity is a subluxation of the first metatarsal phalangeal joint, resulting from the adduction of the first metatarsal and the abduction of the hallux. This deformity progresses throughout a person's lifetime, often leading to hypermobility of the first metatarsal cuneiform joint. The prominence and subluxation can be painful, especially when wearing shoes, because of the pressure applied by the shoes to the bunion deformity.

Chronic hallux valgus deformities are frequently arthritic. These deformities are treated conservatively by adapting the shoe to the deformity, ie, instructing the patient to wear wider shoes with a wider toe box and to use various padding techniques. Surgery may be considered if the deformity is symptomatic and unresponsive to conservative management. The types of procedures undertaken depend on the severity of the deformity and on the patient's health and activity level.

Studies evaluating orthopedic quality-of-life indicators and Short Form-36 after repair of hallux valgus showed that patients experienced a reduction in symptoms and were once again able to wear shoes comfortably. In most instances, this positive outcome was seen regardless of the surgical approach. These findings were consistent over all age ranges (SOE=B).

Hammertoe Deformities

Hammertoes are caused by a muscle-tendon imbalance that occurs around the metatarsal phalangeal joint. Hammertoes involve a buckling or contraction at the proximal interphalangeal joint (PIPJ) or the distal interphalangeal joint (DIPJ) of the lesser toes. In a "classic" hammertoe, there is a flexor contracture at the PIPJ. A mallet toe is a hammertoe that contracts at the DIPJ. A claw toe is a hammertoe that contracts at the PIPJ and the DIPJ.

Hammertoes can be flexible and easily reducible, or they can be rigid and nonreducible. Rigid hammertoes are generally more painful and create problems when the patient is wearing shoes. When hammertoes press against the shoe, a callus or corn is created, causing foot pain. Treatment of hammertoes may include padding of the affected area, a wide toe box in shoes or custom shoes, the debridement of calluses, or surgical correction of the deformity. If irritation occurs on the dorsal toe, extra depth shoes with more height will help alleviate the symptoms. When irritation occurs at the distal end of the tuft or toe, a cress pad can help elevate the front of the digit and reduce pressure (SOE=C).

Neuromas

A neuroma is a benign growth of a peripheral nerve, caused by chronic entrapment. Neuromas are often

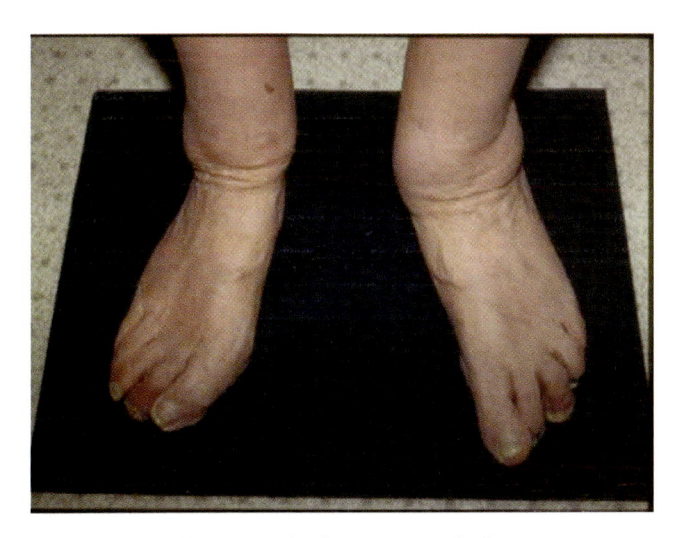

Figure 59.3—Stage III tibialis posterior dysfunction

seen in the foot between the third and fourth metatarsal heads, where they are referred to as Morton neuromas. It is theorized that the metatarsal nerve is entrapped by the deep intermetatarsal ligament as it courses underneath the ligament and forms the digital nerve branches.

Conservative treatment of neuromas may involve metatarsal pads, orthoses, corticosteroid injections, cryotherapy, or alcohol injections. Alternatively, the patient may require surgical release of the intermetatarsal ligament or primary excision of the neuroma. A comparative review of surgical intervention consistently demonstrates favorable results, with 80% of patients reporting a high level of satisfaction after surgery (SOE=B).

Posterior Tibial Tendon Dysfunction

Posterior tibial tendon dysfunction is a foot deformity defined as the gradual tearing and/or rupturing of the tibialis posterior tendon. The tibialis posterior muscle arises from the posterior aspect of the leg, and its tendon runs posteromedially across the ankle joint and inserts primarily into the navicular joint, with small connections to remaining tarsal bones. In a healthy foot, this muscle serves as a powerful inverter and plantar flexor, and the loss of its function creates significant disability, especially in obese patients. This condition causes collapse of the longitudinal arch, which in turn leads to subluxation of the rear-foot tarsal joints, and eventually the ankle joint.

The dysfunction is divided into 4 stages. Stage I is a tendinitis of the tibialis posterior tendon without foot deformity. Stage II is tearing or rupturing of the tibialis posterior tendon, which creates a flexible and fully reducible deformity. Stage III involves a deformity that has become rigid and arthritic (Figure 59.3). Stage IV occurs when the pronatory forces weaken the deltoid ligament, resulting in a valgus ankle deformity. This can be crippling in older adults.

Conservative treatment ranges from using orthoses to place the foot in a supinatory position to bracing with either an ankle-foot orthosis or a custom brace that provides increased foot control. Surgical treatment may vary, depending on the stage of deformity. Stage I deformity is treated with synovectomy and repair of the tendon, Stage II requires calcaneal osteotomies and tendon transfers to reconstruct the foot, Stage III involves arthrodesis of the rear foot, and Stage IV requires a plantar arthrodesis. Stage I and II repairs can improve function and reduce symptoms (SOE=B).

Plantar Fasciitis and Heel Pain

Heel pain is common in older adults, with studies demonstrating that up to 1 in 7 patients will present with a painful heel. Patients generally have two different symptoms: a painful heel on waking or after rest, or a painful plantar heel while walking.

The first condition, commonly referred to as plantar fasciitis, involves the plantar fascial ligament pulling from the medial tuberosity of the calcaneus as the medial arch collapses. As this process becomes chronic, osseous bleeding causes calcification of the ligament and is seen as a bone spur on radiographic examination. A tight Achilles tendon causes equinus and predisposes patients to this process. Initial treatments include reducing inflammation through the use of oral NSAIDs, steroid injections, and/or physical therapy. Second and more preventive therapies include reducing ligamental strain with inserts, night splints, and stretching exercises such as rolling the arch of the foot over a frozen water bottle.

Heel pain while walking is associated with fat pad atrophy. As the plantar cushion thins, direct bone-to-skin contact occurs because of the lack of the intermediary cushion, causing pain. Direct palpation demonstrates lack of the fat pad, and possible keratotic lesions may be present at pressure points. Symptoms increase during barefoot ambulation and decrease with the use of cushioned shoes or inserts. The only treatment for fat pad atrophy is accommodative shoes and inserts, which act as external shock absorbers.

General Treatment Strategies

Orthoses

Orthoses are external devices placed either on the foot or into the shoe to accommodate for a foot deformity or to alter the function of the foot to relieve physical stress on a certain portion of the foot. Orthoses placed on the foot include temporary felt padding or silicone/putty spacers to accommodate for structural deformities (eg, hallux valgus, hammertoes, tailor's bunion).

Orthoses placed in the shoe can be either OTC or custom made. OTC devices are generally made of lightweight polyethylene foam, soft plastics, or silicone, and

Table 59.2—Other Common Foot Disorders

Disorder	Definition or Description
Cystic erosion	Areas of radiolucency usually noted with arthritic changes, such as rheumatoid arthritis, and usually seen in the metatarsal heads with associated joint changes
Entrapment syndrome	Occurs when a nerve is compressed by ligamentous or other soft-tissue inflammation, resulting in pain and possibly numbness and neuropathic symptoms; most common sites are the posterior tibial nerve and the intermetatarsal nerve, plantarly.
Periostitis	Inflammation of the periosteum
Subluxation	Deviation of a joint's position
Tenosynovitis	Inflammation of the synovial sheath of a tendon complex, sometimes associated with a tendon tear

Table 59.3—Shoe Terms

Term	Definition or Description
Custom-made molded shoes	Made from an impression of the foot either by a plaster cast or foam imprint
Extra depth shoe	Provides additional space in the toe box
Heel counter	Back of the shoe that the heel fits in; shoes with a stiffer and higher heel counter have more stability
Rocker bottom sole	Modification of the sole
Shock-absorbing heel	Hard but absorbent material that provides shock absorption; good for patients with a cavus foot and for obese patients
Thomas heel modification	A distal medial extension of the heel that provides stability of the arch
Toe box	Part of the shoe that contains the toes
Velcro® lacing	Hook and loop tape used to secure the shoe closed, rather than conventional laces

are produced for a certain size of foot. A custom-made device is constructed from an impression of a person's foot. In the past, impressions were made by plaster casting the foot in a subtalar joint neutral position; currently, impressions are made through computerized assessment or through a foam box. The devices are then made to the impression, taking into account the patient's structural deformities. These devices are generally made from a variety of flexible and rigid plastics. Orthotics require a prescription, which allows for the rigidity, materials, posting (angle degree of foot correction), and accommodative modifications.

When structural changes do not improve with shoe changes or OTC modifications, a referral to an orthopedic surgeon or podiatrist may be necessary.

Shoes

Because of physical changes that develop in the foot with age, shoes usually do not fit well in older adults and can be a source of foot pain. Studies have indicated that approximately 75% of adults ≥65 years old wear shoes that are too small. It is common for feet to flatten and widen with age, and feet should be measured routinely. Older adults should be advised to purchase a well-fitting shoe that has a sturdy heel counter, a firm beveled sole, and good traction. With the expansion of the wider shoe size market, shoes that fit well and are structurally sound are available OTC. Athletic and walking sneakers also offer older adults accommodative shoes with structural support.

Narrow high heels should be avoided. A wide heel that is <6 cm high can be appropriate for women who have tight heel cords and have been wearing high-heeled shoes all their lives. Older adults wearing heels that are >6 cm high are at a greater risk of falls. Proper shoes and inserts that reduce pressure can decrease pain, protect the foot from injury, and improve function in older adults (SOE=B). See Table 59.3.

Most patients can be fitted with OTC shoes, except when significant structural changes occur or systemic diseases change the foot. Extra-depth shoes can help accommodate foot changes that prevent regular use of shoe wear. In diabetes, intrinsic muscle weakness causes hammering of the digits and bunion formation. Extra-depth shoes have one-and-a-half times the toe box height and soft leather material, which prevents irritation to the dorsal contracted digits. When structural changes are severe, as seen in patients with end-stage rheumatoid arthritis, a custom molded shoe may be required. These shoes are manufactured from plaster molds of the patient's feet to allow for the severe changes and to prevent skin breakdown.

Surgical Considerations of Foot Deformities

Foot surgery in older adults has increased substantially in the past 30 years, mainly because of the growth of this population segment. Studies have shown that poor surgical outcomes usually reflect the overall health of an individual rather than his or her chronological age. When relief of pain and restoration of function are the goals, surgery may be a better alternative for foot problems that are not alleviated by conservative methods. Most podiatric surgical procedures for older adults can be performed under local anesthesia with monitored sedation, thereby minimizing surgical risk.

SKIN AND NAIL DISORDERS

Skin Lesions

Skin lesions on the foot are common in older adults but are rarely malignant. Suspicious lesions require biopsy. Common benign lesions include the following:

- Keratotic lesions: These calluses or corns are often seen over sites of pressure. Common types are heloma durum (hard corn), heloma molle (soft corn), and tyloma (widespread callus). Treatment options include surgical debridement by a podiatrist or medical professional with experience. In older adults, over-the-counter treatments are limited because of the acid base of these products. Self-care can include using a pumice stone or foot file after bathing to help reduce the thickness of these lesions.

- Plantar verruca: This is the most common skin disorder of the foot, although these lesions dramatically reduce in incidence with age. This viral infection of the plantar aspect is caused by a strain of the human papilloma virus. Lesions are circular, punctated, flat, and commonly contain thrombosed vessels. It is important to differentiate these lesions from keratotic lesions. Clinically, verrucae demonstrate interrupted skin lines, pinpoint bleeding with debridement, and increased lateral compression pain when compared with keratosis. A cluster of the lesions is referred to as a mosaic wart. Treatments include application of topical salicylic acid, bleomycin injections, cryotherapy, CO_2 laser treatment, and surgical excision, which must be used with caution in older adults who have reduced circulation and impaired healing. Treatment of verrucoid lesions in older adults may require mixing approaches and treating associated complications, eg, treating hyperkeratosis with keratolytic agents such as urea (SOE=B).

- Epidermal inclusion cysts: These cysts are created by a portion of the epidermis proliferating in the dermis.

- Dermatofibromas: These flat-topped, raised, and firm lesions are generally not treated unless located across a joint or irritated by shoe wear. Recurrence rate after excision is high.

- Hemangioma: These common vascular tumors manifest as flat-topped, red lesions that contain abundant capillaries and are typically seen on the plantar aspect of the foot.

Malignant lesions are uncommon in the foot but can easily go undiagnosed and generally have a poor outcome. Pigmented lesions of the foot should be fully evaluated, and any suspicious lesions biopsied. Characteristics of a potentially malignant lesion include a new lesion in a patient ≥60 years old, or a lesion that changes in shape, color, or diameter. Lesions not responding to conservative therapy and slow or nonhealing ulcerations of the foot should be biopsied to exclude a potential underlying neoplasm. Morbidity associated with these lesions increases at age 60 and beyond. Malignant lesions identified in the foot include basal cell carcinoma, Bowen disease, squamous cell carcinoma, and malignant acral lentiginous melanoma.

Xerosis

Excessive dryness, or xerosis, is associated with a lack of hydration and lubrication. The number of sebaceous and sweat glands decrease in older adults and plantar skin lacks sebaceous glands, so it is common for fissures to develop on the heel, resulting in dryness and increased stress in that area.

The goal in managing xerosis is to prevent infection and other complications. Urea cream or solution (10%, 20%, or 40%) or ammonium lactate (12%) may be helpful as a mild and safe keratolytic. A heel sleeve or pad made with mineral oil or a heel cup can help minimize trauma to the heel, thereby reducing the potential for complications. Urea and/or lactic acid–based emollients have been shown to be effective but must be used daily and applied after bathing (SOE=C).

Eczema

Eczema is inflamed skin that is not infected. The most common types in older adults are xerotic eczema, venous stasis eczema, and drug-induced eczema. Treatment is generally a combination of emollients and steroid creams, with or without occlusive dressings.

Nail Disorders

Ingrown Nails and Paronychia

Nail disorders are the most common disorders of the foot.

Onychocryptosis, the incurvation of the edge of the nail plate into the nail groove, is generally seen in the distal portion of the nail groove. This condition can result from long-term improper nail cutting (too short), narrow shoes, and/or genetically incurvated nail matrixes. In determining the best treatment option, the physician should consider the need for antibiotics and foot soaking to treat the ingrown nail. A chronically ingrown nail is best treated either with a partial nail avulsion or a permanent matricectomy.

Paronychia, a localized infection caused by the nail embedding into the nail groove, requires incision and drainage of the abscess with removal of the nail spicule.

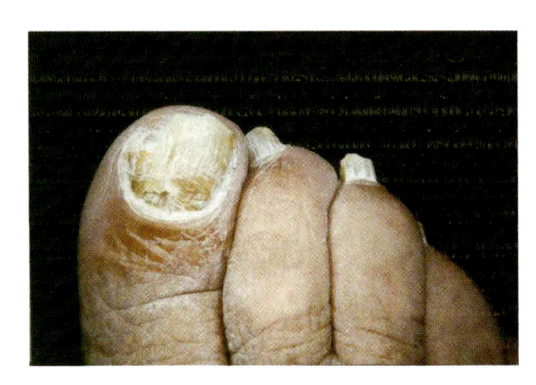

Figure 59.4—Onychomycosis. Nails infected by fungi are often yellow, thickened, and friable, with yellow-brown debris under the nail plate.

All infected granulation tissue is resected. Depending on the presence of cellulitis or comorbidities, antibiotic treatment may be needed. Toes with chronic paronychia should be radiographed to exclude underlying osteomyelitis, especially in patients with diabetes or peripheral arterial disease.

Onychomycosis

Approximately one-third of the older population has onychomycosis, a fungal infection of the nail plate. An increased incidence is seen in older adults with obesity, immunodeficiency, diabetes, peripheral arterial disease, chronic tinea pedis, and/or psoriasis. By the age of 65, approximately 20% of men and 10% of women are affected; these values are doubled in those with diabetes. Dermatophytes account for 80% of infections, with the remainder caused by saprophytes or yeast.

Onychomycosis results in thickening of the nail plate and can cause pain (Figure 59.4). In patients with neuropathy, onychomycosis can be a source of nail bed ulcerations. Treatment includes topical and oral antifungal medications, as well as permanent excision of the nail plate. A decision to treat is usually made because of one of the following: the cosmetic concern of a yellow friable nail, other comorbidities (particularly diabetes mellitus, in which the break in the epidermal barrier due to the fungal infection can serve as a route for bacterial infections), and occasionally pain.

Topical antifungal treatments with amorolfine, ciclopirox, and tioconazole have exhibited efficacy in improving and curing onychomycosis (SOE=C) but require 24–48 weeks of treatment, often at considerable out-of-pocket expense, for cure rates that are <50%. Oral antifungals such as terbinafine, fluconazole, and itraconazole are effective for onychomycosis, but their duration of treatment, adverse-event profile, and high rate of relapse after discontinuation warrant careful consideration for use in older adults. These agents are primarily metabolized by the liver and can interact with many medications that are commonly administered to older adults. Treatment can take 3–4 months, and the rate of relapse is high. Comorbidities such as diabetes, secondary fungal infections, and quality of life should be considered before starting treatment.

SYSTEMIC DISEASES AFFECTING THE FOOT AND ANKLE

Diabetes Mellitus

Diabetes is the number one disease affecting foot health in older adults. Complications of diabetes can cause loss of limbs and significant disability. It has been estimated that 50%–75% of all amputations in patients with diabetes could be prevented by foot health education, periodic clinician assessment, and early intervention. The ocular complications of diabetes can adversely impact the ability of patients to see ingrown toenails, corns, and ulcers. Other complications of diabetes that contribute to poor foot health include neuropathy, vascular insufficiency, dermopathy, atrophy of the muscles and soft tissues, and deformity. Neuropathy, especially sensory impairment, is a precursor to ulcers. Paresthesias, decreased vibratory sense, and loss of sensation are among the most important neuropathic changes that contribute to ulcer formation in older diabetic patients.

Arterial insufficiency causes pallor, a loss or decrease in the posterior tibial and dorsalis pedis pulse, dependent rubor, and decreased capillary filling time in the toes. Severe vascular disease can result in rest pain that typically occurs at night. A loss of the plantar metatarsal fat pad is associated with vascular insufficiency and predisposes to ulcerations at the site of bony prominences or deformities of the foot.

Foot ulcers are a common result of the multiple pathologies found in patients with diabetes. Prevention and early recognition are the most important strategies in managing foot ulcers. Clinicians should ensure that older diabetic patients have their feet examined at least annually. Diabetic patients are often instructed to remove their shoes at all visits so that the clinician can visually inspect the feet and the areas between the toes to ensure there has been no skin breakdown. Patients and caregivers should be instructed in the importance of daily foot inspections. Preventive strategies include optimizing glycemic control, and monitoring and treating peripheral neuropathy, arterial disease, limited joint mobility, bony deformities, hyperkeratosis, and onychodystrophy (SOE=C).

Prevention of foot ulcers in diabetic patients is both cost-effective and limb saving in this high-risk population (SOE=A). Assessing vibratory sensation using the Semmes-Weinstein monofilament and monitoring reflex changes help the clinician determine a patient's risk of development of ulcers. If a diabetic patient's risk is high, appropriate steps should be taken to prevent ulcers, including reducing excessive pressure, shock, and shear by accommodating, stabilizing, and supporting deformities through weight diffusion and dispersion (SOE=C). Early intervention with proper shoes and foot care reduces complications in high-risk feet, as demonstrated by the Lower Extremity Amputation Prevention (LEAP) program and Medicare Loss of Protective Sensation (LOPS) program.

When an ulcer develops despite preventive efforts, the history should focus on duration, inciting event or trauma, prior ulcerations, previous attempts at wound care, and use of pressure off-loading procedures. The examination should include an assessment of the location and depth of the ulcer, the presence of infection, ischemic or neuropathic changes, edema, and the presence of a Charcot joint. Imaging should be performed to exclude osteomyelitis (SOE=B) and may include plain radiography, CT, technetium bone scans, indium scans, and MRIs. Noninvasive vascular studies include Doppler and transcutaneous oxygen tension. Consultation with a vascular specialist may be needed when vascular insufficiency is severe or the wounds are nonhealing.

The general principles of high-risk foot management include debridement, pressure relief, off-loading, avoidance or limitation of weight bearing, proper dressings, treatment of infection with antibiotics, management of ischemia, medical management of comorbidities, and hospitalization and surgical management when necessary. Weight bearing can be modified by the use of crutches and wheelchairs as well as contact casts, walkers, boots, braces, total contact orthotics, modified surgical shoes and boots, and appropriate dressings. Wounds should be reduced by 50% within a 4-week period. If a wound is reducing as planned, then regular follow-up care and prevention are required. Nonreducing wounds require reassessment of the patient's medical condition, and well as his or her vascular, infectious, and nutritional statuses. Adjunctive therapies should be used if there is no response to treatment or correction of medical status.

A wide variety of dressings and topical agents is available; selection is guided by the nature of the ulcer and its complications. Topical agents include saline, antiseptics, topical antibiotics, enzymes, growth factors, and dermal skin substitutes. Vacuum-assisted closure and hyperbaric oxygen chambers can also aid in closure of difficult-to-heal wounds in diabetic patients (SOE=B). Empiric antibiotic therapy should be started early when infection is suspected. Hospitalization is usually indicated in cases involving osteomyelitis or limb-threatening infection. The choice of antibiotic is based on the clinical symptoms; culture and sensitivity; presence of deep infection, bone exposure, or sepsis; and whether soft tissue or bone is infected (SOE=B).

Peripheral Arterial Disease

Older adults with peripheral arterial disease demonstrate many of the same signs and symptoms as those with diabetes mellitus. In contrast to neuropathic ulcers, vascular ulcers are extremely painful.

Arthritis

Osteoarthritis is common in older adults. It causes pain, swelling, stiffness, limitation of movement, and deformity in weight-bearing joints. It may be worsened by chronic trauma, strain, or obesity. Gouty arthritis is monoarticular and is most common in the first metatarsal phalangeal joint. In its early stages, it results in intense pain and erythema, followed later by joint damage.

Rheumatoid arthritis affects the hands and feet equally and is usually symmetric in its presentation. It can result in muscle wasting and marked deformity. The metatarsal phalangeal joints become dislocated or subluxed; there is increased protrusion of the metatarsal heads, and walking becomes painful. If conservative treatment with orthotics and special shoes do not relieve the pain, surgery may help to allow less painful ambulation.

REFERENCES

- Edmonds ME, Foster AV. *Managing the Diabetic Foot*. 3rd ed. Chichester, UK: John Wiley & Sons, Ltd.; 2014.

    This article is a good review of treatment options for the diabetic foot.

- Goff JD, Crawford R. Diagnosis and treatment of plantar fasciitis. *Am Fam Physician*. 2011;84(6):676–682.

    This article is a good overview of the diagnosis and treatment of plantar fasciitis.

- Scheffer N. *21 Things You Need To Know About Diabetes and Your Feet*. American Diabetes Association; 2012.

    This excellent review text is a comprehensive analysis of podiatric pathology in the geriatric population. It covers epidemiology, physiologic changes, assessment, skin disorders, nail disorders, and structural disorders of the foot. It also reviews orthotic therapy and footwear considerations.

- Vernon W, Borthwick A, Walker J. The management of foot problems in the older person through podiatry services. *Rev Clin Gerontology*. 2011;21(4):331–339.

    This article defines podiatry and its integration with geriatrics. Comprehensive foot care may involve additional disciplines beyond podiatry because there may be serious systemic sequelae that require multidisciplinary approaches.

- Yates B, ed. *Merriman's Assessment of the Lower Limb*. 3rd ed. Philadelphia, PA: Churchill Livingstone; 2012.

    This text provides excellent coverage of diagnosis and evaluation of foot conditions.

Douglas A. Albreski, DPM

CHAPTER 60—NEUROLOGY

KEY POINTS

- New-onset seizures in late life are frequently a symptom of an underlying brain disease or injury. Recurrent seizures can be prevented with medications. Newer anticonvulsant drugs are better tolerated.

- Parkinson disease and other common movement disorders seen in older patients are diagnosed clinically and can be effectively managed medically.

- Peripheral neuropathy is common in older adults, and diabetes is the most common cause in the United States. Several medications are approved by the FDA for the treatment of painful diabetic neuropathy.

- New onset of headaches in older adults should prompt a search for a secondary cause, including brain tumor, systemic illness, temporal arteritis, or medication-induced causes.

Neurologic diseases and disorders are increasingly common with advancing age. The most prevalent neurologic disorders include Alzheimer disease (AD) and related dementias, gait disorders, cerebrovascular disease, epilepsy, Parkinson disease (PD), and peripheral neuropathy. In the United States, almost half (40%–50%) of the population >85 years old suffer from dementia, and a similar percentage of hospitalized patients of this age have a gait disorder caused by a neurologic condition. Other U.S. population data include the following: 7.5% of adults 60–79 years old and 15% of those ≥80 years old have had a stroke, 1% of adults >60 years old and 3% of those >80 years old have been diagnosed with PD, 3% of adults by age 75 and close to 10% of the nursing-home population have epilepsy, and up to 10% of adults >65 years old have some signs of a peripheral polyneuropathy. This chapter will cover epilepsy in older adults, PD and other movement disorders, and other common neurologic conditions, including neuromuscular disorders, myelopathy, and headaches.

Individual neurologic disorders in older adults can be challenging to diagnose, given that it is common for a patient to have more than one such disorder or sequela when examined. Pharmacologic treatment of neurologic disorders must account for the unique metabolism of older adults and the potential for drug-drug interactions. Furthermore, because neurologic disorders add substantially to the burden of functional dependency, acknowledging the psychosocial aspects of these conditions is vital in constructing treatment plans to improve functional abilities and quality of life.

EPILEPSY IN OLDER ADULTS

A seizure is caused by excessive and synchronous discharges of cortical neurons producing a transient change in brain function. Recurrent seizures are the defining feature of epilepsy. Seizures are broadly classified as partial or generalized, depending on whether the seizure discharges involve only a portion of the cortex or the entire cortex. Partial seizures are subdivided on the basis of whether the seizure is associated with impaired consciousness. Simple partial seizures do not impair consciousness, but complex partial seizures do. Most commonly, simple partial seizures involve focal rhythmic motor twitching. Complex partial seizures are often preceded by an aura, followed by loss of awareness and responsiveness typically manifested as staring off into space. Automatisms and other minor motor manifestations may occur with complex partial seizures. After the event, patients display postictal confusion and amnesia for the seizure. Generalized seizures involve the entire cortex and typically cause tonic-clonic convulsions (ie, generalized tonic-clonic, or "grand mal," seizures). A seizure may start as a complex partial seizure and secondarily progress into a generalized seizure. In critical care settings, a generalized seizure may manifest as a nonconvulsive continuous seizure (ie, nonconvulsive status epilepticus) in which a patient shows persistent alteration in mental status without convulsive movements.

The incidence of epilepsy follows a bimodal pattern with respect to age, with an initial peak within the first year of life and a second peak after the age of 60. The annual incidence of epilepsy peaks at 135 per 100,000 in those >80 years old. Secondary causes of seizures, ie, those with an underlying discernible cause, are more common among older adults. In this demographic group, about 70% of new-onset seizures are secondary. Common causes include cerebrovascular disease, space-occupying lesions, brain trauma, neurodegenerative diseases, and alcohol withdrawal. It is estimated that cerebrovascular disease causes 50% of known causes of late-onset seizures, with tumors, trauma, and degenerative dementias each causing 10%–20% of cases. Cortical or hemorrhagic strokes are more likely to cause seizures. AD increases the risk of seizures, although seizures in AD are relatively uncommon, occurring in 2%–5% of patients. Seizures in AD are seen more often in advanced stages of dementia and in young-onset AD. The incidence of partial epilepsy (which frequently has an underlying cause) increases in older adults, whereas the incidence of primary generalized epilepsy

Table 60.1—Newer Antiepileptic Drugs Commonly Used In Older Populations

Antiepileptic Drug	Advantages	Disadvantages	Titration Schedule
Lamotrigine	Studied in older adults Broad spectrum[a] Well tolerated	Slow titration Possible adverse effects: drug rash, insomnia	25 mg q12h × 14 days, 50 mg q12h × 14 days, then 50 mg in am and 100 mg in pm
Gabapentin	Studied in older adults No drug interactions Other uses (eg, pain, mood stabilizer)	Three times a day dosing Possible adverse effects: sedation, dizziness, weight gain Must dose-adjust for renal function	300 mg per day for 3 days, then increase by 300 mg every 3 days until 1,500 mg total per day on q8h schedule (eg, 300 mg, 600 mg, 600mg)
Levetiracetam	Studied in older adults Broad spectrum[a] No drug interactions Fast titration Can be given IV or po	Possible adverse effects: irritability, sedation	250 mg q12h × 7 days, then 500 mg q12h

[a]Effective for treatment of both partial and generalized epilepsies.

(generally idiopathic or genetic) is more common in pediatric populations.

It is important that older adults with new-onset seizures undergo diagnostic evaluation to exclude an underlying treatable condition. The neurologic history and examination should aim to clinically characterize the seizure and localize its source, as well as to elicit other signs of a focal lesion or a metabolic disturbance (eg, uremia, hepatic failure). Blood studies (comprehensive metabolic panel, magnesium, calcium), brain imaging (MRI is preferable to CT), and electroencephalography play important roles. Brain imaging should be obtained with and without contrast to identify and characterize structural brain lesions.

Once the appropriate evaluation has been done, the decision to begin an anticonvulsant drug should be made carefully to maximize benefit and minimize risk. On average, 30% of patients with a single unprovoked seizure have another seizure, but 70% do not. The presence of a focal brain abnormality on brain imaging or epileptic changes on an electroencephalogram (EEG) raises the likelihood of recurrence and should prompt consideration of pharmacologic therapy. If a patient has a second unprovoked seizure, then the probability of further seizures increases to 70%, and pharmacologic therapy should generally be initiated.

There have been only 3 randomized, double-blind, comparative clinical trials in older adults with newly diagnosed epilepsy. In the Veterans Administration (VA) study, lamotrigine, gabapentin, and carbamazepine were compared. Seizure control was similar among these three antiepileptic drugs, but carbamazepine was significantly less well tolerated than the other two. Discontinuation rates due to adverse events were 12% with lamotrigine, 22% with gabapentin, and 31% with carbamazepine in this 52-week study. Two other trials compared lamotrigine to carbamazepine. As in the VA trial, both drugs effectively prevented recurrent seizures, but lamotrigine was significantly better tolerated. This difference in tolerability was completely negated in a third study in which a controlled-release form of carbamazepine and flexible dosing design were used. Several of the other newer antiepileptic drugs have been examined in open-label trials in older populations, including studies with oxcarbazepine, levetiracetam, and low-dose topiramate. These agents have demonstrated good seizure control and tolerability. Thus, there is growing evidence that use of one of the newer antiepileptic drugs described above is preferred to the use of older antiepileptic drugs in the older population, because of improved tolerability and compliance (SOE=A).

The incidence of adverse effects and drug-drug interactions increases with age. This is particularly true of the older antiepileptic drugs, such as phenobarbital, carbamazepine, phenytoin, and valproate. For example, phenobarbital can cause cognitive adverse effects, phenytoin can cause ataxia, carbamazepine can cause hyponatremia, and valproate can cause weight gain, tremors, and parkinsonism. Many of the older antiepileptic drugs, including phenobarbital, phenytoin, and carbamazepine, are potent inducers of the cytochrome P450 system, which increases the risk of drug-drug interactions. Also, each of these three agents has been associated with increased bone loss with age. Finally, changes in hepatic function or binding protein levels in older adults can alter the metabolism of older antiepileptic drugs, active drug levels, and risk of adverse effects. Clinical pharmacists can help to resolve complex issues of drug interactions, dosages, and adverse events, especially when using older antiepileptic drugs.

Table 60.1 describes advantages, disadvantages, and titration schedules for 3 of the newer antiepileptic drugs that have been studied in older adults (lamotrigine, gabapentin, levetiracetam). Antiepileptic drug doses are best started at low levels and increased very slowly in older adults to avoid problematic adverse effects. Older adults may have difficulty with adherence to antiepileptic drug schedules for a variety of reasons. It is particularly important when treating older adults to involve caregivers so that the goals of the treatment, adverse events, and monitoring of response are understood. Final medication dose is determined by consideration of seizure control and adverse events. Ideally, drug doses are escalated to a level that assures elimination of seizures, but not so high that adverse effects arise. Newer antiepileptic drugs, such as those described in Table 60.1, do not require laboratory monitoring. Common causes of breakthrough seizures in individuals known to be epileptic are systemic infections, metabolic disturbances, sleep deprivation, and medication noncompliance. Providers should consider discontinuing antiepileptic drugs if a patient has not had a seizure for ≥2 years, particularly if the original seizure was a single or poorly characterized event, and if a recent EEG does not show epileptic activity.

Epilepsy surgery has become an increasingly common choice of younger patients whose seizures have proved refractory to pharmacologic management. The utility of epilepsy surgery in older adults is not known.

MOVEMENT DISORDERS IN OLDER ADULTS

A simple definition of movement disorder is the presence of abnormal involuntary movements. These movements result not from weakness or sensory deficits but from dysfunction of the extrapyramidal motor systems. Movement disorders can be classified as hypokinetic (paucity of movement) or hyperkinetic (excessive movement). The hypokinetic movement disorders include PD and the related Parkinson-plus syndromes (eg, multiple system atrophy, progressive supranuclear palsy). Hyperkinetic movement disorders include conditions that produce chorea (eg, Huntington disease), dyskinesias (eg, tardive dyskinesias), dystonia, and tremor (eg, essential tremor). Movement disorders are especially common among older adults.

Parkinson Disease (PD)

PD is a progressive neurodegenerative disease that results in neuronal dysfunction and neuronal loss in pathways of the brainstem, basal ganglia and cerebral cortex. The pathologic hallmark of the disease is the Lewy body, an intracellular inclusion body originally found in dopaminergic neurons of the substantia nigra. These neurodegenerative changes cause a constellation of clinical signs, including tremor at rest, bradykinesia, rigidity, and postural instability. As the disease progresses, neurodegeneration and Lewy body pathology extends into the cortex (limbic region and neocortex), causing neuropsychiatric and cognitive symptoms (ie, PD with dementia).

The incidence and prevalence of PD increase with age. Prevalence rates in the United States rise from 1% of the population at age 60 to 3% at age 80. Aging, environmental factors, and genetics are thought to be involved in the pathogenesis of PD. Risk factors associated with increased risk of PD include exposure to pesticides, welding as a profession, exposure to manganese, age, and family history. Smoking and caffeine consumption have been associated with decreased risk. A small proportion of PD cases (5%–10%) are the result of a causative genetic mutation, while a larger proportion of patients may have inherited a susceptibility gene that increases risk. Approximately 10 genes have been associated with PD, either as causative mutations or susceptibility genes. Idiopathic PD (ie, parkinsonism not attributable to strokes, medications, or other primary causes) most commonly appears clinically between the ages of 50 and 79 years. Dementia in PD occurs in 30%–40% of PD patients and is more common with longer duration of disease, more severe motor symptoms, an akinetic-rigid presentation, and older age of onset of motor symptoms.

Diagnosis of PD

Recent clinical diagnostic criteria continue to highlight the central role of the motor signs of PD and the importance of the physical examination in making a clinical diagnosis. To make a diagnosis of PD, there should be evidence of parkinsonism, defined as the presence of bradykinesia in combination with either resting tremor, rigidity, or both. The term *bradykinesia* describes either a slowness in initiating movement (ie, a paucity of spontaneous movements) or slow movements themselves. This can be manifested clinically as reduced frequency and amplitude of fine finger movements, decreased facial expression or blinking, and micrographia (small handwriting). The resting tremor in PD is generally asymmetric and has a slow frequency (usually 4–6 Hz). It is present at rest and typically resolves or decreases with active, purposeful movement. Muscular rigidity is usually readily evident on passive movement of a limb when the patient is relaxed. Passive movement may demonstrate a smooth resistance ("lead pipe" rigidity) or superimposed ratchet-like jerks (ie, "cogwheel" phenomenon, which is caused by tremor superimposed on the rigidity). The fourth cardinal motor feature of PD is impaired postural reflexes, which can be elicited with a pull test (pulling a standing patient backward and assessing his or her ability to maintain balance). Impaired postural balance is a feature present later in the course of idiopathic PD; the presence of early postural imbalance and frequent falls often signals a Parkinson-plus syndrome.

Additional clinical features are supportive (not required) of a diagnosis of idiopathic PD, while other features are exclusionary or serve as "red flags" that suggest an alternative cause of parkinsonism. A unilateral resting tremor supports a diagnosis of idiopathic PD, whereas bilateral symmetric parkinsonism is a "red flag" for the presence of a different diagnosis. A clear and dramatic improvement in motor symptoms with dopaminergic medications is similarly supportive, as is the presence of levodopa-induced dyskinesia, and lack of response after a proper trial of a dopaminergic medication raises the question of an alternative cause. Loss of the sense of smell is an early and sensitive marker of PD pathology, and standardized tests are available (eg, University of Pennsylvania Smell Identification Test [UPSIT]) to quantify a patient's olfactory function. However, loss of sense of smell is not specific to PD and can be seen in other neurodegenerative disorders (including AD), or in those with paranasal sinus disease or a history of head trauma.

Many features on examination suggest an alternative cause of parkinsonism. Examples include the presence of unequivocal cerebellar findings, downward vertical supranuclear gaze palsy, parkinsonism limited to only the legs for >3 years, cortical sensory loss, limb ideomotor apraxia, and progressive aphasia. Treatment with a dopamine-receptor blocker (eg, antipsychotic agents) in a dose high enough to produce extrapyramidal features also excludes PD as the diagnosis. Other findings very atypical of PD are rapid progression of gait impairment or recurrent falls early in the disease course, early bulbar dysfunction, early severe autonomic failure, unexplained pyramidal tract signs, and the absence of progression of motor symptoms for >5 years.

It is appropriate to refer patients to a neurologist with movement disorder expertise if atypical features are present or the diagnosis is unclear.

Treatment of PD

Patients who are functionally disabled by tremors, bradykinesia, or rigidity should be offered pharmacologic treatment. Drug therapy is effective in reducing these symptoms but does not improve postural instability or nonmotor symptoms of PD. Patients who respond well to initial pharmacologic treatment are generally well managed by geriatricians or other primary care providers, but those with advanced disease or suboptimal response to drug therapy may benefit from referral to neurologists with movement disorder expertise, who are familiar with the increasing variety of available treatments. Nonpharmacologic therapy should include a regular exercise program. Many older adults benefit from a course of physical therapy aimed at restoring their confidence in walking and maintaining balance, often with instruction in PD-focused physical therapy programs (eg, "BIG" program) or symptom-focused therapy (eg, disabling freezing episodes). Physical therapists can also help, when needed, with selection of appropriate canes or walkers. A home visit by an occupational therapist can help to evaluate safety and equipment needs in the home, such as appropriate placement of wall rails, grab bars, and other such assistive devices that reduce the possibility of falling.

Levodopa therapy for PD motor symptoms: The most effective pharmacologic treatment of patients with PD is levodopa combined with carbidopa (SOE=A). Levodopa is converted to dopamine in both the CNS and the periphery via dopa decarboxylase. Peripheral conversion is reduced by combining levodopa with carbidopa (a dopa decarboxylase inhibitor), which does not cross the blood-brain barrier. This formulation decreases adverse events associated with peripheral conversion. Treatment usually begins with a half tablet of the 25/100 combination (ie, 25 mg carbidopa to 100 mg levodopa) administered every 8 to12 hours. Every 1 to 2 weeks, the dose can be increased by one-half tablet, to reach a dosage of one full tablet three times a day (commonly 30 minutes before meals). The duration of action of this formulation is typically 4 hours. If disabling bradykinesia, rigidity, or resting tremor is still present, the dosage can be gradually increased further, with cautious observation for adverse events. Older adults, particularly those who are cognitively impaired, rarely tolerate total levodopa doses of greater than 1,000 mg/d. The controlled-release form (25/100 and 50/200) generally requires a slightly higher total daily dose. Common adverse events of levodopa-carbidopa include nausea, abdominal cramping, orthostatic hypotension, and visual hallucinations.

Managing PD symptoms with medications becomes more challenging as the disease progresses, because the therapeutic window narrows, making it difficult to control motor symptoms without undesirable side effects. After 5 years of treatment for PD, up to 50% of patients develop motor fluctuations or dyskinesias (involuntary choreiform movements). PD patients are commonly described as "on" (symptoms well controlled), "on with dyskinesias" (symptoms controlled but complicated by dyskinesias), or "off" (parkinsonism not well controlled). End-of-dose "off" symptoms are common and can be treated by increasing the dosing frequency of levodopa to every 3–4 hours or by adding an enzyme inhibitor such as rasagiline or entacapone (both described below) to increase the duration of action of levodopa. Peak dose "on" dyskinesias are common and are treated by increasing the interval between levodopa doses or lowering the total daily dose of dopaminergic medications. The incidence and severity of dyskinesias can be reduced by introducing a dopamine agonist (described below) early in the treatment of PD, either as monotherapy or in combination with levodopa when daily dosages exceed 400 mg/d. This is an important consideration in younger patients (<75 years old) expected to have a long duration of disease and treatment.

Other medications for PD motor symptoms: Medications other than levodopa that can be used to treat PD motor symptoms include enzyme inhibitors, amantadine and anticholinergic medications, and dopamine agonists. Enzyme inhibitors include the catechol-O-methyl-transferase (COMT) inhibitor entacapone. COMT inhibitors block breakdown of levodopa, thereby increasing bioavailability at the synapse. Entacapone increases the duration of action of levodopa, resulting in greater "on" time for a given dose of levodopa, but it can also exacerbate dyskinesias (SOE=A). Adverse events of COMT inhibitors are similar to those of levodopa. A second class of enzyme inhibitors are the monoamine oxidase B (MAO-B) inhibitors, which also block one of the enzymes responsible for dopamine breakdown. Rasagiline is a newer selective MAO-B inhibitor that has been approved by the FDA as early monotherapy or as adjunct therapy (SOE=A). Selegiline, an older MAO-B inhibitor, was shown in controlled trials to delay the need for additional antiparkinsonian agents (SOE=A). A neuroprotective role of MAO-B inhibitors in PD has been investigated but not established. Although chemically related to nonselective monoamine oxidase inhibitors, the selective MAO-B inhibitors, rasagiline and selegiline, do not require dietary restrictions. MAO-B inhibitors are generally well tolerated, although some patients can experience adverse events, including nausea, insomnia, confusion, or anxiety. Other medications used to treat motor symptoms of PD include amantadine and anticholinergic medications such as trihexyphenidyl. Amantadine, which has multiple pharmacologic properties, can provide mild improvement in PD motor symptoms and decreased dyskinesias (SOE=B). Older adults, especially with impaired renal clearance, can develop confusion and hallucinations with amantadine. Anticholinergic medications can modestly improve some PD symptoms, but adverse events such as dry mouth, urinary retention, and confusion outweigh benefits in most older adults.

Dopamine agonists may be used initially as monotherapy to treat motor symptoms of PD, or may be added to levodopa when its dosage exceeds 400 mg/d. The agents may be particularly useful for younger PD patients with milder disease and no signs of dementia (SOE=A). A slow titration is required with dopamine agonists, because nausea, sleepiness, orthostatic hypotension, and hallucinations are common adverse events. When compared with levodopa, dopamine agonists are less effective in controlling motor symptoms and are associated with more adverse events. However, early use of dopamine agonists can delay the emergence of levodopa-induced dyskinesias (SOE=A). Commonly used dopamine agonists include ropinirole, pramipexole and rotigotine transdermal patch. All dopamine agonists, and to a lesser extent levodopa, have been associated with sudden sleep attacks in which patients may doze off abruptly while driving. Additionally, dopamine agonists have been associated with compulsive behaviors such as pathologic gambling. Patients should be warned of these rare but potentially serious adverse events, and clinicians should ask about these behaviors during routine follow-up visits.

Deep brain stimulation: Surgical options can be considered for patients with PD who initially demonstrated a good response to dopaminergic medications, but over time develop suboptimal motor response, medication adverse effects, motor fluctuations, or dyskinesias that cannot be controlled by adjustments in medical therapy. Deep brain stimulation (DBS) of the globus pallidus or subthalamic nucleus is effective in controlling rest tremor, rigidity, bradykinesia, motor fluctuations, and dyskinesias. A documented good response to dopaminergic medications is the best predictor of good response to DBS. DBS significantly increases "on" time and decreases troubling dyskinesias and motor fluctuations (SOE=A). Complications of DBS include surgical site infection, intracranial hemorrhage, death (about 1%), cognitive and speech problems, and an increased risk of falls. Although there is no age cut-off, DBS is typically performed in patients <80 years old.

Nonmotor Symptoms of PD

Nonmotor symptoms are common in PD and can be a target of treatment. These include urinary incontinence, constipation, drooling, seborrhea, anxiety, depression, visual hallucinations, sleep disorders, and cognitive impairment. PD patients are also at higher risk of melanoma and may benefit from routine screening for the condition. For PD patients who develop visual hallucinations or delusions, dopaminergic medications should be adjusted and doses reduced. If symptoms are severe, the addition of low-dose clozapine or quetiapine may be considered; these atypical antipsychotic agents are least likely to exacerbate PD motor symptoms. PD patients who develop dementia symptoms can be treated with a cholinesterase inhibitor. Rivastigmine has been FDA approved for treatment of the dementia associated with PD (SOE=A).

"Parkinson-plus" Syndromes

"Parkinson-plus" or parkinsonian syndromes are a group of disorders with some motor features of PD (ie, resting tremor, bradykinesia, rigidity, postural imbalance) but that also have additional distinct and distinguishing features. As a group, these disorders are much less responsive to pharmacologic treatment with dopaminergic medications than idiopathic PD. The parkinsonian syndromes described in some detail below include multiple system atrophy (MSA) and progressive supranuclear palsy (PSP). Other Parkinson-plus syndromes include dementia with Lewy bodies (DLB); vascular parkinsonism, in which small-vessel ischemic strokes in the basal ganglia produce parkinsonism; and medication-induced parkinsonism, in which dopamine-receptor blocking medications (typically antipsychotic or antiemetic drugs) produce parkinsonism.

Multiple System Atrophy

A histopathologic understanding of 3 parkinsonian syndromes, olivopontocerebellar atrophy, Shy-Drager syndrome, and striatonigral degeneration, has permitted these overlapping syndromes to be included within the rubric of one disease called multiple system atrophy (MSA). MSA produces degeneration in 3 distinct neuronal systems, the basal ganglia, cerebellum, and autonomic nervous system. MSA is characterized by parkinsonism, autonomic failure (eg, severe orthostatic hypotension, constipation, incontinence, impotence, impaired sweating or temperature control), and cerebellar dysfunction (eg, ataxia, dysmetria). Other features that can accompany MSA are upper motor neuron signs, severe dysarthria, stridor, dystonia, and restless legs syndrome. The diagnosis is clinical, and MSA can initially be indistinguishable from idiopathic PD, but the degree of autonomic dysfunction, disappointing response to levodopa, and cerebellar signs all support a diagnosis of MSA. The mean age of onset for MSA is 55 years; it is slightly more common in men, and it progresses to death in approximately 7 years on average. MSA accounts for approximately 3% of cases of parkinsonism. Orthostatic hypotension is often the most disabling symptom of MSA. Nonpharmacologic management of autonomic dysfunction includes eating small meals, arising to standing position slowly, use of compressive elastic stockings, and increased salt and fluid intake. Medications may be needed to treat severe orthostatic hypotension and include midodrine, fludrocortisone, and droxidopa (SOE=A). Use of these medications may result in supine hypertension, which requires close blood pressure monitoring and medication adjustments. Levodopa may initially help with some symptoms of rigidity and bradykinesia, but the improvement is not as significant as in idiopathic PD, and dopamine replacement may worsen orthostatic hypotension.

Progressive Supranuclear Palsy

Progressive supranuclear palsy (PSP) accounts for approximately 4% of cases of parkinsonism. PSP is marked by an akinetic-rigid form of parkinsonism with early loss of postural balance causing frequent falls (afflicted persons typically fall backward). As the disease progresses, supranuclear gaze palsy (described below) becomes apparent, and patients eventually develop spasticity, dystonia, dysarthria, dysphagia, and a subcortical-frontal dementia. Usual age of onset is the late 50s or early 60s. The pathogenesis is unknown. The disease typically progresses rapidly, with marked incapacity occurring within 3–5 years and death within 6–8 years, generally as a result of aspiration, infection, or complications of immobility. Progressive supranuclear palsy derives its name from progressive impairments of voluntary, vertical gaze. Most patients develop eye movement restrictions approximately 3–4 years into the disease course. Patients are unable to voluntarily look downward or upward (upward gaze is less severely involved). Resting tremor is typically absent and the rigidity is more pronounced in the neck and trunk (axial rigidity). Patients with PSP often have a fixed facial expression due to facial dystonia that causes them to keep their eyebrows elevated in a look of surprise or furrowed in a persistent scowl. The dysarthria of PSP is distinct from that of PD, with mixed spastic (strangled) and hypophonic features. Gait is disturbed early in the course, and falls are frequent in most patients. Cognition, particularly involving executive function or judgment, is often affected, and personality changes may arise as well. Treatment with levodopa may partially reduce the rigidity, but the dramatic response to levodopa seen in patients with early PD is lacking.

Hyperkinetic Movement Disorders

Chorea

Chorea is a flowing, continuous, random movement that migrates from one part of the body to another. A variety of conditions are associated with chorea in older adults. The pathologic basis for chorea is dysfunction of the striatum. Huntington disease (HD) is the most common cause of chorea in adults. In HD, a patient's family history will suggest an autosomal dominant mode of inheritance, and other family members may have a genetically confirmed diagnosis. Sometimes, however, suggestive family history is lacking, or the patient may be the first family member to display a late onset of the disease with mild features. The diagnosis of HD can be made by genetic testing of the huntingtin gene, which entails a search for increased number of CAG repeats. Other causes of choreiform movements include drug-induced chorea (eg, from levodopa, anticonvulsants, estrogen), which is common and optimally treated by reducing or removing the offending agent. Chorea may arise from ischemic injury to the basal ganglia (ie, vascular chorea). Idiopathic choreiform movements may occur as an isolated symptom in adults ≥60 years old, a condition termed senile chorea if other causes of chorea have been excluded. Chorea can be treated with dopamine receptor–blocking medications (eg, risperidone[OL], haloperidol[OL]), but possible benefit must be weighed against adverse effects, including risk of development of tardive dyskinesia (SOE=B). Tetrabenazine blocks the storage and transport of dopamine presynaptically; it is currently approved by the FDA for the treatment of chorea in Huntington disease (SOE=A) and has be used to treat other causes of chorea. It is not associated with an increased risk of tardive dyskinesia. Patients taking tetrabenazine need to be monitored closely for signs of depression and parkinsonism.

Dystonia

Dystonia is a hyperkinetic movement disorder that results in sustained muscle contractions causing twisting movements or abnormal postures. Dystonia may occur as an isolated disorder, on a genetic basis, or as part of another movement disorder (eg, PD, corticobasal degeneration). Common focal dystonias seen in older adults include cervical dystonia (spasmodic torticollis), blepharospasm, spasmodic dysphonia, or focal hand dystonia (writer's cramp). Medications such as anticholinergics (eg, trihexyphenidyl) or muscle relaxants (eg, baclofen) may be tried, but improvement in symptoms is typically limited (SOE=B). Botulinum toxin injections into contracted muscle can provide effective, but temporary, relief of dystonia (SOE=A).

Drug-Induced Movement Disorders

Several different types of involuntary movements can arise as a result of the use of medications. It is important to distinguish among medication effects that are acute, chronic but reversible, and chronic and irreversible. One acute effect that may occur with antipsychotic medications is an acute dystonic reaction resulting in oral, lingual, or neck dystonia. If the dystonia is severe enough, treatment with intravenous diphenhydramine or lorazepam may be required, although this approach in older adults should be exercised with caution due to risk of adverse effects. Chronic reversible drug effects (effects that resolve when the causative medication is discontinued) include action tremor (eg, lithium, theophylline, valproic acid), parkinsonism (eg, antipsychotic or antiemetic medications), chorea (eg, anticonvulsant medications, estrogen, levodopa), or dystonia (dopamine replacement therapy in PD). Chronic irreversible drug effects or tardive phenomena often begin after the medication (usually an antipsychotic medication) has been used for weeks to months. Movements can include orobuccal dyskinesias, dystonia, akathisia (sensation of needing to move), myoclonus, and tics. Advanced age and duration of treatment with antipsychotic medications are the only well-established risk factors for developing tardive movement disorders. Once the diagnosis of a tardive phenomenon is established, the dosage of medication should be reduced, or the medication should be discontinued. Treatment for tardive dyskinesia or tardive dystonia includes anticholinergic agents (eg, trihexyphenidyl[OL]), baclofen[OL], and tetrabenazine[OL], all of which must be used with caution in older adults. In cases of severe tardive dystonia, intramuscular injections of botulinum toxin can reduce the frequency and severity of abnormal movements.

Essential Tremor

Essential tremor (ET) is the most common form of tremor. The tremor of ET is an action tremor, which is present when the limbs are in active use (eg, while writing or holding a cup). The tremor most commonly involves the arms, although the head and voice may be affected also. Other commonly affected areas of the body include the chin, tongue, and legs. Typically, the tremor in ET is symmetric, but it may be slightly worse in one arm than the other. The severity of the action tremor may vary significantly depending on the type of movement. The tremor disappears when the arms are relaxed, such as when the person is sitting with hands at rest in the lap, or standing with arms held at the sides. Functionally, the tremor may interfere with many daily activities, such as eating, writing, or fastening buttons. Stress or anxiety often exacerbates the tremor. The frequency of the tremor is in the range of 4–12 Hz, which is faster than the rest tremor of PD. The prevalence of ET increases with advancing age, with as many as 5% of adults >60 years old affected. The age of onset seems to have a bimodal distribution, with peaks in the teens through 20s and in the 50s through 70s. Prevalence rates among men and women are similar. Affected individuals commonly report they have an affected relative, suggesting a familial or genetic cause. Familial forms of the tremor have been linked to regions on chromosomes 2p and 3q. Familial and sporadic forms of ET have no apparent clinical differences. Alcohol may decrease the severity of ET.

The main indication for treatment of ET is functional disability due to the tremor (eg, difficulty writing, using a cup or spoon, trouble holding objects). It is important to educate the patient about exacerbating factors such as caffeine, stress, and fatigue. The first-line options for pharmacologic treatment of ET are nonselective β-blockers (propranolol, nadolol[OL]) or primidone[OL]

(SOE=A). Propranolol is the only drug approved by the FDA for treatment of ET. Each of these drugs improves the severity of tremor in most patients by approximately 30%–50%. Other medications, including baclofen[OL], gabapentin[OL], mirtazapine[OL], pregabalin[OL], and topiramate[OL], have been described as effective in some patients, but results have not been consistent (SOE=B/C). Occupational therapy may provide complementary benefit for patients whose tremor threatens function. Some patients with severe, medically refractory tremor may undergo DBS. DBS stimulation in the ventral intermediate nucleus of the thalamus provides significant improvement in tremor control in most patients (SOE=A). Potential adverse events are similar to those of DBS in PD (described above).

Restless Legs Syndrome

Restless legs syndrome (RLS) is a condition in which a patient feels an uncontrollable urge to move the legs at night, usually accompanied by an uncomfortable and unpleasant sensation of the legs that worsens with inactivity and improves with movement. The symptoms occur while the person is awake, and symptoms may also involve the arms. The diagnosis is based on the patient's description of the symptoms; polysomnography is not required. There may be a family history of the condition, particularly in patients with an earlier age of onset of RLS. Some patients have an associated, underlying medical disorder (eg, anemia, or renal or neurologic disease). RLS is 1.5 times more common in women than men, and evidence suggests that RLS prevalence increases with age. Periodic limb movements of sleep (PLMS), which entail involuntary limb movements while asleep, occurs in most (80%–90%) patients with RLS, but the presence of PLMS is not specific for RLS. RLS may also be seen in demented patients who may not be able to adequately describe the symptoms. Such patients may demonstrate behaviors such as rubbing or massaging of legs, increased motor activity (eg, pacing, wandering), and evidence of leg discomfort that occurs in the evening and/or with inactivity; improvement is evident with movement of the legs. Many medications may aggravate or induce RLS symptoms, such as antiemetics, antipsychotics, SSRIs, tricyclic antidepressants, and diphenhydramine. Clinicians should carefully review the medication regimens of patients with new or worsening RLS.

If pharmacologic treatment for RLS or PLMD is indicated (because of severity of symptoms or significant effects on quality of life), dopaminergic agents are the initial agent of choice. An evening dose of a dopamine agonist (eg, pramipexole or ropinirole, about 1–2 hours before bedtime) is effective in the treatment of RLS and PLMD (SOE=A). A nighttime dose of carbidopa-levodopa[OL] may also be effective (SOE=A) and can be used for patients who need medication infrequently (ie, for as-needed use). However, some patients describe a shift of their symptoms to daytime hours with successful treatment of symptoms at night; this problem (termed augmentation) appears more frequently when carbidopa-levodopa is selected as treatment for RLS. Recently, an extended-release form of gabapentin (gabapentin enacarbil) and pregabalin[OL] have been shown to be effective in improving RLS symptoms (SOE=A). The extended-release form of gabapentin has received FDA-approval for treatment of RLS. In a blinded, head-to-head comparison, pregabalin was as effective as the dopamine agonist pramipexole in controlling RLS symptoms but less likely to produce augmentation. RLS has been associated with iron deficiency, and RLS symptoms may improve with iron replacement therapy in such patients (SOE=B). Patients with RLS should be screened for iron deficiency. Benzodiazepines[OL] and opioids[OL] have also been used for RLS, but likely have more adverse events in older adults than the FDA-approved agents.

NEUROMUSCULAR DISORDERS, PERIPHERAL NEUROPATHY, AND MYELOPATHY

The prevalence of peripheral neuropathy in older adults has been estimated to be as high as 10%. Peripheral neuropathy can be particularly devastating in older adults, because it may cause gait impairment from sensory and motor deficits with a resulting propensity to fall. In developed countries, diabetic neuropathy is the most common form of the condition; up to 30%–60% of diabetic patients >60 years old have peripheral neuropathy. Several types of neuropathy are associated with diabetes mellitus, including a distal symmetric neuropathy; asymmetric neuropathies that may involve cranial nerves, roots, or plexi; and mononeuropathy multiplex. Other common causes of peripheral neuropathy in older adults are medications (eg, amiodarone, colchicine, phenytoin, lithium, vincristine, isoniazid), alcohol abuse, nutritional deficiencies (eg, deficiencies of vitamins B_6 and B_{12}, thiamine, folate, and niacin), renal disease (ie, uremia), monoclonal gammopathy (eg, multiple myeloma or monoclonal gammopathy of undetermined significance), hereditary forms of neuropathy, and neoplasia (eg, infiltration of peripheral nerves by malignant cells or paraneoplastic syndromes).

The history and physical examination are the most important tools in diagnosis of a peripheral neuropathy. Questions from the history should be geared toward identifying possible causes and risk factors. If the patient is not known to be diabetic, risk factors for diabetes or insulin resistance should be assessed. The past history and review of systems may give clues to a systemic disease that could contribute to a peripheral nerve disorder. A history of gastric bypass, eating disorder, or hemodialysis could indicate a possible nutritional deficiency. A thorough medication history should be taken to look for possible causes. The social history may uncover evidence of a possible exposure, such as alcohol or an occupational toxin. The family history should include inquiries for possible genetic forms of peripheral neuropathy. The neurologic examination focuses on establishing evidence of a length-dependent loss of sensory and/or motor function that is maximal distally in the limbs, associated with decreased reflexes and atrophy in affected regions.

Electrodiagnostic studies (ie, electromyography and nerve conduction studies) are considered an extension of the neurologic examination. They may yield valuable information in classifying the neuropathy, which may help to narrow a complicated differential diagnosis. First, these studies can differentiate between lesions affecting a single nerve, a nerve root, or a peripheral polyneuropathy. Next, they can help classify a polyneuropathy as axonal, demyelinating, or mixed. This distinction is important because certain neuropathies affect nerves in characteristic ways. For instance, a diabetic neuropathy is predominantly axonal, as are many of the toxic neuropathies such as alcohol and heavy metal exposure. In contrast, the hereditary and immune-mediated neuropathies more commonly cause peripheral demyelination. Acute, atypical, rapidly progressive, or severe forms of neuropathy should be referred to a neurologist with neuromuscular medicine expertise, who may perform tests of small fiber function, tests of autonomic function, peripheral nerve biopsy, and epidermal skin biopsy.

Treatment of the neuropathy depends on the underlying cause and ranges from withdrawal of the causative agent (eg, alcohol, medications) to nutritional supplementation (in the case of nutrient deficiency), to treatment of a primary cancer (in the setting of paraneoplastic neuropathy). There is evidence that optimizing glucose control can lessen the severity of diabetic neuropathy. Treatment of neuropathic pain may include the use of tricyclic antidepressants[OL] or anticonvulsant medications such as gabapentin and pregabalin. Gabapentin and pregabalin are approved for use in treatment of post-herpetic neuralgia, and pregabalin is also approved for use in diabetic neuropathy and fibromyalgia (SOE=A). Two other FDA-approved medication options for use in patients with diabetic neuropathic pain are duloxetine, which is a serotonin-norepinephrine reuptake inhibitor antidepressant, and tapentadol, which also blocks reuptake of serotonin and norepinephrine but also has additional agonist effects at mu-opioid receptors (SOE=A). In addition, tramadol[OL], which has properties similar to those of tapentadol, and opioids[OL] may be used to treat neuropathic pain (SOE=B). Topical agents such as capsaicin cream and local anesthetic medications (eg, lidocaine patch) may provide pain relief for some patient with peripheral neuropathy (SOE=B). Combination therapy with effective medications that have different mechanisms of action are often needed to control symptoms adequately.

Radiculopathy

Radiculopathy results from compression of a spinal root as it exits the spinal canal. Among older adults, this can be the result of herniated discs or osteophyte formation. Symptomatic nerve root compression may result in complaints of pain radiating down the neck, back, arm, or leg, and on neurologic examination, this can be accompanied by motor and sensory deficits as well as by diminution of reflexes in the distribution of a particular spinal root or roots. MRI imaging of the involved nerve root may determine a structural cause of radiculopathy. Progressive involvement of lumbosacral nerve roots may be seen in meningeal carcinomatosis. MRI imaging with contrast and lumbar puncture with cytology may help to make this diagnosis. An acute, immune-mediated form of polyradiculopathy is acute inflammatory demyelinating polyradiculoneuropathy (AIDP), also termed Guillain Barré syndrome. AIDP is treated with immunotherapy acutely, using either plasma exchange or intravenous immunoglobulin therapy (IVIG). Chronic inflammatory demyelinating polyneuropathy is a chronic form of AIDP and requires long-term immunotherapy. Patients with diabetes may present with diabetic amyotrophy, which is a lumbosacral polyradiculitis and plexopathy that starts with subacute onset of severe neuropathic pain in the thighs, which is often asymmetric, followed by proximal muscle weakness in the legs and eventual atrophy. Referral to a neuromuscular specialist is recommended for atypical and severe cases of radiculopathy.

Myopathy

Myopathies are characterized by proximal limb weakness, muscle wasting, and diminished or absent reflexes. They can be accompanied by increases in serum concentrations of muscle enzymes (eg, creatine kinase), a myopathic pattern on electromyogram, and abnormalities on muscle biopsy. Older adults may attribute mild to moderate muscle weakness to aging and therefore may not immediately consult a clinician. Proximal muscle weakness, which results in difficulty rising from a chair, climbing stairs, or washing one's hair, is particularly likely to be falsely attributed to aging or arthritis.

The most common myopathies in older adults are polymyositis, endocrine myopathies, and toxic myopathies. Polymyositis, a disorder of skeletal muscle with diverse causes, is characterized by lymphocytic infiltration of the muscles. Muscle biopsy usually shows signs of myocyte degeneration and regeneration as well. Immunotherapy with prednisone is considered the treatment of choice in polymyositis, but it should be used with caution in older adults because of adverse effects of chronic steroid use. In thyrotoxic myopathy, weakness and wasting are greatest in the pelvic girdle muscles and, to some extent, in the muscles of the shoulder region. Reflexes can be normal, and diagnosis is based on the distribution of muscle weakness in an individual with thyrotoxicosis. The myopathy improves with successful treatment of the underlying endocrine disorder. Hypothyroidism may cause a myopathy that improves with thyroid replacement therapy. Creatine kinase levels are significantly increased in the myopathy associated with hypothyroidism. Finally, several medications are known to cause myopathy, including corticosteroids, lipid-lowering agents, colchicine, and procainamide. The treatment of choice for drug-induced myopathy is cessation of the offending medication.

Motor Neuron Disease

Motor neuron disease, also called amyotrophic lateral sclerosis (ALS), is a neurodegenerative condition involving the cell bodies of both upper and lower motor neurons. It is characterized clinically by progressive weakness and wasting of skeletal muscles, often in combination with dysarthria, dysphagia, and respiratory failure. The incidence increases with age but reaches a plateau in the seventh decade of life. To date, age remains the single most clearly identifiable risk factor for this progressive and fatal disorder. Genetic causes of ALS are thought to occur in 5%–10% of patients. Four genes have been identified that can cause ALS. The gene C9ORF72 is the most common cause of familial ALS, accounting for 25%–40% of such cases. Mutations in this gene can also cause frontotemporal dementia or a combination of ALS and frontotemporal dementia.

Patients with ALS commonly present with gait disturbance, falls, foot drop, weakness in grip, dysphagia, or dysarthria. On neurologic examination, patients may have a combination of upper motor neuron signs (eg, hyperreflexia, clonus, extensor plantar responses) and lower motor neuron signs (eg, weakness, atrophy, fasciculations). Weakness of the face, tongue, and palate are common, but extraocular muscles are usually spared. The electromyogram demonstrates findings consistent with diffuse denervation and poor recruitment of motor units. The differential diagnosis includes lesions at the level of the foramen magnum, a combination of cervical myelopathy associated with cervical and lumbar polyradiculopathies, or a motor predominant peripheral polyneuropathy in a patient with CNS lesions. The prognosis is poor with survival time averaging 2–3 years. The presence of bulbar weakness carries a poorer prognosis. Although most new cases of ALS are in older adults, it is less common than several other neurologic disorders in this population. Therefore, gait disturbance and focal motor weakness may frequently be incorrectly attributed to the more common conditions. Older adults are also more likely to have coexisting neurologic disorders that might explain symptoms of weakness, adding to the challenge of and delay in diagnosing ALS. In one study, afflicted individuals >65 years old were diagnosed after 19 months, while those <65 years old were diagnosed after 3 months.

Treatment of ALS is predominantly supportive. Riluzole, which has demonstrated modest effects on survival or time to tracheostomy (SOE=A), is in widespread use. Riluzole is thought to protect against glutamate toxicity, which may be involved in the pathogenesis of ALS. Follow-up in a dedicated multidisciplinary ALS or muscular dystrophy clinic has also been shown to improve quality of life of ALS patients and may improve survival (SOE=B). In these settings, patients may receive multidisciplinary care from a team, including a neuromuscular subspecialist; respiratory, physical, occupational, and speech therapists; and a social worker. Noninvasive support of ventilation, such as bilevel intermittent positive-airway pressure (BiPAP), has been shown to improve survival in ALS patients with respiratory compromise (SOE=A).

Myelopathy

In older adults, myelopathy or spinal cord dysfunction can be the result of extrinsic compression of the spinal cord or intrinsic spinal cord lesions. The cervical region is affected most commonly. Intrinsic spinal cord lesions may include spinal cord tumors, vascular events (eg, infarcts or hemorrhages), or trauma (eg, central cord syndrome). Extrinsic compressive lesions are more prevalent; common causes among older adults are cervical spondylosis (with resultant osteophyte formation and degenerative disc disease), disc prolapse or herniation, rheumatoid arthritis with vertebral body subluxation, meningioma, or spinal metastases. Nearly 80% of adults ≥70 years old have radiographic evidence of osteophyte formation with some narrowing of the spinal canal, but most are asymptomatic. Cervical spinal stenosis most often arises from spondylosis but may be worsened by disc protrusion or a congenitally narrow canal. Narrowing of the cervical canal can lead to neck stiffness and pain; radicular pain, sensory loss, or weakness in the arms; and weakness and upper motor neuron signs (eg, hyperreflexia, spasticity, Babinski sign) in the legs. Narrowing of the lumbar canal may lead to lower back pain; radicular pain, sensory loss, or weakness in the legs; and lower motor neuron signs in the legs. Lumbar spinal stenosis causes neurogenic claudication, manifested by increasing pain with weakness and numbness while walking, relieved by flexion at the waist or sitting.

MRI can be helpful for diagnosis of myelopathy, but results must be viewed with caution as abnormal MRI findings are common in asymptomatic older adults. If the patient cannot tolerate MRI because of the presence of an implanted metallic object (such as a pacemaker) or severe claustrophobia, then spinal CT with intrathecal contrast may be performed. Conservative management includes activity modification, neck immobilization with a cervical collar, massage, heat treatment, physical therapy, and analgesics. Decompressive surgery is recommended for patients with persistent pain or progressive neurologic deficit. Older adults are more prone to have multiple levels of involvement, and some studies have suggested the prognosis after surgery of older adults is poorer than that of younger patients.

HEADACHES

The prevalence of headaches appears to diminish with age. One study demonstrated that although 74% of men and 92% of women 21–34 years old have headaches, these proportions drop to 22% and 55% after the age of 75 years. Headache is one of the most common medical complaints in young persons, and yet one study suggests that it is the tenth most common symptom in older women and the fourteenth most common symptom in older men. The incidence of migraine, the most common cause of headaches in younger adults, also declines with age, with only 2% of people developing their first migraine after age 50.

New-onset or persistent headaches in older adults are more likely to represent systemic illness or intracranial lesions (ie, secondary causes). In one study, 10% of headaches among younger patients represented systemic illness or intracranial lesions; in older adults, this proportion was 34%. These secondary causes include intracranial masses (eg, primary or secondary tumors, subdural hematomas), cervical spondylosis, chronic obstructive pulmonary disease, obstructive sleep apnea, carbon monoxide poisoning, and giant cell arteritis. Brain imaging with contrast (ie, head CT or brain MRI) is indicated in older patients with new-onset or progressive headaches to exclude structural causes. An important secondary cause of headache specific to older adults is giant cell (temporal) arteritis. Temporal arteritis does not appear to develop in those <50 years old and peaks in incidence between the ages of 70 and 80.

Women are affected twice as often as men. Pain may be centered at the temporal or occipital arteries. Palpation of the scalp arteries may reveal focal tenderness and nodularity. Complaints of visual changes, low-grade fever, polymyalgia, and constitutional symptoms further suggest the diagnosis. Typically, the serum sedimentation rate is significantly increased, and the diagnosis is made with a temporal artery biopsy. If the diagnosis is suspected and biopsy is planned within a few days, then corticosteroids may be initiated to prevent vascular complications (eg, loss of vision or stroke). In addition to structural and systemic causes of headaches, many commonly used medications may cause headaches that are dull, diffuse, and nondescript, including vasodilators (eg, nitrates), antihypertensives, antidepressant medications, and stimulants.

The common primary headache disorders can be classified into migraine (with or without aura), tension-type headaches, cluster headache, and chronic daily headaches. Migraines are headaches of moderate to severe intensity associated with nausea, vomiting, or photophobia. Half of the time they are unilateral and throbbing, but commonly the pain is bilateral. Auras, when they occur, usually precede the headache and are manifested by transient neurologic symptoms that can be localized to the cerebral cortex or brain stem. Visual phenomena are among the most common types of auras. Migraine headaches in older adults typically present as they do in younger people, but atypical presentations have been described. These include migraine auras without headache (acephalic migraine). The occurrence of an isolated visual or sensory aura in the absence of a headache can be diagnostically challenging, because it can mimic signs of a transient ischemic attack. In contrast to migraines, tension-type headaches typically are more diffuse in distribution, less severe in intensity, have a pressing or a tight quality, and are much less often associated with nausea or vomiting. Cluster headaches are much more common in men, may be associated with tearing and rhinorrhea, are of shorter duration (15 minutes commonly but up to 3 hours) than migraines, but are severe in intensity and tend to recur in clusters during an interval of time (eg, within a day or within a few weeks). Chronic daily headaches are persistent, often bilateral, and have features that overlap with those of both migraine and tension-type headaches.

The treatment of migraine headaches can be categorized as either abortive (treating an attack that has already begun) or preventive. Other than various OTC preparations that contain NSAIDs, migraine-specific abortive therapies include ergotamines or triptans (eg, sumatriptan), which act by central serotonergic mechanisms. These medications are mild vasoconstrictors and contraindicated in patients with uncontrolled hypertension, stroke, or coronary artery disease. Generally, safety data in geriatric populations are lacking. Preventive therapies for migraine include nonselective β-blockers (eg, propranolol[OL]), valproic acid, topiramate, tricyclic antidepressants[OL], and calcium channel blockers (eg, verapamil[OL]). Preventive therapies decrease the frequency and severity of migraine over time and should be considered in patients who have disabling migraine headaches ≥2 times per month. The choice of agent should be guided by an effort to avoid adverse events and drug interactions. Treatment of muscle tension headaches includes NSAIDs[OL] as abortive agents and low doses of tricyclic antidepressants[OL] as preventive medication in chronic muscle tension headaches. Muscle relaxants, such as tizanidine[OL], have shown some effectiveness in treating chronic muscle tension headaches in open-label studies. Each of the medications above may be contraindicated by comorbidities or existing medication regimens. A referral to a headache specialist should be considered for patients with either cluster headaches or chronic daily headaches.

REFERENCES

- Ferreira JJ, Katzenschlager R, Bloem BR, et al. Summary of the recommendations of the EFNS/MDS-ES review on therapeutic management of Parkinson's disease. *Eur J Neurol.* 2013;20(1):5–15.

    This is an extensive review of therapeutic options for the treatment of Parkinson's disease, including disease modification and symptomatic pharmacotherapy for motor symptoms and non-motor symptoms. A very thorough list of references is provided.

- Postuma RB, Berg D, Stern M, et al. MDS clinical diagnostic criteria for Parkinson's disease. *Mov Disord.* 2015;30(12):1591–1599.

    This paper outlines the criteria required to make a clinical diagnosis of Parkinson's disease, including required features, supportive features, exclusion criteria and "red flags". References are provided on the medical literature supporting these diagnostic criteria.

- Roberson ED, Hope OA, Martin RC, et al. Geriatric epilepsy: Research and clinical directions for the future. *Epilepsy Behav.* 2011;22(1):103–111.

    This article summarizes the scope of the problems posed by epilepsy in older adult populations and discusses diagnostic and treatment issues. In addition, the article highlights the work of two young investigators in the field. One studies basic mechanisms of epileptic activity in Alzheimer's disease animal models, and the second focuses on defining and measuring the quality of geriatric epilepsy care.

- Watson JC, Dyck PJ. Peripheral neuropathy: a practical approach to diagnosis and symptom management. *Mayo Clin Proc.* 2015;90(7):940–951.

    This article describes how to screen for a peripheral neuropathy in the office setting, how to determine which patients should be referred to a specialist for further evaluation, and how to treat symptoms of painful peripheral neuropathy.

- Wrobel Goldberg S, Silberstein S, Grosberg BM. Considerations in the treatment of tension-type headache in the elderly. *Drugs Aging.* 2014;31(11):797–804.

    This paper provides a review of the most common primary headache type in the elderly, tension-type headaches. The authors discuss diagnostic criteria, the epidemiology of tension-type headaches in older adults, and treatment options.

Daniel L. Murman, MD, MS, FAAN

CHAPTER 61—STROKE AND CEREBROVASCULAR DISEASE

KEY POINTS

- Cerebrovascular disease is a leading cause of disability and death among older adults.

- Acute stroke treatments can effectively improve outcomes in patients, especially when care is provided soon after stroke symptoms begin and in a multidisciplinary stroke center.

- Primary and secondary stroke prevention can significantly decrease the burden of cerebrovascular disease in older populations.

IMPACT OF CEREBROVASCULAR DISEASE

Stroke is a leading cause of disability and death among older adults. The incidence of stroke increases with advancing age, approximately doubling with each decade. At younger ages, incidence of stroke for women is 25%–30% lower than that for men in comparable age groups, but it surpasses that of men ≥85 years old. Approximately 795,000 new strokes occur each year in the United States, and there are an estimated 6.8 million adults who are stroke survivors. Long-term disability is very common in stroke survivors. Six months after a stroke in those ≥65 years old, 26% are dependent in their activities of daily living and 46% have measurable cognitive deficits. Although older age is associated with worse functional recovery (measured by independence in performing activities of daily living), stroke patients at any age can benefit from formal rehabilitation.

Besides being the most common acute, serious neurologic disease, stroke is also a leading cause of death. The fatality rate within 1 month of an acute stroke is 20%–30% across all age groups. Survival in part depends on the anatomic location and severity of the stroke. Neurologic causes of death include the brain injury itself or resultant brain edema. Common medical causes of death associated with stroke are myocardial infarction, arrhythmia, heart failure, aspiration pneumonia, and pulmonary embolism.

ISCHEMIC STROKE

Ischemic strokes are caused by occlusion of a cerebral blood vessel causing interruption of blood flow and infarction of the brain. Approximately 80%–85% of strokes are ischemic. Epidemiologic studies suggest that approximately 27% of ischemic strokes are due to cardiac emboli, 19% are due to large vessel disease, 17% are due to small vessel disease, and 35% cannot be classified. These proportions vary by 5%–10% among different study populations because of differences in risk factors, diagnostic studies performed, and race. Knowing the cause of the ischemic stroke helps to guide treatment decisions and to estimate risk and prognosis.

Small Vessel Disease

Small vessel disease causes occlusion of small penetrating vessels due to lipohyalinosis (lipid deposition and hyalinization) or local arteriolosclerosis. Small vessels supply deep white and gray matter structures such as the internal capsule, basal ganglia, thalamus, and pons. Occlusion of these small vessels can result in several well-defined clinical syndromes, including pure motor hemiplegia, pure hemisensory stroke, ataxic hemiparesis, and dysarthria–clumsy hand syndrome. Small vessel disease causes ischemic strokes that are typically less than one centimeter in size and are termed lacunar infarcts. Risk factors include hypertension, diabetes mellitus, and smoking. Lacunar strokes can occur independently or concurrently with large vessel cerebrovascular disease or other mechanisms of ischemic stroke.

Large Vessel Disease

Large vessel disease is most commonly caused by atherosclerosis and can cause progressive occlusion of cerebral vessels in the anterior and posterior circulation. Ischemic stroke in the setting of large vessel disease is often caused by emboli generated by the atherosclerotic lesion. Complete occlusion of large cerebral vessels can lead to severe and often life-threatening strokes. Strokes caused by large vessel disease can cause recognizable clinical syndromes that are consistent with anatomical distribution of major cerebral vessels (eg, hemiparesis or hemisensory loss associated with aphasia, apraxia, neglect, or visual field deficits). In addition, a lesion at the origin of the internal carotid artery can lead to transient monocular blindness (amaurosis fugax) or a cerebral hemispheric deficit, because both the retina and cerebral hemispheres derive their blood supply from the internal carotid artery. Syndromes associated with vascular lesions in the posterior circulation (vertebral and basilar arteries) can result in dysfunction of the cranial nerves, descending motor or ascending sensory tracts within the brain stem, cerebellar and vestibular pathways, and visual cortex. Signs and symptoms can include crossed cranial nerve and long-tract findings (eg, complete facial palsy ipsilateral to the lesion and hemiparesis involving the contralateral arm and leg), vertigo, double vision, ataxia, dysarthria, hemianopia or cortical blindness, Horner syndrome (ipsilateral miosis, anhidrosis, and mild ptosis), stupor, or coma. Large vessel disease can be identified by noninvasive imaging of the carotid arteries (Doppler ultrasonography, computer tomography angiography, or magnetic resonance angiography) or conventional angiography. Risk factors for large vessel disease include hypertension, hyperlipidemia, diabetes, and smoking.

Cardioembolic and Cryptogenic Stroke

Cardioembolic strokes are an important, potentially preventable cause of ischemic stroke. Atrial fibrillation is the most common cause of cardioembolic stroke, associated with a 4-to 5-fold increased risk because of thrombus formation in the left atrial appendage and cardioembolism to cerebral vessels. Cardioembolic stroke due to atrial fibrillation accounts for 25%–30% of all ischemic strokes. The estimated stroke risk is similar for persistent and paroxysmal atrial fibrillation. Emboli from the heart tend to occlude medium-sized cerebral vessels (eg, branches of the middle cerebral artery) and often cause multiple cerebral infarcts that involve more than one vascular territory. Cardioembolic strokes often occur without preceding transient ischemic attack (TIA).

A substantial proportion of ischemic strokes do not have a clearly identifiable cause and are classified as cryptogenic. Brain and vascular imaging should, however, provide an indication of the size of the vessel(s) involved. Atypical causes of stroke should be considered in the setting of cryptogenic stroke (eg, vasculitis, coagulopathy, mitochondrial disorder), and prolonged cardiac monitoring is sometimes needed to capture intermittent atrial fibrillation as a potential cause of cryptogenic stroke.

Treatment of Acute Ischemic Stroke

In the setting of acute stroke symptoms, it is important to quickly determine whether the patient is suffering from an ischemic or hemorrhagic event with head CT imaging, and then to assess the severity and pattern of neurologic deficits. The NIH Stroke Scale (NIHSS) is a standardized rating scale used for this assessment (Table 61.1). The severity of deficits on this scale can help to make therapeutic decisions acutely and to determine long-term prognosis during the recovery phase. In general, a NIHSS score of <5 is associated with a very good prognosis. Individuals with a score >20 have a very poor prognosis and a high likelihood of major complications. In the immediate evaluation, non-stroke causes of acute neurologic dysfunction, such as migraine, seizure, and drug intoxication, need to be identified. Recent meta-analyses suggest that patients who are evaluated and treated in a multidisciplinary stroke center have better survival and functional outcomes than those who are not (SOE=B).

Table 61.1—Components of the National Institutes of Health Stroke Scale[a]

Stroke Scale Item	Item Score[b]
Level of consciousness	0–7
Best gaze	0–2
Visual fields	0–3
Facial palsy	0–3
Motor: arms	0–8
Motor: legs	0–8
Limb ataxia	0–2
Sensory	0–2
Best language	0–3
Dysarthria	0–2
Extinction and inattention	0–2
Total	**0–42**

[a] Full details of criteria for scoring each item can be obtained at www.ninds.nih.gov/doctors/NIH_Stroke_Scale.pdf (accessed Jan 2016).
[b] Greater score reflects increased impairment.

The current protocol for acute care of the older stroke patient includes optimizing hydration status; controlling blood pressure while avoiding hypotension; preventing deep-vein thrombosis; detecting and treating coronary ischemia, heart failure, and cardiac arrhythmias; and starting long-term treatment with antiplatelet agents or oral anticoagulation (depending on the presumed cause) to prevent recurrent stroke. Body temperature and blood glucose should be normalized in the acute setting. Dehydration on presentation is common, but rehydration should occur gradually to reduce the risk of cerebral edema. To prevent aspiration pneumonia, all ischemic stroke patients should receive a formal dysphagia evaluation before allowing oral intake. Immediately after an ischemic cerebral infarction, treatment of hypertension should be delayed (unless blood pressure is very high, eg, >220/120 mmHg) until the situation stabilizes. The eventual goal is to reduce blood pressure gradually (eg, a goal of 15% reduction over the first 24 hours) while avoiding hypotension. The target systolic blood pressure should be 10–20 mmHg higher than the baseline pressure; if the baseline is unknown, systolic pressure should not be lowered below 160 mmHg. Patients treated with thrombolytic agents (see below) require careful blood pressure monitoring, especially during the first 24 hours of treatment. Patients with a history of ischemic heart disease or arrhythmia, and patients with embolic strokes should be monitored with telemetry for at least 48 hours. For large, ischemic strokes (eg, involving most of the middle cerebral artery territory, or that of both middle and anterior cerebral arteries) in the setting of atrial fibrillation, anticoagulation therapy is not initiated for 7–14 days after onset because of a high risk of hemorrhagic transformation. Earlier anticoagulation does not improve outcome in these patients.

Recombinant tissue-plasminogen activator (rt-PA, alteplase) is approved for treatment of acute, ischemic stroke by the FDA. Infusion of this medication within 3 hours of stroke onset approximately doubles the chances of a favorable outcome at 3 months (SOE=A; very limited data in older adults). However, the benefits of rt-PA must be weighed against the increased risk of intracranial hemorrhage, which can be fatal or result in worsened neurologic status. Overall, the literature suggests that approximately one-third of patients treated with thrombolytic therapy have a better outcome, as measured by >1-point improvement in the modified Rankin scale (ie, a clinically meaningful improvement), when compared with placebo. Intracerebral hemorrhage occurs in 6% of patients and is fatal in approximately half of these individuals. Most hemorrhagic events occur among patients with severe strokes (eg, NIHSS score >20).

Use of rt-PA requires careful assessment by a clinician experienced in treatment of stroke. rt-PA should be considered in all patients who present within 3 hours of onset of neurologic deficit and in whom CT confirms the absence of intracranial hemorrhage. Major contraindications include major surgery within the previous 2 weeks, previous intracranial hemorrhage, sustained systolic blood pressure >185 mmHg or diastolic >110 mmHg despite treatment, symptoms of subarachnoid hemorrhage, recent uncontrollable source of bleeding, coagulopathy, thrombocytopenia (platelet count <100,000 mm^3), or INR >1.7. The American Heart Association (AHA) has recommended an increase in the window for use of rt-PA in acute stroke to 3–4.5 hours after symptom onset in patients ≤80 years old who have an NIHSS score of ≤25 and no prior history of stroke or diabetes. This AHA recommendation was based on results from the European Cooperative Acute Stroke Study 3 (ECASS 3), which identified continued benefit in this time window (SOE=B).

Four recent randomized clinical trials have shown that endovascular thrombectomy in patients with proximal, large vessel occlusions of the anterior cerebral circulation provides significant benefit when treatment begins within 6 hours of stroke onset. In these studies, most patients received rt-PA (given IV) before endovascular thrombectomy. This combination therapy is best delivered in a coordinated, comprehensive stroke center. The benefits of this therapy were seen at 24 hours, with a 50% reduction in stroke severity as measured by the NIHSS, and again at 90 days with improvements in functional outcomes as measured by the modified Rankin Scale (mRS). The number needed to treat for a mRS of 0–2 (functional independence) at 90 days ranged between 2 and 4 in these trials (SOE=A).

Transient Ischemic Attack (TIA)

Special consideration should be given to those suffering a TIA, which is defined as a brief episode of neurologic dysfunction caused by focal ischemia to the brain or spinal cord that does not result in acute infarction. The traditional definition suggested that these deficits could last up to 24 hours, but with newer imaging it is clear that a TIA typically lasts <1–2 hours, and longer episodes are commonly associated with acute infarction. TIA is a major risk factor for subsequent stroke. A patient with TIA symptoms should be evaluated emergently. Brain imaging, ideally with MRI, is important to determine whether there has been an acute stroke and, if one is found, its location and type. Noninvasive imaging of the carotid arteries (Doppler ultrasonography or magnetic resonance angiography), electrocardiogram, and an echocardiogram are important tests to obtain to better determine the most likely cause of ischemia. Fasting glucose and lipid levels should be measured, blood pressure monitored, and patients asked about tobacco use to look for modifiable risk factors. Treatment for patients with TIA is focused on completion of diagnostic tests and initiation of treatments for secondary stroke prevention based on the results of the evaluation.

Primary and Secondary Ischemic Stroke Prevention

Throughout the latter half of the 20th century, the incidence of stroke declined in the United States, Canada, and Western Europe. In the past four decades, stroke incidence rates have fallen by 42% in high-income countries but have remained the same or increased in low and middle-income countries. The drop in incidence in high-income countries is attributable in part to better control of modifiable risk factors, including hypertension, heart disease, diabetes mellitus, cigarette smoking, and increased blood lipids. Hypertension is the most prevalent risk factor for stroke, and its treatment substantially reduces that risk. Treatment of isolated systolic hypertension in older adults reduces the risk of stroke by nearly 40% (SOE=A). Initiation of blood pressure (BP) therapy to maintain the systolic BP <140 mmHg and diastolic BP <90 mmHg is recommended for secondary stroke prevention (SOE=A) and for primary prevention in those with other risk factors such as diabetes. Dyslipidemia is another independent risk factor for stroke. Treatment with an HMG coenzyme-A reductase inhibitor ("statin") is recommended for the primary prevention of ischemic stroke in patients estimated to have a high 10-year risk of cardiovascular events based on AHA guidelines (SOE=A). In patients who have had a TIA or stroke believed to be of atherosclerotic origin, high-intensity statin therapy is recommended, regardless of the LDL-C level, to prevent future TIA or stroke (SOE=B). Several studies have confirmed a 2- to 4-fold increased risk of stroke in individuals with diabetes mellitus (SOE=A). Some research suggests that tight control of blood glucose levels in healthier adults might reduce the risk of stroke in individuals with diabetes mellitus, although the evidence for reduction of other vascular complications (eg, retinopathy, nephropathy) is more compelling. Additionally, aggressive treatment of hypertension and hyperlipidemia in the diabetic population is a crucial component in lowering the risk of stroke. Cigarette smoking independently increases the risk of stroke as much as 3-fold (SOE=A). Nevertheless, the incidence of stroke declines significantly even after 2 years of smoking cessation, and after 5 years the level of risk returns to that of nonsmokers. Thus, counseling and assisting patients to stop smoking is important.

For patients with valvular and nonvalvular atrial fibrillation (AF) at high risk of stroke and low risk of hemorrhagic complications, long-term oral anticoagulation therapy is recommended (SOE=A). Risk stratification scales developed for patients with AF, such as the CHADS2 or CHA2DS2-VASc risk scores, can help determine risk. Scores ≥2 points imply high risk. A meta-analysis of stroke prevention trials in the setting of nonvalvular atrial fibrillation has shown an average relative risk reduction of 64% for warfarin and 19% for aspirin when compared with placebo. Warfarin dosed to a target INR of 2.0–3.0 is recommended for valvular AF (SOE=A). For nonvalvular AF, first-line anticoagulant options are warfarin with INR 2.0–3.0 (SOE=A) or the novel oral anticoagulants apixaban, edoxaban, and rivaroxaban, with dabigatran as an alternative (SOE=B). For patients with nonvalvular AF and low risk of stroke, aspirin can be considered (SOE=C). If possible, oral anticoagulation should be initiated within 14 days of the TIA or stroke in those with AF.

Aspirin is the mainstay of antiplatelet therapy for secondary stroke prevention in patients with noncardioembolic ischemic stroke (SOE=A; relative risk reduction 15%–20%; NNT approximately 60 for prevention of one stroke over 1 year of therapy). Studies on the use of aspirin in stroke prevention suggest that dosages >325 mg/d do not add therapeutic benefit, but the minimal necessary dosage has not been definitively determined. Many clinicians routinely prescribe 81–325 mg/d, although even the lower dosage can cause GI irritation and blood loss. Other antiplatelet medications are available but have not shown consistent superiority to aspirin. These agents include sustained-release dipyridamole combined with aspirin (SOE=A) and clopidogrel (SOE=B). Clopidogrel 75 mg/d is an alternative for patients who cannot tolerate aspirin. Combining clopidogrel and aspirin does not provide additional benefit in the secondary prevention of stroke when initiated days to years after a stroke or TIA (SOE=B). In two large trials, no benefit was found for the use of warfarin over aspirin for secondary stroke prevention (SOE=A) in the setting of large vessel disease, including intracranial atherosclerotic disease.

For all patients with cerebral atherosclerotic disease, medical management should target modifiable risk factors and should include daily use of an antiplatelet agent and a statin (SOE=B). For patients with ≥70% symptomatic carotid stenosis, carotid endarterectomy (CEA) significantly reduces subsequent stroke risk, provided that endarterectomy is performed at an institution and by a surgeon with extensive experience with the procedure and perioperative risk of morbidity and mortality <6% (SOE=A). For patients with recent TIA or ischemic stroke and ipsilateral moderate (50%–69%) carotid stenosis, CEA can be considered if the patient is a good surgical candidate and the perioperative morbidity and mortality risk is <6%. In this setting, the number needed to treat [NNT] is 15 to prevent one ipsilateral stroke over 5 years of follow-up (SOE=B). Endovascular treatment with carotid artery angioplasty and stenting (CAS) using an embolic-protection device has been shown to demonstrate similar efficacy and safety, with less procedural morbidity, than endarterectomy for significant stenosis (SOE=B), making this procedure an attractive option in patients with significant comorbidities (especially those at high risk of general anesthesia or with prior neck radiation exposure, prior carotid endarterectomy, or contralateral carotid occlusion). It is reasonable to consider performing CEA or CAS in *asymptomatic* patients who have >70% stenosis of the internal carotid artery if the perioperative risk of stroke, myocardial infarction, and death is very low (< 3%, SOE=B). CEA or CAS is not recommended for asymptomatic carotid stenosis <70%.

Treatment of cryptogenic stroke includes evaluating and treating modifiable stroke risk factors and initiating antiplatelet therapy. Atypical causes of stroke should be considered, including coagulopathies, vasculitis, metabolic or genetic causes, and a referral to a vascular neurologist may be helpful in diagnosis and management. If a cardioembolic cause is suspected, then prolonged (eg, 30 days) cardiac rhythm monitoring for AF is reasonable (SOE=B), and oral anticoagulant therapy should be initiated if intermittent AF is found. There are insufficient data to establish whether anticoagulation is equivalent or superior to aspirin for secondary stroke prevention in patients with a patent foramen ovale (PFO) but without AF (SOE=B). However, in the setting of PFO and venous source of embolism, oral anticoagulation is recommended (SOE=A). If anticoagulation is contraindicated in such a patient, then an inferior vena cava filter (SOE=C) or transcatheter PFO (SOE=C) closure can be considered. In a patient with cryptogenic

TIA or stroke who has a PFO but no venous source of embolism, available evidence does not support a benefit for PFO closure (SOE=B).

HEMORRHAGIC STROKE

Hemorrhagic strokes (intracranial hemorrhages) account for 15%–20% of all strokes. There are 4 main subtypes: intracerebral hemorrhage, subarachnoid hemorrhage, subdural hematoma, and epidural hematoma. Intracerebral hemorrhages outnumber subarachnoid hemorrhage by approximately 2 to 1. Subdural hematomas and epidural hematomas are less common than subarachnoid hemorrhages and most commonly caused by trauma. Intracranial hemorrhages present with abrupt onset of focal neurologic symptoms and often are associated with severe headache, vomiting, very high blood pressure, and coma or decreased level of consciousness. However, none of these features is specific enough to distinguish the syndrome from ischemic stroke on the basis of clinical features alone. For this reason, emergent brain imaging (eg, head CT) is needed to determine whether a stroke is hemorrhagic or ischemic. Hemorrhagic strokes carry a higher risk of mortality than ischemic strokes and are best treated in comprehensive stroke centers with neurosurgical expertise and neurointensive care units.

Intracerebral Hemorrhage

The most common risk factor for spontaneous intracerebral hemorrhage (ICH) is uncontrolled hypertension, which is present in 75%–80% of cases. Excessive use of alcohol is also associated with a higher incidence. The incidence of ICH increases with age, from 36 per 100,000 person-years in those aged 55–64 to 196 per 100,000 person-years in those older than 84. Common locations for "hypertensive bleeds" are the putamen, thalamus, cerebellar hemisphere, pons, and cerebrum. These are structures supplied by small penetrating vessels that are prone to rupture in the setting of uncontrolled hypertension. Another important cause of spontaneous ICH in older adults is lobar hemorrhage caused by cerebral amyloid angiopathy, which can be visualized as microbleeds on brain MRI scans and can be associated with Alzheimer disease. Intracranial bleeds tend to be recurrent in patients with cerebral amyloid angiopathy. The risk of spontaneous ICH can also be increased by oral anticoagulants, especially warfarin when the INR exceeds 3.

For patients presenting with acute ICH who have a systolic BP between 150 and 220 mmHg, acute lowering of the systolic BP to 140 mmHg is safe and recommended (SOE=A). Patients on warfarin should receive intravenous vitamin K and therapy to replace vitamin K–dependent clotting factors to normalize the INR (SOE=B). Patients with severe coagulation factor deficiency or severe thrombocytopenia should receive appropriate factor replacement therapy or platelets as needed (SOE=B). All anticoagulant and antiplatelet therapies should be stopped in the acute period. Initial management of ICH patients should occur in an intensive care unit or dedicated stroke unit with neurologic acute care expertise (SOE=B). All patients with ICH should have intermittent pneumatic compression stockings placed on admission to prevent deep-vein thrombosis (SOE=A) and receive formal screening for dysphagia before oral intake to reduce the risk of pneumonia (SOE=B). Patients with cerebellar hemorrhage who are deteriorating neurologically, who have brain-stem compression, or ventricular obstruction should undergo surgical removal of the hemorrhage as soon as possible (SOE=B). In addition, some large hemorrhages with intraventricular extension may also require neurosurgical intervention.

The most important intervention to prevent recurrent ICH is long-term blood pressure control with a goal of <130 mmHg systolic and <80 mmHg diastolic (SOE=B). The decision to restart anticoagulation or antiplatelet medications after ICH can be difficult. The choice depends on many factors, including but not limited to the reason the medications were started, the cause of the hemorrhage, the risk of future ischemic events, and the neurologic state of the patient. In those at high risk of future ischemic cerebrovascular events, such as those with mechanical heart valves and prior ischemic stroke, restarting anticoagulation may be needed within 2 weeks of the hemorrhage, but in all others it is not recommended to restart oral anticoagulation for at least 4 weeks to prevent recurrent hemorrhage (SOE=B).

Subarachnoid Hemorrhage

Subarachnoid hemorrhage (SAH) is caused by a rupture of an intracranial aneurysm (80%–85% of the time) or another abnormality of a cerebral vessel (eg, arteriovenous malformation). Some subgroups are at higher risk of developing intracranial aneurysms, including those with autosomal dominant polycystic kidney disease (3- to 10-fold increase in risk), connective tissue diseases (eg, Marfan syndrome, Ehlers-Danlos syndrome), and some genetic disorders (Klinefelter syndrome, neurofibromatosis type 1, α_1-antitrypsin deficiency). The incidence of intracranial saccular aneurysms increases with age from 21 per 100,000 person-years at age 60 to 41 per 100,000 person-years at age 80. These aneurysms are more common in women in each age range after age 45. High-risk groups (eg, polycystic kidney disease, strong family history of aneurysm or SAH) should be offered noninvasive screening for saccular aneurysms with CT or MR angiography (SOE=B).

Unruptured cerebral aneurysms are relatively common, with prevalence estimates of 2000–4000 per

100,000, but the incidence of SAH is 10 per 100,000 person-years. Thus, determining what factors increase the risk of rupture is important to effectively manage these unruptured cerebral aneurysms. Meta-analyses have shown that risk of rupture is associated with the size of the aneurysm, age, female gender, posterior circulation location, change in size of aneurysm over time, and prior SAH. The importance of aneurysm size was shown by a large prospective longitudinal study which documented that the annual risk of rupture was ≤0.5% for aneurysms <7 mm, 1.69% for those 7–9 mm, 4.37% for those 10–24 mm and 33.4% for those >25 mm. Patients with aneurysms at higher risk of rupture should be referred to a neurosurgeon with expertise in management of cerebral aneurysms. Treatment options for unruptured cerebral aneurysm in high-risk patients include surgical clipping or endovascular coil embolization of the lesion. Location and size of the aneurysm and patient characteristics are considered when deciding on the best approach.

The acute management of SAH is similar to that of ICH but includes both medical and surgical interventions to prevent additional bleeding, and focuses on detection and treatment of arterial vasospasm that commonly complicates SAH. As in ICH, treatment in a multidisciplinary stroke center with neurosurgical expertise and an ICU with neuroscience expertise is needed for best outcomes.

Subdural Hematoma

A subdural hematoma is a collection of blood between the dura and the arachnoid. It is usually due to head trauma, although the trauma may be mild, particularly in older adults. In approximately 15% of cases, the hematomas are bilateral. Some older adults suffer from chronic subdural hematoma that may be symptomatic. The incidence of chronic subdural hematoma increases with age, from 0.13 per 100,000 person-years for those in their 20s to 7.4 per 100,000 person-years for those in their 70s. In 50% of chronic subdural hematomas, there is no history of head injury, and other risk factors include clotting disorders, shunting procedures, and seizures. Symptoms of chronic subdural hematoma are headache, slight to moderate cognitive impairment, and focal neurologic signs (eg, hemiparesis, hemisensory loss). Neuroimaging studies reveal an extra-axial collection of blood or fluid (eg, subdural hygroma). Treatment varies depending on whether the hematoma is symptomatic or an incidental finding on a neuroimaging study. If the patient is symptomatic and clinically worsening, removal of the clot may be attempted. If the patient is asymptomatic or improving, then clinical monitoring is appropriate, because the hematoma may resolve without surgery. Some individuals may develop seizures with or after a subdural hematoma. A history of subdural hematoma may increase the risk of developing normal pressure hydrocephalus.

CHOOSING WISELY® RECOMMENDATION
Stroke and Cerebrovascular Disease

- Do not recommend carotid endarterectomy for asymptomatic carotid stenosis unless the complication rate is low (<3%).

REFERENCES

- Hemphill JC III, Greenberg SM, Anderson CS, et al. Guidelines for the management of spontaneous intracerebral hemorrhage: a guideline for healthcare professionals from the American Heart Association/American Stroke Association. *Stroke*. 2015;46(7):2032–2060.

  This paper provides evidence-based recommendations related to the acute management of patients with spontaneous intracerebral hemorrhages. The literature is reviewed critically and areas in which there is a lack of evidence or guidelines are discussed.

- Kernan WN, Ovbiagele B, Black HR, et al. Guidelines for prevention of stroke in patients with stroke and transient ischemic attack: a guideline for healthcare professionals from the American Heart Association/American Stroke Association. *Stroke*. 2015;45(7):2160–2236.

  This review of the literature related to secondary prevention of stroke included guidelines related to control of stroke risk factors, antiplatelet therapy, and recommendations regarding surgical interventions for patients with extra-cranial carotid stenosis. It contains extensive references and rates the strength of the evidence for each recommendation.

- Meschia JF, Bushnell C, Boden-Albala B, et al. Guidelines for the primary prevention of stroke: a statement for healthcare professionals from the American Heart Association/American Stroke Association. *Stroke*. 2014;45(12):3754–3832.

  This extensive, well-referenced review of the literature concerning the primary prevention of stroke lists clinical guidelines based on the current evidence and rates the strength of the evidence for each guideline.

- Powers WJ, Derdeyn CP, Biller J, et al. 2015 AHA/ASA Focused update of the 2013 guidelines for the early management of patients with acute ischemic stroke regarding endovascular treatment: a guideline for healthcare professionals from the American Heart Association/American Stroke Association. *Stroke*. 2015 June 29. (*e-pub ahead of print*)

  This guideline reviews the results of recent clinical trials of endovascular therapy in acute ischemic stroke caused by proximal occlusions of cerebral vessels and provides guidelines for use of this therapy in addition to the acute stroke guidelines published in 2013.

- Thompson BG, Brown RD Jr, Amin-Hanjani S, et al. Guidelines for the management of patients with unruptured intracranial aneurysums: a guideline for healthcare professionals from the American Heart Association/American Stroke Association. *Stroke*. 2015;46(8):2368–2400.

  This paper provides an extensive review of available literature related to the development of cerebral aneurysms and risk of rupture. Evidence-based guidelines are given for screening and management of unruptured cerebral aneurysms.

Daniel L. Murman, MD, MS, FAAN

CHAPTER 62—INFECTIOUS DISEASES

KEY POINTS

- Immune function wanes with age, and resistance is compromised in older adults not only as a consequence of age-related declines in immunity (ie, immune senescence), but more importantly because of comorbid disease and increased exposure to nosocomial pathogens.

- Accepted thresholds for "fever" generally do not apply in infected older adults because of their altered febrile response to infection. Fever can be redefined in frail older adults (temperature >2° F over baseline, single oral temperature >100° F, or repeated oral temperatures >99° F) to enhance its diagnostic utility.

- Applying minimal criteria for starting antibiotic therapy in residents of long-term care facilities is likely to reduce inappropriate antibiotic use without jeopardizing patient safety.

- Overtreatment of asymptomatic bacteriuria with antibiotics leads to development of multidrug resistant organisms. Providers should be cognizant of susceptibility patterns for urinary isolates, especially when treating urinary tract infections in long-term care residents.

- Vaccinations play an important role in prevention of life-threatening illnesses in older adults, especially influenza and invasive pneumococcal disease. Vaccination rates for herpes zoster in older adults is extremely low at 16%.

Infection is the major cause of mortality in 40% of those ≥65 years old, and it contributes to death in many older adults. Infection is also a significant cause of morbidity in older adults, often exacerbating underlying illness or leading to hospitalization. Pneumonia and other respiratory tract infections, urinary tract infection, and sepsis are all in the top 20 diagnosis-related groups paid by Medicare. Furthermore, older adults are often a "sentinel" population in which new infections (eg, West Nile virus), more virulent strains (*Clostridium difficile* colitis), or the return of annual epidemics (eg, influenza) are first noted. Associations of infection and inflammation with age-related chronic diseases suggest that infectious diseases may play an even larger role in the morbidity and mortality of the older adult population than previously realized. This chapter explores the biological, cultural, and societal factors that influence susceptibility to infection, the presentation of disease, and management suggestions for several common infectious disease syndromes in older adults.

PREDISPOSITION TO INFECTION

The immune system undergoes an age-related decline, often termed immunosenescence, putting older adults at higher risk of development of infectious diseases, which are also more severe in course. Vaccine efficacy is also lower in older adults because of this phenomenon. Changes in adaptive immunity because of thymic involution involve depressed T-cell functions. B cells in older adults can produce antibodies with lower affinity, leading to weakened immunogenicity of vaccines. Deficits of innate immunity include decreased macrophage activity, causing infections to have a longer course. Macrophages also regulate the adaptive immune response, which can be dysfunctional in older adults (Table 62.1).

Although age itself influences immune function, nonspecific host-resistance factors that change with age also increase the risk of infection in older adults. For example, poor skin integrity predisposes to skin and soft-tissue infection, impaired cough or gag reflexes increase the risk of pneumonia, and increased gastric pH and decreased GI motility predispose to diarrheal illnesses. However, all of these changes associated with aging have far less influence on risk of infection than comorbid diseases. Diabetes mellitus, chronic kidney disease, heart failure, chronic edema due to venous insufficiency, COPD, and stroke are but a few examples of age-related comorbid illnesses that increase risk of infection. Comorbidity further influences the outcomes of and management strategies for infection in older adults. For example, community-acquired pneumonia in otherwise healthy adults <50 years old is typically treated on an outpatient basis and rarely causes mortality; however, in older adults with community-acquired pneumonia and multiple comorbid conditions, the increased risk of morbidity and mortality often necessitates hospitalization. In addition, cognitive impairment and other barriers to adherence may make treating older patients more difficult, increasing complications and costs.

A major influence on immune function in older adults is nutritional status. Protein and calorie malnutrition is present in 30%–60% of adults ≥65 years old on admission to the hospital. Among outpatients, 11% of older adults are malnourished, 90% of which is due to reversible underlying conditions such as depression, poorly controlled diabetes mellitus, and adverse effects of medication (SOE=B). Delayed wound healing, increased risk of nosocomial infection, extended lengths of hospital stay, and increased mortality are all

Table 62.1—Changes in Immune Function Associated with Aging

Type of Immunity	Change With Age	Comment
Innate immunity		
Skin, mucous membranes	↓↓↓	Skin thins and dries with aging
Polymorphonuclear neutrophils		
Adherence, chemotaxis	—	
Ingestion	—	
Intracellular killing	↓	Most changes are due to comorbidity
Adaptive immunity		
Thymic hormones	↓↓↓	
Lymphocyte subsets		
T cells	↓↓↓	Shift from naive to memory subtypes
Natural killer cells	↓↓	Number increases but function declines
Lymphocyte functions		
Proliferative responses	↓↓	
Senescent phenotype	↑↑↑	Refers to oligoclonal expansion of CD8 cells that have replicative senescence, are CD28 negative, and secrete high quantities of proinflammatory cytokines
Cytokine production, secretion		
IL-2, IL-2 receptor	↓↓↓	After stimulation
Interferon-γ	↑	Primarily basal secretion
Prostaglandin E_2	↑↑	Basal and stimulated
Delayed-type hypersensitivity	↓↓	
Autoimmunity	↑↑	Autoantibodies common but of unclear significance

NOTE: — = no age-related changes; ↑ = mild increase; ↑↑ = moderate increase; ↑↑↑ = marked increase; ↓ = mild decrease; ↓↓ = moderate decrease; ↓↓↓ = marked decrease; IL = interleukin

associated with malnutrition. Even mildly malnourished older adults (ie, those with a serum albumin of 3–3.5 g/dL) have evidence of immune compromise, poor vaccine responses, and diminished cytokine responses to specific challenges. Nutritional interventions may boost immune function in some older adults, but this practice remains controversial. Some studies suggest a clinical benefit, particularly in older adults with subclinical nutritional deficiencies, whereas others do not. Differences in study design, population enrolled, duration of follow-up, and definitions of infection (self-reported versus physician diagnosed) may account for many of these differences.

Residing in long-term care or nursing facilities also places older adults at increased risk of epidemic diseases such as influenza. Widespread antibiotic use in these settings increases the likelihood of acquiring diseases caused by multidrug resistant organisms (MDROs); methicillin-resistant *Staphylococcus aureus* (MRSA), vancomycin-resistant enterococci (VRE), and extended spectrum β-lactamase–producing gram-negative rods (ESBLs) are more common causes of infection in institutionalized than in community-dwelling older adults. Resistance issues are augmented in long-term care facilities by debilitated hosts, close proximity of residents, poor staff compliance with prevention strategies (eg, influenza immunization), overutilization of antibiotics, and difficulties in implementing infection-control measures in long-term care.

DIAGNOSIS AND MANAGEMENT OF INFECTIONS

Presentation

Older adults often present without typical signs and symptoms of infection. Fever, the most readily recognized feature of infection, may be absent in 30%–50% of frail older adults with serious infections, even bacteremia, pneumonia, or endocarditis. The cause of impaired febrile responses in older adults is incompletely understood, but diverse mechanisms of thermoregulation are involved, including a reduced basal body temperature in many older adults and blunted thermogenesis by brown adipose tissue.

Given the sensitivity, specificity, and positive and negative predictive values, fever in older long-term care residents can be redefined appropriately as a temperature >2° F (1.1° C) over baseline (if a baseline is available), an oral temperature >99° F (37.2° C) or a rectal temperature >99.5° F (37.5° C) on repeated measures, or a single oral temperature >100° F (37.8° C) (SOE=B). This definition of fever has a sensitivity of 82.5% in long-term care residents, and the specificity remains high at 89.9% (Table 62.2). These data were generated

Table 62.2—Defining Fever in Frail, Older Residents of Long-Term Care Facilities

Definition	Sensitivity	Specificity	(+) Likelihood Ratio	(−) Likelihood Ratio
T >101°F (38.3°C)	40.0%	99.7%	133	0.6
T >100°F (37.7°C)	70.0%	98.3%	41	0.3
T >99°F (37.2°C)	82.5%	89.9%	8	0.2

NOTE: (+) Likelihood ratio = sensitivity / (1− specificity); (−) Likelihood ratio = (1− sensitivity) / specificity; T = temperature

SOURCE: Data from Castle SC, Yeh M, Toledo S, et al. Lowering the temperature criterion improves detection of infections in nursing home residents. *Aging Immunol Infect Dis*. 1993;4(2):67–76.

in a cohort of frail, older, male veterans in a nursing home. It would seem reasonable to apply the same definitions to frail, older adults of either sex in the community, although the performance characteristics of this definition of fever in otherwise healthy older adults have not been validated.

The absence of fever is only one way that infectious diseases can present atypically in older adults. For example, pneumonia can be signaled by a nonspecific decline in baseline functional status, such as confusion or falling, without cough, sputum production, or shortness of breath. Symptoms of a urinary tract infection may include atypical symptoms such as change in character of the urine and change in mental status. Anorexia and decreased oral intake may be the primary manifestation of infection, or exacerbation of an underlying illness (eg, atrial fibrillation) may become the predominant feature. Cognitive impairment, when present, further contributes to the often confusing presentation of infections in older adults. Many cognitively impaired older adults are unable to communicate symptoms accurately, and clinicians must be ready to pursue objective assessments such as laboratory and radiologic evaluations at a lower threshold, unless advance directives indicate otherwise. Because of the challenges involved with diagnoses of infections in long-term care residents, surveillance definitions have been developed to assist with clinical decision making (Table 62.3).

Antimicrobial Management

Drug distribution, metabolism, excretion, and interactions can be altered with age. Aging in the absence of any comorbid disease is associated with decreased renal function, and antibiotic dosages may need to be reduced in older adults. Furthermore, antibiotics interact with many other medications commonly prescribed for older adults. Digoxin, warfarin, oral hypoglycemic agents, theophylline, antacids, lipid-lowering agents, antihypertensive medications, and H_2-receptor antagonists all have significant interactions with commonly prescribed antimicrobials. Drug concentrations can increase (eg, enhanced digoxin toxicity associated with macrolides, tetracyclines, and trimethoprim) or decrease (eg, reduced absorption of some fluoroquinolones with antacids) with concomitant medication administration.

Atrophic gastritis, a common problem in older adults, and H_2-blockers or proton-pump inhibitors can reduce the absorption of some antimicrobials, such as ketoconazole or itraconazole. Furthermore, chronic use of proton-pump inhibitors, often prescribed in older adults, has been associated with an increased risk of community-acquired pneumonia (SOE=C). Finally, adherence to prescribed regimens may be limited as a consequence of poor cognitive function, impaired hearing or vision, multiple medications, and financial constraints.

The choice and timing of antibiotics may also be important. In sepsis, pneumonia, and other severe infections, an increasing body of evidence suggests that broad coverage is warranted initially because outcomes (ie, mortality, length of stay in intensive care) are improved when the offending organism is covered by the initial antibiotic regimen. In older adults with pneumonia, data suggest that delaying the start of therapy for ≥4 hours after admission to the hospital is associated with an increased risk of mortality (SOE=B). "De-escalation," a narrowing of antibiotic choice to specific therapy if the offending organism is identified by culture or other diagnostic studies, is essential for antibiotic stewardship and should be done whenever possible. Unfortunately, diagnostic studies (eg, obtaining sputum) are often difficult in older adults or are unavailable in long-term care settings. These factors and the atypical presentation of infection noted above often lead to early initiation of antimicrobials in older adults, particularly in long-term care. However, this practice results in inappropriate use of antibiotics in up to 75% of cases in this setting. The use of strict, minimal criteria for initiation of antimicrobials in long-term care is most likely to reduce inappropriate antibiotic use without jeopardizing patient safety (SOE=C). In addition, because prompt initiation of antibiotics is important, discontinuing antibiotics when no longer indicated is an equally important practice for geriatricians.

IMMUNIZATIONS

Immunizations are particularly important for prevention of infection in adults ≥65 years old, because this population is at increased risk of severe complications from vaccine preventable illnesses, particularly influenza and pneumococcal disease. Immunization rates for

Table 62.3—Surveillance Definitions of Infections in Long-Term Care Facilities: Revisiting the McGeer Criteria

Condition	Minimal Criteria
Urinary tract infection, without catheter	Positive urine culture plus at least 1 of the following: ■ Acute dysuria or acute pain, swelling, or tenderness of the testes, epididymis, or prostate ■ Fever or leukocytosis plus 1 of the following: acute costovertebral angle pain or tenderness, suprapubic pain, gross hematuria, new or marked increase in incontinence, frequency, or urgency ■ In the absence of fever or leukocytosis, then 2 of the following symptoms: acute costovertebral angle pain or tenderness, suprapubic pain, gross hematuria, new or marked increase in incontinence, frequency, or urgency
Urinary tract infection, with catheter	Positive urine culture plus at least 1 of the following: ■ Fever, rigors, or hypotension ■ Change in mental status or functional decline ■ New-onset suprapubic pain or costovertebral angle pain or tenderness ■ Purulent discharge from catheter site or acute pain swelling or tenderness of testes, epididymis, or prostate
Skin and soft-tissue infection	At least 1 of the following must be present: ■ Pus present at a wound, skin, or soft-tissue site ■ New or increasing presence of at least 4 of the following: heat, redness, swelling, tenderness or pain, serous drainage or 1 constitutional criteria such as fever, leukocytosis, acute change in mental or functional status from baseline
Pneumonia	All 3 criteria must be present: ■ Interpretation of a chest radiograph showing new infiltrate ■ At least 1 of the following: new or increased cough, sputum production, O_2 saturation <94% on room air or reduction in O_2 saturation of >3% from baseline, new or changed lung examination, pleuritic chest pain, respiratory rate ≥25 breaths/min ■ At least 1 of the following: fever, leukocytosis, acute change in mental status or function status from baseline

SOURCE: Data from Stone ND, Muhammad S, Ashraf, et al. Surveillance definitions of infections in long-term care facilities: revisiting the McGeer Criteria. *Infect Control Hosp Epidemiol*. 2012;33(10):965–977.

both influenza and pneumococcus in adults ≥65 years old have improved significantly, although rates are still estimated at 65% for influenza and 60% for pneumococcus. Estimated rates of vaccination for herpes zoster (shingles) in older adults are unacceptably low at 16%.

Influenza Vaccine

In 2009, the FDA approved a high-dose seasonal influenza vaccine for use in adults ≥65 years old, based on data suggesting improved immune response (ie, antibody production) with the high-dose vaccination, which contains 4 times the dose of the same antigens used in the standard-dose vaccine. In a study evaluating the efficacy of the high-dose influenza vaccine for prevention of laboratory-confirmed influenza, the high-dose vaccine provided enhanced protection compared with the standard-dose. In this randomized, controlled trial, adults without moderate or severe illness, ≥65 years old, were assigned to receive either high-dose or standard-dose influenza vaccine. The percentage of adults with laboratory-confirmed influenza who received the high-dose vaccine was 1.4% compared with 1.9% in the standard-dose group (relative efficacy, 24.2%; 95% CI, 9.7–36.5) (SOE=A). Currently, the Advisory Committee on Immunization Practices (ACIP) of the CDC continues to recommend yearly influenza vaccination with either standard or high-dose inactivated influenza vaccine for adults ≥65 years old, although this recommendation may change given the recent findings (Table 62.4).

Pneumococcal Vaccine

The incidence of invasive pneumococcal disease and pneumococcal pneumonia continues to be higher in older adults than in younger ones, especially in those with chronic medical comorbidities. Currently, ACIP continues to recommend vaccination with 23-valent pneumococcal polysaccharide vaccine (PPSV23) in all adults ≥65 years old. Adults who received PPSV23 before age 65 should receive another dose of the vaccine at age 65 or older if at least 5 years have passed since their previous dose (Table 62.4).

Although most professional societies continue to endorse vaccination of older adults with PPSV23 per ACIP guidelines, studies evaluating efficacy of the vaccine, especially in preventing pneumococcal pneumonia in older adults, have demonstrated conflicting results. A meta-analysis published in 2013 sought to evaluate the efficacy of PPSV23 in prevention of invasive pneumococcal disease and pneumococcal pneumonia. The authors found that PPSV23 did reduce the

Table 62.4—Immunization Schedule for Adults ≥65 Years Old[a]

Vaccine	Dose Recommendation
Influenza	1 dose annually of standard or high-dose inactivated influenza vaccine
Tetanus, diphtheria, pertussis (Td/Tdap)	Administer Tdap then boost with Td every 10 years
Varicella	2 doses unless immune or previous receipt of 2-vaccine series
Zoster	1 dose in adults ≥60 years old regardless of history of herpes zoster[b]
Pneumococcal (conjugate) (PCV13)	1 dose in adults ≥ 65years old before receiving PPSV23[c] or in those ≥19 years old with certain comorbid conditions[d]
Pneumococcal (polysaccharide) (PPSV23)	1 dose in adults ≥65 years old or 5 years after previous dose if given before age 65
Meningococcal	1 or more doses based on risk factors[e]
Hepatitis A	2 doses based on risk factors[f]
Hepatitis B	3 doses based on risk factors[g]
Haemophilus influenzae type b	1 or 3 doses based on risk factors[h]

[a] Recommendations from the CDC Advisory Committee on Immunization Practices 2014

[b] Excludes patients with severe acquired or primary immunodeficiency

[c] PCV13 should be given before PPSV23 in vaccine-naive adults ≥65 years old, or at least 1 year after adults ≥ 65 years old who have previously received PPSV23.

[d] Only in older adults with chronic renal failure, asplenia, CSF leaks, or cochlear implants.

[e] Risk factors include functional asplenia, persistent complement component deficiencies, travelers to endemic countries.

[f] Risk factors include men who have sex with men, persons who use illicit drugs, persons with chronic liver disease or who receive clotting factor concentrates, travelers.

[g] Risk factors include sexually active persons not in a monogamous relationship, injection drug users, men who have sex with men, those being evaluated for a sexually transmitted infection, diabetic patients, those potentially exposed to blood or body fluids (eg, health care workers), persons with end-stage renal disease (including those on hemodialysis), HIV infection, persons with chronic liver disease, household contacts and sex partners of hepatitis B–positive persons, travelers, all adults in institutions and nonresidential daycare facilities, or persons with developmental disabilities.

[h] One dose should be administered to older adults who have functional or anatomic asplenia, sickle cell disease, or are undergoing elective splenectomy and have not previously received *Haemophilus influenzae* type b vaccination. Vaccination should occur 14 days before splenectomy. Patients receiving hematopoietic stem cell transplant should be vaccinated with 3 doses 6–12 months after transplant in 4-week intervals.

risk of invasive pneumococcal disease (OR 0.26, 95% CI, 0.14–0.45) in the general population, including the subgroup of healthy individuals in high-income countries, which included many older adults (OR 0.20, 95% CI, 0.10–0.39). They did not, however, find a reduction in all-cause pneumonia or all-cause mortality in this subgroup.

Given the lack of known efficacy for PPSV23 in preventing pneumococcal pneumonia, the pneumococcal conjugate vaccine (PCV13), previously indicated only in younger children, was approved by the FDA in 2011 for use in adults ≥50 years old, after a few studies demonstrated increased antibody production after vaccination. In addition, a randomized placebo-controlled trial of approximately 85,000 adults ≥65 years old demonstrated efficacy of the PCV13 vaccine against vaccine-type pneumococcal pneumonia, vaccine-type non-bacteremic pneumonia, and vaccine-type invasive pneumococcal disease in this population. These results, along with immunogenicity studies demonstrating immune responses as good as or better than those seen with PPSV23, prompted ACIP to recommend vaccination with PCV13 for all adults ≥65 years old. Adults ≥65 years old who have not previously received pneumococcal vaccine should receive PCV13 followed by a dose of PPSV23 approximately 12 months later. Adults previously vaccinated with PPSV23 should receive a dose of PCV13 at least 1 year after immunization with PPSV23 (Table 62.4). Immunization of children with PCV13 has reduced the incidence of pneumococcal pneumonia, with serotypes present in this vaccine even in older adults. Therefore, by adhering to vaccination guidelines for children in close contact with older adults, there may be herd immunity that older adults can benefit from as well.

Varicella-Zoster Virus Vaccine

Varicella-zoster virus vaccine is a live, attenuated vaccine used to prevent herpes zoster in older adults. ACIP recommends a single dose of zoster vaccine for adults ≥60 years old, even in those with a history of herpes zoster. The recommendation is based on results from a large placebo-controlled clinical trial of almost 40,000 adults ≥60 years old, in which the vaccine reduced the incidence of herpes zoster by 51.3% (95% CI, 47.5–79.2). In addition, the vaccine decreased the duration of pain and discomfort in patients who developed zoster and decreased the incidence of post-herpetic neuralgia (SOE=A). It should be noted that older adults with cognitive impairment, significant functional impairment, and <5 years of remaining life expectancy were excluded from the study. In 2012, a follow-up study conducted to assess ongoing efficacy of the vaccine in older adults found that the vaccine continued to decrease the incidence of herpes zoster by 39.6% (95% CI, 18.2–55.5) through year 5 after vaccination.

The herpes zoster vaccine has been shown to be safe and well tolerated in adults with a prior history of herpes zoster. Contraindications for vaccination include a history of severe allergic reaction to gelatin or the antibiotic neomycin, severe primary or acquired immunodeficiencies, solid organ transplantation, and current chemotherapy or high-dose corticosteroid therapy. Patients receiving low-dose immunosuppression may still be eligible for vaccination. Primary Care Guidelines for Management of Persons Infected with HIV, published in 2013 by the Infectious Diseases Society of America, recommend clinicians consider zoster vaccination in HIV-infected adults >60 years old with CD4 counts ≥200 cells/μL (SOE=C). Ongoing studies evaluating safety and efficacy of the vaccine in HIV-infected older adults are still under investigation. ACIP has not yet recommended this vaccine for adults ≥50 years old, although data supporting its efficacy in this population have been published.

Tetanus, Diphtheria, Acellular Pertussis Vaccine

ACIP recommends the use of tetanus, diphtheria, acellular pertussis (Tdap) vaccine in older adults to protect children from pertussis infection (Table 62.4).

INFECTIOUS SYNDROMES

Bacteremia and Sepsis

Bacteremia is a common cause of hospitalization in older adults. Older adults with bacteremia are less likely than their younger counterparts to have chills or sweats, and fever is often absent. Gastrointestinal and genitourinary sources of bacteremia are more common; thus, the causative bacteria are more likely to be gram-negative rods or enterococci in older adults versus younger patients.

Bacteremia carries a poor prognosis in older adults. For example, nosocomial gram-negative bacteremia carries a mortality rate of 5%–35% in young adults, but 37%–50% in older adults. Major contributing factors include coexisting diseases that reduce physiologic reserve and the more common use of invasive devices (eg, intravenous or urinary catheters) that make eradication of organisms difficult.

The management of bacteremia and sepsis in older and younger patients is similar. Rapid administration of appropriate antibiotics aimed at the most likely sources is essential, and early "goal-directed" therapy for volume resuscitation has proven benefit in populations of all ages with sepsis (SOE=B).

Pneumonia

Patients aged ≥65 years old account for >50% of all pneumonia cases, and annual hospitalization rates for pneumonia range from 12 per 1,000 among community-dwelling adults ≥75 years old to 32 per 1,000 among long-term care residents. In fact, the cumulative 2-year risk of pneumonia for long-term care residents is approximately 30%. Mortality caused by pneumonia in older adults is 3–5 times that in young adults, but the rate is profoundly influenced by comorbidity. Comorbidity, defined in one study as cancer, collagen vascular disease, or advanced liver disease, was the strongest independent predictor of mortality in community-acquired pneumonia in older adults, with a relative risk (RR) of 4.1. Other independent risk factors for pneumonia-related mortality include age ≥85 years old; debility (decreased motor function); serum creatinine >1.5 mg/dL; and the presence of hypothermia (<36.1°F), hypotension (<90 mmHg systolic), or tachycardia (>110 beats per minute) on admission (SOE=A). Long-term follow-up data also suggest that community-acquired pneumonia in older adults indicates a higher risk of subsequent all-cause mortality over the next 12 years, as a consequence of both recurrent pneumonia (RR 2.1; 95% CI, 1.3–3.4]) and cardiovascular disease (RR 1.4; 96% CI, 1.0–1.9]) (SOE=A).

The causes of pneumonia in younger and older adults differ. In older patients, *Streptococcus pneumoniae* is still the predominant organism, but gram-negative bacilli (eg, *Haemophilus influenzae, Moraxella catarrhalis, Klebsiella* spp) are much more common than in younger adults, particularly in patients with COPD or who reside in long-term care facilities. *Staphylococcus aureus* and respiratory viruses are also common causes of community-acquired pneumonia in long-term care residents. Obtaining a microbiologic diagnosis is often difficult in older adults who rarely produce sputum. Blood cultures should be obtained before antimicrobial therapy but are positive in only 10%–15% of patients. Urinary antigen testing for *S pneumoniae* (sensitivity 70%–80%; specificity 77%–97%) or *Legionella pneumophila* (sensitivity 70%–80%; specificity 77%–97%) can be useful diagnostic tests to perform in older adults that are unable to produce sputum. Importantly, the sensitivity of these tests is not affected for up to 24 hours after initiation of antimicrobial therapy. The test for legionellosis detects only serogroup 1, which causes 80% of all *Legionella* infection.

Guidelines for pneumonia therapy have evolved to account for emergence of resistant bacteria, particularly drug-resistant *S pneumoniae*, and for the recognition of comorbidities, health care setting versus community-acquired illness, and specific pathogens of interest in certain settings (eg, *S aureus* after viral influenza infection). Because of their ease of administration and broad activity versus respiratory pathogens, respiratory fluoroquinolones are used often in older adults, and they are one of the first-line therapies suggested by various guidelines. Guidelines of the Infectious Diseases Society of

America for treatment of community-acquired pneumonia suggest the following as first-line therapy in adults ≥60 years old with or without comorbidity: a β-lactam/β-lactamase combination or advanced-generation cephalosporin (eg, ceftriaxone or cefotaxime) with or without a macrolide. Alternatively, one of the fluoroquinolones with enhanced activity against S pneumoniae (eg, levofloxacin, moxifloxacin) may be used. However, several notes of caution are needed regarding fluoroquinolone use in older adults: first, fluoroquinolones kill bacteria better at higher concentrations, and outcomes are better in older adults when high drug concentrations are present (SOE=B). Thus, full-dosage therapy should be provided (ie, the adage of "start low, go slow" often invoked for drug therapy in older adults is *not* appropriate for this class of drugs). Second, if tuberculosis is a realistic possibility, fluoroquinolone use should be reserved. Use of fluoroquinolones to treat community-acquired pneumonia can lead to delayed diagnosis of tuberculosis (by an average of >40 days) and to fluoroquinolone resistance in the organism. Finally, significant adverse events, including dizziness, cardiac conduction abnormalities (QT prolongation), and risk of Achilles tendon rupture may limit the use of fluoroquinolones in certain older adults. However, fluoroquinolone use in older adults without underlying conduction abnormalities or specific contraindications is quite safe (SOE=B).

Long-term care facility–acquired pneumonia or hospital-acquired pneumonia in older adults requires broader initial therapy than does community-acquired pneumonia because of the broader spectrum of organisms causing infection. In the long-term care setting, polymicrobial infection, often due to aspiration and S aureus, is much more common than in the community setting. In the hospital setting, gram-negative bacilli predominate, but S aureus is more common as well and is more likely to affect specific antibiotic choices because of resistance. Outcomes data suggest that response to therapy is greater when the initial antibiotic regimen covers the offending agent. Thus, initial regimens should be broadly inclusive, followed by step-down therapy to more narrow coverage if the causative agent is identified. Importantly, if patients are known to be colonized with methicillin-resistant *Staphylococcus aureus* (MRSA), initial regimens should include vancomycin or linezolid until MRSA is excluded as the causative agent. Daptomycin should not be used to treat MRSA pneumonia due to high failure rates, because the drug binds to surfactant and thus is not an effective treatment. Further, data suggest that patients with clinically improving hospital-acquired pneumonia not caused by nonfermenting gram-negative bacilli (eg, *Pseudomonas, Stenotrophomonas*) can be treated with shorter courses of antibiotics (7 or 8 days, rather than the 2 weeks commonly used in the past). Shorter courses (8 days versus 15 days) of antibiotics are associated with equivalent efficacy and less antibiotic resistance (SOE=A).

Prevention of pneumonia in older adults is a complex issue, and a multipronged approach is most likely to be effective. Immunization of at-risk individuals is by far the most well-studied measure. Annual influenza vaccine and pneumococcal vaccine should be administered to all older adults. In addition to vaccines, smoking cessation and aggressive treatment of comorbidities (eg, minimizing aspiration risk in patients after stroke, limiting use of sedative hypnotics) can reduce the risk of infection. Finally, system changes with attention to infection control (isolation, cohorting, skin testing for tuberculosis with purified-protein derivative or interferon-gamma release assays, and immunization policies for staff and visitors) can be particularly effective in long-term care facilities.

Influenza

Influenza results in approximately 40,000 deaths annually in the United States, nearly all of which are in the older adult population. The clinical syndrome of influenza is easily recognized by most clinicians, particularly in the setting of local activity or an outbreak frequently seen in long-term care facilities. Although some controversy exists with regard to the effectiveness of influenza vaccine in frail older adults, most data suggest the vaccine is 60%–80% efficacious in older adults for preventing severe disease, hospitalization, and death. Therefore, annual immunization is recommended for all adults (SOE=A).

Several medications are available for treatment and prophylaxis of influenza. M2 inhibitors (amantadine and rimantadine) block the M2 ion channel of influenza and are effective only against influenza A; their use is limited by widespread resistance (>90% of the most virulent strains). Further, amantadine is particularly difficult to use in older adults because of the extensive dosage adjustments required for small changes in kidney function and marked adverse events, particularly CNS symptoms. In contrast, neuraminidase inhibitors (zanamivir and oseltamivir) are effective against both influenza A and B; they inhibit the virus by interfering with an essential enzyme, neuraminidase, that cleaves sialic acid to expose host cell receptors for the virus. Oseltamivir, a capsule, is preferred over zanamivir in older adults because zanamivir must be inhaled, and it is difficult for many older adults to properly use the product. Treatment of influenza is effective if started in the first 48 hours, but it is most effective if started within 24 hours of symptom onset (SOE=A). Oseltamivir and zanamivir can also be used for prevention in outbreak situations (eg, in long-term care) when combined with appropriate vaccination strategies (SOE=A).

Urinary Tract Infection

Urinary tract infection (UTI) is among the most common of clinical illnesses in older adults, with an incidence of 10.9 per 100-person years in men and 14 per 100 person-years in women ≥65 years old. Gram-negative bacilli (eg, *Escherichia coli*, *Enterobacter* spp, *Klebsiella* spp, *Proteus* spp) are most common, but there is an increase in more resistant isolates, such as *Pseudomonas aeruginosa*, and in gram-positive organisms, including enterococci, coagulase-negative staphylococci, and *Streptococcus agalactiae* (group B strep). In patients with indwelling catheters, the microbes listed still predominate, but it is also common to encounter additional organisms, including enterococci, *S aureus*, and fungi, particularly *Candida* spp. The organisms colonizing urinary catheters commonly develop biofilms, and infections are difficult to resolve with the same urinary catheter in place.

Asymptomatic Bacteriuria

Asymptomatic bacteriuria (ASB) in women is defined as the presence of two consecutive urine specimens positive for the same bacterial strain in quantities of ≥10^5 colony-forming units/milliliter (CFU/mL), in the absence of symptoms. Up to 20% of women in the community and 50% of women in nursing homes have ASB. In men, ASB is defined as one voided urine specimen with ≥10^5 CFU/mL in the absence of symptoms. The incidence in men is approximately half that in women. Rates of ASB are even higher with the use of condom catheters (87%) or Foley catheters (nearly 100%). Numerous studies have suggested that there is no clinical benefit from the treatment of ASB, and that treatment is associated with significant adverse events, expense, and potential for selection of resistant organisms. Thus, routine screening and treatment of ASB are not recommended in older adults (SOE=A).

Urinary Tract Infection in Community-Dwelling Older Women

In contrast to ASB, symptomatic UTI requires therapy. Diagnosis of UTI in cognitively intact older adults is similar to that in younger adults and is made based on a combination of genitourinary symptoms (eg, new or worsening urgency, frequency, suprapubic pain, gross hematuria) along with evidence of a urine culture growing no more than 2 urinary pathogen in quantities ≥10^5 CFU/mL.

Therapy is based on the location of infection (upper versus lower tract disease) and the likely causative agent. Lower-tract UTI (ie, cystitis) is often treated in young women for 1–3 days, and 3–7 days of therapy is probably sufficient for uncomplicated cystitis in older women (SOE=B). Upper UTI (ie, pyelonephritis), characterized by fever, chills, nausea, and flank pain, is commonly accompanied by lower-tract symptoms and requires a longer period of therapy (7–21 days). According to the International Clinical Practice Guidelines by the Infectious Diseases Society of America and the European Society for Microbiology, first-line therapy for treatment of uncomplicated UTI includes nitrofurantoin 100 mg twice daily for 5 days, or trimethoprim-sulfamethoxazole (TMP-SMX) 160/800 mg twice daily for 3 days, if local resistance rates do not exceed 20%. Nitrofurantoin is contraindicated by the FDA for use in patients with chronic kidney disease (creatinine clearance <60 mL/min), but it has been shown to be safe to administer in patients with creatinine clearance ≥40 mL/min and can be considered for treatment of cystitis in older adults. TMP-SMX is the preferred empiric treatment for UTI in older adults but caution is warranted in those concurrently receiving warfarin or in those with renal disease. Fluoroquinolones, although highly effective for sensitive organisms, are not recommended empirically because of high resistance rates (SOE=C).

Intravenous administration of antibiotics remains the standard of care for patients with suspected urosepsis, those with upper-tract disease due to relatively resistant bacteria such as enterococci, or those unable to tolerate oral medications. Culture and sensitivity data are more useful in guiding antimicrobial therapy in upper-tract UTIs than in lower-tract disease and should be obtained in most cases (SOE=A).

Urinary Tract Infection in Community-Dwelling Older Men

Prostatic disease (primarily hyperplasia) or functional disability, such as autonomic neuropathy from diabetes mellitus with incomplete bladder emptying, account for most lower and upper UTIs in older men. Therapy should last at least 7–14 days, and if prostatic involvement is suspected (ie, acute or chronic prostatitis), at least 6 weeks (SOE=B). The causative organisms and treatment choices are similar to those outlined above for older women. Fluoroquinolones and TMP-SMX are most widely used when prostatic involvement is suspected and culture data confirm the organism's susceptibility because, of the available agents, these two penetrate the prostate best. Because treatment for all UTIs in men is generally longer than in women and the prostate is a common reservoir of organisms responsible for recurrent UTIs, culture and sensitivity data should guide therapy for virtually all UTIs in men (SOE=C).

Urinary Tract Infection in Long-Term Care Residents

Distinguishing symptomatic UTI from ASB in long-term care residents is challenging, because many long-term care residents suffer from cognitive impairment, which limits their ability to effectively communicate genitourinary symptoms. Antibiotics are often inappropriately prescribed for treatment of UTI when residents develop nonspecific symptoms such as changes in functional status. Overuse of antibiotics in this situation has led to the development of multidrug resistant organisms. Several professional societies have developed guidelines to assist clinicians with the diagnosis and treatment of UTI in this population. In 2012, the Society for Healthcare Epidemiology of America updated the current guidelines for diagnosis of UTI to include a combination of genitourinary signs and symptoms, fever or leukocytosis, and a positive urinary culture (SOE=C) (Table 62.3).

Antibiotic Prophylaxis
Prophylactic antibiotics intended to prevent recurrent UTIs in older women are not preferred because of the risk of development of highly resistant organisms; however, if other preventive strategies are ineffective, this treatment modality can be effective. Few small studies have shown benefit of intravaginal estrogen replacement to reduce the recurrence of UTI in postmenopausal women. Cranberry juice has been shown to be efficacious in older adults and has been used for prevention of UTI for several decades, but it is not always well tolerated. More recently, use of cranberry capsules, which contain at least 36 mg of proanthocyanidin, the active ingredient thought to prevent adherence of *E coli* to uroepithelial cells, has been shown to reduce bacteriuria and pyuria in nursing-home residents. Additional studies evaluating efficacy of cranberry formulations in reducing UTI recurrence are underway.

Tuberculosis

Worldwide, approximately 1.7 billion people are infected with *Mycobacterium tuberculosis*; 16 million are in the United States. Adults ≥65 years old account for one-fourth of all active tuberculosis (TB) cases in the United States, most in community-dwelling older adults. However, the rate of infection with TB in long-term care residents is much higher than in community-dwelling adults. Tuberculin skin-test (TST) studies show prevalence rates of skin-test reactivity in the range of 30%–50%. This high prevalence is because of exposure to *M tuberculosis* in the early 1900s, when it was estimated that 80% of all individuals were infected by age 30. Most active cases of TB in older adults are, therefore, due to reactivated disease, but primary infection may account for 10%–20% of cases and is of particular concern in outbreaks in long-term care facilities.

A decline in T-cell mediated immune response in older adults increases the risk that latent TB will become active. Other factors that contribute to the reactivation of TB include chronic comorbid illness (eg, COPD, chronic renal failure, malnutrition) and increased exposure to the health care system, particularly chronic institutionalization.

As with most other infections, TB may not present in the classical fashion (ie, cough, sputum, hemoptysis, fever, night sweats) in older adults. Often, fatigue, anorexia, decreased functional status (eg, changes in activities of daily living, cognitive decline), or low-grade fever are presenting manifestations. Thus, the diagnosis of TB is often mistaken for other more common age-related diseases such as malignancy or failure to thrive. Most tuberculous disease in older adults occurs with lung involvement (75%) and pneumonic processes. Disease that occurs in a subacute manner should particularly raise a high index of suspicion for *M tuberculosis* infection. Older adults are more likely than younger ones to have extrapulmonary disease. Other sites include miliary (disseminated) disease, tuberculous meningitis or osteomyelitis, and urogenital disease, but virtually any body structure or organ system can be involved and can account for the major presenting symptom.

A diagnosis of active disease usually requires isolation of the organism from sputum, urine, or other clinical specimen. Current techniques have improved the speed of diagnosis, particularly for identifying the species of *Mycobacterium* after isolation. This is now typically accomplished within 24 hours of obtaining a positive culture by use of DNA probes. Direct polymerase chain reaction of clinical specimens or other rapid diagnostic techniques are not available or reliable in most local laboratories, but such tests can be available in research settings. They are most likely to be helpful for establishing a diagnosis from cerebrospinal or pleural fluid, which yields positive cultures in only 10%–15% of cases.

The most confusing area of TB diagnostics is typically interpretation of the results of the tuberculin skin test (TST) using 0.1 mL of purified-protein derivative (PPD). In all populations, induration of ≥15 mm 48–72 hours after placement of a 5-tuberculin–unit PPD indicates a positive test. Induration ≥10 mm is considered a positive test in long-term care residents, recent converters (previous PPD <5 mm), immigrants from countries with high endemicity of *M tuberculosis* infection, underserved populations in the United States (homeless people, and black, Hispanic, and Native Americans), and those with specific risk factors (eg, gastrectomy, >10% below ideal body weight, chronic kidney failure, diabetes mellitus, or immunosuppression, including that caused by corticosteroids or malignancy). In individuals infected with HIV, those with a history of close contact with people with active *M tuberculosis*, and those with chest radiographs consistent with *M tuberculosis* infection, ≥5 mm induration is considered a positive PPD test. Anergy panel testing in conjunction with PPD testing is of little value and is not recommended (SOE=C).

More recently, the use of interferon gamma release assays (IGRAs) have been developed to detect latent TB in most populations. The benefit of using IGRAs instead of TSTs is the ability to have results within 24 hours, without the need for a follow-up visit 2 days later. Thus, IGRAs may be an attractive alternative for older outpatient adults, who often have functional limitations and/or difficulty with transportation. Currently, the CDC recommends use of either the TST or IGRA in most clinical situations.

Long-term care facilities should always screen patients for TB on admission. If residents have a documented negative TST done within the previous 12 months, only a single TST is needed. If there is no report of a prior TST, a two-step procedure for PPD testing should be performed during the initial evaluation of residents (SOE=C). Two-step testing requires retesting of patients with <10 mm induration within 2 weeks. If the second skin test results in ≥10 mm of induration or the increase in the size of the induration from the first to the second skin test is ≥6 mm, the patient is considered PPD positive. Alternatively, a single IGRA should be done. If TST/IGRA is positive, the resident should have a chest radiograph and evaluation as soon as possible.

The treatment of active TB in older adults is similar to that in younger adults. Four-drug therapy (usually isoniazid [INH], rifampin, pyrazinamide, and ethambutol or streptomycin) is recommended as initial therapy, with tapering to one of several two- or three-drug regimens once susceptibility testing is available. The most common regimen is INH, rifampin, and pyrazinamide for 2 months, followed by INH and rifampin for an additional 4 months. However, adjustments in routine drug treatment protocols are often needed because of comorbidities and drug tolerance in older patients.

Prophylaxis with 9 months of INH for asymptomatic individuals with a positive PPD or IGRA should be provided regardless of age in adults who are recent converters (defined in adults >35 years old as those having a PPD that has gone from <10 mm to ≥15 mm within 2 years), or regardless of duration of PPD positivity if an individual has any of the specific risk factors highlighted above. Patients with a positive PPD or IGRA of unknown duration should receive INH prophylaxis, even those >35 years old (as opposed to recommendations in the 1990s). Older adults should be monitored closely for symptoms and signs of peripheral neuropathy (due to INH and preventable by coadministration of pyridoxine) and hepatitis (due to treatment with INH, rifampin, or pyrazinamide). Shorter-course therapy with 2 months of rifampin and pyrazinamide is effective but has a much higher incidence of hepatotoxicity than INH treatment and thus should be used only in very specific circumstances (SOE=B).

Infective Endocarditis

Since the early part of the 20th century, infective endocarditis has undergone a transformation from a disease of young adults primarily due to rheumatic or congenital valve anomalies to one of older adults associated with degenerative valvular disorders and prosthetic valves. Viridans streptococci and *S aureus* typically cause native-valve endocarditis, and occasional infections are due to HACEK organisms (a group of typically nonfermenting gram-negative rods that primarily inhabit the oral cavity and include the genera *Haemophilus, Actinobacillus, Cardiobacterium, Eikenella,* and *Kingella*). Gastrointestinal and genitourinary organisms, such as enterococci and gram-negative rods, are more common in native-valve infective endocarditis in older adults, and coagulase-negative staphylococci are a common cause of prosthetic-valve endocarditis, particularly in the first 60 days after placement of the valve.

The diagnosis of endocarditis is often difficult in older adults. Fever is less common in older adults than in younger ones, occurring in 55% versus 80%, respectively, as is leukocytosis, occurring in 25% versus 60%. Rates of positive blood cultures do not vary by age; however, degenerative, calcific valvular lesions and prosthetic valves lower the sensitivity of transthoracic echocardiography to 45% in older patients (from 75% in younger patients). Transesophageal echocardiography (TEE) improves the diagnostic yield for infective endocarditis, but the lack of positive findings on TEE never excludes it. TEE is of particular value in resolving *S aureus* bacteremia. Positive findings on TEE support prolonged antibiotic administration (4–6 weeks) versus short-course (2 weeks) therapy. However, TEE is invasive and expensive. Interestingly, age does not appear to play a major role in mortality risk, with a 2-year survival of 75% for infective endocarditis in all age groups unless major comorbidities are also present.

Antibiotic treatment of infective endocarditis is directed at the identified pathogen or at the most likely causes if blood cultures are negative. Therapy is administered intravenously for 2–6 weeks. Surgical therapy should be considered in cases of severe valvular dysfunction, recurrent emboli, marked heart failure, myocardial abscess formation, fungal endocarditis, or when appropriate antibiotic treatment does not yield negative blood cultures.

Recommendations for endocarditis prophylaxis for dental procedures were revised in 2007, focusing on providing prophylaxis only in the highest-risk patients and eliminating recommendations for prophylaxis for those undergoing gastrointestinal or genitourinary procedures.

Prosthetic Device Infections

Permanent implantable prosthetic devices are common in older adults. Prosthetic joints, cardiac pacemakers, artificial heart valves, intraocular lens implants, vascular grafts, penile prostheses, and a variety of other devices are placed more often in older than in younger adults. A discussion of all prosthetic device infections (PDIs) is beyond the scope of this chapter, but several general concepts can be summarized.

PDIs are usually separated into early versus late infections, because the causative agents differ significantly. Early PDIs, most commonly defined as occurring <60 days after device implantation, are primarily due to contamination at the time of implantation or to events associated with the acute hospitalization (eg, occult bacteremia caused by intravenous catheters). Thus, coagulase-negative staphylococci predominate, and *S aureus* and diphtheroids are common as well; gram-negative bacilli and fungi are relatively rare causes of early PDI. Late PDIs are usually caused by organisms that commonly cause transient bacteremia (in older adults this is most often skin, respiratory, gastrointestinal, or genitourinary organisms). Staphylococci, including coagulase-negative staphylococci, play a major role in both early and late PDIs, although their relative importance is greater in early PDIs. Thus, empiric staphylococcal therapy should be provided in either early or late PDIs if a specific causative agent is not identified.

In general, hardware removal is required to clear PDIs. However, early antibiotic treatment, in some instances combined with aggressive surgical drainage, can be successful. Small studies in prosthetic joint infection suggest that initial debridement and culture and a brief course (2 weeks) of intravenous antibiotics followed by combination oral two-drug therapy that includes rifampin may obviate the need for device removal. Until more definitive data are available, it is prudent to restrict this approach to patients with a short duration of symptoms (<3 weeks), those who are likely to have difficulty tolerating another surgical procedure, or those in whom return to full functional status is not a realistic goal because of comorbidities. In those older adults in whom full function is the goal, the best chance for cure is a two-stage procedure in which the device is removed and antibiotics are given for an extended period (6–8 weeks), followed by delayed reimplantation. Of course, for life-saving devices, such as mechanical valves or implantable defibrillators, this is not an option. Infected prosthetic devices are usually surrounded by microbial biofilms, such as microbe-derived glycocalyx. Biofilms reduce antibiotic penetration and thus greatly increase the concentrations of antibiotic needed for bactericidal activity. Furthermore, many conditions associated with infected prostheses are also accompanied by poor blood flow to the area. Therefore, it is preferable to use bactericidal antibiotics, often in combination with a second agent that penetrates biofilms and poorly perfused areas (eg, rifampin for staphylococci).

Bone and Joint Infections

Native bone and joint infections in the absence of prostheses occur in older adults. Septic arthritis is more likely to occur in joints with underlying pathology (eg, rheumatoid changes, gout, osteoarthritis), and early arthrocentesis is indicated in any mono- or oligo-articular syndrome to exclude infection. *S aureus* is the most likely pathogen; infections are only rarely due to gram-negative bacilli and streptococci. Aggressive antibiotic therapy combined with serial arthrocentesis may be as effective as open surgical drainage in uncomplicated septic arthritis, while also preserving better joint function. Surgical drainage is required if this more conservative strategy is not successful.

Osteomyelitis in older adults can be due to hematogenous seeding from a bacteremia or contiguous spread from an adjacent focus. *S aureus* is the predominant organism, but gastrointestinal and genitourinary flora are again more common in older adults, emphasizing the advantage of a specific microbiologic diagnosis to guide therapy. Pressure ulcer infections and diabetic foot infections are very common, particularly in institutionalized older adults, and such infections commonly require surgical consultation combined with aggressive antimicrobial therapy aimed at mixed aerobic and anaerobic bacteria. Osteomyelitis requires definitive treatment with aggressive debridement/amputation of the infected bone with up to 8 weeks of appropriate (and often intravenous) antimicrobial therapy in consultation with an infectious diseases specialist.

HIV Infection and AIDS

HIV infection in older adults was initially limited to those who had received blood transfusions for surgical procedures. However, increasing numbers of older Americans with HIV have acquired their infection via sexual activity. In addition, improvements in treatment have resulted in a large population of adults aging with HIV infection. By 2015, >50% of U.S. adults infected with HIV will be ≥50 years old. Older adults constitute approximately 10% of all new diagnoses of AIDS in the United States, but this group and their clinicians often suffer from a lack of HIV awareness. Nonspecific symptoms such as forgetfulness, anorexia, weight loss, and recurrent pneumonia are often dismissed as age related, delaying HIV testing.

Untreated HIV infection in older adults tends to pursue a more rapid downhill course, perhaps because of impaired T-cell replacement mechanisms with advanced age and the impact of additional comorbidities. However, if older adults are treated with aggressive highly active antiretroviral therapy (HAART), the antiviral response is similar to that seen in young adults. In fact, older adults often are more adherent with complicated HAART regimens than young adults. However, despite this response, increasing data suggest immune reconstitution is less robust in older adults with HIV infection. Recommendations are becoming more aggressive with regard to threshold for initiation of HAART; however, these recommendations have been in a state of flux for the past several years, and it is suggested that all patients with HIV be under the care of an infectious diseases specialist to decide when to begin therapy and what agents are most appropriate.

Treatment regimens and prophylaxis of opportunistic infections with HAART are similar to those used in younger patients. Indications that HIV therapies can accelerate atherosclerosis and glucose intolerance suggest that an aggressive approach to prevention of cardiovascular disease in older HIV-infected adults is warranted and may lead to specific recommendations in older adults if associations of metabolic changes with specific HIV therapies become clearer. Other age-related comorbidities are also more common in HIV-infected individuals, even those with well-controlled viral replication (ie, a peripheral blood viral load <50 copies/mL). Many types of cancer, osteoporosis, and cirrhosis are all more prevalent in this population and appear to develop about a decade earlier in HIV-infected individuals versus appropriately matched, uninfected controls. Older adults appear to be more susceptible to specific complications associated with HIV infection, such as encephalopathy. Finally, older HIV-infected adults are more likely than uninfected, age-matched adults to have multiple comorbidities, which increases the complexity of their care and the potential for medication interactions.

HIV prevention is rarely discussed in the geriatric community but is important if the trend of increasing sexual acquisition of HIV in older adults is to be reversed. Most older women do not believe they are at risk of HIV infection, yet heterosexual activity is the primary mode of infection in this group. The concept of HIV-risky behavior is not well known among older adults, because HIV was not a problem during their adolescence or young adulthood. Older adults must be included in educational programs aimed at ensuring safe sexual practices and increasing awareness of the benefits of testing and effective HIV therapy.

Miscellaneous Infectious Syndromes

Hepatitis C

Hepatitis C is one of the leading causes of end-stage liver disease in the United States and the most common indication for liver transplantation. Most adults who harbor the hepatitis C virus are asymptomatic and unaware of their infection status. Over the past several years, more effective, better tolerated treatments for hepatitis C have become available and have led to improvement in virologic cure (ie, sustained virologic response). Data from population based studies have shown that three-fourths of adults who are infected with hepatitis C were born between 1945 and 1965, many of which remain asymptomatic. Based on this data, the U.S. Preventive Services Task Force (USPSTF) recently updated their recommendations in 2013 to include 1-time screening for hepatitis C virus infection to adults born between 1945 and 1965. Adults in this age group are at potential risk because of possible exposure before universal blood screening (B recommendation). The USPSTF concluded that early detection and intervention for hepatitis C virus infection in this group with antiviral regimens resulted in sustained virologic response and improved clinical outcomes, although there was no direct evidence for reducing overall morbidity and mortality.

Infections of the Central Nervous System

Bacterial meningitis is most common at the age extremes of life, and most meningitis-associated fatalities are in older adults. *Streptococcus pneumoniae* remains the most common cause in older adults, but gram-negative bacilli (20%–25%), *Listeria* spp (up to 10%), and tuberculosis are more common than in young adults. Because many *S pneumoniae* are resistant to β-lactam antibiotics (up to 30% penicillin resistance and 10% ceftriaxone resistance nationwide), ceftriaxone or cefotaxime *plus* vancomycin are recommended as empiric therapy for bacterial meningitis in older adults until a specific isolate can be tested for antimicrobial susceptibility. Ampicillin is the drug of choice for *Listeria* spp and is appropriate to add to the empiric antibiotic regimen in older adults, and more resistant gram-negative rods (eg, *Pseudomonas* spp) require ceftazidime or an extended-spectrum penicillin with or without intrathecal aminoglycoside therapy.

Neurosyphilis remains one of the most perplexing diagnoses in medicine. It is often raised as a possible underlying process in stroke or dementia in older adults. Syphilis should also be considered in unilateral deafness, gait disturbances, uveitis, and optic neuritis. In reality, there is no gold-standard test to exclude neurosyphilis. Neurosyphilis can only be "ruled in" by such

Table 62.5—Evaluation of Fever of Unknown Origin in Older Adults

Sequential Step	Details
1. Confirm fever	Temperature >38° C for ≥3 weeks
2. Comprehensive history	Specifically include travel history, other possible exposures to *Mycobacterium tuberculosis*, place of residence (eg, long-term care facility), and current/past sexual history (often not obtained in older adults). Review all medications, including OTC medications and recently discontinued medications (eg, antibiotics).
	Detailed review of systems should focus on new-onset or recent changes in symptoms, including constitutional symptoms, and symptoms of giant cell arteritis (ie, scalp pain and tenderness, vision loss, jaw pain).
	Consider obtaining history from family members or caregivers, especially if patient has cognitive impairment.
3. Comprehensive physical examination	Include detailed dental examination, temporal arteries and shoulders if symptoms are suggestive of polymyalgia rheumatica, abdomen (tenderness may subtle), skin (including back and sacrum to evaluate for pressure ulcers), and lymph nodes.
4. Initial laboratory evaluation	CBC with differential, liver enzymes, erythrocyte sedimentation rate, blood cultures × 3, procalcitonin, chemistry panel, chest radiograph, urinalysis, antinuclear antibody, C reactive protein, HIV-antibody, PPD skin testing, or IGRA.
If no obvious source based on history and all nonessential or concerning medications have been discontinued:	
5. Initial imaging evaluation	Chest or abdomen CT; can consider FDG-PET/CT scan or indium-111 labeled WBC scan.
6. Further testing	If CT or WBC scan is positive, consider biopsy of identified pathology. If no pathology identified, consider empiric diagnostic tests listed below: ■ Temporal artery biopsy should be obtained if any symptoms or signs are consistent with giant cell arteritis or polymyalgia rheumatica (eg, increased erythrocyte sedimentation rate or tenderness on palpation of temporal arteries). ■ Consider liver biopsy if liver function tests are abnormal. Bone marrow biopsy if abnormal CBC (include Gram stain and cultures [acid-fast bacilli, fungal, and bacterial]).

tests. However, suspicion is often first raised when a serum rapid plasma reagent or Venereal Disease Research Laboratory test (VDRL) is positive. A reasonable diagnostic evaluation after discovery of such a positive test includes confirmation of nonspecific tests (rapid plasma reagent and VDRL) with a specific test (microhemagglutination-*Treponema pallidum*, or fluorescent treponemal antibody absorption); if tests are confirmed, lumbar puncture should be performed for cell counts, glucose, protein, and cerebrospinal fluid (CSF) VDRL. A positive VDRL on CSF is diagnostic of neurosyphilis, but the sensitivity of this test is approximately 75% in most series. Other diagnostic tests are controversial. The ratio of intrathecal to serum-specific treponemal antibody (standardized to the total IgG in CSF and serum) may also be helpful, with ratios ≥3 indicating likely infection. In the absence of these tests, it must be the judgment of the clinician as to whether minor abnormalities in CSF (eg, low-level pleocytosis) and the clinical picture support the diagnosis and warrant therapy for neurosyphilis. Optimal treatment of neurosyphilis remains penicillin G, but a study in HIV-infected patients suggests that ceftriaxone may be an acceptable alternative.

Facial nerve palsy (Bell's palsy) is common in older adults and associated with at least three infectious causes: herpes simplex virus, varicella zoster virus, and *Borrelia burgdorferi* (which causes Lyme disease). There are no strong data at present to suggest benefit of antiviral therapy for facial nerve palsies due to herpes simplex virus, but trials are underway. If facial nerve palsy is seen as part of an episode of varicella zoster virus, treatment is indicated. If Lyme disease is suspected clinically, the patient should receive oral amoxicillin 500 mg q6h for 14 days, oral doxycycline 100 mg q12h for 14 days, or intravenous ceftriaxone 2 g/d for 14 days.

Gastrointestinal Infections

Gastrointestinal infections are common among older adults. Diverticulitis, appendicitis, cholecystitis, intra-abdominal abscess, and ischemic bowel can present diagnostic dilemmas in the absence of fever or increased WBC counts. A high index of suspicion is necessary in older adults. CT of the abdomen and pelvis is most likely to be of value in establishing the diagnosis of intra-abdominal infection, and ultrasonography is an easy, readily available tool to assist in diagnosing cholecystitis, appendicitis, or abscess. Ischemic bowel often requires angiography.

Infectious diarrhea is also common in older adults. Older patients with achlorhydria are at particular risk, because a lower bacterial inoculum is necessary to cause disease. Decreased intestinal motility associated with specific medications and advanced age may further increase susceptibility to infection. Epidemics occurring in the long-term care setting are commonly due to *E coli*, viruses, *Salmonella* spp, or *Shigella* spp. Frequent use of antimicrobials in older adults also increases the risk of *Clostridium difficile* colitis, and the risk of severe disease is greatest in this age group.

Clostridium difficile Infection and Pseudomembranous Colitis

Clostridium difficile infection (CDI) is becoming increasingly recognized among older hospitalized patients and is the source of epidemics in hospitals and long-term care facilities for older adults. The reasons for this trend are uncertain but likely relate to spread of more virulent strains, widespread use of fluoroquinolone antibiotics, and use of proton-pump inhibitors (SOE=B).

A hypervirulent strain, NAP1/BI/027, has been implicated as the responsible pathogen in selected CDI outbreaks and is capable of enhanced production of toxins A and B. The infection is often precipitated by use of antibiotics, particularly clindamycin, third-generation cephalosporins, and fluoroquinolones.

Older adults often present with watery diarrhea and abdominal cramps, with or without fever. Constipation or ileus can sometimes be the presenting symptom, especially in postoperative patients. Other signs include significant leukocytosis (often >20,000 WBCs/μL), hypoalbuminemia, fecal WBCs, and a distinctive fecal odor.

In many clinical settings, diagnosis is made using polymerase chain reaction for B toxin gene. Alternatively, a combination approach, using antigen detection (enzyme immunoassay method) for the *C difficile* antigen followed by A/B toxin assay, may be used. A negative test excludes the presence of *C difficile*, but a positive test must be interpreted in the context of clinical assessment, because up to 50% of hospitalized patients can be colonized. Testing for *C difficile* should be performed only on unformed stool and should not be repeated during the same episode of diarrhea.

Treatment of CDI, most importantly, begins with discontinuing offending antimicrobial agents as soon as possible. Initiation of oral metronidazole 500 mg q8h is considered first-line therapy for mild or moderate illness, even in older adults. However, older adults often present with more severe disease (WBC counts ≥15,000/μL or a serum creatinine level ≥1.5 times baseline), in which case oral vancomycin 125 mg q6h for 10–14 days is recommended (SOE=B). Metronidazole should not be used beyond the first recurrence of CDI because of the risk of neurotoxicity. Fidaxomicin 200 mg q12h for 10 days has been shown to reduce the rate of relapse compared with oral vancomycin in patients with recurrent CDI; however, it is expensive and often not covered by insurance plans. Multiple relapses of CDI are more common in older adults and can occur in >25% of patients. Fecal microbiota transplantation (FMT) has recently been used for treatment of recurrent CDI in those with severe recurrent infection not responsive to antibiotic therapy. In a 2013 study, 91% of patients who received FMT reported either complete resolution or improvement in diarrhea, with no definite adverse effects. Thus, restoration of normal flora with FMT may be a safe, effective method for resolving CDI in patients with severe, recurrent CDI (SOE=C).

Prevention of transmission of CDI, particularly in hospitals and long-term care facilities is of utmost importance, because this population is at greatest risk of complications from CDI. The mainstay of CDI prevention is compliance with hand washing with soap and water after contacting patients with CDI (SOE=A). Other strategies include contact precautions with gloves and gowns on entry into a patient room and the use of private rooms for patients infected with *C difficile*.

FEVER OF UNKNOWN ORIGIN

Fever of unknown origin (FUO) is defined as temperature >101°F (38.3°C) that lasts for at least 3 weeks and is undiagnosed after 1 week of medical evaluation. Several studies have examined this syndrome in older patients and demonstrated differences between older and younger adults. The presence of fever is more likely to be related to a serious infection or illness in older adults than in younger adults or children.

The cause of FUO can be determined in 70%–90% of cases in older adults, and one-third have treatable infections, such as intra-abdominal abscess, bacterial endocarditis, tuberculosis, perinephric abscess, dental abscess, or occult osteomyelitis, with an incidence of infection similar to that in younger patients. In contrast, collagen vascular diseases are more common causes of FUO in older than in younger patients. These are primarily due to giant cell arteritis, polymyalgia rheumatica, and polyarteritis nodosa, but rarely to granulomatosis with polyangitis, (formerly known as Wegner granulomatosis). In several published series, 28% of all FUOs in older adults were due to collagen vascular diseases. Neoplastic disease accounts for another 20%, but with rare exceptions, fever due to cancer is primarily caused by hematologic malignancies (eg, lymphoma and leukemia) and not solid tumors. Medications are another cause of FUO in older adults. Rare causes in this age group include deep-vein thrombosis with or without recurrent pulmonary emboli and hyperthyroidism.

For a diagnostic approach to FUO in older adults, see Table 62.5.

Choosing Wisely® Recommendations

Infectious Diseases

- Don't use antimicrobials to treat bacteriuria in older adults unless specific urinary tract symptoms are present.

REFERENCES

- DiazGranados CA, Dunning AJ, Kimmel M, et al. Efficacy of high-dose versus standard-dose influenza vaccine in older adults. *N Engl J Med.* 2014;371(7):635–645.

    This randomized controlled study compared the standard-dose inactivated influenza vaccine to a high-dose inactivated influenza vaccine in protection against laboratory-confirmed influenza illness in adults ≥65 years old. The authors found an overall improved efficacy of approximately 25% in adults who received the high-dose vaccination, suggesting that approximately one-quarter of influenza illnesses could be prevented if high-dose vaccination is used in this population. However, the study excluded patients with moderate or severe acute illnesses.

- Moberley S, Holden J, Tatham DP, et al. Vaccines for preventing pneumococcal infection in adults. *Cochrane Database Syst Rev.* 2013 Jan 31;1:CD000422.

    This 2013 systematic review and meta-analysis reviewed the efficacy of pneumococcal polysaccharide vaccine in preventing invasive pneumococcal disease and pneumococcal pneumonia. A subgroup analysis, which included many older adults, found significant evidence in reduction of invasive pneumococcal disease but not in overall mortality or all-cause pneumonia.

- Morison VA, Oxman MN, Levin MJ, et al. Safety of zoster vaccine in elderly adults following documented herpes zoster. *J Infect Dis.* 2013;208:559–563.

    This study evaluated the safety of zoster vaccine in adults with a prior history of herpes zoster. Using patients from the large Shingles Prevention Study, 420 patients with a prior history of herpes zoster received the vaccine; mean time from zoster to vaccine was approximately 4 years. There was no significant difference in significant adverse events after receiving the vaccine in patients who had a history of herpes zoster compared with those who did not.

- Moyer V. Screening for hepatitis C virus infection in adults: U.S. Preventive Services Task Force Recommendation Statement. *Ann Intern Med.* 2013;159(5):349–357.

    This update by the USPSTF makes new recommendations for one-time hepatitis C screening for all adults who were born between 1945 and 1965 because of the higher prevalence of hepatitis C virus infection in this age group (three-fourths of patients in the United States with hepatitis C were born during this period). The increased risk is possibly secondary to blood transfusions before the introduction of screening in 1992 (SOE=B).

- Surveillance definitions of infections in long-term care facilities: revisiting the McGeer criteria. *Infect Control Hosp Epidemiol.* 2012;33(10):965–977.

    This comprehensive review updates the 1991 infection surveillance definitions for long-term care residents. Most notably, changes to the definition for urinary tract infection include the need for microbiologic confirmation in patients with and without a Foley catheter. The definition for diagnosis of pneumonia or lower respiratory tract infection requires all 3 of the following findings: positive radiography results, respiratory signs or symptoms, and constitutional criteria.

- Tomczyk S, Bennett NM, Stoecker C, et al. Use of 13-valent pneumococcal conjugate vaccine and 23-valent pneumococcal polysaccharide vaccine among adults aged ≥65 years: recommendations of the Advisory Committee on Immunization Practices (ACIP). *Morb Mortal Wkly Rep.* 2014;63(37):822–825.

    This report discusses recommendations from ACIP that both PCV13 and PPSV23 should be routinely administered to all adults aged ≥65 years old. This recommendation is based on a randomized placebo-controlled trial of approximately 85,000 adults ≥65 years old demonstrating clinical benefit of PCV13 in prevention of vaccine-type pneumococcal pneumonia, vaccine-type nonbacteremic pneumococcal pneumonia, and vaccine-type invasive pneumococcal disease. Recommendations for routine PCV13 use in this population will be reevaluated in 2018.

Manisha Juthani-Mehta, MD
Theresa A. Rowe, DO

CHAPTER 63—ENDOCRINOLOGY

KEY POINTS

- Thyrotropin (thyroid-stimulating hormone) is an adequate screening test for thyroid function in a healthy older adult outpatient population, but both free T_4 and thyrotropin should be used to evaluate thyroid status in sick older adults.

- Chronic adrenal insufficiency presents with nonspecific symptoms such as anorexia, nausea, weight loss, abdominal pain, weakness, hypotension, and impaired function. It should be considered as a cause of unexplained cachexia, mobility disability, and hypotension, even in the absence of hyponatremia and hyperkalemia.

- Vitamin D deficiency is common and not only contributes to bone loss due to osteoporosis and osteomalacia but also has been associated with muscle weakness and falls.

- The most common causes of hypercalcemia are primary hyperparathyroidism in outpatients, and malignant hypercalcemia (eg, caused by squamous cell cancers, breast cancer, myeloma, and lymphoma) in the inpatient setting.

- There is little evidence of long-term clinical benefit from supplementation with dehydroepiandrosterone (DHEA), testosterone, and growth hormone in older adults.

Impaired homeostatic regulation, a hallmark of aging, occurs in many endocrine systems but may become manifest only during stress. For example, fasting blood glucose concentrations change little with normal aging, increasing 1–2 mg/dL per decade of life. In contrast, glucose concentrations after glucose challenge (eg, postprandially) increase much more in healthy older adults than in young adults. In some cases, a loss of function in one aspect of endocrine function can result in a compensatory change in endocrine regulation and be associated with changes in catabolism that maintain homeostasis. For example, decreased testosterone production by the testes, which is seen in many older men, may be partially compensated for by an increase in secretion of pituitary luteinizing hormone and offset by a decrease in metabolism of testosterone. In other instances, compensatory changes or changes in hormone catabolism do not fully offset age-related impairment in endocrine functions, as illustrated by the age-related decline in basal serum aldosterone concentrations. In this case, a decline in aldosterone clearance fails to offset the decrease in aldosterone secretion.

As with diseases in other organ systems, endocrine disorders in older adults often have nonspecific, muted, or atypical symptoms and signs. Some of these presentations are well-defined syndromes that are seen almost exclusively in older adults, such as apathetic thyrotoxicosis or hyperosmolar nonketotic state in patients with type 2 diabetes mellitus. However, more commonly, endocrine disorders present with subtle, nonspecific symptoms, such as cognitive impairment or reduced functional status, or an absence of any complaints. Indeed, the diagnosis of endocrinopathies such as primary hyperparathyroidism, type 2 diabetes mellitus, hypothyroidism, and hyperthyroidism in older adults is commonly established as a result of abnormalities found on routine laboratory testing.

Laboratory evaluation of older adults for endocrine disorders can be complicated by coexisting medical illnesses and medications. For example, the presence of serious acute or chronic nonthyroidal illness can lead to the mistaken impression of a thyroid disorder because of the increase or decrease in T_4 concentrations and sometimes increased or decreased thyrotropin concentrations in sick but euthyroid older adults. As a result of biological and assay variability, hormone concentrations may vary considerably in the short term. Therefore, abnormal hormone measurements should always be repeated to confirm endocrine dysfunction, and a stimulatory or suppression test may be required to firmly establish a diagnosis of endocrine hypofunction or hyperfunction, respectively. Furthermore, ranges of normal laboratory values for endocrine testing are commonly established in younger adults, and even age-adjusted norms for laboratory tests may be confounded by the inclusion of older adults who are ill. Consequently, normal ranges for healthy older adults are not available for many laboratory tests.

THYROID DISORDERS

With aging, a decrease in T_4 secretion is balanced by a decrease in T_4 clearance, resulting in unchanged circulating T_4 concentrations. T_3 concentrations are unchanged until extreme old age, when they decrease slightly, possibly reflecting a decrease in 5′-deiodinase activity with aging. T_3 concentrations are also commonly decreased in nonthyroidal illness because of decreased peripheral conversion of T_4 to T_3. The distribution of thyrotropin concentrations shifts toward a higher level with increasing age, with the 97.5th percentile of thyrotropin distribution of 6.3–7.5 mIU/L in adults ≥80 years old, contributing to the higher prevalence of biochemical hypothyroidism. This shift toward higher thyrotropin concentrations with age appears also to apply to extremely long-lived individuals. Nonspecific, atypical, or asymptomatic presentations of thyroid disease are common in older adults. Laboratory testing in the stable outpatient using thyrotropin measurements is the most reliable way to identify hypothyroidism or hyperthyroidism in older adults who are not acutely ill. There is no consensus regarding screening asymptomatic older adults for hypo- and hyperthyroidism. However, the prevalence of hypothyroidism and hyperthyroidism is sufficiently high to warrant thyrotropin testing in all older adults with a recent decline in clinical, cognitive, or functional status, or on admission to a nursing home. The results of thyroid function testing can be confusing in euthyroid patients with significant concurrent illnesses (discussed below).

Hypothyroidism

Most prevalence estimates of hypothyroidism in older adults range from 0.5% to 5% for overt disease, depending on the population studied. As in younger people, most cases of hypothyroidism in older adults are due to chronic autoimmune thyroiditis (Hashimoto disease). Symptoms of hypothyroidism are often atypical in older adults. Some clinical features of hypothyroidism (eg, dry skin, decreased skin turgor, slowed mentation, weakness, constipation, anemia, hyponatremia, arthritis, paresthesias, peripheral neuropathy, gait disturbances, edema, and increased myocardial fraction of creatine kinase) can misleadingly suggest other diseases. Furthermore, these symptoms usually have an insidious onset and a slow rate of progression. As a result, the diagnosis of hypothyroidism is recognized on clinical examination in only 10%–20% of cases in older adults, and laboratory screening is necessary to detect most cases of hypothyroidism in this population. In addition, older adults with mild hypothyroidism who develop serious nonthyroidal illness may rapidly become severely hypothyroid, a situation that increases susceptibility to myxedema coma. Demented older adults with hypothyroidism rarely recover normal cognitive function with thyroid replacement, but cognition, functional status, and mood may improve with treatment of the hypothyroidism.

Subclinical hypothyroidism, characterized by increased serum thyrotropin and normal free T_4 concentrations, has been reported in up to 15% of people ≥65 years old, and is more common in women. However, up to 70% of these individuals actually have values within their age-specific 97.5th percentile, and those with exceptional longevity have higher thyrotropin levels than those aged 70 years. These findings suggest that using an age-specific TSH reference range would reduce the risk that many older adults will be mislabeled as having subclinical hypothyroidism. Epidemiologic studies in older adults have not found a consistent association between subclinical hypothyroidism and risk of coronary heart disease mortality or total mortality. In a meta-analysis of studies involving 55,287 participants, no effect of subclinical hypothyroidism on all-cause mortality was observed, although coronary heart disease mortality increased with serum thyrotropin levels ≥7 mIU/L and especially with levels ≥10 mIU/L. The exception among the included studies was the Leiden-85-Plus Study that involved participants ≥85 years old exclusively, whereas in all other studies the mean age was lower; in the Leiden study, increased thyrotropin was associated with decreased all-cause mortality.

Levothyroxine supplementation has not been shown to have beneficial effects in older adults with mildly increased TSH levels. Furthermore, in octogenarians, higher endogenous free T_4 levels are independently associated with mortality. Randomized controlled trials (RCTs) of T_4 supplementation in older adults with subclinical hypothyroidism have not shown a consistent improvement in symptoms, although those with thyrotropin concentrations ≥10 mIU/L may derive symptomatic benefit. Based on the foregoing, T_4 supplementation in older adults with mildly increased thyrotropin levels may be of limited clinical benefit or possibly even harmful. However, adults with thyrotropin levels ≥10 mIU/L may manifest symptoms of hypothyroidism and are at increased risk of congestive heart failure and cardiovascular mortality regardless of age and should be considered for levothyroxine supplementation for relief of symptoms. It is unknown whether these risks can be ameliorated with thyroxine replacement.

By itself, an increased thyrotropin concentration is usually due to primary hypothyroidism, but thyrotropin concentrations may be transiently increased during recovery from acute illnesses. Therefore, the diagnosis of hypothyroidism should be confirmed by the combination of a persistently increased thyrotropin concentration and a decreased free T_4 or free T_4 index (total T_4 × thyroid uptake [an estimate of thyroid hormone binding]). Potentially confusing scenarios in the diagnosis of hypothyroidism may occur in the *nonthyroidal illness syndromes*, which may present with low serum total T_4 levels ("low T_4 syndrome") without increased thyrotropin concentrations in euthyroid patients with severe nonthyroidal illnesses. Free T_4 concentrations are usually normal in the low T_4 syndrome, with increased concentrations of reverse T_3. Serum thyrotropin levels may also be low in nonthyroidal illness syndrome. However, the most common alteration in thyroid hormone levels in nonthyroidal illness is a decrease in serum T_3 levels *(low T_3 syndrome)*, occurring even in mild nonthyroidal illnesses. In the past, patients with the nonthyroidal illness syndrome were thought to be euthyroid, but some may actually have developed *transient* secondary hypothyroidism. Thyroid hormone supplementation has not been shown to be beneficial in these patients, and it may be harmful. An inappropriately normal or low thyrotropin concentration found in conjunction with a low free T_4 concentration suggests *secondary hypothyroidism*, which may be differentiated from the low T_4 syndrome by the presence of hypopituitarism (deficiencies in other pituitary hormones) and decreased reverse T_3 concentrations (versus increased reverse T_3 in nonthyroidal illness). Rarely, older adults with primary hypothyroidism can also have inappropriately normal thyrotropin concentrations resulting from suppression of thyrotropin by fasting, acute illnesses, and medications such as dopamine, phenytoin, or glucocorticoids. To minimize confusion between thyroid disease and the nonthyroidal illness syndrome, thyroid function testing in seriously ill patients should be performed only if thyroid dysfunction is strongly suspected, with repeat testing performed after recovery from acute illnesses.

T_4 replacement is usually started at a low dosage in older adults (eg, 25 mcg/d, or 50 mcg/d in those without evidence of coronary heart disease), increasing the dosage every 4–6 weeks until thyrotropin concentrations reach the normal range. However, in patients with severe cardiac disease, it is sometimes prudent to begin replacement therapy at even lower dosages (eg, 12.5 mcg/d) if patients are asymptomatic or have minimal symptoms of hypothyroidism (SOE=D). In these patients, thyroid replacement should not be withheld for fear of exacerbating cardiac disease; instead, the goal is to reduce or eliminate symptoms of hypothyroidism while minimizing the potential for exacerbating cardiac symptoms, such as angina. Older adults who are severely hypothyroid at presentation should receive higher initial T_4 replacement doses of 50–100 mcg orally, or as high as 200 mcg IV followed by 100 mcg IV daily until oral intake is possible for those with myxedema stupor or coma, even if there is preexisting heart disease (SOE=D). Older adults with severe hypothyroidism or myxedema stupor or coma should also be tested to exclude concomitant adrenal insufficiency as well as given stress doses of glucocorticoids before receiving T_4 to avoid precipitating an adrenal crisis with T_4 replacement.

Thyroid hormone requirements decrease with aging because of a decreased clearance rate, and T_4 replacement dosages are as much as a third lower in older than in younger adults. The average T_4 replacement dosage in older adults is approximately 110 mcg/d. However, in many older hypothyroid patients, low T_4 doses (25–50 mcg/d) are sufficient to normalize serum thyrotropin levels. Thyroid hormone is best taken fasting to avoid reduced absorption related to food and other medications (eg, calcium, iron, or soy). The target thyrotropin level should be higher in older than in young adults (4–7 mIU/L). Over-replacement of thyroid hormone should be avoided, because osteopenia related to increased bone turnover and exacerbation of heart disease may occur. With correction of the hypothyroid state, the clearance rate of medications such as anticonvulsants, digoxin, and opioid analgesic agents may be affected, necessitating dosage adjustments.

Hyperthyroidism

Hyperthyroidism develops in 0.5%–2.3% of older adults, and 15%–25% of all cases of thyrotoxicosis are in adults ≥60 years old. In the United States, most cases in older adults are due to Graves disease, but toxic multinodular goiter and autonomously functioning adenomas are more common in older than in young adults, especially in populations with low iodine intake.

Hyperthyroidism often presents with vague, atypical, or nonspecific symptoms in frail older adults. Many findings that are common in younger adults (eg, tremor, hyperkinesis, heat intolerance, tachycardia, frequent bowel movements, ophthalmopathy, increased perspiration, goiter, brisk reflexes) are less common or absent in older adults, whereas other manifestations, such as atrial fibrillation, heart failure, weight loss, muscle atrophy, and weakness, are more common in older adults. Older adults more often present with a paucity of symptoms than young adults, which may lead to delays in treatment and poorer outcomes. Older adults can present with *apathetic thyrotoxicosis*, a well-known clinical presentation of hyperthyroidism that is rarely seen in younger adults, in which the usual hyperkinetic presentation is replaced by depression, inactivity, lethargy, or withdrawn behavior, often in association with symptoms such as anorexia, weight loss, constipation, muscle weakness, or cardiac symptoms. A low thyrotropin concentration is associated with a 3-fold higher risk of developing atrial fibrillation within 10 years, and hyperthyroidism is present in 13%–30% of older adults with atrial fibrillation. Hyperthyroidism is a cause of secondary osteoporosis and should be considered in the evaluation of patients with decreased bone mass.

A highly sensitive thyrotropin test is adequate as an initial test for hyperthyroidism in relatively healthy older adults, but the diagnosis should be confirmed with free T_4 and T_3 tests. Most asymptomatic older adults with low serum thyrotropin concentrations are clinically euthyroid and have normal T_4 and T_3 concentrations, with normal thyrotropin on repeat testing 4–6 weeks later. T_3 *thyrotoxicosis*, with increased T_3 but normal T_4 concentrations, is seen in a minority of hyperthyroid patients, but it is more common with aging, especially in older adults with toxic adenomas or toxic multinodular goiter. However, in contrast to young adults, many older adults with hyperthyroidism do not have increased T_4 or T_3 concentrations, probably because of decreased conversion of T_4 to T_3 associated with aging and concomitant nonthyroidal illness. The reduction in T_4 to T_3 conversion in nonthyroidal illness is mediated by a decrease in T_4-5′-deiodinase activity, although the specific factors mediating changes in enzymatic activity are unknown. Diagnostic confusion can occasionally occur in euthyroid patients with nonthyroidal illness or medications causing increased T_4 concentrations (*high T_4 syndrome*). The high T_4 syndrome can develop with medications or illnesses that decrease the conversion of T_4 to T_3 (high-dose glucocorticoids or β-blocking agents, acute fasting) or that increase circulating concentrations of thyroid-binding globulin (estrogens, clofibrate, hepatitis). Uncommonly, a critically ill patient with hyperthyroidism may have low serum thyrotropin levels together with normal to low total and free T_4 and/or T_3 levels, which may be very difficult to distinguish from nonthyroidal illness in critically ill but euthyroid patients. In these cases, a free T_4 level well within the normal range and/or an undetectable serum thyrotropin level suggest the patient may be hyperthyroid. Finally, clinicians may encounter otherwise healthy older adults with low serum thyrotropin levels together with low-normal free T_4 and T_3 levels and no evidence of thyroid or pituitary disease. These individuals are thought to have an altered set point of the pituitary-thyroid axis; subclinical hyperthyroidism may be excluded in such cases by radioactive iodine uptake (RAIU) testing to detect autonomous thyroid function. When the etiology of hyperthyroidism is unclear, a RAIU test and thyroid scan should be performed (SOE=C) (Figure 63.1). It is important to identify hyperthyroid patients with low RAIU, because these patients do not respond to radioactive iodine therapy or antithyroid medications and are treated symptomatically.

Subclinical hyperthyroidism, defined as a low or undetectable serum thyrotropin level with normal free T_4 and T_3 levels, with or without signs and symptoms consistent with thyroid hormone excess, is present in approximately 2% of older adults without known thyroid disease. However, its prevalence is as high as 10% in iodine-deficient regions, and exogenous subclinical hyperthyroidism is present in 20%–40% of patients on levothyroxine supplementation. Over hyperthyroidism develops in 1%–2% of patients (per year) with a thyrotropin concentration of <0.1 mIU/L but is uncommon in those with thyrotropin concentrations of 0.1–0.45 mIU/L. Thyrotropin concentrations normalize over time in many of these patients, although in those with undetectable thyrotropin levels, persistence of subclinical hyperthyroidism is the most common outcome.

There is good evidence for an association between subclinical hyperthyroidism and atrial fibrillation in those with thyrotropin concentrations <0.45 mIU/L, especially when concentrations are <0.1 mIU/L (SOE=A), as well as in people with thyroid function in the high-normal range. Subclinical hyperthyroidism can increase left ventricular mass and cardiac contractility and can cause delayed diastolic relaxation, but these effects are of uncertain clinical importance. It is unknown whether subclinical hyperthyroidism increases the risk of cardiovascular and all-cause mortality. Subclinical hyperthyroidism can accelerate bone mineral density (BMD) loss, especially in people with a thyrotropin concentration <0.1 mIU/L, but even thyroid function within the high-normal range is associated with reduced BMD and increased risk of hip and other nonvertebral fractures. In postmenopausal women, ongoing bone losses associated with thyrotropin concentrations <0.1–0.2 mIU/L are stabilized by treating the hyperthyroidism. A systematic review found that low serum thyrotropin levels were associated with cognitive impairment or dementia in 14 of 23 studies, all but 2 of which involved participants >60 years old. It is unknown whether antithyroid therapy can prevent cognitive decline in these individuals.

Treatment of hyperthyroidism should be strongly considered in all older adults with persistently low thyrotropin concentrations <0.1 mIU/L and considered in older adults with thyrotropin levels of 0.1–0.45 mIU/L. These recommendations are based on the increased risk of atrial fibrillation in these patients and evidence of progressively increased mortality risk with age in patients with subclinical hyperthyroidism who are >60 years old (SOE=C).

Radioactive iodine (RAI) therapy is the treatment of choice for most older adults with hyperthyroidism caused by Graves disease or toxic nodular thyroid disease. RAI treatment is usually curative in patients with toxic adenoma, but higher or repeated doses are often necessary for patients with toxic multinodular goiter. Antithyroid drugs such as methimazole may be given before RAI (SOE=B); eg, beginning 4–6 weeks before and stopping 3 days before RAI, resuming 3 days afterward, and tapering off over 1–3 months, to control symptoms and to avoid a worsening of thyrotoxicosis due to transient release of thyroid hormone after RAI. However, some experts believe the risk of exacerbating thyrotoxicosis is sufficiently low that the risks of antithyroid drugs may outweigh the anticipated benefit. β-Blocking agents are helpful to manage symptoms such as tachycardia, tremor, and anxiety[OL] (SOE=B), but patients should be monitored for changes in cardiopulmonary function. These patients may also require treatment of coexisting congestive heart failure, myocardial ischemia, and atrial arrhythmias, including atrial fibrillation. Treatment with β-blocking agents may be sufficient to manage cardiovascular morbidity due to subclinical hyperthyroidism, notably atrial fibrillation.

After RAI therapy, patients should be monitored by serial measurements of thyrotropin concentration for eventual development of hypothyroidism and for persistent or recurrent hyperthyroidism. With resolution of hyperthyroidism, the clearance rate of other medications may decrease, necessitating dosage adjustments to avoid excessive drug concentrations.

Nodular Thyroid Disease and Thyroid Cancer

The incidence of multinodular goiter increases with age. Multinodular goiters often have autonomously functioning areas, so that administration of exogenous thyroid hormone to suppress these goiters can cause iatrogenic hyperthyroidism. Older adults with multinodular goiter can develop iodine-induced thyrotoxicosis after receiving radiocontrast or amiodarone.

Approximately 90% of women ≥70 years old and 60% of men ≥80 years old have thyroid nodules. Most of these nodules are nonpalpable but are detected incidentally on highly sensitive ultrasound or imaging studies done for other reasons (eg, carotid duplex ultrasound to assess carotid artery atherosclerosis). Thyroid nodules are more likely to be malignant in adults ≥60 years old, especially men. Thyroid cancer is present in 4%–6.5% of thyroid nodules, and incidentally discovered nonpalpable nodules are as likely to be malignant as palpable nodules. The incidence of differentiated thyroid cancers is similar in older and younger adults, whereas thyroid lymphomas are more common and anaplastic thyroid carcinomas are found almost exclusively in older adults. However, even well-differentiated papillary and follicular carcinomas are more aggressive and are associated with increased mortality in older adults.

Ultrasound is the most sensitive test to detect thyroid nodules. Screening ultrasonography of the thyroid is not indicated in the general population, but ultrasonography and a serum thyrotropin are indicated in all patients with known or suspected thyroid nodules or multinodular goiter (SOE=A) (Table 63.1). Autonomously functioning thyroid nodules are rarely malignant, so no further evaluation for cancer is required in patients with low thyrotropin concentrations and a "hot" nodule on radionuclide thyroid scanning that corresponds to a palpable nodule. Radionuclide thyroid scanning is not indicated in individuals with normal or increased thyrotropin levels; these scans cannot conclusively distinguish whether a "cold" (nonfunctioning) nodule is benign or malignant, and fine-needle aspiration (FNA) is needed to exclude malignancy. FNA for cytology is the diagnostic procedure of choice to detect cancer in thyroid nodules (SOE=A), with ultrasound guidance for nodules that are nonpalpable, primarily cystic, posteriorly located, or nondiagnostic after FNA guided by palpation (SOE=B). Current guidelines call for varying size thresholds for aspiration depending on the clinical and sonographic characteristics of the nodule. In general, in individuals without known thyroid cancer risk factors, only nodules >1 cm require evaluation for malignancy because of their potential to be clinically significant cancers. Ultrasonographic features suspicious for cancer appear to be more accurate in predicting malignancy than nodular size alone. However, nodules >5 mm should be evaluated if a known thyroid cancer risk factor is present, or if findings on ultrasound are suspicious. Nodules that are purely cystic do not require FNA. Benign thyroid nodules on FNA should be followed with serial ultrasonography 6–18 months after the initial aspiration (SOE=D). FNA should be repeated when the results are nondiagnostic. If cytology is diagnostic or suspicious for a malignancy, surgery should be performed (SOE=A). Nodules with indeterminate cytology and without evidence of autonomous function on ^{123}I or ^{99m}Tc pertechnetate scanning have a 5%–32% risk of malignancy, and surgical resection should be considered. Alternatively, repeat FNA may be performed within 3–6 months, with surgery for nodules with persistent atypia on cytology (SOE=B). Molecular testing may help to reduce the number of diagnostic thyroid surgeries in patients ultimately found to have benign thyroid nodules.

Postsurgical treatment with RAI decreases the risk of cancer recurrence and death in older patients with large tumors (>4 cm), any size tumor with gross extrathyroidal extension, or distant metastases. Selected older patients with intrathyroidal tumors 1–4 cm in size who have lymph node metastases or other high risk histologic features may benefit from RAI after treatment (SOE=B). Levothyroxine suppressive therapy is indicated to reduce the risk of cancer recurrence and mortality for patients with thyroid cancer after near-total or total thyroidectomy (SOE=B), but adverse events on the heart and osteoporosis can occur with long-term thyroid suppression. β-Blocking agents^{OL} and bone antiresorptive agents^{OL} can

Table 63.1—Indications for Thyroid Ultrasonography

Screening
- History of head and neck irradiation
- Multiple endocrine neoplasia type 2
- Family history of thyroid cancer

Diagnosis
- Unexplained cervical lymphadenopathy
- All patients with known or suspected thyroid nodules or multinodular goiter
- Selection of thyroid nodule(s) for biopsy
- Guidance for fine-needle aspiration of single or multiple thyroid nodules
- Identification of nodular characteristics suspicious for cancer
- Thyroid nodule discovered incidentally on CT, MRI, or PET scanning

Table 63.2—Causes of Age-Related Changes in Calcium Homeostasis

Decreased concentrations of 25(OH)D and 1,25(OH)D
    Decreased renal 1α-hydroxylase activity
    Decreased vitamin D synthesis by the skin
    Decreased sunlight exposure (housebound and institutionalized older adults)
Decreased intestinal absorption of dietary calcium
    Inadequate dietary calcium and vitamin D intake
    Decreased intestinal responsiveness to 1,25(OH)D
    Decreased gastric acid secretion
    Lactase deficiency (avoidance of dairy products)
Increase in serum parathyroid hormone concentrations
    Slight decrease in serum calcium concentrations
    Decreased renal clearance of parathyroid hormone
Decreased parathyroid hormone responsiveness

help minimize these untoward effects (SOE=D). Thyrotropin should be suppressed to <0.1 mU/L for intermediate- or high-risk patients with thyroid cancer (aggressive tumor histology, ^{131}I uptake outside thyroid bed on post-resection scan, incomplete tumor resection, large tumor [>4 cm], extrathyroidal extension [capsular and blood vessel invasion], cervical lymph node metastases, or distant metastases [SOE=B]), while a lesser degree of thyrotropin suppression at or slightly below normal (0.3–2 mU/L) is appropriate for low-risk patients (SOE=B). Patients with heart disease and low BMD may also require less thyrotropin suppression.

DISORDERS OF PARATHYROID AND CALCIUM METABOLISM

Important changes occur with aging in several systems that regulate calcium homeostasis, ultimately leading to decreased bone mass and, in some cases, osteoporosis in older adults (Table 63.2). The net effect of these changes is to increase circulating concentrations of parathyroid hormone (PTH), which increases 30% between 30 and 80 years of age. Serum calcium concentrations remain normal as a result of the increase in PTH, but the balance between bone resorption and bone formation is changed in favor of resorption, resulting in decreased bone mass and increased risk of osteoporosis with aging.

Vitamin D Deficiency

Vitamin D deficiency, defined as a circulating 25(OH)D level <20 ng/mL, is extremely common. In the National Health and Nutrition Examination Survey (NHANES) 2000–2004, 26.6% of men and 33.6% of women of all races >70 years old had serum 25(OH)D levels <20 ng/mL. Exposure to natural sunlight is the major source of vitamin D, but many older adults do not receive adequate sunlight to maintain sufficient vitamin D and, even with adequate exposure to sunlight, the synthesis of vitamin D in skin declines progressively with aging. In addition, dietary calcium intake is inadequate in most older adults. However, as a consequence of factors mentioned in Table 63.2, older adults are less able than younger adults to compensate by increasing their intestinal absorption of ingested calcium. Increased bone turnover and bone loss, especially of cortical bone, is a major consequence of secondary hyperparathyroidism in vitamin D–deficient older adults. Furthermore, vitamin D deficiency is associated with muscle weakness and can contribute to fall risk in some individuals.

Although population screening for vitamin D deficiency is not recommended in current guidelines, 25(OH)D levels should be obtained in older adults at high risk of vitamin D deficiency, including those with obesity, malnutrition, weight loss, a history of falls, non-traumatic fractures, osteoporosis, or who take medicines such as corticosteroids and anticonvulsant drugs. Obese people are at high risk of vitamin D deficiency likely because vitamin D is fat soluble and sequestered in body fat. As a consequence, the increment in 25(OH)D levels after either cutaneous sunlight exposure or oral vitamin D supplementation is less in obese adults than in non-obese adults, and longer periods of vitamin D supplementation may be required to normalize 25(OH)D levels in obese vitamin D-deficient individuals. The main form of vitamin D in circulation, 25(OH)D, is measured in serum to evaluate vitamin D status. Measurements of 1,25(OH)$_2$D$_3$, the active metabolite of vitamin D, are not useful to assess vitamin D status in most individuals, because levels are normal or increased in vitamin D–deficient individuals with secondary hyperparathyroidism. Levels of 1,25(OH)$_2$D$_3$ are mostly used clinically in patients with late-stage chronic kidney disease.

In 2010, the Institute of Medicine (IOM) recommended dietary reference intakes for calcium and vitamin D intended to optimize bone health in the general population. The IOM recommended maintaining 25(OH)D concentrations >20 ng/mL, with the goal of assuring vitamin D levels adequate for bone health in at least 97.5% of the population. There is general agreement that 25(OH)D levels <20 ng/mL are suboptimal for bone health, and that optimal serum 25(OH)D concentrations for outcomes other than bone health have not been established. However, other experts, including the American Geriatrics Society (AGS) Workgroup on Vitamin D Supplementation for Older Adults advocate a minimum level of 30 ng/mL in older adults. In contrast to the IOM recommendations for the population at large, the AGS recommendations are intended to provide clinical guidance for the care of older, frail adults, many of whom have osteoporosis and are at risk of falls, injuries, and fractures.

Serum 25(OH)D levels <30 ng/mL are associated with impaired balance and lower extremity function, muscle weakness, decreased BMD, and increased fall rates, yet >75% of older adults in the United States have 25(OH)D concentrations below 30 ng/mL. A meta-analysis of 9 RCTs of vitamin D supplementation in community-dwelling older adults reported a 17% reduction in falls risk in studies with a median dose of 800 IU/d. Another meta-analysis of 8 RCTs found a 19% reduction in falls risk with vitamin D doses of 700–1,000 IU/d and a 23% reduction in falls with achieved 25(OH)D levels >24 ng/mL, but no significant reduction in falls risk with doses of ≤600 IU/d or achieved 25(OH)D levels <24 ng/mL. Of note, 4 RCTs within this meta-analysis with achieved 25(OH)D levels >24 ng/mL had lower fall rates than all RCTs with levels <24 ng/mL. Additionally, RCTs with the highest achieved 25(OH)D concentrations showed the greatest reduction in falls risk.

With regard to fracture risk, a meta-analysis of 12 double-blind RCTs for nonvertebral fractures and 8 RCTs for hip fractures comparing vitamin D with or without calcium supplementation versus calcium or placebo found a pooled RR of 0.86 (95% CI, 0.77–0.96) for prevention of nonvertebral fractures and 0.91 (95% CI, 0.78–1.05) for hip fracture prevention. The effect on fracture reduction was seen only at dosages >400 IU/d of vitamin D, which reduced nonvertebral fractures by 29% in community-dwelling older adults and 15% in institutionalized older adults. Furthermore, an 18% reduction in hip fracture risk was seen in patients receiving >400 IU/d of vitamin D (95% CI, 0.69–0.97). Antifracture efficacy increased significantly with greater achieved 25(OH)D levels. Based on the foregoing, the AGS Workgroup concluded that higher doses of vitamin D supplementation and achieved 25(OH)D concentrations ≥25 ng/mL confer greater protection against falls and fractures.

How much vitamin D should be prescribed for older adults? The IOM recommends dietary intakes of cholecalciferol (vitamin D_3) of 800 IU/d for men and women >70 years old. However, the AGS Workgroup strongly advised that older adults receive a dosage of vitamin D of at least 1,000 IU/d, along with calcium supplementation to reduce risk of falls and fractures (SOE=A). In establishing this recommendation, AGS noted the preponderance of benefits over harm with supplementation at this level in older adults. Maintaining adequate calcium intake (1,000–1,500 mg/d from the diet and supplements) is also important for bone health and prevention of secondary hyperparathyroidism. In this regard, it is important to consider daily dietary intake of calcium (primarily in dairy products), which in some individuals may be considerable, obviating the need to use calcium supplements. High-dose vitamin D supplementation may cause vitamin D intoxication with hypercalciuria (the initial manifestation of toxicity), hypercalcemia, impairment of kidney function, and bone loss, but dosages of 10,000 IU/d do not cause toxicity when taken for up to 5 months. The maximum tolerable intake for maintenance therapy in the general population is 4,000 IU/d. Vitamin D–deficient older adults (25(OH)D <20 ng/mL) should be treated with 50,000 IU/week of vitamin D_2^{OL} or vitamin D_3 for 8–12 weeks or an equivalent daily dose of 6,000 IU of vitamin D_2 or vitamin D_3 with the goal of achieving a blood level of 25(OH)D >30 ng/mL, followed by 1,000–1,500 IU/d (occasionally higher dosages) for maintenance therapy (SOE=A). Obese individuals (BMI >30 kg/m^2), people taking medications that accelerate vitamin D metabolism such as phenytoin and phenobarbital, and those with malabsorption syndromes who are vitamin D–deficient may require vitamin D dosages 2- to 3-fold higher, ie, at least 6,000–10,000 IU/d of vitamin D to achieve a 25(OH)D level >30 ng/mL, followed by maintenance therapy of 3,000–6,000 IU/d (SOE=A). Monitoring of 25(OH)D levels should be considered in these situations. A few patients who are unable to take daily oral supplements may benefit from oral vitamin D_3 at 100,000 IU every 6 months with minimal risk of hypercalcemia.

Hypercalcemia

Primary hyperparathyroidism and malignancy are the most common causes of hypercalcemia in older adults. The annual incidence of primary hyperparathyroidism is approximately 1 per 1,000, and the disease is 3-fold more prevalent in women than in men. Most patients with primary hyperparathyroidism are asymptomatic, and the diagnosis is made after an incidental finding of hypercalcemia. When the disease is symptomatic, older adults are more likely than younger adults to present with neuropsychiatric symptoms such as depression and cognitive impairment, neuromuscular symptoms such as proximal muscle weakness, hypertension, and osteoporosis. For typical laboratory findings in primary hyperparathyroidism and other common causes of hypercalcemia, see Table 63.3. The diagnosis of primary hyperparathyroidism is confirmed with an increased or high normal PTH concentration, by the use of an assay for intact PTH, in the presence of hypercalcemia. A low 24-hour urinary calcium excretion distinguishes familial hypocalciuric hypercalcemia from primary hyperparathyroidism. Familial hypocalciuric hypercalcemia is associated with longstanding mild hypercalcemia, does not respond to parathyroidectomy, and is generally not associated with complications. Normocalcemic primary hyperparathyroidism may be identified during the evaluation of older adults with reduced BMD. Causes of secondary hyperparathyroidism

Table 63.3—Typical Laboratory Results in the Differential Diagnosis of Hypercalcemia

Laboratory Test	Primary Hyperparathyroidism	Humoral Hypercalcemia of Malignancy	Local Osteolytic Hypercalcemia
Serum calcium	↑	↑ or ↑↑	↑ or ↑↑
Serum phosphate	↓ or low-normal	↓	↑
Urine calcium	↑	↑	↑
Parathyroid hormone	↑	↓↓	↓↓
Parathyroid hormone-related peptide	0	↑	0

NOTE: The diagnosis of malignancy-related hypercalcemia is normally straightforward, and extensive diagnostic testing is rarely required.
↑ = increased; ↑↑ = markedly increased; ↓ = decreased; ↓↓ = markedly decreased; 0 = undetectable

should be excluded in these patients, including renal failure, vitamin D deficiency, calcium malabsorption (eg, from celiac disease), and urinary calcium loss due to the use of loop diuretics.

Parathyroid surgery is the treatment of choice for symptomatic primary hyperparathyroidism and for asymptomatic patients with total serum calcium concentrations >1 mg/dL above the normal range; creatinine clearance <60 mL/min; markedly decreased BMD (T score below −2.5 at lumbar spine, hip, or distal 1/3 of radius on bone densitometry); vertebral fracture, nephrolithiasis or nephrocalcinosis on imaging; or 24-hour urine calcium >400 mg/d, together with increased stone risk by biochemical stone risk analysis. Many older adults with primary hyperparathyroidism who do not meet these criteria have subtle symptoms such as apathy, depression, fatigue, irritability, sleep disorders, and impaired cognition that may improve after successful parathyroidectomy, although it is not currently possible to predict which patients with cognitive and neuropsychiatric symptoms will improve after surgery. In RCTs evaluating parathyroidectomy and medical management in patients with mild, apparently asymptomatic disease (note: some neurocognitive manifestations may be subtle), BMD and other measures that may be relevant to quality of life improved after parathyroidectomy. Asymptomatic patients not meeting guidelines for surgery can safely be followed without surgery, at least for several years; many of these patients remain stable without deterioration of biochemical indices or BMD for up to 10 years. However, by 8–10 years, about 25% of these patients develop progressive disease, including worsening hypercalcemia, hypercalciuria, and reductions in BMD, and BMD eventually declines in most patients followed for 10–15 years. Parathyroidectomy can be performed safely in older adults, who may experience improvements in symptoms after the procedure comparable to those in younger adults, as well as improvements in function (SOE=B). However, it remains unclear whether the potential benefits of surgery outweigh the risks in frail older adults with asymptomatic or mildly symptomatic disease.

Some manifestations of primary hyperparathyroidism such as reduced BMD and fracture risk are exacerbated by vitamin D deficiency and improve with vitamin D repletion. However, increased hypercalcemia and hypercalciuria may occur during vitamin D repletion in patients with primary hyperparathyroidism, so vitamin D supplementation should be undertaken cautiously (eg, vitamin D_3 starting dose of 600–1,000 IU/d). The optimal dose for supplementation in this situation is unknown, although a recent meta-analysis of 10 small studies provided reassurance that vitamin D supplementation at doses well above this range are highly unlikely to exacerbate hypercalciuria or to cause hypercalcemia. Asymptomatic patients who are managed conservatively should avoid lithium carbonate, thiazide diuretics, volume depletion, and immobilization. Baseline assessment in these patients should include blood pressure; serum calcium, phosphate, and creatinine; creatinine clearance; and bone densitometry. Follow-up assessments should include serum calcium and creatinine every 12 months, and bone densitometry (at 3 sites) every 12–24 months (SOE=C). Moderate calcium (eg, 1,200 mg/d) and vitamin D supplementation (with a goal of 25(OH)D level ≥20–30 ng/mL) should be maintained. In addition, these patients should be followed clinically for development of nephrolithiasis, fractures caused by minimal trauma, and neuropsychiatric or neuromuscular symptoms.

Medical management options for primary hyperparathyroidism are appropriate when it is desirable to lower the serum calcium level, increase BMD, or both. Options for patients with low BMD include the bisphosphonate alendronate, which improves BMD in patients with primary hyperparathyroidism without consistently affecting calcium or PTH concentrations[OL] (SOE=A). However, it is unknown whether alendronate or other bisphosphonates reduce fracture risk in these patients. Cinacalcet, a calcimimetic agent that inhibits parathyroid cell function, reduces or normalizes serum calcium concentrations and reduces PTH concentrations during long-term treatment of primary hyperparathyroidism (SOE=A), but BMD is not increased. Accordingly, the role of cinacalcet is limited to management of symptomatic or severe hypercalcemia in patients who are unable to undergo parathyroid surgery. Limited data suggest that combined therapy with cinacalcet and a bisphosphonate may accomplish both calcium lowering and improvement in BMD in people who have both low BMD and severe hypercalcemia (SOE=B). Estrogen–progestin therapy increases BMD in postmenopausal women with primary hyperparathyroidism but without consistent effects on serum calcium or PTH levels. Estrogen-progestin therapy may be a useful option for women who are not surgical candidates, especially those with menopausal symptoms, but the benefits and risks must be considered in light of contraindications to this therapy (see estrogen replacement therapy, below).

In hospitalized patients, the most common cause of hypercalcemia is a malignancy that produces PTH-related peptide (PTHrp), often referred to as humoral hypercalcemia of malignancy, with hypercalcemia resulting primarily from increased net bone resorption. The presence of an underlying cancer is usually evident on examination and routine diagnostic testing. Squamous cell cancers of the lung or head and neck are common causes of hypercalcemia due to PTHrp production. Other common malignancies associated with hypercalcemia include breast cancer, lymphoma, and myeloma, although the mechanisms of the hypercalcemia associated with these malignancies are usually not PTHrp-mediated and may be responsive to glucocorticoid treatment. Acute treatment for hypercalcemia of malignancy includes volume replacement with intravenous saline. A parenteral bisphosphonate such as pamidronate or zoledronic acid should be given, along with treatment for the underlying malignancy, if possible. In addition to their usefulness in treatment of hypercalcemia, high-potency bisphosphonates such as zoledronic acid may decrease bone pain and the risk of pathologic fractures in patients with osteolytic bone metastases from a variety of cancers (SOE=A). Nephrotoxicity associated with these agents may be minimized by adhering to recommended dosages and infusion times. However, these agents should be used cautiously if at all in people with a creatinine clearance of ≤30 mL/min. Cancer patients receiving repetitive dosing of parenteral bisphosphonates who have had recent dental extractions, dental implants, poorly fitting dentures, or preexisting disease, or receiving high-dosage glucocorticoid treatment are at increased risk of osteonecrosis of the jaw. Denosumab is an approved alternative to bisphosphonates for treatment of hypercalcemia of malignancy refractory to bisphosphonates, and to prevent skeletal-related events (eg, fractures, pain from bone metastases) in people with bone metastases from solid tumors but not for patients with multiple myeloma.

Paget Disease of Bone

Paget disease is characterized by localized areas of increased bone remodeling, resulting in a change in bone architecture and an increased tendency to deformity and fracture. Its prevalence increases with aging, affecting 2%–5% of people ≥50 years old. Paget disease is usually asymptomatic and is often diagnosed as an incidental finding on radiographs or during evaluation for an unexplained increase in serum alkaline phosphatase. The most commonly affected sites are the pelvis, spine, femur, tibia, and skull. When Paget disease is symptomatic, pain is the most common presenting symptom, either localized to the affected bones or resulting from secondary osteoarthritic changes, often in the hips, knees, and vertebrae. When bone deformities occur, the long bones of the legs are usually affected, often with bowing. Skull involvement may result in sensorineural hearing loss, thought to be due to cochlear damage rather than to compression of the eighth cranial nerve. Paraplegia or quadriplegia occurs rarely as a result of spinal stenosis from vertebral involvement and vascular steal, and is often reversible with timely treatment. The most devastating complication of Paget disease is malignant transformation of the affected bone, especially development of osteosarcoma.

When Paget disease is suspected, plain radiographs should be obtained of areas of suspected involvement. After the diagnosis is made, a radionuclide bone scan may be useful to determine the extent of the disease, along with serum alkaline phosphatase (SAP) or bone-specific alkaline phosphatase (BAP) to determine the level of metabolic activity. It is not usually necessary to measure other markers of bone turnover such as serum osteocalcin or urinary N-telopeptide. The primary indication for treatment in asymptomatic patients is active disease in areas where complications may occur, including the skull, weight-bearing bones, and bone adjacent to major joints, which may increase the risk of secondary osteoarthritis (SOE=C). Bisphosphonates suppress the accelerated bone turnover and bone remodeling that is characteristic of Paget disease and are the treatment of choice for most patients with active disease who are at risk of complications (SOE=A). Increasing evidence indicates that a single dose of zoledronic acid 5 mg IV is superior to other bisphosphonates for patients without contraindications, eg, glomerular filtration rate <35 mL/min; it is more likely to achieve a complete and sustained response to therapy, including improved pain and quality of life than with other bisphosphonates (SOE=A). Osteoarthritis commonly occurs in weight-bearing joints such as the hip or knee, adjacent to Paget-affected bones. Bisphosphonates may help to prevent or slow the development of hearing loss and osteoarthritis in joints adjacent to Paget disease (SOE=C), although joint replacement may be necessary in some individuals to restore function and relieve joint pain. Pretreatment with an aminobisphosphonate may be advisable 1–4 months before elective total joint replacement to minimize the risks of intraoperative bleeding due to increased blood flow to Pagetic bone, and postoperative loosening of the prosthesis (SOE=B).

Calcium and vitamin D should be administered concomitantly with bisphosphonates to prevent hypocalcemia[OL]. NSAIDs may be useful in treating secondary osteoarthritis for short periods (eg, several weeks), although even short courses of treatment with NSAIDs exposes older adults to known risks, including increased risk of heart attack and stroke, GI bleeding, renal dysfunction, and other adverse effects. During treatment, patients should be monitored clinically for changes in bone pain, joint function, and neurologic status. SAP or BAP levels should be monitored to assess the initial and ongoing response to bisphosphonate therapy.

DISORDERS OF THE ANTERIOR PITUITARY

It is challenging to separate the effects of aging per se on pituitary hormone secretion from the effects of comorbid illnesses, medications, body composition, physical activity, and other confounding factors. Additionally, aging effects on pituitary hormone secretion may not be apparent in the basal state and may become evident only in response to stimulatory (or inhibitory) influences (Table 63.4).

As noted above, basal serum thyrotropin levels tend to increase with aging (Table 63.4). A decrease in thyrotropin-releasing hormone (TRH) stimulation of thyrotropin release with aging has been better documented in men than in women. TRH stimulation testing is of limited value in distinguishing between hypothalamic and pituitary causes of secondary (central) hypothyroidism; furthermore, TRH is unavailable at present in the United States. Patients with suspected secondary hypothyroidism require neuroimaging of the hypothalamus and pituitary as well as measurement of other pituitary hormones with special attention to exclude secondary adrenal insufficiency before T4 administration that could result in adrenal crisis.

Hypothalamic-pituitary-adrenal (HPA) axis function is relatively intact with aging. Basal adrenocorticotropic hormone (ACTH) levels are unchanged with aging, whereas the effects of aging on the ACTH response to stress vary depending on the type of stress. Increases in cortisol and ACTH levels in response to metyrapone, ovine corticotropin-releasing hormone (CRH), and insulin-induced hypoglycemia are normal or slightly prolonged with aging. Inhibition of ACTH secretion by cortisol is unchanged with aging, indicating that feedback sensitivity to cortisol is unchanged. However, in healthy older women, ACTH escape after suppression by cortisol, and recovery of cortisol levels, are attenuated compared with those in older men (Table 63.4). The dose-dependent suppression of corticotropin-releasing hormone–induced ACTH release by dexamethasone is blunted with aging.

Growth hormone (GH) secretion is decreased during sleep, as well as in response to fasting, exercise, and most secretagogues. However, GH secretion in response to insulin-induced hyperglycemia is unchanged with aging (Table 63.4). Age-related changes in circulating gonadotropin levels in men are described below (see testosterone).

Hyperprolactinemia and Pituitary Adenomas

Prolactin secretion decreases with aging in healthy men and postmenopausal women, with decreases in both basal prolactin secretion and the amplitude of pulsatile prolactin release from the pituitary (Table 63.4). The nocturnal rise in pulsatile prolactin secretion is blunted with aging. Some older adults develop mild hyperprolactinemia due to causes such as renal failure, primary hypothyroidism, hypothalamic diseases that interfere with synthesis of dopamine (prolactin-inhibitory factor), and medications that inhibit dopamine activity (eg, antipsychotics, opioids, and metoclopramide). The clinical manifestations of hyperprolactinemia often go unrecognized in older adults and are usually subtle, including sexual dysfunction, gynecomastia, and rarely galactorrhea. Hyperprolactinemia should be considered in evaluation of secondary causes of osteoporosis in older men, because the antigonadotropic actions of prolactin may cause hypogonadism and accelerated bone loss.

When hyperprolactinemia is detected in asymptomatic patients, macroprolactinemia due to less bioactive dimeric and polymeric forms of prolactin should be excluded to avoid further unnecessary evaluation and management in these patients. In patients with true hyperprolactinemia, imaging of the hypothalamus and pituitary (eg, with MRI) may be indicated to exclude a tumor or other lesion (eg, when prolactin level is >150–200 ng/mL). Treatment of underlying secondary causes of hyperprolactinemia or discontinuation of medications such as antipsychotics often result in normalization of hyperprolactinemia. Hyperprolactinemia due to a pituitary microadenoma (defined as <10 mm in size) may be managed with observation if the patients is asymptomatic, or with a dopamine agonist if secondary osteoporosis or symptoms such as sexual dysfunction are present. Dopamine agonists are first-line treatment for hyperprolactinemia from any cause and are effective in reducing

Table 63.4—Alterations in Anterior Pituitary Function and Circulating Target Organ Hormone Levels with Aging

Endocrine Parameter	Effect of Aging
Hypothalamic-Pituitary-Thyroid Axis	
Thyroxine (T_4)	Unchanged
Triiodothyronine (T_3)	Decreased, especially if systemic illness or debilitation
Thyrotropin	Unchanged; increased in women
Suppression of thyrotropin by T_4	Increased (ie, smaller T_4 dose required to suppress thyrotropin)
Hypothalamic-Pituitary-Adrenal Axis	
Cortisol	Unchanged
Adrenocorticotropic hormone (ACTH)	Unchanged
Diurnal rhythm of cortisol and ACTH	Decreased (reduced amplitude and phase advance of cortisol variation)
ACTH stimulation of cortisol	Unchanged
Feedback suppression of ACTH by cortisol	Unchanged
Stimulation of ACTH and cortisol by insulin-induced hypoglycemia, corticotropin-releasing hormone (CRH), metyrapone	Unchanged; increased (CRH)
Recovery of ACTH and cortisol after stress	Decreased (peak cortisol levels higher, remain increased longer)
Growth Hormone (GH) Axis	
Insulin-like growth factor 1 (IGF-1)	Decreased
GH secretion during sleep	Decreased
GH secretion with fasting and exercise	Decreased
Amplitude of pulsatile GH secretion	Decreased
Frequency of pulsatile GH secretion	Unchanged
GH response to insulin-induced hypoglycemia	Unchanged
GH response to GH-releasing hormone	Decreased
Hypothalamic-Pituitary-Testicular Axis	
Total testosterone	Decreased
Free and bioavailable testosterone	Markedly decreased
Sex hormone binding globulin	Increased (usually within normal range until advanced age)
Luteinizing hormone (LH)	Unchanged/increased (usually within normal range until advanced age)
Follicle-stimulating hormone (FSH)	Unchanged/increased (may remain within normal range until advanced age)
Frequency of pulsatile LH secretion	Decreased
LH response to gonadotropin-releasing hormone (GnRH)	Unchanged
Prolactin	
Prolactin	Decreased
Nocturnal prolactin secretion	Decreased
Amplitude of pulsatile prolactin secretion	Decreased

prolactin concentrations. Older adults are at risk of adverse effects of these agents, including hallucinations and GI symptoms, so dopamine agonists should be started at low doses and the dose increased slowly. Cabergoline is the preferred dopamine agonist for its efficacy in lowering prolactin levels and reducing the size of pituitary macroadenomas (ie, ≥10 mm), and its lower likelihood of causing adverse effects. The increased risk of valvular heart disease seen with high doses of cabergoline used in Parkinson disease does not appear to occur at the lower doses typically used to treat hyperprolactinemia. Dosing of dopamine agonists should be titrated to normalize prolactin levels, with MRI repeated in 1 year or sooner if hyperprolactinemia or symptoms worsen despite treatment. Serial visual field testing is indicated for patients with macroadenomas near the optic chiasm. Trans-sphenoidal surgery or radiation therapy is occasionally necessary in patients with macroprolactinomas and persistent visual field defects or who cannot tolerate dopamine agonists.

The incidence of pituitary adenomas increases with aging, but most of these tumors remain asymptomatic, even in those of advanced age. Most pituitary adenomas are nonfunctioning adenomas, with smaller numbers of prolactinomas and GH-secreting tumors. Nonsecreting and gonadotropin- or α-subunit-secreting adenomas are typically large at the time of diagnosis because of the absence of symptoms associated with hormone excess. Symptoms in these patients are generally due to mass effect, eg, headache, visual field abnormalities due to pressure on the optic chiasm, and panhypopituitarism.

Increasingly, pituitary "incidentalomas" are being found on imaging studies to evaluate comorbid illnesses in older adults. When pituitary incidentalomas are identified, careful clinical evaluation and measurement of pituitary and end-organ hormones should be performed to exclude hypopituitarism and hormone hypersecretion, along with a visual field examination when the tumor is adjacent to the optic chiasm or optic nerves. Pituitary microadenomas may be managed expectantly. Patients with macroadenomas other than prolactinomas should be referred for trans-sphenoidal surgery if there are visual field abnormalities due to compression of optic chiasm or optic nerves; if there is hypersecretion of thyrotropin, ACTH, or GH; or if other neurologic symptoms are present. Hypopituitarism (if present) may persist after pituitary adenomas are surgically removed, so hypopituitarism by itself is not an indication for surgery. The risks of transsphenoidal surgery have been reported to increase with advancing age, but postoperative hypopituitarism and other complications are less likely and outcomes are similar to those in younger adults when these surgeries are performed at specialized centers by surgeons with extensive experience in these procedures.

Hypopituitarism and the Empty Sella Syndrome

Hypopituitarism has been reported to develop in 1/3 to 1/2 of older adults with diagnosed pituitary tumors. Other causes of hypopituitarism in older adults include traumatic brain injury (TBI), infections such as tuberculosis, metastatic cancer, prior irradiation or surgery for pituitary tumors, and vascular disorders such as pituitary infarction or carotid artery aneurysms. Manifestations of *panhypopituitarism* include fatigue, hypogonadism and loss of libido, hypotension, weight loss, hypoglycemia, and hyponatremia. When the diagnosis is suspected, concurrent measurement of pituitary and target organ hormone levels is indicated to determine whether hormonal axis responses are appropriate. Dynamic testing of the HPA axis with ACTH stimulation testing is also indicated to evaluate for secondary adrenal insufficiency. However, the standard dose (250 mcg) ACTH stimulation test may be misleading when acute or recent onset of hypopituitarism is present, because the adrenal glands may still be able to mount a normal response to ACTH challenge. Instead, the low dose (1 mcg) ACTH test or metyrapone test should be considered when acute or recent onset hypopituitarism is a possibility.

After a fall with head injury in an older adult, acute hypopituitarism is common even in those with mild TBI. In the acute phase of TBI (first 7–10 days) potentially life-threatening glucocorticoid sufficiency may develop, and serial morning cortisol measurements should be obtained especially when signs such as hypotension, hypoglycemia, and hyponatremia are present. Acute diabetes insipidus may also occur. Evaluation of GH, thyroid, and gonadal axis function is unnecessary in the acute phase. After the acute phase of TBI, some hormonal deficiencies that were manifest initially may resolve and others may develop. Although the natural history of hypopituitarism after TBI is not well described, it is appropriate to monitor for signs and symptoms and obtain hormone measurements 3–6 months after TBI, again at 1 year, and annually thereafter, and to reevaluate hormonal status whenever concerning symptoms develop.

Cases of empty sella syndrome are increasingly being detected as neuroimaging procedures performed for another indication have increased. Pituitary height and volume tend to diminish with aging in healthy adults, and empty sella has been observed in 19% of older subjects. Most cases of *primary empty sella syndrome* (ie, not associated with pituitary tumors or their treatment) occur in obese middle-aged women with hypertension. In contrast to men, most women with this condition do not have significant pituitary hormone hypofunction. It is unknown whether an incidental finding of empty sella in otherwise healthy older adults has any functional significance. Therefore, conservative management is appropriate in these cases, with visual field testing and pituitary and target organ hormone measurements to detect abnormalities in pituitary hormones.

DISORDERS OF THE ADRENAL CORTEX

Basal serum cortisol concentrations do not change with aging, because decreased cortisol secretion is balanced by a decrease in clearance, although cortisol levels vary considerably with aging from person to person. Stimulation of cortisol production by adrenocorticotropic hormone (ACTH) is unchanged, and cortisol and ACTH responses to stress and secretagogues are unimpaired with aging. Clinically, acute cortisol responses to stress may be higher and more prolonged in older than in younger adults, possibly due to reduced clearance of cortisol in older adults. Accordingly, in nonemergent situations, adrenal function testing should be deferred at least 48 hours after major stressors, such as surgery or trauma. In older adults with a normal ACTH stimulation test in whom adrenal insufficiency is suspected, endocrinology consultation is recommended to assist with further testing.

Hypoadrenocorticoidism

Chronic glucocorticoid therapy is the most common cause of adrenal failure in older adults because of chronic suppression of adrenal function. Recovery of

Table 63.5—Diagnostic Evaluation of Hormone Hypersecretion in Patients with Adrenal Incidentalomas

Indications	Test and Result Supporting Diagnosis	Diagnosis
Cushing syndrome manifestations, before major surgery	1 mg overnight dexamethasone suppression test showing failure to suppress cortisol 24-hour urine free cortisol ↑	Functional adrenocortical adenoma
All patients with incidentaloma	24-hour urine for fractionated metanephrines ↑ or plasma free metanephrines ↑	Pheochromocytoma
Before major surgery	Plasma free metanephrines ↑	Pheochromocytoma
Hypertension with or without hypokalemia	Ratio of morning plasma aldosterone concentration to plasma renin activity ↑	Primary aldosteronism

adrenal axis function is variable and may take several months to a year. Autoimmune-mediated adrenal failure is less common in older than in younger adults, but tuberculosis, adrenal metastases, and adrenal hemorrhage in anticoagulated patients are more common causes of adrenal insufficiency in older adults. Additionally, prolonged use of megestrol acetate (eg, as an appetite stimulant) may cause ACTH suppression and hypoadrenocorticoidism.

Older adults with chronic adrenal insufficiency may present with nonspecific symptoms such as anorexia, nausea, weight loss, abdominal pain, weakness, hypotension, or impaired functional status, and hyponatremia and hyperkalemia may not always be present. Accordingly, a high index of suspicion is required to make the diagnosis. Chronic adrenal insufficiency should be considered in patients with unexplained cachexia, mobility impairment, and hypotension. When adrenocortical insufficiency is suspected, the ACTH stimulation test should be performed (SOE=A) and therapy initiated (SOE=D). A normal serum cortisol (basal or 30–60 minutes after administration of 250 mcg of ACTH [cosyntropin]) is 18–20 mcg/dL. A serum ACTH concentration should be obtained before administration of cosyntropin to distinguish secondary adrenal insufficiency (decreased pituitary ACTH secretion), which is characterized by a low or normal ACTH concentration, from primary adrenal insufficiency, which is associated with a high ACTH concentration. Patients with recent onset ACTH deficiency (eg, within 4 weeks of pituitary surgery) may still be capable of mounting a response to ACTH stimulation. The low-dose (1 mcg) ACTH stimulation test with cortisol measurement 30 minutes after ACTH may be superior to standard dose ACTH testing to diagnose mild or recent onset secondary adrenal insufficiency and mild primary adrenal insufficiency (eg, from chronic use of inhaled glucocorticoids), although this remains controversial. In older adults who are stopping chronic glucocorticoid therapy, the replacement regimen should be tapered gradually (SOE=D), and stress dose coverage given for major surgery and other acute physiologic stresses until adrenocortical function has returned to normal (SOE=D). Recovery of the hypothalamic-pituitary-adrenal axis may take >9 months.

Hyperadrenocorticoidism

Exogenous glucocorticoids are the most common cause of hyperadrenocorticism in older adults, often causing adverse events, including psychiatric and cognitive symptoms, osteoporosis, myopathy, and glucose intolerance. Notably, the use of 10 mg/d of prednisone continuously for >90 days is associated with a 7-fold increase in hip fractures and a 17-fold increased risk of vertebral fractures. For patients beginning long-term glucocorticoid therapy, baseline and follow-up bone densitometry measurements are indicated, and calcium, vitamin D, and antiresorptive treatments such as bisphosphonates should be started as appropriate in patients at high risk of fractures for prevention or treatment of glucocorticoid-induced osteoporosis (or teriparatide in cases of severe bone loss). Hormone replacement therapy may also be appropriate in some cases to counteract corticosteroid-induced suppression of sex hormones. Management of subclinical glucocorticoid hypersecretion is discussed below.

Adrenal Neoplasms

In autopsy studies, the prevalence of clinically inapparent adrenal masses (adrenal incidentalomas) ranges from <1% in people <30 years old to ≥10% in older adults. Most adrenal incidentalomas are benign adrenocortical adenomas, although pheochromocytomas and adrenocortical carcinomas are also found. It is important to exclude pheochromocytoma, because it is not uncommon and potentially life threatening.

The goals of assessment are to determine whether the tumor is functional (hormone-secreting) (Table 63.5) and whether it is benign or malignant. Many adrenocortical adenomas have a degree of functional autonomy, and subclinical glucocorticoid hypersecretion is present in 5%–24% of cases of adrenal incidentalomas. Some of these patients are at increased risk of new vertebral fractures, hypertension, insulin resistance, and other metabolic derangements. An overnight low dose dexamethasone suppression test together with measurement of a morning serum ACTH level are appropriate tests to exclude subclinical Cushing syndrome. However, it is unclear whether subclinical glucocorticoid hypersecretion is associated with long-term morbidity in older adults, or whether the long-term outcomes of adrenalectomy are superior to medical management of metabolic derangements. Moreover, screening all older adults with adrenal incidentalomas for glucocorticoid hypersecretion would yield a high proportion of false-positive results. Accordingly, it may be best to limit testing for hyperadrenocorticoidism to younger individuals, those with a symptom complex suggesting hyperadrenocorticoidism, and patients scheduled for major surgery (eg, thoracic and intra-abdominal procedures under general anesthesia) who are at risk of postoperative adrenal crisis due to diminished HPA axis reserve from chronic glucocorticoid excess (SOE=D).

The most useful initial tool in assessment of malignancy risk in patients with adrenal incidentaloma is the attenuation coefficient in Hounsfield units (HU) on non-contrast CT imaging. Lesions with attenuation values of ≤10 HU are likely to represent benign adenomas. For adrenal masses with values >10 HU, size <4 cm identifies masses likely to be benign adenomas. Surgical resection may be appropriate for masses ≥4 cm, especially for lesions >6 cm and masses with other imaging characteristics suggesting malignancy, including irregular shape, unilaterality, tumor calcification, and rapid growth rate (SOE=B). However, the patient's treatment preferences and clinical condition must be considered before recommending treatment. In patients followed expectantly for masses >2 cm without clearly benign features, imaging should be repeated in 3–6 months to identify rapidly growing tumors that are more likely to be malignant (SOE=B).

Adrenal Androgens

Adrenal production of dehydroepiandrosterone (DHEA) and its sulfate (DHEA-S) is the main source of androgens in women, whereas in men the adrenals contribute very little to overall androgen production. DHEA and DHEA-S are often thought of as adrenal androgens, but they are actually prohormones that are converted to more active androgens (and estrogens) in the adrenal glands and peripheral tissues. In contrast to the changes seen in cortisol concentrations with aging, circulating concentrations of DHEA decline progressively with aging, and in octogenarians are only 10%–20% of concentrations in young adults. Low DHEA concentrations are associated with poor health, whereas DHEA concentrations are positively correlated with some measures of longevity and functional status.

Given these associations, there has been interest in the potential therapeutic "anti-aging" effects of DHEA administration in older adults. However, enthusiasm for DHEA as an anti-aging intervention has waned as RCTs of DHEA supplementation for up to 2 years have not found clear evidence of clinically meaningful benefits on body composition, lipids or carbohydrate metabolism, cognition, strength, physical function, or quality of life in middle-aged and older adults. In one RCT in frail older women, exercise together with DHEA supplementation improved some measures of lower extremity strength and function, but the clinical significance of this finding is unknown. BMD improved with DHEA supplementation in older adults with low DHEA levels in some but not all studies. However, the incremental increase in bone density with DHEA is small by comparison to standard therapy for osteoporosis, and there are no data indicating whether fracture risk improves with DHEA.

Potential risks of DHEA treatment include decreased circulating high-density lipoprotein cholesterol levels in older women, raising the possibility of potential long-term atherogenic effects. Furthermore, DHEA is metabolized to estrogens and to androgens such as testosterone and dihydrotestosterone, and its effects on the risk of breast cancer in women and prostate cancer in men are unknown. Finally, higher dosages of DHEA can cause androgenization in some women and gynecomastia in men. Thus, the safety and efficacy of DHEA supplementation in older adults have not been established, and its use is inappropriate other than in clinical studies.

Women with adrenal insufficiency or who are surgically menopausal develop severe androgen deficiency and may present with symptoms of decreased libido, energy, and well-being despite optimal glucocorticoid and (in primary adrenal insufficiency) mineralocorticoid replacement. A recent guideline advised against routine supplementation with DHEA in women with adrenal insufficiency, citing inadequate efficacy and safety data. However, a meta-analysis of RCTs of DHEA supplementation reported modest improvements in mood and health-related quality of life in women with adrenal insufficiency. Some experts suggest offering DHEA therapy[OL] only to women with adrenal insufficiency who have marked impairments in mood and subjective well-being that persist after glucocorticoid and (if necessary) mineralocorticoid replacement, while monitoring for occurrence of androgenic adverse effects, including hirsutism and acne (SOE=B). A role for DHEA supplementation has not been established for men with adrenal insufficiency.

DHEA is not approved for use in the United States for any indication, and it is available over-the-counter only as a dietary supplement. The potency and purity of these preparations is unreliable, and the long-term safety of DHEA supplementation has not been established. Accordingly, DHEA is not recommended for use in older adults with normal adrenal function.

TESTOSTERONE

Total and free testosterone levels and testosterone secretion are lower in healthy older men than in younger men. Many healthy older men exhibit moderate primary testicular failure, with decreased sperm production, testosterone levels, and testosterone secretory responses to gonadotropin administration. In addition, many of these men also have inappropriately normal (ie, not increased) gonadotropin levels in the presence of low testosterone levels, suggesting secondary (hypothalamic or pituitary) testicular failure. Overt testicular failure is common in chronically ill and debilitated older men or in men receiving chronic glucocorticoids or opioids, manifested by testosterone levels well below the normal range and symptoms suggesting androgen deficiency, including decreased libido and impotence, gynecomastia, and hot flushes. Testosterone replacement therapy is generally warranted in these severely clinically and biochemically androgen-deficient patients, as it would be in hypogonadal young men. However, it is more common to encounter older men with low-normal or mildly decreased serum testosterone levels and nonspecific manifestations, such as decreased libido and potency, reduced energy, depressed mood, weakness, decreased muscle mass, osteopenia, metabolic syndrome, and memory loss. In most cases, these manifestations have multiple causes, but it has been hypothesized that declining testosterone levels with aging contribute to their development and that testosterone supplementation can help to prevent or treat these disorders. At present, it remains uncertain whether declining testosterone levels in older men are simply a biomarker of poor health or whether they represent a deficiency state in need of treatment.

In the European Male Aging Study, symptoms of poor morning erections, diminished sexual desire, and erectile dysfunction were found to correlate with low testosterone levels in middle-aged and older men. Men with these findings had lower BMD, hemoglobin, and muscle mass, and poorer physical performance, than men without sexual symptoms who had higher testosterone levels. These results suggest there may be an identifiable low testosterone syndrome associated with male aging, but only a small percentage of men >70 years old meet these criteria. In the United States, the use of testosterone supplementation by older men has increased nearly 10-fold in the past 15 years, driven at least in part by direct-to-consumer advertising campaigns and the availability of testosterone gel and transdermal patch formulations. Many men who are started on testosterone supplementation have not had recent measurement of serum testosterone concentrations, indicating that inappropriate prescribing is very common.

Age-related male hypogonadism should be diagnosed only in men with signs and symptoms suggesting androgen deficiency, as well as unequivocally low serum testosterone levels. Men with suspected hypogonadism should be evaluated initially with a morning serum total testosterone level using a reliable assay. The diagnosis should be confirmed by repeating measurement of morning total testosterone, or preferably, if available, a morning serum free or bioavailable (non–sex hormone–binding globulin-bound) testosterone level either measured by equilibrium dialysis or calculated from measurements of total testosterone and sex hormone–binding globulin (SHBG) (SOE=C). Concentrations of SHBG, the main circulating binding protein for testosterone, increase with age. Therefore, the age-related decline in serum free or bioavailable testosterone is greater than that of total testosterone, and total testosterone measurements do not accurately reflect the decrease in biologically active testosterone with aging. Furthermore, common conditions such as moderate obesity, low-protein states (eg, nephritic or nephrotic syndrome), hypothyroidism, and use of glucocorticoids lower SHBG concentrations and, therefore, may result in low total testosterone but normal free testosterone levels. Direct "analogue" immunoassays for free testosterone are widely used but not recommended, because they are affected by changes in SHBG and can thus be inaccurate, overestimating androgen deficiency in men with low SHBG concentrations (eg, moderately obese men) and underestimating androgen deficiency in older men with higher SHBG concentrations. Because of the extreme variability in the accuracy of testosterone assays, a consensus statement with an implementation timeline recommended testosterone assay standardization, patient and provider education, and other interventions to improve the accuracy of testosterone testing, and an accuracy-based quality control program has been instituted by the CDC and by the American College of Pathologists.

If abnormally low testosterone levels are confirmed, concentrations of luteinizing hormone and follicle-stimulating hormone should be obtained to determine whether low testosterone is due to a primary disorder of the testes (primary hypogonadism) or is secondary to a hypothalamic-pituitary disorder (secondary hypogonadism). In addition, a review (and if possible, discontinuation) of medications that can suppress gonadotropins (eg, glucocorticoids, opioids, and other medications with CNS activity) and a prolactin concentration are indicated if gonadotropins are low-normal or low in the presence of low testosterone levels. High prolactin concentrations inhibit gonadotropin secretion and could be due to a pituitary adenoma, a hypothalamic disorder, or medications. Further studies may be warranted in such patients, including measurement of iron saturation, MRI of the pituitary fossa, and assessment of other pituitary functions (eg,

Table 63.6—Potential Short-Term Benefits and Risks of Testosterone Supplementation in Older Men with Low-Normal or Mildly Decreased Testosterone Concentrations

Study End Point	Effect of Testosterone
Lean body mass	Increased
Fat mass	Decreased
Bone mineral density	Variable; increased at lumbar spine and hip in some studies
Strength	Improved grip strength in some studies; inconsistent effect on leg muscle strength
Physical function	Inconsistent effects; improved performance of functional tasks in some studies; improvement more likely in older, more frail men in one study
Sexual function	Variable; most consistent findings are activation in sexual behavior and increased libido
Mood	Variable; mood and subjective well-being improved in some studies; inconsistent effects on depression, although some studies showed improvement on Hamilton Depression Rating Scale
Cognitive	Inconsistent effects; in some studies, some cognitive domains improved (eg, verbal memory, visual memory, spatial ability, executive function); worsened effect of practice on verbal fluency
Quality of life	Inconsistent effects; some studies show significant improvement of physical function domain and improvement in subjects with more somatic symptoms at baseline
Lipid profile	Variable; total, low-density lipoprotein cholesterol and high-density lipoprotein cholesterol unchanged or decreased
Coronary heart disease	May increase risk of cardiovascular events in older men with extensive history of cardiovascular disease and immobility
Prostate	Prostate-specific antigen (PSA) increased slightly in many men; significantly higher incidence of prostate-related event (increased PSA, prostate cancer, prostate biopsy) in testosterone-treated men than in placebo-treated men, possibly due to ascertainment bias
Hematocrit	Increased 2.5%–5% versus baseline
Long-term clinical outcomes	Unknown

NOTE: This table summarizes results of placebo-controlled studies.

cortisol response to ACTH and free T_4), and referral to an endocrinologist is recommended. Baseline bone densitometry measurements should be obtained in older men with decreased testosterone levels to exclude osteoporosis.

Testosterone supplementation should be considered only after potentially reversible functional causes of hypogonadism are optimized, including discontinuation of medications that may cause clinical manifestations of hypogonadism. The potential short-term benefits and risks of testosterone supplementation in older men with low-normal or mildly decreased serum testosterone levels in RCTs of up to 3 years' duration are summarized in Table 63.6. However, it is unknown whether these potential benefits and risks are clinically important or whether longer-term potential benefits outweigh risks. A meta-analysis of trials of testosterone supplementation reported an increased risk of cardiovascular events in participants receiving testosterone, although a second meta-analysis that included many of the same trials did not find increased cardiovascular risk. Based on these uncertainties, until adequately powered, long-term trial results are available, the U.S. FDA cautioned that testosterone replacement therapy may be associated with increased cardiovascular risk. Accordingly, caution is suggested when using testosterone treatment in frail older men with established cardiovascular disease or cardiovascular risk factors.

After explicit discussion of the uncertain risks and benefits of testosterone therapy, including potential increased cardiovascular risk, a trial of testosterone supplementation may be appropriate in older men with unequivocally low serum total testosterone levels (eg, <2.8 ng/mL or more conservatively, <2 ng/mL) and/or decreased free or bioavailable testosterone levels, and clinical features suggesting hypogonadism (eg, osteoporosis, muscle wasting or weakness, mild anemia of unclear cause, loss of libido)[OL] (SOE=C). Clinicians should aim to achieve total testosterone levels in the lower part of the normal range for young men (eg, 400–500 ng/dL). Androgen replacement therapy is inappropriate in asymptomatic older men with low-normal total or free testosterone levels who do not have clinical manifestations consistent with androgen deficiency. Notably, bisphosphonates are clearly efficacious in treating older men with low testosterone and osteoporosis, so testosterone therapy is not appropriate in older men without manifestations of hypogonadism other than osteoporosis. Furthermore, testosterone administration is contraindicated in patients with prostate cancer and breast cancer, and should be avoided in men with an undiagnosed prostate

Table 63.7—Testosterone Preparations Available in the United States for Hypogonadal Older Men

Preparation	Initial Treatment Dosage
Testosterone enanthate or cypionate	75 mg IM every week, or 150 mg IM every 2 weeks
Testosterone undecanoate	750 mg IM initially, followed by 750 mg IM 4 weeks later, then 750 mg every 10 weeks thereafter
Nonscrotal transdermal patch	2 or 4 mg transdermal every night
Gel	1% gel: 25–100 mg transdermal every day 1.62% gel: 20.25–81 mg every day 2% gel: 10–70 mg every day
Solution	30–120 mg applied to axilla once daily
Intranasal gel	5.5 mg (1 actuation) each nostril 3 times daily
Buccal tablet	30 mg applied to buccal mucosa every 12 hours
Testosterone pellets	150–450 mg SC every 3–6 months

nodule or induration on digital rectal examination, consistently increased prostate-specific antigen (PSA), erythrocytosis, severe lower urinary tract symptoms due to benign prostatic hyperplasia, or uncontrolled severe heart failure (SOE=C). For available preparations of testosterone, see Table 63.7.

Men should be monitored closely for efficacy as well as for adverse events of testosterone treatment, including new or worsening snoring, observed apnea during sleep, or excessive daytime sleepiness that may suggest obstructive sleep apnea syndrome. Routine monitoring for efficacy and potential adverse effects should be performed before initiation of therapy, 3–6 months after initiation, and then annually thereafter (SOE=C). Monitoring should include measurement of serum hematocrit (to check for erythrocytosis), and inquiry about lower urinary tract symptoms and gynecomastia (tender breast enlargement). Serum PSA and digital rectal examination should be performed before and 3–6 months after starting testosterone (to detect the presence of prostate cancer at baseline or shortly after starting testosterone therapy) and then yearly in older men at high risk of prostate cancer. Serum testosterone levels should also be monitored to assess the adequacy of delivery, especially in men receiving transdermal testosterone formulations (patch or gel). An increase in the PSA concentration to >4 ng/mL or an increase of >1.4 ng/mL over baseline within any 12-month period after starting testosterone therapy can indicate the presence of previously undetected prostate cancer, and testosterone should be discontinued until the prostate has been fully evaluated (SOE=C). However, there is no direct evidence that testosterone therapy increases risk of prostate cancer or symptomatic benign prostatic hyperplasia.

Testosterone Therapy in Older Women

Many experts believe it is inappropriate to diagnose androgen deficiency in healthy older women because of the lack of a clearly defined clinical syndrome, data regarding the long-term safety of testosterone therapy, age-based normative data for serum testosterone concentrations, and correlation between serum androgen levels and sexual function or symptoms in women, among other concerns. These concerns notwithstanding, androgen treatment for menopausal and postmenopausal women with diminished libido has become widespread. Several RCTs of testosterone therapy for female sexual interest/arousal disorder in postmenopausal women or women with pituitary or ovarian failure found that testosterone supplementation into the normal range for young adult women improved libido and several measures of sexual function. Accordingly, a 3- to 6-month trial of testosterone treatment may be warranted in selected postmenopausal women with female sexual interest/arousal disorder (hypoactive sexual desire disorder) in whom nonpharmacologic management is unsuccessful and who have no contraindications to testosterone[OL] (SOE=A). However, testosterone preparations suitable for use in women are unavailable in some countries, including the United States. It is inappropriate to treat women with testosterone preparations designed for use in men, because this may result in markedly supraphysiological testosterone levels and androgenization. A recent guideline advised against use of testosterone for sexual dysfunction other than female sexual interest/arousal disorder, or to optimize metabolic, cognitive, bone, or cardiovascular health. The long-term risks of testosterone treatment, eg, on breast and endometrial cancer, are unknown and, therefore, long-term treatment is not advisable.

ESTROGEN THERAPY

Many of the symptoms and signs of hormone deficiency mimic physiologic changes associated with aging. The fact that many hormones also decline with aging has led to an enthusiasm for attempting to reverse unwanted changes associated with aging by use of hormonal replacement. Based on very compelling epidemiologic data, replacement of estrogen, with or without progesterone, was once the standard of care for postmenopausal women, but is no longer because of more recent data from randomized clinical trials demonstrating significant adverse events from such therapy. Estrogen therapy is now largely limited to treatment of menopausal symptoms.

Early observational work suggested a reduction in heart disease with estrogen. Long-term prospective studies did not confirm these findings. The most recent review of the use of estrogen for primary or secondary prevention of cardiovascular disease, outlined in a Cochrane review, adding 6 new trials since the publication of the large, randomized trial, to 19 other well-designed trials, evaluating approximately 40,000 postmenopausal women demonstrated no protective effect for all-cause mortality, cardiovascular death, nonfatal myocardial infarction, angina, or revascularization. As has been seen before, the risk of stroke was increased (RR 1.24, 95% CI 1.10–1.41) (SOE=A). The analysis also confirmed increased risk of venous thrombosis and pulmonary emboli. Similar to the post-hoc analysis of the Women's Health Initiative (WHI) trial, the risk of cardiovascular events was increased in older women and with increased years since menopause. There was suggestion of decreased risk in postmenopausal women starting therapy <10 years after menopause (RR 0.70, 95% CI 0.52–0.95) (SOE=B), although there were still increased risk of venous thrombosis and not enough evidence to make clear statements about risk of stroke.

Although observational studies also suggested that estrogen may have a role in preventing dementia, a placebo-controlled trial of estrogen replacement given for 1 year to 120 women with early to moderate Alzheimer dementia found no improvement in affective or cognitive outcomes. In the WHI, in a study to assess primary prevention, women in the estrogen arm had clinically important declines in their Mini–Mental State Examination scores or transition to mild cognitive impairment or dementia. There was question of whether these findings were due to timing of estrogen therapy after menopause (WHI began therapy at age 65 years). In two studies in which estrogen was administered much closer to the start of menopause, no improvement or decline in cognitive function was found.

The risks of breast cancer, endometrial cancer, and deep-vein thrombosis/pulmonary emboli associated with use of estrogen have been well established; these results were confirmed in the WHI trial. A recent study to assess change in risk approximately 3 years after the conclusion of the WHI trial demonstrated continued increased risk with previous estrogen use because of fatal and nonfatal malignancies. The risk of breast cancer was similar to that in the nontreatment arm at the 3-year follow-up, and the previously demonstrated beneficial effects on colon cancer had dissipated, but risk of lung cancer was higher than in the nontreatment arm. Overall mortality was similar in the estrogen and placebo groups. In further follow-up, most risk and benefits of the WHI intervention dissipated after intervention (on average, 13 years of follow-up), but the increase in breast cancer risk persisted (HR 1.28, 95% CI 1.11–1.48). There were some mixed results, suggesting that those who used estrogen earlier after menopause had some potential benefits in all-cause mortality and global index (composite of adverse effects) compared with women >70 years old.

GROWTH HORMONE

Growth hormone (GH) secretion declines with aging, and by 70–80 years of age, about half of adults have no significant GH secretion over 24 hours. A corresponding decline occurs in concentrations of insulin-like growth factor 1, which mediates most of the effects of GH; in 40% of adults 70–80 years old, it falls to concentrations comparable to those in GH–deficient children.

Adults with GH deficiency due to hypothalamic-pituitary disease exhibit decreased muscle strength, lean body mass, and bone density; increased fracture risk and abdominal obesity; unfavorable lipid profiles; and an increased risk of cardiovascular disease. Many of these clinical consequences of GH deficiency improved with GH replacement in small trials of up to 15 years' duration. Insulin resistance tends to increase with GH treatment, and the prevalence of metabolic syndrome has been reported to increase after 10 years of GH supplementation, although the risk of type 2 diabetes mellitus does not appear to increase. At this time, the effects of GH supplementation on cardiovascular risk and mortality are unknown.

Older adults without hypothalamic-pituitary disease have many of the same conditions, which leads to the hypothesis that GH supplementation may have a beneficial effect on these clinically important age-related disorders. RCTs of short-term GH supplementation in older adults have reported increased lean body mass and decreased fat mass. However, GH was not found to augment improvements in muscle strength achieved with exercise alone, no improvements in functional status were demonstrated, and there were no significant improvements in bone density or lipid levels after adjustment for body composition changes (SOE=A). Furthermore, significant adverse events were common, including carpal tunnel syndrome, arthralgias, edema, and gynecomastia. The long-term efficacy and safety of GH administration in older adults are unknown. Short-term GH supplementation may improve nitrogen balance in older adults with severe illness and catabolic states. However, GH is very expensive, and it is not recommended for clinical use in older adults without established hypothalamic-pituitary disease.

MELATONIN

Melatonin, a hormone secreted by the pineal gland, is thought to be involved in the regulation of circadian and seasonal biorhythms. Melatonin secretion is inhibited by exposure to light, resulting in a marked circadian variation in circulating melatonin concentrations. Its sedative effects suggest a role in sleep induction. Most studies show that plasma melatonin concentrations decline throughout life after early childhood, but the physiologic significance of this decline in melatonin secretion is unclear. Numerous claims have been made in the lay press regarding the "antiaging" benefits of melatonin supplementation for various conditions, including insomnia, immune deficiency, cancer, and the aging process itself. In placebo-controlled trials up to 6 months, sustained-release melatonin improved several parameters of sleep quality and was well tolerated in older adults with insomnia, and 2 days of treatment with sustained-release melatonin did not impair psychomotor function, memory recall, and driving skills in older adults. In patients with dementia, a Cochrane review did not find evidence that melatonin is effective for cognitive impairment, although a systematic review found that melatonin supplementation in people with dementia improved sundowning and agitated behavior in 2 of 3 RCTs. The incidence of delirium improved with prophylactic melatonin treatment in RCTs involving hospitalized older patients, but studies of delirium incidence after hip fracture repair have not shown consistent improvement. The longer-term risks and benefits of melatonin supplementation have not been established for insomnia or any other indication.

REFERENCES

- American Geriatrics Society Workgroup on Vitamin D Supplementation for Older Adults. Recommendations abstracted from the American Geriatrics Society Consensus Statement on Vitamin D for Prevention of Falls and Their Consequences. *J Am Geriatr Soc*. 2014;62(1):147–162.

    This consensus statement is intended to provide clinical guidance regarding use of vitamin D supplements to prevent falls and fractures in older adults. Its focus is to maximize the likelihood of benefit in this population without risk of toxicity. As a result, some of its recommendations, including a higher minimum vitamin D supplement of 1,000 IU/d in older adults, differ from those of the Institute of Medicine, which recommended dietary reference intakes for vitamin D and calcium in the general population. The AGS Workgroup recognized that this dose is higher than doses used in most intervention trials showing protection from falls or fractures. It was noted that in practice, adherence to supplementation is likely lower than in these trials, that most older adults require higher supplementation to achieve minimum desirable 25(OH)D levels, and that there is no known risk of daily vitamin D supplementation at this level for people without disorders that increase the risk of hypercalcemia. The Workgroup concluded that routine measurement of serum 25(OH)D concentrations is not necessary for older adults in the absence of underlying conditions that increase hypercalcemia risk. The referenced article is a summary presenting key points from the full consensus statement. The full-length document is available online at www.geriatricscareonline.org.

- Boardman HM, Hartley L, Eisinga A, et al. Hormone therapy for preventing cardiovascular disease in post-menopausal women. *Cochrane Database Syst Rev*. 2015 Mar 10;3:CD002229.

    This comprehensive overview of the current literature on estrogen use for primary and secondary prevention of cardiovascular risk highlights some of the newer studies and findings that suggest that early use of estrogen is not harmful and may confer some benefit to women 50–59 years old, but that risk of cardiovascular adverse effects are even greater in women >70 years old.

- Freda PU, Beckers AM, Katznelson L, et al. Pituitary incidentaloma: an Endocrine Society clinical practice guideline. *J Clin Endocrinol Metab*. 2011;96(4):894–904.

    The Endocrine Society Task Force recommendations for patients with pituitary incidentalomas include laboratory screening for hormone hypersecretion and hypopituitarism, along with visual field examination for lesions adjacent to optic nerves or chiasm. The approach to follow-up for patients not meeting criteria for surgical removal is described, along with indications for surgical intervention.

- Manson JE, Chlebowski RT, Stefanick ML, et al. Menopausal hormone therapy and health outcomes during the intervention and extended poststopping phases of the Women's Health Initiative randomized trials. *JAMA*. 2013;310(13):1353–1368.

    This most recent analysis of the women involved in the WHI outlines a comprehensive overview of the primary and secondary outcome measures with extended follow-up (an average of 13 years). Primary efficacy and safety outcomes were coronary heart disease and invasive breast cancer, respectively. A global index also included stroke, pulmonary embolism, colorectal cancer, endometrial cancer, hip fracture, and death. The findings reveal a complex pattern of risks and benefits that do not support use of estrogen for chronic disease prevention, although it is appropriate for vasomotor symptoms in some women.

- Matsumoto AM. Testosterone administration in older men. *Endocrinol Metab Clin North Am*. 2013;42(2):271–286.

    The only indication for testosterone supplementation in older men is replacement therapy for male hypogonadism, evidenced by symptoms and signs of androgen deficiency together with consistently low serum testosterone levels. This monograph provides detailed information on the clinical manifestations and approach to the biochemical diagnosis of hypogonadism in older men. Functional and organic causes of androgen deficiency are reviewed, along with treatment of functional causes. The importance of patient-centered treatment goals is discussed. Precautions and monitoring parameters during testosterone treatment are reviewed, as well as considerations in choosing testosterone formulations.

- McCarrey AC, Resnick SM. Postmenopausal hormone therapy and cognition. *Horm Behav*. 2015;74:167–172.

    This is an up-to-date review article on estrogen therapy and cognition that highlights findings from the large-scale WHI Memory Study (WHIMS), the "critical window hypothesis," which suggests that a window of opportunity may exist shortly after menopause during which estrogen treatments are most effective, and evidence that potential adverse effects on cognition are more likely in women with higher disease burden such as diabetes.

- Waring AC, Arnold AM, Newman AB, et al. Longitudinal changes in thyroid function in the oldest old and survival: the Cardiovascular Health Study All-Stars Study. *J Clin Endocrinol Metab.* 2012;97(11):3944–3950.

    Few data are available on thyroid function in the oldest old, and studies of the relationship between thyroid function and mortality in this age group have yielded conflicting results. This multicenter, population-based study described longitudinal changes in thyroid function in a cohort of 843 older adults (mean age 85 years) and assessed the relationship between thyroid function and mortality. The main outcome measures were serum thyrotropin, free T_4, total T_3, and thyroid peroxidase antibody status measured in 1992–1993 and 2005–2006. Mortality data were obtained from medical records, death certificates, autopsy reports, and coroners reports through early 2011. Over the 13-year study period, thyrotropin increased 13%, free T_4 increased 1.7%, and total T_3 decreased 13%. No associations were found between death and subclinical hypothyroidism, and thyrotropin level, but higher free T_4 levels were associated with death. These findings add to concerns about treating mildly increased thyrotropin levels with thyroid supplementation in the oldest old.

David A. Gruenewald, MD
Anne M. Kenny, MD
Alvin M. Matsumoto, MD

CHAPTER 64—DIABETES MELLITUS

KEY POINTS

- Diabetes mellitus, one of the most common chronic conditions in older adults, results in decreased life expectancy, numerous complications and comorbidities, a higher risk of other common geriatric conditions (eg, polypharmacy, urinary incontinence, falls, cognitive impairment, depression, chronic pain), functional impairment, and disability.

- Lifestyle modifications, such as exercise and weight loss can prevent diabetes in high-risk patients and can help in management of hyperglycemia in patients with diabetes.

- Because of the great heterogeneity in the older population, treatment goals for older diabetic patients must be carefully individualized.

- Although the target blood pressure is debated, attempts to lower blood pressure are important for older hypertensive diabetic patients.

- Diabetes self-management is an important part of diabetes care, and annual self-management training is a covered benefit under Medicare Part B.

Diabetes mellitus (DM) is a group of metabolic disorders characterized by hyperglycemia due to abnormalities in insulin secretion, insulin action, or both. It is one of the most common chronic diseases affecting older adults. The CDC estimates that among people ≥65 years old, 27% have diagnosed or undiagnosed diabetes. Because the general population is aging and rates of obesity are increasing among middle-aged adults, people ≥65 years old will constitute the majority of diabetic adults in the United States and in other developed countries in the coming decades. In the coming years, the largest percent increase in diabetes prevalence in any age group will be among those >75 years old.

The age-adjusted prevalence of DM is higher among black Americans and Hispanic Americans than white Americans. Further, black Americans suffer from complications of diabetes at disproportionately higher rates than white Americans. Research is only starting to decipher the effects of race on diabetes development and outcomes.

DM in older adults leads to higher rates of vascular complications and geriatric syndromes, which in turn lead to increased morbidity and mortality. Older adults with diabetes can expect a 10-year reduction in life expectancy and a mortality rate nearly twice that of people without diabetes. In addition, older adults disproportionately experience the vascular complications such as atherosclerosis, neuropathies, loss of vision, and renal insufficiency. Older adults with diabetes are at higher risk than those without diabetes for geriatric syndromes, including incontinence, falls, frailty, cognitive impairment, and depressive symptoms; they also have a higher prevalence of functional impairment and disability. Mobility problems are about 2–3 times more likely, and disability in activities of daily living is about 1.5 times more likely in older adults with diabetes than in those without.

PATHOPHYSIOLOGY OF DIABETES IN OLDER ADULTS

More than 90% of older adults with diabetes have type 2 DM, which is generally characterized by insulin resistance, increased insulin requirements to maintain euglycemia, and ultimately, relative insulin deficiency when the pancreatic beta cells are unable to meet the higher insulin requirements. The prevalence of type 2 DM increases with age. The reasons for this are not fully known; there appears to be an interaction among several factors, including increasing rates of obesity and decreased physical activity. An altered inflammatory environment with aging can also contribute to the higher rates of diabetes in older adults.

In addition to intrinsic physiologic mechanisms, external factors can contribute to glucose intolerance and type 2 DM. Some medications commonly taken by older adults—diuretics, sympathomimetics, glucocorticoids, niacin, and olanzapine—change carbohydrate metabolism and increase glucose concentration. Concurrent illnesses, such as infections, myocardial infarction, and stroke, as well as other physiologic stresses can lead to worsened hyperglycemia.

Less than 10% of older adults with diabetes have type 1 DM, which is characterized by autoimmune destruction of pancreatic beta cells, resulting in an absolute insulin deficiency. Unlike most patients with type 2 DM, all patients with type 1 DM require exogenous insulin.

Physiologic changes that develop with diabetes and its complications can interact with physiologic changes associated with aging to further decrease physiologic reserve. Type 2 DM and obesity are associated with inflammatory dysregulation, which can also be associated with aging and lead to clinical sequelae such as sarcopenia. Aging is associated with decreased physiologic reserve in multiple organ systems (eg, renal, cardiovascular, CNS), which may interact with end-organ damage due to diabetes, resulting in increased vulnerability to physiologic stressors.

DIAGNOSIS AND EVALUATION

In 2009, an international group of diabetes experts recommended using a hemoglobin A_{1c} (HbA_{1c}) level of ≥6.5% to diagnose diabetes; the American Diabetes Association (ADA) participated in that decision and formally adopted this recommendation in 2010. This decision was based on the ease of performing the HbA_{1c} test, which can facilitate diagnosis of more people with diabetes. None of the diagnostic criteria include any adjustments for age. The 4 ways to establish the diagnosis of diabetes mellitus are summarized below; each must be confirmed, on a subsequent day, preferably by the same method.

- HbA_{1c} ≥6.5% using an assay standardized to the national glycohemoglobin standardization program

- Symptoms of polyuria, polydipsia, and unexplained weight loss, plus a random plasma glucose concentration of ≥200 mg/dL (11.1 mmol/L)

- A plasma glucose concentration after an 8-hour fast of ≥126 mg/dL (7 mmol/L)

- A plasma glucose concentration of ≥200 mg/dL (11.1 mmol/L) measured 2 hours after ingestion of 75 g of glucose in 300 mL of water administered after an overnight fast

Older adults with a fasting blood glucose of 100–125 mg/dL (5.6–6.9 mmol/L), a 2-hour plasma glucose of 140–199 mg/dL (7.8–11 mmol/L) after a 75-g oral glucose tolerance test, or an HbA_{1c} of 5.7%–6.4% are considered to have prediabetes. Prediabetes appears to confer increased risk of atherosclerotic complications, as well as increasing the risk of subsequently developing DM.

PREVENTION

Several diabetes prevention trials demonstrated that in people with impaired glucose tolerance at high risk of developing type 2 DM, lifestyle modification that focuses on diet, exercise, and weight loss can delay or prevent progression to diabetes (SOE=A). The largest of these studies was the Diabetes Prevention Program, which tested whether metformin or lifestyle modification decreased progression to diabetes in high-risk adults. In older adults (>60 years), lifestyle modification was especially powerful, decreasing the incidence of diabetes 71% compared with usual care in 2.8 years of follow-up. Metformin, however, decreased the incidence of diabetes by only 11% in older adults, compared with 44% in younger adults (25–44 years old).

Thus, for obese older adults at high risk of diabetes, the focus of diabetes prevention should be on lifestyle modification (diet, exercise, and weight loss) rather than on metformin.

MANAGEMENT

General Principles

Older adults with diabetes require a comprehensive evaluation, which in the primary care setting may be done over several patient visits. For patients with significant functional impairments and comorbidities, including those with psychosocial problems and caregiver requirements, a formal, comprehensive geriatric assessment may be needed. Regardless of how the comprehensive evaluation of an older adult with DM is handled, 3 issues deserve special attention.

First, the history and physical examination must include evaluation of risk factors for atherosclerotic disease and the presence of all comorbid diseases. Diabetes is a well-established risk factor for atherosclerotic cardiovascular disease, so other risk factors such as smoking, family history, hypertension, and hyperlipidemia should also be explored. Diabetes is also associated with multiple vascular complications that may be subclinical or clinical. The presence of coronary artery disease, peripheral vascular disease, neuropathy, foot problems, and medical eye disease must be determined. In many cases, subspecialty consultation (as for retinopathy) and laboratory or diagnostic testing is indicated. In addition, older adults with diabetes are also likely to have prevalent chronic diseases that are not necessarily associated with their diabetes, such as osteoarthritis.

Second, a thorough medication history is important. As previously stated, certain medications can contribute to hyperglycemia. More often, older adults may be on multiple medications for multiple comorbidities and may experience adverse drug events or trouble with medication management or finances. A medication review will help minimize polypharmacy and help in formulating an optimal treatment plan.

Third, an assessment of common geriatric syndromes is critical. Multiple studies have shown that functional impairment, urinary incontinence, falls, pain, cognitive impairment, and depression are more common in older adults with diabetes (SOE=B). An assessment of geriatric syndromes will help identify important factors that will affect treatment plans. For example, a functional assessment will help identify a patient's ability to increase physical activity. A cognitive and depression assessment will help identify a patient's ability to self-manage his or her diabetes.

Goals of Diabetes Care in Older Adults

The clinician develops goals for diabetes management and individualized clinical targets with each older adult with diabetes, involving the caregiver when appropriate. The goals of diabetes management in older adults include the following:

- Control of hyperglycemia and its symptoms
- Evaluation and treatment of associated risks for atherosclerotic and microvascular disease
- Evaluation and treatment of diabetes complications
- Avoiding hypoglycemia

Although these goals are similar for older and younger people with diabetes, the management of older patients is complicated by the medical and functional heterogeneity of this group. In fact, this heterogeneity is a key consideration in developing individualized diabetes management interventions and clinical targets for older patients with diabetes. Some may have developed diabetes in middle age and have developed multiple related comorbidities. Others may have just converted from impaired glucose tolerance to diabetes and may have few complications or comorbidities. In addition to medical heterogeneity, older adults with diabetes are heterogeneous in their functional status. Many are active with excellent function. Others may be disabled and frail, with advanced cognitive impairment, multiple comorbidities and complications, and significant functional limitations. Many others are in between, with mild or early functional limitations, several related comorbidities, and multiple risks for worsening morbidity.

Another consideration in treating older adults with diabetes is life expectancy and the time needed for clinical benefit from a specific intervention. Clinical trials have demonstrated that >8 years are needed before the benefits of glycemic control are reflected in reduced microvascular complications such as diabetic retinopathy or kidney disease but that only 2–3 years are required to see benefits from better control of blood pressure and lipids (SOE=A). It is important to remember that the median remaining life expectancy for a 70-year-old woman is 14 years, which is plenty of time for development of diabetes complications. Therefore, for a person in his or her early 70s who is newly diagnosed or highly functional, diabetes management is no different from that of younger people. However, management must be designed to fit the clinical status of older adults who are significantly functionally impaired or who have multiple comorbidities that limit life expectancy or that significantly increase the risks of hypoglycemia. In all cases, patient preferences and quality of life must be considered.

Patient preferences must be elicited and considered, because the patient is the one who will ultimately manage his or her diabetes and comorbid conditions. Some patients do not want to follow some management recommendations. Some fear dependency and the need for assistance more than death. Some find certain medications or monitoring activities burdensome.

Therefore, it is important to establish individual goals for diabetes management and clinical targets with patients; to reevaluate the patient's clinical, functional, and social status if these goals and targets are not being met; and to determine if caregiver support or specialty input is needed. A practical clinical method of individualizing and prioritizing diabetes care is to assess goals and preferences, assess patient longevity and functional status, consider the time needed for treatment impact, screen for geriatric syndromes, and assist patients with decision making and prioritization of treatment strategies.

The American Geriatrics Society developed guidelines for improving the care of older adults with diabetes mellitus in 2003 and published updated guidelines in 2013. The ADA also published guidelines for older adults in 2012. Both guidelines stress that older adults with diabetes are remarkably heterogeneous, requiring clinicians to individualize both treatment goals and therapies to achieve optimal patient outcomes.

INTERVENTIONS

Overview

Solid evidence supports the effectiveness of several components of diabetes care, including control of lipids and blood pressure, smoking cessation, appropriate eye and foot care, diabetes education and self-management support for medication adherence, appropriate nutrition, weight loss if indicated, and increased physical activity (SOE=A). Studies suggest that these interventions decrease vascular complications, including myocardial infarctions and strokes (macrovascular outcomes) and nephropathy and retinopathy (microvascular outcomes). Home monitoring of blood glucose has not been found to be cost-effective (SOE=A). Very few of the data supporting these interventions were obtained from research studies of older adults, adding uncertainty to whether these conclusions are appropriate for geriatric patients. In addition, debates continue about the targets for glycemic and blood pressure control; there is less debate about low-density lipoprotein (LDL) targets (discussed below, under "Lipid Control"). It is likely that many management guidelines can be generalized to many older adults with diabetes, particularly those who are healthy and functional. For some older patients, particularly those with severe comorbidities and disabilities, aggressive management is not likely to provide benefit and may even result in harm, such as hypoglycemia with aggressive glycemic control or hypotension with aggressive blood pressure control.

Older adults with diabetes should undergo age-appropriate prevention interventions such as influenza and pneumococcal vaccinations. In addition, because lower extremity infections and amputations are more common among older adults with diabetes than those without diabetes, careful annual foot examination is recommended. To screen for kidney disease, a test for the presence of albuminuria should be performed at diagnosis and annually (SOE=C). If a patient is taking an ACE inhibitor or angiotensin-receptor blocker, there is no need for continued screening (SOE=D).

Diabetes Education and Self-Management Support

Because diabetes is a disease for which the patient and/or caregivers bear the primary responsibility for management and ultimate control, it is imperative that the patient understands the mechanisms and management of the metabolic derangements and becomes fully involved in diabetes self-management. Therefore, education about diabetes, and particularly diabetes self-management, are key components of effective care. Often, basic education can be accomplished in the primary care setting. Patients with diabetes and other comorbidities may need referral to a diabetes educator for one-on-one counseling or group classes, enrollment in a comprehensive diabetes disease management program, or specialty physician care. Annual diabetes self-management training is a covered benefit under Medicare Part B. DM education programs may be particularly important in older adults with diabetes who are members of minority groups, particularly black Americans or Hispanic Americans. It is extremely important to recognize when caregiver involvement in diabetes self-management activities is required. The caregiver must be highly involved and educated about diabetes and its self-management when the patient is cognitively impaired, is significantly disabled or frail, or when communication issues exist, eg, the patient has limited proficiency in English.

Diabetes self-management and support must cover several important areas. The older patient, and caregiver if appropriate, must be educated about hypo- and hyperglycemia, including precipitating factors, prevention, symptoms, monitoring, treatment, and indications for notifying the clinician. For patients requiring insulin, the patient and caregiver should be taught blood-glucose self-monitoring, and their technique should be reassessed and reinforced periodically.

Diet and physical activity remain important components of the initial and ongoing management of patients with diabetes. Specific dietary recommendations must be tailored for each individual and include assessment of cholesterol intake and weight management. Physical activity programs should also be individualized. The patient should be assessed regularly for level of physical activity and informed about the benefits of exercise and available resources for becoming more active.

An older adult with diabetes who is prescribed a new medication, and a caregiver, should be educated on the purpose of the medication, how to take it, and the common or important adverse events, with reassessment and reinforcement periodically as needed. Finally, every older adult with diabetes and a caregiver should be educated about risk factors for foot ulcers and amputation. Physical ability to provide foot care should be evaluated, with periodic reassessment and reinforcement.

For patient education to be an effective tool in diabetes management, it must take into account the level of adjustment to the disease. In addition, it is critical that the patient and/or caregivers understand not only "what" needs to be done but "why" it needs to be done. Self-efficacy strengthening and coping skills training should also be addressed. Support groups, such as those available through the ADA, can be extremely helpful for the older patient and/or caregivers.

Smoking Cessation

Meta-analyses of studies suggest that smoking cessation reduces cardiovascular events 3–5 times in patients with diabetes compared with patients without diabetes. Further, smoking cessation leads to greater reductions in mortality than control of blood pressure or lipids. Thus, smoking cessation counseling and pharmacologic intervention should be offered to any older adult with diabetes who smokes.

Aspirin for Primary Prevention of Cardiovascular Disease

It is unclear whether older adults with diabetes but no other history of cardiovascular disease would benefit from aspirin. In 2010, the American Diabetes Association, American Heart Association, and the American College of Cardiology suggested that low-dose aspirin (75–162 mg daily) may be considered in adults with diabetes if they have a 10-year risk of cardiovascular events >10%. In contrast, the 2012 European Guidelines on Cardiovascular Disease Prevention recommends against aspirin use for primary prevention.

Blood Pressure Control

A number of randomized controlled trials provide strong evidence that management of hypertension in older adults with diabetes reduces cardiovascular events and mortality; some of these studies included substantial numbers of older adults with diabetes (SOE=A). The best target blood pressure for older diabetic patients is not clear, but the preponderance of evidence suggests that for healthier patients with few comorbidities and functional limitations, a blood pressure target of 120–140 systolic and 70–80 diastolic may be ideal. In the ADVANCE trial, with 11,140 people in multiple sites around the world with a mean age of 66 years, a mean blood pressure of 136/73 mmHg was achieved in the intensive treatment group, in which the relative risk of cardiovascular death decreased 18%; the relative risk of all-cause death decreased 14% (ARR=1.3%, NNT=79 for all-cause mortality over 5 years) (SOE=A). In the ACCORD study, a blood pressure of <119/70 mmHg was achieved in the intensive treatment arm versus 140/70 mmHg in the standard treatment arm. No significant benefit of intensive blood pressure on cardiovascular outcomes was observed (SOE=A).

Some older adults may not be able to tolerate aggressive blood pressure lowering; thus, hypertension treatment should be advanced gradually. If a patient develops orthostasis, then falls, fractures, and functional limitations may result. Thus, for patients with orthostatic hypotension, the harms of treatment may outweigh the benefits, and relaxing the blood pressure target may be most appropriate. Evidence for medication choice in older adults with diabetes suggests that most classes chosen (diuretics, ACE inhibitors, β-blockers, and calcium channel blockers) have comparable effectiveness in reducing cardiovascular disease and mortality. ACE inhibitors (SOE=A) and angiotensin II receptor blockers (SOE=B) have additional cardiovascular and renal benefit for people with diabetes.

Lipid Control

Randomized controlled trials and a meta-analysis have confirmed the benefit of the statin drugs, particularly for secondary prevention of cardiovascular events (SOE=A). In general, most studies with statin management suggest that patients with diabetes benefit more from cholesterol lowering than those without diabetes, and secondary prevention is particularly beneficial. Analyses have calculated NNTs of 14 to 46 for prevention of one major cardiovascular event over 5 years of lipid-lowering treatment in diabetic patients.

In contrast to secondary prevention, there is conflicting data on whether primary prevention of hyperlipidemia decreases cardiovascular events in patients with diabetes. In 2013, the American Heart Association, American College of Cardiology, and the National Heart, Lung and Blood Institute published new guidelines for cholesterol treatment to decrease atherosclerotic disease. They suggested that although LDL levels are beneficial in risk stratifying patients, there is little evidence that treating to a specific LDL target is beneficial. For older adults with diabetes age 40–75 and LDL between 70–189 mg/dL, high-dose statins are recommended for those with 10-year atherosclerotic cardiovascular disease (ASCVD) risk >7.5% and moderate-dose statins for those with ASCVD risk <7.5%. Further, they suggest that although continuation of statins beyond age 75 is warranted, it is unclear whether starting statins for primary prevention is beneficial for those >75 year old.

Alanine aminotransferase concentration should be measured within 12 weeks of starting or changing the dosage of a statin or niacin to assess adherence and response to the drug. Statins can cause a range of muscle injury, ranging from rhabdomyolysis (<0.5% of patients) to myalgias (9.3% among healthy, young volunteers). More potent statins at higher doses appear to increase the risk of adverse effects.

Glycemic Control

Control of hyperglycemia in diabetes is important to prevent the symptoms of uncontrolled hyperglycemia, such as weight loss, fatigue, sometimes the classic polyuria and polydipsia, and possibly increased infections. Treatment of hyperglycemia in type 2 DM to prevent vascular complication is more controversial. Control of hyperglycemia to near-normal levels may prevent retinal and renal complications, but the effects are modest and lead to a 1.5- to 3-fold increase in the risk of serious hypoglycemia (SOE=A). Three large, randomized trials of intensive versus moderate control of hyperglycemia, the VADT, ADVANCE, and ACCORD, did not demonstrate any benefit of intensive control (targeting HbA_{1c} to <6.5%) on cardiovascular outcomes (SOE=A). The glycemic control arm of ACCORD was terminated early because of excess mortality in the intensively controlled group (1.41% versus 1.14% per year; hazard ratio 1.22 [95% CI, 1.01–1.46]). All three studies investigated patients with long-standing diabetes and included older patients with comorbidities (mean ages were 60 ± 6 years VADT, 62 ± 6 years ACCORD, 66 ± 6 years ADVANCE; <1% of enrolled patients were ≥80 years old at baseline). Long-term follow-up (10–20 years) of the UK Prospective Diabetes Study (UKPDS) suggested an effect of more intensive control on cardiovascular outcomes, but UKPDS targeted younger adults (mean age 54) with newly diagnosed diabetes.

The VADT and ADVANCE trials found that control of hyperglycemia to a target HbA_{1c} <7% in patients with long-standing diabetes reduced microalbuminuria, and analyses of ACCORD also show lower rates of microvascular complications (SOE=A). Given these conflicting

Table 64.1—Non-Insulin Agents for Treating Diabetes Mellitus

Medication Class Individual Agents	Percent of HbA_{1c} Lowering	Comments (Metabolism)
Oral Agents		
Biguanide Metformin	1–2	Decreases hepatic glucose production; does not cause hypoglycemia
2nd-Generation Sulfonylureas Glimepiride, glipizide, glyburide	1–2	Increase insulin secretion; can cause hypoglycemia and weight gain
α-Glucosidase Inhibitors Acarbose, miglitol	0.5–1	Delay glucose absorption; can cause hypoglycemia and weight gain
DPP-4 Enzyme Inhibitors Alogliptin, linagliptin, sitagliptin, saxagliptin	0.5–1	Protect and enhance endogenous incretin hormones; do not cause hypoglycemia, weight neutral
Meglitinides Nateglinide, repaglinide	1–2	Increase insulin secretion; can cause hypoglycemia and weight gain
Thiazolidinediones Pioglitazone, rosiglitazone	0.5–1.5	Insulin resistance reducers; increased risk of heart failure; avoid if NYHA Class III or IV cardiac status; discontinue if any decline in cardiac status; weight gain
SGLT2 Inhibitors Canagliflozin, dapagliflozin, empagliflozin	0.5–1.5	Decreases glucose reabsorption from kidney
Other Bromocriptine, colesevelam	0.5	
Injectable Agents		
GLP-1 receptor agonist Exenatide, liraglutide, albiglutide, dulaglutide	0.7–1	Less likely to cause hypoglycemia than insulin or sulfonylureas; can cause weight loss; risks include acute pancreatitis and possibly medullary thyroid cancer
Amylin analogue Pramlintide	0.4–0.7	Nausea common; reduce pre-meal dose of short-acting insulin by 50%

SOURCE: Adapted with permission from Reuben DB, Herr KA, Pacala JT, et al. *Geriatrics At Your Fingertips*, 17th ed. New York: American Geriatrics Society; 2015:100–103.

findings, glycemic targets for all patients with diabetes are unclear and continue to be debated. Most guidelines and experts strongly recommend individualizing glycemic targets, with healthier older adults with excellent self-management capability striving for HbA_{1c} targets near 7% and more frail patients aiming for an HbA_{1c} level closer to 8.5%–9% (SOE=C).

Medications to Lower Glucose

There are many options for drug therapy in older adults with type 2 DM, with no clearly preferred algorithm. Few comparisons of the medications are available, and most studies have focused on decreasing hyperglycemia, an intermediate outcome. Little information is available about adverse drug events other than hypoglycemia.

Hyperglycemia-lowering regimens can consist of any of several classes of drugs (Table 64.1 and Table 64.2), used alone or in combination. The regimen should be adjusted over the course of the illness as goals change, the disease progresses, or complications develop. Sulfonylurea preparations have a long record of safety and effectiveness. Hypoglycemia is a serious adverse event, and these medications must be used cautiously in older adults with significant hepatic and renal insufficiency, because the liver is the primary site of metabolism and excretion is via the kidneys. Meglitinides are similar to sulfonylureas in terms of mechanism of action but may have a slightly lower hypoglycemia risk. α-Glucosidase inhibitors impair the breakdown of carbohydrates in the gut and limit absorption; the residual carbohydrates in the intestinal lumen are responsible for diarrhea observed in about 25% of older adults who use these medications. The biguanide preparations also have GI adverse events and can theoretically cause lactic acidosis in older adults with renal insufficiency. However, a Cochrane review of metformin found no significantly increased risk of lactic acidosis. In older adults taking metformin, serum creatinine concentration should be measured at least annually and with any increase in dosage. For those ≥80 years old or suspected to have reduced muscle mass, renal function should be assessed thoroughly, either through a timed urine collection or application of a formula that corrects serum creatinine for age.

Another class of drugs, the thiazolidinediones, although apparently well tolerated by most patients, carries black box warnings because of a risk of worsening

Table 64.2—Insulin Preparations

Preparations	Onset	Peak (hours)	Duration (hours)	Number of Injections or Inhalations/day
Rapid-acting				
Insulin glulisine (Apidra)	20 min	0.5–1.5	3–4	3
Insulin lispro (HumaLog)	15 min	0.5–1.5	3–4	3
Insulin aspart (NovoLog)	30 min	1–3	3–5	3
Inhaled (Afrezza)[a]	15 min	1	3–4	3
Regular (eg, Humulin, Novolin)[a]	0.5–1 h	2–3	5–8	1–3
Intermediate or long-acting				
NPH (eg, Humulin, Novolin)[b]	1–1.5 h	4–12	24	1–2
Insulin detemir (Levemir)	3–4 h	6–8	6–24 depending on dose	1–2
Insulin glargine (Lantus)[c]	2–4 h	—	24	1
Combinations				
Isophane insulin and regular insulin injectable (Novolin 70/30)	See individual drugs	2–12	24	1–2
Insulin lispro protamine suspension and insulin lispro (HumaLog mix 50/50; 75/25)	See individual drugs			

NOTE: NPH = neutral protamine Hagedorn (insulin)
[a] Available as 4-unit and 8-unit single-use cartridges administered by inhalation.
[b] Also available as mixtures of NPH and regular in 50:50 proportions.
[c] To convert from NPH dosing, give same number of units once a day. For patients taking NPH q12h, decrease the total daily units by 20% and titrate on basis of response. Starting dosage in insulin-naive patients is 10 U once daily at bedtime.
SOURCE: Reuben DB, Herr KA, Pacala JT, et al. *Geriatrics At Your Fingertips*, 17th ed. New York: American Geriatrics Society; 2015:104. Reprinted with permission.

of heart failure. Because of the concern about increased cardiovascular events, access to rosiglitazone was restricted from 2010–2014. However, analysis of data from the Rosiglitazone Evaluated for Cardiovascular Outcomes and Regulation of Glycemia in Diabetes (RECORD) trial suggested that rates of cardiovascular events were not different between participants taking rosiglitazone versus other agents. RECORD study results led the FDA to lift the restrictions on rosiglitazone prescription.

The DPP-4 enzyme inhibitors, and newer injectable agents such as exenatide, are effective in lowering glucose but have a limited role in routine care of older adults with diabetes. These drugs are contraindicated in significant chronic kidney disease, and exenatide is associated with hypoglycemia. Both are expensive and confer no benefit over the usual oral antidiabetics.

Sodium glucose co-transporter 2 (SGLT2) inhibitors promote renal excretion of glucose to lower increased blood glucose levels. Hypoglycemia risk is low, and SGLT2 inhibitors may decrease weight and blood pressure through osmotic diuresis. However, SGLT2 inhibitors may lead to dehydration and orthostatic hypotension as well as an increased risk of vulvovaginal candidiasis and urinary tract infections.

Finally, insulin can be used effectively in older adults with type 2 DM. Good glycemic control can often be achieved with one or two injections a day of an intermediate-acting insulin preparation. The greatest risk of insulin therapy is hypoglycemia; frail older adults are at higher risk of serious hypoglycemia than healthier, more functional older adults. The management plan for an older adult with diabetes who experiences severe or frequent hypoglycemia should be evaluated, and an appropriate higher glycemic target set. Hypoglycemia is increasingly being recognized as a relatively uncommon but important problem among older adults with diabetes. Longer-acting sulfonylureas (such as glyburide) more commonly cause hypoglycemia than shorter-acting sulfonylureas (such as glipizide). In patients with a history of hypoglycemia, or those with multiple comorbidities and poor functional status who are at risk of hypoglycemia, short-acting sulfonylureas or oral antidiabetics that do not cause hypoglycemia should be used. Psychosocial reasons for hypoglycemia must be investigated and treated, such as an inability to understand self-management because of cognitive problems, inadequate diabetes knowledge, difficulty in implementing therapy because of disability, or lack of caregiver support.

Choosing Wisely® Recommendations

Diabetes Mellitus

- Avoid using medications to achieve HbA_{1c} <7.5% in most adults ≥65 years old; moderate control is generally better.

- There is no evidence that using medications to achieve tight glycemic control in most older adults with type 2 diabetes is beneficial. Among non-older adults, except for long-term reductions in myocardial infarction and mortality with metformin, using medications to achieve glycated hemoglobin levels less than 7% is associated with harms, including higher mortality rates. Tight control has been consistently shown to produce higher rates of hypoglycemia in older adults. Given the long timeframe to achieve theorized microvascular benefits of tight control, glycemic targets should reflect patient goals, health status, and life expectancy. Reasonable glycemic targets would be 7.0 – 7.5% in healthy older adults with long life expectancy, 7.5 – 8.0% in those with moderate comorbidity and a life expectancy < 10 years, and 8.0 – 9.0% in those with multiple morbidities and shorter life expectancy.

REFERENCES

- AGS Expert Panel on Care of Older Adults with Diabetes Mellitus. AGS Guidelines for Improving the Care of Older Adults with Diabetes Mellitus: 2013 Update. *J Am Geriatr Soc.* 2013;61(11):2020–2026.

    In 2003, the California Healthcare Foundation and the AGS convened an expert panel to develop guidelines for the optimal care of older adults with diabetes. In 2013, an expert panel was convened to update these guidelines. In addition to reviewing the evidence for interventions appropriate for all adults with diabetes (eg, smoking cessation, blood pressure control, lipid control, etc), the panel highlighted the importance of geriatric syndromes such as polypharmacy, cognitive impairment, and urinary incontinence in the care of older adults with diabetes.

- Hemmingsen B, Lund SS, Gluud C, et al. Targeting intensive glycaemic control versus targeting conventional glycaemic control for type 2 diabetes mellitus. *Cochrane Database Syst Rev.* 2013 Nov 11;11:CD008143.

    In this Cochrane systematic review of randomized clinical trials that compared intensive glycemic control with standard glycemic control, no differences in all-cause or cardiovascular mortality were seen. However, intensive glycemic control appeared to reduce the risk of nonfatal myocardial infarction, lower extremity amputations, and microvascular complications, as well as episodes of severe hypoglycemia. These results were driven in large part by studies in younger patients with diabetes, casting doubt on whether similar benefits would be seen in older adults.

- Kirkman MS, Briscoe VJ, Clark N, et al. Diabetes in older adults. *Diabetes Care.* 2012;35(12):2650–2664.

    In this summary of a February 2012 conference sponsored by the American Diabetes Association, experts in the field outlined issues regarding diabetes in older adults. Authors outlined 6 questions focusing on the epidemiology, pathogenesis, prevention, treatment, and guidelines about diabetes in older adults and the factors that should be considered when individualizing treatment.

- Moreno G, Mangione CM. Management of cardiovascular disease risk factors in older adults with Type 2 diabetes mellitus: 2002–2012 literature review. *J Am Geriatr Soc.* 2013;61(11):2027–2037.

    The AGS expert panel convened to update the Guidelines for the Care of Older Adults with Diabetes conducted a review of interventions to decrease cardiovascular risk. This report summarizes the evidence behind blood pressure control, lipid control, glycemic control, and aspirin for primary prevention.

- Pogach L, Hobbs C. VA/DoD Clinical Practice Guideline for the Management of Diabetes Mellitus. 2010 Aug; Version 4.0. www.healthquality.va.gov/guidelines/CD/diabetes/ (accessed Jan 2016).

    This evidence-based review of diabetes management highlights numerous aspects of diabetes care, including aspirin, hypertension, dyslipidemia, kidney disease, screening, glycemic control, eye care, foot care, and self-management and education.

Sei J. Lee, MD, MAS

CHAPTER 65—HEMATOLOGY

KEY POINTS

- The reserve capacity of hematopoiesis diminishes with advancing age.

- The possibility of a multifactorial cause should be considered when a patient with anemia of chronic disease has a hemoglobin (Hb) of <10 g/dL.

- Data from the National Health and Nutrition Examination Survey III (NHANES III) indicate that about 35% of all anemias among older adults in the United States result from nutrient deficiencies (iron, vitamin B_{12}, and/or folate), 45% is attributable to chronic disease(s), and 20% is unexplained despite an exhaustive evaluation.

- Coagulation enzyme activity increases with advancing age. This biochemical hypercoagulability can lead to increased thrombotic events in older adults.

- The incidence of myelodysplasia and acute myeloid leukemia increases with age. Age-related defects in lymphopoiesis are thought to be the basis of the myeloid dominance of adult leukemia.

- Polycythemia vera, essential thrombocythemia, and idiopathic myelofibrosis occur primarily in older adults and have a slow rate of spontaneous transformation to leukemia.

HEMATOPOIESIS

Hematopoietic Stem Cells and Aging

The hematopoietic system derives from a small pool of hematopoietic stem cells (HSCs) that can either self-renew or differentiate along one of several lineages to form mature RBCs, WBCs, or platelets. HSCs differentiate into mature cells through an intermediate set of committed progenitors and precursors, each with decreasing self-renewal potential and increasing lineage commitment. Hematopoiesis is tightly regulated by a complex series of interactions between HSCs, their stromal microenvironment, and diffusible regulatory molecules, the hematopoietic growth factors (HGFs) that effect cellular proliferation. The orderly development of the hematopoietic system in vivo and the maintenance of homeostasis require that a strict balance be maintained between self-renewal, differentiation, maturation, and cell loss.

A major question with regard to the aging hematopoietic system is whether the pluripotent HSC has a finite replicative capacity. Studies of long-term bone marrow culture show that maintenance of hematopoiesis varies inversely with age of the donor. Studies in mice have shown that with aging, HSCs demonstrate a reduced ability to regenerate the hematopoietic system and an increased propensity for myeloid differentiation and a decreased ability to generate mature lymphocytes. This skewed pattern of myeloid-lymphoid differentiation is not influenced by the aging marrow microenvironment and is thought to be an inherent attribute of the aging HSC. Thus, it has been postulated that the myeloid dominance of adult human leukemia may in part be driven by age-related deficient lymphopoiesis. Gene expression analysis supports this hypothesis by revealing a 2- to 12-fold down-regulation of lymphoid lineage genes; a 2- to 6-fold up-regulation of myeloid genes; and a 2- to 5-fold up-regulation of the leukemic proto-oncogenes *Aml 1, Pml,* and *Eto* with aging in HSCs. Accumulated DNA damage has been proposed as the principal and unifying mechanism underlying age-dependent decline of HSCs. This accumulated DNA damage appears to be mediated by Batf (basic leucine zipper transcription factor, ATF-like). Batf induces differentiation in cells of lymphoid and myeloid lineage and restricts the self-renewal of HSCs with deficient telomeres. HSCs lacking Batf have evidence of persistent DNA damage, a finding consistent with that reported to occur in HSCs of old mice and older adults.

Hematopoietic Response with Aging

Human aging is associated with reduced reserve capacity for hematopoiesis. This hematopoietic property appears to be caused by a series of factors that coincide with changes across all HSC lineages. Age-related deficient hematopoiesis is characterized by decreased competence in the innate immune system (decreased natural-killer activity, decreased phagocytic ability of neutrophils and macrophages, and a proinflammatory state) and the adaptive immune system (decreased numbers of memory B and T cells), the expansion of myeloid elements, and the occurrence of a mild to moderate normocytic anemia. Diminished adaptive immune response is one of the more common consequences of the aging of the hematopoietic system. This is thought to be due to an imbalance of two functionally different subsets of HSCs, one predisposed to lymphoid differentiation (CD-150^{Lo}) and the other more predisposed to myeloid differentiation (CD150^{hi}). With aging, the CD150^{hi} population predominates in the HSC pool, thus explaining the loss of lymphoid potential previously described. Because CD150^{Lo} HSCs that are DNA damaged or telomere deficient are directed toward lymphoid differentiation, they forgo self-renewal.

Numerous animal studies have shown a reduced ability of the aged hematopoietic system to respond to stimulation. Studies in people have not been as conclusive. Some of these abnormalities, not evidenced in the basal state, become apparent in the stimulus-driven state. In addition to being of a lower magnitude, the aged response is also more variable. Given a comparable stress, hematologic abnormalities are likely to occur earlier and to be of greater severity in older than in younger adults. Thus, the rate of return of the hemoglobin to normal after phlebotomy is blunted, and the ability to mount a granulocyte response to infection is reduced. The relative contributions of age per se and age-related comorbidities to this suboptimal response are unclear. Retrospective analysis of bone marrow transplantations has established donor age to be the only donor parameter significantly associated with survival of the human recipients, which is consistent with presence of an age-related defect in the donor HSCs. This finding is also consistent with the decrease in the number of functionally competent HSCs seen in aging mice.

Although there is no significant change in basal blood cell counts with aging, the prevalence of anemia tends to increase modestly. This is more evident in men ≥75 years old, which in cross-sectional studies have lower hemoglobin values than their younger counterparts (≤65 years old). The mechanism for the difference is unclear but is thought to reflect the presence of comorbid illness or reduced erythropoietin drive, or both, as a result of declines in androgen. Androgens enhance the degradation of hepcidin, a plasma protein that is synthesized in the liver and serves as a major regulator of ferroportin. Ferroportin is a transmembrane protein that transports iron across the mucosa of the GI tract and from macrophages of the reticuloendothelial system (RES) into plasma. Androgen excess results in decreased plasma hepcidin levels, which in turn increase the availability of iron to red cell precursors. This is thought to be the primary pathophysiologic mechanism for the secondary polycythemia seen in patients receiving exogenous androgen therapy. Inversely, androgen deprivation appears to be associated with increased hepcidin levels, which could contribute to the occurrence of anemia. Older adults do not appear to have an impaired ability to increase hematocrit in response to exogenous erythropoietin or to increase granulocyte count after administration of granulocyte colony–stimulating factor. The severity of neutropenia after chemotherapy in older cancer patients is greater in those who are underweight and malnourished than in those who are not. Although aging reduces hematopoietic reserve, it is of clinical relevance only in the presence of comorbidities.

Aging does not appear to affect the circulating concentrations of erythropoietin and most other HGFs; the increase in response to anemia or infection in older adults is equivalent to that in their younger counterparts. However, in response to stress, the blunted hematopoietic response seen with age has been attributed to an impaired ability to release HGFs. This might explain the age-related reduced neutrophil response to infection seen in animal studies and may contribute to increased infection-induced morbidity with aging. The production of certain growth factors, particularly interleukin-6 (IL-6) and growth differentiation factor 15 (GDF15), appears to increase with aging, leading to the notion that aging is accompanied by dysregulation of growth factor production, with overproduction of some cytokines and underproduction of others. GDF15 is derived from erythroid progenitor cells. Increases have been associated with the presence of ineffective erythropoiesis in other hematologic disorders and may imply that this also exists in older adults with anemia. GDF15 has been associated with both increases and decreases in serum hepcidin levels. This effect appears to depend on the concentration of GDF15 in vitro and may or may not reflect an actual physiologic effect.

ANEMIA

Anemia, clearly the most common age-related hematologic abnormality, is seen in both older men and women. According to World Health Organization criteria, anemia is diagnosed if the hemoglobin concentration is <13 g/dL in men and <12 g/dL in women. Studies have shown a high prevalence of anemia in older hospitalized adults, those seen in geriatric clinics, or in nursing homes. However, if stringent criteria are used to select healthy participants, the prevalence drops. Results from NHANES III in the United States indicated that the prevalence of anemia in community-dwelling adults >65 years old was 11% in men and 10.2% in women. In several studies, the prevalence of anemia in the population >80 years old is reported as being 18%–22% in men and 12%–16% in women.

In the general population, the annual incidence of anemia is estimated to be 1%–2%. In contrast, the incidence of anemia in a well-defined population of white people >65 years old attending the Mayo Clinic was reported to be 4- to 6-fold higher. The Mayo Clinic investigators found that in every age group >65 years old, the incidence of anemia was higher in men than in women.

The anemia seen among NHANES III participants was mild; 2.8% of women and 1.6% of men had a hemoglobin concentration of <11 g/dL. Among older adults in the United States, 35% of cases of anemia resulted from deficiencies of iron, vitamin B_{12}, and/or folate (nutritional deficiencies), 45% was attributable to chronic

Table 65.1—Physiologic Classification of Anemia

Hypoproliferative	Ineffective	Hemolytic

■ Iron-deficient erythropoiesis
  Iron deficiency
  Chronic disease
	■ Macrocytic
	  Vitamin B_{12}
	  Folate
	  Myelodysplastic syndrome (refractory anemia)
		■ Immunologic
		  Idiopathic
		  Secondary

■ Erythropoietin lack
  Renal
  Endocrine
	■ Microcytic
	  Thalassemia
	  Sideroblastic
		■ Intrinsic
		  Abnormal hemoglobin
		  Metabolic

■ Stem-cell dysfunction	■ Normocytic
	  Myelodysplastic syndrome
		■ Extrinsic
		  Mechanical

■ Aplastic anemia		

SOURCE: Data from Chatta GS, Lipschitz DA. Aging and hematopoiesis. In: Hazzard WR, Blass JP, Ettinger WH Jr., et al., eds. *Principles of Geriatric Medicine and Gerontology.* 5th ed. New York: McGraw-Hill Health Professions Division; 2003:763–770.

disease(s), and 20% was unexplained. Possible etiologies for these cases of unknown cause include reduced pluripotent HSC reserve, decreased production of HGFs, reduced sensitivity of HSCs to HGFs, marrow microenvironment abnormalities, unrecognized anemia of chronic disease, occult renal failure, and undiagnosed myelodysplasia. It is also possible that age-associated increases in levels of proinflammatory cytokines, such as IL-6, may reduce the responses of stem cells to growth factors, including erythropoietin. Results from the InChianti study examined levels of hemoglobin, erythropoietin, and inflammatory molecules (C-reactive protein, IL-6, IL-1, IL-1b, and tumor necrosis factor alpha [TNF-α]) in 1,453 older adults. In this population, the proinflammatory markers increased with age, with a commensurate increase in the serum erythropoietin concentration in those with a normal hemoglobin and an inappropriately low serum erythropoietin concentration in those with anemia. Patients whose anemia was categorized as "unexplained" characteristically had lower than expected proinflammatory markers and low (not increased) erythropoietin levels.

The importance of anemia in older adults has implications not only relative to the underlying cause but also to its consequence. Studies have shown that morbidity and mortality outcomes are worse with hemoglobin concentrations both <12 g/dL and >15 g/dL. Despite this observation, a direct causality between anemia and mortality and morbidity has not been satisfactorily established. It is postulated that even mild anemia in older adults leads to decreases in cardiac output, local tissue hypoxia, aggravation of already existent comorbidities, and functional decline. Along these lines, anemia in older adults is associated with impaired performance-based mobility function such as walking speed or ability to rise from a chair, impaired cognitive performance, the occurrence of depressive symptoms, and a decrease in quality of life. Of great physical consequence is that anemia is associated with increases in muscle weakness, severity of frailty, impaired balance, risks of falls, and mortality. Women >65 years old with hemoglobin concentrations <11 g/dL have a higher risk of all-cause mortality than those whose hemoglobin concentrations were ≥12 g/dL. This increased risk of mortality is independent of the presence of other comorbidities.

Evaluation of Anemia

The presence of multiple pathologies in older adults often makes evaluation of anemia challenging. Attempting to define the cause of anemia when the hemoglobin concentration is 12–13 g/dL is rarely helpful. A decision as to how aggressively to evaluate these patients depends on clinical judgment. Once a decision has been made to investigate a low hemoglobin concentration, the principles involved in assessment and evaluation are similar to those used in patients of any age.

For a summary of the causes of the various anemias seen in older adults, see Table 65.1. Thus, patients with anemia should be evaluated for renal, hepatic, endocrine, and marrow function. The initial evaluation should include a medication, alcohol, and dietary history; physical examination; a CBC with an absolute reticulocyte count; and fecal blood testing. Results may reveal pale conjunctiva, chronic indigestion, and dark stools or urine. A specific inquiry should be made about medications that increase risk of bleeding such as anticoagulants and NSAIDs. Microcytosis (mean corpuscular volume [MCV] <84 fL) indicates an impairment of hemoglobin synthesis, and macrocytosis (MCV >100 fL) can be caused by an abnormality in nuclear maturation (eg, deficiencies in folate and vitamin B_{12} or the presence of myelodysplasia). Although reticulocytosis may result in some enlarged red cells, rarely is the MCV significantly increased because of this.

Iron deficiency and vitamin B_{12} deficiency can coexist, resulting in confusing RBC indices. RBC production can be estimated by interpreting the absolute reticulocyte count as determined on an automated cell counter. The use of the absolute reticulocyte count rather than the

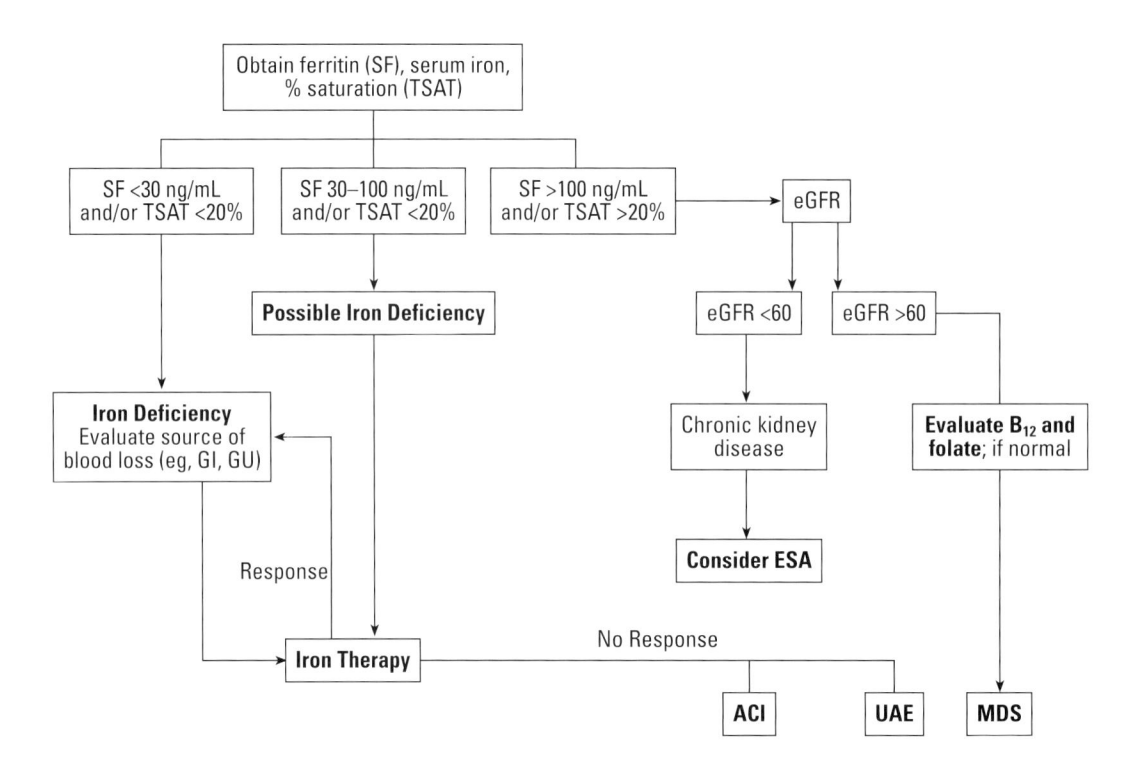

Figure 65.1—Evaluation of Possible Iron-Deficiency Anemia

SOURCE: Adapted from Reuben DB, Herr K, Pacala JT, et al. *Geriatrics At Your Fingertips*, 17th ed. New York: American Geriatrics Society; 2015. Reprinted with permission.

absolute reticulocyte percentage (proportion of reticulocytes present per a fixed number of red cells) is more accurate, does not require correction for differences in the hemoglobin concentration or hematocrit, and does not require correction for the presence of polychromasia seen on a peripheral blood smear. In the absence of anemia, the normal absolute reticulocyte count is between 25,000 and 75,000/µL. Hemolytic anemia usually has an absolute reticulocyte count ≥100,000/µL, whereas anemia caused by a lack of production of circulating red cells is indicated by an absolute reticulocyte count <75,000/µL. Absolute reticulocyte counts between 75,000 and 100,000/µL should be interpreted in the context of the clinical presentation. Decreased production of circulating red blood cells is caused by hypoproliferative anemias or by ineffective erythropoiesis. An increased serum lactate dehydrogenase (LDH) concentration and indirect hyperbilirubinemia result from the increased destruction of RBC precursors in the marrow and can be used to distinguish ineffective erythropoiesis from hypoproliferative anemia. For an approach to the laboratory evaluation of anemia, see Figure 65.1 and Figure 65.2. An absolute reticulocyte count ≥100,000/µL, indirect hyperbilirubinemia, and an increased serum LDH concentration are indicative of hemolytic anemia. An absolute reticulocyte count <75,000/µL, increased indirect bilirubin, and an increased serum LDH concentration suggest ineffective erythropoiesis. In older adults with ineffective erythropoiesis, macrocytosis strongly suggests vitamin B_{12} or, less commonly, folate deficiency, and microcytosis suggests sideroblastic anemia.

The Hypoproliferative Anemias

Conflicting information exists in regard to the proportion of anemias caused by various underlying conditions. According to NHANES III, among community-dwelling older adults in the United States, the causes of anemia can be divided into 4 broad categories: nutrient deficiencies (iron deficiency, folate deficiency, and vitamin B_{12} deficiency), anemia secondary to renal disease, anemia of chronic inflammation, and anemias that are otherwise unexplained.

Iron-Deficiency (or Iron-Restricted) Anemia

Iron is the only nutrient that limits the rate of erythropoiesis alone. Thus, an inadequate iron supply for erythropoiesis is the most common cause of anemia in

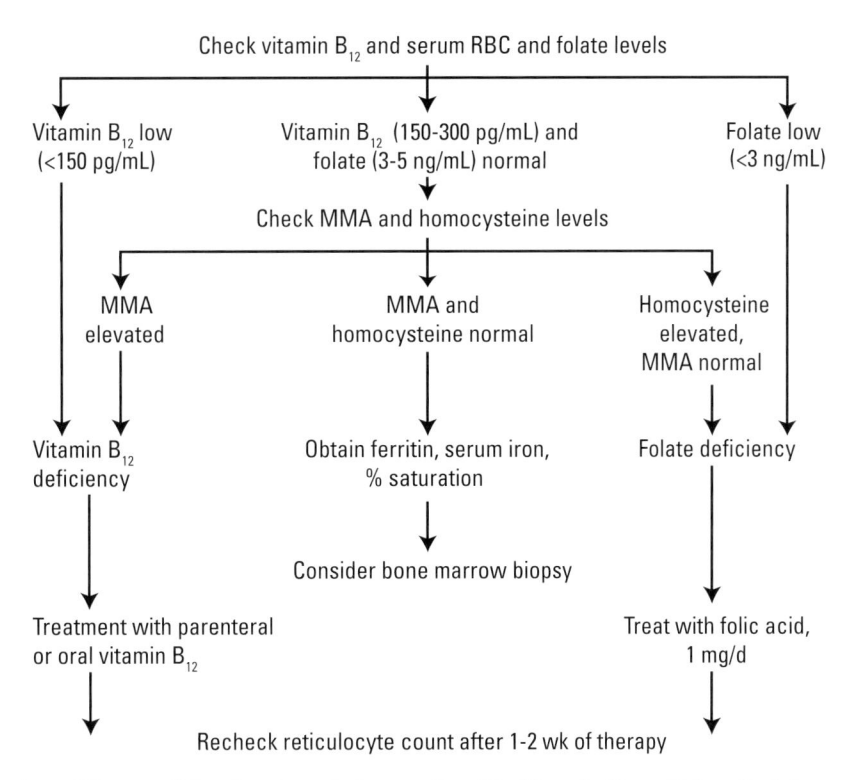

```
                    Check vitamin B₁₂ and serum RBC and folate levels
                                          │
          ┌───────────────────────────────┼───────────────────────────────┐
          ▼                               ▼                               ▼
   Vitamin B₁₂ low            Vitamin B₁₂ (150-300 pg/mL) and        Folate low
   (<150 pg/mL)                folate (3-5 ng/mL) normal              (<3 ng/mL)
                                          │
                               Check MMA and homocysteine levels
                                          │
                        ┌─────────────────┼─────────────────┐
                        ▼                 ▼                 ▼
          ┌──────►   MMA            MMA and            Homocysteine
          │        elevated         homocysteine        elevated,
          │                          normal             MMA normal
          │           │                 │                  │
          ▼           ▼                 ▼                  ▼
      Vitamin B₁₂              Obtain ferritin,        Folate
      deficiency               serum iron,            deficiency
                                % saturation
                                      │
                                      ▼
                            Consider bone marrow biopsy

      Treatment with parenteral                     Treat with folic acid,
      or oral vitamin B₁₂                           1 mg/d
                      │                                    │
                      └──────────────┬─────────────────────┘
                                     ▼
                  Recheck reticulocyte count after 1-2 wk of therapy
```

Figure 65.2—Evaluation of Hypoproliferative Anemia Due to Possible Vitamin B_{12} or Folate Deficiency

SOURCE: Balducci L. Epidemiology of anemia in the elderly: Information on diagnostic evaluation. *J Am Geriatr Soc.* 2003;51(3 Suppl):S2-9. Reprinted with permission.

older adults, resulting in a hypoproliferative anemia. This iron restriction is diagnosed by the presence of a decreased serum iron, a decreased transferrin saturation (serum iron concentration divided by the serum total iron binding capacity or serum transferrin concentration, expressed as a percentage), and a normal or increased serum ferritin concentration. Serum iron levels and transferrin saturation are regulated by the release of iron from its storage sites (macrophages in the RES). Absolute iron deficiency (another kind of iron-restricted anemia usually caused by blood loss, malabsorption, or nutritional deficiency) is the most common cause of iron-deficient erythropoiesis in younger people. Blood-loss anemia, the anemia of inflammation or chronic disease, and the anemia associated with protein-energy malnutrition are the most prevalent anemias in older populations. Nutritional iron deficiency is very rare in the older age group, despite the prominence of other nutritional problems.

When unexplained iron deficiency occurs, it is almost exclusively due to blood loss from the GI tract. Typical findings in blood-loss anemia are low iron, low serum ferritin, and high total iron binding capacity, reflecting absent iron stores. It is important to note, that in the presence of both iron deficiency and anemia of chronic inflammation, the serum ferritin may be within the normal range. Medication-related gastritis, angiodysplasia, and benign tumors are common causes but should be considered only after a malignancy has been excluded. Rarely, iron deficiency can result from malabsorption or urinary losses of iron, which occurs in the face of intravascular hemolysis.

Iron deficiency can be treated with either parenteral or oral iron preparations. Some of the parenteral preparations can be administered intramuscularly; however, this mode of administration is often painful, may leave unsightly blue-black discoloration at the injection site, and requires a significant muscle mass for the target injection site. Intravenous administration is indicated in patients receiving an erythrocyte-stimulating agent during dialysis, or if the use of oral iron preparations is untenable. Multiple intravenous iron products are available, with similar efficacy and a reasonable safety profile. The choice of agent is based on the patient's allergy history and the length of infusion course desired. Newer agents have shorter courses of administration but are costly and also may be complicated by iron overload, hypertension, and hypophosphatemia, compared with iron sucrose, sodium ferric gluconate, or low-molecular-weight iron dextran preparations. Published reviews of safety differences between the different intravenous agents do not conclude absolute differences in safety because of the voluntary nature of adverse event reporting. Intravenous ferumoxytol is a commonly used preparation, administered as two doses of 510 mg, given 3–7 days apart.

As first-line, the oral route is preferred for iron supplementation, using ferrous sulfate 325 mg three times daily, given 1 hour before or 2 hours after a meal, which will provide 195 mg of elemental iron. Ferrous gluconate is another option that provides less elemental iron per dose. There is no significant difference among the oral iron preparations in regard to either efficacy or adverse-event profile, although one type of preparation may be better tolerated than another by an individual patient. Oral iron absorption requires that the upper portion of the small bowel be intact and appropriately acidified by gastric secretions. In the presence of achlorhydria from gastric resection or atrophic gastritis, or medications that suppress gastric acid secretion, medicinal iron absorption may be impaired. Often, supplementation with orange juice or oral vitamin C preparations will correct their malabsorption defect. Although unusual, the incidence of celiac disease, which is characteristically associated with iron malabsorption, is increased in the older population. Common dose-related adverse events of oral iron preparations include mild nausea and constipation. For this reason, the frequency and dosage of administration may require adjustment to ensure compliance. Tablets containing a lower elemental dose of iron (15–20 mg), such as ferric gluconate, may be better tolerated than higher dose preparations. Iron elixir and liquid iron drops may be better absorbed; however, the adverse-event profile is similar to that for tablet preparations. Treatment may need to continue for ≥6 months to adequately replace iron stores.

Anemia of Inflammation/Anemia of Chronic Disease

The terms *anemia of inflammation* or *anemia of chronic disease* are often used to explain an anemia associated with some other major disease process. Examples include cancer, collagen vascular disorders, rheumatoid arthritis, and inflammatory bowel disease. Occasionally, the anemia may be the initial manifestation of an occult disease. It is critical that this condition be distinguished from iron-deficiency (blood-loss) anemia to avoid unnecessary GI tests and to prevent inappropriate prescribing of oral iron therapy.

The pathophysiology of the anemia of chronic disease is complex and is due to an inability of RES macrophages to release iron from the breakdown of senescent RBCs to the plasma. As a consequence, serum iron decreases and, as with blood-loss anemia, the iron supply is inadequate for erythropoiesis. In contrast to blood-loss anemia with absent iron stores, iron stores are normal or increased in anemia of chronic disease. Laboratory features include a mild anemia, a low serum iron, low serum transferrin saturation, and normal to increased iron stores (ferritin >100 ng/mL). However, laboratory parameters often can be equivocal, and it may be difficult to distinguish between iron deficiency and defective iron utilization. In this setting, measuring an erythrocyte sedimentation rate or C-reactive protein level may be helpful, because these will often be increased in the presence of an occult inflammatory condition. Hepcidin, a 25 amino acid peptide produced in the liver, has been implicated in the pathogenesis of anemia of chronic inflammation. Hepcidin functions as a direct mediator of iron homeostasis, regulating both intestinal iron absorption as well as release of RES macrophage iron to erythroid progenitors. Although hepcidin levels have been reported to be increased nearly 100-fold in association with anemia of chronic inflammation, studies on the clinical utility of hepcidin are limited by the availability of a suitable clinical assay. The possibility of a multifactorial causation, including blood loss, malnutrition, or hemolysis, should always be considered when anemia of chronic disease is associated with a hemoglobin concentration of <10 g/dL. In this circumstance, laboratory investigations commonly have equivocal results; hence, a bone marrow examination may be required. Clinical judgment is critically important in deciding how aggressive the evaluation for anemia ought to be. Treatment is directed toward the underlying disease, although there is some evidence that patients with profound fatigue may benefit transiently from iron infusions. Sometimes, patients respond to erythropoietin replacement therapy; however, this is often not the case, because increased inflammatory cytokines render bone marrow erythroid precursors resistant to the effect of erythropoietin.

Anemia from Decreased Erythropoietin Production

Decreased erythropoietin production accounts for the anemia of end-stage renal disease and is implicated in some anemias of cancer and chronic diseases. Many cancer patients have anemia independent of myelosuppressive therapy. The anemia is characterized by an inability to use iron stores and an inadequate erythropoietin response, indicated by inappropriately low erythropoietin levels. In addition, a component of the erythroid suppression is mediated by cytokines such as IL-1, TNF-α, and transforming growth factor beta. Although the precise incidence of cancer-related anemia is not known, a number of studies have documented a decrease in transfusion frequency after treatment with erythropoietin. Depending on symptoms, erythroid support may be indicated for patients with hemoglobin concentrations <10 g/dL (SOE=B). The currently available alternative to packed red cell transfusions is the use of erythropoiesis-stimulating agents, including epoetin alfa, epoetin beta, and darbopoietin. All of these products are types of recombinant human erythropoietin that bind to erythropoietin receptors on red cell precursors, which results in the increased proliferation and production of mature RBCs. Erythropoietin treatment can be started after excluding hemolysis, iron deficiency, and bleeding, especially in symptomatic older adults. Their use is controversial: studies and national guidelines caution their use because of increased cardiovascular events and mortality with hemoglobin increased >11 mg/dL. Iron stores should be evaluated monthly in patients receiving erythropoietin supplementation. Iron replacement should be added to the regimen if ferritin levels fall to <100 ng/mL or transferrin saturation to <20%. Serum ferritin concentrations should not exceed 500 ng/mL, because serum ferritin concentration greater than this has been associated with an increased risk of bacterial infection. A temporary cessation of therapy followed by a 25% dosage reduction in erythropoietin therapy is indicated if the hemoglobin concentration approaches 12 g/dL or if the rate of rise is >1 g/dL every 2 weeks. If the hemoglobin concentration remains <10 g/dL and does not increase by 1 g/dL after 4 weeks, or if the hemoglobin concentration falls to <10 g/dL, a 25% increase in dosage is in order. If the target range of hemoglobin >10 g/dL is not achieved after appropriate dosage adjustments over 12 weeks, the patient should be reevaluated for infection, iron restriction, or the presence of an anemia not responsive to epoetin alpha. If after reassessment and iron replacement, the anemia remains refractory to treatment, epoetin alfa therapy should be discontinued. Although it is difficult to prospectively identify nonresponders, it has been reported that patients with endogenous erythropoietin levels >500 mU/mL are unlikely to respond.

Marrow Failure

Marrow failure due to interference with the proliferation of hematopoietic cells is seen in older adults. The disorder is generally associated with suppression of all marrow elements and is suggested by presence of peripheral pancytopenia. Common causes include medications, immune damage to the stem-cell population, intrinsic marrow lesions, and marrow replacement by malignant cells or fibrous tissue. The latter is usually associated with a myelophthisic blood picture (nucleated RBCs, giant platelets, and metamyelocytes) as a reflection of the disruption of marrow stromal architecture. The presence of pancytopenia and the absence of iron-deficient erythropoiesis is an indication for bone marrow aspiration and biopsy. Occasionally, isolated suppression of erythropoiesis occurs, which is referred to as pure red cell aplasia. This disorder can be related to medication or caused by benign or malignant abnormalities of lymphocytes, including thymoma, or by presence of a viral infection (eg, parvovirus B19). These patients have isolated anemia, an increased serum iron, and an absence of erythroid precursors on bone marrow examination. Patients with parvovirus infection typically have reduced red cell precursors, which, if present, may have peculiar intranuclear inclusion bodies. Parvovirus-related pure red aplasia often responds to intravenous immunoglobulin infusions and sometimes antivirus therapy.

Ineffective Erythropoiesis

Macrocytic Anemias

Macrocytic anemias in older adults result from vitamin B_{12} and folate deficiency and myelodysplasia. The prevalence of pernicious anemia increases with advancing age. Pernicious anemia results from malabsorption of vitamin B_{12} as a consequence of the action of antibodies against gastric parietal cells and intrinsic factor. Atrophic gastritis and decreased secretion of intrinsic factor occur, resulting in failure of vitamin B_{12} absorption. Pernicious anemia is most common in adults >60 years old and is more common in women and patients with autoimmune thyroid disease. Although vitamin B_{12} deficiency is common with aging, anemia secondary to this is rare (see the discussion on vitamin B_{12}, folate, and homocysteine, below). The presence of macrocytosis, hypersegmented neutrophils in the peripheral smear, a decreased reticulocyte index, an increased serum LDH level, and indirect hyperbilirubinemia suggest a diagnosis of megaloblastic anemia. The bone marrow classically shows giant metamyelocytes, hypersegmented neutrophils, and enlarged erythroid precursors with more hemoglobin than would be expected from the immaturity of their nuclei (nuclear-cytoplasmic dissociation).

Chronic pancreatitis and diseases of the distal ileum (blind-loop syndrome) can cause vitamin B_{12} deficiency. An increased prevalence of B_{12} deficiency also has been reported in patients with diabetes taking metformin, chronic use of proton-pump inhibitors, and those on strict vegetarian diets. Folate deficiency of sufficient severity to cause anemia in older adults is rare. Alcohol and various drugs (eg, metformin, valproic acid) interfere with folate absorption and metabolism. Vulnerability to deficiency is significantly greater when folate requirements are increased as a result of inflammation, neoplastic disease, or hemolytic anemia.

Microcytic Anemias

The major causes of ineffective erythropoiesis and microcytosis are thalassemia and the sideroblastic anemias. Although thalassemia is generally diagnosed at an earlier age, there are reports of its initial detection in older adults. Mild anemia, a disproportionately low MCV, and the absence of iron deficiency usually point to a diagnosis of thalassemia trait, a condition of little or no clinical consequence. Iron supplements have no role in the treatment of thalassemia trait; on the contrary, they can be detrimental. Acquired sideroblastic anemia, which is primarily a disease of older adults, is a heterogenous group of disorders characterized by presence of iron deposits in the mitochondria of normoblasts. It is a consequence of impaired heme synthesis, and it usually reflects an intrinsic marrow lesion (idiopathic) but may be secondary to inflammation, neoplasia, or drug ingestion. The common finding is the presence of a dimorphic RBC population, in part markedly hypochromic and in part normochromic. The diagnosis is made by demonstration of ringed sideroblasts in the bone marrow as well as by presence of maturation abnormalities of myeloid and erythroid precursors. Older adults with sideroblastic anemia may show some response to pyridoxine (200 mg q8h). This dosage should be given for 3 months until it becomes apparent that hemoglobin concentration will not increase. For patients who are unresponsive to pyridoxine, the anemia should be treated symptomatically.

Myelodysplastic Syndromes

The myelodysplastic syndromes (MDS) are a group of stem-cell disorders characterized by disordered hematopoiesis that occur primarily in the older age group. This group of disorders is classified as refractory cytopenia with unilineage dysplasia (eg, refractory anemia, refractory neutropenia, refractory thrombocytopenia), refractory anemia with ringed sideroblasts, MDS with isolated del (5q), refractory cytopenia with multilineage dysplasia, refractory anemia with excess blasts-1 (5%–9% bone marrow blasts) or with excess blasts-2 (10%–19% bone marrow blasts), and MDS unclassifiable. Refractory anemia and refractory anemia with ringed sideroblasts account for 25%–30% of MDS. Refractory anemia commonly presents as a macrocytic anemia with marrow erythroid hyperplasia and relatively normal myeloid and megakaryocytic lineages. Cytogenetic abnormalities are relatively common in MDS, and one of particular interest in older adults is deletion of the long arm of chromosome 5 (5q–). The median age at presentation is 66 years, and the 5q– syndrome is characterized by macrocytic anemia, modest leukopenia, normal or increased platelet counts, and marrow erythroid hypoplasia or hyperplasia; it is also more common in women.

Treatment of MDS in older adults has historically been primarily supportive. However, MDS is a heterogenous group of disorders, and increasingly, a risk-adapted approach has been used to treat patients. Thus, based on the percentage of marrow blasts, the presence or absence of cytogenetic abnormalities, and the number of peripheral cytopenias, patients are assigned a score using the International Prognostic Scoring System (IPSS) and categorized as having low-, intermediate-, or high-risk disease. Advances into the molecular basis of MDS have led to the use of hypomethylating agents for treatment. Thus far, 5-azacytidine and decitabine (both hypomethylating agents) and lenolidomide (a more potent derivative of thalidomide) have been approved by the FDA for treatment of MDS. They appear to improve the outcome for patients with intermediate- and poor-risk MDS (IPSS scores ≥1.5) by ameliorating the cytopenias of MDS, decreasing the percentage of blasts in the bone marrow, and reducing transfusion dependence. Lenolidomide, in particular, appears to be the drug of choice in patients with 5q– syndrome.

Prognosis in MDS correlates with the IPSS: median survival for low, intermediate, and high risk disease being ≥10 years, 2–5 years, and <12 months respectively.

Clonal expansion of an HSC is a necessary step for development of MDS. Whole-exome sequencing information from 2 large population-based studies (n approximately 30,000) involving persons not known to have hematologic disorders revealed mutations leading to clonal hematopoiesis in 5.6% of those 60–69 years old, 9.5% of those 70–79 years old, 11.7% of those 80–89 years old, and 18.4% of those ≥90 years old. Remarkably, most mutations driving clonal expansion were noted in 3 genes previously associated with the myelodysplastic syndrome, myeloproliferative disorders, and acute myeloid leukemia: ASXL1 (encoding additional sex combs–like transcriptional regulator 1, which modifies chromatin) and DNMT3A and TET2 (which influence DNA methylation). There are several reasons why normal aging might confer a predisposition to clonal hematopoiesis: processes that maintain metabolic integrity age, telomere length decreases, and the numbers of mutations per cell division increase. Cells acquiring ASXL1, DNMT3A, or TET2 mutations would expand sufficiently to be considered clonal hematopoiesis. Clonal hematopoiesis is common with aging, and its prevalence greatly exceeds the age specific incidence of leukemias. Hence, its clinical import is likely similar to that of MGUS and B-cell monoclonal lymphocytosis—processes that also occur more commonly with aging.

Hemolytic Anemias

The causes of hemolytic anemia in older adults are different than those in younger people. Although most patients with congenital disorders will have been previously identified, an occasional older adult with congenital hemolytic anemia (such as G6PD or pyruvate kinase deficiency or hereditary spherocytosis) can present for the first time with symptoms related to cholelithiasis. Autoimmune hemolysis is the most common kind of hemolytic anemia in the older age group. The diagnosis is made by finding spherocytes or red cell clumping on a peripheral blood smear, a high serum LDH, a low plasma haptoglobin, and a positive direct antiglobulin test. In younger patients, a cause of the autoimmune hemolysis is only rarely identified. In contrast, in older adults, the anemia is more likely to be associated with a lymphoproliferative disorder (non-Hodgkin lymphoma or chronic lymphocytic leukemia), collagen vascular disease, or drug ingestion. Corticosteroids and splenectomy are usually effective in patients with red cell antibodies of the IgG type that most frequently cause a warm autoimmune hemolysis. Patients with red cell antibodies of the IgM variety usually have cold reactive antibodies and are typically refractory to splenectomy and corticosteroids. These patients can usually be treated by simply keeping them warm and administering warmed blood products. In the case of cold reactive antibody disease that is difficult to manage, physical removal of the IgM antibodies by plasmapheresis may be indicated. Long-term responses have been seen with administration of the anti-CD20 antibody rituximab or anti-C'5 antibody eculizimab. Rarely, patients can have cold-reactive IgG antibodies that may be responsive to treatments similar to those used in patients with warm-reactive antibodies.

Microangiopathic hemolytic anemia occurs secondary to either disseminated intravascular coagulation (DIC) or as a manifestation of the syndrome of thrombotic thrombocytopenic purpura-hemolytic uremic syndrome (TTP-HUS). DIC is usually associated with severe infections or disseminated cancer and presents with not only intravascular hemolysis but also a consumptive coagulopathy. The presence of red cell fragmentation, thrombocytopenia, a prolonged prothrombin time, a prolonged partial thromboplastin time, and hemosiderinuria suggests this diagnosis. Treatment of DIC entails treating the underlying disorder as well as providing blood product support, including fresh frozen plasma and cryoprecipitate (if the fibrinogen is <100 ng).

TTP-HUS is characterized by microangiopathic hemolysis and thrombocytopenia. Neurologic symptoms and renal dysfunction are seen in patients with TTP, whereas HUS is characterized by renal involvement. In adults, it is often difficult to distinguish between TTP and HUS at presentation, and the initial treatment tends to be the same. In contrast to DIC, in TTP-HUS both the prothrombin time and partial thromboplastin time are usually normal. Making the specific diagnosis early is imperative, because TTP responds to treatment with plasmapheresis and plasma exchange, whereas HUS is relatively unresponsive to this therapeutic option. Childhood HUS is usually preceded by episodes of diarrhea, is commonly associated with the presence of Shiga toxin–producing *E coli* or pneumococcal infection, and tends to be self-limited. With adult TTP-HUS, a diarrheal prodrome occurs in only 8% of patients. The disorder is thought to be idiopathic in about 40% of the patients, with the remaining cases thought to be due to autoimmune causes, infection, or cancer (27%), drug-induced (12%), pregnancy (7%), and hematopoietic stem cell transplantation (6%). Adult TTP is often associated with a markedly decreased plasma ADAMTS13 concentration and the presence of an ADAMTS13 antibody and is responsive to aggressive plasma exchange with or without corticosteroid support. ADAMTS 13 is an enzyme, synthesized in the liver, that degrades von Willebrand factor in the plasma. It is believed that the presence of large amounts of nonprocessed large-molecular-weight multimers of von Willebrand factor plays a pathophysiologic role in this disease. It is presumed that plasma exchange replaces the deficient ADAMTS13 and also removes the antibody. In adult patients with more clearly defined HUS, the ADAMTS 13 tends to be normal, or at least not as severely deficient, and no ADAMTS13 antibody is detected. As is the case in childhood HUS, this disorder tends to be self-limited. There does exist an atypical HUS that is not preceded by a prodrome, has a normal or near normal ADAMTS13 concentration and no detectable ADAMTS13 antibody, but may be characterized by defects in the complement cascade. Atypical HUS tends not to be responsive to plasma exchange but may be responsive to eculizumab, a monoclonal antibody that interferes with formation of the membrane attack complex of complement on the red cell surface.

Hemolysis is frequently associated with implantation of prosthetic heart valves. In different series, the incidence of hemolysis varied from 5% to 35% and is affected by a variety of factors, mostly related to the type of valve implanted and to the hemodynamic conditions after implantation. In a report of 278 patients, mild subclinical hemolysis was identified at 12 months in 26% of patients with a mechanical prosthesis and in 5% with a bioprosthesis. On multivariate analysis, independent predictors of the presence of subclinical hemolysis were mitral valve replacement, use of a mechanical prosthesis, and double valve replacement. Among mechanical valve recipients, double versus single valve replacement and mitral versus aortic valve replacement were correlated with the presence of hemolysis; double valve recipients also showed a more severe degree of hemolysis. Valve-associated anemia is seldom severe. The amount of hemolysis is assessed based on serum levels of LDH and haptoglobin and on the presence and amount of reticulocytes and schistocytes in the peripheral blood. Treatment of hemolysis includes the supplementation of iron and folate when their deficiency is evident. The use of β-blockers appear to decrease the severity of hemolysis, likely through induction of bradycardia and negative inotropic effects.

Vitamin B_{12}, Folate, and Homocysteine

Older adults are more likely than younger adults to have lower concentrations of serum vitamin B_{12} and folate. In epidemiologic studies, approximately 10% of apparently healthy adults ≥70 years old were found to have low serum vitamin B_{12} levels, and 5%–10% were found to have low serum folate concentrations. Low serum vitamin B_{12} and serum folate concentrations are not necessarily accompanied by macrocytosis or evidence of megaloblastic anemia. Atrophic gastritis leading to vitamin B_{12} malabsorption is the likely cause in most cases of vitamin B_{12} deficiency. Surgery in the GI tract, such as resection of the terminal portion of the small intestine or gastrectomy, also causes malabsorption of vitamin B_{12}. Although gastritis can also contribute to low folate levels in older adults, alcohol abuse, drug interactions with folate absorption, and inadequate dietary intake, in particular strict vegan diets without appropriate vitamin supplementation, are the most common causes of low folate levels. Some evidence suggests that low serum vitamin B_{12} levels may contribute to cognitive decline in older adults. There is no question that severe vitamin B_{12} deficiency can result in cognitive loss and significant neurologic deficits. However, in most demented patients, vitamin B_{12} deficiency is not the cause of their dementia. Nevertheless, aggressive replacement should always be undertaken when a patient with dementia presents with low serum vitamin B_{12} or low serum folate concentrations.

Even in patients with atrophic gastritis, oral vitamin B_{12} is generally adequate; 1%–2% of orally administered vitamin B_{12} will be absorbed by mass action alone and does not require the presence of intrinsic factor. Thus, patients with vitamin B_{12} concentrations in the low-to-normal range should receive a daily oral dose of 1 mg (1,000 mcg). Oral vitamin B_{12} is equally effective as parenteral replacement, and it also provides a significant cost-advantage. In patients with severe vitamin B_{12} deficiencies (ie, concentrations <100 pg/mL) or with neurologic symptoms, parenteral replacement of 1,000 mcg/d for 1 week initially via intramuscular (or deep subcutaneous) route, then 1,000 mcg/week for 1 month, and then reduced to 1,000 mcg/month for maintenance, should be used. In older adults with low-normal serum vitamin B_{12} concentrations (<300 pg/mL), measuring methylmalonic acid (MMA) concentrations has been suggested to exclude metabolically active B_{12} deficiency. Kidney failure can artificially increase the serum MMA concentration. In those patients with low-normal serum vitamin B_{12} concentrations and macrocytosis (with or without anemia) or neurologic changes, vitamin B_{12} replacement should be considered, particularly if the MMA concentration is increased. Levels of serum vitamin B_{12} should be checked at 4 weeks to assess repletion. Folic acid can be replaced in dosages ranging from 1 to 5 mg/d for 3–4 months (1 mg/day is usually sufficient). At these dosages, homocysteine concentrations decrease (analogous to the decrease in MMA when vitamin B_{12} is replaced).

Low concentrations of serum vitamin B_{12} or folate are accompanied by increased concentrations of homocysteine. Epidemiologic studies initially found that B_{12} and folate deficiencies with high levels of homocysteine are associated with cardiovascular disease; however, subsequent trials of homocysteine lowering through vitamin therapy did not reduce end points such as stroke and myocardial infarction, and may increase cancer risk. Increased serum homocysteine concentrations are common in patients with renal impairment and, for this reason, should be interpreted with caution.

Platelets and Coagulation

Bleeding diatheses are not uncommon in older adults. Unexplained bruises, recurrent nosebleeds, GI blood loss, or excessive blood loss during surgery or after dental extraction are common presentations. In these patients, screening platelet counts and coagulation studies should be obtained. Tests of platelet aggregation are useful in detecting disorders of platelet function.

Thrombocytopenia is a common cause of bleeding problems in older adults. For diagnostic purposes, a platelet count <150,000/μL may be significant, but bleeding usually occurs at much lower levels. Common causes include decreased production of platelets in the bone marrow, sequestration in enlarged spleens, and increased peripheral destruction. Decreased production of platelets occurs in the leukemias, marrow aplasia, or most commonly in older adults in association with medications that suppress platelet production. The major cause of increased peripheral destruction is immune thrombocytopenia. The incidence of immune thrombocytopenia peaks in patients >60 years old. Although most cases remain idiopathic, lymphoma, collagen vascular disease, or drug-induced causes are more common in older adults with autoimmune thrombocytopenia than in younger individuals. Treatment of thrombocytopenia depends on the cause. For decreased production, platelet transfusion should be considered if there is significant blood loss, irrespective of the platelet count. Generally, nontraumatic bleeding occurs when the platelet count drops to ≤10,000/μL. Because immune thrombocytopenia is often secondary to some other underlying disorder in older adults, the initial approach is to identify and treat the primary cause. If no cause is found, a trial of corticosteroids is warranted. Isolated thrombocytopenia in older adults should prompt an evaluation to exclude MDS, particularly when the low platelet count is thought to be secondary to inadequate production. DIC and TTP-HUS are also important causes of thrombocytopenia in the older age group, and they should be recognized and treated appropriately. Patients with TTP-HUS seldom bleed, even when the platelet count is profoundly low. Platelet replacement in this disorder has a strong relative contraindication because of the increased risk of thrombosis.

Platelet function disorders, although uncommon, can cause bleeding in older adults receiving aspirin or nonaspirin NSAIDs. However, platelet dysfunction may be severe enough to cause bleeding without drug exposure. Also, platelet-inhibiting drugs may cause bleeding in the absence of a primary platelet disorder. Platelets exposed to aspirin (an irreversible inhibitor of cyclooxygenase) are impaired for their lifetime. In contrast, platelets exposed to nonaspirin NSAIDs (reversible cyclooxygenase inhibitors) are only transiently affected. For this reason, bleeding risk may be higher in patients receiving aspirin than in those receiving nonaspirin NSAIDs. In addition to these analgesic medicines, platelet function can be impaired by administration of drugs used to prevent or treat acute cardiovascular events. Dipyridamole (an adenosine deaminase inhibitor) is used in combination with aspirin and may increase bleeding risk beyond that seen in patients treated with aspirin alone.

P_2Y_{12} is a platelet receptor for ADP that plays a role in platelet release and aggregation. Clopidogrel and prasugrel are irreversible P_2Y_{12} inhibitors that are used either alone or with aspirin, impair platelet function, are associated with occurrence of TTP, and may predispose to bleeding. Ticagrelor is a reversible inhibitor of P_2Y_{12} and has an adverse-event profile similar to that of prasugrel. It is unknown whether ticagrelor is associated with TTP. Platelet glycoprotein IIb/IIIa inhibitors (abciximab, eptifibatide, tirofiban) are used in patients with acute coronary syndromes and can be associated with immediate onset of profound and transient thrombocytopenia and may cause life-threatening bleeding. In the rare circumstance, spontaneous bleeding occurs or is precipitated by injury or surgery. In this case, platelet transfusions may be needed.

Hereditary von Willebrand disease (vWD) can first present in older adults and is categorized as type 1, 2, or 3. Type 1 vWD, the most common type, is usually mild and is frequently the type found in the older population, because these patients may not have previously had a hemostatic challenge sufficient enough to cause bleeding. It is caused by a reduced concentration of von Willebrand factor (vWF) accompanied by a reduced concentration of factor VIII. Type 2 vWD has 4 subtypes (2A, 2B, 2M and 2N) and is associated with a qualitative defect in vWF, whereas type 3 vWD, the most rare type, occurs when there is a severe deficiency in vWF and is characterized by bleeding similar to that seen in patients with severe hemophilia. Acquired von Willebrand syndrome, although rare, is a disease of older adults. It is commonly associated with monoclonal gammopathies, lymphomas, hypothyroidism, myeloproliferative diseases, or myeloma. These patients tend to have phenotypes similar to those seen in patients with hereditary type 1 and type 2A vWD. When treatment is necessary, desmopressin acetate may be used for patients with type 1 vWD. Desmopressin is relatively contraindicated in patients with type 2A disease and strongly contraindicated in the other types of vWD.

Bleeding can also occur because of clotting factor deficiencies, which in older adults are usually acquired and caused by the presence of circulating clotting factor inhibitors. Rarely, older male patients may present for the first time with mild hemophilia and, even more rarely, older female patients may present as hemophilia carriers with minimal decreases in coagulation factor VIII or factor IX levels. The most common acquired factor deficiency is caused by an inhibitor to factor VIII. The onset is often sudden. Titers of antifactor VIII antibodies can be very high, and presentation is with bleeding into soft tissue and muscle. This is in contrast to the presentation of a patient with congenital hemophilia, which is commonly hemarthrosis. Treatment involves factor replacement or activated factor VII concentrate, or factor VIII inhibitor bypassing activity concentrate (FEIBA®); depending on the severity, prednisone or cyclophosphamide may also be needed.

Deficiency of the vitamin K–dependent clotting factors tends to occur in older adults with major illnesses. Disorders of the hepatobiliary tree, antibiotics that neutralize bowel bacteria (a major source of vitamin K), malabsorption, and severe malnutrition are the common causes. The deficits are readily treated with vitamin K. All patients requiring reversal of warfarin should receive vitamin K replacement either orally or intravenously, depending on the acuity of the circumstance. The subcutaneous administration of vitamin K is discouraged because of a slower time to correction of the prolonged INR and variable absorption. In patients receiving warfarin with severe bleeding and who are unable to receive fresh frozen plasma or in those in need of urgent reversal, a 4-factor prothrombin complex concentrate (Kcentra®) or 3-factor prothrombin complex concentrate plus recombinant activated factor VIIa (Profilnine® + rHFVIIa) may be administered. Patients with previous episodes of immune-mediated heparin-induced thrombocytopenia should not receive Kcentra®, because it contains trace amounts of heparin.

Liver disease must always be considered in patients who present with excessive bleeding. The prothrombin time is prolonged even in mild to moderate liver disease because of the short plasma half-life of factor VII. The partial thromboplastin time remains normal until liver disease becomes severe, because the half-lives of the coagulation factors effecting the partial thromboplastin time are more prolonged. Except for factor VIII (which is produced by endothelial cells), all clotting factors are eventually reduced. The degree of these reductions depends on the severity of liver impairment. Liver disease is also associated with DIC; fibrin degradation products are not cleared as well, platelet function can be affected, and tissue plasminogen activator and plasmin remain in the circulation longer, which adds to the predisposition toward bleeding, and, paradoxically, these same patients may have an increased risk of venous thrombosis. The treatment of a bleeding diathesis in liver disease is fresh frozen plasma or a nonactivated prothrombin complex concentrate. Sometimes, the platelet function defect is responsive to cryoprecipitate infusion or administration of desmopressin.

CHRONIC MYELOPROLIFERATIVE NEOPLASMS

The Philadelphia chromosome–negative chronic myeloproliferative neoplasms—polycythemia vera (PV), essential thrombocythemia (ET), and idiopathic myelofibrosis (IMF)—have overlapping clinical features but exhibit different natural histories and different therapeutic requirements. All 3 disorders are seen primarily in the older age group and are characterized by involvement of a multipotent hematopoietic progenitor cell, marrow hypercellularity, overproduction of one or more marrow lineages, thrombotic and hemorrhagic diatheses, exuberant extramedullary hematopoiesis, and a slow rate of spontaneous transformation to acute leukemia. The diagnostic criteria for PV, ET, and IMF adopted by the World Health Organization include the identification of clonal markers. JAK2 V617F is present in about 95% of patients with PV and in about half of patients with ET and IMF. In JAK2 V617F–negative patients, JAK2 mutations are found in 2%–4% of patients with PV but have not been identified in patients with either IMF or ET. Other mutations of significance include the MPL (myeloproliferative leukemia) W515 mutation and the calreticulin mutation. Somatic MPL mutations (eg, W515L and W515K) have been detected in a small percentage of patients with ET and IMF. The calreticulin gene has been described in 50%–71% of patients with ET, and 56%–88% of patients with IMF that are JAK2 and MPL mutation negative. The presence of a calreticulin mutation and mutations of JAK2 or MPL are mutually exclusive. Patients with a calreticulin mutation have a superior outcome when compared with that or patients with JAK2-mutated or MPL-mutated ET or IMF.

Polycythemia vera, ET, and IMF have a long natural history, distinguishing them from chronic myeloid leukemia, the Philadelphia chromosome–positive myeloproliferative disorder, which progresses and transforms much more rapidly. The main cause of morbidity and mortality in PV and ET is thrombosis, which occurs more commonly in older adults or in those with previous vascular complications. Severe bleeding is rare and limited to patients with a very high platelet count or to those taking antiplatelet drugs. Cytotoxic therapy is effective in preventing thrombosis but increases the risk of leukemic transformation. Because there is no curative therapy for PV and ET, the goals of therapy are to minimize thrombotic risk and to prevent progression to marrow fibrosis or acute leukemia, or both.

Several different treatment strategies for PV have been tested in randomized clinical trials. In the PV Study Group (PVSG-01) trial, 431 patients were randomized to one of the following: phlebotomy alone, 32P (a myelosuppressive agent) plus phlebotomy, or chlorambucil plus phlebotomy. The median survival time in the three arms was 13.9 years, 11.8 years, and 8.9 years, respectively. In the phlebotomy-only arm, thrombotic deaths were higher, particularly in the first 2–3 years. In the other two arms, the incidence of leukemic transformation was higher. The risk of thrombotic events is highest in those ≥60 years old and in those with a prior history of thrombosis. Given these findings, current treatment recommendations include the following:

- Phlebotomy in all patients to maintain hematocrit <0.45

- Myelosuppressive agents like hydroxyurea in patients at high risk of thrombosis (>60 years old) and in those with excessive phlebotomy requirements

- Hydroxyurea and an antiplatelet agent for symptomatic thrombocytosis

32P, busulfan, pegylated interferon, and anagrelide remain as viable options in these patients; however, they are usually reserved for patients with disease that is difficult to control. Patients receiving anagrelide have been reported to have an increased risk of developing myelofibrosis and arterial thrombosis. Pegylated interferon is effective but may not be well tolerated. Additionally, given the results of the European Collaboration on Low-dose Aspirin in Polycythemia Vera trial, low-dose aspirin is recommended for all patients with PV. In this trial, 531 patients with PV were randomized to receive either no aspirin or low-dose aspirin. In those treated with aspirin, cardiovascular mortality was reduced by 59%, with a nonsignificant risk of increased bleeding.

The incidence of thrombotic and hemorrhagic complications in ET was analyzed in 1,850 patients from 21 retrospective cohort studies. Rates of thrombosis ranged from 7% to 17%, and rates of hemorrhage from 8% to 14%. Age >60 years, a prior thrombotic event, and a long duration of thrombocytosis are the major risk factors for thrombotic events. Consensus-based practice guidelines for ET include observation in asymptomatic low-risk patients with platelet counts <1,500 × 10^9/L, and hydroxyurea plus aspirin in high-risk patients with platelet counts ≥1,500 × 10^9/L. Anagrelide is also very effective at reducing high platelet counts. However, a randomized trial comparing hydroxyurea plus aspirin to anagrelide plus aspirin demonstrated that hydroxyurea was more effective and associated with less adverse events. Hydroxyurea appears to be associated with a better overall survival, less serious hemorrhagic events, and fewer fibrotic transformations than anagrelide. ET, like PV, has a long natural history with a low incidence of leukemic transformation. In contrast, IMF progresses much more rapidly, with median survival of 3.5–5.5 years. Roxuolitinib, a JAK1 and JAK2 inhibitor, has been approved for treatment of symptomatic patients with IMF or myelofibrosis developing as a result of ET, or PV. Although this therapy does not offer a cure, it does considerably reduce spleen size and untoward symptoms in selected patients.

REFERENCES

- Ganz, T. Hepcidin and iron regulation, 10 years later. *Blood.* 2011;117(17):4425–4433.

    This review explains how iron metabolism is regulated and the pathophysiology of iron-restricted anemias.

- Garcia-Manero G. Myelodysplastic syndromes: 2014 update on diagnosis, risk-stratification, and management. *Am J Hematol.* 2014;89(1):97–108.

    This review updates the current approach to diagnosis and makes treatment recommendations based on risk stratification.

- Geiger H, de Haan G, Florian MC. The ageing haematopoietic stem cell compartment. *Nat Rev Immunol.* 2013;13(5):376–389.

    This review describes the effect of time on the hematopoietic stem cell. It speculates on the pathophysiology of anemia in older adults at a molecular and biochemical level.

- Nemeth E, Ganz T. Anemia of inflammation. *Hematol Oncol Clin North Am.* 2014;28(4):671–681.

    This review provides a thorough explanation of the pathophysiology of the anemia of chronic disease.

- Pang WW, Schrier SL. Anemia in the elderly. *Curr Opin Hematol.* 2012;19:133–140.

    Using data from NHANES III and studies of more comprehensive hematologic evaluation, this article describes the epidemiology of anemia in older adults. The authors find that myelodysplastic syndromes are an important cause of anemia in older adults and that up to 50% of anemia in the older age group is unexplained.

- Powers JM, Buchanan GR. Diagnosis and management of iron deficiency anemia. *Hematol Oncol Clin North Am.* 2014;28(4):729–745.

    This article does not target iron deficiency specifically in older adults but provides an excellent review of the topic, which also applies to the aged.

Roy E. Smith, MD, MS
Gurkamal S. Chatta, MD

CHAPTER 66—ONCOLOGY AND HEMATOLOGIC MALIGNANCIES

KEY POINTS

- Older adults and black Americans of all ages are more likely to develop cancer and present with more advanced disease.

- Older age has a variable association with the aggressiveness and growth rate of malignant tumors.

- Surgery, radiation, chemotherapy, and biologic therapies are safe and effective treatment interventions for older cancer patients when appropriate precautions are taken based on the patient's comorbidities, vital organ functions, and medications.

- There has been no demonstrated age-associated resistance to chemotherapy.

- Although some acute toxicities (eg, nausea, vomiting, and hair loss) of chemotherapy are less prominent in older adults, other toxicities such as diarrhea and neuropathy are more common.

- Geriatric assessment can help determine which older patients are more likely to benefit from aggressive cancer treatment and which are most likely to experience toxicity from cancer treatment.

Cancer is a disease associated with aging—most cancer diagnoses and deaths are in people >65 years old. Currently, the median age of patients with a new cancer diagnosis is 70 years. On the basis of the aging of the U.S. population and the known association between cancer and aging, a dramatic increase in the number of new cancer diagnoses is projected for the next 20 years. It is anticipated that patients ≥65 years old will account for 70% of all cancer diagnoses by the year 2030.

According to the National Cancer Institute's Surveillance, Epidemiology and End Results data, over 70% of cancer deaths were in people >65 years old. One in four deaths in the United States is caused by cancer. Overall cancer incidence rates decreased in the most recent time period in both men (1.3% per year from 2000 to 2006) and women (0.5% per year from 1998 to 2006), largely due to decreases in the three major cancer sites in men (lung, prostate, and colorectum) and two major cancer sites in women (breast and colorectum). Among men, death rates for all races combined decreased by 21.0% between 1990 and 2006, with decreases in lung, prostate, and colorectal cancer rates accounting for nearly 80% of the total decrease. Among women, overall cancer death rates between 1991 and 2006 decreased by 12.3%, with decreases in breast and colorectal cancer rates accounting for 60% of the total decrease. Although progress has been made in reducing incidence and mortality rates and improving survival, cancer still accounts for more deaths than heart disease in people <85 years old. After age 85, heart disease becomes the number one killer, and the risk of cancer declines for reasons that are not defined. Because of the paucity of older adults in clinical trials, it is not clear how much of the improvement in treatment has translated to the benefit of older patients. However, when such data have been evaluated (eg, for colon cancer, breast cancer) within clinical trials, it appears that treatment that is effective in younger patients is also effective in older patients (SOE=A). The older patients in clinical trials, however, tend to be healthy (ie, other than having cancer) and are therefore without significant comorbidities or functional impairment.

Although cancer has long been recognized as a disease of older people, emphasis on the interactions of cancer and aging is a recent development. Experimental data and clinical experience have indicated that tumors are not resistant to treatment by virtue of age alone. However, age is associated with reductions in certain organ functions, and these deficiencies in physiologic reserve might be magnified by comorbid conditions. Cancer treatments can therefore be associated with an increase in adverse events, and treatment should be tailored to the individual, taking into consideration potential increased toxicities and balancing this with expectations of survival in the context of comorbidities. Although we have much to learn about providing optimal management of cancer in older adults, especially those who are vulnerable or frail, some research has shown that geriatric assessment can help identify older patients who would most benefit from aggressive treatment and those who are at most risk of toxicities from cancer treatment.

Four questions form the basis of this new emphasis: Why are tumors more common in older adults? Is there a difference in tumor aggressiveness with advancing age? Should treatment be different for older patients? How can cancer treatment be best individualized for older patients?

CANCER BIOLOGY AND AGING

Numerous explanations have been offered as to the biologic connection between cancer and aging, including extended exposure to carcinogens, increased DNA instability resulting in a higher mutation potential, telomere shortening, immune dysregulation, and increased susceptibility to oxidative stress. Although these explanations for the link between cancer and aging are plausible, they do not pinpoint the reason why one older adult is more susceptible to cancer than another. Furthermore, the association between cancer and aging is complex. Population-based studies demonstrate a steady rise in the probability of developing cancer across the strata of age, but few studies have examined cancer prevalence and mortality in the highest age groups.

Explaining the Increased Prevalence of Cancer with Age

The prevalence of cancer increases with age for at least three reasons. First, cancers, particularly those that occur in people >65 years old, are thought to develop over a long period, perhaps decades. This is best exemplified by the current understanding of colon cancer, which has been shown to develop because of an accumulation of several damaging genetic events occurring in a stochastic manner over time. Colon cancer, which occurs via an intermediate precursor (the adenomatous polyp), is an example of the multi-step genetic changes required over time for cancer development. In colon cancer, mutations in tumor suppressor genes such as inactivation of the *APC* and *DCC* genes and subsequent additional genetic defects in the oncogenes such as *K-Ras* promote the accumulation of mutations that lead to carcinogenesis. If mutations are acquired at a constant rate, older people are more likely to have lived long enough to develop the 8 to 10 genetic lesions it takes to develop a malignancy. In contrast, lymphomas are just as likely to occur in young as in old people. Lymphocytes normally undergo gene rearrangements and mutations to generate antigen receptors, and these processes appear to be particularly vulnerable to errors that can lead to lymphoma at any age.

A second reason for the greater prevalence of cancer with advancing age is that DNA repair mechanisms are thought to decline with age. As a consequence, cells can accumulate damage. Normally, a dividing cell pauses in G1 (the gap after mitosis [M] and before DNA replication [S]) and in G2 (the gap after S and before M) to take inventory and repair any damage before proceeding to the next phase. These are the G1 and G2 checkpoints. Older cells may fail to detect or repair damage and fail to accurately control DNA replication. This leads to aneuploidy and uncontrolled proliferation. In younger people, these aberrations can trigger the death of the cell; in older people, the errors may be tolerated and fail to signal cell death. Cells without functioning checkpoints are vulnerable to loss of growth control. Telomere dysfunction and increased epigenetic gene silencing have also been implicated in the pathogenesis of cancers. Telomeres are essential for chromosomal stability; with aging, their length progressively shortens, which interferes with cell division. This instability at the cellular level increases the rate of somatic mutations that predispose to cancer and other disorders like aplastic anemia. Paradoxically, human cancers have developed mechanisms to maintain telomere length for survival. Autophagy is interrupted with aging, which leads to the accumulation of damaged proteins and mitochondria, which in turn are a source of reactive oxygen species and contribute to cancer.

A third contribution to increased cancer incidence in older people may be a decline in the function of the immune system, particularly in cellular immunity. A number of findings suggest that the immune system can recognize and control certain cancers. A decline in immune function may lead to the emergence of a cancer in an older adult that was controlled when that person was younger.

The Different Characteristics of Cancer with Age

A long-held but incompletely documented clinical dogma that cancers in older people are less aggressive or slower growing has not been consistently supported by epidemiologic data from tumor registries or large clinical trials. Such data can be confounded by geriatric problems that shorten survival independently of the cancer (eg, comorbidity, multiple medications, clinician or family bias regarding diagnosis and treatment in older adults, and age-associated life stresses). These factors may counter any primary influence that aging might have on tumor aggressiveness. Despite these uncertainties, however, there is experimental support for the contention that tumor aggressiveness declines with age. Data obtained from laboratory animals with a wide range of tumors under highly controlled circumstances demonstrate slower tumor growth, fewer experimental metastases, and longer survival in old mice. Tumor growth involves several levels of interaction between the tumor and the host. It may be that tumor angiogenesis is impaired in older people, thereby controlling the rate of tumor growth. The clinical importance of this work is limited, inasmuch as it is difficult to know in any given individual whether the course of the disease will be characterized by an indolent or aggressive pattern of growth.

Breast cancer is the most notable clinical example of an age-associated decline in tumor aggressiveness. Older patients are more likely to have more favorable histologic types, higher levels of estrogen- and progesterone-receptor expression, lower growth fraction, and less frequent metastases. In a published series on breast cancer patients with primary tumors ≤1 cm in diameter, the single most important predictor of metastasis to axillary nodes has consistently been found to be patient age: patients <50 years old have the highest likelihood of spread, whereas those >70 years old have the lowest likelihood of spread. Stage for stage in breast cancer, older patients seem to have longer survival times than younger patients (SOE=A).

By contrast, Hodgkin disease seems to be a more aggressive disease in older patients. The most likely reason for the age-associated differences in prognosis is that Hodgkin disease is a different disease in patients ≥45 years old than in younger patients. Incidence data demonstrate two distinct peak incidence rates, one at age 32 years and one at age 84 years. The frequency of particular histologic subtypes of Hodgkin disease is different in younger and older patients: nodular sclerosis is the most common subtype in younger patients, whereas mixed cellularity is the most common in older patients. In all reported treatment series, older age is an independent prognostic factor. Additional study is necessary to document age-associated differences in tumor cell biology.

Acute leukemia, like Hodgkin disease, appears to be a different disease in older people; the MDR1 drug resistance pump (which eliminates toxins, including certain cancer chemotherapy agents, from the cell) is more commonly expressed, response to treatment is less, and survival time is shorter than in younger patients.

However, for most cancer types, the molecular biology and clinical behavior of the tumor is similar across the age span.

Ethnic Differences in Cancer Incidence and Mortality

As the demographics of the U.S. population changes, additional information is needed on incidence and on natural history differences in cancers that develop in different ethnic and racial groups. There is a lack of basic data about aging minority populations. This is largely because of small sample sizes of these populations and to language barriers that prevent certain racial and ethnic groups from participating in survey research. The U.S. Census Bureau estimates that by 2050, Hispanic Americans will account for nearly 25% of the population, and black Americans, Asian Americans, and Native Americans combined will total another 25%. By the year 2050, under current projections, U.S. numbers in minority populations are expected to outpace the number of white Americans. Although the number of older white Americans is anticipated to double to 62 million, the number of older black Americans will nearly quadruple to over 9 million. Older Hispanics will total about 12 million, 11 times as many as in 1990. The number of American Indian and Alaska Natives will grow to 562,000, and the number of older Asian and Pacific Islanders will approach 7 million.

Cancer incidence and death rates are lower in other racial and ethnic groups than in white and black Americans for all cancer sites combined and for the four most common cancer sites. Overall, black Americans have the highest cancer incidence and mortality rates. Cancer incidence among black Americans is 10% higher than among white Americans, 50%–60% higher than among Hispanic Americans and Asian Americans, and more than twice as high as among Native Americans. Black Americans with cancer have shorter survival times than white Americans at all stages of diagnosis. Relative 5-year survival rates are higher among people diagnosed at younger ages (52% among black Americans diagnosed before age 45) than in those diagnosed at older ages (43% among those diagnosed after age 75). The cancer death rate for black Americans is about 30% higher than for white Americans and more than twice as high as for Hispanic Americans, Asian Americans, and Native Americans.

The factors contributing to the ethnic differences are not defined. However, certain data suggest that when the quality of the health care delivered to white and black Americans is similar, disease outcomes in the two groups are comparable (SOE=B).

PRINCIPLES OF CANCER MANAGEMENT

Randomized clinical trials are the most reliable method of studying medical intervention, and treatment decisions are best founded on their results. However, despite efforts from the cooperative oncology groups, patients entered into trials are by and large younger and presumably healthier than the typical older patient with the same disorder. Only 3% of older patients are treated in clinical trials. There is little evidence of efficacy and tolerability of cancer treatment in older patients, especially those who are >75 years old and/or vulnerable because of comorbidities. Furthermore, common endpoints of these trials are length of survival (for therapeutic interventions) or disease-specific deaths (for prevention studies), which are not always the most appropriate outcomes for older patients (because of their inherently limited remaining life expectancies on the basis of age alone). More and more, clinical researchers are addressing issues of geriatric oncology. New, geriatrics-oriented trials are focusing more on symptom reduction and quality-of-life outcomes than on life expectancy. Surveys have indicated that many older adults, when fully informed, most often choose life-extending treatments, even at the risk of toxicity. Because of physiologic changes in older adults, there is potential for an increase in adverse events associated with standard chemotherapy and other cancer management options. However, for the most part, tumors are not more resistant to treatment in older adults (SOE=B), and acute toxicities (eg, nausea, vomiting, hair loss) may be less prominent in this population (SOE=B). Thus, although quality of life remains a primary treatment consideration, older adults should not be denied efforts at extending life on the basis of age alone.

Oncologists are often faced with the challenge of making management decisions in older adults in the absence of evidence-based guidelines. Aging is associated with a multitude of physiologic changes, which in turn are magnified by medical comorbidities and other geriatric problems. Appropriate treatment for cancer can be safe and effective in older adults if an adequate assessment is done and appropriate precautions are undertaken. Unfortunately, the fear of treatment-related adverse events and lack of evidence-based data leads to the undertreatment of cancer and decreased survival in this population. Life expectancy based on chronologic age is heterogeneous, with comorbidities, disability, and geriatric syndromes having a substantial impact. After estimating the life expectancy, it should be determined whether the benefit of the suggested treatment is likely to be realized in the remaining life span. This consideration is important when making treatment decisions about adjuvant therapy. Assessment of underlying health status is also important for older patients with advanced cancer, for whom the benefits of treatment may be low and the toxicity of treatment high. The geriatric assessment is the gold standard for evaluation of the older patient; it provides an assessment of the global health of the patient, including an evaluation of functional status, comorbid medical conditions, cognition, nutrition, polypharmacy, psychological status, social support, and geriatric syndromes. Each domain is an independent predictor of morbidity and mortality in older patients.

Guidelines for both the assessment of the older patient with cancer and treatment algorithms are in progress, with the National Comprehensive Cancer Network's Senior Adult guidelines being the most well developed (www.nccn.org/professionals/physician_gls/f_guidelines.asp [accessed Jan 2016]).

Assessment of the Older Cancer Patient

Data regarding the application of the geriatric assessment to patients with cancer and the use of it to determine the capacity of patients to tolerate treatment are growing. Several abbreviated versions of geriatric assessment are being evaluated for their ability to predict treatment tolerability. Even these tools need to be applied and interpreted with good clinical judgment. An 85-year-old man who was mowing his lawn last month but now presents with a tumor-related decline in function is much more likely to tolerate therapy than a person whose baseline level of activity was poor.

Although the commonly used Karnofsky Performance Status and Eastern Cooperative Oncology Group (ECOG) performance measures do correlate with treatment toxicity, these tools alone do not predict outcomes as well as geriatric assessment in older adults.

Although data are growing, few oncology trials that have provided evidence for cancer treatment in older adults have included geriatric assessment. Geriatric assessment can detect issues pertinent to cancer management that would go unrecognized otherwise. Dependence on others for assistance with basic activities and instrumental activities of daily living (ADLs, IADLs) has been shown to be predictive of mortality in geriatric oncology patients, and it has been observed that older patients with cancer have a higher incidence of ADL and IADL deficiencies than age-matched controls. The prevalence of comorbidity increases with age and can affect survival of patients with advanced cancer. Polypharmacy can complicate cancer treatment and increase the risk of adverse events from chemotherapy. Weight loss is a marker of declining nutritional status and is often observed in the geriatric population, particularly in those who are frail. Studies of community-dwelling geriatric patients found a 2-fold increased risk of mortality in those patients with weight loss of 5% of body weight. Approximately 20% of community-dwelling older adults screen positive for some degree of cognitive disorder. The presence of cognitive disorders, particularly more advanced disease, may limit life expectancy and influence the decision to institute cancer-related treatment. Additionally, patients with cognitive disorders may have more difficulty reporting treatment-related adverse effects. In addition, studies have identified depression as a significant prognostic factor in patients undergoing treatment for cancer. In both geriatric and oncology literature, social isolation has been associated with increased risk of mortality. Older cancer patients, in general, require considerable support from a caregiver. Research has also found that social support, such as marital status, can independently affect cancer outcomes. In studies that have evaluated the impact of geriatric assessment on survival in older cancer patients, factors that were independently associated with overall survival have included low albumin, ECOG performance status ≥2, positive geriatric depression screen, advanced stage disease, malnutrition, and advanced age.

Geriatric assessment domains can also help estimate the risk of severe toxicity from chemotherapy. In one study of 500 patients, geriatric assessment factors were associated with grade 3–5 toxicity. Patients ≥65 years old with cancer (and from seven institutions) completed a prechemotherapy geriatric assessment. Grade 3–5 toxicity occurred in 53% (50% grade 3, 12% grade 4, 2% grade 5). Risk factors for grade 3–5 toxicity included age ≥73 years, cancer type (gastrointestinal or genitourinary), standard dose, poly-chemotherapy, falls in last 6 months, assistance with IADLs, and decreased social activity. In a second study, which developed The Chemotherapy Risk Assessment Scale for High-Age Patients (CRASH) Score, over 500 patients ≥70 years old who were starting chemotherapy completed a geriatric assessment. Severe toxicity was observed in 64% of patients. The best model for hematologic toxicity included IADL score, LDH level, diastolic blood pressure, and chemotherapy toxicity. The best predictive model for nonhematologic toxicity included performance status, Mini–Mental score (cognition), Mini-Nutritional Score, and chemotherapy. Overall, these predictive risk stratification schemes allow clinicians to identify which patients are at highest risk of chemotherapy toxicity, and could be used in further research to identify and apply interventions to reduce development of chemotherapy toxicity in vulnerable older populations.

Geriatric assessment requires a multidisciplinary approach and analysis of the data to create a personalized plan. Incorporation of a geriatric assessment into care of older adults improves outcomes by preventing disability and reducing hospitalizations, and it may prove beneficial for older cancer patients. Recent studies have shown that geriatric assessment is feasible in oncology clinical assessment and cooperative group clinical trials, and that factors within geriatric assessment can predict toxicity from chemotherapy. Geriatric assessment can help stratify patients into "fit," "vulnerable," and "frail" subgroups. This stratification scheme can help to identify patients who would most benefit from standard treatments and those who would be at highest risk of toxicity. More data are necessary to examine whether geriatric assessment and interventions can improve outcomes. It is likely that support from a multidisciplinary expertise, including social work, physical therapy, occupational therapy, and nutrition can help develop geriatric assessment–guided interventions for an at-risk older adult with cancer. For example, studies have shown review of medication usage by a pharmacist can decrease suboptimal prescribing and potentially lead to a decrease of adverse drug events.

Treatment Options for Older Patients with Cancer

Current forms of cancer treatment include surgery, radiation, chemotherapy, hormone manipulation, and biologic therapy. Age alone does not preclude any of these approaches, but because of normal changes with age in certain organs and also age-associated conditions (comorbidities), special considerations are warranted.

Cancer Screening

Screening for breast, colon, and (in some cases) cervical cancer is recommended. Prostate cancer screening is controversial at any age and is unlikely to benefit someone with <10 years of remaining life expectancy. Lung cancer screening for current or former heavy smokers may have some mortality benefit but is not yet widely endorsed and is not considered standard of care. The American Board of Internal Medicine's Choosing Wisely® recommends considering life expectancy and the risks of testing, overdiagnosis, and overtreatment when recommending cancer screening for older adults. Assessing remaining life expectancy should involve a comprehensive evaluation of health status and include disability, comorbidity, and geriatric syndrome. The trajectory and expected survival from cancer should be balanced with other health status issues to identify the patients most likely to benefit from screening.

Chemotherapy

Aging can be associated with changes in key pharmacologic parameters of antineoplastic agents and in the susceptibility to end-organ toxicity (Table 66.1). Understanding the physiologic aspects of aging is important, because these changes have implications for efficacy and tolerance to chemotherapy. With aging, there are anatomical and structural changes that can adversely impact physiologic reserve in all organ systems. Cancer treatment should be tailored to minimize toxicity, because the loss of reserve is variable. Several changes are important to consider. Older patients have decreased cardiac reserve. Both conventional chemotherapies like doxorubicin and targeted agents like trastuzumab can potentiate heart failure. Older adults are more susceptible to mucositis secondary to change in the mucosal protective mechanism. Intestinal motility, absorptive surface area, and GI blood flow are also decreased and may increase GI toxicity. A decrease in the vital capacity of the lungs, along with impaired gas exchange can increase the toxicity of radiation. The older population is especially susceptible to confusion, syncope, and falls because of change in arterial pressure, cerebral blood flow, and dysequilibrium. The time to recovery from physiologic compromise is also prolonged and is particularly relevant to tissues such as the bone marrow. A dysregulated bone marrow can increase the risk of infection, anemia, and thrombocytopenia, with adverse impact on prognosis.

The most consistent pharmacokinetic change of aging is a progressive delay in the elimination of renally excreted medications because of a reduced glomerular

Table 66.1—Chemotherapy Issues in Geriatric Oncology

Issue	Comments
General	■ Comorbidities and multiple medications add complexity.
Pharmacokinetic changes	■ A progressive delay with age in the elimination of renally excreted medications, due to a reduction in glomerular filtration rate, can account in part for more severe toxicity.
Pharmacodynamic changes	■ Possible enhanced resistance with age to antitumor agents. ■ Increased expression of the multidrug resistance gene has been reported in some older adults. ■ Other proteins that result in drug efflux have been shown to have prognostic importance, but age-associated changes have not been described. ■ Increased tumor hypoxia with age has been observed in a murine model.
Toxicity	■ Mucositis, cardiotoxicity, and peripheral and central neurotoxicity become more common and more severe with aging (SOE=B). ■ Cardiotoxicity is a complication of anthracyclines and anthraquinones, mitomycin C, and high-dose cyclophosphamide; incidence of cardiotoxicity increases with age. ■ Peripheral neurotoxicity with vincristine is more common and more severe in older adults. ■ The incidence of cerebellar toxicity from high-dose cytosine arabinoside increases with age.
Myelotoxicity	■ Chemotherapy-related myelotoxicity can become more severe and more prolonged with aging, but moderately toxic treatment regimens, such as CMF (cyclophosphamide, methotrexate, fluorouracil), cisplatin and fluorouracil, and cisplatin and etoposide are tolerated by many patients ≥70 years old without life-threatening neutropenia or thrombocytopenia (SOE=A). ■ However, infections are markedly increased among older patients with acute leukemia who are undergoing intensive induction treatment; in these cases, it is possible that the disease itself, rather than an age-associated change in "marrow reserve," is responsible for the depletion of hematopoietic stem cells.
Recent advances	■ Granulocyte colony-stimulating factor and granulocyte-macrophage colony-stimulating factor have reduced the incidence of neutropenic infections in patients receiving intensive treatment, and their effectiveness does not appear to be diminished with advancing patient age. ■ Certain new medications or new formulations may be particularly suitable for older patients, eg, oral etoposide and fludarabine, gemcitabine, vinorelbine, capecitabine, paclitaxel protein-bound particles, and liposomal doxorubicin.

filtration rate. The prolonged half-life of these agents can account in part for more severe toxicity. Several chemotherapy agents (eg, cisplatin and capecitabine) are contraindicated or need to be dose-adjusted in renal insufficiency. It is possible to reduce toxicity with appropriate dosing. For example, in a study of women ≥65 years old with metastatic breast cancer, dosages of methotrexate and cyclophosphamide were modified according to creatinine clearance. As a consequence, myelotoxicity was markedly reduced without compromise of therapeutic effect.

Owing to differences in their pharmacokinetics and pharmacodynamics, certain chemotherapy agents can be particularly suitable for treating older patients. Oral etoposide provides valuable palliation for small-cell cancer of the lung and large-cell lymphoma, with minimal risk of complications. Fludarabine, which is very active in lymphoproliferative neoplasms, induces apoptosis of cancer cells, a process that can be altered in malignancies occurring in older adults. Vinorelbine, gemcitabine, and docetaxel are agents that are active against lung and breast cancer and are well tolerated and effective in older adults.

Possible toxicities from chemotherapy should be considered before initiation. Some toxicities occur in higher frequencies in older patients. As mentioned, geriatric assessment can also help identify which patients are at highest risk of toxicities. Toxicities that occur with commonly used chemotherapy agents include neuropathy, GI adverse events such as diarrhea and mucositis, and fatigue. Chemotherapy toxicity can have significant functional consequences in older adults. Neuropathy may have significant consequences for older patients who have other physical performance problems and may increase the risk of falls. Diarrhea can lead to dehydration and delirium. Because older patients may have less resilience in returning to baseline physiologic status after chemotherapy toxicity, "starting low and going slow" is a reasonable approach with chemotherapy, especially for those with metastatic disease for whom chemotherapy is palliative only. In other words, starting therapy with a single agent versus combination agents or starting at a dose reduction may allow for decreased toxicity. More data are needed regarding the balance of efficacy and toxicity with these approaches. Other supportive care practices should be undertaken for an older patient on chemotherapy including frequent visits, close attention to medications (including supportive care medications), evaluation for appropriate social support, and consideration for growth factor use.

Hormonal Therapy

Hormonal treatment is effective in cancers of the breast, prostate, and endometrium. Most of these are well tolerated by older adults and commonly are the treatment of choice in this age group. However, adverse events of hormonal therapies should be considered in older patients. Tamoxifen, a selective estrogen-receptor modulator, has antagonistic and partial agonistic effects. It is a useful therapy in adjuvant treatment of breast cancer and also has estrogen-like positive effects on cardiovascular risk factors and bone disease. Aromatase inhibitors are oral medications that have been proved to be more efficacious than tamoxifen in the adjuvant and metastatic treatment for breast cancer. Although well-tolerated, osteoporosis and fractures are more common in patients on aromatase inhibitors. Treatment with aromatase inhibitor therapy does not negatively impact cognitive function. Hormonal therapies are the first-line of treatment for patients with systemic prostate cancer. The most commonly used hormonal therapies significantly decrease testosterone levels. Because prostate cancer can be an indolent and chronic disease, older men can be subjected to adverse events of hormonal therapies for many years. Growing evidence shows that hormonal therapy is associated with metabolic syndrome, cardiovascular disease, osteoporosis/fractures, and physical performance issues in older men. The decision to start hormonal treatment should not be taken lightly and should include an assessment of life expectancy, prostate cancer severity, and overall health status.

Biologic and Targeted Therapies

Over the last decade, the options for biologic and targeted therapies for cancer have grown significantly. These options have significantly changed the field of oncology. Immunotherapy, or modulation of immune response, is a particularly attractive option in treating older adults, whose natural defenses against cancer can be impaired by immune senescence. Only a limited number of options are clinically available, and these are still clearly inadequate to restore a normal immune response in older adults. Targeted therapies involve options that influence the activity of a specific receptor involved in cancer signaling. These options, including monoclonal antibodies or small molecule inhibitors, are used with chemotherapy or as a single agent, depending on the stage and type of cancer. Adverse-event profiles tend to be different for these agents. For example, many agents (such as the monoclonal antibody bevacizumab and the oral agents sunitinib and sorafenib) target the vascular endothelial growth factor (VEGF) receptor, thereby limiting tumor-related angiogenesis. These agents are associated with hypertension and thromboembolism, which can be a significant issue in patients who already have a history of these conditions. Hypertension can be particularly hard to control, and close interdisciplinary care and communication are necessary to prevent complications.

Several immunotherapy options are available for selected cancers. Recombinant α-interferon at moderate dosages is reasonably well tolerated by patients of all ages. At higher dosages, α-interferon causes myelosuppression, severe fatigue, flu-like illness, malaise, fever, neuropathy, and abnormalities of liver enzymes. Delirium, depression, and dementia after α-interferon use have been reported in patients ≥65 years old. More information on the safety of α-interferon in older patients is needed, particularly because interferon has been shown to be effective therapy for chronic myeloid leukemia, hairy cell leukemia, and multiple myeloma, hematologic malignancies that are more common among older adults (SOE=A). It may also prolong survival after chemotherapy for follicular lymphoma and has been used in renal cell carcinoma. It is being tested at higher, more toxic dosages in patients with stage II melanoma after surgical resection of the primary lesion. About 15% of patients with metastatic melanoma can experience a partial response from α-interferon. However, because of adverse events, interferon is often not chosen as a first-line treatment.

Interleukin-2 is used to treat metastatic melanoma and renal cancer. When administered daily, it may produce partial responses in about 15% of patients and complete remissions, many of which are long lasting, in about 5% of patients. Interleukin-2 can produce severe dose-related toxicity, including capillary leak syndrome, hypotension, adult respiratory distress syndrome, cardiac arrhythmias, peripheral edema, renal failure (prerenal), cholestatic liver dysfunction, skin rashes, and thrombocytopenia. These complications can be life-threatening in any patient, and initiation (especially when other options are available) should be undertaken cautiously.

Recent advances in cancer therapeutics have introduced several new agents in immune therapy. In advanced melanoma, two new immunologic agents are available including ipilimumab, a monoclonal antibody directed at cytotoxic T lymphocyte–associated antigen-4 (CTLA-4), and pembrolizumab, a monoclonal antibody against the programmed death receptor-1 (PD-1). These immunologic agents have unique and significant adverse effect profiles, such as autoimmune-mediated colitis and endocrinopathies. Limited data exist regarding their safety and efficacy in older patients; however, small studies suggest that in fit older patients, safety and efficacy are similar to that in younger counterparts.

Monoclonal antibodies directed against CD20 (rituximab) expressed on B-cell lymphomas and against HER-2/*neu* (trastuzumab) expressed on breast cancer and other epithelial malignancies are effective treatments. These humanized antibodies generally have mild toxicities. Patients can develop hypotension or shortness of breath with the first infusion because of complement fixation. Symptoms abate when the infusion rate is slowed, and such symptoms rarely recur. Although monoclonal antibodies and targeted therapies are thought to be safer than chemotherapy because of decreased risk of myelosuppression, toxicities do occur and supportive mechanisms for older patients should be considered. Of note, many of the newer agents are administered as oral agents. Nonadherence is linked to adverse cancer outcomes, and therefore close monitoring is important.

Antibody-drug conjugates have also been developed in cancer therapeutics. These agents combine a monoclonal antibody directed at a specific cancer target with a cytotoxic agent. An example of this is ado-trastuzumab emtansine (TDM-1), which combines trastuzumab, a monoclonal antibody targeting the her-2/*neu* receptor in breast cancer, with DM-1, a cytotoxic chemotherapeutic. These therapies provide more directed anticancer therapy, although they can still elicit systemic adverse effects.

Radiation Therapy

Radiation therapy provides palliation for virtually all cancers, and it may be part of a treatment plan for lymphomas and cancers of the prostate, bladder, cervix, esophagus, breast, and head and neck area. In combination with cytotoxic chemotherapy, radiation therapy has allowed organ preservation in cancers of the anus, bladder, and larynx, and in extremity sarcomas. A central issue for radiation therapy in older adults is safety. There has been a trend for almost five decades to use radiation therapy as an alternative to surgery in poor surgical candidates, mainly patients ≥65 years old, with the implied expectation that such an approach is less toxic. In fact, published reports have indicated that radiation therapy is both safe and effective in older patients (SOE=A). However, concern remains when treatment involves irradiation of the whole brain (fear of neurologic sequelae, including dementia) or pelvis (fear of marrow aplasia, myelodysplasia, or radiation enteritis), but no systematic investigation has categorically substantiated these concerns.

Advances in radiation therapy include techniques that allow a more restricted radiation field (such as stereotactic techniques for brain and lung), new applications of brachytherapy (insertion of radiation sources into the tumor bed), the development of radiosurgery (gamma ray knife, a precisely focused external beam of radiation) that allows destruction of small lesions (diameter ≤4 cm) of the CNS without craniotomy, and the development of new radiosensitizers.

Surgery

Concerns related to cancer surgery in older adults are safety and rehabilitative potential. Several reports indicate that age itself is not a risk factor for elective cancer surgery, but the length of hospital stay and the time to full recovery become longer with advancing age. Similar results have been reported both from referral centers and community hospitals.

Advances in anesthesia and surgery have benefited older patients. Included among these are endoscopic procedures that provide valuable palliation for the many tumors of the GI tract, and the more widespread use of spinal anesthesia for major abdominal interventions, with a substantial decline in perioperative complications and mortality. More widespread use of laparoscopic surgical techniques and application of laser and photodynamic therapy is also broadening the surgical armamentarium and providing more older patients with potential palliation and cure.

The trend to manage cancer without deforming surgery can preclude the need for complex rehabilitation and can be of special value for older adults. Organ preservation without compromise of treatment outcome is obtainable for cancer of the anus and larynx, and is being studied for cancers of the oropharynx, esophagus, bladder, and vulva. Also, the use of initial (neoadjuvant) chemotherapy before primary surgery has been effective in patients with large primary breast and lung cancers. Such an approach results in less extensive and potentially more curative surgical procedures.

Quality-of-Life Issues

Several studies have determined that the perception of quality of life is highly subjective and poorly reproduced by external observers, even by those who have close relationships with the patient or by health care providers who are very familiar with the patient's physical condition. Furthermore, there is considerable discrepancy between the physician's determination of the patient's quality of life and the patient's own assessment, with physicians tending to underestimate the patient's quality of life (SOE=B).

Early assessments of quality of life focused on functional status and freedom from pain, but these factors, although important, are inadequate for evaluating far-reaching consequences of serious diseases on all domains of life. In the past decade, several instruments for measuring quality of life have been validated and used successfully to study specific problems, such as the effects on quality of life of intensive care, the consequences of limb amputation or of partial and total mastectomy, and iatrogenic impotence. These instruments are questionnaires querying an individual to rate his or her own well-being in several dimensions with a categorical or a visual analog scale. Several scales have been used and validated for older patients with cancer (eg, Functional Assessment of Cancer Therapy and EORTC Quality of Life Questionnaire Core). Unfortunately, these instruments have not been adjusted to the special needs of older adults, and the relationship between geriatric assessment and quality-of-life measurement tools remains unclear. Although it is reasonable to assume that the importance of some factors, such as professional or job satisfaction, may decline with age, the importance of others, including social support and perception of family burden, can become more prominent.

Other problems related to assessing quality of life include the complexity of some questionnaires, which can overwhelm some older adults. In addition, little progress has been made in assessment of quality of life in cognitively impaired individuals. Studies of pain in individuals with dementia have demonstrated the reliability of repetitive behavioral testing in assessing discomfort, even in patients with cognitive impairment. Perhaps the same principles can be applied to assessing quality of life in dementia patients.

At present, the main application of quality-of-life assessment in clinical decision making concerns the choice between interventions yielding comparable survival. An area of potential use is in medical decisions involving limited survival benefits at the price of a decline in quality of life. At present, the value of this trade-off is evaluated with measures known as "quality-of-life adjusted survival" or "quality-adjusted time without symptoms or toxicity," both of which may be important to consider for adults ≥70 years old. Research is needed in the melding of geriatric assessment and quality-of-life instruments.

SPECIFIC CANCERS

Among women, the three most commonly diagnosed types of cancer are cancers of the breast, lung and bronchus, and colorectum, accounting for 50% of estimated cancer cases. Breast cancer alone is expected to account for 29% of all new cancer cases among women. Among men, cancers of the prostate, lung and bronchus, and colorectum account for 48% of all newly diagnosed cancers. Prostate cancer alone accounts for 26% of incident cases in men. Based on cases diagnosed between 1999 and 2005, an estimated 92% of these new cases of prostate cancer are expected to be diagnosed at local or regional stages, for which the 5-year relative survival approaches 100%.

Breast Cancer

Worldwide, nearly a third of breast cancer cases are seen in patients >65 years old; in more developed countries, this proportion rises to more than 40%. Advanced age at diagnosis of breast cancer is associated with more favorable tumor biology as indicated by increased hormone sensitivity and lower grades and proliferative indices. However, older patients are more likely to present with larger and more advanced tumors. Furthermore, there seem to be no major differences in outcomes in stage-matched patients as age increases. Nevertheless, older patients are less likely to be treated according to accepted treatment guidelines, and undertreatment can have an adverse impact on overall outcome. The explanation for these age-related differences in approach to treatment is complex and includes physician and patient bias, psychosocial issues, cost, and proximity to treatment centers. Underlying complexities due to health status also influence decision-making for treatment. Despite the fact that breast cancer occurs mainly in older patients, this population is under-represented in clinical trials. Less than 5% of participants included in clinical trials that evaluate adjuvant chemotherapy are ≥75 years old. Age is a significant predictor of whether older patients with breast cancer are offered entry into clinical trials, when in fact older patients are just as likely as younger patients to participate if given the opportunity. Because comorbidities and functional status significantly affect prognosis and treatment choice, thorough consideration must be given to the overall health of older patients.

For patients with localized cancer, the evidence supports surgical treatment versus primary hormonal treatment. Breast conservation treatment, consisting of breast-conserving surgery (lumpectomy or partial mastectomy) and postoperative radiotherapy, is now recommended as the standard of care for patients of all ages with early disease. As in younger patients, total mastectomy remains a surgical option for older patients who prefer it over breast conservation treatment and for those who decline or are not candidates for postoperative breast radiotherapy. Mastectomy is also indicated in patients with large primary lesions. Axillary lymph node dissection should be done in patients with clinical evidence of axillary lymph node involvement. However, for those without clinical lymph node involvement, the indication for upfront axillary lymph node dissection has been less clear in the older population. Sentinel lymph node dissection has been introduced as an alternative to axillary lymph node dissection. Sentinel lymph node biopsy has been shown to be a safe and accurate method of predicting axillary status in patients with breast cancer, including those ≥70 years old. It is now widely considered an acceptable treatment option in patients of all ages with tumor size <2–3 cm and no clinical evidence of axillary involvement. Findings from such biopsies in older patients with breast cancer could significantly affect subsequent treatment decisions, including adjuvant systemic treatment. Controversy exists regarding the need for complementary axillary lymph node dissection after a positive sentinel lymph node is found. Data suggest that sentinel node sampling is just as accurate as axillary dissection but considerably less toxic (SOE=A).

Controversy surrounds several critical issues in the management of this most common malignancy in older women. These issues include postoperative irradiation after lumpectomy, adjunct hormonal treatment, and initial management of metastatic breast cancer.

Postoperative Irradiation after Lumpectomy

Although irradiation after lumpectomy is safe in women ≥65 years old, it may be a source of significant inconvenience and cost. The value of postoperative irradiation has been questioned because the local recurrence rate of breast cancer may decrease with age, and the inconvenience of daily radiation treatment protocols may outweigh the limited benefits for some. In patients ≥70 years old who receive breast-conserving therapy followed by adjuvant hormonal therapy, omission of adjuvant radiation therapy can be considered. Individuals without adjuvant radiation therapy experience higher rates of local/regional recurrence (4% for tamoxifen alone versus 1% for tamoxifen and adjuvant radiation therapy at 5 years, $P<.001$); however, overall survival was not significantly different between the two groups.

Adjunct Hormonal Treatment

Adjuvant hormonal therapy is recommended for estrogen receptor–positive breast cancer. Aromatase inhibitors are used as first-line treatment in women with estrogen receptor–positive tumors, and the medication is given for at least 5 years. Aromatase inhibitors are both more effective and less toxic than tamoxifen (SOE=A). In women currently on tamoxifen, it is recommended that tamoxifen treatment be continued for a 5-year duration, followed by 5 years of an aromatase inhibitor. The benefits and risks of more prolonged treatment, especially for women >70 years old, remain controversial. Evidence suggests that even frail, older women tolerate aromatase inhibitor therapy well, although this treatment is less likely to be offered by oncologists to this group of patients.

Initial Management of Metastatic Breast Cancer

Women ≥65 years old with metastatic, hormone receptor–positive breast cancer are likely to have effective palliation with hormonal therapy. Hormonal treatment has been shown to benefit older women with hormone receptor–poor tumors, but chemotherapy has also been shown to be safe and effective in this group of patients. Generally, single agents are used, and treatment is begun at full dosage for fit older adults with modifications based on any toxicities that develop. In vulnerable older adults, treatment can usually begin safely at 75% of the recommended dosage.

Lung Cancer

Lung cancer is the leading cause of cancer-related death in Western countries for both men and women. More than 40% of patients diagnosed with lung cancer are ≥70 years old. Management options for lung cancer are based on the cell type. Non–small-cell cancer constitutes around 80% of all lung cancers, with small-cell cancer making up the remaining. Most patients with lung cancer present with stage 4 disease, in which the goal of therapy is palliative. Lung cancer is becoming increasingly common in older women for reasons that are not completely understood. The increase may possibly be due to higher smoking rates among women. In addition, some data suggest that women are at greater risk (than men) of developing lung cancer per unit of tobacco exposure. Early recognition and surgical resection remain the best chance for cure. For patients with lesions in a location that precludes surgery, localized radiation can result in long-term survival. Over the past decade, chemotherapy has produced clinical responses and provided effective palliation for a portion of patients with metastatic disease. A meta-analysis of over 50 trials comparing chemotherapy to best supportive care indicated that chemotherapy is not associated with a worse outcome in older adults and thus paved the way for exploration of better suited regimens. Combination chemotherapy with a platinum doublet is the standard of care for treatment of advanced non–small-cell lung cancer. Historically, oncologists have been concerned about tolerability of platinum-based doublets in older lung cancer patients. A randomized phase III study evaluated patients ≥70 years old with advanced lung cancer determined that this population still benefited from doublet chemotherapy regimens (median overall survival 10.3 months for doublet chemotherapy versus 6.2 months for monotherapy, $P<.0001$) (SOE=A). However, toxic adverse effects were noted more frequently in the doublet chemotherapy arm, and most patients enrolled in the study were felt to be fit.

Colon Cancer

Colonoscopy has become the mainstay of prevention of colon cancer, primarily because it enables direct visualization of the entire colon and biopsy. Polyps do not usually cause symptoms, but they may bleed or predispose to cancer. Colonic polyps are usually classified as neoplastic (adenomas) or non-neoplastic (hyperplastic). Approximately 40% of the U.S. population ≥50 years old have one or more adenomas. Detection and removal of adenomas significantly decrease the morbidity and

Table 66.2—Follow-Up Recommendations Based on Polyp Characteristics

Polyp Characteristics	Repeat Colonoscopy Recommendation (years)
Non-neoplastic	
Hyperplastic, all <1 cm, in rectosigmoid	10
Low-risk adenomas	
Tubular adenoma (1–2), all <1 cm	5–10
High-risk adenomas	
Tubular adenomas (3–10), all <1 cm	3
Tubular adenomas (>10)	<3
Tubular adenoma ≥1 cm	3
Villous adenoma	3
Adenoma with high-grade dysplasia	3
Serrated lesions	
Sessile serrated polyps, all <1cm	5
Sessile serrated polyp ≥1cm	3
Sessile serrated polyp with dysplasia	3
Traditional serrated adenoma	3
Serrated polyposis syndrome	1

SOURCE: Data from Lieberman DA, Rex DK, Winawer SJ, et al. Guidelines for colonoscopy surveillance after screening and polypectomy; a consensus update by the US Multi-Society Task Force on Colorectal Cancer. *Gastroenterology*. 2012;143(3):844–857.

mortality associated with colorectal cancer. Old age and male gender are major risk factors. First-degree relatives of patients with adenomas are also at increased risk of colorectal cancer and should undergo screening. Adenomas are most often detected by colon cancer screening tests, primarily sigmoidoscopy. Because adenomas do not typically bleed, the fecal occult blood test is an insensitive screening method. Older age, villous histology, and size >1 cm are independent risk factors for malignancy within an adenoma. The risk of colon cancer also increases with the number of high-risk adenomas present.

Serrated lesions of the colon are precursors for 20%–30% of colorectal cancers. Serrated lesions are classified pathologically according to the World Health Organization criteria as hyperplastic polyp, sessile serrated adenoma/polyp with or without cytologic dysplasia, or traditional serrated adenoma. These lesions are difficult to detect because they may be the same color as surrounding tissue, have indiscreet edges, are nearly always flat or sessile, and may have a layer of adherent mucus that obscures the vascular pattern. At this time, lacking longitudinal studies, recommendations for surveillance after colonoscopy are based on expert consensus.

Colonoscopy with endoscopic polypectomy is the ideal examination for the detection and removal of adenomatous polyps. The examination should be meticulous, with emphasis to mucosal detail to not miss flat or depressed adenomatous lesions. In addition, a minimum of 6 minutes of colonoscopic withdrawal time is associated with increased polyp yield. Large adenomas that cannot be safely or completely resected endoscopically should generally be removed by segmental colectomy. If a polyp is detected by barium enema, colonoscopy is recommended to establish the histology, remove the polyp, and search for other lesions. If a single polyp is detected by sigmoidoscopy, it should be biopsied. If the polyp is hyperplastic, colonoscopy is not required. If the polyp is adenomatous, full colonoscopy is warranted. In patients with a known history of polyps, discontinuation of surveillance should be considered in those >75 years old in whom a follow-up examination is normal or shows only small tubular adenomas. For follow-up colonoscopy recommendations based on polyp characteristics, see Table 66.2.

A 3-year interval for surveillance colonoscopy is safe and cost-effective for most patients with adenomas. If only a small tubular adenoma is found, the interval may be extended to 5 years; in contrast, after removal of a large villous adenoma, a 1-year follow-up is recommended. After a negative screening or surveillance colonoscopy, an examination interval of 5 years appears to be sufficient. Patients with colorectal cancer should also have regular colonoscopic surveillance for adenomas starting 1 year after surgery, because these patients have adenoma or cancer recurrence rates of 25%–30% at 3 years.

Colorectal cancer is the third leading cause of cancer in the United States and the second leading cause of cancer death. The risk of colorectal cancer increases dramatically with age, with >90% of cases occurring in people >50 years old. Two-thirds of patients with colorectal cancer are ≥65 years old. Women are more likely than men to harbor right-sided colonic adenomas. The risk of colorectal cancer in patients with rectal bleeding is age related and may reach 25% in patients ≥80 years old. Up to 40% of colorectal cancer arises proximal to the splenic flexure, and <10% is within reach of digital rectal examination. Because it is impossible to identify the source of bleeding by clinical criteria, a colonoscopy should be performed in all cases of hematochezia, occult GI bleeding, iron-deficiency anemia, or even melena after a negative upper endoscopy (SOE=C). Other symptoms, such as abdominal pain, altered bowel habits, or pencil-thin feces are less predictive of colorectal cancer but do require thorough investigation, starting with a colonoscopy. Typically, right-sided cancers present with iron-deficiency anemia and occult GI bleeding, whereas left-sided cancers lead to obstructive symptoms, changes in bowel habits, and overt hematochezia.

Surgical excision may be adequate for lesions confined to the colon, but if regional nodes are involved, postoperative adjuvant chemotherapy (usually 5-fluorouracil plus leucovorin) has reduced recurrence by 40%–50% (SOE=A). The addition of oxaliplatin to 5-fluorouracil for adjuvant chemotherapy has improved outcomes for younger patients with regional nodes after resection (ie, stage III disease). Trials that have evaluated this regimen for patients included very few older patients, so more data are necessary. Oxaliplatin may not have the same safety and efficacy profile in the adjuvant setting for older patients with colon cancer. For patients with localized rectal cancer, the standard of care involves a multidisciplinary approach, including oncology, radiation oncology, and surgery, because treatment involves chemotherapy combined with radiation, surgery (most often, abdominoperineal resection involving a colostomy), and postoperative chemotherapy.

The standard of care in patients with stage 4 colorectal cancer is systemic chemotherapy with or without targeted therapy and surgical intervention when appropriate for curative intent or symptom management. Survival of patients with metastatic disease in the liver or other organs has improved significantly because of new medications, such as irinotecan and oxaliplatin, that have induced partial remissions in a subset of patients. Survival has increased from 6 months on average to >2 years for patients who can tolerate treatment. Active debate continues on the use of combination therapy versus monotherapy in the management of older patients with metastatic colon cancer because of a similar overall survival benefit noted in several trials. Capecitabine, an oral 5-fluorouracil pro-drug, is an option for older patients, especially those who are wary of infusional regimens. New medications that target a tyrosine kinase (an integral enzyme for cellular proliferation) within tumor cells and neutralize VEGF (thought to promote angiogenesis) have improved outcomes. Bevacuzimab, a VEGF antibody, has been shown to improve overall survival of older adults when used in combination with standard chemotherapy (SOE=A). The incidence of arterial thromboembolic events increased with age, and caution must be used when prescribing this in older adults. For patients whose colorectal cancer is k-ras wild-type, monoclonal antibodies to the epidermal growth factor receptor can improve survival.

Age per se should not be considered a contraindication for surgery. In patients with hepatic metastasis only, hepatic resection can offer a chance of long-term survival. In selected older patients, this procedure is safe and feasible with a similar survival benefit (SOE=B). Unfortunately, older patients who undergo this procedure are less likely to receive perioperative chemotherapy. Surgical excision of solitary hepatic lesions offers a survival advantage for selected patients, primarily those with smaller lesions, five or fewer lesions confined to a single hepatic lobe, and a longer interval from original tumor resection until the diagnosis of hepatic metastasis.

Gastric and Esophageal Cancers

Cancers originating in the lower esophagus, gastroesophageal junction, and gastric area are treated similarly, because they share a common pathogenesis, regardless of histology. Approximately 60% of esophageal and gastric cancers arise in patients ≥65 years old. Fit older patients with resectable disease should be considered for preoperative chemotherapy with radiation or perioperative chemotherapy in conjunction with surgery. A multidisciplinary approach, including oncology, radiation oncology, and surgery, is very important from the beginning of the decision-making process. In older patients with recurrent and metastatic disease, palliative chemotherapy not only improves overall survival but also improves quality of life. The efficacy and tolerability of a platinum-containing regimen in patients ≥70 years old has been established and is comparable to that in younger patients. The major drawback to combination chemotherapy regimens is the need for a central venous line for administration and high incidence of line-related complications. Similar outcomes have been shown when capecitabine (oral pro-drug of 5-fluorouracil) was substituted for infusional 5-fluorouracil, and when oxaliplatin is substituted for cisplatin. In older patients who cannot tolerate combination chemotherapy, single agent 5-fluorouracil or capecitabine are reasonable options.

Esophageal cancer is commonly diagnosed at an advanced, incurable stage in older patients who are not candidates for tumor resection. These patients are plagued by symptoms of esophageal obstruction or fistula formation, dysphagia, aspiration, and weight loss. In such instances, endoscopic palliation can be achieved with either laser therapy or a single, permanent, metal stent placement. Laser therapy with neodymium-yttrium-aluminum-garnet (Nd:YAG) laser fulgurates the malignant obstructing tissue and restores luminal patency in >90% of cases, with a 5% risk of perforation. Relief can last for up to several months; treatments may be repeated. Photodynamic therapy uses a photosensitizing agent in combination with endoscopic laser exposure. It is more effective than Nd:YAG laser for palliation and has fewer complications, but it can cause skin photosensitivity. Stenting with self-expanding metal stents is preferable therapy for patients with a malignant stricture or an esophagobronchial fistula, because it relieves dysphagia and aspiration in up to 95% of patients and has a low complication rate (SOE=B). The disadvantages of stents include their high cost, tumor ingrowth, and stent migration.

Prostate Cancer

Prostate cancer affects older men disproportionately. The estimated prevalence of prostate cancer in men ≥75 years old is over 1 million, with more than 60% of all new cases diagnosed in men >65 years old. Because of the long natural history of the disease, the case fatality rate is low in the young. It is notable, however, that 70% of men who die of prostate cancer are ≥75 years old. Advanced prostate cancer cannot be cured and affects patients whose disease has spread beyond the prostate and/or are symptomatic, as well as patients with biochemical recurrence only (a rise in prostate-specific antigen with no evidence of disease). Androgen-deprivation therapy (ADT) is used in the initial management of these patients and is associated with a multitude of adverse events, including hot flashes, sexual dysfunction, osteoporosis, and metabolic syndrome. ADT consists of gonadotropin releasing–hormone agonist or antagonist as well as an antiandrogen, and their effects lie in their ability to lower the testosterone levels available to the cancer cells. Given the significant consequence of ADT in older men, serious consideration must be undertaken with the patient regarding risks versus benefits before beginning therapy. For older patients with indolent cancer characteristics and no clinical symptoms, active surveillance should be considered.

In older men, when the disease has progressed on ADT (castrate-resistant prostate cancer), standard-dose chemotherapy is docetaxel every 3 weeks. Subset analysis of the index trials has established that men >75 years old had an equivalent response to that of the younger population with a predictable increase in toxicity. A lower weekly dosage of docetaxel has been studied in an attempt to address the issue of myelosuppression and other adverse events seen with standard-dose chemotherapy. Results from these studies indicate that this schedule has a modest effect on the progression-free survival but does not impact overall survival. Several new regimens have been approved for treatment of castrate-resistant prostate cancer. Abiraterone, which selectively blocks the cytochrome P450 C17 and thereby inhibits androgen biosynthesis, has been shown to improve overall survival in this setting. The trial that led to its approval included patients >75 years old (28% of the study population) who had similar benefit. Overall survival was also improved with sipuleucel-T, an autologous active cellular-based immunotherapy, when compared with placebo in a trial in which the median age was 72 years old (SOE=A).

Bladder Cancer

Age is an independent risk factor for development of transitional cell cancer of the bladder. The median age at diagnosis is 69 years for men and 71 years for women, with the peak incidence at 85 years. With advanced age, there is an increased risk of detecting higher stage and higher grade cancers. Treatment is based on whether the disease is muscle invasive and metastatic or not.

Radical cystectomy with pelvic lymph node dissection and urinary diversion remains the standard of care in patients with clinically localized muscle invasive cancer. However, most older patients never actually undergo this procedure because of a multitude of reasons that include high perioperative morbidity. The patients who undergo this procedure can still have poor oncologic outcomes because of inadequate pelvic lymph node dissection and inadequate use of chemotherapy in the neoadjuvant or adjuvant setting. Alternative approaches like extensive transurethral resection and radiation therapy with chemotherapy are at best only palliative. Bladder-sparing approaches can be considered in patients who are high risk for surgery but are associated with worse overall and cancer-specific survival.

Cisplatin-based therapy is the most effective regimen for patients with this cancer in both the adjuvant and metastatic setting but is associated with various toxicities, including renal insufficiency, nausea and vomiting, myelosuppression and neuropathy. Because of the high prevalence of impaired renal function and other comorbidities in this population, >40% of the population is ineligible for a cisplatin-based regimen. In patients who are not eligible for cisplatin, several other regimens have been studied and include single agent gemcitabine, paclitaxel, combination regimens of gemcitabine/paclitaxel and carboplatin and have all demonstrated modest activity with good tolerance. Hence, when considering therapy for an older patient with bladder cancer, overall benefit should be weighed against adverse effects and remaining life expectancy.

Renal Cell Cancer

The average age at presentation of renal cell cancer is 64 years in both sexes. Currently, >60% of cases are diagnosed incidentally compared with the 1970s when only 10% of cancers were found by chance. As a result, more patients are diagnosed with early stage disease. The treatment for local disease can be surgery (radical or partial nephrectomy) or ablative therapies (radiofrequency, cryotherapy). Even if in most cases surgery is safe, complications such as alteration of renal function may occur, especially in older adults, with physiologic renal impairment at baseline. Given that the growth rate of small renal cell cancer is low and that the capacity to induce dissemination of metastases is limited, active surveillance can be proposed in an asymptomatic setting and in patients who are frail with limited remaining life expectancies. The average growth rate is approximately 0.30 cm per year, and 1% of patients develop metastatic disease.

In advanced disease, the role of cytoreductive nephrectomy to significantly prolong survival, delay time to progression, and enhance the response to systemic biologic therapy in the postoperative period is well established in select young patients with metastatic renal cell cancer. Patients ≥75 years old have a higher risk of perioperative mortality. In spite of this increased early death, the median survival is similar in older versus younger patients. Because of the high perioperative mortality, until more data is available in the targeted agent era, it is perhaps reasonable to consider these agents alone.

In contrast to other malignancies, renal cell cancer is not treated with chemotherapy. For a long time, interleukin-2 and interferon were the only available systemic options for management of renal cell cancer. The toxicities of these cytokines (fatigue, edema, depression, cardiovascular adverse effects) were an obstacle to treatment in both the young and old. Agents targeting tumor angiogenesis (VEGF inhibitor) and intracellular pathways mediating proliferation and growth (mammalian target of rapamycin, an mTOR inhibitor) have demonstrated improved efficacy with a favorable toxicity profile in phase III trials and have largely replaced cytokine treatments. The median age of patients in most of these trials was 62 years, and in all of these studies >30% of the study population was older than 65 years.

These targeted agents have unique adverse effects that can adversely impact outcome in older adults, including diarrhea, hand/foot syndrome, hypertension, cardiovascular toxicity (both ischemia and heart failure), mucositis, skin toxicities, and fatigue. Retrospective subgroup analysis of these trials suggested a similar benefit in patients of all age groups, with similar toxicity and a beneficial effect on quality of life. In the absence of prospective controlled comparison between different agents, when selecting an agent, the toxicity profile and implications of specific comorbid conditions should be taken into account. Comanagement with geriatrics and primary care is necessary to manage hypertension and other cardiovascular toxicities.

HEMATOLOGIC MALIGNANCIES, LYMPHOMAS, AND MULTIPLE MYELOMA

Leukemias

Acute myeloid leukemia (AML) is more likely to be refractory to treatment and to have a smoldering course, for which only supportive care is administered. Increasing age is a poor prognostic factor for AML, independent of cytogenetics. What is not clear is whether the prevalence of unfavorable cytogenetic abnormalities and of multilineage neoplastic involvement increases with age in de novo AML. The subset of patients with myelodysplasia who do not have excess blasts or overt leukemia but are neutropenic and have recurrent infections may benefit from intermittent treatment with granulocyte colony-stimulating factor.

In a trial with older patients with AML, delayed treatment was much less effective than immediate treatment. Although this study established the value of timely chemotherapy, the choice of treatment (whether full-dose induction or low-dose cytarabine) remains controversial. In one study, the survival of older patients with leukemia treated with low-dose cytarabine was better than of those receiving standard induction (because of lower treatment-related mortality). However, others have obtained different results and claimed the superiority of standard treatment. Low-intensity therapy with agents such as 5-azacytadine or decitabine may be considered for older patients, particularly those who are unfit or have significant comorbidities.

Chronic lymphocytic leukemia is the most common form of leukemia in the Western world; about 12,500 cases are diagnosed each year in the United States. The incidence is declining for unknown reasons. The median age at diagnosis is 61 years. The diagnosis is most often made incidentally when a peripheral WBC count reveals leukocytosis with a small-lymphocyte count >4,000/μL. Treatment is generally instituted only to control a life-threatening or symptomatic complication. The major complications are infection and marrow failure. Because about 25% of patients develop autoimmune anemia or thrombocytopenia sometime in the course of the disease, it is important to investigate the mechanism of any decline in peripheral blood cell counts. Autoimmune mechanisms can be treated with glucocorticoids or splenectomy, whereas marrow infiltration by tumor cells requires antitumor therapy. Chlorambucil and fludarabine are the two most active agents, although several targeted therapies are emerging for this disease. Median survival varies with the stage of disease. Once anemia or thrombocytopenia develops as a consequence of marrow failure, median survival is about 18 months.

Non-Hodgkin Lymphoma

Although there are about 38 named varieties of lymphoma, the two most common forms (diffuse large B-cell lymphoma and follicular lymphoma) account for about 75% of cases. The prognosis of non-Hodgkin lymphoma worsens with age, but the explanation remains unclear. It is likely that older adults are more susceptible to the complications of intensive treatment.

The treatment of older adults with diffuse large B-cell lymphoma has improved in recent years. In this group, 60%–70% of patients obtain a durable complete remission with combination chemotherapy (eg, cyclophosphamide, doxorubicin, vincristine, prednisone [CHOP]) plus rituximab (a monoclonal antibody against CD20 on B cells). Administration of lower-than-normal dosages results in a poorer outcome. Hematopoietic growth factors can lessen the hematopoietic toxicity of treatment.

The treatment of follicular lymphoma is more controversial. Localized forms of the disease (seen in 15% of patients) are curable with radiation therapy. In the 85% of patients with more advanced disease, single agent and combination chemotherapy can sometimes induce long, complete remissions (median duration 6–7 years). However, in patients with other serious morbidities and a remaining life expectancy of 5 years, treatment may not be needed because of the indolent nature of the disease progression.

Hodgkin Disease

Hodgkin disease exhibits a curious bimodal age-incidence curve, with a second peak late in life. Compared with younger patients, older patients with advanced disease may respond less well to therapy and have poorer survival rates (SOE=C). Several factors can contribute to this poorer prognosis: more extensive disease at presentation, biologic variations from true Hodgkin disease, greater toxicity with standard treatment regimens, and less aggressive treatment. Older adults can usually tolerate full doses of doxorubicin, bleomycin, vinblastine, and dacarbazine (ABVD) without life-threatening bone-marrow toxicity.

Multiple Myeloma and Monoclonal Gammopathy of Uncertain Significance (MGUS)

Multiple myeloma is diagnosed in about 19,900 people each year in the United States. The median age at diagnosis is 68 years; it is rare in people <40 years old. The incidence in black Americans is twice that in white Americans. The classic triad of myeloma is marrow plasmacytosis (>10%), lytic bone lesions, and a serum or urine (or both) monoclonal gammopathy. Monoclonal gammopathy is common in older adults, estimated at 6% of those ≥70 years old. When an abnormal paraprotein is discovered on serum immunoelectrophoresis, the best diagnostic test to distinguish myeloma from MGUS is a skeletal survey. If the skeletal survey is normal, a bone marrow biopsy is still indicated to determine the presence of marrow plasmacytosis. Patients with MGUS have marrow plasma cells constituting <10% of the total cell number; do not have lytic bone lesions; and usually do not have other features of myeloma, including hypercalcemia, renal failure, anemia, or susceptibility to infection. MGUS progresses to multiple myeloma or a related malignancy at a rate of 1% per year (SOE=B).

Patients with myeloma require treatment when the lytic bone lesions become symptomatic or progressive, infections are recurrent, or the serum paraprotein increases. Standard treatment consists of lenalidomide plus dexamethasone for those who will go on to receive high-dose therapy plus an autologous stem-cell transplant. For those who are not transplant candidates, intermittent pulses of an oral alkylating agent (eg, melphalan), prednisone, and lenalidomide are given for 4–7 days every 4–6 weeks. Supportive care includes bisphosphonates to decrease bone turnover, erythropoietin and other hematinics for the anemia, intravenous immunoglobulin for recurrent infections, radiation for specific symptomatic bone lesions, maintenance of hydration to preserve renal function, and adequate analgesia.

PRINCIPLES OF MANAGEMENT

Both the incidence and prevalence of cancer increase with age, and older adults more often present with advanced-stage disease. Screening older populations for colon and breast cancer can lead to early detection of more curable lesions. Older patients can have less physiologic reserve than younger patients, but unless a specific comorbid illness is influencing baseline organ function, cancer treatments with curative or palliative potential should be offered to most patients in most settings, regardless of age. Curative surgical procedures may require more prolonged convalescence, but recovery from most procedures is expected. Radiation therapy is safe and effective in the same settings in which it is used in younger patients. Chemotherapy may need to be adjusted to the individual patient's level of tolerance of the adverse events, but usually the changes should be made in the face of toxicities that actually develop rather than on toxicities anticipated to develop. Biologic therapies also are generally safe.

> **CHOOSING WISELY® RECOMMENDATIONS**
>
> *Oncology*
>
> - Do not recommend screening for breast cancer, colorectal cancer, or prostate cancer (with the PSA test) without considering life expectancy and the risks of testing, overdiagnosis, and overtreatment.
>
> - Assessing remaining life expectancy should involve a comprehensive evaluation of health status and include disability, comorbidity, and geriatric syndrome.

REFERENCES

- Hurria A, Togawa K, Mohile SG, et al. Predicting chemotherapy toxicity in older adults with cancer: a prospective multicenter study. *J Clin Oncol.* 2011;29(25):3457–3465.

    This landmark study reveals that items within a comprehensive geriatric assessment can predict chemotherapy toxicity in older cancer patients.

- Hurria A, Wildes T, Blair SL, et al. Senior adult oncology, version 2.2014: clinical practice guidelines in oncology. *J Natl Compr Canc Netw.* 2014;12(1):82–126.

    This review notes that chronologic age is not a reliable criterion for deciding whether to use effective therapy in older patients with cancer. Toxicities and response rates are often comparable to those in younger patients. This guideline reviews management decisions for older patients with cancer.

- Lieberman DA, Rex DK, Winawer SJ, et al. Guidelines for colonoscopy surveillance after screening and polypectomy: a consensus update by the US multi-society task force on colorectal cancer. *Gastroenterology.* 2012;143(3):844–857.

    This article provides an update to the 2006 guidelines addressing emerging issues including risk of interval colorectal cancer, proximal colorectal cancer, and the role of serrated polyps.

- Mohile S, Dale W, Hurria A. Geriatric oncology research to improve clinical care. *Nat Rev Clin Oncol.* 2012;9(10):571–578.

    This article provides a model for selecting older oncology patients who would benefit from comprehensive geriatric assessment. It also defines functional risk factors (eg, mobility limitation, frailty, and dementia) and relates this information to risk of toxicities and anticipation of ancillary support needs using a case-based format.

- Wildiers H, Heeren P, Puts M, et al. International Society of Geriatric Oncology consensus on geriatric assessment in older patients with cancer. *J Clin Oncol.* 2014;32(24):2595–2603.

    This study is a review of the role of geriatric assessment in the care of older adults with cancer.

Allison Magnuson, DO
Supriya Mohile, MD, MS

INDEX

Page references followed by *t* and *f* indicate tables and figures, respectively.

A

A-a gradient, 438
Abandonment, 121, 122*t*
Abatacept, 551
Abciximab, 639
Abdominal aortic aneurysm (AAA), 464
    indications for repair, 464
    screening for, 88*t*, 91–92
Abdominal ultrasonography, 88*t*
ABI (ankle-brachial index), 290, 422, 463–464
Abiraterone, 654
Abnormal Involuntary Movement Scale (AIMS), 390
Abscesses
    intra-abdominal, 598
    psoas, 542
Abstinence
    from alcohol, 402–403
    from nicotine, 407
    pharmacotherapy support for, 407
Abuse. *See* Mistreatment
ACA (Patient Protection and Affordable Care Act), 27, 28, 33, 35, 41, 52, 172, 472
Acamprosate, 407, 408*t*
Acarbose (Precose), 626*t*
Accountable care organizations (ACOs), 27, 216
Acculturation, 65
Accumulation theories of aging, 8*t*, 10
ACE (Acute Care for Elders), 170
ACE inhibitors. *See* Angiotensin-converting enzyme inhibitors
Acetaminophen (Tylenol)
    for delirium, 355, 355*t*
    for fibromyalgia, 558
    for OA-related pain, 549
    for persistent pain, 152*t*, 155
    for postsurgical pain, 134
N-Acetylcysteine, 444
Achalasia, 484
Acid-base balance disorders, 502
Aclidinium, 441–442, 442*t*
Acne rosacea, 418–419
ACPA (anti-cyclic citrullinated peptide/protein antibodies), 550
Acquired immunodeficiency syndrome (AIDS), 596–597
    nursing-home financing for care for those with, 198
    treatment and care, 74
Acral lentiginous melanoma, 427, 427*f*
Acromioclavicular disease, 540
ACTH (adrenocorticotropic hormone), 610, 611*t*
ACTH (adrenocorticotropic hormone) stimulation test, 612, 613
Actinic cheilitis, 426
Actinic keratoses, 426, 426*f*
Actinobacillus, 458, 595
Action tremor, 574
Active Choices program, 83

Active listening, 145
Active Living Every Day program, 83
Activities of daily living (ADLs), 46, 46*t*
    Barthel ADL Index, 184*t*, 187
    difficulties with, 5
    family support, 55
Activity Measure for Post Acute Care (AM-PAC), 183, 184*t*
Activity theory, 8
Activity therapy, 347
Acupuncture, 115, 117
Acute back pain, 545
Acute bacterial prostatitis, 528
Acute care, 201–202. *See also* Hospital care
Acute Care for Elders (ACE), 170
Acute colonic pseudo-obstruction, 495
Acute confusional state, 349
Acute coronary syndromes (ACS), 448, 452–453
Acute functional decline, 47–48
Acute inflammatory demyelinating polyneuropathy (AIDP), 576
Acute interstitial nephritis, 505
Acute ischemic stroke, 581–582
Acute kidney injury (AKI), 497, 503–504
Acute leukemia, 644
Acute mental status change, 349
Acute myeloid leukemia (AML), 629, 655
Acute nephritic syndrome, 506
Acute pain, 147
Acute tubular necrosis (ATN), 504–505
Acute urinary retention (AUR), 522
Acyclovir, 424
Adalimumab, 551
ADAMTS 13, 637
Adaptive behavioral difficulties, 413
Adaptive methods, 193, 195
Adaptive servo-ventilation (ASV), 363–364
Addictions, 156, 402–409
    alcoholism, 276*t*
    definition of, 148*t*
    magnitude of the problem, 403–404
    pseudoaddiction, 148*t*, 156
    substance abuse, 402–403
    treatment of, 405–407, 408*t*
Additional sex combs–like transcriptional regulator 1 gene (*ASXL1*), 636
Adenocarcinoma, 516
Adenomas
    colonic, 651–652, 652–653
    gonadotropin-secreting, 611
    pituitary, 610–612
    α-subunit-secreting, 611
Adenomatous polyps, 652, 652*t*
ADEs. *See* Adverse drug events
Adhesive capsulitis (frozen shoulder), 540
ADLs. *See* Activities of daily living

Ado-trastuzumab emtansine (TDM-1), 649
Adrenal androgens, 614
Adrenal cortex disorders, 612–614
Adrenal incidentalomas, 613–614, 613*t*
Adrenal insufficiency, 614
    chronic, 601, 613
Adrenal neoplasms, 613–614
α-Adrenergic agonists
    adverse drug events, 238*t*
    and incontinence, 275*t*
    for postural hypotension, 260
β-Adrenergic agonists, 441–442, 442*t*, 443*t*
α-Adrenergic antagonists or blockers
    adverse drug events, 106, 106*t*
    for benign prostatic hyperplasia, 521, 521*t*
    for hypertension, 479
    and incontinence, 275*t*
β-Adrenergic antagonists. *See* β-Blockers
Adrenocorticotropic hormone (ACTH), 610, 611*t*
Adrenocorticotropic hormone (ACTH) stimulation test, 612, 613
Adrogue-Madias formula, 500
Adult day care, 211, 213*t*
Adult foster care, 214
Adult Protective Services (APS), 124, 211
Advance care planning, 24–25, 334
Advance directives, 18, 23–24, 66–67, 269
    recommendations for, 89*t*, 95*t*, 97
Advance Payment ACO Model, 27
Adverse drug events, 106–107, 106*t*, 385. *See also specific drugs*
    in-hospital, 161
    risk factors for, 105*t*, 106
Advocacy organizations, 59*t*
Aerobic activity recommendations, 78, 79–80, 80*t*, 116
Aerobic exercise, 380. *See also* Exercise
Affective disorders, 276*t*
Afferent pupillary defects, 229
Affordable Care Act (ACA). *See* Patient Protection and Affordable Care Act
Aflibercept (VEGF Trap-Eye), 234
Afrezza (inhaled insulin), 627*t*
African Americans
    alcohol use, 404
    cancer, 642, 644
    CVD mortality rates, 448
    dental caries, 431
    depression in, 373
    diabetes mellitus, 621
    dual eligibles, 34–35
    educational attainment, 4
    end-of-life care, 137
    family caregivers, 55
    hypertension, 475
    kidney failure, 507

life expectancy, 3, 3t
median income, 4
multiple myeloma, 656
nursing-home population, 196
oral cancer, 433
osteoporosis, 313
periodontitis, 431
population projections, 3, 268, 644
poverty rates, 4
risk factors for depression, 373
African plum, 117
Age-related changes, 11–15, 12t, 262–263
   in anterior pituitary function, 610, 611t
   in antidiuretic hormone, 498
   in auditory system, 240
   in body composition, 262
   in bone formation, 314
   bone remodeling and bone loss, 314
   in calcium homeostasis, 606, 606t
   cardiovascular, 448–450, 449t
   in eating, 270
   in endocrine system, 601
   in energy requirements, 262
   in female sexuality, 534
   in fluid needs, 263
   in GI tract, 483
   in hematopoietic response, 629–630
   in immune function, 586, 587t
   in kidney function, 497, 498t
   in lower urinary tract, 275–276
   in macronutrient needs, 262
   in male sexuality, 530
   in micronutrient needs, 262–263
   in oral tissues, 429, 430t
   in organ systems, 11–15, 12t
   in pharmacodynamics, 104, 646–647, 647t
   in pharmacokinetics, 101–104, 646–647, 647t
   physiologic, 11–15, 12t
   pulmonary, 438
   in salivary function, 432
   in salivary glands, 429, 430t
   in sexuality, 530
   in skin, 417
   in sleep, 361–362, 362t
   in smell, 435
   in swallowing, 270
   in taste, 435
   in teeth, 429, 430t
   in testosterone, 615
Age-related macular degeneration (ARMD), 230t, 233–235
   rehabilitation for, 239
   symptoms and treatment of, 231t
Age-related pathologies, 16, 16t
Agency for Health Care Policy and Research (AHCPR), 407, 440–441
Aggression
   in dementia, 347
   in intellectual disability, 414
   intermittent, 347
Aging
   accumulation theories of, 8t, 10
   antagonistic pleiotropy theory of, 7–8
   cancer and, 642–643
   concerns about, 75
   definition of, 7
   demography of, 1–6
   endocrine theory of, 8t, 10–11
   epigenetic theory of, 8t, 10
   error catastrophe theory of, 8t, 10
   evolutionary theories of, 7–8
   free radical theory of, 8t, 10
   global trends, 1–2, 1f
   hematopoietic stem cells and, 629
   homeostenosis and, 16–17
   immune theory of, 8t, 11
   mitochondrial DNA (mtDNA) theory of, 8t, 9
   mutation accumulation theory of, 7, 8t
   normal, 15–16
   photoaging, 15, 417
   physiologic theories of, 8–11, 8t
   psychosocial theories of, 8
   rate of living theory of, 8t, 10
   stem cell/progenitor cell theory of, 8t, 11
   target theory of genetic damage, 8t, 9
   telomere theory of, 8t, 9
   theories of, 7–11
   transposable element activation theory of, 8t, 9
   U.S. trends, 2–6
Aging Brain Care Medical Home, 218
Agitated delirium, 356t, 357
Agitation
   Cohen-Mansfield Agitation Inventory (CMAI), 340
   in dementia, 339–340, 347
   intermittent, 347
Agoraphobia, 383, 386t
AGS. See American Geriatrics Society
AIDP (acute inflammatory demyelinating polyneuropathy), 576
AIDS (acquired immunodeficiency syndrome), 596–597
   nursing-home financing for care for those with, 198
   treatment and care, 74
AIDS Community Research Initiative of America, 74
AIMS (Abnormal Involuntary Movement Scale), 390
Akathisia, 574
Albiglutide, 626t
Albumin, 264
Albuminuria, 498
Albuterol, 442, 442t
Alcohol
   and delirium, 355t
   and incontinence, 275t, 276t
   nutrient interactions, 265t
   and risk of osteoporosis, 316, 316t
Alcohol dependence, 404–405, 407, 408t
Alcohol detoxification, 407, 408t
Alcohol intoxication or withdrawal, 392
Alcohol-related dementia, 405
Alcohol use
   abstinence from, 402–403
   at-risk drinking, 404, 407, 408t
   benefits of, 404
   binge drinking, 402
   in clinical settings, 404
   counseling interventions for, 89t, 93
   cultural and demographic factors, 404
   epidemiology of, 403
   heavy drinking, 403
   low-risk or moderate use, 404
   magnitude of the problem, 403–404
   problem drinking, 407, 408t
   recommended upper limit of, 402
   in transgender adults, 74
Alcohol Use Disorders Identification Test (AUDIT), 93
Alcohol withdrawal, 392, 406
Alcoholics Anonymous, 406
Alcoholics Victorious, 406
Alcoholism, 403
   and incontinence, 276t
   screening for, 405
Aldosterone antagonists
   for heart failure, 468, 469, 471
   and hyperkalemia, 501, 501t
Alendronate, 320, 321t, 608
ALFs (assisted-living facilities), 177, 197
Alfuzosin, 521, 521t
Aliskiren, 479
Alkaline phosphatase, 319, 609, 610
Allergic conjunctivitis, 230–232, 237t
Allodynia, 148t
Allopurinol, 552
Alogliptin, 626t
Alosetron, 494
α-Adrenergic agonists
   adverse drug events, 106, 106t, 238t
   and incontinence, 275t
   for postural hypotension, 260
α-Adrenergic antagonists or blockers
   adverse drug events, 106, 106t
   for benign prostatic hyperplasia, 521, 521t
   for hypertension, 479
   and incontinence, 275, 275t
α-Interferon, 648
Alprazolam, 102
Alprostadil, 533t, 534
ALS (amyotrophic lateral sclerosis), 577
Alteplase, 582
Altered mental status, 349
Alternative medicine, 112, 113t. See also Complementary and integrative medicine
Alzheimer disease (AD), 326, 568
   Behavioral Pathology in Alzheimer Disease Rating Scale (BEHAVE-AD), 340
   deaths due to, 6
   delirium and, 352–353
   dementia associated with, 116–117
   diagnostic features and treatment of, 330t

differential diagnosis of, 330
disease management, 218
in Down syndrome, 412–413
etiology of, 327
familial, 327
family caregiver interventions, 56, 57t
gait abnormalities, 298t, 299
general progression of, 333t
personality changes in, 394
prevalence of, 5f
protective factors for, 327–328, 328t
risk factors for, 327–328, 328t
Alzheimer's Association, 59t, 337
   recommendations for brain imaging, 329
   Safe Return, 334
Alzheimer's Disease Education and Referral site (NIA), 59t
AM-PAC (Activity Measure for Post Acute Care), 183, 184t
AMA. See American Medical Association
Amantadine
   and delirium, 355t
   for influenza, 592
   for PD motor symptoms, 572
Ambient bright light therapy, 369
Ambulance services, 31t
Ambulatory blood pressure monitoring, 476
Ambulatory electrocardiographic monitoring, 257t, 258–259
American Academy of Family Practitioners, 265
American Academy of HIV Medicine (AAHIVM), 74
American Academy of Ophthalmology, 229
American Academy of Otolaryngology–Head and Neck Surgery, 438–439
American Association of Clinical Endocrinologists, 322
American Association of Critical-Care Nurses, 26
American Association of Family Physicians (AAFP), 216
American Association of Retired Persons (AARP), 55, 59t
American Association of Sex Educators, Counselors, and Therapists, 537
American Board of Internal Medicine Choosing Wisely® Recommendations. See Choosing Wisely® Recommendations
American Cancer Society, 59t, 523
   recommendations for screening, 87, 90
American College of Cardiology (ACC), 624
   cardiac risk assessment for noncardiac surgery, 127, 128f
   guidelines for preoperative cardiac assessment, 127
   recommendations for screening, 92
American College of Obstetricians and Gynecology (ACOG), 512

American College of Physicians (ACP), 129, 216, 523, 532
American College of Rheumatology (ACR), 553
American College of Sports Medicine (ACSM)
   Exercise is Medicine Initiative, 82
   Exercise Management for Chronic Diseases and Disabilities, 82
   recommendations for physical activity, 79, 80, 81, 82
American College of Surgeons, 127
American Diabetes Association, 623, 624
American Dietetic Association, 265
American Geriatrics Society (AGS), 85
   Beers Criteria, 105, 108t, 161, 487, 536
   clinical practice guidelines for care of nursing-home residents, 207
   guidelines for care of older adults with diabetes mellitus, 623
   guidelines for persistent pain management, 549
   guidelines for preventing falls, 305, 308, 309
   guidelines for prevention and management of postoperative delirium, 358t, 359
   recommendations for calcium and vitamin D supplements, 606–607
   "Recommended Treatment Strategies for Clinicians Managing Older Patients with HIV," 74
American Heart Association (AHA), 624
   cardiac risk assessment for noncardiac surgery, 127, 128f
   guidelines for preoperative cardiac assessment, 127
   recommendations for dental treatment of older adults, 436
   recommendations for physical activity, 79, 80, 81, 82
   recommendations for screening, 92
   recommendations for treatment of acute ischemic stroke, 582
   resources and tools for caregivers, 59t
American Indian and Alaska Natives, 644
   life expectancy, 3, 3t
   population projections, 3, 268, 644
   poverty rates, 4
American Medical Association (AMA), 47
   certification for medical directors (CMD), 203–205
   recommendations for fair process, 167–168
American Medical Directors Association
   clinical practice guidelines for care of nursing-home residents, 207
   competencies for attending physicians in post-acute and long-term care medicine, 200–201, 204t

website, 206
American Osteopathic Association (AOA), 216
American Psychological Association (APA), 58
American Recovery and Reinvestment Act, 41
American Society of Anesthesiologists, 127, 127t
American Stroke Association, 59t
American Urogynecologic Association, 516
American Urological Association, 87, 520, 523
Amiloride
   Beers Criteria for, 108t
   and hyperkalemia, 501, 501t
Amiodarone, 453, 460, 470
Amitiza (lubiprostone), 491t
Amitriptyline, 355t
AML (acute myeloid leukemia), 629, 655
Amotidine, 141t
Amoxicillin
   drug interactions, 102, 107t
   for Lyme disease, 598
Ampicillin, 597
Amputation
   assessment of, 191
   epidemiology of, 191
   leg, 191
   rehabilitation for, 191–192
Amylin analogues, 626t
Amyloid precursor protein (APP), 327
Amyloidosis, 507
Amyotrophic lateral sclerosis (ALS), 577
Amyotrophy, diabetic, 576
Anagrelide, 640–641
Anakinra, 551
Anal cancer, 72
Analgesia. *See also* Pain management; Palliative care
   definition of, 148t
   Pain Ladder (WHO), 155
   patient-controlled analgesia, 134
   preemptive, 134
Analgesics
   and delirium, 355t
   and incontinence, 275t
   medications to avoid, 158
   for myelopathy, 578
   narcotic, 134, 265, 275t
   nonopioid adjuvant, 155, 157–158
   for OA-related pain, 549
Androgen ablation, 526t, 527
Androgen deficiency, 614, 617
Androgen deprivation, 526t, 527, 528, 630
Androgen-deprivation therapy (ADT), 654
Androgen excess, 630
Androgen replacement therapy, 630
Androgens, adrenal, 614
Anemia, 629, 630–637
   of chronic disease, 634
   CKD-associated, 508–509
   classification of, 631, 631t

from decreased erythropoietin
production, 634–635
evaluation of, 631–632, 632f
hemolytic, 505, 631t, 636–637
hypoproliferative, 631t, 632–635, 633f
ineffective, 631t
of inflammation, 634
iron-deficiency (or iron-restricted), 632–634, 632f
laboratory evaluation of, 631–632, 633f
macrocytic, 635
management of, 508–509
microcytic, 635–636
refractory, 636
and rehabilitation, 186
sideroblastic, 635–636
valve-associated, 637
Aneurysms
abdominal aortic (AAA), 88t, 91–92, 464
cerebral, 584–585
intracranial saccular, 584
Angina pectoris
and anxiety, 385
epidemiology of, 452
medical therapy for, 454
Angiodysplasia, 494
colonic, 494–495
Angiogenesis inhibitors, 495
Angiography, renal, 503
Angioplasty
carotid artery, 583
renal artery, 503
Angiotensin-converting enzyme (ACE) inhibitors
for acute coronary syndrome, 452, 453
adverse drug events, 106, 106t
for chronic CAD, 454
drug interactions, 107, 107t
for heart failure, 468, 469t
and hyperkalemia, 501, 501t
for hypertension, 478–479, 478t
and incontinence, 275t
for peripheral arterial disease, 464
for prevention of cardiovascular disease, 625
for renal artery stenosis, 503
Angiotensin-receptor blockers (ARBs)
for acute coronary syndrome, 452, 453
adverse drug events, 106, 106t
for chronic CAD, 454
drug interactions, 107, 107t
for heart failure, 468, 469t, 471
and hyperkalemia, 501, 501t
for hypertension, 478t, 479
for peripheral arterial disease, 464
for prevention of cardiovascular disease, 625
for renal artery stenosis, 503
Angular cheilitis, 434, 434f
Anhedonia, 373–374
Ankle-brachial index (ABI), 290, 422, 463–464
Ankle problems, 559, 566–567

Annual wellness visit (AWV), 36, 94t–95t
Anorectal manometry, 490–491
Anorexia, 142–143
Anserine bursitis, 542, 543
Antabuse reaction, 408t
Antacids
adverse drug events, 106, 106t
drug interactions, 588
for nausea, 141t
nutrient interactions, 265t
Antagonistic pleiotropy theory of aging, 7–8
Antalgic gait, 297t, 298, 298t
Anterior ischemic optic neuropathy, 238, 238f
Anterior pituitary changes, 610, 611t
Anterior pituitary disorders, 610–612
Anterior uveitis, 230
Anthropometrics, 263–264
Anti-CCP (anti-cyclic citrullinated peptide/protein antibodies), 550
Anti-cyclic citrullinated peptide/protein antibodies (anti-CCP or ACPA), 550
Antiandrogens, 347
for prostate cancer, 526t, 527
Antianxiety agents, 398
Antiarrhythmics
for acute coronary syndrome, 453
adverse drug events, 106, 106t, 392
for atrial fibrillation, 459–460
for tachy-brady syndrome, 463
Antibiotics
for COPD exacerbation, 442, 443t
de-escalation of, 588
drug interactions, 588
for foot ulcers, 567
for infections, 588
for infective endocarditis, 429, 436, 458, 595
for irritable bowel syndrome, 493
minimal criteria for initiation in long-term care, 586, 588, 589t
nutrient interactions, 265t
for osteomyelitis, 596
perioperative, 128, 130t
for pneumonia, 592
for prostatitis, 528
for rhinosinusitis, 439
for UTIs, 593, 594
Antibodies, monoclonal, 648–649
Antibody-drug conjugates, 649
Anticholinergics
adverse drug events, 106, 106t, 281
for COPD, 442, 442t, 443t
and delirium, 355, 355t
for drug-induced movement disorders, 574
and incontinence, 275t
for LUTS, 522
for nausea, 141t
for PD motor symptoms, 572
Anticoagulation therapy
adverse drug events, 106, 106t
cessation before surgery, 128, 130t
for intracerebral hemorrhage, 584

novel oral anticoagulants (NOACs), 460, 461
perioperative, 128, 130t
for stroke prevention, 583–584
for VTE, 445–446
Anticonvulsants
adverse drug events, 106, 106t
and delirium, 355t
for fibromyalgia, 558
for persistent pain, 152t, 157
and risk of osteoporosis, 316, 316t
to stabilize mood in mania and bipolar depression, 378–379, 379t
Antidepressants
for abstinence, 407
adverse drug events, 106, 106t, 344
for alcohol detoxification, 407, 408t
for anxiety disorders, 386
and delirium, 355t
for dementia, 336–337
for depression, 377–378, 377t
for depression in terminally ill, 145
for depressive features of behavioral disturbances in dementia, 342–343, 343t
for fibromyalgia, 558
for headaches, 579
and incontinence, 275t
indications to start, 374, 375t
interventions for preventing falls with, 310t
for migraine, 579
for neuropathic pain, 576
for persistent pain, 152t, 157
for personality disorders, 397–398
for psychotic symptoms in mood disorders, 391
sedating, 369t, 370–371
tricyclic, 152t, 275t, 342–343, 343t, 355t, 370–371, 377t, 576, 579
Antidiarrheal medications, 491
Antidiuretic hormone (ADH)
age-related changes in, 498
inappropriate secretion of, 377, 499–500
Antiepileptic drugs, 569–570, 569t
Antifungals, 566
Antihistamines
adverse drug events, 106, 106t
and delirium, 355t
drug interactions, 588
for nausea, 141t
sedating, 366, 371–372
Antihypertensives, 106, 106t
drug interactions, 588
interventions for preventing falls with, 310t
Antimanic medications, 391
Antimicrobial management. See Antibiotics
Antimuscarinics, 280–281
Antineoplastic agents, 392
Antineutrophil cytoplasmic antibody (ANCA)-associated vasculitis, 506
Antiparkinsonian agents
adverse drug events, 106, 106t

and delirium, 355t
Antiplatelet therapy
	for acute coronary syndrome, 453
	adverse drug events, 106, 106t
	dual antiplatelet therapy (DAPT), 453
	for intracerebral hemorrhage, 584
	perioperative, 128, 129
	for stroke prevention, 583
Antipsychotics, 356–357
	adverse drug events, 106, 106t
	for bipolar depression, 378
	black-box warnings, 346
	for delirium, 355, 355t, 356–357
	dosing and adverse events of, 389–390, 390t
	and incontinence, 275t
	interventions for preventing falls with, 310t
	for personality disorders, 397–398
	for psychotic depression, 377–378
	for psychotic symptoms in dementia, 344–346, 345t, 391
	for psychotic symptoms in mood disorders, 391
	second generation, 355t, 391
	sedating, 371
	to stabilize mood in mania and bipolar depression, 378, 379t
Antisecretory medications, 142, 143t
Antisocial personality disorder
	features of, 395, 395t
	long-term course, 396–397
	therapeutic strategies for, 397–398, 398t
Antispasmodic medications, 142, 143t
Antithrombotics
	for ACS, 452
	adverse events, 461
Antiviral agents, 392
Anxiety, 382
Anxiety disorders, 382–387
	classes of, 382–385
	comorbidity, 385
	depression with marked anxiety, 385
	features of anxious or fearful behaviors, 395t
	generalized anxiety disorder (GAD), 384, 386, 386t
	illness anxiety disorder, 399
	and incontinence, 276t
	marked anxiety, 385
	and medical disorders, 385, 386t
	pharmacologic management of, 385–386
	psychologic management of, 386–387
	treatment strategies for, 385–386, 386t
Aortic regurgitation (AR), 456
	clinical features and treatment of, 457t
	diagnosis of, 456
	epidemiology of, 456
Aortic stenosis (AS), 448, 456
	clinical features and treatment of, 457t

diagnosis of, 456
prevalence of, 456
Aortic valve replacement
	surgical (SAVR), 448, 456–458
	transcatheter (TAVR), 448, 456–458
Apathetic thyrotoxicosis, 603
Aphthous ulcers, 434–435, 435f
Apidra (insulin glulisine), 627t
Apixaban
	Beers Criteria for, 108t
	for stroke prevention, 460, 461
	for VTE, 446
Apolipoprotein E gene (APOE), 327
Appendicitis, 598
Appetite stimulants, 267–268
Applied behavioral analysis, 414
Aprepitant, 141t
Aqueous outflow facilitators, 237–238, 238t
Aqueous suppressants, 237–238, 238t
ARBs. See Angiotensin-receptor blockers
Arch disorders, 559–560, 560f
Arcus senilis, 230t
Area Agencies on Aging, 59t, 337
Arformoterol, 442t
Aripiprazole
	for depression, 377
	dosing and adverse events of, 390t
	for psychosis in dementia, 345, 345t
	to stabilize mood in mania and bipolar depression, 379t
ARMD (age-related macular degeneration), 230t, 233–235
	rehabilitation for, 239
	symptoms and treatment of, 231t
ARMD (macular degeneration, age-related), 230t
Aromatase inhibitors, 316, 316t, 648, 651
Aromatherapy, 117, 347, 387
Arrhythmias
	bradyarrhythmias, 462–463
	cardiac, 458–463
	cardiac syncope due to, 254, 255t
	supraventricular, 461–462
	ventricular, 462
Arterial insufficiency, 566
Arterial ulcers, 422–423, 423t
Arteriosclerotic parkinsonism, 299
Arteriovascular disease, 276t
Arteriovenous malformation, 494
Arthritis
	of elbow, 541
	family caregiver interventions, 56, 57t
	of foot, 567
	gouty, 551
	of hand, 548, 549f
	of hip, 542
	of knee, 542, 543, 548, 549f
	osteoarthritis, 542, 543, 548–550, 549f
	prevalence of, 5, 5f
	psoriatic, 421–422
	rheumatoid, 539, 543, 550–551

of wrist, 541
Arthritis Foundation, 151, 548
Arthrocentesis, 552
Arthroplasty, total joint, 190–191, 549
Arthroscopic debridement, 549
Artificial feeding, 269
Artificial saliva, 556
Artificial sphincter, 282–283
Asenapine
	dosing and adverse events of, 390t
	for psychosis in dementia, 345t
Asian Americans
	burning mouth syndrome, 435
	cancer, 644
	CVD mortality rates, 448
	educational attainment, 4
	end-of-life care, 137
	family caregivers, 55
	life expectancy, 3, 3t
	median income, 4
	nursing-home population, 196
	osteoporosis, 313
	population projections, 268, 644
	poverty rates, 4
	urinary incontinence, 274
Aspiration, 271
Aspiration pneumonia, 186, 271
Aspirin therapy
	for acute coronary syndrome, 452, 453
	adverse drug events, 106, 106t
	for atrial fibrillation, 460
	for chronic CAD, 454
	for diabetes mellitus, 624
	perioperative, 128, 130t
	for peripheral arterial disease, 464
	for polycythemia vera, 640–641
	for prevention of cardiovascular disease, 624
	preventive, 89t, 97–98
	for stroke prevention, 460, 583
Assessment, 43–48. See also Screening
	of amputation, 191
	of anxiety, 382
	of behavioral disturbances in dementia, 340–342
	Berg Balance Test, 307
	brown-bag evaluation, 108–109
	of cancer patients, 645–646
	cardiac risk assessment for noncardiac surgery, 127, 128f
	caregiver, 56–58
	cognitive, 45, 94t
	comprehensive eye examination, 229
	comprehensive geriatric assessment (CGA), 95, 187, 218–219
	Confusion Assessment Method (CAM), 161, 349–351
	Confusion Assessment Method for the Intensive Care Unit (CAM-ICU), 350t, 351
	daily evaluation of hospitalized patients, 168–170
	of decisional capacity, 21–22, 22t
	of delirium, 349–351, 350t
	driving, 47, 89t, 334–335
	executive function testing, 45

falls risk assessment, 89t
of frailty, 225–226
of functional status, 184t
General Practitioner Assessment of Cognition, 96
health risk assessment, 94t
of hearing loss, 243
of hip, 187
in home care, 210
home-hazard, 308, 308t
at hospital admission, 164, 165t
of hospitalized older patients, 164–168
kidney, 497
life space, 46–47, 47t
of lower back pain, 544t
Mini-Cog Assessment Instrument for Dementia, 44t, 45, 96, 165, 328, 329t
Mini–Mental State Examination (MMSE), 22, 45, 328, 329t
Mini-Nutritional Assessment (MNA), 265
Mini-Nutritional Assessment, short form (MNA-SF), 262
Montreal Cognitive Assessment (MoCA), 44t, 45, 165, 328, 329t
of nutrition, 263–265
of older drivers, 47
of oropharyngeal dysphagia, 271–272
Outcome and Assessment Information Set (OASIS), 183, 209
Patient Health Questionnaire (PHQ), 44t, 45
Performance-Oriented Mobility Assessment (POMA), 46, 300, 307
of persistent pain, 148–150
physical, 43–45, 121
of physical activity, 82
preoperative, 126–131
of pressure ulcers, 284–286
psychologic, 45
Rapid Assessment of Physical Activity, 82
rapid screening followed by, 43, 44t
rolling, 43
Short Form-36 Health Survey (SF-36), 48
Simplified Nutrition Assessment Questionnaire, 265
skin, 289
social, 46
St. Louis University Mental Status (SLUMS) examination, 44t, 45, 328, 329t
St. Thomas's Risk Assessment Tool (STRATIFY), 307
systematic, 164, 165t
Timed Up and Go (TUG) test, 44t, 46, 300
of urinary incontinence, 282
vertebral fracture assessment (VFA), 318–319

vision testing, 89t, 96, 229
Assessment instruments, 184t
Assisted-living facilities, 177, 197, 213–214, 213t
Assistive devices, 193, 310t, 548
Assistive listening devices, 244–245
costs of, 247, 247t
Asthma, 439–440, 443
Asthma action plans, 440, 441t
At-risk drinking, 404, 407, 408t
At-risk use (of alcohol or other substance), 402
Atenolol
for acute coronary syndrome, 452
for hypertension, 479
Atheroembolism, 505
Atherosclerotic renal artery stenosis, 481
Atherosclerotic renovascular disease, 502–503
Atorvastatin, 452, 454
ATP-binding cassette subfamily A member 7 gene (ABCA7), 327
Atrial fibrillation (AF), 448, 459–461
anticoagulation therapy for, 583
clinical features of, 459
diagnosis and evaluation of, 459
management of, 459–461
prevalence of, 459
Atrial flutter, 461
Atrial tachycardia, 461–462
Atrioventricular block, 462–463, 463t
Atrioventricular-nodal reentrant tachycardia, 461–462
Atrophy
multiple system, 573
urogenital, 512, 513–514, 514f
vaginal, 535, 536
vulvovaginal, 536
Atropine eye drops, 145
Attenuated delirium, 351
Attitudes
regarding disclosure and consent, 66
toward advance directives, 67
toward North American health services, 65
Audiometry screening, 89t, 96–97, 243
AUDIT (Alcohol Use Disorders Identification Test), 93
Auditory system changes, 240
Autism spectrum disorders, 414
Auto-titrating PAP (autoPAP), 364
Autoimmune hemolysis, 636–637
Autoimmune skin conditions, 418–422
Autolytic debridement, 292
Automatisms, 568
Automobile accidents, 47
Autonomic dysfunction, 573
Autonomy, 21
respect for, 18
AutoPAP (auto-titrating PAP), 364
Avanafil, 533, 533t
Avoidant personality disorder
differential diagnosis of, 396
features of, 395t
therapeutic strategies for, 398, 398t
5-Azacytidine, 636

Azathioprine, 420, 444, 555, 557
Azithromycin, 107, 107t
Azotemia, prerenal, 503–504

B

B-CAM, 350t
B-cell lymphoma, 656
B-type natriuretic peptide (BNP), 467
Back disease, 541, 544–545
Back pain, 543–545
acute, 545
CIM for, 115
conditions causing, 543, 544t, 545–547
recommendations for, 545
Back problems, 538
Baclofen, 392, 574, 575
Bacteremia, 591
Bacterial keratitis, 230, 237t
Bacterial meningitis, 597
Bacterial prostatitis, 528
Bacterial vaginosis, 514
Bacteriuria, 283
antibiotic prophylaxis of, 594
asymptomatic, 91t, 586, 593
urinary catheter-associated, 164
Baker cyst, 543
Balance assessment, 46
Berg Balance Scale (Test), 300, 307
Balance impairment, 310t
Balance screening, 89t
Balance training, 78, 80–81, 80t, 308, 308t, 309, 310t
Balanced Budget Act of 1997 (BBA 97), 40, 183, 198
Balanced Budget Revision Act, 40–41
Barbiturates, 355t
Barthel ADL Index, 184t, 187
Basal cell carcinoma, 426, 427f, 516
Baseline activity, 80
Batf (basic leucine zipper transcription factor, ATF-like), 629
Bathing, 368
Beclomethasone diproprionate, 442t
Bedsores. See Pressure ulcers
Beers Criteria (AGS), 105, 108t, 161, 487, 536
BEHAVE-AD (Behavioral Pathology in Alzheimer Disease Rating Scale), 340
Behavior(s)
adaptive, 413
anxious or fearful, 395t
challenging, 411
compulsive, 384
dramatic, emotional, or erratic, 395t
maladaptive, 414
odd or eccentric, 395t
pain behaviors in cognitively impaired, 150–151, 150t
self-injurious, 412, 414
Behavioral disturbances
assessment of, 340–342
clinical features of, 339–340
in delirium, 354t, 356–357
in dementia, 339–348, 343t
differential diagnosis of, 340–342

disorders in aging adults with intellectual disability, 413
management of, 356–357
manic-like features of, 344, 344t
medications to treat depressive features of, 342–343, 343t
recommendations for, 347
treatment of, 342–347
Behavioral health management, 381
Behavioral interventions. *See also* Cognitive-behavioral therapy
for aggression or agitation, 347
for dementia care, 342, 342t
dialectical behavior therapy, 397
for frailty, 227
for insomnia, 346, 346t, 368–370
for urinary incontinence, 279–280, 282
Behavioral Pathology in Alzheimer Disease Rating Scale (BEHAVE-AD), 340
Bell's palsy (facial nerve palsy), 598
Benazepril, 469t
Beneficence, 18, 21
Benign growths, 425–426
Benign paroxysmal positional vertigo (BPPV), 249
diagnostic criteria for, 252
self-treatment of, 252f, 253
Benign prostatic hyperplasia (BPH), 520–522
CIM for, 117
diagnosis of, 520–521
epidemiology of, 520
management options for, 521, 521t
treatment of, 520, 521–522
Benzodiazepines, 403
adverse drug events, 106, 106t
for alcohol detoxification, 407, 408t
for anxiety disorders, 386, 386t
chronic use of, 371
and delirium, 355, 355t, 356–357
dependence on, 406–407
drug interactions, 107, 107t
for insomnia, 367, 369t, 371
interventions for preventing falls with, 310t
for nausea, 141t
for sleep problems, 365, 366
Benzoyl peroxide, 419
Benztropine, 355t
Bereavement, 374
Berg Balance Scale (Test), 300, 307
Berger disease, 506
β-Adrenergic agonists, 441–442, 442t, 443t
β-Blockers
for acute coronary syndrome, 453
adverse drug events, 106, 106t, 238t, 392
for anxiety disorders, 385, 386t
for atrial fibrillation, 459
for chronic CAD, 454
for essential tremor, 574–575
for heart failure, 468–469, 469t, 471
and hyperkalemia, 501, 501t
for hypertension, 479

for migraine, 579
perioperative, 128, 130t
for prevention of cardiovascular disease, 625
for ventricular arrhythmias, 462
β-Carotene, 234, 267
β-Lactam/β-lactamase, 587
β-Lactam/β-lactamase antibiotics, 592
Better Outcomes by Optimizing Safe Transitions (BOOST), 179t
Bevacizumab, 234, 648, 653
Bi-level positive-airway pressure (biPAP), 364, 577
Biceps tendonopathy and tendon rupture, 540
Biguanides, 626, 626t
Biliary disease, 489
Binge drinking, 402
Bio-identical compounded hormonal preparations, 513
Bioavailability, 101
Biofeedback, 116, 490, 491
Biologic therapy, 113t
for cancer, 648–649
for diabetes mellitus, 118
for rheumatoid arthritis, 550–551
safety issues, 113–114
Biological or larval therapy, 292
Biology, 7–17
BiPAP (bi-level positive-airway pressure), 364, 577
Bipolar depression, 375–376
medications to stabilize mood in, 379t
pharmacotherapy for, 378–379
psychosocial interventions for, 380–381
Bipolar disorder, 375–376
type 1, 375, 376
type 2, 375–376
Bisacodyl (Dulcolax), 490t, 491t
Bisexual men. *See also* Lesbian gay bisexual transgender (LGBT) older adults
disease risk, 71–72
sexual risk, 73
Bisexual women. *See also* Lesbian gay bisexual transgender (LGBT) older adults
disease risk, 72
sexual risk, 73
Bisoprolol, 468–469, 469t
Bisphosphonates
adverse drug events, 106, 106t, 320–322, 437
for humoral hypercalcemia of malignancy, 609
for hyperparathyroidism, 608–609
investigational agents, 324
for osteoporosis, 313, 320–322, 321t, 509, 554
for Paget disease of bone, 609–610
for persistent pain, 158, 528
Bivalirudin, 452
Black Americans. *See* African Americans
Black cohosh, 117
Black hairy tongue, 435, 435f

Bladder cancer, 91t, 654
Bladder contractions, uninhibited, 276
Bladder diaries, 278, 279t
Bladder neck slings, 281
Bladder obstruction, 277
Bladder outlet obstruction, 504
Bladder training, 279–280
Bleeding
gastrointestinal, 494
vaginal, 512, 518, 518t
Bleeding diatheses, 638, 639–640
Blepharitis, 230–232, 237t
Blepharochalasis, 229
Blepharoptosis, 229
Blind-loop syndrome, 635
Blindness
causes of, 229, 231t
definition of, 229
irreversible, 231t
reversible, 231t
Blood glucose screening, 88t
Blood pressure. *See also* Hypertension; Hypotension
classification of, 475, 475t
screening, 88t
targets in hypertension, 502
Blood pressure control, 624–625
Blood pressure monitoring
ambulatory, 476
home, 480
indirect or cuff, 476
BMI (body mass index), 93, 263–264
BNP (B-type natriuretic peptide), 467
Board and care, 213t
Body-based methods, 113t
Body composition changes, 262
Body language, 64
Body mass index (BMI), 93, 263–264
Body size classification, 264
Body weight, 81
Bodywork services, 113
Bone
age-related changes, 12t, 13, 314
age-related pathologies, 16t
Bone alkaline phosphatase (BAP), 319, 609, 610
Bone-anchored hearing aids (BAHAs), 247–248
Bone disease, 542
adynamic, 509
CKD-related, 509
Paget disease of bone, 243, 609–610
Bone infections, 596
Bone loss, 314. *See also* Osteoporosis
Bone marrow failure, 635
Bone mineral density
diagnostic criteria for osteoporosis, 313
WHO definitions, 313, 314t
Bone mineral density testing, 317–318
indications for, 317, 318t
recommendations for, 92, 317–318
serial measurement, 324
Bone remodeling, 314
Bone spurs, 562
Bone turnover, 314, 319

BOOST (Better Outcomes by Optimizing Safe Transitions), 179t
Borderline personality disorder
 differential diagnosis of, 396
 features of, 395, 395t
 long-term course, 396–397
 therapeutic strategies for, 397–398, 398t
Bordetella pertussis infection, 439
Boston Naming Test, 331
Botulinum toxin, 281, 417, 574
Bouchard nodes, 548
Bowel incontinence, 490–491
 with developmental disabilities, 415t
Bowel obstruction
 medications for, 142, 143t
 in terminal illness, 142
BPH. *See* Benign prostatic hyperplasia
BPPV. *See* Benign paroxysmal positional vertigo
Brachytherapy, 526t, 527
Braden Scale, 286–287
Bradyarrhythmias, 459, 462–463
 indications for permanent pacemaker implantation, 462–463, 463t
Bradycardia
 management of, 462–463, 463t
 mild, 462
Bradykinesia, 570
Brain imaging studies, 329
Brain injury, traumatic (TBI), 612
Brain tumors, 394
Breast cancer, 650–651
 characteristics of, 643–644
 chemotherapy for, 647, 651
 CIM for, 118
 hormonal therapy for, 648, 651
 incidence rates, 642
 metastatic, 653
 risk in older lesbian and bisexual women, 72
 screening for, 86, 91t, 646
 targeted therapy against, 648–649
Breast Cancer Risk Assessment Tool, 98
Breast self-examination (BSE), 86
Breathing disorders, sleep-related, 363–364
Breathlessness, 143–144
Bridging integrator 1 gene *(BIN1)*, 327
Brief interventions, 407, 408t
Bright light, 368, 368t, 369
Brimonidine, 238t
British Geriatrics Society (BGS), 305, 308, 309
Bromocriptine, 626t
Bronchitis, chronic, 443t
Bronchodilators, inhaled, 442, 442t, 443t
Brown-bag review, 108–109, 353
Budesonide, 442t
Bulk laxatives, 491t
Bullous pemphigoid, 420, 420f
Bundled Payments for Care Improvement initiative, 27, 28t
Bunions, 561t
Buprenorphine, 407, 408t

Bupropion, 343, 343t, 377, 377t, 407
Burch operation (colposuspension), 281
Burning mouth syndrome, 435
Burnout, health professional, 146
Bursitis
 anserine, 542, 543
 olecranon, 540–541
 trochanteric, 541, 542
Buspirone
 for anxiety disorders, 386, 386t
 for depression, 377
Busulfan, 640–641
Butorphanol, 158
Bypass surgery, 455

C

C-reactive protein (CRP), 451, 550
Cachexia, 142–143
Caffeine, 310t
CAGE (Cut down, Annoy, Guilt, Eye-opener) questionnaire, 93, 405
Calcaneal spur, 561t
Calcitonin, 322, 509
Calcium
 abnormalities in CKD, 509
 coronary artery content, 451
 dietary intake, 319–320
 disorders of metabolism of, 606–610
 drug interactions, 265t
 foods that contain, 319–320, 320t
 homeostasis changes, 606, 606t
 RDIs for adults ≥71 years old, 263t, 267
 RDIs for older adults, 606–607
Calcium channel blockers
 adverse drug events, 106, 106t, 265
 for chronic CAD, 454–455
 drug interactions, 107, 107t
 for hypertension, 478t, 479
 and incontinence, 275t, 281
 for migraine, 579
 for prevention of cardiovascular disease, 625
Calcium-containing antacids, 106, 106t
Calcium deficiency, 315
Calcium hydroxylapatite, 417
Calcium pyrophosphate dihydrate deposition disease (CPPD), 550, 552
Calcium receptor antagonists, 322
Calcium supplements
 for hyperparathyroidism, 608
 for osteoporosis, 316, 316t, 319–320
 preventive, 89t, 98, 607
Caloric requirements, 292
Calreticulin, 640
CAM (Confusion Assessment Method), 161, 349–351
CAM-Severity (CAM-S), 351
Canagliflozin, 626t
Canalith repositioning procedure, 252f, 253
Cancer, 642
 anal cancer, 72
 assessment of, 645–646
 back pain due to, 543

biologic therapies for, 648–649
biology of, 642–644
bladder cancer, 654
breast cancer, 72, 86, 642, 643–644, 650–651
cervical cancer, 72, 87
characteristics of, 643–644
chemotherapy for, 646–647, 647t
CIM for, 118
colon cancer, 492, 494, 642, 643, 651–653
colorectal cancer, 86–87, 494, 642, 652–653
endometrial cancer, 518
esophageal cancer, 653–654
ethnic differences in, 644
family caregiver interventions, 56, 57t
gastric cancer, 653–654
guidelines for assessment and treatment of, 645
hormonal therapy for, 648
immunotherapy for, 648
incidence of, 642, 644
lip cancer, 433
lung cancer, 90, 642, 651
management of, 644–650, 656
mortality of, 644
oral cancer, 429, 432–433
ovarian cancer, 89
physical activity recommendations for, 80t
prevalence of, 5, 5f, 643
prostate cancer, 72, 87, 520, 522–528, 642, 654
pseudodisease, 86
quality-of-life issues, 649–650
radiation therapy for, 649
recommendations for, 657
renal cell cancer, 648, 654–655
risk in older gay and bisexual men, 72
risk in older lesbian and bisexual women, 72
skin cancer, 89, 417, 426–428
surgery for, 649
targeted therapies for, 648–649
thyroid cancer, 90, 605–606
treatment options, 646
of vulva, 512, 516
Cancer screening, 646
 counseling on, 98–99
 recommendations for, 85–90, 88t, 99
 tests, 85–90
 in transgender older adults, 72–73
Candesartan, 469t, 471, 471t
Candidiasis
 oral, 434, 434f
 skin, 425
 vulvovaginal, 514
Canes, 193–194, 193t
Cannabinoids, 118–119, 141t
Cannabis (marijuana), 118–119, 392, 403
Capecitabine, 647t, 653
Capsaicin, 151, 549
Capsaicin cream, 421, 576

Capsicum frutescens (cayenne), 115
Captopril, 469*t*
Carbamazepine (Tegretol, Epitol)
    adverse effects of, 106, 106*t*, 569
    for alcohol detoxification, 408*t*
    for behavioral disturbances in dementia with manic-like features, 344, 344*t*
    for dementia, 337
    for persistent pain, 152*t*, 157
    for personality disorders, 397
    to stabilize mood in mania and bipolar depression, 379*t*
Carbidopa-levodopa
    for Parkinson disease, 571
    for periodic limb movement disorder, 365
    for restless legs syndrome, 365, 575
Carbonic anhydrase inhibitors, 238*t*
Carboplatin, 654
Cardiac arrest
    code status discussions, 167–168
    in-hospital (IHCA), 167–168
Cardiac arrhythmias, 458–463
    epidemiology of, 458–459
    syncope due to, 254, 255*t*
Cardiac assessment, preoperative, 127–129
Cardiac asthma, 439
Cardiac disease
    deaths due to, 6
    with developmental disabilities, 415*t*
    prevalence of, 5, 5*f*
Cardiac rehabilitation, 192
    for acute coronary syndrome, 453
    for chronic CAD, 455
    for heart failure, 468
Cardiac resynchronization therapy (CRT), 472
Cardiac risk assessment
    for noncardiac surgery, 127, 128*f*
    Revised Cardiac Risk Index, 127
    surgical risk calculators, 127
Cardiac stress testing, preoperative, 127–128
Cardiac syncope
    due to arrhythmia, 254, 255*t*
    predictors of, 256, 256*t*
Cardiobacterium, 458, 595
Cardioembolic stroke, 581
Cardiology, 448–465
    activity recommendations for, 80*t*
    CIM for, 115–116
    epidemiology of, 448, 448*t*
    and incontinence, 276*t*
    mortality rates, 448
    prevalence of, 448, 448*t*
    prevention of, 624, 625
    recommendations for, 465
    risk factors for, 450–451
    risk in older gay and bisexual men, 71–72
    risk in older lesbian and bisexual women, 72
    screening for, 92
    in transgender older adults, 72

Cardiorenal syndrome, 504
Cardiovascular events, 508
Cardiovascular system
    age-related changes in, 12*t*, 13, 17, 448–450, 449*t*
    age-related pathologies, 16*t*
    indications for revascularization, 127–128, 129*t*
    perioperative therapy to reduce complications, 128, 130*t*
    postoperative management of problems, 131–132
    preoperative assessment and management of, 127–129
Care Area Assessments, 269
Care plans, 52
Care teams, patient-aligned (GERI-PACT), 52
Care transitions, 174–180, 174*f*
    barriers to safety, 175–176
    communication for, 178
    definition of, 174
    discharge destinations, 177
    policy approaches, 176
    questions to assist with, 178
    steps to improve, 178–180
    strategies for, 176–177, 179*t*
    suboptimal, 174–175
    target measures for improvement, 180
    venues of care, 177
Care Transitions Intervention, 176, 179*t*
Caregiver apps, 59*t*
Caregiver burden, 341
Caregivers
    assessment of, 56–58
    communication with, 178
    education of, 332–334
    family caregivers, 54, 55, 56–58, 58–59
    interventions for, 56, 57*t*
    primary caregivers, 57–58
    resources and tools for, 59*t*, 60
    role of older adult with, 123
    support for, 332–334, 337, 347
    treatment of, 58–59
Caregiving, 54–56
    clinical considerations, 56–60
    risk factors for inadequate or abusive caregiving, 120, 121*t*
The Caregiving Resource Center (AARP), 59*t*
CareMore model, 217–218
Carotid artery angioplasty and stenting (CAS), 583
Carotid artery intima-media thickness, 451
Carotid artery stenosis, 91*t*
Carotid endarterectomy (CEA), 583
Carotid sinus hypersensitivity, 310*t*
Carotid ultrasound, 451
Carpal tunnel syndrome, 541
Carvedilol, 469, 469*t*
Case managers, 185*t*
CASES approach to ethical dilemmas, 18, 20*t*
Casuistry, 20
Cataract surgery, 308, 308*t*, 309

Cataracts, 230*t*, 231*t*, 232–233
Catastrophic insurance, 33
Catechol-*O*-methyltransferase inhibitors, 572
Cathespin K inhibitors, 322
Catheter ablation, 460
Catheter-associated urinary tract infections (CAUTIs), 163–164
Catheter care, 282–283
Catheters, 282–283
    urinary, 163–164
Cavus deformity, 559–560, 560*f*
Cayenne *(Capsicum frutescens)*, 115
CDC (Centers for Disease Control and Prevention), 548
Cefotaxime, 592, 597
Ceftriaxone, 592, 597, 598
Celecoxib (Celebrex), 153*t*
Center for Medicare and Medicaid Innovations (CMI), 27, 35, 41
Center of Excellence on Elder Abuse & Neglect, 120
Centers for Disease Control and Prevention (CDC), 548
Centers for Medicare and Medicaid Services (CMS)
    Bundled Payments for Care Improvement initiative, 27–28, 28*t*
    Federal Coordinated Health Care Office, 35
    Hospital Compare, 171–172
    Hospital Readmissions Reduction Program, 472
    Medicare Personal Plan Finder, 35, 40
    Medicare Prescription Drug Plan Finder, 33
    "The National Partnership to Improve Dementia Care in Nursing Homes," 205
    Nursing Home Compare tool, 39, 59*t*
    Quality Indicator Survey (QIS) process, 203
    quality measures for nursing homes, 199*t*, 202–203
    Risk-Standardized-Readmission Rates (RSRR), 172
Central nervous system (CNS) infections, 597–598
Central nervous system (CNS) medications, 403
Central pain, 148*t*
Central retinal artery occlusion, 230, 237*t*
Central sleep apnea, 363–364, 366–367
Cephalexin, 107, 107*t*
Cephalosporins, 592
Cerebellar ataxia, 298*t*
Cerebral aneurysms, 584–585
Cerebral insufficiency, 336
Cerebral palsy, 416
Cerebrospinal fluid (CSF) analysis, 329
Cerebrovascular disease, 568, 580
    deaths due to, 6
    and incontinence, 276*t*
    large-vessel disease, 580–581
    small-vessel disease, 580

Certificate of Terminal Illness, 137–138
Certification for medical directors (CMD), 203–205
Certolizumab, 551
Cerumen impaction, 243
Cervical cancer
　risk in older lesbian and bisexual women, 72
　screening for, 87, 91t, 646
Cervical disc disease, 539
Cervical disc displacement, 539
Cervical myelopathy, 301
Cervical radiculopathy, 539
Cervical stenosis, 539
Cevimeline, 432, 556
CGA. *See* Comprehensive geriatric assessment
CGIC-PF (Clinical Global Impression of Change in Physical Frailty), 226
CHA_2DS_2-VASc score, 460
$CHADS_2$ score, 460
Chalazion, 237t
Charles Bonnet syndrome, 238, 391–392
Checklist of Nonverbal Pain Indicators, 151
Cheilectomy, 562
Chemical restraints, 356
Chemoprophylaxis, 89t, 97–98
Chemosensory perception, oral, 435–436
Chemotherapy, 646–647, 647t
　for breast cancer, 651
　for colon cancer, 653
　for colorectal cancer, 653
　for prostate cancer, 654
　and risk of osteoporosis, 316, 316t
Chemotherapy-induced nausea and vomiting, 118–119
Chemotherapy Risk Assessment Scale for High-Age Patients (CRASH) Score, 646
Cherry angiomas, 425–426
Chest radiography, 467
Cheynes-Stokes breathing, 363
Chiropractic services, 112, 113
Chlamydia trachomatis, 528
Chloral hydrate, 355t
Chlorthalidone, 478
Cholangitis, 488
Cholecalciferol. *See* Vitamin D_3
Cholecystitis, 488, 598
Cholesterol, 264
Cholesterol screening, 88t
Cholestyramine
　adverse drug events, 106, 106t
　for diarrhea, 142
Cholinesterase inhibitors (ChIs)
　adverse drug events, 106, 106t
　for dementia, 335–336, 413
　and incontinence, 275, 275t
　for psychotic symptoms, 392
Chondrocalcinosis, 552, 553f
Chondroitin, 114–115
Choosing Wisely® Recommendations
　for acute back pain, 545
　for behavioral disturbances in dementia, 347

　for cancer screening, 646
　for cardiology, 465
　for cerebrovascular disease, 585
　for coronary artery disease, 465
　for delirium, 359
　for dementia, 337
　for diabetes mellitus, 239, 628
　for feeding and swallowing, 273
　for gastroenterology, 495
　for heart failure/device therapy, 474
　for hospice, 146
　for hospital care, 172
　for hypertension, 481
　for infectious diseases, 600
　for kidney diseases and disorders, 511
　for musculoskeletal pain, 547
　for nephrology, 511
　for neurologic diseases and disorders, 585
　for oncology, 657
　for osteoporosis, 324
　for palliative care, 141, 146
　for perioperative care, 134
　for peripheral arterial disease, 465
　for pharmacotherapy, 110
　for prevention, 99
　for prostate disease, 528
　for rheumatology, 558
　for sleep issues, 372
　for stroke, 585
　for syncope, 260
　for urinary incontinence, 283
　for valvular heart disease, 465
　for visual loss and eye conditions, 239
Chorea, 573–574
Choroidal neovascularization (CNV), 233, 234, 234f
Chromium, 118
Chromosome 5 long arm deletion, 636
Chronic adrenal insufficiency, 601, 613
Chronic bacterial prostatitis, 528
Chronic benzodiazepine use, 371
Chronic bronchitis, 443t
Chronic constipation
　management of, 489–490, 490t
　medications for, 490, 491t
Chronic coronary artery disease, 453–455
　medical therapy for, 454–455
　presentation and diagnosis of, 453–454
Chronic cough, 439, 441t
Chronic diarrhea, 491–492
Chronic disease
　age-related, 15, 16t
　anemia of, 634
　prevalence of, 5, 5f
Chronic dislocated metatarsal phalangeal joint, 560–562, 562f
Chronic hospitalization, 177
Chronic hypnotic use, 371
Chronic inflammatory demyelinating polyradiculoneuropathy (CIDP), 576
Chronic kidney disease (CKD), 497, 507–510

　advanced, 511
　classification of, 507–508, 508t
　definition of, 507
　management of, 508–510
　medication use in, 508
　prevalence of, 5f
　screening for, 91t, 93
Chronic leg ulcers, 417, 422
Chronic lower respiratory disease, 6
Chronic lymphocytic leukemia, 655
Chronic myeloid leukemia, 648
Chronic myeloproliferative neoplasms, 640–641
Chronic obstructive pulmonary disease (COPD), 440–444
　anxiety and, 385
　diagnostic criteria for, 440, 441t
　GOLD guidelines for, 440, 441t
　inhaled bronchodilators and corticosteroids for, 442, 442t
　screening for, 91t
　therapy for, 441–442, 442t, 443t
Chronic pain, 557. *See also* Persistent pain
　definition of, 147–148
　family caregiver interventions, 56, 57t
　nonpharmacologic therapy for, 557–558
　pulsed radiofrequency (PRF) treatment of, 158
Chronic pain syndromes with developmental disabilities, 415t, 416
Chronic prostatitis, 520
Chronic subdural hematoma, 585
Chronic wounds, 285, 285t
　infectious aspects, 293
　palliative care for, 293–294, 293t
Cilostazol, 464
CIM. *See* Complementary and integrative medicine
Cimetidine, 108t, 141t, 531
Cinacalcet, 608–609
Ciprofloxacin
　for diverticulitis, 492
　drug interactions, 107, 107t
Circadian rhythm sleep disorders, 365, 371
Circulatory support, mechanical, 471–472
Circumduction, 297t
Cisplatin, 654
Citalopram, 342, 343, 343t, 377, 377t
　for anxiety disorders, 382
　for depression in CKD, 509
Citrucel (methylcellulose), 491t
CKD. *See* Chronic kidney disease
CKD-Epi equation, 497
Clarithromycin, 107, 107t
Clinical breast examination (CBE), 86
Clinical feasibility, 51–52
Clinical Global Impression of Change in Physical Frailty (CGIC-PF), 226
Clinical management, 49
Clinical practice guidelines (CPGs), 49
Clinical settings

medical director responsibilities for leadership in, 200t, 203–205
promoting physical activity in, 82
rehabilitation services, 182t
Clinker theory, 10
Clobetasol propionate, 515
Clock-drawing test, 45, 96
Clomipramine, 386t
Clonazepam (Klonopin)
for persistent pain, 152t, 157
for REM sleep behavior disorder, 366
Clonidine, 479, 513
Clopidogrel, 639
for acute coronary syndrome, 452, 453
for chronic CAD, 454
for peripheral arterial disease, 462
for stroke prevention, 460, 583
Clostridium difficile infection (CDI), 485, 599
Clotting factor deficiencies, 639–640
Clozapine
and delirium, 355t
dosing and adverse events of, 390t
for Parkinson disease and hallucinations, 392
for psychosis in dementia, 345, 345t, 346
Clubbing, 444
Clusterin gene *(CLU)*, 327
CMAI (Cohen-Mansfield Agitation Inventory), 340
CMI (Center for Medicare and Medicaid Innovations), 27, 35, 41
CMS. *See* Centers for Medicare and Medicaid Services
Coagulation, 638–640. *See also* Anticoagulation
Cocaine, 392, 403
Cochlear implants, 248, 248t
Cockcroft-Gault equation, 103, 129–131, 497
Code of Federal Regulations, 202
Code status discussions, 167–168
Coenzyme Q$_{10}$, 114t, 117
Cognitive assessment, 45
Medicare wellness visits, 94t
Mini-Cog Assessment Instrument for Dementia, 44t, 45, 96, 165, 328, 329t
Mini–Mental State Examination (MMSE), 22, 45, 328, 329t
Montreal Cognitive Assessment (MoCA), 22, 44t, 45, 165, 328, 329t
rapid screening followed by assessment and management, 43, 44t
screening instruments for, 328, 329t
St. Louis University Mental Status (SLUMS) examination, 22, 44t, 45, 328, 329t
Cognitive-behavioral therapy (CBT), 145
for alcohol dependence, 408t
for anxiety disorders, 382, 386, 386t

for chronic benzodiazepine use, 371
for depression, 380, 381
for fibromyalgia, 557–558
for insomnia, 368, 368t
for pain, 151
for personality disorders, 397
for somatic symptom disorders, 400
Cognitive dysfunction, postoperative (POCD), 353
Cognitive enhancers, 336
Cognitive impairment
in dementia, 331–332, 333t
in ED patients, 169–170
in hospitalized patients, 164–166, 165t
interventions for, 164–166, 165t
interventions for preventing falls, 308, 310t
mild, 330, 330t
in nursing-home population, 196–197
pain assessment and treatment in, 150–151
pain behaviors in, 150–151, 150t
postoperative decline, 133–134, 455
screening for, 89t, 96
trends in, 5
Cognitive reconditioning, 354t
Cognitive rehabilitation, 332
Cognitive restructuring, 387
Cognitive training, 332
Cogwheel phenomenon, 570
Cohen-Mansfield Agitation Inventory (CMAI), 340
Cohousing, senior, 213
Colchicine
Beers Criteria for, 108t
for CPPD, 553
for gout, 552
nutrient interactions, 265t
Colesevelam, 626t
Colitis
C difficile, 599
ischemic, 495
lymphocytic and collagenous, 492
microscopic, 492
pseudomembranous, 599
Collagen, 281
Collagen-containing products, 291, 291t
Colon: disorders of, 489–495
Colon cancer, 492, 494, 651–653
CIM for, 118
incidence rates, 642
prevalence of, 643
screening for, 88t, 91t, 646
Colonic adenomas, 651–652, 652–653
Colonic angiodysplasia, 494–495
Colonic ischemia, 495
Colonic polyps, 494, 651
Colonic pseudo-obstruction, acute, 495
Colonic secretagogues, 490, 490t, 491t
Colonoscopy, 86, 88t, 652, 652t
Colorectal cancer, 494, 654–655
incidence rates, 642
screening for, 86–87, 88t
Colposuspension (Burch operation), 281

Comfrey root extract *(Symphytom officinale L.)*, 115
Communication
addressing the healthcare provider, 63
addressing the patient, 63
asking about sexual orientation and gender identity, 71
code status discussions, 167–168
discussing death, 137
discussing serious news, 138–140, 139t
end-of-life decision-making conversations, 139–140
framework for, 139–140, 139t
with hearing-impaired people, 243–244, 244t
key techniques, 63–64
medical director responsibilities for, 200t, 203–205
patient-clinician, 43
respectful nonverbal communication, 64
strategies to enhance, 43, 44t, 243–244, 244t
strategies to facilitate, 43
teach-back method, 63–64
in transitional care, 178
unspoken challenges, 65
Community-acquired pneumonia, 591–592
Community-based care, 209–215
services not requiring change in residence, 211–213
services requiring change of residence, 213–214, 213t
Community Care Transitions Program, 37
Community-dwelling older Americans, 306f
Community Living Centers (VA), 196
Comorbidity
definition of, 49t
and rehabilitation, 185–186
Complementary and integrative medicine (CIM), 112–119
categorization of modalities, 112
definition of, 112
efficacy of, 114
for managing illness in older adults, 114–118
safety issues, 113–114
usage patterns, 112–113, 113t
Complex bereavement disorder, persistent, 374
Complex regional pain syndrome (CRPS), 150
Comprehensive eye examination, 229
Comprehensive geriatric assessment (CGA), 95
in primary care, 218–219
in rehabilitation, 187
Compression, intermittent pneumatic, 446
Compression stockings, 446
Compulsions, 384
Computed tomography (CT), 492
low-dose, 90

COMT (catechol-*O*-methyltransferase) inhibitors, 572
Concierge practice, 30
Conduction disturbances, 462–463, 463*t*
Conductive hearing loss, 241, 242*f*
Confusion Assessment Method (CAM), 161, 349–351
    B-CAM, 350*t*
    CAM-Severity (CAM-S), 351
    3D-CAM, 350*t*
Confusion Assessment Method for the Intensive Care Unit (CAM-ICU), 350*t*, 351
Congestive heart failure, 276*t*
Conjunctivitis
    allergic, 230–232, 237*t*
    viral, 230–232, 237*t*
Consciousness
    altered level of, 351
    sudden loss of, 254, 255*t*
Consent
    attitudes regarding, 66
    informed consent, 21–22
Consequentialism, 20
Constipation, 489–490
    IBS with alternating constipation and diarrhea (IBS-M or IBS mixed), 493
    irritable bowel syndrome with (IBS-C), 493–494
    management of chronic constipation, 489–490, 490*t*
    medications for chronic constipation, 490, 491*t*
    opioid-induced, 156–157
    postoperative, 132–133
    in terminal illness, 141–142
Constraint-induced movement therapy, 188
Consultation
    ethics, 20
    outpatient, 218–219
    proactive, 358
Continuing-care retirement communities (CCRCs), 214
Continuity theory, 8
Continuous passive-motion (CPM) machines, 191
Continuous positive-airway pressure (CPAP), 364, 444
Conversion disorder, 399
COPD. *See* Chronic obstructive pulmonary disease
COPE program, 334
Copper, 265*t*
Corneal ulcers, 230, 232, 237*t*
Coronary artery calcium content, 451
Coronary artery disease (CAD), 451–452
    chronic, 453–455
    epidemiology of, 451–452
    medical therapy for, 454–455
    presentation and diagnosis of, 453–454
    recommendations for, 465
    screening for, 91*t*
Coronary bypass surgery, 455

Coronary revascularization, 127–128, 129*t*
Coronary stents, 129
Corticosteroids. *See also* Glucocorticoids
    adverse drug events, 392
    for bowel obstruction, 142
    for COPD, 442, 442*t*, 443*t*
    for CPPD, 552
    for idiopathic pulmonary fibrosis, 444
    inhaled, 442, 442*t*, 443*t*
    for nausea, 141*t*
    ophthalmic, 232
    for osteoarthritis, 543
    perioperative, 133
    for persistent pain, 157–158
    for PMR, 553–554
    for SLE, 555
    stress doses, 133
    for vulvar lesions, 515
Corticotropin-releasing hormone (CRH), 610, 611*t*
Cortisol, 610, 611*t*
Cosmetic surgery, 417
Costs
    of assisted-living residences, 214
    of assistive listening devices, 247, 247*t*
    of COPD/asthma, 440
    of dementia care, 326
    exercise benefits, 79
    of health care, 27–42
    of hearing aids, 247, 247*t*
    of nursing-home care, 198
    of pressure ulcers, 284
    of preventive health measures, 88*t*–89*t*
    of preventive measures, 85
    of suboptimal care transitions, 174
Cough
    chronic, 439, 441*t*
    in terminal illness, 144
Councils on Aging, 337
Counseling
    on cancer screening and preventive health, 98–99
    family counseling, 357
    healthy lifestyle counseling, 89*t*, 93
    for increasing physical activity, 78, 81–82
    Medicare wellness visits, 94*t*
    nutrition, 268
COX-2 inhibitors, 155
CPAP (continuous positive-airway pressure), 364, 444
Cranberry capsules, 594
CRASH (Chemotherapy Risk Assessment Scale for High-Age Patients) Score, 646
Creatinine clearance, 103, 497, 498
Crohn disease, 492
Cross-over toe deformity, 560, 562*f*
CRP (C-reactive protein), 451, 550
Crutches, 194
Cryptogenic stroke, 581, 583–584
    low-dose, 90
Cultural aspects of care, 21, 62–69
    alcohol use, 404

    caregiving, 60
    nutritional care, 268
    palliative care, 137
Cultural identity, 63
Curanderos, 112–113
Custodial care, 31*t*
Cutaneous horn, 426
Cyclophosphamide, 420, 550
Cyclosporine, 392, 555, 556
Cymbalta (duloxetine), 152*t*
Cyproheptadine, 267
Cystic erosion, 564*t*
Cystitis, 593
Cysts, epidermal inclusion, 565
Cytochrome P450, 102–103, 107*t*
Cytokine-modulating agents, 268

D

D-dimer, 445
Dabigatran
    adverse drug events, 106, 106*t*
    Beers Criteria for, 108*t*
    for stroke prevention, 460, 461
    for VTE, 446
Dabrafenib, 428
Daily evaluation, 168–170
Dakin's solution (hypochlorite), 291*t*
Dance, 310*t*, 332
Dapagliflozin, 626*t*
Daptomycin, 592
Darbopoietin, 634–635
Darifenacin, 280
Day care, 211
Day hospitals, 211
DDAVP (vasopressin), 281
De-escalation, 588
De Quervain tenosynovitis, 541
Death
    with dignity, 25
    leading causes and numbers of, 6
    overall care near, 136–137
    physician-assisted, 25
Death certificate completion, 145–146, 145*t*
Debridement, 291–292, 293
    arthroscopic, 549
    autolytic, 292
    enzymatic, 292
    maggot debridement therapy, 292
    sharp, 292
Decision making
    approach to ethical dilemmas, 18–20, 20*t*
    approaches to, 66
    CASES approach, 18, 20*t*
    cultural aspects, 62–69, 137
    deontological/rights-based approach, 20
    documents to help loved ones or surrogates, 24, 24*t*
    end-of-life, 25–26, 66
    ETHNICS mnemonic, 67
    family decisions, 137–138
    about institutionalization, 211
    sample ethical dilemmas, 19*t*
    shared decision-making, 21
    surgical, 126
    surrogate, 23, 23*t*

Decisional capacity, 18, 21–22
  assessment of, 21–22, 22t
  myths about, 21, 22t
Decitabine, 636
Decompressive surgery, 578
DEED (Discharge of Elderly from the Emergency Department) program, 177, 179t
Deep brain stimulation (DBS)
  for essential tremor, 575
  for PD, 572
Deep tissue injury (DTI), 284t, 285, 287f
Deep venous thrombosis (DVT), 445, 446
Deep venous thrombosis (DVT) prophylaxis
  in hospitalized patients, 164, 167
  Padua Prediction Score, 167
Defecography, 490
Defense of Marriage Act (DOMA), 76
Degenerative joint disease, 415t
Dehydration, 263, 469
Dehydroepiandrosterone (DHEA), 115, 614
  safety issues, 114t
  supplements, 115, 601, 614
Dehydroepiandrosterone sulfate (DHEA-S), 614
Delirium, 349–360, 388
  agitated, 356t, 357
  assessment instruments for, 349–351, 350t
  attenuated, 351
  and dementia, 352–353
  diagnosis of, 349–351
  differential diagnosis of, 331–332, 349–351
  drugs to reduce or eliminate in management of, 354–355, 355t
  evaluation of, 353–359
  guidelines for prevention and management of, 358t, 359
  in hospitalized patients, 161, 172
  incidence of, 349
  and incontinence, 276t
  management of, 353–359, 354t
  management of behavior in, 356–357
  models of care for, 357–359
  neuropathophysiology of, 351–352
  pharmacologic therapy for, 356–357, 356t
  postoperative, 133–134, 353, 358t, 359
  preoperative assessment and management of, 131
  prognosis for, 349
  psychotic symptoms in, 390–391
  quiet, 351
  recommendations for, 172, 359
  in rehabilitation, 186
  reversible causes of, 352, 352t
  risk factors for, 352, 352t
  spectrum of, 351–352
  in terminal illness, 143
DELIRIUM mnemonic for reversible causes of delirium, 352t

Delusional disorder, 390–391
Delusions, 376
  antipsychotic medications for, 344–346, 345t
  definition of, 388
  in dementia, 344–346, 345t
  due to medical conditions, 392
  grandiose, 391
  management of, 389, 391
  mood-congruent, 388, 391
  paranoid, 388
  of poverty, 391
  somatic, 376, 391
Demand ischemia, 449
Dementia, 326–338, 568
  aggression or agitation in, 347
  alcohol-related, 405
  of Alzheimer disease, 116–117
  assessment of, 328–329
  behavioral disturbances in, 339–348
  behavioral interventions for, 342, 342t
  CIM for, 116–117
  definition of, 329
  delirium and, 352–353
  delusions in, 344–346, 345t
  depression in, 339, 342–343, 343t
  diagnostic features of, 329, 330t
  differential diagnosis of, 328–329
  differentiating types of, 329–332
  disease management, 218
  end-stage, 166, 334
  epidemiology of, 326
  etiology of, 327
  frontotemporal, 327, 330t, 331, 394
  gait abnormalities, 298t, 299
  general progression of, 332, 333t
  hallucinations in, 344–346, 345t
  in hospitalized patients, 164–165
  and incontinence, 276t
  with intellectual disability, 412–413
  Lewy body, 326, 327, 330t, 331, 341–342, 388, 392, 573
  management of, 332–337
  manic-like behavioral syndromes in, 340, 344, 344t
  Mini-Cog Assessment Instrument for Dementia, 44t, 45, 96, 165, 328, 329t
  mixed, 326
  mood disturbances in, 342–344
  "The National Partnership to Improve Dementia Care in Nursing Homes," 205
  in nursing-home population, 196–197
  Parkinson, 327
  pharmacologic treatment of, 335–337
  prevalence of, 5f
  prevention of, 88t–89t, 327–328
  protective factors for, 327–328, 328t
  psychosis in, 340, 345t
  psychotic symptoms in, 391
  pugilistic, 412

  recommendations for, 337
  and rehabilitation, 186
  resources for, 337
  risk factors for, 327–328, 328t
  safety concerns, 334–335
  screening for, 96
  sleep changes in, 366
  sleep disturbances in, 346–347
  societal impact of, 326
  supportive therapy for, 332
  treatment of, 330t, 332–337
  and urinary incontinence, 275
  vascular, 326, 330–331, 330t
Demography
  of aging, 1–6, 1f
  of alcohol use, 404
  of nursing-home population, 196–197
Denosumab (RANKL inhibitor), 321t, 323, 609
Dental anatomy, 429, 430f
Dental caries, 429–430, 556
Dental dams, 73
Dental decay, 429–430
Dental/oral conditions with developmental disabilities, 415t
Dental pulp changes, 429, 430t
Dental surgery, 437
Dental treatment, 436–437, 595
Dentistry, 429–437
Denture stomatitis, 434, 434f
Dentures, 429, 431–432
Deontological/rights-based approach, 20
Dependence
  alcohol, 404–405, 407, 408t
  benzodiazepine, 406–407
  definition of, 402
  nicotine, 407, 408t
  opioid, 407, 408t
  physical, 156
  psychological, 156
  substance, 402
Dependent personality disorder
  differential diagnosis of, 396
  features of, 395, 395t
  long-term course, 396–397
  therapeutic strategies for, 398, 398t
Depression, 373–387
  activity recommendations for, 80t
  bipolar, 375–376, 378–379, 379t, 380–381
  in chronic kidney disease, 509
  CIM for, 116
  clinical presentation of, 373–376
  cognitive-behavioral therapy for, 381
  in dementia, 339, 342–343
  with developmental disabilities, 415t
  diagnosis of, 373–376
  differential diagnosis of, 331–332
  electroconvulsive therapy for, 377–378, 379–380
  epidemiology of, 373
  Geriatric Depression Scale (GDS), 45, 374–375
  in hospitalized patients, 165t, 166

indications to start antidepressant therapy based on PHQ-9, 374, 375t
in insomnia, 362–363
interventions for, 165t, 166
interventions for preventing falls, 310t
late-life, geriatric syndrome of, 373–374
major depressive disorder, 373–374, 375, 376, 379–380
major depressive disorder with personality disorder, 397
major depressive disorder without mania but with hypomania, 375
management of, 381
with marked anxiety, 385
minor, 373, 376, 380
in nursing-home population, 197
pharmacotherapy for, 342–343, 343t, 376, 377–378
prescriber response guidelines based on PHQ-9 and the STAR*D studies for, 374, 375t
psychosocial interventions for, 380–381
psychotherapy for, 380
psychotic, 376, 377–378
rapid screening followed by assessment and management of, 43, 44t
recommended preventive measures for, 89t
and rehabilitation, 186
remission of, 374
risk factors for, 373
screening for, 89t, 96, 374–375
with severe anxiety, 386t
subclinical, 376
subsyndromal, 373, 376
suicidal, 376
in terminal illness, 145
treatment of, 376–381
Depressive personality disorder, 394, 396
Dermatitis
neurodermatitis, 419, 515
seborrheic, 418, 418f
stasis, 417
stasis dermatitis, 422
Dermatofibromas, 565
Dermatology, 417–428. See also Skin problems
Dermatomyositis, 556–557
Desensitization, graded, 387
Desipramine (Norpramin)
for depressive features of behavioral disturbances in dementia, 343, 343t
for persistent pain, 152t
Desmopressin, 260, 639
Desvenlafaxine, 343t
DETERMINE checklist, 265
Detoxification, 406, 407, 408t
Detrusor hyperactivity with impaired contractility (DHIC), 274
Detrusor overactivity (DO), 276, 277

Detrusor underactivity, 277
Developmental disabilities, 410–416
comorbidities, 415t, 416
Device therapy, 471–472, 474
Devil's claw *(Harpagophytum procumbens)*, 115
DEXA (dual energy x-ray absorptiometry), 88t, 317, 318, 509
Dexamethasone, 141t
Dextromethorphan-quidine, 347
Dhat, 399
DHEA (dehydroepiandrosterone), 115, 614
safety issues, 114t
supplements, 115, 601, 614
DHEA-S (dehydroepiandrosterone sulfate), 614
Diabetes mellitus (DM), 621–628
activity recommendations for, 80t
and cardiovascular risk, 450
CIM for, 117–118
diagnosis of, 622
education and self-management support, 624
evaluation of, 622
and foot, 566–567
goals of care in older adults, 623
and incontinence, 275, 276t
interventions for, 623–628
management of, 622–623
non-insulin agents for, 626–627, 626t
in nursing-home population, 196
pathophysiology of, 621–622
postoperative management of, 133
prevalence of, 5, 5f, 621
prevention of, 622
recommendations for, 628
and rehabilitation, 186
screening for, 90–91, 91t
self-management of, 621, 624
type 1, 621
type 2, 91t, 621, 626
Diabetic amyotrophy, 576
Diabetic neuropathy, 568, 576
Diabetic retinopathy, 231t, 235–236, 236f
Diagnosis-related groups (DRGs), 162–163, 209
Diagnostic and Statistical Manual of Mental Disorders, 4th edition, Text Revision (DSM IV-TR), 394, 398
Diagnostic and Statistical Manual of Mental Disorders, Fifth Edition (DSM-5), 326, 329, 339, 382, 383, 384, 385
criteria for bipolar disorder type 1, 375
criteria for bipolar disorder type 2, 375
criteria for delirium, 349
criteria for depression, 373, 374
criteria for intellectual disability, 410
criteria for somatic symptom disorders, 398, 399

criteria for substance use disorder, 402
descriptions of personality disorders, 394
Diagnostic imaging, 31t
Diagnostic laboratory tests, 31t
Dialectical behavior therapy, 397
Dialysis, renal, 510, 511
Diarrhea
chronic, 491–492
IBS with (IBS-D), 493, 494
IBS with alternating constipation and diarrhea (IBS-M or IBS mixed), 493
infectious, 598–599
postobstructive, 495
postoperative, 132–133
in terminal illness, 142
Diastolic heart failure, 466
Diazepam, 105
DIC (disseminated intravascular coagulation), 637, 640
Diclofenac sodium, 151, 153t
Dicyclomine, 281
Diet
altered consistencies, 271, 272t
and cancer, 118
for chronic CAD, 454
for CKD, 509–510
for depression, 116
for diabetes mellitus, 624
for gout, 551
for HTN, 478
for IBS, 493
Modified Diet in Renal Disease (MDRD) formula, 103–104, 129–131, 497
for sleep disorders, 117
sodium restriction, 473, 478
Dietary Supplement Health and Education Act (DSHEA), 113
Dietary supplements, 112, 267, 473
for pressure ulcers, 292
safety issues, 113–114, 114t
Dietitians, 184, 185t
Diffuse large B-cell lymphoma, 656
Diffuse peritonitis, 493
Digestive problems. *See* Gastroenterology
Digestive system
age-related changes, 12t, 14, 17
age-related pathologies, 16t
Digit quinti varus, 561t
Digital rectal examination (DRE), 523–524
Dignity therapy, 145
Digoxin
adverse drug events, 106, 106t, 265
drug interactions, 107, 107t, 588
for heart failure, 471, 471t
nutrient interactions, 265, 265t
Dihydropyridines, 265, 454–455
Diltiazem, 453
adverse drug events, 106, 106t
for atrial fibrillation, 459
Diogenes syndrome, 384
Diphenhydramine
adverse drug events, 106, 106t, 366

and delirium, 355t
for insomnia, 371
for nausea, 141, 141t
Diphenoxylate/atropine, 491
Dipivefrin, 238t
Diplopia, 229, 230, 237t
Dipyridamole, 583, 639
Direct thrombin inhibitors, 446
Disability
definition of, 49t
excess, 404–405
hospital-associated, 160–161
International Classification of Functioning, Disability, and Health (ICF) (WHO), 181
preclinical, 46
trends in, 5
Disabled dual eligibles, 34–35
Disalcid (salsalate), 153t
Disc displacement, 539, 544t, 545t
Discharge destinations, 177
Discharge medication regimen, 178
Discharge of Elderly from the Emergency Department (DEED) program, 177, 179t
Disclosure, 66
DISCUS (Dyskinesia Identification System Condensed User Scale), 390
Disease management, 218
Disease-modifying anti-inflammatory drugs (DMARDs), 550
Disease-modifying therapies, 336
Disinhibited impulsive syndrome, 394
Dislocation, metatarsal phalangeal joint, 560–562, 561t, 562f
Disorganized thinking, 351
Disseminated intravascular coagulation (DIC), 637, 640
Distraction techniques, 347
Disulfiram, 407, 408t
Diuretics
adverse drug events, 106, 106t
drug interactions, 107, 107t
for heart failure, 469, 471
for hyperkalemia, 502
for hypertension, 478, 478t
loop, 275t, 469
nutrient interactions, 265t
for prevention of cardiovascular disease, 625
thiazide, 469, 478, 478t, 499
Divalproex sodium
for behavioral disturbances in dementia with manic-like features, 344, 344t
for personality disorders, 397
to stabilize mood in mania and bipolar depression, 378, 379t
Diverticular disease, 492–493
Diverticulitis, 492, 493, 598
mild, 492–493
Diverticulosis, 492
painful, 493
Dix-Hallpike test, 251–252, 299
Dizziness, 249–253
classification of, 249–251, 250t
diagnostic testing for, 252–253
evaluation of, 251–253

history, 251
management of, 253
mixed, 250t, 251
physical examination of, 251–252
prevalence of, 249
DM-1 (emtansine), 649
DMARDs (disease-modifying anti-inflammatory drugs), 550
DNMT3A gene, 636
"Do-not-hospitalize" orders, 207
Docetaxel, 647, 647t, 654
Doctrine of double effect, 25
Documentation
asthma action plans, 440, 441t
death certificate completion, 145–146, 145t
documents to help loved ones or surrogates with decision making, 24, 24t
Durable Power of Attorney (DPOA) documents, 18, 23, 24, 24t, 207
electronic health records, 41
forms that identify patient preferences, 24–25
for house calls, 210
Physician Orders for Life-Sustaining Treatment (POLST), 24–25, 24t, 140
of pressure ulcers, 286–288
wound, 286–288
Docusate sodium, 489–490
Dofetilide, 460
DOMA (Defense of Marriage Act), 76
Donepezil, 335–336, 346, 413
Doorway thoughts in cross-cultural health care, 62
Dopamine agonists
adverse effects of, 611
and delirium, 355t
for hyperprolactinemia, 610–611
for PD motor symptoms, 572
for restless legs syndrome, 575
Dopamine antagonists, 141t
Dopaminergic agents
adverse drug events, 392
for restless legs syndrome, 575
Dorzolamide, 238t
Double effect, doctrine of, 25
Down syndrome, 412–413
Doxazosin, 521, 521t
Doxepin
and delirium, 355t
for insomnia, 369t, 370
Doxorubicin, 647t
Doxycycline, 598
DPOA (Durable Power of Attorney) documents, 18, 23, 24, 24t
DPP-4 enzyme inhibitors, 626t, 627
Dramatic, emotional, or erratic behaviors, 395t, 398
Dressings
for chronic wounds, 294
for foot ulcers, 567
for pressure ulcers, 290, 291t, 292
DRGs (diagnosis-related groups), 162–163, 209
Drinking. *See* Alcohol

Driving accidents: risk factors for, 47
Driving assessment, 47, 334–335
recommendations for, 89t, 97
Dronabinol, 118–119, 141t, 268
Dronedarone, 460
Drop arm sign, 540
Droxidopa, 573
Drug abuse. *See also* Substance abuse
magnitude of the problem, 403
in transgender adults, 74
Drug-drug interactions (DDIs), 107, 107t
Drug holidays, 322
Drug-induced esophageal injury, 486
Drug-induced lupus erythematosus, 555
Drug-induced movement disorders, 573, 574
Drug-induced myopathy, 577
Drug-induced parkinsonism, 573
Drug-nutrient interactions, 264–265, 265t
Drug regimen review, 108–109
Drug resistance, 587
Drugs. *See also* Pharmacotherapy; *specific drugs*
absorption of, 101–102
for addiction treatment, 408t
adverse drug events, 106, 106t, 385
antiepileptic, 569–570, 569t
for anxiety disorders, 385–386, 386t
to avoid in older adults, 158
Beers Criteria for, 105, 108t
for benign prostatic hyperplasia, 521–522, 521t
in chronic kidney disease, 508
clearance of, 103
for constipation, 490, 491t
for delirium, 353–354, 354t
for depressive features of behavioral disturbances in dementia, 342–343, 343t
discontinuing, 109
distribution of, 102
elimination of, 103–104
flexible medication times, 366
guidelines for prevention of falls, 308
half-life of, 103
health insurance coverage for, 31t
hydrophilic, 102
inappropriate/overprescribed and underprescribed medications/classes, 104–105, 105t
for incontinence, 280–281
interventions for preventing falls, 308t, 310t
lipophilic, 102
to lower glucose, 626–627
Medicare Prescription Drug Plan Finder (CMS), 33
medications for insomnia, 369t, 370–371
metabolism of, 102–103
nonadherence to regimens, 109–110
for osteoporosis, 320–324, 321t
outpatient care, 31t

for PD motor symptoms, 571–572
  to reduce or eliminate in management of delirium, 354–355, 355t
  requirements for long-term care facilities, 201t, 205
  to stabilize mood in mania and bipolar depression, 379t
  that can cause or worsen UI, 275, 275t
  that can increase risk of osteoporosis, 316t
  that cause hyperkalemia, 501, 501t
  that interfere with gustation (taste) and olfaction (smell), 435, 436t
Dry eye, 230–232, 230t, 237t
Dry mouth, 432
Dry weight, 468
DSHEA (Dietary Supplement Health and Education Act), 113
Dual antiplatelet therapy (DAPT), 453
Dual eligibles, 34–35, 41, 212
Dual energy x-ray absorptiometry (DEXA), 88t, 317, 318, 509
Dual tasking, 300
Dulaglutide, 626t
Dulcolax (bisacodyl), 491t
Duloxetine (Cymbalta)
  for anxiety, 385, 386
  Beers Criteria for, 108t
  for depression, 377t
  for depressive features of behavioral disturbances in dementia, 343t
  for fibromyalgia, 558
  for incontinence, 281
  for neuropathic pain, 576
  for persistent pain, 152t, 157
Dupuytren contractions, 541
Durable medical equipment, 31t
Durable Power of Attorney (DPOA) documents, 18, 23, 24, 24t, 207
Duragesic (transdermal fentanyl), 154t
Dutasteride, 521–522, 521t
DVT (deep venous thrombosis), 445, 446
Dysequilibrium, 249–251, 250t
Dysesthesia, 148t
Dyskinesia, 570, 571–572
Dyskinesia Identification System Condensed User Scale (DISCUS), 390
Dyslipidemia, 450–451
Dyspareunia, 535, 536, 536t
Dyspepsia, 486–487
Dysphagia, 270–271, 483–484
  classification of, 270
  esophageal, 271
  evaluation of, 484, 484t
  oral, 270
  oropharyngeal, 271–272
  pharyngeal, 270–271
Dyspnea, 439, 441t, 444
  severe, 443, 443t
  in terminal illness, 143–144
Dystonia, 570, 574

E

Ears
  age-related changes, 12t, 14
  age-related pathologies, 16t
Eastern Cooperative Oncology Group (ECOG) performance measures, 645
Eating changes, 270
Eating problems, 270–273
Eccentric behaviors, 395t
Echinacea, 114t
Echocardiography, 257t, 258, 451
  transesophageal (TEE), 458, 595
ECOG (Eastern Cooperative Oncology Group) performance measures, 645
Ectropion, 229, 230t
Eczema, 565
Eczema craquelé, 419, 419f
ED (erectile dysfunction), 530–534
Eden Alternative, 206
Edentulism, 431–432
Edoxaban
  Beers Criteria for, 108t
  for stroke prevention, 460, 461
  for VTE, 446
Education. See also Patient education
  about delirium, 354t
  medical director responsibilities for, 200t, 203–205
Educational attainment, 4
Effexor (venlafaxine), 152t
eGFR (estimated glomerular filtration rate), 497
EGSYS (Evaluation of Guidelines in Syncope Study) score, 256, 256t
Eikenella, 458, 595
Elbow pain, 540–541
Elder Justice Roadmap, 124
Elder mistreatment. See Mistreatment
Eldercare Locator, 59t
Electrical stimulation, 292
Electrocardiography
  ambulatory monitoring, 257t, 258–259
  in heart failure, 467
  implantable loop recorders, 257t, 258
  in syncope, 257–258, 257t
Electroconvulsive therapy
  for depression in terminally ill, 145
  for depressive features of behavioral disturbances in dementia, 343
  for major depressive disorder and mania, 379–380
  for psychotic depression, 377–378
Electrolyte disorders, 132
Electromagnetic field therapy, 114
Electromyography (EMG), 556–557, 576
Electronic health records, 41
Electrophysiologic studies, 257t, 259
Emergency care
  health insurance coverage for, 31t
  hypertensive emergencies and urgencies, 480
Emergency department (ED) care, 169–170

Discharge of Elderly from the Emergency Department (DEED) program, 177, 179t
  geriatric EDs, 169–170
  risk-screening tools, 169, 169t
EMG (electromyography), 556–557, 576
Emotion-oriented psychotherapy, 332
Emotional behaviors, 395t
Empagliflozin, 626t
Employment, 4
Empty can sign, 540
Empty sella syndrome, 612
Emtansine (DM-1), 649
Enalapril, 469t
Encephalopathy
  personality changes in, 394
  toxic or metabolic, 349
End-of-life care
  advance care planning for, 24–25
  controversial procedures, 25–26
  cultural aspects of, 66–67, 137
  family caregiver interventions, 56, 57t
  financing, 40
  for heart failure, 473
  palliative care, 140–145
  preventive health measures, 88t–89t
End-of-life decisions
  conversations, 139–140
  cultural issues, 66, 137
End-stage dementia, 166, 334
End-stage renal disease (ESRD), 509, 510–511
Endocarditis
  infective, 429, 436, 458, 595
  native-valve, 458
Endocrine disorders, 601
  laboratory evaluation for, 601
  postoperative management of, 133
Endocrine myopathy, 577
Endocrine Society, 535
Endocrine system
  age-related changes, 12t, 15, 498t, 601
  age-related pathologies, 16t
Endocrine theory of aging, 8t, 10–11
Endocrinology, 601–620
Endometrial cancer, 518, 648
Endoscopy, 486, 487–488
Endovascular thrombectomy, 582
Endurance exercise training, 192
Enemas, 490, 490t
Energy intake, 264
Energy requirements, 262
Energy therapy, 113t, 118
Enhanced primary care, 216–218
Enoxaparin
  for acute coronary syndrome, 452
  Beers Criteria for, 108t
Entacapone, 572
Entecavir, 551
Entrapment syndrome, 564t
Entropion, 229
Environmental modifications
  for behavioral disturbances, 347
  for delirium, 354t
  for dementia, 334

home care, 210
    for preventing falls, 308, 308t, 310t
    for rehabilitation, 193, 195
    for sleep disorders, 366
Enzymatic debridement, 292
EORTC Quality of Life Questionnaire Core, 650
Epidermal inclusion cysts, 565
Epidural hematoma, 584
Epigenetic theory of aging, 8t, 10
Epilepsy, 568–570
    temporal lobe, 394
Epinephrine, 238t
Eplerenone, 469
Epley maneuver, 252f, 253
Epoetin alfa, 634–635
Epoetin beta, 634–635
Eprosartan, 469t
Eptifibatide, 639
Equinovarus, 297t
Equinus deformity, 560, 561t
Erectile dysfunction (ED), 521, 522, 530–534
    causes of, 530–532, 531t
    evaluation of, 532–533
    treatment options for, 533–534, 533t
Erectile physiology, 530–534
Ergotamines, 578–579
Erratic behaviors, 395t
Error catastrophe theory of aging, 8t, 10
Erythromycin, 281
    drug interactions, 107, 107t
    for rosacea, 419
Erythroplakia, 433, 433f
Erythropoiesis, ineffective, 632, 635–636
Erythropoiesis-stimulating agents (ESAs), 508, 509, 634–635
Erythropoietin production, decreased, 634–635
Erythropoietin therapy
    for anemia, 634–635
    for postural hypotension, 260
ESBLs (extended spectrum β-lactamase–producing gram-negative rods), 587
Eschar, 292
Escitalopram, 343t, 377t
Eskimos, 268
Esophageal cancer, 653–654
Esophageal dysphagia, 271, 483–484, 484t
Esophagitis, pill, 486
Esophagus
    disorders of, 483–486
    drug-induced injury to, 486
    gastroesophageal reflux disease, 484–486
Essential thrombocythemia (ET), 629, 640, 641
Essential tremor (ET), 574–575
Estimated glomerular filtration rate (eGFR), 103–104, 497
Estrogen deficiency, 315
Estrogen-progestin therapy, 609
Estrogen therapy, 617–618
    in chronic kidney disease, 509
    for colonic angiodysplasia, 495
    for female sexual dysfunction, 536
    for incontinence, 275t, 281
    for menopausal symptoms, 512, 513
    for osteoporosis, 321t, 322–323
    for vaginal atrophy, 514, 535
Eszopiclone, 369t, 370
ET (essential thrombocythemia), 629, 640, 641
ET (essential tremor), 574–575
Etanercept, 551
Ethambutol, 595
Ethical issues, 18–26
    approach to ethical dilemmas, 18–20, 20t
    CASES approach, 18, 20t
    in home care, 211
    medical ethics, 21
    related to nutritional status, 268–269
    sample dilemmas, 19t
Ethics and law, 18–26
Ethics consultation, 20
Ethnic differences
    in cancer incidence and mortality, 644
    in depression, 373
    in urinary incontinence, 274
Ethnic minority populations, 3, 644
ETHNICS mnemonic, 67
Etoposide, 647, 647t
European Guidelines on Cardiovascular Disease Prevention, 624
European League Against Rheumatism (EULAR), 553
European Society for Microbiology, 593
Euthanasia, 25–26
Evaluation of Guidelines in Syncope Study (EGSYS) score, 256, 256t
Evidence, 50–51
Evolutionary theories of aging, 7–8
Exalgo (hydromorphone, extended release), 153t
Executive dysfunction, 375
Executive function testing, 45
Exenatide, 626t, 627
Exercise, 355
    benefits of, 451
    for cancer, 118
    counseling for, 89t, 93
    for dementia, 332
    for depression, 380
    for diabetes mellitus, 621, 622
    for DVT, 446
    for gait disorders, 300
    for heart failure, 468
    for hypertension, 478
    Kegel exercises, 516
    for low fitness or low functional ability, 83–84
    for menopausal symptoms, 117
    for neck pain, 539
    for OA-related pain, 543, 548–549
    for osteoporosis, 319
    for pain, 151
    pelvic muscle exercises (PMEs), 279, 280
    for peripheral arterial disease, 464
    for polymyositis, 557
    for preventing falls, 308, 308t, 309, 310t, 311
    recommendations for, 79–81, 80t, 116
    to reduce risk of osteoporosis, 316, 316t
    relative exercise intensity, 78
    for sleep problems, 117, 368–369, 369–370
    total body preoperative exercise, 301
    vestibular rehabilitation therapy (VRT), 253
Exercise: A Guide from the National Institute on Aging, 83
Exercise intensity, 78, 79t
Exercise is Medicine Initiative (ACSM), 82
Exercise Management for Chronic Diseases and Disabilities (ACSM), 82
Exercise stress testing, 258
Exercise training, 192
Exercise volume, 78, 79t
Exploitation, 121, 122t
Exposure with response prevention, 387
Extended spectrum β-lactamase–producing gram-negative rods (ESBLs), 587
Extensivists, 217–218
External beam radiation therapy, 526t, 527
Extracellular fluid volume
    depletion, 499
    normal, 499–500
    overload, 499
Eye conditions, 229–230, 230t, 231t, 237t
    inflammatory conditions, 556
Eye drops, 237–238, 238t
Eyes
    age-related changes, 12t, 14
    age-related pathologies, 16t
    comprehensive examination of, 229

F

F-tags, 202, 282
FACES Pain Rating Scale with Foreign Translations, 149
Faces Pain Scale, 149
Facial nerve palsy (Bell's palsy), 598
Facial volume restoration, 417
Factitious disorder, 399
Factor VII, 639–640
Factor VIIa, recombinant activated (rHFVIIa), 639
Factor VIII, 639
Factor VIII inhibitor bypassing activity concentrate (FEIBA®), 639
Factor Xa inhibitors, 446
Failure to thrive, 227
Fair process, 167–168
Faith/spiritual beliefs, 62
Falls, 303–312
    activity recommendations for, 80t
    causes of, 303–305

clinical guidelines for prevention of, 305, 308
diagnostic approach to, 305–307
history in, 305–307
in hospitalized patients, 163, 165t
interventions for, 163, 165t
interventions for lowering risk of, 307, 308t
laboratory and diagnostic tests for, 307
physical examination in, 305–307
prevalence and morbidity of, 303
prevention of, 95–96, 304, 306f, 307–311, 308t, 310t
risk assessment for, 89t, 95–96, 305, 311
risk factors for, 303–304, 310t, 311
screening for, 307
treatment of, 307–311
Famcyclovir, 424
Familial Alzheimer's disease, 327
Families, 332–334
fictive kin, 66
of LGBT older adults, 75
Familismo, 60
Family Caregiver Alliance, 56–57, 58, 59t
Family Caregiver Navigator, 59t
Family caregivers, 54, 55, 326
assessment of, 56–58
information and referral for, 60
interventions for, 56, 57t
treatment of, 58–59
Family caregiving, 55–56
cultural considerations, 60
Family COPE intervention, 57t
Family counseling, 357
Family decisions, 137–138
Family education, 354t
Family-focused treatment, 380–381
Famotidine, 108t, 141t
Fanconi syndrome, 502
Fasting blood glucose, 601
Fatalism, 268
Fearful behaviors, 395t
Febuxostat, 552
Fecal bulking agents, 491
Fecal impaction, 490
Fecal incontinence, 490–491
with developmental disabilities, 415t
Fecal microbiota transplantation (FMT), 599
Fecal occult blood testing (FOBT), 494
recommendations for, 86–87, 88t
Federal Coordinated Health Care Office, 35
Federal financing of health care, 40–42
Federal health care spending, 29f, 30f
Fee-for-service (FFS) care
discounted FFS, 37
home-health care, 39
inpatient care, 37–38
Medicare, 27, 28–32, 31t, 35–36, 36t
nursing-home care, 39
outpatient care, 35–36
postacute rehabilitation, 38

private plans, 32
readmissions, 172
Feeding, 270–273
artificial, 269
hand, 272–273
recommendations for, 172, 273
tube, 272–273
Feeding assistance, 354t, 355
Feeding problems, 270–273
Feeding tubes, 269, 272, 273
FEIBA® (factor VIII inhibitor bypassing activity concentrate), 639
Female sexual dysfunction, 535
evaluation of, 535–537
treatment options for, 535
Female sexuality, 534–537
Femoral hernia, 542
Femoral neuropathy, 541, 542
FE_{Na} (fractional excretion of sodium), 503–504
Fentanyl, transdermal (Duragesic), 154t
Fermentable oligo-, di- and monosaccharides and polyols (FODMAP diet), 493
Ferric gluconate, 634
Ferritin, 635
Ferrous gluconate, 634
Ferrous sulfate, 634
Ferumoxytol, 633
Fesoterodine, 280, 281
Festination, 297t
Fever
evaluation of, 598t, 599
in frail, older residents, 586, 587–588, 588t
in older nursing-home residents, 587–588
Fever of unknown origin (FUO), 598t, 599–600
Fiber, dietary, 490t
Fiber supplements, 489
FiberCon (polycarbophil), 491t
Fibrinolytic therapy, 452–453
Fibromyalgia, 557–558
FICA (faith and belief, importance, community, and address in care), 68
Fictive kin, 66
Fidaxomicin, 599
FIM (Functional Independence Measure), 183, 184t
Financial assessment, 122–123
Financial mistreatment, 122–123
Financial security challenges, 76
Financing
for assisted living, 214
costs of hearing aids, 247, 247t
end-of-life care, 40
federal, 40–42
health care, 27–42
home-health care, 39
for house calls, 210
inpatient care, 37–38
nursing-home care, 39–40
for nursing-home care, 198
outpatient care, 35–37
postacute rehabilitation, 38–39

for rehabilitation services, 182–183, 182t
Finasteride, 521–522, 521t
Fine-needle aspiration (FNA), 605
Firearms, 374–375
Fish oil, 116
Fitness, low, 83–84
"Five A's" method of smoking cessation, 407, 440–441
5q– syndrome, 636
Flashes, 237t
Flat foot, 559–560, 560f
Flavor enhancement, 435
Flavoxate, 281
Flecainide, 460
Flexibility activity recommendations, 80, 80t
Flexible medication times, 366
Flexible sigmoidoscopy, 86
Flibanserin, 535
Floaters, 229, 230, 230t, 237t
Floating the heels, 289
Florbetapir, 329
Flu. *See* Influenza
Fluconazole, 107, 107t
Fludarabine, 647, 647t
Fludrocortisone, 310t, 573
Fluid needs, 263
Fluid replacement, 489–490, 490t
Fluoride, 430
Fluoroquinolones, 592
5-Fluorouracil, 653
Fluoxetine, 281, 342, 343t
Flutamide, 527
Fluticasone, 442t
Focal segmental glomerulosclerosis, 507
FODMAP diet (fermentable oligo-, di- and monosaccharides and polyols), 493
Folate
drug interactions, 265t
RDIs for adults ≥71 years old, 263t
Folate deficiency, 633f, 635, 638
Folic acid, 267
Follicle-stimulating hormone (FSH), 611t, 615
Follicular lymphoma, 648, 656
Folstein Mini–Mental State Examination (MMSE), 22, 45, 96, 328, 329t
Fondaparinux, 452
Beers Criteria for, 108t
for DVT prophylaxis, 167
for VTE prophylaxis, 446
Food and Nutrition Board, Institute of Medicine, 262
Foods, calcium-containing, 319–320, 320t
Foot care, 559
Foot diseases and disorders, 559
arthritis, 567
associated deformities, 560–563
common deformities, 559–565, 561t, 564t
in diabetes mellitus, 566–567
interventions for preventing falls, 309
nail disorders, 565–566
peripheral arterial disease, 567

skin lesions, 565
surgical considerations for deformities, 564–565
systemic diseases, 566–567
treatment strategies for, 563–565
Foot drop, 297t, 298
Foot slap, 297t
Foot ulcers, 566–567
Footwear
for preventing falls, 309, 310t
shoe terms, 564t
shoes, 309, 310t, 564
Formality, 63
Formoterol fumarate, 442t
Fosinopril, 469t
Foster care, 214
4AT, 350t
400-meter walk test, 300
Fractional excretion of sodium (FE_{Na}), 503–504
Fracture risk assessment model (FRAX™) (WHO), 313, 316, 318, 318t
Fractures
diagnosis of, 316–318
fragility, 313
of hip, 189–190, 313, 607
prediction of, 316–318
risk factors for, 316, 316t
sacral fractures, 543, 544t, 545t, 546
secondary causes of, 316–317
vertebral, 318–319, 324
vertebral compression fractures, 324, 538, 543, 544t, 545t, 546
Fragile X syndrome, 416
Fragility fracture, 313
Frailty, 222–228
activity recommendations for, 80t
assessment of, 225–226
and associated vulnerability, 222
behavioral prevention or treatment of, 227
and cardiovascular disease, 451
causes of, 224, 225f
as clinical syndrome, 223–224
as core clinical concept, 222
criteria that define, 223, 224t
cycle of, 223, 223f
definition of, 49t
evidence-based findings, 222–224
and failure to thrive, 227
fever in frail, older residents of long-term care facilities, 586, 587–588, 588t
hypertension in, 480–481
management strategies for, 226
palliative care for, 227
pharmacologic treatments for, 226–227
pre-frailty, 451
prevention of, 227–228
primary, 222, 224
screening tests for, 225–226
secondary, 222, 224–225
FRAX™ (fracture risk assessment model) (WHO), 313, 316, 318, 318t
Free radical theory of aging, 8t, 10

Free T_3 test, 603
Free T_4 test, 603
Free water deficit, 500
Freezing of gait, 297t, 298
Frequency-volume charts, 278
Frontal lobe disease, 298–299, 298t
Frontal lobe injury, 394
Frontotemporal dementia
diagnostic features and treatment of, 330t
differential diagnosis of, 331
etiology of, 327
personality changes in, 394
Frozen shoulder (adhesive capsulitis), 540
FSH (follicle-stimulating hormone), 611t, 615
Fukuda stepping test, 252
Functional Activities Questionnaire, 328, 329t
Functional Ambulation Classification scale, 300
Functional Assessment of Cancer Therapy, 650
Functional Independence Measure (FIM), 183, 184t
Functional reach test, 307
Functional status
acute decline, 47–48
assessment of, 46–47, 184t
with developmental disabilities, 415t
impairments in hospitalized patients, 165t
International Classification of Functioning, Disability, and Health (ICF) (WHO), 181
interventions for, 165t
low fitness or low functional ability, older adults with, 83–84
of nursing-home population, 196, 199t
performance-based assessment of, 299–300
postoperative decline, 455
rapid screening followed by assessment and management of, 43, 44t
trends in, 5
Fungal infections, 566, 566f
FUO (fever of unknown origin), 598t, 599–600
Furosemide, 265
Futility, 168–169

G

GABAergic agents, 275t
Gabapentin (Neurontin, Gralise, Horizant), 569–570, 569t
for alcohol detoxification, 408t
Beers Criteria for, 108t
for depressive features of behavioral disturbances in dementia, 343t
for essential tremor, 575
and incontinence, 275t
for insomnia, 346–347
for neuropathic pain, 576

for persistent pain, 152t, 157
for restless legs syndrome, 365, 575
for vasomotor symptoms, 513
GAD (generalized anxiety disorder), 384, 386, 386t
Gait abnormalities, 297, 297t, 298t
antalgic gait, 297t, 298, 298t
associated findings, 298t
freezing of gait, 297t, 298
idiopathic, 297
"senile" gait disorder, 297
steppage gait, 297t, 298t
Trendelenburg gait, 297–298, 297t, 298t
Gait and balance screening, 89t, 300
Gait apraxia, 299
Gait disorders, 568
rehabilitation of, 300
Gait impairment, 46, 296–302
assessment of, 297–300
conditions that contribute to, 17, 296–297
epidemiology of, 296
history and physical examination of, 299
interventions for preventing falls, 310t
interventions to reduce disorders, 300–302
laboratory and imaging assessments of, 299
performance-based functional assessment of, 299–300
Gait speed, 46, 300
Gait training, 308, 308t, 309, 310t
Galantamine, 335–336, 346, 413
Gall stones, 489
Gambling, 407–409
Gammopathy, monoclonal, of uncertain significance (MGUS), 656
Gastric cancer, 653–654
Gastroenterology, 483–496
Gastroesophageal reflux disease (GERD), 484–486, 495
Gastrointestinal bleeding, 494
Gastrointestinal diseases and disorders
with developmental disabilities, 415t
and incontinence, 276t
infections, 598–599
recommendations for, 495
Gastrointestinal obstruction, 142
Gastrointestinal system
age-related changes in, 483
postoperative management of, 132–133
Gastrostomy
contraindications to, 273
percutaneous endoscopic, 272
Gastrostomy tube placement, 273
Gay men. *See also* Lesbian gay bisexual transgender (LGBT) older adults
concerns about aging, 75
disease risk, 71–72
sexual risk, 73
GDF15 (growth differentiation factor 15), 630

GDS (Geriatric Depression Scale), 44t, 45, 96, 374–375
GEM (geriatric evaluation and management) units, 170, 218–219
Gemcitabine, 647, 647t, 654
Gender differences
    cultural aspects, 66
    in drug metabolism, 103
    in urinary incontinence, 274
Gender identity, 71
General Practitioner Assessment of Cognition, 96
Generalized anxiety disorder (GAD), 384, 386, 386t
Genetic damage, 8t, 9
Genetic disorders, 416
Genital prolapse, 516, 517
Genu recurvatum, 297t
Geographic distribution of older adults, 4
Geographic tongue, 434
"Geographical Practices Cost Indices," 209–210
GERD (gastroesophageal reflux disease), 484–486
GERI-PACT (patient-aligned care teams) model, 52
Geriatric Depression Scale (GDS), 44t, 45, 96, 374–375
Geriatric EDs, 169–170
Geriatric evaluation and management (GEM) units, 170, 218–219
Geriatric Resource Nurse (GRN) Model, 171
Geriatric Resources for Assessment and Care of Elders (GRACE), 179t, 217
Geriatric specialty care, 219–220
Geriatrics-orthopedics services, 358
Gerotranscendence theory, 8
GFR. *See* Glomerular filtration rate
Giant cell arteritis (GCA), 230, 237t, 554
Gingivitis, 430
Ginkgo biloba, 116
    for dementia, 336
    safety issues, 114t
Glaucoma, 230t, 236–238
    angle-closure, 230, 230t, 237t
    definition of, 236
    eye drops for, 237–238
    narrow-angle, 231t
    open-angle, 231t, 236–237
    screening for, 96, 229
    symptoms and treatment of, 231t
    treatment of, 237t
    types of, 236
Gleason grading system, 524
Glimepiride, 626t
Glipizide, 626t, 627
Global aging trends, 1–2, 1f
Global Initiative for Chronic Obstructive Lung Disease (GOLD), 440, 441t
Glomerular disease, 506
Glomerular filtration rate (GFR), 129–131, 497, 507
    age-related changes in, 103, 498t
    estimated (eGFR), 103–104, 497

Glomerulonephritis, 506
    pauci-immune, 506
    postinfectious, 506
    proliferative, 506
    rapidly progressive, 506
Glomerulosclerosis, focal segmental, 507
GLP-1 receptor agonists, 626t
Glucocorticoid-induced osteoporosis, 316–317, 316t
Glucocorticoids
    adverse drug events, 106, 106t
    for dermatomyositis, 557
    for gout, 552
    for hip OA, 549
    for knee OA, 549
    for polymyositis, 557
Glucosamine, 114, 114t
Glucose screening, 88t
α-Glucosidase inhibitors, 626, 626t
Glyburide, 626t, 627
Glycemic control, 623, 625–626
    medications to lower glucose, 626–627
Glycoprotein IIb/IIIa inhibitors, 452, 639
Glycopyrrolate
    for bowel obstruction, 143t
    for loud respirations, 145
GnRH (gonadotropin-releasing hormone), 611t
GnRH (gonadotropin-releasing hormone) agonists, 316, 316t
Goiter, toxic multinodular, 603
Gold, 550
GOLD (Global Initiative for Chronic Obstructive Lung Disease), 440
Golfer's elbow, 540, 541
Golimumab, 551
Gonadotropin-releasing hormone (GnRH), 611t
Gonadotropin-releasing hormone (GnRH) agonists, 316, 316t
Gonadotropin-secreting adenomas, 611
Gottron papules, 556
Gout, 541, 542, 543, 551–552
GRACE (Geriatric Resources for Assessment and Care of Elders), 179t, 217
GRACE Team Care™, 217
Graded desensitization, 387
Grading of Recommendations Assessment, Development and Evaluation working group (GRADE), 52
Gralise (gabapentin), 152t
Grandiose delusions, 391
Granisetron, 141t
Granulocyte colony-stimulating factor, 647t
Granulocyte-macrophage colony-stimulating factor, 647t
Granulomatosis with polyangiitis, 506
Graves disease, 603, 604
Green House Model, 206
Green Prescription (New Zealand), 82
GRN (Geriatric Resource Nurse) Model, 171

Groin pain, 542
Group homes, 214
Growth differentiation factor 15 (GDF15), 630
Growth hormone (GH), 268, 601, 618
    age-related changes in, 610, 611t, 618
Growth hormone (GH) deficiency, 618
Growth retardation, 415t
Guardianship, 415–416
Guided Care, 176–177, 179t, 216–217
Guillain-Barré syndrome, 576
Gustatory dysfunction
    age-related changes, 435
    medications that cause, 435, 436t
    nonpharmacologic causes of, 435, 436t
Gynecology, 512–519

H
H_2-receptor antagonists
    adverse drug events, 265
    and delirium, 355, 355t
    drug interactions, 588
    for GERD, 485
    for nausea, 141t
HAART (highly active antiretroviral therapy), 597
HACEK (*Haemophilus, Actinobacillus, Cardiobacterium, Eikenella,* and *Kingella*) organisms, 458, 595
Haemophilus, 458, 595
Haemophilus influenzae type b immunization, 590t
Haglund deformity, 561t
Hair, 417
Hairy cell leukemia, 648
Hairy tongue, 435, 435f
HALE (healthy life expectancy), 3
Half-life, 103
Hallucinations, 390
    antipsychotic medications for, 344–346, 345t
    definition of, 388
    in dementia, 344–346, 345t
    due to medical conditions, 392
    isolated, 391–392
    visual, 238, 390, 392
Hallus valgus, 562
Hallux abducto valgus, 561t, 562f
Hallux limitus, 561t, 562
Hallux rigidus, 561t
Hallux valgus, 561t
Haloperidol
    for agitated delirium, 356t, 357
    for chorea, 574
    dosing and adverse events of, 390t
    for nausea, 141, 141t
    for psychosis in dementia, 345t
Hammertoes, 561t, 562
Hand feeding, 272–273
Hand osteoarthritis, 548, 549f
Hand pain, 541
Hand washing, 599
Handoffs, 174
Handovers, 174
Harpagophytum procumbens (devil's claw), 115

Harris Hip Questionnaire, 184t, 187, 190
Hayflick's limit, 9
Head injury, 612
Head-thrust test, 252
Headaches, 568, 578–579
Healers, 112–113
Healing
  caloric requirements, 292
  chronic wounds, 285, 285t
  Pressure Ulcer Scale for Healing, 286
  products that promote, 290–291
  protein requirements, 292
Healing touch, 118
Health beliefs, 65
Health care
  attitudes toward North American health services, 65
  Bundled Payments for Care Improvement initiative, 27–28, 28t
  costs of, 27–42
  coverage of, 27–42
  federal financing of, 40–42
  federal spending on, 29f, 30f
  financing of, 27–42, 29f
  GRACE model, 217
  trends in, 5–6
Health care expenditures, 5–6, 5f
Health care proxy, 97
Health insurance
  coverage for older Americans, 27–42, 31t
  coverage for rehabilitation, 182–183
  trends in, 5–6
Health literacy, 63
Health Maintenance Organizations (HMOs), 32
Health maintenance visits, 332
Health professional burnout, 146
Health risk assessment, 94t
Healthcare Employers' Data Information System (HEDIS), 40
Healthcare providers
  addressing, 63
  primary, 209–210
  response guidelines based on PHQ-9 and STAR*D studies, 374, 375t
  role in home care, 209–210
Healthy life expectancy (HALE), 3
Healthy lifestyle counseling, 89t, 93
Hearing
  age-related changes in, 240
  health insurance coverage for services, 31t
  normal, 240
Hearing aids, 241
  bone-anchored (BAHA), 247–248
  caring for, 247
  costs of, 247, 247t
  styles of, 245–246, 246t
Hearing Handicap Inventory for the Elderly—Screening Version, 243
Hearing loss, 240–248
  assessment of, 44

clinical presentation of, 241–243
conductive hearing loss, 241, 242f
effects of, 245, 245t
epidemiology of, 240–241, 242f
indications for medical evaluation of, 243, 244t
mixed hearing loss, 242f
rapid screening followed by assessment and management of, 43, 44t
recommended preventive measures for, 89t, 96–97
rehabilitation of, 245, 245t
screening for, 89t, 96–97, 243
sensorineural hearing loss, 241, 242f
strategies to improve communication, 243–244, 244t
treatment of, 243–248
trends in, 5
Heart
  age-related changes, 12t, 13
  age-related pathologies, 16t
Heart disease
  deaths due to, 6
  in nursing-home population, 196
  prevalence of, 5, 5f
  and rehabilitation, 186
  valvular, 456, 457t, 465
Heart failure, 466–474
  Cheynes-Stokes breathing pattern of, 363
  classification of, 469, 470t
  clinical features of, 466–467
  device therapy for, 471–472
  diagnosis of, 467
  diastolic, 466
  end-of-life care for, 473
  epidemiology of, 466
  etiology of, 466
  family caregiver interventions, 56, 57t
  and incontinence, 276t
  management of, 467–472
  in nursing-home population, 196
  pathophysiology of, 466
  pharmacotherapy for HFpEF, 471, 471t
  pharmacotherapy for HFrEF, 468–471
  with preserved ejection fraction (HFpEF), 466, 471, 471t
  prognosis for, 473
  recommendations for, 474
  with reduced ejection fraction (HFrEF), 466, 468–471
  systolic, 466
Heart rate abnormalities, 309
Heart transplantation, 471–472
Heart valves
  prosthetic, 637
  valvular heart disease, 456, 457t, 465
Heartburn, 484–485
Heat treatment, 578
Heavy drinking, 403
Heberden nodes, 548

HEDIS (Healthcare Employers' Data Information System), 40
Heel pain, 563
Heel pressure ulcers, 285–286, 331t
  prevention strategies, 289
Heel spur, 561t
Height measurement, 88t, 93
Helicobacter pylori infection, 486–487, 488
HELP (Hospital Elder Life Program), 170–171, 357–358
HELP (Hospitalized Elderly Longitudinal Project), 136
Hemangioma, 565
Hematologic malignancies, 642–657
Hematology, 629–641
Hematoma
  epidural, 584
  subdural, 584, 585
Hematopoiesis, 629–630
Hematopoietic stem cells (HSCs), 629
Hematuria, 503
Hemiparesis, 298t
Hemiplegia, 298t
Hemodialysis, 510
Hemolytic anemia, 505, 631t, 636–637
Hemolytic-uremic syndrome (HUS), 505, 637, 638
Hemorrhage
  intracerebral (ICH), 584
  intracranial, 584
  subarachnoid (SAH), 584–585
  subconjunctival, 230–232, 237t
Hemorrhagic stroke, 584–585
Heparin
  and hyperkalemia, 501, 501t
  LMWH (low-molecular-weight heparin), 128, 130t, 445–446
  and risk of osteoporosis, 316, 316t
  unfractionated, 446, 452
Hepatitis A vaccine, 590t
Hepatitis B vaccine, 590t
Hepatitis C, 597
Hepatitis C screening, 88t, 92–93, 597
Hepcidin, 634
Herbal medicines, 112
  for cancer, 118
  cannabis and cannabinoids, 118–119
  for low back pain, 115
  for menopausal symptoms, 117
  safety issues, 113
  sleeping agents, 371–372
  for vasomotor symptoms, 513
Hernia, 541
  femoral, 542
  inguinal, 542
Herpes simplex, oral, 434–435, 435f
Herpes simplex keratitis, 230, 237t
Herpes zoster (shingles), 232, 237t, 423–424, 424f
Herpes zoster ophthalmicus
  signs and symptoms of, 230, 237t
  treatment of, 232, 237t
Herpes zoster vaccine, 586, 590–591
  immunization schedule for adults ≥65 years old, 590t
  recommendations for, 88t, 97

High T_4 syndrome, 604
Highly active antiretroviral therapy (HAART), 597
Hip disease, 541, 542, 545t
Hip fracture, 189–190, 313
    epidemiology of, 189–190
    prevention of, 190, 607
    rehabilitation after, 190
    surgical care of, 189–190
Hip joint assessment, 184t, 187
Hip osteoarthritis, 548, 549
Hip pain, 549
Hip protectors, 311
Hip surgery
    for hip fracture, 189–190
    rehabilitation after, 301
    total hip and knee arthroplasty, 190–191
Hispanic Americans
    alcohol use, 404
    cancer, 644
    chronic kidney disease, 507
    CVD mortality rates, 448
    dental caries, 431
    diabetes mellitus, 621
    dual eligibles, 34–35
    educational attainment, 4
    family caregivers, 55
    hypertension, 475
    life expectancy, 3, 3t
    median income, 4
    nursing-home population, 196
    periodontitis, 431
    population projections, 3, 268, 644
    poverty rates, 4
    urinary incontinence, 274
History of immigration or migration, 64–65
History of traumatic experiences, 64
Histrionic personality disorder
    differential diagnosis of, 396
    features of, 395t
    long-term course, 396–397
    therapeutic strategies for, 398t
HIV (human immunodeficiency virus) infection, 596–597
    barriers to optimal prevention and detection of, 73
    in LGBT older adults, 73
    nursing-home financing for care for those with, 198
    prevention of, 73, 597
    risk in older gay and bisexual men, 73
    risk in older lesbian and bisexual women, 73
    risk in transgender people, 73
    screening for, 88t, 95, 532
    treatment and care, 74
HMOs (Health Maintenance Organizations), 32
Hoarding disorder, 384
Hodgkin disease, 644, 656
Home blood pressure monitoring, 480
Home care, 209–211
    ethical issues in, 211
    fee-for-service, 39
    financing, 39
    health insurance coverage for, 31t
    interventions for lowering risk of falls in, 308t
    for LGBT older adults, 75–76
    liability and legal issues, 211
    limitations of, 210–211
    managed care, 39
    patient assessment, 210
    physician's role in, 209–210
    preventing falls, 308, 308t, 311
    prospective payment system for, 209
    rehabilitation services, 182t, 183, 184
    technologic innovations in, 212–213
    transition from hospital to, 176
    virtual home visits, 213
Home-delivered meals, 266–267
Home-hazard assessment, 308, 308t
Home Health Compare tool, 209
Home health skilled care, 214, 214t
Home-health–related groups (HHRGs), 209
Home hospital, 171, 212
Homeostasis, 601
Homeostenosis, 16–17
Homocysteine, 638
Homosexuality, 70
Horizant (gabapentin), 152t
Hormonal regulation
    influences in men, 315
    screening tests for hypersecretion, 613–614, 613t
Hormone replacement therapy (HRT)
    for menopausal symptoms, 512, 513
    strategies for risk reduction, 513
Hormone therapy
    for breast cancer, 648, 653
    for cancer, 648
    for colonic angiodysplasia, 495
    for endometrial cancer, 648
    for erectile dysfunction, 534
    estrogen therapy, 617–618
    for female sexual dysfunction, 536
    for incontinence, 275t, 281
    for osteoporosis, 321t, 322–323
    preventive, 89t, 98
    for prostate cancer, 526t, 648
    testosterone replacement therapy, 616–617
    testosterone supplementation, 601, 616–617, 616t, 617t
    for urogenital atrophy, 514
Hospice, 136, 137–138
    for advanced CKD, 511
    cultural aspects, 137
    health insurance coverage for, 31t
    Medicare benefits, 33–34, 40
    recommendations for, 146
    services, 137, 137t
Hospice in a Minute app, 137
Hospital-acquired pneumonia, 592
Hospital-acquired pressure ulcers, 163, 165t, 284
Hospital-associated disability, 160–161
Hospital-at-home care, 171
Hospital care, 157–170
    alternatives to, 171
    daily evaluation, 168–170
    day hospitals, 211
    emergency department (ED), 169–170
    flexible medication times, 366
    geriatric EDs, 169–170
    geriatric evaluation and management (GEM) units, 170, 218–219
    hazards and opportunities commonly overlooked in, 164, 165t
    hazards of hospitalization, 160–162
    health insurance coverage for, 31t
    home hospitals, 212
    intensive care, 168–169
    interventions for lowering risk of falls in, 308t
    never events, 162–163
    readmission, 172
    recommendations for, 172
    recurrent hospitalization, 472–473
    rehabilitation hospitals, 182–183, 182t
    surgical co-management, 171
    for syncope, 259
    systematic assessment on admission, 164, 165t
    transition to home from, 176
Hospital Compare, 171–172
Hospital Elder Life Program (HELP), 170–171, 357–358
Hospital Readmissions Reduction Program, 472
Hospitalists, 200
Hospitalization, chronic, 177
Hospitalized Elderly Longitudinal Project (HELP), 136
Hospitalized patients
    alcohol use, 404
    assessment of, 164–168
    daily evaluation, 168–170
    management of, 164–168
    models of care for, 170–171
    sleep disturbances in, 366–367
Hot flushes, 513
Hounsfield units (HU), 614
House calls, 210
Housing, 75–76, 214
Housing and Urban Development programs, 214
Humalog (insulin lispro), 627t
HumaLog mix (insulin lispro protamine suspension and insulin lispro), 627t
Human growth hormone, 268
Human immunodeficiency virus (HIV) infection. *See* AIDS; HIV infection
Human papillomavirus (HPV) infection, 72
Human papillomavirus (HPV) testing, 87
Humoral hypercalcemia of malignancy, 608t, 609
Humulin (insulin), 627t
Huntington disease (HD), 327, 570, 573
Hurley Discomfort Scale, 151

Hutchinson sign, 232, 423
Hutchison sign, 427
Hwabyeong, 399
Hyaluronic acid, 114–115, 417, 543
Hydralazine, 469–470, 479
Hydrocephalus, normal-pressure (NPH)
　gait abnormalities, 298t
　and incontinence, 276t
　surgery for, 301
Hydrocodone (Lorcet, Lortab, Vicodin, Norco, Vicoprofen)
　opioid equivalent dosages, 155t
　for persistent pain, 153t, 155
　sustained-release (Hysingla ER, Zohydro ER), 153t
Hydromorphone
　extended release (Exalgo), 153t
　opioid equivalent dosages, 155t
　for persistent pain, 153t, 155, 156
Hydrophilic drugs, 102
Hydrotherapy, 292
Hydroxychloroquine, 550, 555
Hydroxyurea, 640, 641
Hydroxyzine, 141t
Hyoscyamine, 281
　for bowel obstruction, 143t
　for loud respirations, 145
Hyperadrenocorticoidism, 613
Hyperalgesia, 148t
Hyperbaric oxygen, 292
Hypercalcemia, 607–609
　causes of, 601
　differential diagnosis of, 607–608, 608t
　and incontinence, 276t
Hypercalciuria, idiopathic, 316
Hyperglycemia
　in diabetes mellitus, 625
　non-insulin agents for, 626–627, 626t
　perioperative, 133
　treatment of, 625
Hypericum perforatum (St. John's wort), 116
　for depression, 116
　safety issues, 114t
Hyperkalemia, 501–502
　medications that cause, 501, 501t
Hyperkinetic movement disorders, 573–575
Hyperlipidemia, 5f, 92
Hypernatremia, 500
Hyperparathyroidism
　differential diagnosis of, 607–608, 608t
　primary, 316, 607–609
　secondary, 315
Hyperpathia, 148t
Hyperprolactinemia, 610–612
Hypersexuality, 347
Hypertension, 475–482
　blood pressure targets, 502
　and cardiovascular risk, 450
　CIM for, 115–116
　classification of, 475, 475t
　clinical evaluation of, 476
　emergencies and urgencies, 480
　epidemiology and physiology of, 475–476
　follow-up visits, 479–480
　in frail older adults, 480–481
　in long-term care settings, 480–481
　pharmacologic treatment of, 478–479, 478t
　prevalence of, 5, 5f
　pseudohypertension, 476
　recommendations for, 481
　recommended preventive measures for, 88t
　refractory or resistant, 480
　screening for, 90
　secondary, 502
　special considerations for, 480–481
　stage 1, 475t
　stage 2, 475t
　treatment of, 476–480, 478t
　white-coat, 476
Hyperthyroidism, 603–605
　screening for, 90
　subclinical, 604
Hypertonic saline, 500
Hypervolemia, 501
Hypnotics
　chronic use of, 371
　and delirium, 355t
　and incontinence, 275t
　interventions for preventing falls with, 310t
　for sleep problems, 367–368, 370
Hypoactive sexual desire disorder (HSDD), 535, 536–537
Hypoadrenocorticoidism, 612–613
Hypoalgesia, 148t
Hypochondriasis, 398, 399
Hypoglycemia, 627
Hypogonadism, 316
　male, 531t, 532, 615–616
Hypokalemia, 501
Hypomania, 375
Hypomethylating agents, 636
Hyponatremia, 498–499
　hypotonic, 499
　with normal extracellular fluid volume, 499–500
　pseudohyponatremia, 499
　severe, 500
　treatment of, 500
　with volume depletion, 499
　with volume overload, 499
Hypopituitarism, 612
Hypoproliferative anemia, 631t, 632–635
　due to vitamin B_{12} or folate deficiency, 633f, 635
　evaluation of, 631–632, 633f
Hypotension, postural (orthostatic), 259–260, 573
　interventions for preventing falls, 309, 310t
Hypothalamic-pituitary-adrenal (HPA) axis, 610
　age-related changes in, 610, 611t
Hypothalamic-pituitary-testicular axis, 611t

Hypothalamic-pituitary-thyroid axis, 611t
Hypothyroidism, 602–603
　screening for, 90
　secondary, 603
　subclinical, 602
　transient secondary, 603
Hypotonic hyponatremia, 499
Hypovolemia, 501
Hypoxis rooperi, 117
Hysingla ER (hydrocodone, sustained-release), 153t

I

IADLs (instrumental activities of daily living), 46, 46t
Ibandronate, 321t, 322
IBS. *See* Irritable bowel syndrome
Ibuprofen, 153t, 155
ICD-9 (International Classification of Diseases), 209
ICD-10 (International Classification of Diseases), 339, 349
ICDs (implantable cardiac defibrillators), 471–472, 473, 474
ICH (intracerebral hemorrhage), 584
Idarucizumab, 446
Identification of Seniors at Risk (ISAR), 169, 169t
Identity, cultural, 63
Idiopathic myelofibrosis (IMF), 629, 640, 641
Idiopathic pulmonary fibrosis (IPF), 444–445
IL-2 (interleukin-2), 648, 655
IL-6 (interleukin-6), 630
Illicit drugs, 403
Illness anxiety disorder, 399
Iloperidone
　dosing and adverse events of, 390t
　for psychosis in dementia, 345t
Imagery, 387
Imaging
　abdominal ultrasonography, 88t
　brain imaging studies, 329
　of gait impairment, 299
Imipramine, 281, 355t
Immigration history, 64–65
Immigration status, 64
Immobility, 165t
Immune system
　age-related changes, 12t, 15, 586, 587t
　age-related pathologies, 16t
Immune theory of aging, 8t, 11
Immune thrombocytopenia, 638
Immunizations, 88t, 97
　for hospitalized patients, 165t, 166–167
　interventions for, 165t
　recommendations for, 97
　schedule for adults ≥65 years old, 590t
Immunoglobulin, intravenous, 420, 557, 576
Immunoglobulin A nephropathy, 506
Immunosenescence, 11, 586

Immunotherapy
    for cancer, 648
    for dementia, 336
    for prostate cancer, 654
    for radiculopathy, 576
IMPACT (Improving Mood—Promoting Access to Collaborative Treatment), 218
Implantable cardiac defibrillators (ICDs), 471–472, 473, 474
Implantable hemodynamic monitoring, 473
Implantable loop recorders (ILRs), 257t, 258
Implants, cochlear, 248
    characteristics of older candidates for, 248, 248t
Improving Mood—Promoting Access to Collaborative Treatment (IMPACT), 218
In-hospital cardiac arrest (IHCA), 167–168
Inattention, 351
Incidentalomas
    adrenal, 613–614, 613t
    pituitary, 612
Inclusion body myositis, 556
Incontinence
    with developmental disabilities, 415t
    fecal, 490–491
    and rehabilitation, 185–186
    urinary, 89t, 96, 117, 274–283
Indacaterol maleate, 442t
Independence at Home Demonstration project, 210
Ineffective anemia, 631t
Ineffective erythropoiesis, 632, 635–636
Infection control, 592
Infections
    antimicrobial management of, 588
    back pain due to, 543–544, 544t, 545t
    bone and joint, 596
    diagnosis and management of, 587–588
    fungal, 566, 566f
    gastrointestinal, 598–599
    HIV and AIDS, 73
    predisposition to, 586–587
    presentation of, 587–588
    in pressure ulcers, 293
    prosthetic device (PDIs), 596
    sexually transmitted, 73, 95
    skin problems, 423–425
    surveillance definitions of, 588, 589t
    vulvovaginal, 514
Infectious diarrhea, 598–599
Infectious diseases, 586–600
    recommendations for, 600
Infectious Diseases Society of America, 591–592, 593
Infectious syndromes, 591–599
Infective endocarditis, 458, 595
    antibiotics for, 429, 436, 458, 595
Infestations, 423–425
Inflammation

    anemia of, 634
    vulvovaginal, 514
Inflammatory bowel disease, 115
Inflammatory skin conditions, 418–422
Inflliximab, 551
Influenza, 592
Influenza vaccine, 5, 165t, 166, 587
    immunization schedule for adults ≥65 years old, 590t
    recommendations for, 88t, 97, 592
Informed consent, 21–22
Ingrown nails, 565–566
Inguinal hernia, 542
INH (isoniazid), 595
Inhaled bronchodilators and corticosteroids, 442, 442t, 443t
Inhalers, 443
Initial Preventive Physical Examination (IPPE), 36, 94t–95t
Injectable agents
    anesthetic, 437
    for diabetes mellitus, 626t, 627
    insulin preparations, 627t
    trigger point injections, 158
Injury. See also specific types of injury
    preventing, 97
Inpatient care
    fee for service, 37–38
    financing, 37–38
    managed care, 38
    rehabilitation care, 183–185
Insomnia, 362–363
    behavioral interventions for, 368–370
    behavioral management of, 346, 346t
    epidemiology of, 361
    management of, 367–372
    nonpharmacologic interventions for, 368–370
    pharmacotherapy for, 370–371
    prescription medications for, 369t, 370
    prevalence of, 362
    treatment of, 346–347
Insomnia disorder, 362
Institute of Medicine
    Food and Nutrition Board, 262
    The Mental Health and Substance Use Workforce for Older Adults: In Whose Hands?, 404
    RDIs for calicum and vitamin D, 606–607
Institutional mistreatment, 123
Institutionalization decisions, 211
Instrumental activities of daily living (IADLs), 46, 46t
Insulin
    for diabetes, 627
    preparations, 627t
Insulin aspart (NovoLog), 627t
Insulin detemir (Levemir), 627t
Insulin glargine (Lantus), 627t
Insulin glulisine (Apidra), 627t
Insulin-like growth factor 1 (IGF-1), 611t
Insulin lispro (Humalog), 627t

Insulin lispro protamine suspension and insulin lispro (HumaLog mix), 627t
Insurance coverage, 27–42, 31t
Integrative medicine, 112. See also Complementary and integrative medicine
Intellectual disability, 410–416
    causes of, 410
    definition of, 410
    developmental disabilities with, 415t, 416
    diagnostic issues, 411–412
    medical disorders with, 414
    mental disorders with, 412–414
    and mental illness, 411
    prevalence of, 410–411
    psychiatric disorders with, 412–414
    social conditions with, 414–416
    treatment issues, 411–412
Intensive care
    Confusion Assessment Method for the Intensive Care Unit (CAM-ICU), 350t, 351
    of critically ill, 168–169
INTERACT (Interventions to Reduce Acute Care Transfers), 177, 179t
Interferon, 392, 640–641, 648, 655
α-Interferon, 648
Interferon gamma release assays (IGRAs), 595
Interleukin-2 (IL-2), 648, 655
Interleukin-6 (IL-6), 630
Intermittent clean catheterization, 283
Intermittent pneumatic compression, 446
International Classification of Diseases (ICD-9), 209
International Classification of Diseases (ICD-10), 339, 349
International Classification of Functioning, Disability, and Health (ICF) (WHO), 181
International Continence Society, 516
International Prostate Symptom Score, 520
International Society of Clinical Densitometry, 318
Interpersonal and social rhythms therapy, 380–381
Interpreters, 64
Interstitial nephritis, acute, 505
Intertrigo, 419–420, 420f
Interventions to Reduce Acute Care Transfers (INTERACT), 177, 179t
Intra-abdominal abscess, 598
Intracerebral hemorrhage (ICH), 584
Intracranial hemorrhage, 584
Intracranial saccular aneurysms, 584
Intraoperative floppy iris syndrome (IFIS), 521
Intravenous fluids, 489
Intravenous immunoglobulin, 420, 557, 576
Invasive mechanical ventilation, 443t
Investigational agents, 324
Iodine, radioactive, 605–606
Ipilimumab, 428, 648

IPPE (Initial Preventive Physical
    Examination), 36, 94t–95t
Ipratropium bromide
    adverse drug events, 265
    for COPD, 441, 442t, 443t
Iraglutide, 626t
Irbesartan, 469t, 471, 471t
Iris prolapse, 521
Iron, 263t
Iron-containing antacids, 106, 106t
Iron deficiency, 509, 633
Iron-deficiency anemia, 632–634
    evaluation of, 631–632, 632f
Iron-restricted anemia, 632–634
Iron supplements, 634
Iron therapy
    for anemia, 509, 633, 634
    drug interactions, 265t
    preparations, 633
    for restless legs syndrome, 575
Irrigation, 292
Irritable bowel syndrome (IBS), 493–494
    with alternating constipation
        and diarrhea (IBS-M or IBS
        mixed), 493
    with constipation (IBS-C),
        493–494
    with diarrhea (IBS-D), 493,
        494
    recommendations for, 495
ISAR (Identification of Seniors at Risk),
    169, 169t
Ischemic bowel, 598
Ischemic optic neuropathy, 230, 237t,
    238, 238f
Ischemic stroke, 580
    acute, 581–582
    prevention of, 582–584
Isoflavones, 117
Isoniazid (INH), 265t, 595
Isosorbide dinitrate, 469–470
Isosorbide mononitrate, 455
Isotonic saline, 500
Isotretinoin, 419
Ivabradine, 454
Ivermectin, 425

J

Jaeger cards, 44, 166
Jaw: osteonecrosis of, 429
Jehovah's Witness, 21
Jejunostomy, percutaneous endoscopic,
    272
Jewett-Whitmore staging system, 524–525, 524t
Johrei, 118
Joint Commission on Accreditation of
    Healthcare Organizations, 68
Joint disease, degenerative, 415t
Joint infections, 596
Joint Principles of the PCMH (AAP,
    ACP, AAFP, AOA), 216, 217t
Joint replacement
    hip replacement, 301
    knee replacement, 301
    rehabilitation after, 300, 301
    total hip and knee arthroplasty,
        190–191, 549
Justice, 18, 21

K

Kadian (morphine, sustained release),
    154t
Karnofsky Performance Status, 645
Kava, 371–372
Kayexalate (sodium polystyrene), 502
Kcentra®, 639
KDOQI (Kidney Disease Outcomes
    Quality Initiative), 103–104,
    507–508
Kegel exercises, 516
Keratitis, bacterial, 230, 237t
Keratitis sicca, 231
Keratoconjunctivitis sicca, 556
Keratotic lesions, 565
Ketoconazole, 281
Ketorolac, 153t
Kidney(s)
    age-related changes, 103, 497, 498t
    assessment of, 497
    functional measures, 497
    preoperative assessment and
        management of, 129–131
Kidney Disease: Improving Global
    Outcomes (KDIGO) CKD Work
    Group 2012 Guidelines, 507–508
Kidney Disease Outcomes Quality
    Initiative (KDOQI), 103–104,
    507–508
Kidney diseases and disorders See
    Nephrology
Kidney transplantation, 510–511
Kingella, 458, 595
Klonopin (clonazepam), 152t
Knee osteoarthritis, 548, 549f
    CIM for, 114
Knee pain, 538, 542–543, 549
Knee replacement
    rehabilitation after, 301
    total hip and knee arthroplasty,
        190–191
Kyphoplasty, 324, 546

L

Labetalol, 479
Labial fusion, 513–514, 514f
Labor force participation, 4
Laboratory testing
    in anemia, 631–632, 633f
    in endocrine disorders, 601
    in falls, 307
    in gait impairment, 299
    health insurance coverage for,
        31t
    in osteoporosis, 316, 317t
Lactulose (Chronulac), 491t
Lamivudine, 551
Lamotrigine, 569–570, 569t
    for behavioral disturbances in
        dementia with manic-like
        features, 344, 344t
    for bipolar depression, 378–379,
        379t
    for personality disorders, 397

Language, 63
    body language, 64
Lansoprazole, 141t
Lantus (insulin glargine), 627t
Larval therapy, 292
Laryngoscopy, nasopharyngeal,
    271–272
Laser therapy, 653
Laser trabeculoplasty, 237
Latanoprost, 238t
Lateral epicondylitis, 541
Latino cultures, 60
Latinos, 268
Laxatives
    bulk, 491t
    for chronic constipation, 489, 490,
        490t
    nutrient interactions, 265t
    osmotic, 489–490, 490t, 491t
    saline, 489–490
    stimulant, 489–490, 490t, 491t
LDL-C testing, direct, 92
Leadership, 200t, 203–205
LEAP (Lower Extremity Amputation
    Prevention) program, 567
Leflunomide, 550
LeFort colpocleisis, 517
Left ventricular assist devices (LVADs),
    472
Left ventricular mass, 451
Leg amputation, 191
Leg-length discrepancies, 299
Leg pain, 542
Leg ulcers, chronic, 417, 422
Legal issues, 18–26
    in home care, 211
    related to nutritional status,
        268–269
Legislation, 202–205
Lenalidomide, 656
Length of stay, 197
Lenolidomide, 636
Lentigo maligna, 427
Lesbian gay bisexual transgender
    (LGBT) older adults, 70–77
    concerns about aging, 75
    family structure, 75
    financial security challenges, 76
    home care for, 75–76
    housing, 75–76
    long-term care for, 75–76
    medical and psychosocial concerns,
        71, 71t
    medical issues, 71–74, 71t
    mental health issues, 74
    palliative care needs, 75
    poverty rates, 76
    sexual health of, 73
    social supports for, 75
    suicide rates, 74
Lesbian women. *See also* Lesbian gay
    bisexual transgender (LGBT) older
    adults
    concerns about aging, 75
    disease risk, 72
    sexual risk, 73
Lesser metatarsal phalangeal joint
    dislocation, 561t

Leukemia, 655
    acute, 644
    acute myeloid (AML), 629, 655
    chronic lymphocytic, 655
    chronic myeloid, 648
    hairy cell, 648
    myeloproliferative, 640
Leukoaraiosis, 299
Leukoplakia, 433, 433f
Leuprolide acetate, 347
Levalbuterol, 442t
Levemir (insulin detemir), 627t
Levetiracetam, 569–570, 569t
    Beers Criteria for, 108t
Levodopa, 265t
    for multiple system atrophy, 573
    for PD motor symptoms, 571–572
    for progressive supranuclear palsy, 573
Levodopa-carbidopa
    and delirium, 355t
    for PD motor symptoms, 571
    for restless legs syndrome, 575
Levofloxacin, 107, 107t, 592
Levothyroxine supplementation, 602
Levothyroxine suppressive therapy, 605–606
Lewy body, 570
Lewy body dementia, 392, 573
    behavioral disturbances in, 341–342
    diagnostic features and treatment of, 330t
    differential diagnosis of, 331
    epidemiology of, 326
    etiology of, 327
LGBT older adults. *See* Lesbian gay bisexual transgender older adults
LH (luteinizing hormone), 611t, 615
LHRH (luteinizing hormone-releasing hormone) agonists, 526t, 527
Liability, 211
Libido, decreased, 535, 536–537, 536t, 617
Lice, 425
Lichen planus, 515
Lichen sclerosus, 514f, 515
Lichen simplex chronicus, 419, 419f, 515
Lid abnormalities, 229, 230t
Lid ectropion or entropion, 229, 230t
Lid malposition/exposure, 230–232, 237t
Lidocaine, 158, 453
Lidocaine patch, 151, 576
Life-course theory, 8
Life expectancy, 3, 3t, 623
    healthy life expectancy (HALE), 3
Life space assessment, 46–47, 47t
Lifestyle modification
    for benign prostatic hyperplasia, 521, 521t
    for cancer, 118
    for diabetes mellitus, 621, 622
    for gout, 551
    healthy lifestyle counseling, 89t, 93
    for hypertension, 477–478
    for urinary incontinence, 279

Light therapy, 292, 368, 368t, 369
Limb movements
    periodic limb movements disorder (PLMD), 575
    periodic limb movements during sleep (PLMS), 364–365, 575
    restless legs syndrome, 364–365
Linaclotide (Linzess), 490, 490t, 491t
Linagliptin (Tradjenta), 626t
Linezolid, 592
Linzess (linaclotide), 491t
Lip cancer, 433
Lipid-binding resins, 265t
Lipid control, 625
Lipid-lowering therapy, 588
Lipohyalinosis, 580
Lipophilic drugs, 102
Lisinopril, 469t
Listeria, 597
Literacy, 63
Lithium
    for behavioral disturbances in dementia with manic-like features, 344, 344t
    for bipolar depression, 378
    drug interactions, 107, 107t
    for personality disorders, 397
    to stabilize mood in mania and bipolar depression, 378, 379t
Living arrangements, 3–4
Living wills, 18, 24, 24t
LMWH (low-molecular-weight heparin), 128, 130t, 445–446
Long lie, 303
Long-term care, 213t. *See also* Assisted-living facilities; Nursing-home care
    competencies for attending physicians in, 200–201, 204t
    fever in frail, older residents, 586, 587–588, 588t
    hypertension in, 480–481
    interface with acute care, 201–202
    for LGBT older adults, 75–76
    managed long-term care programs (MLTC), 212
    minimum criteria for initiation of antibiotic therapy in, 586, 587–588, 589t
    pneumonia in, 592
    pressure ulcers in, 284
    requirements for facilities, 201t, 203–205
    tuberculosis in, 595
    urinary incontinence in, 282
    UTIs in, 593–594
    wound care in, 292
Long-term care specialists, 200
Loop diuretics
    drug interactions, 107, 107t
    for heart failure, 469
    and incontinence, 275t
Loperamide, 491
LOPS (Loss of Protective Sensation) program, 567
Lorazepam, 356t, 357
    for anxiety disorders, 386
    for nausea, 141, 141t

Lorcet (hydrocodone), 153t
Lortab (hydrocodone), 153t
Losartan, 469t
Loss of appetite, 136, 142–143
Loss of consciousness, sudden, 254, 255t
Loss of Protective Sensation (LOPS) program, 567
Louse infestations, 425
Low back pain, 150, 543, 546–547
    assessment of, 544t, 545
    CIM for, 115
    physical examination of, 544, 545t
Low-dose computed tomography (LDCT), 90
Low-molecular-weight heparin (LMWH), 128, 130t, 445–446
Low T_3 syndrome, 602–603
Low T_4 syndrome, 602–603
Low-vision aids, 239
Low-vision rehabilitation, 238–239
Lower extremities: innervation of, 544–545, 545t
Lower Extremity Amputation Prevention (LEAP) program, 567
Lower respiratory disease, chronic, 6
Lower urinary tract
    age-related changes in, 275–276
    pathophysiology in UI, 276–277, 277t
Lower urinary tract symptoms (LUTS), 274, 520
Lubiprostone (Amitiza), 490, 490t, 491t
Lubrication, decreased, 535, 536, 536t
Lumbar spinal stenosis, 301, 538, 543, 544t, 545–546, 545t
Lumbar spine, unstable, 544t, 545t
Lumbar spine disease, 542
Lumpectomy, 651
Lung cancer, 651
    chemotherapy for, 647
    CIM for, 118
    incidence rates, 642
    screening for, 88t, 90, 646
Lung disease
    chronic obstructive pulmonary disease (COPD), 385, 440–444
    with developmental disabilities, 415t
    and incontinence, 276t
Lung transplantation, 444–445
Lupus erythematosus
    drug-induced, 555
    late-onset, 554–555
Lurasidone
    dosing and adverse events of, 390t
    for psychosis in dementia, 345t
Lutein, 118, 234
Luteinizing hormone (LH), 611t, 615
Luteinizing hormone-releasing hormone (LHRH) agonists, 526t, 527
LVADs (left ventricular assist devices), 472
Lyme disease, 598
Lymphadenectomy, pelvic, 525
Lymphocytic and collagenous colitis, 492
Lymphoma

diffuse large B-cell lymphoma, 656
follicular lymphoma, 648, 656
large-cell lymphoma, 647
non-Hodgkin lymphoma, 656
Lyrica (pregabalin), 152t

M

M2 inhibitors, 592
Macrocytic anemia, 635
Macrolides, 592
Macronutrient guidelines, 262
Macronutrient needs, 262
Macronutrient supplements, 267
Macular degeneration, age-related (ARMD), 230t, 233–235
   rehabilitation for, 239
   symptoms and treatment of, 231t
Macular edema, diabetic, 235–236, 236f
Maggot debridement therapy, 292
Magnesium
   drug interactions, 265t
   RDIs for adults ≥71 years old, 263t
Magnesium-containing antacids, 106, 106t
Magnesium hydroxide (Milk of Magnesia), 489–490
Magnetic resonance pulmonary angiography, 445
Magnetic stimulation, repetitive transcranial (rTMS), 380
Major depressive disorder
   diagnosis of, 373–374
   electroconvulsive therapy for, 379–380
   epidemiology of, 373
   with personality disorder, 397
   screening for, 374
   treatment of, 376
   without mania but with hypomania, 375
Maladaptive behaviors, 414
Malassezia furfur, 418
Male hypogonadism, 531t, 532, 615–616
Male sexuality, 530–534
Malignancy
   deaths due to, 6
   hematologic malignancies, 642–657
   humoral hypercalcemia of, 608t, 609
Malnutrition, 262, 586–587
Mammography, 86, 88t
Managed care
   home-health care, 39
   inpatient care, 38
   nursing-home care, 40
   outpatient care, 37
   postacute rehabilitation, 38–39
Managed long-term care programs (MLTC), 212
Mandibular torus, 433–434, 434f
Mania
   DSM-5 criteria for, 375
   electroconvulsive therapy for, 379–380
   hypomania, 375
   late-onset, 376
   medications to stabilize mood in, 379t
   pharmacotherapy for, 378, 379t
Manic-like behavioral syndromes in dementia, 340, 344
   mood stabilizers for, 344, 344t
   treatment of, 344
Manipulation therapy, 115
Manipulative and body-based methods, 113t
Marche a petits pas, 299
Marijuana *(Cannabis)*, 118–119, 392, 403
Marital status, 2, 3–4
Marrow failure, 635
Martel sign, 551
Massage, 112, 115, 578
MAST (Michigan Alcoholism Screening Test)—Geriatric Version, 405
Maze procedure, 460
McGill Pain Questionnaire, 149
MDRD (Modified Diet in Renal Disease) formula, 103–104, 129–131, 497
Meals-on-Wheels, 337
"Meaningful Use" standard, 41
Mechanical circulatory support, 471–472
Mechanical debridement, 292
Mechanical ventilation, 443t
   invasive, 443t
Meclizine, 141t
Medicaid, 27, 28, 31t, 34
   advantages and disadvantages of, 36t
   assisted-living benefits, 214
   benefits for LGBT older adults, 76
   continuing-care retirement community benefits, 214
   day care benefits, 211
   dual eligibles, 34–35, 41
   federal spending, 29f
   future directions, 41–42
   hearing aid benefits, 247
   hospice benefits, 137
   nursing-home care benefits, 36t
   primary care physician reimbursements, 28
   requirements for long-term care facilities, 201t, 205
Medicaid Home and Community-Based Services waiver, 217
Medical cannabis, 118–119
Medical devices, 289
   prosthetic device infections (PDIs), 596
Medical directors
   certification for medical directors (CMD), 203–205
   requirements for long-term care facilities, 201t, 203–204
   roles and responsibilities of, 200t, 203–204
Medical ethics, 21
Medical homes, 217
Medical interpreters, 64
Medical-legal interface, 124
Medical Orders for Life-Sustaining Treatment (MOLST), 25
Medical Orders for Scope of Treatment (MOST), 25
Medical savings accounts (MSAs), 33
Medicare, 5, 28
   ACO programs, 27
   annual wellness visit (AWV), 36, 94t–95t, 95
   assisted-living benefits, 214
   care venues, 177
   cochlear implant coverage, 247
   continuing-care retirement community benefits, 214
   day hospital benefits, 211
   dual eligibles, 34–35, 41
   federal spending, 29f, 30f
   fee-for-service (FFS), 27, 28–32, 31t, 35–36, 36t
   future directions, 41–42
   "Geographical Practices Cost Indices," 209–210
   hearing aid benefits, 247
   home-care benefits, 209, 210
   home-health benefits, 183
   Home Health Compare tool, 209
   hospice benefits, 33–34, 40, 137
   house-call benefits, 210
   Loss of Protective Sensation (LOPS) program, 567
   mobility-related device benefits, 193
   nursing-home care benefits, 36t, 39, 198, 206–207
   nursing services benefits, 210
   out-of-pocket expenses, 32
   Part A, 27, 28–32, 31t, 36t, 181–182, 182–183, 182t
   Part B, 27, 28–32, 31t, 36t, 41, 182, 182t
   Part C, 27, 32–33, 36t. *See also* Medicare Advantage (MA)
   Part D, 27, 28, 31t, 32, 33, 34, 35, 36t, 41
   postacute care benefits, 183
   preventive health benefits, 85, 99
   primary care physician reimbursements, 28
   private contracts, 30, 31
   prospective payment system (PPS), 38, 198, 209
   prospective reimbursement, 183
   readmissions, 172
   rehabilitation benefits, 181–182, 182–183, 182t
   requirements for long-term care facilities, 201t, 205
   requirements for rehabilitation sites, 182t
   Shared Savings Program, 27
   skilled-nursing-facility benefits, 198
   transitions of care, 174
   "Welcome to Medicare" preventive visits, 36, 99
   wellness visits, 94t–95t, 95, 99
Medicare Administrative Contractors, 28

Medicare Advantage (MA), 27, 28, 31t, 32–33
    advantages and disadvantages of, 36t
    discounted FFS, 37
    types of plans, 32–33
Medicare Basics for Caregivers, 59t
Medicare Health Maintenance Organizations (HMOs), 32
Medicare Health Outcomes Survey, 40
Medicare Personal Plan Finder, 35, 40
Medicare Prescription Drug Improvement and Modernization Act, 41
Medicare Prescription Drug Plan Finder (CMS), 33
Medicare SELECT, 34
Medicated urethral system for erection (MUSE), 533t, 534
Medication assessment, 45
Medication-induced parkinsonism, 573
Medication-induced psychotic disorder, 392
Medication Regimen Complexity Index, 52
Medication review, 108–109, 110, 403
    brown-bag evaluation, 108–109
    for delirium, 353
    for diabetes mellitus, 622
    discharge medication regimen, 178
    at hospital admission, 165t
    for preventing falls, 308, 308t
    requirements for long-term care facilities, 201t, 205
Medication trays, 110
Medications. *See* Drugs; Pharmacotherapy; *specific medications*
Medigap, 27, 30, 31t, 34
    advantages and disadvantages of, 36t
Mediterranean diet, 227
Medline Plus, 59t
Megestrol, 267–268
Meglitinides, 626, 626t
Melanoma, 427–428, 427f
    acral lentiginous, 427, 427f
    immunotherapy for, 648
    metastatic, 648
    nodular, 427
    superficial spreading, 427
    vulvar, 516, 516f
Melatonin, 117, 347, 359, 618–619
    safety issues, 114t
    for sleep disorders, 366, 371, 619
Melatonin receptor agonists, 369t, 370
Melphalan, 656
Memantine, 336, 413
Membranous nephropathy, 506–507
Memory Impairment Screen, 96
Memory problems. *See* Cognitive impairment; Dementia
Memory retraining, 332
Men
    alcohol use, 404
    benign prostatic hyperplasia, 117
    cancer, 642
    cardiovascular disease, 448, 448t
    erectile dysfunction, 521, 522, 530–534
    gay and bisexual men, 71–72
    hormonal influences, 315
    indications for osteoporosis screening, 317–318, 318t
    labor force participation, 4
    life expectancy, 3, 3t
    marital status and living arrangements, 3–4
    oral cancer, 432
    population projections, 3
    poverty rates, 4
    prostate cancer, 654
    prostate disease and cancer, 520–529
    RDIs for micronutrients, 262–263, 263t
    recommendations for calcium intake, 319
    recommendations for osteoporosis screening, 317–318
    recommendations for vitamin D intake, 320
    schizophrenia, 388
    sexual dysfunction, 95, 530–534, 531t
    testosterone supplementation for, 616, 616t
    urinary tract infections, 593
Men who have sex with men (MSM). *See also* Bisexual men; Gay men; Lesbian gay bisexual transgender (LGBT) older adults
    anal cancer, 72
    mental health issues, 74
    sexual risk, 73
Mendelson syndrome, 271
Meniere disease, 246, 249
Meningitis, bacterial, 597
Meningococcal vaccination, 590t
Meniscal disease, 543
Menopausal symptoms
    CIM for, 117
    treatment of, 513
Menopause, 513
Mental health
    acute mental status change, 351
    concerns of LGBT older adults, 71, 71t
    health insurance coverage for outpatient care, 31t
    rehabilitation and, 186
    requirements for long-term care facilities, 201t, 205
The Mental Health and Substance Use Workforce for Older Adults: In Whose Hands? (IOM), 404
Mental health problems, 405
    in aging adults with intellectual disability, 411, 412–414
    diagnosis and treatment of, 413–414
    in LGBT older adults, 74
    requirements for long-term care facilities, 201t, 205
Meperidine, 158, 355t
Merit-Based Incentive Payment System (MIPS), 41
Mesh, vaginal, 517
Metabolic acidosis, 502
Metabolic alkalosis, 502
Metabolic disease, 276t
Metabolic disorders, 498–502
Metabolic encephalopathy, 349
Metabolism
    age-associated changes in, 102–103
    of drugs, 102–103
    preoperative assessment and management of, 129–131
Metamucil (psyllium), 491t
Metastatic breast cancer, 653
Metastatic melanoma, 648
Metatarsal phalangeal joint dislocation, 560–562, 561t, 562f
Metatarsalgia, 561t
Metformin
    for diabetes mellitus, 622, 626, 626t
    nutrient interactions, 265t
Methadone, 407, 408t
Methicillin-resistant *Staphylococcus aureus* (MRSA), 587, 592
Methimazole, 604
Methotrexate, 553–554, 555, 557
Methylcellulose (Citrucel), 491, 491t
Methyldopa, 513
Methylmalonic acid (MMA), 637
Methylphenidate, 145, 343
Methylprednisolone
    for dermatomyositis, 557
    for polymyositis, 557
Metoclopramide
    adverse drug events, 106, 106t
    for nausea, 141t
Metolazone, 469
Metoprolol
    for acute coronary syndrome, 452
    adverse drug events, 392
    for heart failure, 468–469, 469t
Metronidazole
    for *C difficile* infection, 599
    for diverticulitis, 492
    for rosacea, 419
Metronidazole gel, 294
Mexican Americans, 313
Mexican *curanderos*, 112–113
Mexiletine (Mexitil), 152t
Michigan Alcoholism Screening Test (MAST)—Geriatric Version, 405
Microadenomas, pituitary, 610–611, 612
Microalbuminuria, 498
Microangiopathy, thrombotic, 505
Microcytic anemia, 635–636
Micrographia, 570
Micronutrient needs
    age-related changes in, 262–263
    recommended dietary intakes, 262–263, 263t
Micronutrient supplements, 267
Microscopic colitis, 492
Microscopic polyangiitis, 506
Midodrine, 310t, 573
Miglitol (Glyset), 626t

Migraine headaches, 578–579
Migration history, 64–65
Migratory glossitis, 434
Mild cognitive impairment
    diagnostic features and treatment of, 330t
    differential diagnosis of, 330
Milnacipran (Savella), 152t, 558
Mind-body interventions, 112, 113t
    for cancer, 118
    for menopausal symptoms, 117
Mineral oil, 265t
Mini-Cog Assessment Instrument for Dementia, 44t, 45, 96, 165, 328, 329t
Mini–Mental State Examination (MMSE), 22, 45, 328, 329t
Mini-Nutritional Assessment (MNA), 265
Mini-Nutritional Assessment, short form (MNA-SF), 262
Minimal change disease (MCD), 507
Minimum Data Set (MDS), 202–203, 282
    definition of significant weight loss, 263
    quality measures for nursing homes based on, 199t, 202–203
    sections related to nutritional status, 268–269
Minor depression, 376
Minority individuals
    depression in, 373
    population projections, 3
Minoxidil, 479
Miotics, 238t
Mirabegron, 281
Miralax (polyethylene glycol), 491t
Mirror therapy, 188
Mirtazapine
    for depression, 377t
    for depressive features of behavioral disturbances in dementia, 343, 343t
    for essential tremor, 575
    for insomnia, 337, 369t, 370
    for sleep disturbances in dementia, 346–347
    for undernutrition, 267
Misoprostol, 155, 487
Mistreatment, 120–125
    definition of, 120
    financial, 122–123
    incidence of, 120
    institutional, 123
    interventions for, 123–124
    medical-legal interface, 124
    physical abuse, 121
    prevalence of, 120
    prevention of, 120
    psychological abuse, 121–122
    questions to guide intervention for, 123–124
    risk factors for, 120, 121t
    screening for, 97, 121, 122t
    signs of abuse, 121, 122t
Mistreatment history, 120–121
Mitochondrial DNA (mtDNA) theory of aging, 8t, 9
Mitral regurgitation, 456, 457t

Mitral stenosis, 456, 457t
Mixed dementia, 326
Mixed hearing loss, 242f
Mixed pain syndromes, 150
Mixed UI, 274, 277
MMA (methylmalonic acid), 637
MMSE (Mini–Mental State Examination), 22, 45, 328, 329t
MNA-SF (Mini-Nutritional Assessment, short form), 262
Mobility aids, 193–195, 193t
    for gait disorders, 301–302
Mobility assessment
    activities of daily living (ADLs), 46, 46t
    Performance-Oriented Mobility Assessment (POMA), 46, 300, 307
    rapid screening followed by assessment and management of, 43, 44t
Mobility difficulty, 5
MoCA (Montreal Cognitive Assessment), 44t, 45, 165, 328, 329t
Modified Diet in Renal Disease (MDRD) formula, 103–104, 129–131, 497
Moexipril, 469t
Moisture-associated skin damage (MASD), 289, 289f
Moisture balance, 290–291
MOLST (Medical Orders for Life-Sustaining Treatment), 25
Mometasone furoate, 442t
Monoamine oxidase (MAO)-B inhibitors, 572
Monoclonal antibodies, 648–649
Monoclonal gammopathy of uncertain significance (MGUS), 656
Montreal Cognitive Assessment (MoCA), 22, 44t, 45, 165, 328, 329t
Mood-congruent delusions, 388, 391
Mood disorders, 373–387
    with developmental disabilities, 415t
    epidemiology of, 373
    psychotic symptoms in, 391
    treatment of, 376–381
Mood disturbances
    in dementia, 342–344
    treatment of, 342–344
Mood stabilizers
    for alcohol detoxification, 407, 408t
    for behavioral disturbances in dementia with manic-like features, 344, 344t
    for bipolar depression, 378
    for mania, 378
    for personality disorders, 397–398
Moral distress, 26
Morbidity, 5
Morpheaform basal cell carcinoma, 426
Morphine
    immediate release (MSIR, Roxanol), 154t
    opioid equivalent dosages, 155t
    for persistent pain, 155
    sustained release (MSContin, Kadian), 154t

Morse Fall Scale, 307
Mortality, 6
Morton neuroma, 561t, 562–563
MOST (Medical Orders for Scope of Treatment), 25
Motor neuron disease, 577
Motorized scooters, 195
Mouse trapping, 541
Movement disorders, 568, 570–575
    drug-induced, 574
    hyperkinetic, 573–575
Moxifloxacin, 592
MRSA (methicillin-resistant *Staphylococcus aureus*), 587, 592
MS Contin (morphine, sustained release), 154t
Multicultural nutrition counseling, 268
Multidrug resistant organisms (MDROs), 587
Multifocal atrial tachycardia, 461–462
Multimorbidity, 49–53
    approach for optimal management of, 50, 50f
    definition of, 49t
    guiding principles, 50–52
    prevalence of, 5
    relevant domains, 50
Multinodular goiter, toxic, 603
Multiple myeloma, 505, 648, 656
Multiple sclerosis, 276t, 394
Multiple system atrophy, 573
Multivitamin supplements, 89t, 98
Muscle energy techniques, 115
Muscle-strengthening activity recommendations, 78, 80, 80t
Musculoskeletal diseases and disorders
    CIM for, 114–115
    and incontinence, 276t
    recommendations for, 547
    regional complaints, 539–547
    and rehabilitation, 186
Musculoskeletal pain, 538–547
Musculoskeletal system
    age-related changes, 11–13, 12t
    age-related pathologies, 16t
Music therapy, 117, 347, 387
Mutation accumulation theory of aging, 7, 8t, 10
Mycobacterium tuberculosis, 594
Mycophenolate mofetil, 555, 557
Myelodysplasia, 629
Myelodysplastic syndromes (MDS), 636
Myelofibrosis, idiopathic (IMF), 629, 640, 641
Myelopathy, 577–578
Myeloproliferative leukemia, 640
Myeloproliferative neoplasms, chronic, 640–641
Myelotoxicity, chemotherapy-related, 646–647, 647t
Myocardial infarction
    and anxiety, 385
    epidemiology of, 452
    indications for permanent pacemaker implantation, 462–463, 463t
    non-ST-elevation (NSTEMI), 452–453

ST-elevation (STEMI), 452–453
Myofascial pain, 151
Myofascial pain syndrome, 149t, 151
Myopathy, 576–577
Myositis, 556–557
MyPlate (USDA), 262
MyPlate for Older Adults (USDA), 268

N

N-terminal pro-BNP (NT-proBNP), 467
Nabilone, 118–119
Nabumetone (Relafen), 153t
Nadolol, 574–575
Nail disorders, 565–566
Nails, ingrown, 565–566
Nalbuphine, 158
Naloxone, 157
Naltrexone, 407, 408t
Naproxen sodium, 153t
Narcissistic personality disorder
    features of, 395t
    long-term course, 396–397
    therapeutic strategies for, 398, 398t
Narcotics
    adverse drug events, 265
    and incontinence, 275t
    for OA-related pain, 549
    for postsurgical pain, 134
Narcotics Anonymous, 406
Nasal pillows, 444
Nasopharyngeal laryngoscopy, 271–272
Nateglinide (Starlix), 626t
National Adult Day Services Association, 59t
National Adult Protective Services Association, 124
National Alliance of Caregiving (NAC), 55
National Cancer Institute (NCI), 59t
National Center for Complementary and Integrative Health (NCCIH), 112
National Center for Ethics in Health Care, 18, 20t
National Center on Caregiving, 58
National Center on Elder Abuse, 124
National Comprehensive Cancer Network (NCCN), 525
    Senior Adult guidelines, 645
National Consensus Guidelines, 138, 139t
National Consensus Project for Quality Palliative Care, 138
National Council on Aging, Inc.
    Nutrition Screening Initiative, 265
    website, 83
National Health and Aging Trends Study/National Survey of Caregiving (NHATS/NSOC), 55
National Health Interview Survey, 112
National Highway Traffic Safety Administration, 47
National Institute on Aging (NIA)
    Alzheimer' Disease Education and Referral site, 59t
    Exercise: A Guide from the National Institute on Aging, 83

recommendations for brain imaging, 329
strategies to facilitate communication with older patients, 43
National Institutes of Health (NIH)
    guidelines regarding body size classification based on BMI, 264
    resources and tools for caregivers, 59t
    Stroke Scale, 188, 581, 581t
National Kidney Foundation (NKF)
    guidelines for management of CKD, 508
    Kidney Disease Outcomes Quality Initiative (KDOQI), 103–104, 507–508
    online calculator, 497
National Osteoporosis Foundation, 317
National PACE Association (NPA), 212, 220
"The National Partnership to Improve Dementia Care in Nursing Homes," 205
National Pressure Ulcer Advisory Panel (NPUAP), 283, 284t, 287f, 289
National Quality Forum, 138
National Transitions of Care Coalition, 178
Native Americans
    burning mouth syndrome, 435
    cancer incidence, 644
    chronic kidney disease, 507
    CVD mortality rates, 448
    population projections, 644
    traditional medicine, 113
Native Hawaiians and Other Pacificic Islanders
    CVD mortality rates, 448
    life expectancy, 3, 3t
    population projections, 3, 268, 644
    poverty rates, 4
Native-valve endocarditis, 458
Natural Death Act (California), 24
Natural products, 112
Nausea and vomiting
    chemotherapy-induced, 118–119
    medications for nausea, 141t
    opioid-induced, 157
    postoperative nausea, 133
    in terminal illness, 141
    Senior Adult guidelines, 645
Nebivolol, 471, 471t
Neck dystonia, 574
Neck pain, 539
Negative-pressure wound therapy (NPWT), 290
Neglect. See also Mistreatment
    risk factors for inadequate caregiving, 120, 121t
    self-neglect, 122t, 123, 384
    signs of, 121, 122t
Neisseria gonorrhea, 528
Neodymium-yttrium-aluminum-garnet (Nd:YAG) laser, 653–654
Neoplasia
    adrenal, 613–614

chronic myeloproliferative neoplasms, 640–641
    vulvar, 515–516
Neostigmine, 495
Nephritis, acute interstitial, 505
Nephrolithiasis, 503
Nephrology, 497–511
    acute kidney injury (AKI), 497, 503–504
    chronic kidney disease (CKD), 91t, 497, 507–510
    end-stage renal disease (ESRD), 509, 510–511
    impaired kidney function, 104
    intrinsic renal disease, 504–506
    metabolic disorders, 498–502
    Modified Diet in Renal Disease (MDRD) formula, 103–104, 129–131, 497
    postoperative management of, 132
    recommendations for, 511
    renal cell cancer, 648, 654–655
    renal function impairment, 104
    vascular disease, 505
    volume disorders, 498–502
Nephropathy, membranous, 506–507
Nephrotic syndrome, 506–507
Nerve conduction studies, 576
Nervous system
    age-related changes, 11, 12t, 17
    age-related pathologies, 16t
Neuraminidase inhibitors, 592
Neurocognitive disorder (NCD), 326, 339
    differential diagnosis of, 331
    differentiating types of, 329–332
    mild, 330
Neurodermatitis, 419, 515
Neurokinin-1 receptor antagonists, 141t
Neurologic diseases and disorders, 568
    CIM for, 116–117
    and incontinence, 276t
    recommendations for, 585
    stroke, 580
Neurologic testing, 257t, 259, 337
Neurology, 568–579
Neuromas, 562–563
Neuromuscular disorders, 575–578
Neurontin (gabapentin), 152t
Neuropathic pain, 149t, 150
Neuropsychiatric concerns, preoperative, 131
Neuropsychiatric Inventory (NPI), 340
Neurosyphilis, 597–598
Neuroticism, 399
Never events, 162–163
New York Heart Association
    classification of HF, 469, 470t
New Zealand, 82
NHATS/NSOC (National Health and Aging Trends Study/National Survey of Caregiving), 55
Niacin
    drug interactions, 265t
    RDIs for adults ≥71 years old, 263t
NICHE (Nurses Improving Care of Health System Elders), 171
Nicotine dependence, 407, 408t

Nicotine replacement, 407, 408t
Nifedipine, 102
NIH Stroke Scale (NIHSS), 188, 581, 581t
Nitrates
  adverse drug events, 106, 106t
  for chronic CAD, 455
  for heart failure, 470
Nitrofurantoin, 593
Nivolombab, 428
Nizatidine, 108t
Nociceptive pain, 149–150, 149t
Nociceptors, 148t
Nocturia, 277, 277t, 281
Nocturnal polyuria, 277t
Nodular basal cell carcinoma, 426
Nodular melanoma, 427
Nodular thyroid disease, 605–606
Non-Hodgkin lymphoma, 656
Nonadherence to medication regimens, 45, 109–110
Nonbenzodiazepine-benzodiazepine receptor agonists (NBRAs), 370
Nonmaleficence, 18, 21
Nonsteroidal anti-inflammatory drugs (NSAIDs)
  adverse effects of, 106, 106t, 265, 487
  for CPPD, 552
  drug interactions, 107, 107t
  gastric complications, 487
  for gout, 552
  for headaches, 579
  and hyperkalemia, 501, 501t
  and incontinence, 275t, 281
  for OA-related pain, 549
  for persistent pain, 153t, 155
  for SLE, 555
Nonthyroidal illness syndromes, 602
Nonverbal communication, respectful, 64
Norco (hydrocodone), 153t
Normal-pressure hydrocephalus (NPH)
  gait abnormalities, 298t
  surgery for, 301
Norpramin (desipramine), 152t
North American Menopause Society, 536
Nortriptyline (Pamelor)
  for depression, 377t
  for depressive features of behavioral disturbances in dementia, 343, 343t
  for persistent pain management, 152t
Novel oral anticoagulants (NOACs), 460, 461
Novolin (insulin), 627t
Novolin 70/30 (isophane insulin and regular insulin injectable), 627t
NovoLog (insulin aspart), 627t
Noxious stimulus, 148t
  gait abnormalities, 298t
  and incontinence, 276t
  surgery for, 301
NPH insulin (Humulin, Novolin), 627t
NPUAP (National Pressure Ulcer Advisory Panel), 283, 284t, 287f, 289

NSAIDs. See Nonsteroidal anti-inflammatory drugs
Nucynta (tapentadol), 154t
Nucynta ER (tapentadol extended release), 154t
Numeric Rating Scale, 149
Nurse practitioners, 31t
  in home care, 210
  in nursing home, 206
  rehabilitation team role, 184, 185t
Nurses Improving Care of Health System Elders (NICHE), 171
Nursing, 214, 214t
Nursing facilities
  medical directors of, 200t, 203–205
  staffing patterns, 198–201
Nursing-home care, 196–208, 213t
  alcohol use, 404
  availability of, 197–198
  clinical practice guidelines for, 207
  demographic characteristics of older adults in, 196–197
  falls risk in, 303
  fee-for-service, 39
  financing, 39–40, 198
  functional characteristics of older adults in, 196, 199t
  health insurance coverage for, 31t, 36t
  interventions for lowering risk of falls in, 308t
  Interventions to Reduce Acute Care Transfers (INTERACT), 177
  involuntary weight loss in, 266
  legislation influencing, 202–205
  length of stay in, 197
  managed care, 40
  medical care issues, 205–206
  occupancy rates, 197
  physician practice in, 206–207
  physician responsibilities in, 206–207
  placement factors, 201
  population, 3–4, 196–197, 199t
  postacute care, 197
  pressure ulcers in, 284
  Quality Assurance and Performance Improvement (QAPI) programs, 205
  quality issues, 202–205
  quality measures for, 199t, 202–203
  recommendations for preventing falls, 311
  sleep in, 367
  staffing patterns, 198–201
  standards of care, 269
  unacceptable weight loss in, 268–269
  urinary incontinence in, 282
  venues of care, 177
Nursing Home Compare, 39, 59t
Nutrition, 262–269
  for chronic kidney disease, 509–510
  culturally appropriate care, 268
  drug-nutrient interactions, 264–265, 265t

  for hospitalized patients, 162, 165t
  intake, 264
  interventions, 165t, 266–268
  oral, 266–267
  for pressure ulcers, 290
  to reduce risk of osteoporosis, 316, 316t
  risk factors for poor status, 265, 265t
  standards of care for, 269
  syndromes, 266
  undernutrition, 267–268
Nutrition assessment, 44–45, 263–265
  multi-item tools for, 265
  rapid screening followed by assessment and management, 43, 44t
  screening evaluations, 95
  threshold to trigger, 269
Nutrition Screening Initiative, 265
Nutritional supplements, 266–267, 355
  for pressure ulcers, 292
  safety issues, 113–114

O

OASIS (Outcome and Assessment Information Set), 183, 209
Obergefell v. Hodges, 76
Obesity, 266
  activity recommendations for, 78, 81
  cardiovascular risk, 451
  definition of, 451, 607
  prevalence of, 5, 266
  recommendations for, 93
OBRA (Omnibus Budget Reconciliation Act), 123, 196, 202–203, 268–269
Obsessions, 384
Obsessive-compulsive disorder (OCD), 384, 386, 386t
Obsessive-compulsive personality disorder
  features of, 395, 395t
  long-term course, 396–397
  therapeutic strategies for, 398, 398t
Obstruction
  acute colonic pseudo-obstruction, 495
  bowel, 142, 143t
  gastrointestinal, 142
Obstructive pulmonary disease, chronic (COPD), 440–444
  anxiety and, 385
  screening for, 91t
Obstructive sleep apnea (OSA), 276t, 363, 364, 366, 444
Obstructive uropathy, 504
Occupational therapy (OT)
  for dementia, 337
  health insurance coverage for, 31t
  for pain, 549
  for preventing falls, 310t
  rehabilitation team role, 183, 185t
OCD (obsessive-compulsive disorder), 384, 386, 386t
Octreotide, 141t, 143t, 260, 495
Ocular surface tumors, 230

Odanacatib, 322
Odd or eccentric behaviors, 395t
Odynophagia, 484
Office visits, 43, 332
Ogilvie syndrome, 495
1,25(OH)D levels, 606, 606t
25(OH)D levels, 320, 606–607, 606t
Olanzapine
    for agitated delirium, 356t, 357
    for depression, 377–378
    dosing and adverse events of, 390, 390t
    for psychosis in dementia, 345, 345t, 346
    to stabilize mood in mania and bipolar depression, 379t
Older Americans Act, 214, 266–267, 337
Oldways®, 268
Olecranon bursitis, 540–541
Olfactory dysfunction
    age-related changes, 435
    medications that cause, 435, 436t
    nonpharmacologic causes of, 435, 436t
Olmesartan, 469t
Olodaterol, 442t
Omalizumab, 440
Omega-3 fatty acids, 114t, 115, 118
Omeprazole, 141t
Omnibus Budget Reconciliation Act (OBRA), 123, 196, 202–203, 268–269
Oncology, 642–657. See also Cancer
    recommendations for, 657
Ondansetron, 141t
Onychocryptosis, 565
Onychomycosis, 566, 566f
Operative therapy. See also Surgical care
    iatrogenic complications, 131
    perioperative care, 126–135
    preoperative assessment and management of, 126–131
Ophthalmic corticosteroids, 232
Opioids
    adverse drug events, 106, 106t, 156–157, 392
    barriers to using, 155–156
    and delirium, 355, 355t
    delivery routes, 155t, 156
    dependence on, 407, 408t
    for dyspnea, 144
    for fibromyalgia, 558
    interconverting, 155t, 156
    for OA-related pain, 549
    for persistent pain, 153t–154t, 155–156
Optic neuropathy, ischemic, 230, 237t, 238, 238f
Optimizing therapies and care plans, 52
Oral appliances, 364
Oral dysphagia, 270
Oral health, 429–437
    cancer, 91t, 429, 432–433
    candidiasis, 434, 434f
    dental decay, 429–430
    with developmental disabilities, 415t

edentulism, 431–432
    lesions, 432–435
Oral hygiene, 429, 436, 556
Oral nutrition, 266–267
Oral tissues, 429, 430t
Orchiectomy, 526t
Oregon: adult foster care, 214
Orexin receptor antagonists, 370
Organ systems
    age-related changes, 11–15, 12t
    age-related pathogies, 16, 16t
Oropharyngeal carcinoma, 432–433
Oropharyngeal dysphagia, 271–272, 483
    evaluation of, 484t
    treatment of, 484
Orthoses
    for foot disorders, 563–564
    for gait disorders, 301–302
    for osteoarthritis, 548
    for rehabilitation, 193, 195
Orthostatic (postural) hypotension, 259–260, 573
    interventions for preventing falls, 309, 310t
Orthotists, 184t
Oseltamivir, 592
Osmotic laxatives, 489–490, 490t
Ospemifene, 536
Osteoarthritis (OA), 548–550, 549f
    activity recommendations for, 78, 80t
    CIM for, 114–115
    of hand, 548, 549f
    of hip, 542, 549
    interventions for preventing falls, 310t
    of knee, 542, 543, 549, 549f
Osteoblasts, 314
Osteolytic hypercalcemia, local, 607–608, 608t
Osteomyelitis, 596
Osteonecrosis, 429, 437
Osteopenia, 314t, 415t
Osteophytes, 548
Osteoporosis, 313–325, 509
    activity recommendations for, 80t
    CIM for, 115
    definition of, 313, 314t, 317
    with developmental disabilities, 415t
    diagnosis of, 313
    epidemiology of, 313–314
    impact of, 313–314
    investigational agents for, 324
    laboratory testing in, 316, 317t
    modifications to reduce risk of, 316, 316t
    pathogenesis of, 314–315
    pharmacologic options for, 320–324, 321t
    physical examination in, 317
    prevention of, 313, 319–324, 554
    recommendations for, 324
    risk factors for, 316, 316t
    sacral fractures of, 543, 544t, 545t, 546
    screening for, 88t, 92, 313, 317, 318t

    secondary, 313, 316–317, 316t
    treatment of, 319–324
    vertebral compression fractures of, 543, 546
Ottawa Hospital Research Institute, 59t
Outcome and Assessment Information Set (OASIS), 183, 209
Outpatient care
    alcohol use, 404
    fee-for-service (FFS) care, 35–36
    financing, 35–37
    health insurance coverage for, 31t
    managed care, 37
    medications, 31t
    mental health care, 31t
    patient selection for interventions, 220
    rehabilitation services, 182t, 184
    for substance abuse, 406–407
    systems of care, 216–221
Outpatient consultation, 218–219
Outreach, 75–76
Ovarian cancer, 89, 91t
Overactive bladder, 274
Overprescribing, 104–105, 105t, 108
Overweight
    activity recommendations for, 79, 81
    definition of, 451, 454
Oxaliplatin, 653
Oxandrolone, 268
Oxazepam, 386
Oxybutynin
    and delirium, 355t
    for incontinence, 280, 281
Oxycodone
    immediate release (OxyIR, Roxicodone, Percocet, Percodan, Tylox), 154t
    opioid equivalent dosages, 155t
    for persistent pain, 154t, 156
    sustained release (OxyContin), 154t
Oxygen, hyperbaric, 292
Oxygen therapy
    for COPD, 442–443, 443t
    for dyspnea, 144
OxyIR (oxycodone, immediate release), 154t

P

P_2Y_{12} inhibitors, 452, 639
PACE (Program of All-inclusive Care of the Elderly), 39, 211–212, 219–220
Pacemakers, 260
    indications for, 462–463, 463t
    and preventing falls, 308, 309
Pacific Islanders. See Native Hawaiians and Other Pacificic Islanders
Paclitaxel, 647t, 654
Padua Prediction Score, 167
Paget disease of bone, 243, 609–610
Pain
    acute, 147
    back pain, 543–545, 544t
    central, 148t
    chronic, 56, 57t, 147–148, 158, 415t, 416, 557–558

in cognitively impaired adults, 150–151, 150t
definition of, 147
dyspareunia, 535, 536, 536t
elbow pain, 540–541
family caregiver interventions, 56, 57t
gait abnormalities, 298, 298t
in groin, 542
guidelines for management of, 549
hand and wrist pain, 541
heel pain, 563
hip pain, 549
knee pain, 538, 542–543, 549
leg pain, 542
low back pain, 544t, 546
lumbar spinal stenosis, 538
mixed or unspecified, 150
musculoskeletal, 538–547
myofascial, 151
neck pain, 539
neuropathic, 149t, 150, 576
nociceptive, 149–150, 149t
persistent, 147–148, 549
phantom limb pain, 192
shoulder, 539–540
somatic, 149–150, 149t
terms used in care of patients in, 147–148, 148t
thigh pain, 541–542
types of, 149–150, 149t
visceral, 149–150, 149t
wind-up, 148t
Pain Disability Scale, 149
Pain disorder (somatic pain), 149–150, 149t, 398
Pain intensity scales, 149–150
Pain Ladder (WHO), 155
Pain management, 147–159
in cognitively impaired adults, 150–151
in debridement, 292
for delirium, 354t
interventional, 158
nonpharmacologic therapy, 151
in osteoarthritis, 548–549
pharmacologic therapy, 151–158
in post-herpetic neuralgia, 424
postoperative, 134
pulsed radiofrequency (PRF) treatment, 158
in terminal illness, 140
trigger point injections, 158
in vertebral compression fractures, 324
Pain maps, 149
Painful diabetic neuropathy, 568
Painful diverticulosis, 493
Paliperidone
dosing and adverse events of, 390t
for psychosis in dementia, 345t, 346
Palliative care, 136–146
for COPD and dyspnea, 444
cultural aspects of, 137
ethnographic data, 137
for frailty, 227
guidelines for, 138, 139t

hospice, 137–138
for LGBT older adults, 75
overall care near death, 136–137
quality indicators for, 138
recommendations for, 141, 146
in terminal illness, 140–145
of wounds, 293–294, 293t
Palliative Performance Scale, 136–137
Palliative sedation, 25, 26
Palsy, progressive supranuclear (PSP), 573
Pamelor (nortriptyline), 152t
Pancreatic cancer, 91t
Pancreatitis, 488–489, 635
Panhypopituitarism, 612
Panic attacks, 382–383
Panic disorder, 382–383
treatment strategies for, 386, 386t
Pantothenic acid, 263t
PaO_2, 438
Pap smear, 88t
Papaverine, 533t, 534
Paranoid delusions, 388
Paranoid personality disorder
features of, 395, 395t
long-term course, 396–397
therapeutic strategies for, 398, 398t
Paraparesis, 298t
Paraplegia, 298t
Parathyroid disorders, 606–610
Parathyroid hormone (PTH)
age-related changes in, 606, 606t
and renal bone disease, 509
secondary hyperparathyroidism, 315
Parathyroid hormone (teriparatide), 321t, 323
Parathyroid hormone-related peptide (PTHrp), 609
Parathyroid surgery, 608
Parkinson dementia, 327
Parkinson disease (PD), 568, 570–572
CIM for, 117
diagnosis of, 570–571
gait abnormalities, 299
interventions for preventing falls, 310t
motor symptoms of, 571–572
nonmotor symptoms of, 276t, 572
psychotic symptoms of, 392
treatment of, 571–572
"Parkinson-plus" syndromes, 572–573
Parkinsonian syndromes, 298, 572–573
Parkinsonism, 570
arteriosclerotic, 299
gait abnormalities, 298, 298t
medication-induced, 573
vascular, 573
Paronychia, 565–566
Paroxetine
for depression, 342
for depressive features of behavioral disturbances in dementia, 343t
drug interactions, 107, 107t
Passive-aggressive personality disorder, 394
Past medical history, 165t

Patellofemoral pain, 542–543
Patent foramen ovale, 583–584
Patient-aligned care teams (GERI-PACT), 52
Patient-centered medical homes (PCMHs), 27, 216
Joint Principles of the PCMH (AAP, ACP, AAFP, AOA), 216, 217t
Patient-clinician communication, 43
Patient-controlled analgesia, 134
Patient education
cultural appropriate nutrition materials, 268
about diabetes, 624
for fibromyalgia, 557–558
medical director responsibilities for, 200t, 203–205
for persistent pain, 151
for preventing falls, 308
Patient Health Questionnaire (PHQ-9), 44t, 45, 375
indications to start antidepressant therapy based on, 374, 375t
initial two questions (PHQ-2), 374
prescriber response guidelines based on, 374, 375t
Patient preferences, 50
code status discussions, 167–168
cultural aspects, 66
for diabetes care, 623
for end-of-life-care, 140
formality, 63
forms that identify, 24–25
promoting individual preferences for future care, 23–25
Patient Protection and Affordable Care Act (ACA), 27, 28, 33, 35, 41, 52, 172, 175, 205, 472
Independence at Home Demonstration project, 210
Patient safety. See Safety
Patient Self-Determination Act (PSDA), 24, 40
Patient surveillance, 332
Pauci-immune glomerulonephritis, 506
Pay-for-performance (P4P), 41, 203
Peak expiratory flow meters and inhalers, 443
Pediculosis capitis, 425
Pediculosis corporis, 425
Pediculosis pubis, 425
Pegylated interferon, 640–641
Pelvic examination, 512, 513
Pelvic floor retraining, 490
Pelvic floor support disorders, 516–517
Pelvic lymphadenectomy, 525
Pelvic muscle exercises (PMEs), 279, 280
Pelvic organ prolapse, 516, 516f
Pelvic Organ Prolapse Quantification (POPQ), 516
Pelvic physical therapy, 490t, 491
Pelvic reconstruction, 517
Pembrolizumab, 428, 648
Penicillamine, 550
Penile-brachial pressure index, 532
Penile prosthesis, 533t, 534
Pentamidine, 501, 501t

Pentoxifylline, 464
Peptic ulcer disease (PUD), 487–488
Percocet (oxycodone, immediate release), 154t
Percodan (oxycodone, immediate release), 154t
Percutaneous coronary intervention (PCI)
　for acute coronary syndrome, 452–453
　for chronic CAD, 455
Percutaneous endoscopic gastrostomy or jejunostomy, 272
Performance-based functional assessment, 299–300
Performance-Oriented Mobility Assessment (POMA), 46, 300, 307
Perindopril, 469t, 471, 471t
Periodic limb movements disorder (PLMD), 575
Periodic limb movements during sleep (PLMS), 364–365, 575
Periodontal anatomy, 429, 430f
Periodontal disease, 430–431
Periodontal ligament, 430
Periodontitis, 429, 430, 431
Periodontium, 430–431
Perioperative care, 126–135
　recommendations for, 134
Periostitis, 564t
Peripheral arterial disease (PAD), 448, 463–464
　diagnosis of, 463–464
　and foot, 567
　recommendations for, 465
　screening for, 91t, 93
　and thigh pain, 542
　treatment of, 464
Peripheral neuropathy, 568, 575–578
　gait abnormalities, 298, 298t
Peripheral vascular disease, 186
Peripheral venous insufficiency, 276t
Peritoneal dialysis, 510
Peritonitis, diffuse, 493
Permethrin cream, 425
Perphenazine
　dosing and adverse events of, 390t
　for nausea, 141t
　for psychosis in dementia, 345t
Persistent complex bereavement disorder, 374
Persistent pain
　assessment of, 148–150
　definition of, 147–148
　guidelines for management of, 549
　nonopioid adjuvant medications for, 157–158
　pharmacotherapy for, 151–156, 152t–154t
　treatment of, 151–158
Personality changes, 394, 395
Personality disorders, 394–398
　definition of, 394
　diagnostic challenges, 396
　differential diagnosis of, 396
　epidemiology of, 395–396
　features of, 394, 395t
　long-term course, 396–397

organic, 394
other specified, 394
therapeutic strategies for, 397–398, 398t
unspecified, 394
Pes anserine, 543
Pes cavus, 559–560, 560f
Pes plano valgus, 559–560, 560f
Pes planus, 559–560, 560f
Pessaries, 281, 512, 516–517
Phalen maneuver, 541
Phantom limb pain, 192
Pharmacodynamics
　age-associated changes in, 104, 646–647, 647t
　chemotherapy issues, 646–647, 647t
Pharmacokinetics
　age-associated changes in, 101–104, 646–647, 647t
　chemotherapy issues, 646–647, 647t
Pharmacotherapy, 101–111
　adverse drug events, 105t, 106, 106t, 385
　for agitated delirium, 356t
　for anxiety disorders, 385–386
　for benign prostatic hyperplasia, 521–522, 521t
　for bipolar depression, 378–379, 379t
　for bipolar disorder, 376
　brown-bag evaluation of, 108–109
　for constipation, 490, 491t
　for delirium, 353–354, 354t, 356–357
　for dementia, 335–337
　for depression, 342–343, 343t, 376, 377–378
　for diabetes mellitus, 626–627, 626t
　drugs to reduce or eliminate in management of delirium, 354–355, 355t
　flexible medication times, 366
　for frailty, 226–227
　for HFpEF, 471, 471t
　for HFrEF, 468–471
　for hypertension, 478–479, 478t
　inappropriate prescribing, 104–105, 105t
　for insomnia, 369t, 370–371
　investigational agents for osteoporosis, 324
　to lower glucose, 626–627
　for mania, 378, 379t
　medications to avoid, 158
　nonadherence to regimens, 109–110
　optimizing, 52, 104–105
　for osteoporosis, 320–324, 321t
　for pain, 151–158
　for persistent pain, 151–156, 152t–154t
　polypharmacy, 52
　prescribing cascade, 107
　principles of prescribing, 108–109, 109t

　recommendations for, 110
　for schizophrenia and schizophrenia spectrum syndromes, 389–390
　for somatic symptom and related disorders, 394
　suboptimal, 161–162, 165t
　for substance abuse, 407
　for undernutrition syndromes, 267–268
Pharyngeal dysphagia, 270–271
Phenobarbital, 355t, 569
Phentolamine, 533t, 534
Phenytoin
　adverse effects of, 265, 569
　and delirium, 355t
　drug interactions, 107, 107t
　nutrient interactions, 265, 265t
Phlebotomy, 640
Phobia
　social (social anxiety disorder), 383–384, 386t
　specific, 383, 386t
　treatment strategies for, 386t, 387
Phosphatidylinositol-binding clathrin assembly protein gene (PICALM), 327
Phosphodiesterase inhibitors
　adverse events of, 106, 106t
　for COPD, 442, 443t
　for erectile dysfunction, 532, 533
　for HFpEF, 471, 471t
　for LUTS in BPH, 521t, 522
　for PAD, 464
Phosphorus, 509
Photoaging, 15–16, 417
Photodynamic therapy, 653–654
Photographs, 288
PHQ-2 (Patient Health Questionnaire), 374
PHQ-9 (Patient Health Questionnaire), 44t, 45, 374, 375, 375t
Physical activity, 78–84. See also Exercise
　assessing, 82
　baseline activity, 80
　for behavioral disturbances, 347
　benefits of, 78–79, 116
　and cardiovascular disease, 451
　for chronic constipation, 489–490, 490t
　for chronic pain syndromes, 557–558
　counseling for, 81–82, 89t, 93
　for dementia, 332
　for diabetes mellitus, 624
　economic benefits of, 79
　for fibromyalgia, 557–558
　guidelines for plans, 82
　for heart failure, 468
　for hypertension, 478
　for OA-related pain, 548–549
　for pain, 151
　prescription for, 82
　preventive health benefits of, 78–79
　promoting, 78, 81–84
　providing assistance in increasing, 83

Rapid Assessment of Physical Activity, 82
recommendations for, 78, 79–81, 80t
relative exercise intensity, 78
risks of, 83
screening for, 81
for sleep issues, 369–370
therapeutic benefits of, 79
Physical Activity Guidelines Advisory Committee, 81
2008 Physical Activity Guidelines for Americans (HHS), 79, 80, 81
Physical assessment, 43–45, 121
Physical dependence, 156
Physical disability
excess, 404–405
International Classification of Functioning, Disability, and Health (ICF) (WHO), 181
Physical examination
daily evaluation, 168
digital rectal examination, 523–524
gynecologic, 512–513
at hospital admission, 164, 165t
Initial Preventive Physical Examination (IPPE), 36, 94t–95t
of lower back pain, 544, 545t
in mistreatment, 121
in musculoskeletal pain, 538
in osteoporosis, 317
pelvic examination, 512, 513
with urinary incontinence, 278
Physical mistreatment, 121
Physical restraints, 356
Physical status, 127, 127t
Physical therapy (PT)
for delirium, 354t
for dementia, 337
for gait disorders, 301
health insurance coverage for, 31t
for myelopathy, 578
for pain, 151, 549
for Parkinson disease, 117
pelvic, 490t, 491
for preventing falls, 310t
rehabilitation team role, 183, 185t
Physician aid-in-dying (PAD), 25
Physician assistants, 206
Physician-assisted death, 25
Physician-assisted suicide, 25
Physician Orders for Life-Sustaining Treatment (POLST), 24–25, 24t, 140
Physician Orders for Scope of Treatment (POST), 25
Physician Quality Reporting System (PQRS), 41
Physicians
competencies for attending physicians in post-acute and long-term care medicine, 200–201, 204t
health insurance coverage for, 31t
in nursing home, 206–207
rehabilitation team role, 184, 185t

requirements for long-term care facilities, 201t, 205
responsibilities in nursing home, 206–207
role in home care, 209–210
The Physician's Guide to Assessing and Counseling Older Drivers (AMA), 47
Physiologic theories of aging, 8–11, 8t
Phytoestrogens, 117
Pick disease, 341
Pilates, 80t
Pill esophagitis, 486
Pilocarpine, 237t, 432, 556
Pink eye, 232
Pioglitazone (Actos), 626t
Pioneer ACO Model, 27
Pirbuterol, 442t
Pirfenidone, 444
Pituitary adenomas, 610–612
Pituitary gland
anterior pituitary changes, 610, 611t
anterior pituitary disorders, 610–612
Plantar fasciitis, 561t, 563
Plantar verruca, 565
Plaque, 430
Plasma exchange, 576
Platelets, 638–640
Pneumatic compression, intermittent, 446
Pneumococcal pneumonia, 271
Pneumococcal vaccine, 589–590, 592
in hospitalized patients, 5, 165t, 166–167
immunization schedule for adults ≥65 years old, 590t
recommendations for, 88t, 97
Pneumonia, 591–592
aspiration, 186, 271
community-acquired, 591–592
guidelines for therapy, 591–592
hospital-acquired, 592
institution-acquired, 429
long-term care facility–acquired, 592
pneumococcal, 271
and rehabilitation, 186
surveillance definition of, 589t
Podagra, 551
Podiatry, 559–567
Polarity, 118
Policy issues, 75–76
POLST (Physician Orders for Life-Sustaining Treatment), 24–25, 24t, 140
Poly-l-actic acid, 417
Polyangiitis
granulomatosis with, 506
microscopic, 506
Polycarbophil (FiberCon), 491t
Polycythemia vera (PV), 629, 630, 640–641
Polyethylene glycol (Miralax), 489–490, 490t, 491t
Polymyalgia rheumatica (PMR), 539, 550, 552–554

Polymyositis, 556–557, 577
Polypharmacy, 45, 52
Polyps
adenomatous, 652, 652t
colonic, 494, 651
Polysomnography, 362
Polyunsaturated fatty acids (PUFAs), 115, 118
Polyuria, nocturnal, 277t
POMA (Performance-Oriented Mobility Assessment), 46, 300, 307
Poor metabolizers (PMs), 102–103
Popeye sign, 540
Popliteal cyst, 543
POPQ (Pelvic Organ Prolapse Quantification), 516
Population projections, 2–3
Positional vertigo, benign paroxysmal (BPPV), 249
diagnostic criteria for, 252
self-treatment of, 252f, 253
Positive-airway pressure (PAP), 363–364
auto-titrating PAP (autoPAP), 364
bi-level (biPAP), 364, 577
continuous (CPAP), 364
Positron emission tomography (PET), 329
POST (Physician Orders for Scope of Treatment), 25
Post-herpetic neuralgia (PHN), 232, 423–424
Postacute care, 183
AM-PAC (Activity Measure for Post Acute Care), 184t
competencies for attending physicians in, 200–201, 204t
health insurance coverage for, 31t
nursing-home care, 197
Postacute care specialists, 200
Postacute rehabilitation
fee-for-service (FFS) care, 38
financing, 38–39
managed care, 38–39
Posterior tibial tendon dysfunction, 563, 563f
Posterior uveitis, 230, 237t
Postobstructive diarrhea, 495
Postoperative cognitive dysfunction (POCD), 353
Postoperative delirium, 133–134, 353, 358t, 359
Postoperative infections, 230
Postoperative management, 131–134
Posttraumatic stress disorder (PTSD), 384–385, 386, 386t
Postural (orthostatic) hypotension, 259–260, 573
interventions for preventing falls, 309, 310t
Postvoid residual (PVR)
increased, 274, 278, 279
testing, 278
Potassium, 263t
Potassium balance disorders, 501–502
Potassium-sparing diuretics
adverse drug events, 106, 106t
drug interactions, 107, 107t

Index **693**

Potassium supplements
　　adverse drug events, 106, 106t, 265
　　drug interactions, 265, 265t
　　for hypertension, 478
Poverty: delusions of, 391
Poverty rates, 4, 76
Power mobility devices, 194–195
PPD (purified-protein derivative) skin tests, 595–596
Pra (Probability of Repeated Admission) Questionnaire, 220
Pramipexole
　　for PD motor symptoms, 572
　　for periodic limb movement disorder, 365
　　for restless legs syndrome, 365, 575
Pramlintide (Symlin), 626t
Prasugrel, 452, 453, 639
Prazosin, 386t, 521, 521t
Pre-frailty, 451
Prealbumin, 264
Preclinical disability, 46
Prednisolone, 107
Prednisone
　　for dermatomyositis, 557
　　for GCA, 554
　　for gout, 552
　　for multiple myeloma, 656
　　for nausea, 141t
　　for PMR, 553–554
　　for polymyositis, 557
　　for rheumatoid arthritis, 551
Preferred behavior programs, 414
Preferred provider organizations (PPOs), 32
Pregabalin (Lyrica)
　　Beers Criteria for, 108t
　　for essential tremor, 575
　　for fibromyalgia, 558
　　and incontinence, 275t
　　for neuropathic pain, 576
　　for persistent pain, 152t, 157
　　for restless legs syndrome, 575
　　for vasomotor symptoms, 513
Prehabilitation, 301
Prehabilitative approach, 170
Preoperative assessment and management, 126–131
Preoperative exercise, total body, 301
Prerenal azotemia, 503–504
Presbycusis, 241
Presbyesophagus, 270
Prescribing
　　Beers Criteria for, 105, 108t
　　inappropriate, 104–105, 105t
　　optimizing, 52, 104–105
　　principles of, 108–109, 109t
Prescribing cascade, 107
Prescription drugs. See Drugs; Pharmacotherapy
Presenilin 1 (PS1), 327
Presenilin 2 (PS2), 327
Pressure Sore Status Tool, 286
Pressure stockings, 310t
Pressure Ulcer Scale for Healing, 286
Pressure ulcers, 282–293, 423
　　assessment of, 284–286
　　Braden Scale, 286–287
　　characteristics of, 423, 423t
　　classification of, 285–286
　　definition of, 283–284
　　documentation of, 286–288
　　dressings for, 290, 291t, 292
　　hospital-acquired, 163, 165t, 284
　　incidence of, 284
　　infectious aspects, 293
　　nutritional recommendations for, 292
　　prevalence of, 284
　　prevention of, 163, 165t, 288–290, 331t
　　and rehabilitation, 185
　　risk-assessment scales, 286–287
　　risk factors for, 287, 288t
　　staging system for, 283, 284t, 287f
　　support surfaces for older adults at risk of, 287–288
　　surgical repair of, 284
　　treatment of, 290–292
　　unavoidable, 283
　　unstageable, 285, 286t, 287f
Presyncope, 249, 250t
Prevention, 85–100
　　aspirin therapy, 89t, 97–98
　　available health measures, 85, 88t–89t
　　of cardiovascular disease, 624, 625
　　counseling on, 98–99
　　of diabetes mellitus, 622
　　of falls, 95–96, 304, 306f, 307–311, 308t, 310t
　　of frailty, 227–228
　　health insurance coverage for services, 31t
　　of hip fracture, 607
　　of hip fracture recurrence, 190
　　HIV, 597
　　Initial Preventive Physical Examination (IPPE), 36, 94t–95t
　　of migraine headache, 579
　　of mistreatment, 120
　　of osteoporosis, 313, 319–324
　　physical activity benefits for, 78–79
　　of pneumonia, 592
　　of pressure ulcers, 163, 165t, 288–290, 331t
　　recommendations for, 99
　　recommended measures, 85, 88t–89t
　　of stroke, 582–584
　　of UTIs, 594
　　of venous thromboembolism, 165t, 167
　　"Welcome to Medicare" preventive visits, 36, 99
Preventive services plan, 94t
Primary care
　　CareMore model of, 217–218
　　comprehensive geriatric assessment (CGA) in, 218–219
　　enhanced, 216–218
　　geriatrics in, 216–219
　　GRACE model of, 217
Primary care physicians (PCPs), 28, 216–217
Primary caregivers, 57–58
Primary providers, 209–210
PRIME-MD, 374
Primidone, 355t, 574–575
Principlism, 20
Private contracts, 30, 32
Private FFS plans, 32
Pro-anthocyanidin, 594
Probability of Repeated Admission Questionnaire (Pra), 220
Probenecid
　　Beers Criteria for, 108t
　　for gout, 552
Probiotics, 493
Problem drinking, 407, 408t
Problem-solving therapy, 380
Problem substance use, 402
Procainamide, 460
Prochlorperazine, 141t
Profilnine®, 639
Progesterone, 347, 495
Progestins, 513
Prognosis, 51
Program at Home (VA), 212
Program of All-inclusive Care of the Elderly (PACE), 39, 211–212, 219–220
Progressive supranuclear palsy (PSP), 573
Project RED (Re-Engineered Discharge), 176, 179t
Prokinetic agents, 141t
Prolactin
　　age-related changes in, 610, 611t
　　hyperprolactinemia, 610–612
Prolapse
　　genital, 516, 517
　　iris, 521
　　uterine, 516, 516f
　　vaginal, 516, 516f, 517
Promethazine, 141t
Prompted voiding, 280, 282
Propafenone, 460
Propantheline, 281
Propranolol, 574–575, 579
Proprioceptive deficits, 298, 298t
Propulsion, 297t
Prospective payment system (PPS), 38, 198, 209
Prostaglandin analogues, 155
Prostaglandins, 238t
Prostate: transurethral vaporization of, 521t, 522
Prostate cancer, 522–528, 654
　　advanced/metastatic, 526t, 527–528
　　CIM for, 118
　　diagnostic tests, 523–524
　　grading, 524
　　hormonal therapy for, 648
　　incidence and epidemiology of, 522–523
　　incidence rates, 642
　　localized, 525–526, 526t
　　locally advanced, 526t, 527
　　management approaches for, 525, 526t

risk in older gay and bisexual men, 72
screening for, 87, 91t, 523–524, 646
staging, 524–525, 524t
symptoms of, 523
treatment of, 520
Prostate disease, 520–529
recommendations for, 528
Prostate-specific antigen (PSA) testing, 520, 523–524
recommendations for, 87, 88t
Prostatectomy
open, 521t, 522
radical, 525–527, 526t
Prostatic hyperplasia, benign (BPH), 520–522
CIM for, 117
Prostatism, 520
Prostatitis, 520, 528
Prostheses, penile, 533t, 534
Prosthetic device infections (PDIs), 596
Prosthetic heart valves, 637
Prosthetic rehabilitation, 193
Prosthetists, 184, 185t
Protein deposition diseases, 507
Protein-energy malnutrition, 266
Protein excretion: measures of, 497–498
Protein requirements, 292
Proteinuria, 497–498
Proton-pump inhibitors (PPIs), 549
adverse drug events, 265
Beers Criteria for, 487
drug interactions, 588
for GERD, 485–486
for nausea, 141t
for persistent pain, 155
for PUD, 488
Provider-sponsored organizations (PSOs), 32
Pruritus, 420–421
PS1 (presenilin 1), 327
PS2 (presenilin 2), 327
PSA (prostate-specific antigen) testing, 520, 523–524
recommendations for, 87, 88t
Pseudo-obstruction, acute colonic, 495
Pseudoaddiction, 148t, 156
Pseudodisease, 86
Pseudogout, 541, 542, 543, 552
Pseudohypertension, 476
Pseudohyponatremia, 499
Pseudomembranous colitis, 599
Pseudomonas, 597
Pseudothrombophlebitis, 543
Psoas abscess, 542
Psoriasis, 421–422, 421f
Psychiatric disorders
in aging adults with intellectual disability, 411, 412–414
CIM for, 116
diagnosis and treatment of, 413–414
and incontinence, 276t
Psychoactive medications, 308, 337
Psychogenic ED, 531, 531t, 534
Psychologic assessment, 45
Psychological abuse, 121–122

Psychological assessment, 121–122
Psychological dependence, 156
Psychological mistreatment, 121–122
Psychosis
antipsychotic medications for, 344–346, 345t
in dementia, 340, 344–346, 345t
and incontinence, 276t
late-onset, 388
Psychosocial functioning, 201t, 205
concerns of LGBT older adults, 71, 71t
interventions for depression, 380–381
Psychosocial theories of aging, 8
Psychotherapy
for abstinence, 407
for alcohol dependence, 408t
for anxiety disorders, 386–387
for bipolar disorder, 376
for depression, 376, 380
emotion-oriented, 332
for personality disorders, 397
for somatic symptom and related disorders, 394
Psychotic depression, 376, 377–378
Psychotic disorders, 392
due to another medical condition, 392
substance/medication-induced, 392
Psychotic symptoms, 390–391
in delirium and delusional disorder, 390–391
in dementia, 391
in depression, 388
in mood disorders, 391
Psychotropic medications, 397–398
Psyllium (Metamucil), 491t
PTH. *See* Parathyroid hormone
PTHrp (parathyroid hormone-related peptide), 609
Ptosis, 229, 230t
PTSD (posttraumatic stress disorder), 384–385, 386, 386t
PubMed, 59t
PUFAs (polyunsaturated fatty acids), 115, 118
Pugilistic dementia, 412
Pulmonary diseases, 439–446
chronic obstructive pulmonary disease (COPD), 91t, 385, 440–444
with developmental disabilities, 415
guidelines for risk assessment and perioperative management of, 129
and incontinence, 276t
Pulmonary embolism (PE), 445
recurrent thromboembolism, 446
Pulmonary fibrosis, idiopathic, 444–445
Pulmonary rehabilitation, 192, 442–443, 443t
Pulmonary system
age-related changes, 12t, 13–14, 17, 438
age-related pathologies, 16t

Pulmonary thromboembolism, recurrent, 446
Pulmonology, 438–447
Pulsed lavage, 292
Pulsed radiofrequency (PRF), 158
Pumpkin seed extracts, 117
Pupillary defects, afferent, 229
Purified-protein derivative (PPD) skin tests, 595–596
Pyelonephritis, 593
Pyrazinamide, 595
Pyridostigmine, 260
Pyridoxine, 636
Pyuria, 594

Q

Qi gong, 118
Quality Assurance and Performance Improvement (QAPI) programs, 205
Quality Improvement System for Managed Care (QISMC), 40
Quality Indicator Survey (QIS), 203
Quality of care
medical director responsibilities for, 200t, 203–205
nursing-home care, 202–205
requirements for long-term care facilities, 201t, 203–205
Quality of life
assessment of, 48
with cancer, 649–650
Quetiapine
for agitated delirium, 356t, 357
dosing and adverse events of, 390, 390t
for Parkinson disease and hallucinations, 392
for psychosis in dementia, 345, 345t, 346
to stabilize mood in mania and bipolar depression, 379t
Quinapril, 469t
Quinidine, 460, 470
Quinlan, Karen Ann, 23

R

Radiation therapy. *See also specific diseases and disorders*
for cancer, 649
external beam, 526t, 527
postoperative, after lumpectomy, 651
for prostate cancer, 526t, 527–528
Radiculopathy, 576
Radioactive iodine (RAI) therapy, 604, 605–606
Radioactive iodine uptake (RAIU) testing, 604
Radiofrequency treatment, pulsed (PRF), 158
Radiography, chest, 467
Raloxifene, 321t, 322
Ramelteon, 359, 369t, 370
Ramipril, 469t
Ramping technique, 444
Ramsay Hunt syndrome, 423
Randomized controlled trials (RCTs), 85

Ranibizumab, 234, 236
Ranitidine, 108t, 141t, 531
RANKL (receptor activator of nuclear factor kappa-B ligand), 315
RANKL inhibitor (denosumab), 321t, 323
Ranolazine, 455
Rapid Assessment of Physical Activity, 82
Rapid screening, 43, 44t
Rapidly progressive glomerulonephritis (RPGN), 506
Rasagiline, 572
Rate of living theory of aging, 8t, 10
Rational Recovery, 406
Raynaud phenomenon, 555, 556
RDAs (recommended dietary allowances), 262–263
RDIs (recommended dietary intakes), 262–263, 263t
Re-Engineered Discharge (Project RED), 176, 179t
REACH program, 334
Reality orientation, 332
Receptor activator of nuclear factor kappa-B ligand (RANKL), 315
Recombinant tissue-plasminogen activator (rt-PA) (alteplase), 582
Recommended dietary allowances (RDAs), 262–263
Recommended dietary intakes (RDIs), 262–263, 263t
"Recommended Treatment Strategies for Clinicians Managing Older Patients with HIV," 74
Recurrent caries, 429, 430
Red eye, 229, 230–232, 231t, 237t
RED (Re-Engineered Discharge) initiative, 176, 179t
5α-Reductase inhibitors, 520, 521–522, 521t
Reflex syncope, 259–260
Reflux, gastroesophageal, 484–486, 495
Refractive error, 232–233
Refusal of treatment, 21
Regular appointments, 332
Rehabilitation, 181–195
    adaptive methods for, 195
    for amputation, 191–192
    approaches and interventions, 186–187
    cardiac, 192, 453, 455, 468
    cognitive, 332
    comorbid conditions and, 185–186
    comprehensive assessment of, 187
    conceptual model for, 181
    coverage and services, 182–183
    environmental modifications for, 193, 195
    of gait disorders, 300
    goals of, 186, 187–188
    of hearing loss, 245, 245t
    after hip fracture, 190
    after joint replacement, 301
    low-vision, 238–239
    outcomes, 183–184
    postacute, 38–39
    prosthetic, 193
    pulmonary, 192, 442–443, 443t
    sites of care, 181–184, 182t
    for stroke, 187–189
    teams and roles, 184–185, 185t
    total hip arthroplasty, 191
    vestibular rehabilitation therapy (VRT), 253
Rehabilitation Engineering and Assistive Technology Society of North America Wheelchair Service Guide, 194
Rehabilitation hospitals, 182–183, 182t
Reiki, 118
Relafen (nabumetone), 153t
Relative exercise intensity, 78
Relaxation techniques
    for anxiety disorders, 387
    for menopausal symptoms, 117
    for sleep problems, 368t
Relaxation therapy, 116
Relaxation training, 386, 386t
Religious beliefs, 66, 67–68
Religious identity, 63
REM sleep behavior disorder (RBD), 365–366
Reminiscence therapy, 332, 347
Remitting seronegative symmetrical synovitis with pitting edema (RS3PE) syndrome, 550
Renal angiography, 503
Renal artery angioplasty, 503
Renal artery disease, 502–503
Renal artery occlusion, 505
Renal artery stenosis, 481, 502–503
Renal bone disease, 509
Renal care, nonaggressive, 511
Renal cell cancer, 648, 654–655
Renal replacement therapy, 510
Renal tubular acidosis (RTA)
    type II, 502
    type IV, 501, 502
Renin inhibitors, 471, 479
Renovascular disease, 502–503
Repaglinide, 626t
Reperfusion therapy, 452–453
Repetitive transcranial magnetic stimulation (rTMS), 380
Reset osmostat, 499–500
Resident Assessment Protocols, 269
Resistance training
    for preventing falls, 310t
    recommendations for, 78, 80t
Resource utilization group system (RUGS), 38
Respectful nonverbal communication, 64
Respiration, loud, 144–145
Respiratory depression, opioid-induced, 157
Respiratory diseases and disorders
    chronic lower respiratory disease, 6
    preoperative assessment and management of, 129
    pulmonary diseases, 439–446
Respiratory failure, 167–168
Respiratory symptoms and complaints, 438–439
Respiratory system. See Pulmonary system
Respite care, 213t, 334
Restless legs syndrome (RLS), 364–365, 575
Restraints, 347, 356
Resuscitation, 167–168
Retinal detachment, 230, 237t
Retinal tears, 230t
Retinopathy, diabetic, 231t, 235–236, 236f
Retropulsion, 297t
Revascularization
    for chronic CAD, 455
    for peripheral arterial disease, 464
Review of systems at hospital admission, 164, 165t
Revised Cardiac Risk Index, 127
Rheumatic mitral stenosis, 456
Rheumatoid arthritis (RA), 539, 543, 550–551
    CIM for, 115
    of feet, 567
Rheumatoid factor (RF), 550
Rheumatologic disease, 558
Rheumatology, 548–558
Rhinopyma, 418
Rhinosinusitis, 438–439
Rhythm abnormalities, 309
Riboflavin, 263t
Rifampin, 595
Rifaximin, 493
Rights-based approach, 20
Rigidity, 570
Riluzole, 577
Rimantadine, 592
Risedronate, 320, 321t, 322
Risk-Standardized-Readmission Rates (RSRR), 172
Risperidone
    for agitated delirium, 356t, 357
    for chorea, 574
    dosing and adverse events of, 390, 390t
    for psychosis in dementia, 345, 345t, 346
    to stabilize mood in mania and bipolar depression, 379t
Rituximab, 420, 551, 648–649
Rivaroxaban
    adverse drug events, 106, 106t
    Beers Criteria for, 108t
    recommended dosage, 461
    for stroke prevention, 460, 461
    for VTE, 446
Rivastigmine
    for dementia, 335–336
    for dementia with intellectual disability, 413
RLS (restless legs syndrome), 364–365, 575
Roflumilast, 442
Rollators, 193t, 194
Rolling assessment, 43
Romberg test, 299
Ropinirole
    for PD motor symptoms, 572

for periodic limb movement disorder, 365
for restless legs syndrome, 365, 575
Rosacea, 418–419, 418f
Rosalynn Carter Institute for Caregiving, 59t
Rosiglitazone, 626t, 627
Rosuvastatin, 454
Rotator cuff tendonopathies and tears, 540
Rotigotine transdermal patch, 572
Rowland test, 169, 169t
Roxanol (morphine, immediate release), 154t
Roxicodone (oxycodone, immediate release), 154t
Roxuolitinib, 641
RS3PE (remitting seronegative symmetrical synovitis with pitting edema) syndrome, 550
RSRR (Risk-Standardized-Readmission Rates), 172
rTMS (repetitive transcranial magnetic stimulation), 380
RUGS (resource utilization group system), 38
Runciman test, 169, 169t
Rye pollen, 117

S

S-adenosylmethionine (SAM-e), 114t
Saccular aneurysms, intracranial, 584
Sacral fractures, 543, 544t, 545t, 546
Sacral nerve neuromodulation, 281
Sacrocolpopexy, 517
Safe Return, 334
Safety, 97
    attention to, 334–335
    of CIM therapies, 113–114
    and dementia, 334–335
    of dietary supplements, 113–114, 114t
    preventing injury, 97
    in transitions, 175–176
Salicylates, 155, 265t
Saline
    hypertonic, 500
    isotonic, 500
Saline enemas, 490t
Saline laxatives, 489–490
Saliva, artificial, 556
Salivary function, 432
Salivary glands, 429, 430t
Salix alba (white willow bark), 115
Salmeterol, 442, 442t
Salsalate (Disalcid), 153t, 155
SAM-e (S-adenosylmethionine), 114t
SAMHSA (Substance Abuse and Mental Health Services Administration), 407
Saractinib, 322
Sarcoma, 516
Sarcopenia, 270, 438
    activity recommendations for, 80t
    definition of, 270
Sarcoptes scabiei var *hominis*, 425
Savella (milnacipran), 152t

Savvy Caregiver program, 334
Saw palmetto *(Serenoa repens)*
    for benign prostatic hyperplasia, 117, 522
    safety issues, 114t
Saxagliptin (Onglyza), 626t
Scabies, 425
Scheduled toileting, 354t
Schizoid personality disorder
    features of, 389, 395t
    long-term course, 396–397
    therapeutic strategies for, 398t
Schizophrenia and schizophrenia spectrum syndromes, 388–390
    clinical characteristics of, 389
    definition of, 388
    epidemiology of, 389
    late-onset schizophrenia, 388, 389
    negative symptoms, 388
    positive symptoms, 388
    treatment and management of, 389–390
Schizophrenia-like conditions, late-onset, 388
Schizophrenia-like psychosis
    diagnosis of, 388
    very-late-onset, 388
Schizotypal personality disorder
    differential diagnosis of, 396
    features of, 395t
    long-term course, 396–397
    therapeutic strategies for, 398t
Sciatica, 544t, 546
Scissoring, 297t
Scleritis, 230, 237t
Sclerostin antibody, 322
Scooters, motorized, 193t, 195
Scopolamine
    for bowel obstruction, 143t
    for nausea, 141t
Score Hospitalier d'Evaluation du Risque de Perte d'Autonomie (SHERPA), 169, 169t
Screening, 90–91
    for alcoholism, 405
    for cancer, 72–73, 85–90, 99, 646
    for cognitive assessment, 328, 329t
    criteria for recommending, 85
    for depression, 374–375
    ED risk-screening tools, 169, 169t
    for frailty, 225–226
    for glaucoma, 229
    for hearing loss, 243
    HIV, 532
    for hormone hypersecretion in adrenal incidentalomas, 613–614, 613t
    for mistreatment, 121, 122t
    nutrition, 95, 263–265
    oral cancer, 429
    for osteoporosis, 313, 317, 318t
    PHQ-9 questions, 374
    physical activity, 81
    for prostate cancer, 523–524
    rapid, 43, 44t
    recommendations for, 85, 88t, 99
    for risk of falls, 307
    in transgender older adults, 72–73

for urinary incontinence, 89t, 277, 282
for vitamin D deficiency, 267
Seborrheic dermatitis, 418, 418f
Seborrheic keratoses, 425, 426f
Section 8, Housing and Urban Development programs, 214
Sedating antidepressants, 369t, 370–371
Sedating antihistamines, 366, 371–372
Sedating antipsychotics, 371
Sedation, palliative, 25, 26
Sedative/hypnotics
    adverse drug events, 106, 106t
    chronic use, 371
    and incontinence, 275t
    for insomnia, 369t, 371
    interventions for preventing falls with, 310t
    for sleep problems, 367–368
Seizures, 568
    antiepileptic drugs for, 569–570, 569t
    with developmental disabilities, 415t, 416
    signs and symptoms of, 254, 255t
Selective estrogen-receptor modulators (SERMs), 321t, 322, 536
Selective norepinephrine-reuptake inhibitors (SNRIs)
    for anxiety disorders, 386, 386t
    for depression, 377t
    for depressive features of behavioral disturbances in dementia, 343t
    for vasomotor symptoms or hot flushes, 513
Selective serotonin-reuptake inhibitors (SSRIs)
    adverse drug events, 106, 106t, 265
    for alcohol abuse, 407
    for anxiety disorders, 382, 386, 386t
    for depression, 377, 377t
    for depression in CKD, 509
    for depressive features of behavioral disturbances in dementia, 342, 343t
    for postural hypotension, 260
    for vasomotor symptoms or hot flushes, 513
Selegiline, 572
Selenium, 116, 263t
Self-care, 46, 46t
Self-care difficulty, 5
Self-injurious behavior, 412, 414
Self-neglect, 122t, 123, 384
Self-prayer, 112, 113t
"Senile" gait disorder, 297
Senile squalor syndrome, 384
Senior Adult guidelines (NCCN), 645
Senior cohousing, 213
Senior health clinics (SHCs), 219
Senior villages and cohousing, 213
Senna (Senokot), 490t, 491t
Sensorineural hearing loss, 241, 242f
Sensory deprivation, 354t

Sensory impairment
    with developmental disabilities, 415t
    hearing loss, 240–248
    in hospitalized patients, 165t, 166
    interventions for, 165t
    and rehabilitation, 186
    smell dysfunction, 435, 436t, 571
    taste dysfunction, 435, 436t
    vision loss, 229–239
Sepsis, 591
Sequenced Treatment Alternatives to Relieve Depression (STAR*D), 374, 375t
Serenoa repens (saw palmetto)
    for benign prostatic hyperplasia, 117, 522
    safety issues, 114t
Serotonin antagonists, 141t
Serotonin syndrome, 377, 377t
Sertraline, 342, 343t, 377–378, 377t
    for anxiety disorders, 382
    for depression in CKD, 509
Serum alkaline phosphatase (SAP), 609, 610
Sex hormone-binding globulin (SHBG), 611t, 615
Sex therapy, 533t, 534
Sexual activity, 95, 530
Sexual behavior, inappropriate, 347
Sexual desire disorders, 535, 536–537
Sexual dysfunction
    counseling for, 89t, 95
    in older men, 530–534, 531t
    in older women, 530, 535, 536t
Sexual health of LGBT older adults, 73
Sexual orientation, 71
Sexual risk
    in older gay and bisexual men, 73
    in older lesbian and bisexual women, 73
Sexuality, 530–537
    female, 534–537
    male, 530–534
Sexually transmitted infections (STIs), 95
    barriers to optimal prevention and detection of, 73
    prevention of, 73
SF-36 (Short Form-36 Health Survey), 48, 187
SGLT2 (sodium glucose co-transporter 2) inhibitors, 626t, 627
Shared decision-making, 21
Shared Savings Program (Medicare), 27
Sharp debridement, 292
Sheltered housing, 214
Shenkui, 399
SHERPA (Score Hospitalier d'Evaluation du Risque de Perte d'Autonomie), 169, 169t
Shingles (herpes zoster), 232, 237t, 423–424, 424f
    vaccine against, 88t, 97, 586, 590–591, 590t
Shoe terms, 564t
Shoes, 309, 310t, 564

Short Form-36 Health Survey (SF-36), 48, 187
Shoulder pain, 539–540
SIADH (syndrome of inappropriate antidiuretic hormone), 377, 499–500
Sick sinus syndrome, 449, 459, 463
Sideroblastic anemia, 635–636
Sight problems. *See* Visual loss
Sigmoidoscopy, 86
Sildenafil, 444
    for dysphagia, 484
    for erectile dysfunction, 532, 533, 533t
    for heart failure, 471, 471t
Silodosin, 521, 521t
Simplified Nutrition Assessment Questionnaire, 265
Sinusitis, 438–439
Sipuleucel-T, 654
Sitagliptin (Januvia), 626t
Sitaxsentan, 471, 471t
Sites of care, 177
Sitz marker study, 489
6-minute walk test, 299–300
Sjögren syndrome, 432, 555–556
Skeletal system
    age-related changes, 12t
    age-related pathologies, 15–16, 16t
Skilled nursing facilities (SNFs), 31t, 182t, 184
Skin
    age-related changes, 12t, 13, 417
    age-related pathologies, 16t
Skin assessment, 289
Skin lesions, 565
Skin problems
    autoimmune conditions, 418–422
    benign growths, 425–426
    cancer, 89, 91t, 417, 426–428
    dermatology, 417–428
    on foot, 559, 565
    infections, 423–425, 589t
    infestations, 423–425
    inflammatory conditions, 418–422
    moisture-associated skin damage (MASD), 289, 289f
SLE (systemic lupus erythematosus), 554–555
Sleep attacks, 572
Sleep hygiene, 354t, 358–359
Sleep issues, 361–372
    age-related changes, 361–362, 362t
    causes of nocturia, 277t
    central sleep apnea, 363–364, 366–367
    CIM for, 117
    circadian rhythm disorders, 365, 371
    in dementia, 346–347, 366
    epidemiology of, 361
    evaluation of, 362
    in hospitalized patients, 162, 165t, 366–367
    interventions for, 165t
    management of, 367–372
    measures to improve sleep hygiene, 367, 367t

    nonpharmacologic interventions for, 368, 368t
    in nursing home, 367
    obstructive sleep apnea (OSA), 276t, 363, 364, 366, 444
    periodic limb movements, 364–365
    recommendations for, 372
    sleep apnea, 363–364, 366–367
    treatment of, 346–347
Sleep-related breathing disorders, 363–364
Sleep restriction, 368t
Sleeping medications, 366, 371–372
Slings, 281
SLUMS (St. Louis University Mental Status) examination, 22, 44t, 45, 328, 329t
Small molecular inhibitors, 648
Smell dysfunction
    age-related changes, 435
    assessment of, 571
    medications that cause, 435, 436t
    nonpharmacologic causes of, 435, 436t
Smoking, 5, 405
Smoking cessation, 406
    and cardiovascular risk, 451
    for COPD, 440–441, 443t
    for diabetes mellitus, 624
    "Five A's" method, 407, 440–441
    for peripheral arterial disease, 464
    to reduce risk of osteoporosis, 316, 316t
Smoking cessation counseling, 93–95
    recommendations for, 89t
Snellen charts, 44
SNRIs. *See* Selective norepinephrine-reuptake inhibitors
Social anxiety disorder (social phobia), 383–384, 386t
Social assessment, 46
Social conditions, 414–416
Social history, 164, 165t
Social phobia (social anxiety disorder), 383–384
Social Services Block Grant programs, 214
Social support, 71, 71t, 75
Social workers, 184, 185t, 337
Socially detached personality, 389
Sodium, 499
    fractional excretion of sodium (FE_{Na}), 503–504
Sodium balance disorders, 501
Sodium conservation, 498t
Sodium excretion, 498t
Sodium glucose co-transporter 2 (SGLT2) inhibitors, 626t, 627
Sodium polystyrene (Kayexalate), 502
Sodium restriction, 473, 478
Soft-tissue augmentation, 417
Soft-tissue infections, 589t
Solifenacin, 280, 281
Somatic delusions, 376, 391
Somatic pain (pain disorder), 149–150, 149t, 398
Somatic symptom and related disorders, 394, 398–400

clinical characteristics and causes of, 399–400
prevalence of, 399
treatment of, 400
Somatization disorder, 398
Somatoform disorders, undifferentiated, 398
Sorafenib, 648
Sorbitol 70%, 491t
Sotalol, 460
Soy products, 117
Spasticity, 298
SPECIAL mnemonic for palliative care of wounds, 293–294, 293t
Special needs, 41
Special needs plans, 32
Specialty care, geriatric, 219–220
Speech, 241, 242f
Speech therapy, 31t
rehabilitation team role, 183, 185t
Spinal cord dysfunction, 577–578
Spinal cord injury, 276t
Spinal deformities, 415t
Spinal manipulation, 115
Spinal stenosis, 276t
cervical, 539
Spine osteoarthritis, 548
Spirituality, 62, 66, 67–68, 137
Spironolactone
Beers Criteria for, 108t
for heart failure, 469, 471, 471t
Squamous cell carcinoma, 427
oral, 432–433
oropharyngeal, 432–433
of vulva, 515, 516
Squamous hyperplasia, 515
src kinase inhibitors, 322
SSRIs. *See* Selective serotonin-reuptake inhibitors
St. John's wort *(Hypericum perforatum),* 116
for depression, 116
safety issues, 114t
St. Louis University Mental Status (SLUMS) examination, 22, 44t, 45, 328, 329t
St. Thomas's Risk Assessment Tool (STRATIFY), 307
Stabilization, 406
Staffing patterns, 198–201
Staphylococcus aureus, 458
methicillin-resistant (MRSA), 587, 592
STAR*D (Sequenced Treatment Alternatives to Relieve Depression), 374, 375t
Stasis dermatitis, 417, 422
State Veterans Homes, 196
Statin therapy
for acute coronary syndrome, 453
for chronic CAD, 454
perioperative, 128, 130t
recommendations for, 92
for stroke prevention, 583
toxicity, 556
Stem cell/progenitor cell theory of aging, 8t, 11
Stem cells, hematopoietic, 629

Stenson's papillae, 434
Stenting, 481, 503
for BPH, 521t, 522
carotid artery angioplasty and, 583
coronary stents, 129
Steppage gait, 297t, 298t
Stimulant laxatives, 489–490, 490t
Stimulus control, 368t, 369–370
Stinging nettle, 117
STIs (sexually transmitted infections), 95
Stomach disorders, 486–487
Stomatitis, denture, 434, 434f
Stool softeners, 489–490
STRATIFY (St. Thomas's Risk Assessment Tool), 307
Strength training, 308, 308t, 309, 310t
Streptococcus pneumoniae, 458
Streptomycin, 595
Stress incontinence, 274
behavioral therapies for, 279, 280
and impaired urethral sphincter support, 276
management of, 279
minimally invasive procedures for, 281
surgery for, 281–282
Stress management, 118
Stress-reduction techniques, 478
Stress testing, preoperative, 127–128
Stroke
approach to management of, 188–189
cardioembolic, 581
cryptogenic, 581, 583–584
family caregiver interventions, 56, 57t
fatality rate, 580
goals of rehabilitation after, 187–188
guidelines for rehabilitation after, 188–189
hemorrhagic, 584–585
incidence of, 580
and incontinence, 276t
ischemic, 580, 582–584
NIH Stroke Scale, 189, 581, 581t
in nursing-home population, 196
prevention of, 460–461, 582–584
rehabilitation after, 187–189
risk factors for, 582–583
Stroke Impact Scale, 184t, 187
Strontium ranelate, 324
Subarachnoid hemorrhage, 584–585
Subclinical depression, 376
Subclinical hyperthyroidism, 604
Subclinical hypothyroidism, 602
Subconjunctival hemorrhage, 230–232, 237t
Subdural hematoma, 584, 585
Subluxation, foot, 564t
Suboptimal care transitions, 174–175
Substance abuse
counseling interventions for, 89t
in LGBT older adults, 74–75
in transgender adults, 74

Substance Abuse and Mental Health Services Administration (SAMHSA), 407
Substance-induced psychotic disorders, 392
Substance use disorders
brief interventions for, 407
definition of, 402–403
diagnostic criteria for, 402
epidemiology of, 404
identifying disorders, 405
magnitude of the problem, 403–404
outpatient management of, 406–407
pharmacotherapy for, 407
risks and benefits of, 404–405
treatment of, 405–407
Subsyndromal depression, 376
Suicidal depression, 376
Suicide
in LGBT older adults, 74
physician-assisted, 25
in transgender adults, 74
Sulfasalazine, 550
Sulfonylureas, 626, 626t, 627
Sumatriptan, 578–579
Sunitinib, 648
Sunscreens, 417
Superficial basal cell carcinoma, 426
Superficial spreading melanoma, 427
Supplemental Poverty Measure (SPM), 4
Supplemental Security Income (SSI), 214
Supplements, 267
for pressure ulcers, 292
safety issues, 113–114, 114t
Supplies, 31t
Support surfaces, 287–288
Supraventricular arrhythmias, 458, 461–462
Supraventricular tachycardia, 458, 461–462
Surgical aortic valve replacement (SAVR), 448, 456–458
Surgical care. *See also specific diseases and disorders; specific procedures*
bypass surgery, 455
cardiac risk assessment for, 127, 128f
cosmetic, 417
decompressive, 578
dental, 437, 595
iatrogenic complications, 131
pelvic reconstruction, 517
perioperative care, 126–135
postoperative cognitive dysfunction (POCD), 353
postoperative delirium, 133–134, 353, 358t, 359
postoperative management, 131–134
preoperative assessment and management, 126–131
total hip and knee arthroplasty, 190
transsphenoidal, 612
Surgical co-management, 171
Surgical decision making, 126

Surrogate decision-making, 23
  documents to help with, 24, 24t
  state hierarchies of surrogates, 23, 23t
Surveillance, 525
  active, 525, 526t
Suspiciousness, isolated, 391
Susto, 399
Suvorexant, 370
Swallowing, 270–272
Swinging flashlight test, 229
Symphytom officinale L. (comfrey root extract), 115
Syncope, 254–261
  cardiac, 255t
  causes of, 254, 255t
  diagnosis of, 254
  diagnostic evaluation of, 257–258, 257t
  evaluation of, 256–259
  history in, 256
  hospital admission for, 259
  indications for permanent pacemaker implantation, 462–463, 463t
  medical management of, 260
  natural history of, 254
  pathophysiology of, 255–256
  physical examination of, 256–257
  predictors of, 256, 256t
  prognosis for, 254
  recommendations for, 260
  reflex, 259–260
  risk factors for adverse prognosis in, 259, 259t
  signs and symptoms of, 254, 255t
  treatment of, 259–260
  vasovagal, 254, 255t
Syndrome of inappropriate antidiuretic hormone (SIADH), 377, 499–500
Synthetic somatostatin analogues, 141t
Syphilis, 597–598
Systematic assessment, 164, 165t
Systemic lupus erythematosus (SLE), 554–555
Systems review, 164, 165t
Systolic heart failure, 466

T

T-score, 313, 317, 318
T_3. *See* Triiodothyronine
T_4. *See* Thyroxine
Tachy-brady syndrome, 463
Tachycardia
  atrial, 461–462
  AV-nodal reentrant, 461–462
  supraventricular, 461–462
Tadalafil, 521t, 522, 532, 533, 533t
Tai Chi
  for frailty, 227
  for pain, 151
  for preventing falls, 81, 308, 308t, 310t
  recommendations for, 80t, 93
Tailor's bunion, 561t
Tamoxifen, 107, 107t, 648, 651
Tamsulosin, 521, 521t
Tapentadol (Nucynta), 154t, 158, 576

Tapentadol extended release (Nucynta ER), 154t
Tardive dyskinesia (TD), 389–390, 570, 574
Tardive dystonia, 574
Target theory of genetic damage, 8t, 9
Tarsal tunnel syndrome, 561t
Task Force on Community Preventive Services, 82
Task-specific training, 300
Taste dysfunction
  age-related changes, 435
  medications that cause, 435, 436t
  nonpharmacologic causes of, 435, 436t
Td/Tdap (tetanus, diphtheria, acellular pertussis) vaccine, 97, 590t, 591
TDM-1 (ado-trastuzumab emtansine), 649
Teach-back method, 63–64
Teams
  patient-aligned care teams (GERI-PACT), 52
  rehabilitation teams, 184–185, 185t
Technology, in-home, 212–213
TEE (transesophageal echocardiography), 458, 595
Teeth
  age-related changes in, 429, 430t
  anatomy of, 429, 430f
Tegretol (carbamazepine), 152t
Telangiectasias, 494
Telecoil, 246
Telemedicine, 213
Telephone quit lines, 89t
Telmisartan, 469t
Telomere theory of aging, 8t, 9
Telomeres, 643
Temazepam, 369t, 370
Temporal arteritis, 578
Temporal lobe epilepsy, 394
Tender points, 149
Tennis elbow, 540, 541
Tenosynovitis, 564t
TENS (transcutaneous electrical nerve stimulation), 114
Terazosin, 521, 521t
Teriparatide (parathyroid hormone), 321t, 323
Terminal illness
  anorexia in, 142–143
  bowel obstruction in, 142
  cachexia in, 142–143
  constipation in, 140–141
  cough in, 144
  delirium in, 143
  depression in, 145
  diarrhea in, 142
  dyspnea in, 143–144
  nausea and vomiting in, 141
  palliative care, 141–146
Terminology
  glossary of gait abnormalities, 297t
  preferred terms for cultural or religious identity, 63
  shoe terms, 564t
  terms used in care of patients in pain, 147–148, 148t

  terms used to describe older adults who need a geriatric approach to care, 49t
Testosterone, 611t, 615–617
Testosterone replacement therapy, 615, 616–617
Testosterone supplementation, 615
  available preparations, 617, 617t
  benefits and risks, 601, 616, 616t
  for erectile dysfunction, 534
  for hypoactive sexual desire disorder, 536–537
  for older women, 617
TET2 gene, 636
Tetanus: vaccine against, 88t
Tetanus, diphtheria, acellular pertussis (Td/Tdap) vaccine, 97, 590t, 591
Tetrabenazine, 574
Thalassemia, 635–636
Thalassemia trait, 635–636
Thalidomide, 495
Theophylline
  adverse drug events, 265
  for COPD, 442, 443t
  drug interactions, 107, 107t, 588
  for refractory COPD, 442
Theories of aging, 7–11
Therapeutic touch, 118
Thiamine, 263t
Thiamine supplements, 469
Thiazide, 469
Thiazide diuretics, 478, 478t, 499
Thiazolidinediones
  for diabetes mellitus, 626–627, 626t
  and incontinence, 275t
Thigh pain, 541–542
Thinking problems. *See* Cognitive impairment
32P, 640–641
Thought disorder, 388
3D-CAM, 350t
Thrombectomy, endovascular, 582
Thrombocythemia, essential (ET), 629, 640, 641
Thrombocytopenia, 638–639
Thromboembolism, venous (VTE), 128, 130t, 445–446
Thrombopathy, 664
Thromboprophylaxis
  guidelines for, 128, 130t, 167
  in hospitalized patients, 165t, 167
Thrombotic microangiopathy, 505
Thrombotic thrombocytopenic purpura (TTP), 505
Thrombotic thrombocytopenic purpura-hemolytic uremic syndrome (TTP-HUS), 637, 639
Thrush, 434, 434f
Thyroid disorders, 601–606
  cancer, 90, 91t, 605–606
  with developmental disabilities, 415t
  nodular thyroid disease, 605–606
  screening for, 90
  toxic nodular thyroid disease, 604
Thyroid hormone replacement, 603
  and risk of osteoporosis, 316, 316t

Thyroid hormone requirements, 603
Thyroid scans, 604
Thyroid-stimulating hormone (thyrotropin), 90, 601
    age-related changes in, 611t
    screening test, 88t
Thyroid ultrasonography, 605, 605t
Thyrotoxic myopathy, 577
Thyrotoxicosis
    apathetic, 603
    triiodothyronine (T_3), 603–604
Thyrotropin (thyroid-stimulating hormone), 90, 601
    age-related changes in, 611t
    screening test, 88t
Thyrotropin-releasing hormone (TRH), 610
Thyroxine (T_4), 601
    age-related changes in, 611t
    free T_4 test, 603
    high T_4 syndrome, 604
    low T_4 syndrome, 602–603
Thyroxine (T_4) replacement therapy, 603
Thyroxine (T_4) suppplementation, 602
Tibialis posterior dysfunction, 561t, 563, 563f
Ticagrelor, 452, 639
Tilt-table testing, 257t, 258
Timed Up and Go (TUG) test, 44t, 46, 95, 300
Timolol, 238t
Tinel test, 541
Tinnitus, 241
Tiotropium bromide, 441–442, 442t, 443t
Tirofiban, 639
Tissue plasminogen activator (tPA), recombinant (rt-PA) (alteplase), 582
Tizanidine, 579
TMP (trimethoprim), 265t, 501, 501t
TMP-SMX (trimethoprim-sulfamethoxazole)
    drug interactions, 107, 107t
    for UTIs, 593
α-Tocopherol (vitamin E)
    for dementia, 116–117, 336
    RDIs for adults ≥71 years old, 263t
Tofacitinib, 551
Toileting, scheduled, 354t
Tolerance, 156
Tolterodine, 280, 281
Tolvaptan, 499
Tongue, black hairy, 435, 435f
Toothlessness, 431–432
Topiramate, 408t
    for essential tremor, 575
    for migraine, 579
Torus (tori), 433–434, 434f
Total body preoperative exercise, 301
Total body water, 500
Total hip and knee arthroplasty, 190–191, 549
    cause and surgical care of, 190
    management of, 190–191
    rehabilitation after, 191
Toxic encephalopathy, 349
Toxic multinodular goiter, 603
Toxic myopathy, 577

Toxic nodular thyroid disease, 604
Toxicity
    chemotherapy, 646–647, 647t
    statin therapy, 556
Tradition, 65
Traditional Chinese medicine, 112
Traditional Native American medicine, 113
Tramadol (Ultram), 154t, 158
    Beers Criteria for, 108t
    for fibromyalgia, 558
    for neuropathic pain, 576
    for OA-related pain, 549
Trametinib, 428
Trandolapril, 469t
Transcatheter aortic valve replacement (TAVR), 448, 456–458
Transcranial magnetic stimulation, repetitive (rTMS), 380
Transcutaneous electrical nerve stimulation (TENS), 114
Transdermal fentanyl (Duragesic), 154t
Transdermal lidocaine patch, 151, 576
Transdermal rotigotine patch, 572
Transesophageal echocardiography (TEE), 458, 595
Transfer dysphagia, 483
Transfer skills impairment, 310t
Transfers, 174
Transgender adults, 70
    medical needs of, 72–73
    mental health issues, 74
    sexual risk, 73
Transient ischemic attack (TIA), 582
Transient secondary hypothyroidism, 603
Transitional Care Model, 176, 179t
Transitions of care, 174–180, 174f
    barriers to safety, 175–176
    communication for, 178
    discharge destinations, 177
    policy approaches, 177
    questions to assist with, 178
    steps to improve, 178–180
    strategies for, 176–177, 179t
    suboptimal, 174–175
    target measures for improvement, 180
    venues of care, 177
Transplantation
    fecal microbiota (FMT), 599
    heart, 471–472
    kidney, 510–511
    lung, 444–445
Transposable element activation theory of aging, 8t, 9
Transsphenoidal surgery, 612
Transurethral incision of the prostate (TUIP), 521t, 522
Transurethral resection of the prostate (TURP), 521t, 522
Transurethral vaporization of prostate, 521t, 522
Trastuzumab, 648–649
Trauma
    history of traumatic experiences, 64
    posttraumatic stress disorder (PTSD), 384–385, 386, 386t

Traumatic brain injury (TBI), 612
Trazodone
    adverse drug events, 106, 106t
    for depressive features of behavioral disturbances in dementia, 343t
    for insomnia, 337, 369t, 370
    for sleep disturbances in dementia, 346–347
Treatment decisions. *See also* Decision making
    ETHNICS mnemonic, 67
Tremors, 570
    action tremor, 574
    essential tremor (ET), 574–575
Trendelenburg gait, 297–298, 297t, 298t
Trends, 2–6
Tretinoin, 419
TRH (thyrotropin-releasing hormone), 610
Triage Risk Stratification Tool (TRST), 169, 169t
Triamcinolone, 515
Triamterene, 106, 106t
    Beers Criteria for, 108t
    and hyperkalemia, 501, 501t
Tricyclic antidepressants (TCAs)
    adverse drug events, 106, 106t, 344
    and delirium, 355t
    for depression, 377t
    for depressive features of behavioral disturbances in dementia, 343, 343t
    for headaches, 579
    and incontinence, 275t
    for insomnia, 370–371
    for migraine, 579
    for neuropathic pain, 576
    for persistent pain, 152t, 157
Trigger finger, 541
Trigger point injections, 158
Trigger points, 149
Triggering receptor expressed on myeloid cells 2 gene *(TREM2)*, 327
Trihexyphenidyl, 574
Triiodothyronine (T_3), 601
    age-related changes in, 611t
    free T_3 test, 603
    low T_3 syndrome, 602–603
Triiodothyronine (T_3) thyrotoxicosis, 603–604
Trimethoprim (TMP), 265t, 501, 501t
Trimethoprim-sulfamethoxazole (TMP-SMX)
    drug interactions, 107, 107t
    for UTIs, 593
Triptans, 578–579
Trochanteric bursitis, 541, 542
Trospium, 280
TRST (Triage Risk Stratification Tool), 169, 169t
Truth telling, 22–23
TTP (thrombotic thrombocytopenic purpura), 505
TTP-HUS (thrombotic thrombocytopenic purpura-hemolytic uremic syndrome), 637, 639
Tube feeding, 272–273

Tuberculin skin test (TST), 594–595
Tuberculosis (TB), 594–595
Tubular necrosis, acute (ATN), 504–505
Tubulointerstitial disease, 504–505
TUG (Timed Up and Go) test, 44t, 46, 300
TUIP (transurethral incision of the prostate), 521t, 522
Tumor, regional node, metastasis (TNM) staging system, 524–525, 524t
Tumors
    back pain due to, 543, 544, 544t, 545t
    ocular surface, 230
Turn en bloc, 297t
TURP (transurethral resection of the prostate), 521t, 522
Tylenol (acetaminophen), 152t
Tylox (oxycodone, immediate release), 154t

U

uHear (Unitron), 243
Ulcers, 422–423
    aphthous ulcers, 434–435, 435f
    arterial ulcers, 422–423, 423t
    chronic leg ulcers, 417, 422
    corneal, 230, 232, 237t
    foot ulcers, 566–567
    NSAID-induced, 487
    peptic ulcer disease, 487–488
    pressure ulcers, 282–293, 423, 423t
    venous ulcers, 422–423, 423t
Ulnar neuropathy, 541
Ultram (tramadol), 154t
Ultrasound
    abdominal, 88t
    carotid, 451
    thyroid, 605, 605t
Umeclidinium, 441–442, 442t
Undernutrition, 266, 267–268
Underprescribing, 105, 105t
Underweight, 451
United Network for Organ Sharing (UNOS), 510–511
United States
    aging trends and demographics, 2–6
    geographic distribution of older adults, 4
    life expectancy, 3, 3t
University of Pennsylvania Smell Identification Test (UPSIT), 571
Unspoken challenges, 65
Unstable lumbar spine, 544t, 545t
Ureteral obstruction, 504
Urethral mucosal atrophy, 513–514
Urethral sphincter support, impaired, 276
Urge incontinence, 274
    behavioral therapies for, 279, 280
    with detrusor overactivity (uninhibited bladder contractions), 276
    medications for, 280–281
    minimally invasive procedures for, 281
Urgencies, hypertensive, 480
Urinary catheter use, 163–164
Urinary incontinence (UI), 274–283
    assessment of, 282
    behavioral therapies for, 279–280, 282
    CIM for, 117
    comorbid conditions that can cause or worsen, 275, 276t
    with developmental disabilities, 415t
    evaluation of, 277–278
    functional, 274
    history in, 277–278
    with impaired bladder emptying, 277
    from incomplete emptying, 274
    lower urinary tract pathophysiology in, 276–277
    management of, 279–282
    medications that can cause or worsen, 275, 275t
    minimally invasive procedures for, 281
    mixed UI, 274, 277
    in nursing-home residents, 282
    pathophysiology of, 275–277
    physical examination with, 278
    prevalence and impact of, 274
    prevention of, 96
    recommendations for, 283
    red flag symptoms, 277
    risk factors for, 275
    screening for, 89t, 277, 282
    stress UI, 274, 276
    supportive care for, 282
    surgery for, 281–282
    testing for, 278
    transient, 274
    treatment of, 279–282
    types of, 274
    urge UI, 274, 276
Urinary protein excretion: measures of, 497–498
Urinary retention, acute (AUR), 522
Urinary system
    age-related changes, 12t, 14–15
    age-related pathologies, 16t
Urinary tract infections (UTIs), 593–594
    antibiotic prophylaxis of, 594
    antibiotic therapy for, 593, 594
    catheter-associated (CAUTIs), 163–164
    guidelines for diagnosis of, 589t, 594
    in long-term care residents, 593–594
    in men, 593
    surveillance definition of, 589t
    in women, 593
Urinary tract obstruction, 504
Urine dipsticks, 497–498
Urodynamic testing, 278
Urogenital atrophy, 512, 513–514, 514f
U.S. Department of Agriculture (USDA), 262, 268
U.S. Department of Health and Human Services (HHS), 79
U.S. Preventive Services Task Force (USPSTF), 81, 83, 85, 90
    indications for osteoporosis screening, 317, 318t
    recommendations for BMD testing, 317–318
    recommendations for cancer screening, 87, 90
    recommendations for depression screening, 96
    recommendations for hepatitis C screening, 597
    recommendations for HIV screening, 532
    recommendations for lung cancer screening, 90
    recommendations for prostate cancer screening, 523
    recommendations for screening for STIs, 95
    recommendations to promote sustained weight loss, 93
    tests not recommended for screening asymptomatic older adults, 91t, 93
USPSTF. See U.S. Preventive Services Task Force
Uterine prolapse, 516, 516f
Utilitarianism/consequentialism, 20
Uveitis, 230, 237t

V

Vaccinations, 586
    herpes zoster, 88t, 97, 586, 590–591, 590t
    for hospitalized patients, 165t, 166–167
    immunization schedule for adults ≥65 years old, 590t
    influenza, 5, 88t, 97, 166, 589, 590t, 592
    in nursing-home care, 207
    pneumococcal, 5, 88t, 97, 165t, 166–167, 589–590, 592
    tetanus, 88t
    tetanus, diphtheria, acellular pertussis (Td/Tdap), 97, 590t, 591
    zoster, 424
Vacuum tumescence devices, 533–534, 533t
Vaginal atrophy, 535, 536
Vaginal bleeding, 512
Vaginal bleeding, postmenopausal, 518, 518t
Vaginal dryness, 117
Vaginal prolapse, 516, 516f
    classification of, 516
    surgery for, 517
Valacyclovir, 424
Valerian, 371
Valerian root, 117
Valgus position, 561t
Validation therapy, 347
Valproic acid (valproate, divalproex), 337, 569, 579

Valsartan, 469t
Values, 18, 19t
Valve-associated anemia, 637
Valvular heart disease, 456
    clinical features and treatment of, 457t
    diagnosis of, 456
    epidemiology of, 456
    recommendations for, 465
Vancomycin, 504, 597
    for *C difficile* infection, 599
    for CNS infection, 597
    for pneumonia, 592
Vancomycin-resistant enterococci (VRE), 587
Vardenafil, 532, 533, 533t
Varenicline, 407, 408t
Varicella zoster virus (VZV), 423
Varicella-zoster virus (VZV) vaccine, 586, 590–591
    immunization schedule for adults ≥65 years old, 590t
    recommendations for, 88t, 90
Varus position, 561t
Vascular dementia
    diagnostic features and treatment of, 330t
    differential diagnosis of, 329, 330–331
    epidemiology of, 326
    gait abnormalities, 298t
Vascular disease
    arteriovascular disease, 276t
    cardiovascular disease, 448–465
    cerebrovascular disease, 6, 276t
    in kidneys, 505
    peripheral vascular disease, 186
    renovascular disease, 502–503
Vascular ectasia, 494
Vascular endothelial growth factor (VEGF) inhibitors, 234, 235–236, 648, 655
Vascular insufficiency, 541
Vascular parkinsonism, 573
Vasculature
    age-related changes, 12t, 13
    age-related pathologies, 16t
Vasculitis, ANCA-associated, 506
Vasodilators, 479
Vasomotor symptoms, 513
Vasopressin (DDAVP), 281
Vasovagal syncope, 254, 255t
VDRL (Venereal Disease Research Laboratory) test, 598
VEGF (vascular endothelial growth factor) inhibitors, 234, 235–236, 648, 655
Vemurafenib, 428
Venereal Disease Research Laboratory (VDRL) test, 598
Venlafaxine (Effexor)
    for anxiety disorders, 386
    for depression, 377, 377t
    for depressive features of behavioral disturbances in dementia, 343, 343t
    for persistent pain, 152t, 157
Venous insufficiency, 417
Venous thromboembolic disease (VTED), 445–446
Venous thromboembolism (VTE), 445–446
Venous thrombosis prophylaxis
    guidelines for, 128, 130t
    in hospitalized patients, 165t, 167
Venous ulcers, 422–423, 423t
Ventilation/perfusion scans, 445
Ventricular arrhythmias, 458, 462
Venues for care, 177
Verapamil, 453, 470
    adverse drug events, 106, 106t
    adverse effects of, 454–455
    for atrial fibrillation, 459
    drug interactions, 107, 107t
    for migraine, 579
Verbal Descriptor Scale, 149
Vertebral compression fractures, 324, 538, 543, 544t, 545t, 546
Vertebral fracture assessment (VFA), 318–319
Vertebral fracture management, 324
Vertebroplasty, 324, 546
Vertigo, 249, 250t
    benign paroxysmal positional vertigo (BPPV), 249, 252, 252f, 253
VES-13 (Vulnerable Elders Survey-13), 220
Vestibular disorders, 298t
Vestibular rehabilitation therapy (VRT), 253
Veterans Administration (VA)
    Community Living Centers, 197
    GERI-PACT (patient-aligned care teams) model, 52
    medical benefits, 35, 76
    Program at Home, 212
    State Veterans Homes, 196
    Surgical Quality Improvement Program, 129
Veterans Affairs, Department of
    guidelines for rehabilitation after stroke, 188–189
    hearing aid benefits, 247
Vicodin (hydrocodone), 153t
Vicoprofen (hydrocodone), 153t
Videofluoroscopic deglutition examination (VDE), 270, 271–272
Vilazodone, 343t
Vinorelbine, 647, 647t
Viral conjunctivitis, 230–232, 237t
Virtual home visits, 213
Virtual reality, 188
Visceral pain, 149–150, 149t
    referred, 544, 544t, 545t
Vision services, 31t
Vision testing, 89t, 96, 229
Visual hallucinations, 238, 390, 392
Visual imagery, 387
Visual loss, 229–239
    assessment of, 44
    definition of, 229
    gait abnormalities, 298t
    interventions for preventing falls, 309, 310t
    low-vision rehabilitation, 238–239
    rapid screening followed by assessment and management of, 43, 44t
    screening for, 89t, 96
    signs and symptoms requiring immediate referral, 230, 237t
    sudden decrease in vision, 230, 237t
    symptoms and treatment of common eye diseases, 231t
    trends in, 5
Vitamin A
    for dementia, 116
    drug interactions, 265t
    RDIs for adults ≥71 years old, 263t
Vitamin B_1, 265t
Vitamin B_2, 265t
Vitamin B_6
    drug interactions, 265t
    RDIs for adults ≥71 years old, 263t
Vitamin B_6 supplements, 266
Vitamin B_{12}
    drug interactions, 265t
    RDIs for adults ≥71 years old, 263t
Vitamin B_{12} deficiency, 635, 638
    hypoproliferative anemia due to, 633f, 635
    and incontinence, 276t
Vitamin B_{12} supplements, 266, 638
Vitamin C
    for AMD, 234
    for dementia, 116
    RDIs for adults ≥71 years old, 263t
Vitamin D
    dietary sources, 320
    drug interactions, 265t
    preventive, 89t, 98
    RDIs for adults, 320
    RDIs for adults ≥71 years old, 263t, 267
    RDIs for older adults, 606–607
Vitamin D deficiency, 315, 601, 606–607, 608
    in hospitalized patients, 162
    screening for, 93, 267
Vitamin D supplements, 267
    for CKD-related bone disease, 509
    for hyperparathyroidism, 608
    for osteoporosis, 319, 320
    for preventing falls, 308, 308t, 309, 311
    recommendations for, 607
Vitamin D_3 (cholecalciferol) supplements
    for hyperparathyroidism, 608
    recommendations for, 607
    to reduce risk of osteoporosis, 316, 316t
Vitamin E (α-tocopherol)
    for ARMD, 234
    for dementia, 116–117, 336
    drug interactions, 265t
    for vasomotor symptoms, 513
Vitamin K
    drug interactions, 265t
    for intracerebral hemorrhage, 584
    RDIs for adults ≥71 years old, 263t

Vitamin therapy
    for ARMD, 234
    multivitamin supplements, 89t, 98
Volume depletion, 499
Volume overload, 499
Vomiting. *See* Nausea and vomiting
von Willebrand disease (vWD), 639
Vortioxetine, 343t, 377t
Vulnerability, 222
Vulnerable Elders Survey-13 (VES-13), 220
Vulvar disorders, 514–516
    cancer, 512, 516
    excoriation, 515
    melanoma, 516, 516f
    neoplasia, 515–516
    nonneoplastic lesions, 515
Vulvar intraepithelial neoplasia (VIN), 515–516
Vulvodynia, 515
Vulvovaginal atrophy, 536
Vulvovaginal infection and inflammation, 514
vWD (von Willebrand disease), 639
VZV (varicella zoster virus), 423
VZV (varicella-zoster virus) vaccine, 586, 590–591
    immunization schedule for adults ≥65 years old, 590t
    recommendations for, 88t, 90

W
Walkers, 193t, 194
Walking, 80t, 116
    for DVT, 446
    400-meter walk test, 300
    limitations in, 296
    pulmonary rehabilitation, 192
    6-minute walk test, 299–300
Walking sticks, 260
Warfarin therapy
    for acute coronary syndrome, 453, 454
    adverse drug events, 106, 106t
    for atrial fibrillation, 454, 460
    drug interactions, 107, 107t, 588
    recommendations for cessation before surgery, 128, 130t
    for stroke prevention, 583
    for VTE, 445–446
Watchful waiting, 525, 526t
Water balance disorders, 498–500
Wegener's granulomatosis, 506, 599
Weight loss
    anorexia, 142–143
    for chronic CAD, 454
    for diabetes mellitus, 621, 622
    for gout, 551
    involuntary, 266
    for pain management, 548
    recommendations to promote, 93
    significant, 263
    unacceptable, 268–269
    for urinary incontinence, 279
Weight management, 81
    daily weight, 468
    dry weight, 468
Weight screening, 88t, 93

Wellspring Model, 205
Wheelchairs, 193t, 194
Wheezing, 439
Whisper Test, 243
Whisper-voice test, 44, 97
White Americans
    alcohol use, 404
    cancer, 644
    CVD mortality rates, 448
    dental caries, 430
    diabetes mellitus, 621
    educational attainment, 4
    end-of-life care, 137
    family caregivers, 55
    life expectancy, 3, 3t
    median income, 4
    nursing-home population, 196
    oral lesions, 433
    osteoporosis, 313
    periodontitis, 431
    population projections, 3, 644
    poverty rates, 4
    urinary incontinence, 274
White-coat hypertension, 476
White willow bark *(Salix alba)*, 115
WHO. *See* World Health Organization
Widower's syndrome, 531, 531t
Wind-up pain, 148t
Withdrawal, alcohol, 392, 406
Women
    adrenal insufficiency, 614
    alcohol use, 404
    androgen deficiency, 614, 617
    cancer, 642, 650
    cardiovascular disease, 448, 448t
    colonic adenomas, 652–653
    drug metabolism, 103
    dual eligibles, 34–35
    estrogen deficiency, 315
    fecal incontinence, 490
    gynecologic diseases and disorders, 512–519
    history and physical examination, 512–513
    hypertension, 475
    indications for osteoporosis screening, 317–318, 318t
    labor force participation, 4
    lesbian and bisexual women, 72
    life expectancy, 3, 3t, 623
    marital status and living arrangements, 3–4
    menopausal symptoms, 117
    population projections, 3
    poverty rates, 4
    preventive hormone therapy, 89t
    RDIs for micronutrients, 262–263, 263t
    recommendations for BMD testing, 317–318
    recommendations for calcium intake, 319
    recommendations for vitamin D intake, 320
    schizophrenia, 388, 389
    sexual dysfunction, 95, 530, 535, 536t
    stroke, 580

temporal arteritis, 578
testosterone therapy for, 617
urinary incontinence, 274, 275
urinary tract infections, 574
vertebral compression fractures, 538, 546
Wong-Baker FACES Pain Rating Scale with Foreign Translations, 149
World Health Organization (WHO)
    BMD definitions, 313, 314t
    definition of osteoporosis, 313, 314t
    fracture risk assessment model (FRAX™), 313, 316, 318, 318t
    healthy life expectancy (HALE), 3
    International Classification of Functioning, Disability, and Health (ICF), 181
    International Prostate Symptom Score, 520
    Pain Ladder, 155
Wound bed preparation, 290
Wound care, 281–292
    adjunctive therapies, 292
    infectious aspects, 293
    palliative care, 293–294, 293t
    products that promote healing, 290–291
    treatment modalities, 290, 291t
Wound documentation, 286–288
Wound healing
    caloric requirements, 292
    chronic wounds, 285, 285t
    Pressure Ulcer Scale for Healing, 286
    protein requirements, 292
Wrist pain, 541
    chondrocalcinosis of, 552, 553f

X
Xerophthalmia, 556
Xerosis, 419, 565
Xerostomia, 556

Y
Yoga, 80, 80t, 310t

Z
Z-drugs, 304
Z-score, 317, 440
Zaleplon
    for insomnia, 369t, 370
    for sleep disturbances in dementia, 347
Zanamivir, 592
Zeaxanthin, 234
Zinc
    for AMD, 234
    drug interactions, 265t
    RDIs for adults ≥71 years old, 263t
Ziprasidone
    dosing and adverse events of, 390t
    for psychosis in dementia, 345, 345t, 346
Zohydro ER (hydrocodone, sustained-release), 153t
Zoledronic acid
    for humoral hypercalcemia of malignancy, 609

for osteoporosis, 320, 321, 321*t*, 322
for Paget disease of bone, 609–610

Zolpidem
and delirium, 355*t*
drug interactions, 107, 107*t*
for insomnia, 369*t*, 370
for sleep disturbances in dementia, 347